Stress Consequences: Mental, Neuropsychological and Socioeconomic

Stress Consequences: Mental, Neuropsychological and Socioeconomic

EDITOR-IN-CHIEF

GEORGE FINK

Professorial Research Fellow (formerly Director)
Mental Health Research Institute of Victoria
Parkville, Melbourne, Victoria
Australia
Formerly Director, MRC Brain Metabolism Unit
Edinburgh, Scotland
UK

ELSEVIER

Amsterdam • Boston • Heidelberg • London • New York • Oxford
Paris • San Diego • San Francisco • Singapore • Sydney • Tokyo
Academic Press is an imprint of Elsevier

ACADEMIC PRESS

Academic Press is an imprint of Elsevier
525 B Street, Suite 1900, San Diego, CA 92101-4495, USA
Linacre House, Jordan Hill, Oxford, OX2 8DP, UK

British Library Cataloguing in Publication Data
A catalogue record for this book is available from the British Library

Library of Congress Catalog Number
A catalog record for this book is available from the Library of Congress

ISBN: 9780123751744

For information on all Elsevier publications
visit our website at books.elsevier.com

Printed and bound by CPI Group (UK) Ltd, Croydon, CR0 4YY

GENERAL INTRODUCTION

Stress is not something to be avoided. Indeed, it cannot be avoided, since just staying alive creates some demand for life-maintaining energy. Complete freedom from stress can be expected only after death. *Hans Selye*

"Stress" is one of the most frequently used but ill-defined words in the English language. Stress is a phenomenon that has quite different meanings at different times and under different circumstances for different individuals. Stress is a function of three main interactive and often interdependent variables: *(i) excitability/arousal; (ii) perceived aversiveness;* and *(iii) uncontrollability.* We all know when we are stressed – e.g. late for an important meeting and stuck in dense traffic or in a plane that shows no sign of push-back for reasons unknown – but find it difficult rationally to define our feelings. The definition proposed by the distinguished Berkeley psychologist, Richard Lazarus, is perhaps apposite for many stressful situations in man – that is, "a condition or feeling experienced when a person perceives that demands exceed the personal and social resources the individual is able to mobilize."

Hans Selye, sometimes called the "father of stress," coined and defined "stress" as "the nonspecific response of the body to any demand." For some, Selye's definition is "too biological" and ignores cognitive and psychological factors, a criticism that seems to stem from the misconception that cognition is not a function of the brain. For others, Selye's definition is too general. However, Selye's publications show that he understood psychological or cognitive stress. Furthermore, the generality of Selye's definition makes it pertinent for the molecular, genotypic and phenotypic analysis of stress and stress responses across all species from bacteria to man.

The contributions of Walter Bradford Cannon, working at Harvard in the 1920s and 30s, are arguably of equal importance for our understanding of the stress response. Thus, Cannon first proposed the term *homeostasis* (from the Greek homoios, or similar, and stasis, or position) for the coordinated physiological processes that enable the organism to cope with the stressful challenge by maintaining or quickly restoring steady state within the organism. Cannon also coined the term "fight or flight" to describe an animal's response to threat. *Homeostasis*, 'stability through constancy,' which has dominated physiological and medical thinking since 1859 (Claude Bernard's "milieu intérieur") seems in several circumstances (e.g. work-induced increase in cardiovascular load) to be giving way to *allostasis,* which provides 'stability through change.' *Homeostasis* depends on negative feedback control systems: *allostasis* refers to the dynamic maintenance of *homeostasis* by appropriate central nervous regulation of the cybernetic set points that adjust physiological parameters to meet various stresses/challenges.

The purpose of *Stress Science* and this companion volume *Stress Consequences* is to package key up-to date concepts and information regarding stress and its consequent and/or associated adverse effects on human health into a systematically formatted and reader friendly handbook. *Stress Science* is focused on the fundamental neuroendocrine response to stress and its adverse effects on several key somatic systems. The mental, neuropsychological and socioeconomic consequences of stress are covered in this companion volume on *Stress Consequences.*

Note on Terminology of Corticotropin Releasing Factor/Hormone and the Catecholamines

The central nervous regulation of the anterior pituitary gland is mediated by substances, mainly peptides, which are synthesized in the hypothalamus and transported to the gland by the hypophysial portal vessels. Because these compounds are transported by the blood, the term "hormone" or "neurohormone" gained acceptance in the neuroendocrine literature. The major hypothalamic peptide involved in the stress response is the 41-amino acid corticotropin releasing factor (CRF). The Endocrine Society (USA), following convention, adopted the term corticotropin releasing hormone (CRH). However, this nomenclature has been challenged. Hauger et al. (2003), in liaison with the International Union of Pharmacology Committee on Receptor Nomenclature and Drug Classification, argued that the function of CRF extends well beyond the biology of a hormone, and that it should therefore be termed corticotropin releasing factor (CRF) rather than hormone. Since the terminology of CRF versus CRH has yet to be resolved, the two terms and abbreviations are here used interchangeably, depending on author preference.

Adrenaline and *noradrenaline* are catecholamines that play a pivotal role in the stress response. These terms are synonymous with *epinephrine* and *norepinephrine*, respectively. Both sets of terms are used interchangeably in the endocrine, neuroendocrine and stress literature, and this principle has been adopted here. Style has depended on author preference, but wherever possible within-article consistency has been ensured. The adjectival forms, "adrenergic" and "noradrenergic," are used universally.

Reference

Hauger, R. L., Grigoriadis, D. E., Dallman, M. F., Plotsky, P. M., Vale, W. W., and Dautzenberg, F. M. (2003). International Union of Pharmacology. XXXVI. Current status of the nomenclature for receptors for corticotropin-releasing factor and their ligands. *Pharmacological Reviews* 55(1), 21–26.

George Fink

INTRODUCTION TO STRESS CONSEQUENCES

"his mind is walking up and down, walking up and down, in his old prison"
(Description of Dr Manette, from a *Tale of Two Cities* by Charles Dickens)

Stress Consequences, the clinical sequel to the largely basic science-focused *Stress Science*, starts with a chapter by Harrison and Critchley that outlines the impact of modern brain imaging on our understanding of cognition, emotions and mind. The second chapter by Monroe and Slavich reminds us, with examples, that "It is also commonly assumed that with the accelerating progress of civilization, more and more people are afflicted with mental and physical disorders. Historical accounts, however, suggest that such ideas about stressors, civilization, and disease have been common for quite some time."

The present work covers most stress consequences – mental, neuropsychological, psychosocial and socioeconomic – that are likely to be of relevance to psychiatrists, psychologists, psychotherapists, sociologists, epidemiologists, economists, stress researchers and students. *Stress Consequences* will also prove of interest to physicians and other health care workers, endocrinologists and neuroendocrinologists, policy and lawmakers and to the lay reader interested in the impact of stress on humans and human society.

The selection of topics and articles that comprise *Stress Consequences* was based on their importance for understanding stress and its impact, their relevance for psychiatry, medicine and health care delivery, psychology, sociology and economics, their timeliness, and the robustness of their concepts and data. Most of the articles are derived from the recently published *Encyclopedia of Stress*. Readers are referred to the earlier companion volume, *Stress Science*, for reviews of the relationship between stress and circadian and seasonal rhythms, neural plasticity and memory, inflammation and immunity, fetal stress and the "thrifty phenotype" hypothesis, feeding, obesity and the metabolic syndrome, disorders of the cardiovascular system and reproductive disorders. *Stress Science* also reviews some aspects of genetics and genomics, such as the article by Craig on "Genetic Polymorphisms in Stress Response", which are relevant to *Stress Consequences*.

Obesity and cardiovascular disorders, introduced in *Stress Science* and frequently referred to as "epidemics", receive further coverage in the present volume on *Stress Consequences*, especially in the sections on "Neuropsychological" and "Socioeconomic".

What follows is a brief outline of a few points of interest or controversy that perhaps deserve editorial comment.

Some caveats and points of controversy or interest

Posttraumatic Stress Disorder and Hypocortisolemia? Science is a debate, especially when data are subjective as is often the case with symptoms of mood and mental state and when hormonal and neurotransmitter changes may be relatively subtle. This uncertainty problem is exemplified by posttraumatic stress disorder (PTSD). Thus, early studies by Mason and associates (1986) found that urinary-free cortisol levels during hospitalization were significantly lower in PTSD than in major depressive disorder, "bipolar I, manic", and undifferentiated schizophrenia, but similar to those in paranoid schizophrenia. Mason et al underscored the fact that the low, stable cortisol levels in PTSD patients (Vietnam combat veterans) are remarkable because the overt signs of anxiety and depression in PTSD would usually be expected to be associated with cortisol elevations. Mason et al (1986) conclude that "the findings suggest a possible role of defensive organization as a basis for the low, constricted cortisol levels in PTSD and paranoid schizophrenic patients".

As explained by Rachel Yehuda (see "HPA Alterations in PTSD" in the present work, and also Yehuda 2006), the apparently low cortisol levels in PTSD are thought to reflect hyper-responsiveness of the hypothalamic-pituitary-adrenal system (HPA) to cortisol (glucocorticoid) negative feedback inhibition (for explanation see *Stress Science: Neuroendocrinology*). The observation of low cortisol in a disorder – PTSD – precipitated by extreme stress directly contradicts the popular "glucocorticoid cascade hypothesis" which posits that stress-induced increased plasma cortisol concentrations (hypercortisolemia) result in damage to areas of the brain, such as the hippocampus, that are involved in memory and cognition (see articles by BS McEwen, RM Sapolsky and the section on "Neuronal Plasticity-Memory" in *Stress Science*: McEwen 2007). But of greater concern is the fact that the data of Mason et al (1986) have not been universally replicated. Thus, when compared with levels in normal controls, ambient cortisol concentrations in PTSD over a 24-h period have been reported differently in several different publications as significantly lower, significantly higher, and not significantly different (e.g. Yehuda 2006, and "HPA Alterations in PTSD" in the present work; Young & Breslau 2004). Furthermore, most cortisol levels, high or low, in persons with PTSD are within the normal endocrine range, not suggestive of endocrine pathology.

There is, therefore, room for healthy skepticism about accepting hypocortisolemia as a universal and canonical feature of PTSD or other chronic conditions, such as chronic fatigue syndrome and fibromyalgia. As Rachel Yehuda stresses, the clinical significance of cortisol alterations within the normal endocrine range awaits to be determined by more sophisticated and rigorous neuroendocrine follow-up studies that are likely to involve genetics, genomics, molecular biology and brain imaging.

A different slant on within-normal range cortisol levels is offered by a recent study of 4000 former or current British civil servants (Michael Marmot's Whitehall II study). Kumari et al (2009) report that statistically low salivary cortisol concentrations at waking predicted new-onset of reported fatigue during an approximately 2.5-year follow-up. It is not clear whether the low cortisol levels are an effect or cause of fatigue. The authors speculate that their findings might also be relevant for conditions such as chronic fatigue syndrome and burnout (see Maslach and Leiter, present volume). However, although statistically significant (over a relatively huge N), it is not clear whether the seemingly small effect size of the difference between the fatigued and non-fatigued groups would enable salivary cortisol to be used to predict fatigue within individuals.

Human hippocampus - does size matter? Much is often made of hippocampal volume (determined in man by magnetic resonance imaging: MRI) and major depressive disorder – indeed, a Medline search draws down nigh on 270 papers on the subject. This issue is dealt with in the present volume by Rubin and Carroll ("Depression and Manic-Depressive Illness") and Harrison and Critchley ("Neuroimaging and Emotion"). The clear signal that emerges from both of these detailed reviews is that reduction in hippocampal volume, thought by some to reflect the effect of prolonged depression, PTSD or chronic stress (e.g. Lupien et al 2009) is not a consistent finding in major depression. The literature shows that reduction in hippocampal volume cannot be attributed to high levels of cortisol: indeed, reduced hippocampal volume has also been reported in PTSD patients in whom cortisol levels are assumed to be lower than normal (Lupien et al 2009), and in patients with cardiovascular disease (Rubin and Carroll). In a meta-analysis of 2418 patients with major depressive disorder and 1,974 healthy individuals, Koolschijn et al (2009) reported that the MRI data in patients with major depressive disorder showed large volume reductions in frontal regions, especially in the anterior cingulate and orbitofrontal cortex, with smaller reductions in the prefrontal cortex. The hippocampus, the putamen and caudate nucleus showed moderate volume reductions. In a monumental review of the literature, Savitz and Drevets (2009) conclude that "a significant number of studies have failed to find evidence of hippocampal atrophy in depressed patients, and based on these data, we suggest that the following caveat obtains: the majority of studies reporting evidence of hippocampal atrophy have made use of elderly, middle-aged or chronically ill populations". Clearly, much more research is required to improve our understanding of the relationships between mental symptoms, changes in regional brain volumes and neuroendocrine data.

Corticotropin releasing factor antagonists – novel potential anxiolytics and antidepressants: Numerous studies have shown that major depressive disorder often requires more than one step of treatment to elicit a remission of symptoms. Frequently, a second medication needs to be added to augment the first, which nowadays is usually a selective serotonin reuptake inhibitor [SSRI] (Trivedi et al 2006). Current data raise the question of whether to use augmentation agents (or other treatment combinations) as first-line treatment in an attempt to achieve greater remission rates sooner and in more patients than those associated with the use of SSRIs alone (Trivedi et al 2006). According to Trivedi and Daly (2008), treatment-resistant depression (TRD) is a common problem in the management of major depressive disorder, with 60% to 70% of all patients meeting the criteria for TRD. Non-pharmacological treatments, such as collaborative therapy, are being tested in clinical trials, but there remains an unmet need for new anxiolytic and antidepressant agents. This point was underscored by the first Advances in Neuroscience for Medical Innovation Symposium (Agid et al 2007), which recommended that "We should not pursue improved selective serotonin- or noradrenaline-reuptake inhibitors (SSRIs/SNRIs), or the other classes of drugs that have reached their limits". For reasons explained by Gutman and Nemeroff (in the present volume), small molecule antagonists of the corticotropin releasing factor-1 receptor (CRF-R1) might provide suitable alternatives to the classical monoamine targeted anxiolytic and antidepressant drugs. Several novel CRF-R1 antagonists are currently under investigation (Gilligan et al 2009).

Incidental to drug discovery, the finding that the CRF family of peptides and receptors may play a key role in mood and stress-induced behavior is an important spin-off of the CRF-41 story (see review by Gutman and Nemeroff here and many papers in *Stress Science: Neuroendocrinology*)

Alzheimer's Dementia, the aging brain, chaperone proteins and diabetes type 2: No modern work on stress and mental disorder would be complete without a discussion of the aging brain, Alzheimer's Disease and vascular dementia. The five papers on this subject in *Stress Consequences* comprise two on chaperone proteins – mainly heat shock proteins that tend to minimize cellular stress across all species from archaea to man. A relatively new twist to this theme is the paper by Convit, Rueger and Wolf on the impact of diabetes type 2 and stress on memory and the hippocampus, and the relationship between diabetes type 2, glucocorticoids, Alzheimer's Disease and cognitive impairment.

Gastro-duodenal (peptic) ulcers – Stress-Helicobacter pylori interactions: The etiology of gastric and duodenal ulceration and the conceptual switch from *only stress* to *only bacteria* as the cause of ulceration, followed by a sober realization that both factors may play a role, has heuristic value for our understanding of disease pathogenesis. As explained by Murison and Milde in the present volume, "Ulcerations played a key role in Hans Selye's description of the general adaptation syndrome and constituted one of the elements of this nonspecific response to diverse nocuous agents, together with shrinkage of the thymus and enlargement of the adrenal glands" (see also Fink, "Stress: Definition and History" in *Stress Science: Neuroendocrinology*). The (2005 Nobel Prize winning) discovery by Marshall and Warren that 80% of gastric and 90% of duodenal ulcers appeared to be caused by or were associated with *Helicobacter pylori* (Marshall and Warren 1984: Cover and Blaser, 2009) overturned the long-held view that stress was the cause of peptic ulceration. However, several studies reviewed by Murison and Milde and also by Creed in the present volume show that stress may still play a significant role in peptic ulceration, either alone, or as a factor that predisposes to ulcer induction by *H. pylori*. This is exemplified by the fact that the Hanshin-Awaji earthquake that occurred on January 17, 1995 was followed by a significant increase in the number of people with peptic ulceration (see Creed in the present volume, and Matsushima et al 1999). In most of these people ulceration developed in conjunction with *H.Pylori*, but among the physically injured, stomach ulcers developed independently of this infectious agent. Thus, argues Creed, there is a clear relationship with stress, which must be considered alongside other risk factors for peptic ulcer – *H. pylori* infection, non-steroidal anti-inflammatory drugs, smoking, and an inherited predisposition. In her critical review of the interaction between stress and *H. pylori* in the causation of peptic ulcers, Susan Levenstein concludes, "Peptic ulcer is a valuable model for understanding the interactions among psychosocial, socioeconomic, behavioral, and infectious factors in causing disease. The discovery of *H. pylori* may serve, paradoxically, as a stimulus to researchers for whom the concepts of psychology and infection are not necessarily a contradiction in terms" (Levenstein 2000).

Biology of psychosocial and socioeconomic stress consequences: The biological basis for most of the psychosocial and socioeconomic consequences of stress is outlined in many articles in the present volume, as well as in the earlier companion volume, *Stress Science: Neuroendocrinology*. For further information, the reader might wish to consult the *Encyclopedia of Stress*, 2nd edition (Editor in Chief, George Fink, 2007, Academic Press) and recent reviews such as those by Marmot & Bell (2009), McEwen (2007) and Shonkoff et al (2009).

Conclusion and Observations

Stress research has made huge advances since Hans Selye's note to Nature in 1936 and the publication of Walter Cannon's *The Wisdom of the Body* (1932). This is especially the case with respect to the fundamental neuroendocrinology of the stress response (see *Stress Science: Neuroendocrinology*). However, there are still many unknowns. Thus, for example, in spite of the power of modern structural and functional human brain imaging, our understanding of the relationships between the changes in the nervous system and the signals in the endocrine system remain poor. In fact, as outlined above, we appear to have no clue as to the significance of stress neuroendocrinology for changes in hippocampal volume, which can be reduced under conditions of either presumed low or presumed high HPA activity. The glucocorticoid vunerability and neurotoxicity hypothesis seems to have achieved canonical status. But is the hypothesis correct for man – does it apply invariably to all humans under all conditions? What precisely does a change in the volume of the hippocampus or other brain regions signify functionally? Are MRI-determined changes in hippocampal and amygdala volume, trait, or, as seems to be the case in schizophrenia (Velakoulis et al 2006), state dependent? Are we missing some major conceptual or factual points that are staring us in the face?

In terms of understanding stress, cognitive performance and behavior, have we progressed significantly beyond the century-old Yerkes-Dodson Law which, simply put, states that the relationship between arousal and behavioral performance can be linear or curvilinear depending upon the difficulty of the task (Diamond et al 2007)?

This skeptical view has an optimistic side in that the stress field offers numerous opportunities and challenges for future researchers. This seems especially to be the case with respect to the interactions between emotion, cognition, memory, mental state and behavior, and how they translate into the nano-world of the synapse on the one hand and society, culture and economics on the other. Inextricably bound to this are gene-environment interactions (GxE) that are thought to play a role in stress-induced disorders of mood, mental state and behavior. Touched on in Section II of the present volume, and also in *Stress Science*, GxE together with its cognate disciplines is a crucial field under intense investigation. The present volume on *Stress Consequences* shows that there is an exciting future for bright sparks interested in clinically relevant stress research.

Acknowledgements

I am grateful to Ann Elizabeth Fink for putting up with yet another round of stress, and to Mica Haley, Elsevier Neuroscience Acquisitions Editor for her continuing support. I should also like to thank Professors Robert Rubin and Bernard (Barney) Carroll for the helpful discussions regarding post-traumatic stress disorder. Any errors are mine.

Bibliography and Further reading

Agid, Y., et al. (2007). How can drug discovery for psychiatric disorders be improved? *Nature Reviews Drug Discovery* **6**, 189–201(March 2007). doi:10.1038/nrd2217.

Cannon, W. B. (1932). The Wisdom of the Body. New York: Norton.

Cover, T. L. and Blaser, M. J. (2009). Helicobacter pylori in Health and Disease. *Gastroenterology* **136**, 1863–1873.

Diamond, D. M., Campbell, A. M., Park, C. R., Halonen, J. and Zoladz, P. R. (2007). The Temporal Dynamics Model of Emotional Memory Processing: A Synthesis on the Neurobiological Basis of Stress-Induced Amnesia, Flashbulb and Traumatic Memories, and the Yerkes-Dodson Law. Neural Plast. 2007; 2007: 60803. Published online 2007 March 28. doi: 10.1155/2007/60803.

Gilligan, P. J., et al. (2009). 8-(4-Methoxyphenyl)pyrazolo [1,5-a]-1,3,5-triazines: Selective and Centrally Active Corticotropin-Releasing Factor Receptor-1 (CRF_1) Antagonists. *J Med Chem.* **52**, 3073–3083.

Huber, T. J. and Wildt te, B. T. (2005). Charles Dickens' A tale of Two Cities: A case Report of Posttraumatic Stress Disorder. Psychopathology **38**, 334–337.

Koolschijn, P. C., van Haren, N. E., Lensvelt-Mulders, G. J., Hulshoff Pol, H. E. and Kahn, R. S. (2009). Brain volume abnormalities in major depressive disorder: A meta-analysis of magnetic resonance imaging studies. *Hum Brain Mapp.* 2009 May 13. [Epub ahead of print]. doi.10.1002/hbm.20801.

Kumari, M., et al. (2009). Cortisol secretion and fatigue: Associations in a community based cohort. Psychoneuroendocrinology. doi:10.1016/j.psyneuen.2009.05.001 (in press).

Levenstein, S. (2000). The Very Model of a Modern Etiology: A Biopsychosocial View of Peptic Ulcer. *Psychosomatic Medicine* **62**, 176–185.

Lupien, S. J., McEwen, B. S., Gunnar, M. R. and Heim, C. (2009). Effects of stress throughout the lifespan on the brain, behavior and cognition. *Nature Rev Neurosci* **10**, 434–445.

McEwen, B. S. (2007). Physiology and Neurobiology of Stress and Adaptation: Central Role of the Brain. *Physiol Rev* **87**, 873–904.

Marmot, M. G. and Bell, R. (2009). How will the financial crisis affect health? *BMJ* **338**, b1314. doi: 10.1136/bmj.b1314.

Marshall, B. J. and Warren, J. R. (1984). "Unidentified curved bacilli in the stomach of patients with gastritis and peptic ulceration". *Lancet* **1**(8390), 1311–1315.

Mason, J. W., et al. (1986). Urinary free-cortisol levels in posttraumatic stress disorder patients. *J. Nerv. Ment. Dis.* **174**, 145–149.

Matsushima, Y., et al. (1999). Gastric Ulcer Formation after the Hanshin-Awaji Earthquake: A Case Study of Helicobacter pylori Infection and Stress-Induced Gastric Ulcers. *Helicobacter* **4**, 94–99.

Savitz, J. and Drevets, W. C. (2009). Bipolar and major depressive disorder: Neuroimaging the developmental degenerative divide. *Neuroscience and Biobehavioral Reviews* **33**, 699–771.

Selye, H. (1936). A syndrome produced by diverse nocuous agents. *Nature* **138**, 32.

Shonkoff, J. P., Boyce, W. and McEwen, B. S. (2009). Neuroscience, Molecular Biology, and the Childhood Roots of Health Disparities: Building a New Framework for Health Promotion and Disease Prevention. *JAMA* **301**, 2252–2259.

Trivedi, M. H., et al. (2006). Medication Augmentation after the Failure of SSRIs for Depression. *N Engl J Med* **354**, 1243–1252.

Trivedi, M. H. and Daly, E. J. (2008). Treatment strategies to improve and sustain remission in major depressive disorder. *Dialogues Clin Neurosci.* **10**, 377–384.

Velakoulis, D., et al. (2006). Hippocampal and Amygdala Volumes According to Psychosis Stage and Diagnosis: A Magnetic Resonance Imaging Study of Chronic Schizophrenia, First-Episode Psychosis, and Ultra–High-Risk Individuals. *Arch Gen Psychiatry* **63**, 139–149.

Yehuda, R. (2006). Advances in Understanding Neuroendocrine Alterations in PTSD and their Therapeutic Implications. *Ann. N.Y. Acad. Sci.* **1071**, 137–166.

Young, E. A. and Breslau, N. (2004). Cortisol and catecholamines in posttraumatic stress disorder: an epidemiologic community study. *Arch. Gen. Psychiatry* **61**, 394–401.

George Fink

CONTRIBUTORS

T Åkerstedt
Karolinska institutet, Stockholm, Sweden

K J Ajrouch
Eastern Michigan University, Ypsilanti, MI, USA

R A Allison
American Medical Association, Phoenix, AZ, USA

O Almkvist
Karolinska Institutet and University of Stockholm, Stockholm, Sweden

T C Antonucci
University of Michigan, Ann Arbor, MI, USA

L E Arnold
Ohio State University, Columbus, OH, USA

B Ataca
Bogazici University, Istanbul, Turkey

N E Avis
Wake Forest University School of Medicine, Winston-Salem, NC, USA

W R Avison
University of Western Ontario, London, ON, Canada

S Ayers
University of Sussex, Brighton, UK

M W Baldwin
McGill University, Montreal, Quebec, Canada

J C Ballenger
Medical University of South Carolina, Charleston, SC, USA

M Barad
University of Los Angeles, Los Angeles, CA, USA

M Bartley
University College London Medical School, London, UK

D Benedek
Uniformed Services University of the Health Sciences, Bethesda, MD, USA

M Berk
University of California, Los Angeles, CA, USA

L F Berkman
Harvard School of Public Health, Boston, MA, USA

J W Berry
Queen's University, Kingston, ONT, Canada

D Blackwood
University of Edinburgh, Edinburgh, UK

D C Blanchard
University of Hawaii, Honolulu, HI, USA

R J Blanchard
University of Hawaii, Honolulu, HI, USA

S R Bornstein
University Hospital, Duesseldorf, Duesseldorf, Germany

K Bottigi
University of Minnesota, Minneapolis, USA

A B Butler
University of Northern Iowa, Cedar Falls, IA, USA

M van den Buuse
The Mental Health Research Institute of Victoria, Parkville, Victoria, Australia

B J Carroll
Pacific Behavioral Research Foundation, Carmel, CA, USA

R A Catalano
University of California, Berkeley, CA, USA

T Chandola
University College London, London, UK

G Chapman
University of Nevada, Las Vegas, NV, USA

A Christensen
University of California, Los Angeles, Los Angeles, CA, USA

G P Chrousos
University of Athens, Athens, Greece

P J Clayton
American Foundation for Suicide Prevention, New York, NY, USA

E F Coccaro
University of Chicago, Chicago, IL, USA

J A Cohen
Drexel University College of Medicine, Philadelphia, PA, USA

J K Cohen
Pittsburgh, PA, USA

A Convit
Department of Psychiatry, New York University School of Medicine, Millhauser Laboratories, New York, and Nathan Kline Institute, Orangeburg, NY, USA

E Conway de Macario
New York State Department of Health and The University of Albany (SUNY), Albany, NY, USA

L C Cook
University of Nevada, Las Vegas, NV, USA

D Copolov
The Mental Health Research Institute of Victoria, Parkville, Victoria, Australia

I W Craig
King's College London, London, UK

F Creed
University of Manchester, Manchester, UK

H D Critchley
University College London, London, UK

P Csermely
Semmelweis University, Budapest, Hungary

M Dascalu
Washington University School of Medicine, St. Louis, MO, USA

T Dawood
Baker Heart Research Institute and Monash University, Alfred Hospital, Melbourne, Victoria, Australia

A DeLongis
University of British Columbia, Vancouver, BC, Canada

M Devich-Navarro
University of California, Los Angeles, CA, USA

M A Dew
University of Pittsburgh School of Medicine and Medical Center, Pittsburgh, PA, USA

Laura J Dietz
University of Pittsburgh Medical Center, Pittsburgh, PA, USA

A F DiMartini
University of Pittsburgh School of Medicine and Medical Center, Pittsburgh, PA, USA

J E Dimsdale
University of California, San Diego, CA, USA

B Donohue
University of Nevada at Las Vegas, Las Vegas, NV, USA

J Drescher
New York, NY, USA

W W Dressler
University of Alabama, Tuscaloosa, AL, USA

E K Englander
Bridgewater State College, Bridgewater, MA, USA

N C Feeny
Case Western Reserve University, Cleveland, OH, USA

R M Fernquist
Central Missouri State University, Warrensburg, MO, USA

M H Fernstrom
University of Pittsburgh Medical Center, Pittsburgh, PA, USA

J E Ferrie
University College London Medical School, London, UK

E B Foa
University of Pennsylvania, Philadelphia, PA, USA

E Ford
University of Sussex, Brighton, UK

N Frasure-Smith
Centre Hospitalier de l'Université de Montréal Research Center, University of Montreal, McGill University, and Montreal Heart Institute Research Center, Montreal, Canada

J E Gaugler
University of Minnesota, Minneapolis, USA

E L Gibson
Roehampton University, London, UK

M R Gignac
Pittsburgh, PA, USA

D G Gilbert
Southern Illinois University-Carbondale, Carbondale, IL, USA

L Giner
Fundacion Jimenez Diaz and Universidad Autonoma de Madrid. Madrid. Spain

G M Goodwin
University of Oxford, Oxford, UK

W M Greenberg
Nathan S. Kline Institute for Psychiatric Research, Orangeburg, NY, and New York University School of Medicine, New York, NY, USA

T Grieger
Uniformed Services University of the Health Sciences, Bethesda, MD, USA

L M Groesz
University of Texas at Austin, Austin, TX, USA

J G Grzywacz
Wake Forest University School of Medicine, Winston-Salem, NC, USA

M A Gupta
University of Western Ontario and Mediprobe Research Inc., London, Canada

D A Gutman
Emory University School of Medicine, Atlanta, GA, USA

D Hamaoka
Uniformed Services University of the Health Sciences, Bethesda, MD, USA

N A Harrison
University College London, London, UK

P Haynes
University of Arizona, Tucson, AZ, USA

M Hebert
University of Hawaii, Honolulu, HI, USA

D H Hellhammer
University of Trier, Trier, Germany

H Hill
University of Nevada at Las Vegas, Las Vegas, NV, USA

K N Hipke
Wisconsin Psychiatric Institute and Clinics, Madison, WI, USA

M Hirshkowitz
Baylor College of Medicine and Michael E. DeBakey Veteran Affairs Medical Center, Houston, TX, USA

G R J Hockey
University of Sheffield, Sheffield, UK

C J Holahan
University of Texas at Austin, Austin, TX, USA

A Holen
Norwegian University of Science and Technology, Trondheim, Norway

C P Holstege
University of Virginia, Charlottesville, VA, USA

H Holstege
Calvin College, Grand Rapids, MI, USA

P Huezo-Diaz
King's College London, London, UK

K Iley
Canterbury Christ Church University, Canterbury, UK

M Ingram
University of Arizona, Tucson, AZ, USA

M R Irwin
UCLA Semel Institute for Neuroscience, Los Angeles, CA, USA

S Jain
University of California San Diego, San Diego, CA, USA

K D Jennings
University of Pittsburgh, Pittsburgh, PA, USA

D C Jimerson
Beth Israel Deaconess Medical Center and Harvard Medical School, Boston, MA, USA

S Joseph
University of Nottingham, Nottingham, UK

I M A Joung
Erasmus University, Rotterdam, Netherlands

J Juvonen
University of California, Los Angeles, Los Angeles, CA, USA

G Kaltsas
University of Athens, Athens, Greece

A A Kaptein
Leiden University Medical Center, Leiden, The Netherlands

M Karataraki
Penn State University College of Medicine, Hershey, PA, USA

R Kastenbaum
Arizona State University, Tempe, AZ, USA

I Kawachi
Harvard School of Public Health, Boston, MA, USA

C A Kearney
University of Nevada, Las Vegas, NV, USA

C Kirschbaum
Technical University of Dresden, Dresden, Germany

R P Kluft
Temple University, Philadelphia, PA, USA

H Knight
University of Edinburgh, Edinburgh, UK

H W Koenigsberg
Bronx VA Medical Center, Bronx, NY, USA

W J Kop
Uniformed Services University of the Health Sciences, Bethesda, MD, USA

M S Kopp
Semmelweis University, Budapest, Hungary

R L Kormos
University of Pittsburgh School of Medicine and Medical Center, Pittsburgh, PA, USA

M P Koss
University of Arizona, Tucson, AZ, USA

L Kovács
Babes-Bolyai University, Clvj-Napoca, Romania

B M Kudielka
University of Trier, Trier, Germany

A M La Greca
University of Miami, Coral Gables, FL, USA

G W Lambert
Baker Heart Research Institute, Melbourne, Victoria, Australia

J E Lansford
Duke University, Durham, NC, USA

M Le Moal
Université de Bordeaux, Bordeaux, France

M P Leiter
Acadia University, Wolfville, Nova Scotia, Canada

F Lespérance
Centre Hospitalier de l'Université de Montréal Research Center, University of Montreal, and Montreal Heart Institute Research Center, Montreal, Canada

D Lester
Richard Stockton College of New Jersey, Pomona, NJ, USA

J D Levine
University of California, San Francisco, CA, USA

T J Linares
Case Western Reserve University, Cleveland, OH, USA

M Lindau
Uppsala University, Uppsala, Sweden

G Lindbeck
Karolinska institutet, Stockholm, Sweden

R L Lindsay
Arizona Child Study Center, Phoeniz, AZ, USA

P A Linley
University of Leicester, Leicester UK

U Lundberg
Stockholm University, Stockholm, Sweden

A J L Macario
New York State Department of Health and The University of Albany (SUNY), Albany, NY, USA

D F MacKinnon
Johns Hopkins University School of Medicine, Baltimore, MD, USA

T Maier-Paarlberg
University of Nevada at Las Vegas, Las Vegas, NV, USA

H M Malin
Institute for Advanced Study of Human Sexuality, San Francisco, CA, USA

A P Mannarino
Allegheny General Hospital, Pittsburgh, PA, USA

J J Mann
Columbia University and New York State Psychiatric Institute, New York, NY, USA

E C Manning
University of Chicago, Chicago, IL, USA

J R Mantsch
Marquette University, Milwaukee, WI, USA

V March
University of Pittsburgh Medical Center, Pittsburgh, PA, USA

M Marmot
University College London, London, UK

P Martikainen
University of Helsinki, Helsinki, Finland

C Maslach
University of California, Berkeley, CA, USA

F J McClernon
Duke University Medical Center, Durham, NC, USA

P T McFarland
University of California, Los Angeles, Los Angeles, CA, USA

A M McMurtray
West Los Angeles Veteran's Affairs Medical Center and University of California, Los Angeles, CA, USA

M F Mendez
West Los Angeles Veteran's Affairs Medical Center and University of California, Los Angeles, CA, USA

A M Milde
University of Bergen, Bergen, Norway

P J Mills
University of California San Diego, San Diego, CA, USA

I Mino
Harvard University, Cambridge, MA, USA

J Mirowsky
University of Texas at Austin, Austin, TX, USA

A H Mohammed
Karolinska Institutet, Stockholm, and Växjö University, Växjö, Sweden

S A Mohammed
University of Michigan Ann Arbor, MI, USA

S M Monroe
University of Oregon, Eugene, OR, USA

R H Moos
Dept. of Veterans Affairs Health Care System and Stanford University Medical Center, Palo Alto, CA, USA

M E Mor Barak
University of Southern California School of Social Work and Marshall School of Business, Los Angeles, CA, USA

R Murison
University of Bergen, Bergen, Norway

M W Nash
King's College London, London, UK

J Y Nazroo
University of Manchester, Manchester, UK

C B Nemeroff
Emory University School of Medicine, Atlanta, GA, USA

R Norbury
Warneford Hospital and University of Oxford, Oxford, UK

R W Novaco
University of California, Irvine, CA, USA

S Nowakowski
San Diego State University/University of California, San Diego, CA, USA

A Öhman
Karolinska Institutet, Stockholm, Sweden

M A Oquendo
Columbia University and New York State Psychiatric Institute, New York, NY, USA

S Packer
New School for Social Research, New York, NY, USA

K Pajer
The Ohio State University, Columbus, OH, USA

B L Parry
University of California, San Diego, CA, USA

S Pejovic
Penn State University College of Medicine, Hershey, PA, USA

Avril Pereira
Mental Health Research Institute of Victoria, Melbourne, Australia

P V Piazza
Université de Bordeaux, Bordeaux, France

C M Pierce
Harvard University, Cambridge, MA, USA

M L Pilati
Rio Hondo College, Whittier, CA, USA

N Pomara
Nathan S. Kline Institute for Psychiatric Research, Orangeburg, NY, and New York University School of Medicine, New York, NY, USA

L H Powell
Rush University Medical Center, Chicago, IL, USA

W E Profit
Los Angeles, CA, USA

P Prolo
University of California, Los Angeles, and Veterans Administration Greater Los Angeles Health Care System, Los Angeles, CA, USA

J C Pruessner
McGill University, Montreal, Quebec, Canada

E Puterman
University of British Columbia, Vancouver, BC, Canada

N M Ramadan
Rosalind Franklin University of Medicine and Science, North Chicago, IL, USA

D de Ridder
Utrecht University, Utrecht, The Netherlands

N J Rinehart
Monash University, Clayton, Victoria, Australia

I Robbins
St. George's Hospital, London, UK

G M Rooker
Pittsburgh, PA, USA

C E Ross
University of Texas at Austin, Austin, TX, USA

A E Roth
Nathan S. Kline Institute for Psychiatric Research, Orangeburg, NY, USA

R T Rubin
VA Greater Los Angeles Healthcare System, Los Angeles, CA, USA

M Rueger
New York University School of Medicine, New York, NY, USA

L Saldana
Medical University of South Carolina, Charleston, SC, USA

F M Saleh
University of Massachusetts Medical School, Worcester, MA USA

S Sandberg
University College London, London, UK

I N Sandler
Arizona State University, Tempe, AZ, USA

A Sharafkhaneh
Baylor College of Medicine and Michael E. DeBakey Veteran Affairs Medical Center, Houston, TX, USA

W S Shaw
University of Massachusetts, Worcester, MA, USA

J Siegrist
University of Duesseldorf, Duesseldorf, Germany

L J Siever
Bronx VA Medical Center, Bronx, NY, USA

E K Simon
Rosalind Franklin University of Medicine and Science, North Chicago, IL, USA

S M Skevington
University of Bath, Bath, UK

G M Slavich
University of Oregon, Eugene, OR, USA

R G Smart
Centre for Addiction and Mental Health, Toronto, Canada

D Spiegel
Stanford University, Stanford, CA, USA

M N Starkman
University of Michigan, Ann Arbor, MI, USA

M Steinberg
Northampton, MA, USA

A Steptoe
University College London, London, UK

L R Stines
Case Western Reserve University, Cleveland, OH, USA

H J Strausbaugh
University of California, San Francisco, CA, USA

S V Subramanian
Harvard School of Public Health, Boston, MS, USA

R Suddath
University of California, Los Angeles, CA, USA

K Sugden
Social, Genetic and Developmental Psychiatry Centre, London, UK

S Sundram
Mental Health Research Institute of Victoria, Northern Psychiatry Research Centre, and University of Melbourne, Melbourne, Australia

P Surtees
Strangeways Research Laboratory and University of Cambridge, Cambridge, UK

D Svrakic
Washington University School of Medicine, St. Louis, MO, USA

G N Swanson
Allegheny General Hospital, Pittsburgh, PA, USA

C C Swenson
Medical University of South Carolina, Charleston, SC, USA

A N Taylor
University of California, Los Angeles, and Veterans Administration Greater Los Angeles Health Care System, Los Angeles, CA, USA

B J Tonge
Monash University, Clayton, Victoria, Australia

D J Travis
University of Southern California School of Social Work, Los Angeles, CA, USA

R J Ursano
Uniformed Services University of the Health Sciences, Bethesda, MD, USA

J Ventura
University of California, Los Angeles, CA, USA

A N Vgontzas
Penn State University College of Medicine, Hershey, PA, USA

N Wainwright
Strangeways Research Laboratory and University of Cambridge, Cambridge, UK

R L Walker
University of South Carolina, Columbia, SC, USA

J Wardle
University College London, London, UK

A A Weinstein
Uniformed Services University of the Health Sciences, Bethesda, MD, USA

D L Whitehead
University College London, London, UK

H S Willenberg
University Hospital, Duesseldorf, Duesseldorf, Germany

D R Williams
University of Michigan Ann Arbor, MI, USA

K Williams
Rush University Medical Center, Chicago, IL, USA

S A Wolchik
Arizona State University, Tempe, AZ, USA

O T Wolf
University of Bielefeld, Bielefeld, Germany

C M Wong
Mt. Sinai School of Medicine and Bronx Veterans Affairs, New York, NY, USA

S Wuethrich
McGill University, Montreal, Quebec, Canada

M Yang
University of Hawaii, Honolulu, HI, USA

R Yehuda
Mt. Sinai School of Medicine and Bronx Veterans Affairs, New York, NY, USA

J W Younger
Arizona State University, Tempe, AZ, USA

N P Yuan
University of Arizona, Tucson, AZ, USA

S H Zarit
Pennsylvania State University, University Park, PA, USA

A J Zautra
Arizona State University, Tempe, AZ, USA

CONTENTS

VI. SOCIOECONOMIC

I. GENERAL - BACKGROUND

Neuroimaging and Emotion

N A Harrison and H D Critchley
University College London, London, UK

Glossary

Amygdala	An almond-shaped cluster of interrelated nuclei and associated cortex in the anterior medial temporal lobe.
Arousal	A dimension of emotion that varies from calm to excitement and predicts behavioral activity level.
Blood–oxygen level-dependent (BOLD) signal	T2*-weighted signal in functional magnetic resonance imaging (fMRI) that reflects hemodynamic changes in regional perfusion evoked by neural activity.
Functional magnetic resonance imaging (fMRI)	A non-invasive technique with good spatial resolution that detects changes in regional blood flow associated with neural activity.
Interoception	A representation of visceral activity; the afferent limb of homoeostatic neural control of bodily organs.
Magnetoencephalography (MEG)	A non-invasive technique with high temporal resolution that detects the changing magnetic fields associated with neural activity.
Valence	A dimension of emotion that varies from unpleasant (negative) to pleasant (positive) to reflect motivational value.

Emotion

Emotion is central to our everyday human experience. Emotional events or objects within our environment are assigned value, bias our attention, and enhance our subsequent memory. Neuroimaging techniques, perhaps more than other approaches, have led to a growing awareness that emotion, unlike many other psychological functions, is relatively unencapsulated and interacts with and influences multiple other areas of functioning. In addition to effects on attention, perception, memory, and learning, emotion also forms the backbone of our social relationships and is an important component of empathetic understanding of others. Emotional cues also act as powerful reinforcers, have a marked influence on our thoughts and reasoning, and serve to bias our ongoing behavior. Although emotions come in many flavors that may equally serve to bias multiple psychological functions, much of the contemporary research on emotional neuroscience has focused on the processing of fear. For the purposes of this article, we follow this focus, which also accords with an emphasis on stress responses.

Consistent with a broad role in human functioning are the wide-ranging manifestations associated with disorders of emotion regulation. Emotion disequilibrium underlies not just anxiety and stress-related illness but the entire range of mental disorders and acts as the common denominator in much of human unhappiness. This article reviews the contributions of neuroimaging studies to our developing understanding of the neurobiology of human emotion. One particular aim is to highlight how emotion interacts with and influences other areas of cognition and to illustrate how an understanding of the mechanisms underlying these interactions can enable a greater understanding of stress-related disorders.

Definition of Emotion

Differences in definition can lead to markedly different conceptualizations of emotion and underlie seemingly contradictory theories of emotion in the literature. A prevalent view conceptualizes emotion as a transient perturbation in an organism's functioning evoked by a triggering (i.e., emotive) stimulus (either external or internal). Most accounts of emotion also subscribe to a multicomponential description with physiological arousal, motor expression, and subjective feelings forming the reaction triad of emotion. However, the extent to which changes in these various components are necessary and sufficient to define an episode as emotional is more controversial. For the purposes of this article, we use the following definition: emotions are transient events, produced in response to external or internal events of significance to the individual; they are typically characterized by attention to the evoking stimulus and changes in neurophysiological arousal, motor behavior, and subjective feeling state that engender a subsequent biasing of behavior.

Emotion Perception and Attention

Implicit within this definition is that events of significance to the individual (emotive stimuli) are susceptible to preferential perceptual processing. One mechanism through which this is achieved is through the emotional biasing of attentional processes. This is illustrated in behavioral studies using visual search paradigms, in which target items are discriminated from an array containing a variable number of distracter items. Emotionally valenced items or objects are indeed identified more rapidly than non-emotional items. Furthermore, in spatial tasks, the presentation of an emotional cue on one side of the visual space increases the speed of identification of nonemotional stimuli subsequently presented on the same side (i.e., attention is drawn to the location of the preceding emotive stimulus). Neuroimaging studies investigating the neural basis of this emotional capture of attention in spatial orientation tasks show that it is correlated with activity in regions of the frontal and parietal cortices as well as the lateral orbitofrontal cortex.

Evidence from patient studies, neuroimaging, and electroencephalography suggests that even unattended emotional stimuli are more likely to enter awareness, suggesting further mechanisms through which emotional stimuli influence perception. Neuroimaging studies continue to delineate the brain mechanisms through which unattended emotional stimuli gain enhanced access to awareness. One influential hypothesis suggests that the emotional salience of a stimulus is rapidly detected by the amygdala after cursory representational processing. The amygdala subsequently facilitates attention and perception via projections to the sensory cortices to enable more detailed sensory processing. Convergent anatomical studies suggest that this is mediated by both direct and indirect amygdala influences on sensory cortices; reciprocal direct connections exist between the amygdala and sensory cortices, and a projection from the central nucleus of the amygdala to the cholinergic nucleus basalis of Maynert enables indirect ascending cholinergic neuromodulatory influences to be exerted on the same cortical regions.

Functional neuroimaging studies have tested this hypothesis using visual backward-masking paradigms in which briefly presented visual targets are rendered invisible by subsequently presented stimuli. Unseen emotional stimuli, presented in this subliminal manner, can nevertheless still evoke neural responses in the amygdala, compared to nonemotional (neutral) stimuli. Moreover, masked presentations of face stimuli portraying fearful (vs. neutral) facial expressions enhances activation within the fusiform cortex (an extra-striate visual area containing a region implicated as being specialized for processing faces). This activation of the fusiform face area (FFA) is predicted by the magnitude of amygdala activation. Further evidence that emotional processing in the amygdala may enhance activity within sensory cortex comes from the observation that patients with amygdala damage fail to show this enhancement of activity within the face-processing visual cortex when tested on the same paradigm. The presentation of fearful face cues has also been shown to enhance even early perceptual functions such as contrast sensitivity, which is consistent with the suggestion that the amygdala may modulate even activity within the primary visual cortex.

Preattentive processing of emotional stimuli indicates early representational discrimination between emotional and nonemotional events. Studies in humans using magnetoencephalography (MEG), a neuroimaging technique with high temporal resolution, showed discriminatory responses to emotional faces as early as 100–120 ms. This compares to characteristic face-related responses that occurs much later, at 170 ms. Electrophysiological studies in humans using intracranial electrodes also showed an early, 120- to 160-ms response to aversive stimuli. The early recognition of emotionally valenced stimuli accords with animal data suggesting that the amygdala may be activated by a rapid subcortical pathway. Neuroimaging studies in both normal and brain injury subjects highlight subcortical amygdala activation in humans. One study exploited two separate findings: (1) that low- and high-spatial frequency information is processed by separate visual neural pathways and (2) that coarse emotional cues are carried in low-frequency components. When subjects were presented low-frequency (blurred) face stimuli fearful (vs. neutral face stimuli), enhanced activity was seen in the amygdala, pulvinar nucleus of the thalamus, and superior colliculus, components of a proposed subcortical circuit (**Figure 1**). In contrast, the presentation of the same faces at high spatial frequency activated the cortical regions, including the fusiform (face-identity-specific) cortex. Implicit processing of emotional valence can be demonstrated in patients with damage to the primary visual cortex, who are not consciously aware of stimuli presented in their blind hemifield (i.e., blindsight). These patients show amygdala activation to fearful faces presented in their blind hemifield, illustrating the presence of the subcortical visual processing of emotion to the level of the amygdala.

Together these lesion and functional imaging studies provide mechanistic insight into the role of amygdala, through interactions with the sensory cortices, in facilitating enhanced attention and perception of visually presented emotional stimuli. The preferential early processing of emotionally valenced material, illustrated most powerfully with fearful stimuli, sets up a primary bias in subsequent information processing that underpins the regulation of ongoing and prospective behavior.

Neuroscientific studies of human emotion have tended to focus on the visual processing of emotional facial expressions. Nevertheless, this visual communication of emotional state through changes in the facial musculature is only one part of a richer

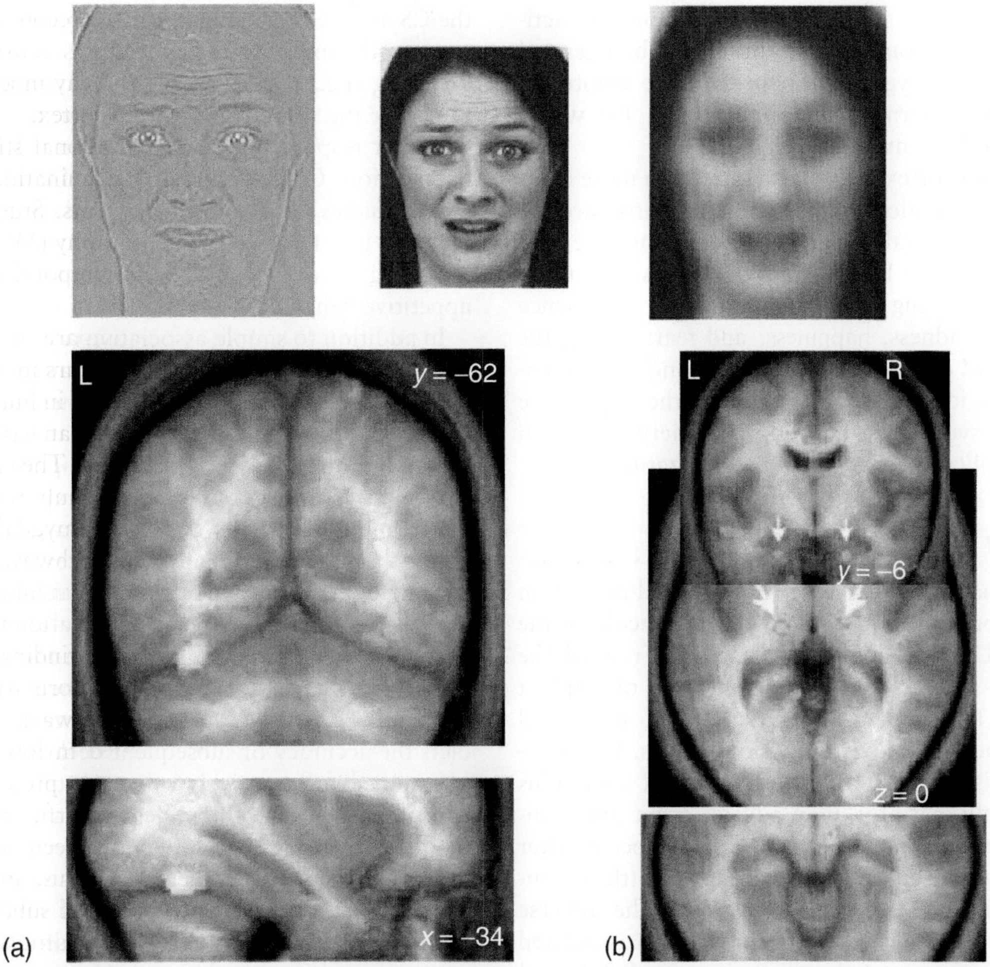

Figure 1 Neural activity in response to viewing facial expressions. a, High-spatial frequency information; b, low-spatial frequency information. High-spatial frequency images activated the fusiform cortex, specialized for the processing of facial identity. Fearful (vs. neutral) facial expressions activated the amygdala bilaterally (vertical arrows) with greater response to low-spatial frequency images. Low-spatial frequency fearful images also activated the posterior inferior thalamus bilaterally (diagonal arrows) and the superior colliculus on the right suggesting that low-spatial frequency images containing emotion information activate a subcortical pathway to the amygdala. Reprinted by permission from Macmillan Publishers Ltd: *Nature Neuroscience;* Vuilleumier, P., Armony, J. L., Driver, J., et al., Distinct spatial frequency sensitivities for processing faces and emotional expressions, **6**, 624–631, copyright (2003).

multimodal vocabulary of affect. Information signaling emotional state is also conveyed by autonomic changes in the skin (leading to color change and sweating) and pupils, by posture and bodily movements, and by content and prosody of speech. Low-level auditory processing of emotional signals are the primary source of emotional information in speech. The prioritized processing of emotional sounds, particularly non-speech intonations of emotional state (gasps, screams, etc.), is illustrated within the primary and accessory auditory cortices. As with the visual system, amygdalo-cortical interactions are implicated in enhanced auditory attention to emotive sounds. Moreover, specificity in emotional processing may cross sensory modalities, such that ventral insular regions implicated in disgust-processing may be activated by auditory and visual expressions of disgust as well as by disgusting stimuli.

A degree of regional specialization in human emotional processing is suggested from the convergence of lesion and neuroimaging studies. Acquired damage to the amygdala impairs the recognition and behavioral experience of fear. Similarly, the neuroimaging literature emphasizes a predominant sensitivity of amygdala responses to threat and fear signals. As previously indicated, other studies implicate regions of insula and striatum in the selective processing of disgust. The impaired recognition of facial expressions of disgust was reported in a patient with damage to these regions, whereas the stimulation of the insula may evoke feelings of nausea or a perception of unpleasant tastes. These lines of evidence for specialized emotion-specific processing within different brain regions are generally circumscribed to fear/threat (amygdala), disgust (insula and striatum), and, to a lesser extent, sadness (subgenual cingulate activity). Many neuroimaging studies highlight a general sensitivity of amygdala responses to the emotional intensity of external emotional stimuli, for which threat is perhaps most arousing.

The insula cortex also appears to play a more complex role in emotion perception, apparently through relating perceptual information with interoceptive representations of bodily states. Thus, insula activity is engaged during the recognition and experience of disgust, sadness, happiness, and fear; during the learning and expression of threat; during the perception of noxious stimuli; and during the experience of phobic symptoms, hunger, and satiety; and even during explicit facial emotion categorization.

Memory and Learning

Emotion has a striking and well described impact on memory processes. Animal studies, particularly the work of LeDoux, highlight the central role of the amygdala in fear conditioning, a form of implicit memory. The same is true in humans, illustrated in many neuroimaging and lesion studies. Fear conditioning is a rapid form of learning that a stimulus is potentially harmful. If an adverse event (unconditioned stimulus, US; e.g., a painful shock) occurs after a relatively innocuous stimulus, the latter (the conditioned stimulus, CS) comes to predict the adverse event and will engender arousal responses associated with the presence of threat. Patients with bilateral amygdala damage do not acquire conditioned fear responses (autonomic or motor), despite having an intact explicit knowledge of the association between the CS and US. Functional neuroimaging studies also confirm the importance of the amygdala in fear conditioning (i.e., the learning of CS–US associations). However the role of the amygdala in the expression of threat responses is more time-limited and shows habituation. Consistent with animal data, neuroimaging studies also describe amygdala engagement in more general associative reinforcement learning, including operant stimulus–reward learning and appetitive behavior.

In addition to simple associative responses, human memory is characterized by declarative richness in episodic and semantic memory. These domains of memory, typically supported both at encoding and recollection by activity within the hippocampus, are strongly modulated by emotional experience. Typically, emotional events and stimuli are remembered better than nonemotional occurrences. Animal studies highlight noradrenergic mechanisms enhancing amygdalo-hippocampal connectivity in preferential encoding of emotional objects. Brain-imaging studies in humans have gone much further, highlighting amygdala activation during encoding actually predicts the accuracy of subsequent declarative memory of positively or negatively valenced stimuli (**Figure 2**) and in delineating the functional architecture for mood-congruency effects (in which negative information is encoded and recalled to a greater extent when the subject is in a negative mood and, likewise, positive material is encoded and recalled to a greater extent in positive mood states). However, the role of the amygdala extends beyond encoding processes; it is also engaged during the retrieval of emotional items and contexts.

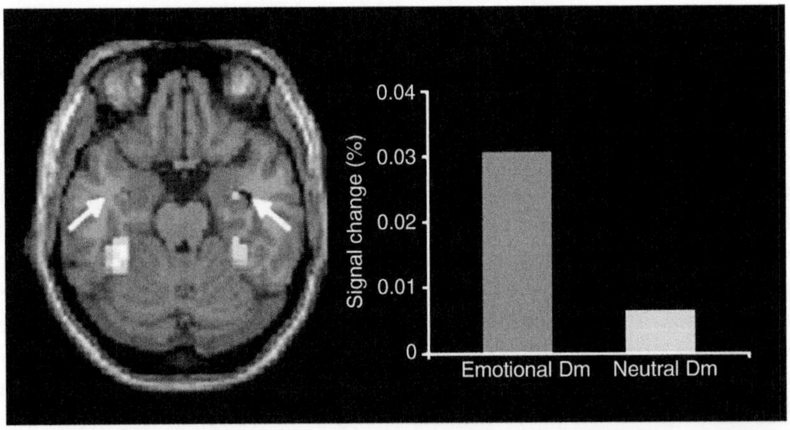

Figure 2 Level of activity within the amygdala (arrows) during the encoding of emotional images predicts whether a subject is subsequently able to recall emotional pictures (emotional Dm) but not neutral pictures (neutral Dm). Reprinted from *Neuron* **48**, E. A. Phelps & J. E. LeDoux, Contributions of the amygdala to emotion processing: from animal models to human behavior, pp. 175–187, Copyright 2005, and adapted from *Neuron*, **42**, F. Dolcos, K. S. LaBar & R. Cabeza, Interaction between the amygdala and the medial temporal lobe memory system predicts better memory for emotional events, pp. 855–863, Copyright (2004), with permission from Elsevier.

Interoception and Subjective Feeling States

Changes in bodily state, reflected in both physiological arousal and motor behavior, are obligatory defining characteristics of emotion. James and Lange, and more recently Damasio, argued that emotional feeling states must have their origin in the brain's representation of the bodily (arousal) state. Without changes in bodily arousal, there is no emotion. This peripheral account of emotion predicts that afferent feedback signals from muscles and viscera associated with physiological arousal are integral to emotional experience. These mechanisms have been illuminated in a number of neuroimaging experiments examining central representation and rerepresentation of autonomic arousal states and homoeostatic sensations, such as temperature.

The role of the insula cortex in this context is particularly interesting. In a positron emission tomography (PET) study, activation within the viscerosensory mid-insula cortex correlated closely with the actual stimulus temperature, yet the subjective ratings of the perceived intensity or pleasantness of hot and cold stimuli correlated with activity in the right anterior insula and orbitofrontal cortex. This finding suggests a dissociation between a primary central representation of viscerosensory information, within mid-insula, and subjective feelings of warmth or cold, represented in the right anterior insula and orbitofrontal cortex. A general role for these regions in the representation of emotional feelings is also supported by their activation observed during generated states of sadness and anger, anticipatory anxiety and pain, panic, disgust, sexual arousal, trustworthiness, and even subjective responses to music.

Behavioral and neuroimaging studies in patients with selective peripheral autonomic denervation (pure autonomic failure, PAF) lend further support to the importance of viscerosensory feedback to emotional feelings. These patients, who do not have autonomic (e.g., heart-rate or skin-conductance) changes in response to emotional stimuli or physiological stressors, show a subtle blunting of subjective emotional experience. In a fear conditioning study of PAF subjects and controls, both groups showed amygdala activity during the learning of threat (face stimuli, CS, were paired with an aversive blast of white noise, US). However, compared to controls, the right insula cortex showed attenuated responses to threat stimuli in the PAF patients, suggesting this region is sensitive to the presence and absence of autonomic responses generated during emotional processing. Moreover, when the threat stimuli were presented unconsciously (using backward masking), the same insula regions (including the right anterior insula) were sensitive to both the conscious awareness of emotion events and induced bodily arousal reactions. This study, particularly, suggests that the right insula is a neural substrate for the contextual integration of external emotional events with feeling states arising from bodily reactions.

The notion that subjective emotional feelings arise from central representations of bodily arousal states predicts that people who are more aware of their bodily responses may experience more intense emotions and feelings. Investigations examining individual differences in interoceptive awareness suggest that patients with anxiety disorders are more attuned to bodily reactions such as their own heartbeat or stomach motility. One such interoceptive task was translated into a neuroimaging study. Subjects were played a series of notes, presented in groups of 10, either synchronously or out of phase with their own heartbeats (see **Figure 3a**). In half the trials, subjects had to judge the timing of their heartbeat in relation to the notes (the control condition was a detection of a rogue note in the sequence). When subjects focused interoceptively to the timing of their own heartbeat, there was enhanced activity in the somatomotor, insula, and cingulate cortices. However, only one region, the right anterior insula cortex, reflected a conscious awareness of internal bodily responses (i.e., how accurately subjects performed the interoceptive task). Significantly, activity in this region, and even the relative amount of right anterior gray matter here (**Figure 3b**), predicted day-to-day awareness of bodily reaction and the subjective experience of negative emotions, particularly anxiety symptoms across individuals. Together these studies suggest that the right anterior insula is a principal neural substrate supporting conscious emotional feelings arising from interoceptive information concerning bodily arousal state (**Figure 4**).

Social Interaction

A characteristic of our social interactions is an intuitive ability to understand other people's mental and emotional states. Humans show a marked tendency to mimic one another's gesticulations, emotional facial expressions, and body postures, suggesting that this mirroring of activity mediates and facilitates emotional understanding among individuals. At a neural level, cells in monkey premotor cortex have been described that respond to observing or performing the same motor actions. Corresponding human imaging studies of action observation also illustrate premotor cortical activity when observing the actions of others, and magnetoencephalography (MEG) studies report resynchronization in the primary motor cortex. Significantly,

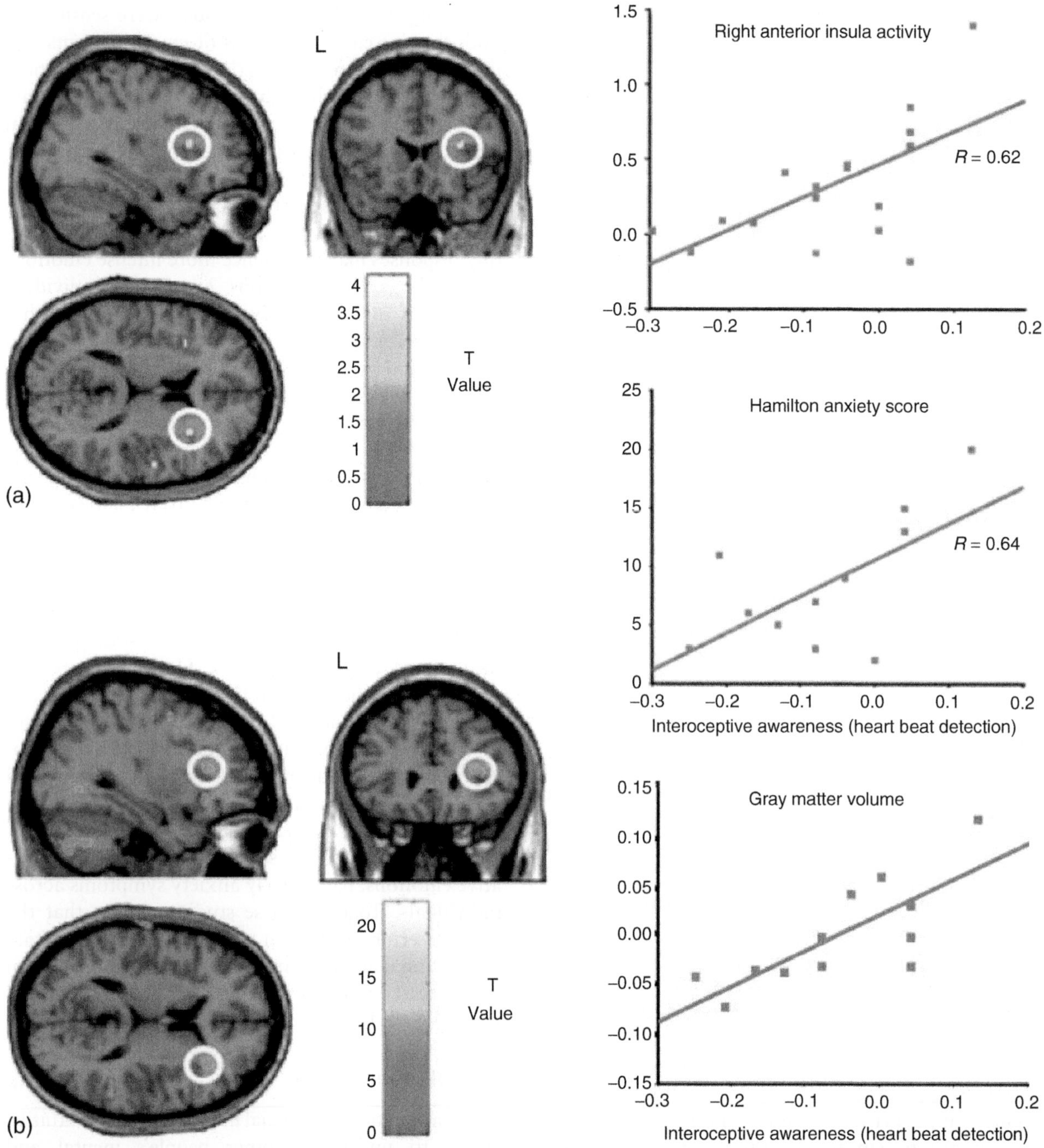

Figure 3 Interoceptive awareness (measured as accuracy on a heartbeat detection task). a, Association with increased neural activity in the right anterior insula/operculum; b, correlation with the gray matter volume of the right anterior insula region. Further subjects with greater interoceptive awareness also showed greater neural activity in this region during interoceptive trials. Activity in this region also correlated with anxiety scores, suggesting that emotional feeling states are supported by explicit interoceptive representations within right insula cortex. Reprinted by permission from Macmillan Publishers Ltd: *Nature Neuroscience*; Critchley, H. D., Wiens, S., Rotshtein, P., et al., Neural systems supporting interoceptive awareness, **7**(2), 189–195, copyright (2004).

these mirror activations are somatotopic with respect to the body part performing the action.

Accumulating evidence supports the extension of these action-perception mechanisms to emotions and feeling states. A common neural representation is proposed for the perception of actions and feelings in others and their experience in self. Thus, viewing emotional facial expressions in others activates automatically mirrored expressions on one's own face (surprisingly, even when the observed facial expressions are masked, hence unavailable to conscious awareness). Significantly, this automatic mimicking

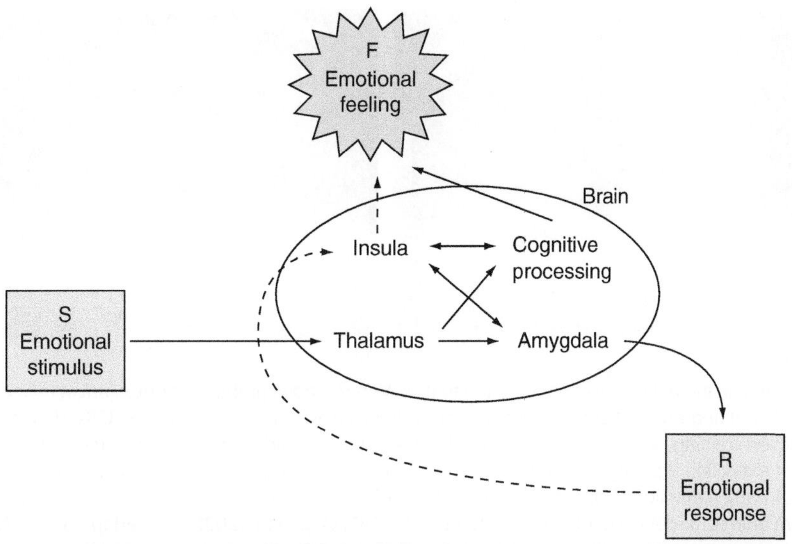

Figure 4 A functional neuroanatomical modification of William James's (1884) model of emotional responses. Emotional stimuli (S) elicit automatic emotional responses (R) via thalamus–amygdala pathways (solid line arrows). This low-level processing occurs independently of conscious cognitive processing. Peripheral autonomic responses are fed back to the mid-insula and then are remapped to the right anterior insula where they interact with higher-level cognitive processing. Emotional feeling states therefore result from peripheral-central interaction in the right anterior insula. Reprinted from *Trends in Cognitive Sciences*, **6**(8), J. S. Morris, How do you feel?, pp. 317–319, Copyright (2002), with permission from Elsevier.

of emotional expressions also extends to autonomic expressions of emotional states such as pupil size in expressions of sadness. Neuroimaging studies show shared neural activation in the somatosensory cortex when a subject experienced or observed another being touched, right insula activity when a subject experienced disgusting odors or observed expressions of disgust, and the activation of a common matrix of regions when a subject experienced or observed pain. The imitation or observation of emotional facial expressions also activates a largely similar network of brain regions including the premotor areas that are critical for action representation. There is also selectivity; compared to nonemotional facial movements, emotional expressions activate the right frontal operculum and anterior insula, and regions such as the amygdala, striatum, and subgenual cingulate are differentially responsive when imitating happy or sad emotions.

Emotion Regulation

Understanding the adaptive mechanisms through which we can control the expression of our emotions is clinically and socially important. Unlearning established emotional reactions is difficult. Many studies have examined the modulation of previously learned emotional responses with experimental extinction; the repeated presentation of a previously CS without its associated US rapidly leads to a diminished emotional response. Nevertheless, the relationship between the two stimuli is not forgotten but inhibited and can be rapidly reinstated. Neuroimaging of extinction learning (or the inhibition of emotional responses) shows increased amygdala activity in early extinction; however, retention after a day was associated with activity in the subgenual anterior cingulate and ventromedial prefrontal cortices, which suggests a role for this region in the longer-term recall of extinction learning (**Figure 5**).

Emotional responses may also be regulated volitionally, using cognitive control or reappraisal. For example, an image of a woman crying may be interpreted as one of sadness, but, if the subject is then told that the picture was taken after her daughter's wedding, it may be reappraised as one of great joy. Neuroimaging studies of emotional reappraisal demonstrate an attenuation of activity in the amygdala associated with enhanced activity in the left middle frontal gyrus, suggesting that activity within the lateral prefrontal cortex modulates emotional reactivity of the amygdala, possibly via connections to medial prefrontal cortex. Similar cognitive emotion-regulation techniques can powerfully diminish responses acquired through fear conditioning, and neuroimaging studies using this paradigm again show increased activity in the left middle frontal gyrus with cognitive control. Taken together, these studies suggest that cognitive emotion regulation and lower-level extinction learning recruit similar overlapping neural mechanisms for the regulation of the amygdala to control primary emotional responses.

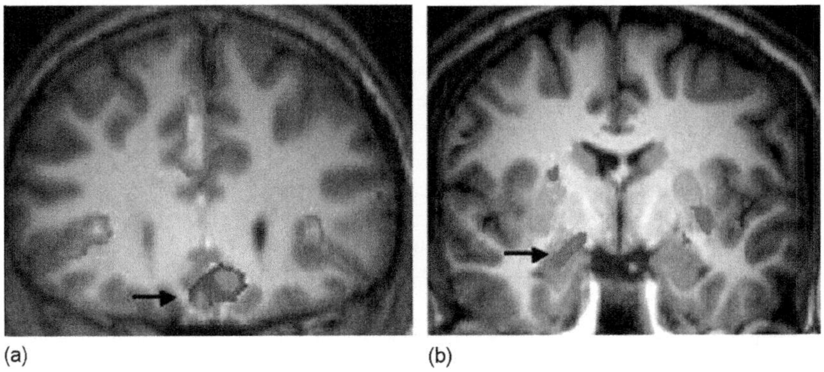

Figure 5 Regions activated in the extinction of conditioned fear. a, Ventromedial prefrontal cortex (arrow) showing less response to the conditioned stimulus (CS+) during acquisition; b, amygdala activation (arrow) in response to the CS+ during acquisition versus early extinction. During extinction training, ventromedial prefrontal cortex activity gradually increased, and the magnitude of this increase predicted the retention of extinction learning. Extinction training resulted in a reduction of amygdala activity in response to the CS+ and predicted the success of early extinction. Reprinted from *Neuron*, **48**, E A. Phelps & J. E. LeDoux, Contributions of the amygdala to emotion processing: from animal models to human behavior, pp. 175–187, Copyright (2005), and adapted from *Neuron*, **43**, E. A. Phelps et al., Extinction learning in humans: role of the amygdala and vmPFC, pp. 897–905, Copyright (2004), with permission from Elsevier.

Emotion Dysregulation

The wide-ranging influences of emotion on other psychological functions may also be seen in the variety of symptoms and presentations associated with emotional disorders. Posttraumatic stress disorder (PTSD), resulting from exposure to a highly traumatic emotional event and usually associated with injury or risk of injury to self or others, is frequently associated with symptoms in multiple psychological domains. Enhanced arousal and startle responses to previously innocuous stimuli are common, as are intrusive traumatic memories (flashbacks) of the triggering event, the numbing of emotional feelings, and impairments to social relationships. The identification of brain regions that show increased activation associated with the enhanced perception and memory for emotional events and associated feeling states enables the linkage of psychological mechanisms in conditions such as PTSD and phobias with their underlying neural substrates.

Abnormal cortisol regulation and adrenergic stress responses are also seen in PTSD, as is a reduction in hippocampal volume. Imaging studies showing a similar reduction in hippocampal volume in endocrine disorders associated with chronically elevated cortisol levels, such as Cushing's disease, suggest an etiological role for stress hormones such as cortisol in this reduction in hippocampal volume. These conclusions are further supported by a recent study of healthy postmenopausal women, which showed a strong correlation between hippocampal volume and lifetime levels of perceived stress, suggesting an influence of stress on regional brain volumes even in the normal population.

Maladaptive cognitive interpretations of situations or events are central components of many emotional disorders such as depression and the anxiety disorders and are a feature focused on by many of the psychological therapies used in their treatment. Understanding the neural mechanisms mediating the modulation of emotional responses will be essential to developing a comprehensive neurobiological understanding of these disorders. Furthermore, a better understanding of these mechanisms offers the opportunity to develop more targeted approaches specifically focused on changing these maladaptive emotional reactions.

Further Reading

Calder, A. J., Keane, J., Manes, F., et al. (2001). Impaired recognition and experience of disgust following brain injury. *Nature Neuroscience* 3(11), 1077–1078.

Craig, A. D. (2002). How do you feel? interoception: the sense of the physiological condition of the body. *Nature Reviews Neuroscience* 3, 655–667.

Critchley, H. D., Mathias, C. J. and Dolan, R. J. (2001). Neuroanatomical basis for first and second order representations of bodily states. *Nature Neuroscience* **4**(2), 207–212.

Critchley, H. D., Mathias, C. J. and Dolan, R. J. (2002). Fear conditioning in humans: the influence of awareness and autonomic arousal on functional neuroanatomy. *Neuron* 33(4), 653–663.

Critchley, H. D., Wiens, S., Rotshtein, P., et al. (2004). Neural systems supporting interoceptive awareness. *Nature Neuroscience* 7(2), 189–195.

Damasio, A. R. (1994). *Descartes error: emotion, reason and the human brain.* New York: Grosset/Putnam.

Damasio, A. R. (1999). *The feeling of what happens: body and emotion in the making of consciousness.* New York: Harcourt Brace.

Darwin, C. (1872). *The expressions of emotion in man and animals.* London: John Murray. (Reprinted 1998 (3rd edn.), Ekman, P. (ed.). London: Harper Collins.)

Dimberg, U., Thunberg, D. and Elmehed, K. (2000). Unconscious facial reactions to emotional facial expressions. *Psychological Science* **11**(1), 86–89.
Dolan, R. J. (2002). Emotion, cognition, and behavior. *Science* **298**, 1191–1194.
Dolcos, F., LaBar, K. S. and Cabeza, R. (2004). Interaction between the amygdala and the medial temporal lobe memory system predicts better memory for emotional events. *Neuron* **42**, 855–863.
Gallese, V. (2003). The manifold nature of interpersonal relations: the quest for a common mechanism. *Philosophical Transactions of Royal Society London B* **358**(1431), 517–528.
Gianaros, P. J., Jennings, J. R., Sheu, L. K., et al. (2007). Prospective reports of chronic life stress predict decreased grey matter volume in the hippocampus. *NeuroImage* **35**(1), 220–232.
Harrison, N. A., Singer, T., Rotshtein, P., et al. (2006). Pupillary contagion: central mechanisms engaged in sadness processing. *Social and Affective Neuroscience* **1**, 5–17.
James, W. (1884). Physical basis of emotion. *Psychological Review* **1**, 516–529.
LaBar, K. S. and Cabeza, R. (2006). Cognitive neuroscience of emotional memory. *Nature Reviews Neuroscience* **7**, 54–64.
Lange, C. (1885/1922). *The emotions*. Haupt, I. A. (trans.). Baltimore, MD: Williams & Wilkins.
LeDoux, J. E. (1996). *The emotional brain: the mysterious underpinnings of emotional life*. New York: Simon & Schuster.
Morris, J. S. (2002). How do you feel? *Trends in Cognitive Sciences* **6**(8), 317–319.
Morris, J. S., DeGelder, B., Weiskrantz, L., et al. (2001). Differential extrageniculostriate and amygdala responses to presentation of emotional faces in a cortically blind field. *Brain* **124**, 1241–1252.
Morris, J. S., Friston, K. J., Buchel, C., et al. (1998). A neuromodulatory role for the human amygdala in processing emotional facial expressions. *Brain* **121**, 47–57.
Morris, J. S., Ohman, A. and Dolan, R. J. (1998). Conscious and unconscious emotional learning in the human amygdala. *Nature* **393**, 467–470.
Ochsner, K. N. and Gross, J. J. (2005). The cognitive control of emotion. *Trends in Cognitive Sciences* **9**(5), 242–249.
Penfield, W. and Faulk, M. E. (1955). The insula: further observations on its function. *Brain* **78**(4), 445–470.
Phelps, E. A. and LeDoux, J. E. (2005). Contributions of the amygdala to emotion processing: from animal models to human behavior. *Neuron* **48**, 175–187.
Phillips, M. L., Young, A. W., Senior, C., et al. (1997). A specific neural substrate for perception of facial expressions of disgust. *Nature* **389**, 495–498.
Scherer, K. R. (2000). Psychological models of emotion. In: Borod, J. C. (ed.) *The neuropsychology of emotion*, pp. 137–162. New York: Oxford University Press.
Singer, T., Seymour, B., O'Doherty, J., et al. (2004). Empathy for pain involves the affective but not sensory components of pain. *Science* **303**(5661), 1157–1162.
Vuilleumier, P., Armony, J. L., Driver, J., et al. (2003). Distinct spatial frequency sensitivities for processing faces and emotional expressions. *Nature Neuroscience* **6**, 624–631.
Vuilleumier, P., Richardson, M. P., Armony, J. L., et al. (2004). Distant influences of amygdala lesions on visual cortical activation during emotional face processing. *Nature Neuroscience* **7**, 1271–1278.
Wicker, B., Keysers, C., Plailly, J., et al. (2003). Both of us disgusted in my insula: the common neural basis of seeing and feeling disgust. *Neuron* **40**, 655–664.

Psychological Stressors, Overview

S M Monroe and G M Slavich
University of Oregon, Eugene, OR, USA

This is a revised version of the article by S M Monroe, Encyclopedia of Stress First Edition, volume 3, pp 287–293, © 2000, Elsevier Inc.

Glossary

Catecholamines — Neurotransmitters, including epinephrine, norepinephrine, and dopamine, that promote sympathetic nervous system activity. They may be released in substantial quantities during stressful times.

Corticosteroids — Complex chemical compounds produced in the outer layer of the adrenal gland, which include both mineralocorticoids and glucocorticoids. Mineralocorticoids maintain salt and fluid balance in the body, while glucocorticoids have metabolic and anti-inflammatory effects and are important mediators of the stress response.

Neuroendocrine — Relating to the nervous and endocrine system, which produces endocrine secretions that help to control bodily metabolic activity.

Stress sensitization The enhanced and progressive sensitivity of an organism to stress given repeated exposure to stressors.

Historical and General Considerations

Historical Matters

It is frequently assumed that psychological stressors are a concern of especially modern origins, or at least that they have become more prominent with recent advances in society and technology. It is also commonly assumed that with the accelerating progress of civilization, more and more people are afflicted with mental and physical disorders. Historical accounts, however, suggest that such ideas about stressors, civilization, and disease have been common for quite some time. Sir Clifford Albutt (1895: 217) expressed such sentiments quite clearly well over 100 years ago:

> To turn now... to nervous disability, to hysteria... to the frightfulness, the melancholy, the unrest due to living at a high pressure, the world of the railway, the pelting of telegrams, the strife of business ... surely, at any rate, these maladies or the causes of these maladies are more rife than they were in the days of our fathers?

The tendency to view life in stressful terms may be even more basic to human cognition than is readily apparent. The Greek myth of Sisyphus is enlightening in this regard. The perpetual work of pushing a boulder up a mountain – only to have gravity bring it back down after each and every effort – captures some of the qualities and characteristics linked to modern views of psychological stressors. Perhaps there is something fundamental about the human condition and psyche that fosters a perception of the world as a place rife with unrelenting demands that can never be fully met, resulting in subjective states of fatigue and distress and eventually leading to ill health. Each era may bring its unique colorations to such perceptions and its own attributions regarding their origins.

It is against this psychological backdrop of belief and possible bias in thinking that modern work on psychological stressors must be examined. Psychological stressors and related concepts have been popular explanatory constructs throughout recent, and perhaps not so recent, history. As a result of their subjective allure and apparent explanatory power, these ideas have often been loosely formulated. Owing to conceptual fuzziness and ambiguity, not only has progress in science been slowed, but nonscientific issues, ideas, and biases have been permitted to masquerade as scientific truths.

The concept of psychological stressors is rich with possibilities for shedding light on important matters in adaptation, dysfunction, and disease. The concept is paralleled, though, by the potential pitfalls that accompany its intuitive appeal. The challenge is to translate the fertile ideas about psychological stressors into more precise concepts, definitions, and operational procedures. With more sound definitional and methodological procedures in place, the utility of stress concepts for understanding adaptation and maladaptation, mental and physical disorder and disease, will be better understood.

Early Ideas and Research

A broad foundation for understanding the organism's reactions to challenging environmental circumstances was laid down by Claude Bernard and Charles Darwin during the nineteenth century. Each of these two influential individuals in his own way touched on issues deriving from the tension resulting from ongoing adaptation to changing and challenging environmental circumstances. Yet it was not until the early to mid-twentieth century that such generality and complexity began to be translated into more specific terminology and technology. These efforts can be traced to at least three different lines of thought and research.

The early work of Walter Cannon dealt with ideas about common emotions and their physiological consequences, particularly with respect to the body's maintenance of homeostasis. This line of study was complemented shortly thereafter by the animal laboratory studies of Hans Selye, wherein acute and severe stressors were systematically investigated. It was in Selye's work that the concept of stress most forcefully emerged. Stress was defined as "the nonspecific response of the body to any demand" (Selye, 1976: 74). Stressors, in turn, were defined as "that which produces stress" (Selye, 1976: 78). Finally, from another vantage point, Adolph Meyer popularized the life chart methodology. This approach emphasized the importance of the dynamic interplay between biological, psychological, and social factors, such that important events within the person's biography became foci of attention for studying health and disease. Collectively, these activities, and the multiple lines of research they generated, served to initiate specific awareness of, and interest in, psychological stressors.

Arising outside of the more purposeful activities of science was another influential development that contributed to the emerging idea that psychological stressors cause both mental and physical disorders. Prior to World War II, psychopathology was commonly attributed to genetic factors or acquired biological propensities; so-called normal people devoid of such taints were thought to be largely invulnerable to mental illness. The experiences during and after World War II dramatically shifted thinking in medical and psychiatric circles to incorporate the idea that severe stress could precipitate breakdown in a previously healthy individual. Once this conceptual shift began, it underscored the multiplicity of health consequences that could be caused by severe stressors. It also opened the door for enlarging conceptual perspectives on psychological stressors by considering how less severe, yet still noxious, aspects of the social and physical environment could contribute to, or precipitate, pathology.

Conceptual Progress

Upon the foundations of stress research and theory laid down by Selye, Cannon, and Meyer, along with the influences of experiences of World War II, modern inquiry into the effects of psychological stressors became a topic of increasing interest and, eventually, of extensive empirical inquiry. Two general themes may be discerned that have underpinned advances in theory: (1) characteristics of psychological stressors and (2) individual differences in response to psychological stressors.

Stressor Characteristics

Despite general agreement about the importance of psychological stressors for health and well-being, determining exactly what it is about stressful circumstances that is deleterious has proven challenging. An initial question of considerable theoretical importance involved the basic nature of psychological stressors: are they best viewed in a unitary manner as nonspecific demands on the organism (as postulated by Selye), or are psychological stressors more effectively viewed as a class of conditions harboring specific component characteristics of importance? Investigators from two traditions – animal and human research – have addressed this issue, with parallel and sometimes intersecting developments. Although considerable progress has been made, the general topic of elaborating stressor characteristics remains one of central importance in current thinking on psychological stressors.

Animal Laboratory Research

A great deal of work in the 1960s and 1970s was performed to determine whether specific psychological characteristics of stressors possess qualitatively distinct implications for the organism. Initially this work revealed how particular features associated with the environmental stressors might be important for predicting adverse outcomes (as opposed to the more psychologically neutral notion proposed by Selye of general or nonspecific adaptive demands). Such research went on to probe the types of psychological stressors and their effects. It became of central interest to understand in a more differentiated way the effects of diverse psychological stressors.

Animal laboratory studies adopted ingenious designs to differentiate psychological components associated with environmental stressors, with the findings from these studies demonstrating that distinctive psychological characteristics were responsible for many immediate behavioral or physiological responses. For example, specific psychological characteristics of stressors, such as undesirability or controllability, were particularly pertinent for the development of various disorders. It became clear, too, that other characteristics of stressors were important. For example, different parameters of shock administration (acute, intermittent, or chronic) produced different physiological effects in animals. Further, such differences might increase, decrease, or not influence the development of particular diseases. Finally, psychological stressors not only could influence immediate psychobiological functioning, but also could have long-term ramifications through permanent alteration of the organism.

As the importance of specificity of stressor characteristics became more apparent and accepted, questions about the specificity of stress responses also arose. What were the implications of specific stressor characteristics for different facets of psychological and physiological functioning? Such theoretical developments greatly extended the framework for inquiry, requiring attention to multiple characteristics of stressors in relation to multiple psychological and biological processes and outcomes. Relatively simple, singular response indices (e.g., corticosteroids, catecholamines) were replaced by patterns of behavioral and biological effects or profiles of neuroendocrine responses. More recently, other levels of conceptualization have been proposed. For example, psychological stressors may promote fundamental disruptions in oscillatory regulation of basic biological functions or reversions to earlier modes of functioning.

Overall, research on psychological stressors from animal research has moved beyond unidimensional and linear concepts of stressors and their effects. More recent thinking has adopted a larger framework for understanding the diverse characteristics of stressors that influence particular and varied response systems of the organism. The response systems of interest have expanded from single systems to patterns or profiles of response across multiple indices.

Human Experimental and Field Studies

Investigators of psychological stressors in humans also conducted innovative and insightful studies, both in the laboratory and in the field. Early work tended to focus on the aversive subjective attributes, particularly perception or appraisal, of psychological stressors as evaluated in an experimental setting. Yet at about this same time research on stressful life events began. It is in this area of stress research that activity on psychological stressors perhaps reached its pinnacle, in terms of both productivity and popular interest.

Extrapolating from animal laboratory studies on the one hand, and integrating with Meyer's life chart procedures on the other, Thomas Holmes and Richard Rahe first formulated the idea that distinctive changes in one's life circumstances – specific and documentable life events – could be defined and assessed in an objective manner. The work was initially based on case histories of some 5000 tuberculosis patients, from which they derived a list of 43 life events "empirically observed to occur just prior to the time of onset of disease, including, for example, marriage, trouble with the boss, jail term, death of spouse, change in sleeping habits, retirement, death in the family, and vacation" (Holmes, 1978: 46). The Schedule of Recent Experiences (SRE) was developed and published, and by 1978 more than 1000 publications had utilized this convenient method for probing a vast range of questions pertaining to stress and illness.

The common feature associated with these disparate life changes – the stressor characteristic of primary concern – was thought to be the degree of social readjustment entailed by the event: "The relative importance of each item is determined not by the item's desirability, by the emotions associated with the item, nor by the meaning of the item for the individual; it is the amount of change that we are studying and the relationship of the amount of change to the onset of illness" (Holmes, 1978: 47). This viewpoint is consonant with Selye's ideas about stressors and stress. Hence, the psychologically neutral notion of the readjustment required of life changes was conceptualized as the characteristic responsible vulnerability to a wide variety of psychological and physical maladies.

Much as the emphasis in animal laboratory studies shifted from psychological neutral concepts of any demand, viewpoints within the stressful life events literature began to shift away from the concept of readjustment and toward emphasizing the undesirable characteristics of events. Human studies of life events consequently began to focus on the particular characteristics of psychological stressors and their potentially unique effects. The principle of specificity also was extended from the characteristics of stressors to the specific consequences of such experiences, elaborating theory about the importance of specific psychological stressors for specific responses and eventually for specific types of disorder or disease. A vast literature on this topic has appeared over the past two decades, with diverse conceptualizations of psychological stressors and myriad methods designed to measure them.

The issue of desirability of events, however, along with the more general issue involving stressor characteristics, brought into focus another important subject in the study of psychological stressors: individual differences. What might be viewed or experienced as undesirable by one person could be viewed or experienced as desirable by another. As discussed next, a variety of considerations are invoked to explain variability in effects and outcomes in relation to psychological stressors.

Individual Differences

Despite progress in conceptualizing the component characteristics of psychological stressors, and despite progress in prediction afforded by such work, considerable variability in response to psychological stressors occurs. Even under the most dire of stressful conditions, all animals or individuals do not necessarily break down. Although a refined understanding of stressor characteristics still may account for some variability in outcomes, other factors may be useful to effectively model effects of psychological stressors. Progress in understanding this issue has again come from both the basic laboratory and human studies of psychological stressors.

Animal Laboratory Research

Although there were characteristic features of physiological responses to the stressors employed in the early paradigm adopted by Selye, not all animals responded to stress in an identical manner. Further, individual differences in response were even more pronounced when the less severe types of stressors were used.

Such variables as prior experience, availability of coping responses, and other aspects of the social and experimental context were found to moderate the influence of psychological stressors. For example, when rats are exposed to electric shock, animals that cannot predict shock occurrence (via warning tones) develop a sixfold increase in gastric ulceration compared to their yoked counterparts (who receive the warning tones). Work along these lines demonstrated the delicate and often subtle interplay among stressor, social context, and resources available to the organism in determining response outcomes. These lines of study, too, suggested that individual differences in susceptibility to psychological stress could be viewed within a developmental perspective in terms of stress sensitization. Laboratory animals repeatedly exposed to severe psychological stressors can become neurobiologically sensitized to the stressors, such that relatively minor degrees of stress eventually acquire the capability of triggering pathogenic responses.

Human Life Stress Research

The importance of individual differences was perhaps more apparent in studies of human life stress and its consequences. A consistent criticism of life events research was the relatively weak association between psychological stressors and disorder. It was assumed that other considerations moderated stress effects, and the elucidation of such factors would increase the predictive capability of disorder following stressful events. Again, there were a number of factors that were believed to moderate the impact of psychological stressors, ranging from environmental factors such as social support to more individual factors such as prior experience and coping. Developmental considerations have also been important in recent theorizing about individual differences in responsivity to psychological stressors, with the idea that prior exposure to severe psychological stressors renders the individual more susceptible to increasingly lower levels of psychological stress.

A major arena for understanding individual differences in stress susceptibility has been perception. The early and elegant laboratory studies of human stress had indicated the importance of such individual differences in perception, or appraisal, of stressors, and such thinking was readily incorporated into theory and method. Studies of life events, for example, used subjective weights of events experienced by the study participants. Once this avenue of inquiry was opened, it also brought to the forefront a variety of influences on perception, along with other factors that might influence stress responsivity. Thus, research began to focus not only on appraisal of stressors, but also on coping, social support, personality, and other considerations that in theory could moderate the effects of psychological stressors.

As research progressed along these lines, it became clear that making some of these distinctions was easier to do in theory than in method. For example, while it made good sense theoretically to consider an individual's subjective perception of psychological stressors, it was more difficult to employ such information in a scientifically sound manner. When it came to operationalization, serious problems became apparent. For example, owing to depression-based perceptual biases, a depressed person might have a skewed perception of events and rate them as particularly negative (irrespective of the objectively stressful qualities *per se*). Generally, such concerns raised an important paradox for investigations of psychological stressors. Namely, although a large part of the desired knowledge pertained to the individual's idiosyncratic appraisal of psychological stressors, methodological concerns cautioned against direct assessment of such information. Instead, alternative approaches were developed to avoid the pitfalls of using subjective reports in research on psychological stressors, as well as to avoid other problems with these methods that eventually came to light.

Methodological Considerations and Recent Developments

While concepts and methods often intertwine and, united, nurture progress, at times one or the other component may unduly influence development (for good or for bad). This situation appears applicable to research on psychological stressors, in which the methods adopted in animal laboratory research have constrained theory and methods adopted in human life stress research have misled theory on psychological stressors.

Animal Laboratory Research

The original work of Selye typically employed situations that were overpowering or unavoidable for the animal. Such conditions did not permit an evaluation of behavioral responses or other moderating influences that could influence an animal's adaptation to stressors. Further, it was realized that this methodological paradigm was not informative about psychological stressors that might be of greater ecological and evolutionary relevance (i.e., more typical with respect to the animal's natural environment and evolutionary history). Thus, such an approach readily masked the implications of less severe psychological stressors on physiology and behavior, which in turn might represent a more fertile area of inquiry into stressor effects. Finally, the nature of the stressor employed in the early stress laboratory studies also contributed to the aforementioned difficulty in differentiating physical from psychological effects, which inhibited progress in the arena of conceptual development.

Overall, the range of psychological stressors was constrained by the methods adopted. Theory, in turn, was constrained to account for the consequences of stressors under such restricted and relatively unnatural stressor conditions. More recent research has benefited from methods that encourage assessment of diverse characteristics of psychological stressors and their severities and incorporate the assessment of a wide variety of behavioral and biological response possibilities. Current perspectives based on these broader methodological approaches suggest that the organism's responses are often exquisitely specific nuances of stressors encountered.

Human Studies of Stressful Life Events

The bulk of empirical work on human life stress has been based on self-report checklist methods. The prototype of this approach is the SRE, the instrument that catalyzed research in this area. The popularity of the SRE was likely due to the combination of the intuitive appeal of the stress concept, the apparent objectivity of the method, and the overall impression of scientific legitimacy.

The methodological paradigm launched by the SRE, however, embodied several problems. It became clear that subjects did not report life events in a reliable manner over time and that investigators did not adequately control for the directionality of effects in research designs (e.g., being depressed initially could bring about life events such as trouble at work, difficulties with spouse, and so on). Indeed, many of the initial items on the SRE were direct indicators of disorder or illness. For example, some of the key criteria for defining clinical depression were represented in the original SRE (e.g., major change in eating habits, major change in sleeping habits). If measures of life events were directly confounded with the presence of disorder or were contaminated by the effects of pre- or coexisting disorder, then clearly general theory about psychological stressors, as well as theory about the characteristics of psychological stressors, rested on flawed information.

In response to these methodological concerns, other investigators designed semistructured interview protocols and developed explicit guidelines, decision rules, and operational criteria for defining and rating life events. These developments further highlighted serious problems with self-report checklist methods. For example, there was too much subjective leeway permitted in defining what constitutes an event with self-report procedures, resulting in considerable variability of content within ostensibly uniform categories of events. In order to have a more firm methodological foundation, the more elaborate and extensive interview and rater-based procedures were employed, which helped to standardize measurement across individuals.

In general, such interview and rater-based approaches have been found to enhance the reliability of life event assessments and to provide stronger predictions of particular kinds of disorders following the occurrence of psychological stressors. Procedures such as these also provide a solid foundation upon which to build in terms of developing taxonomies of psychological stressors and their effects. Although such approaches are more time- and labor-intensive to implement, they represent the current-day gold standard for assessing psychological stressors.

Human Studies Employing Other Measures of Psychological Stressors

There have been other methods in which psychological stressors have been defined and studied. None of these approaches has received the degree of attention devoted to the work on life events, yet each may have useful properties for the study of psychological stressors. Two lines of investigation are noteworthy.

Many investigations have targeted people who experience a specific life event and compared these individuals with controls who do not experience the event. For example, individuals who become unemployed are compared to individuals who do not experience this event in relation to a variety of psychological and physical processes and outcomes. Such work is useful for examining a potentially more homogenous process with more readily identifiable outcomes. On the other hand, such studies may oversimplify the psychological stressors associated with an event and not specifically articulate the different components within the general event that are most pernicious for health and well-being. For example, the effects can be partitioned into a variety of stressful themes that, although often intercorrelated, may not have uniform effects. Thus, although people who become unemployed in general may experience a loss of self-esteem, loss of income, loss of daily schedule, and so on, each particular situation may pull more or less for heightened responses along these different dimensions. Work sensitive to such variability in the component characteristics will be most useful for research on psychological stressors.

Finally, there also have been efforts to measure psychological stressors through questionnaire or diary methods, inquiring about minor but common daily events, chronic conditions, appraisal processes, and other indicators or correlates of psychological stressors. A promising recent avenue of research involves ecological momentary assessment, where subjects can be prompted throughout the day to respond to queries about their circumstances and psychological states. Such procedures help minimize problems with standard retrospective methods.

In closing, it is appropriate to return to the concerns and caveat with which the article began. The specter of possible biases in the measurement of psychological stressors must be consistently borne in mind, and methods employed must be rigorously attentive to such concerns, to provide a solid empirical foundation upon which theory and research can build for this important area of investigation.

Further Reading

Allbutt, C. (1895). Nervous diseases and modern life. *Contemporary Review* **67**, 217.

Brown, G. W. and Harris, T. O. (1989). *Life events and illness.* London: Guilford Press.

Cohen, S., Kessler, R. C. and Gordon, L. U. (eds.) (1995). *Measuring stress: a guide for health and social scientists.* New York: Oxford University Press.

Dohrenwend, B. P. (ed.) (1998). *Adversity, stress, and psychopathology.* New York: Oxford University Press.

Holmes, T. H. and Rahe, R. H. (1967). The social readjustment rating scale. *Journal of Psychosomatic Research* **11**, 213–218.

Lazarus, R. S. (1966). *Psychological stress and the coping process.* New York: McGraw-Hill.

Monroe, S. M. and Harkness, K. L. (2005). Life stress, the 'kindling' hypothesis, and the recurrence of depression: considerations from a life stress perspective. *Psychological Review* **112**, 417–445.

Post, R. M. (1992). Transduction of psychosocial stress into the neurobiology of recurrent affective disorder. *American Journal of Psychiatry* **149**, 999–1010.

Selye, H. (1976). *The stress of life* (2nd edn.). New York: McGraw-Hill.

Stone, A. A., Shiffman, S. S. and DeVries, M. W. (1999). Ecological momentary assessment. In: Kahneman, D., Diener, D. & Schwarz, N. (eds.) *Well-being: the foundations of hedonic psychology.* New York: Russell Sage Foundation.

Weiner, H. (1992). *Perturbing the organism: the biology of stressful experience.* Chicago, IL: University of Chicago Press.

Weiss, J. M. (1972). Psychological factors in stress and disease. *Scientific American* **226**, 104–113.

Life Events and Health

P Surtees and N Wainwright
Strangeways Research Laboratory and University of Cambridge, Cambridge, UK

Glossary

Annual prevalence The proportion of people identified with a disease or other characteristic at any time during the period of a year.

Life event A discrete incident or circumstance that may disrupt life, may require adaptation, and may be associated with, or result in, physical and/or emotional health change.

Major depressive disorder A health state characterized by sustained feelings of sadness, hopelessness, helplessness, and worthlessness that is often also accompanied by suicidal thoughts, an inability to concentrate or to take pleasure in activities that were once enjoyable, and sleep, appetite, and memory problems.

Prospective cohort study A study population defined according to risk factor exposure and prospectively followed up, for example, to ascertain incident disease endpoints.

Record linkage study A study that brings together information included in two or more records based upon a unique identifying system.

On January 17, 1995, at 5:46:52 a.m., the southern part of Hyogo Prefecture in Japan was struck, without warning, by the Hanshin-Awaji earthquake, which measured 7.2 on the Richter scale and lasted for around 20 s. During the 3 months following this unexpected catastrophic natural disaster, in the districts of Awaji Island near the earthquake epicenter, heart attack rates increased by 50% and stroke rates by 90% in comparison with the same observation period during the previous year. Survivors in areas with the greatest loss and destruction of housing experienced the highest subsequent heart attack rates. While the occurrence of a profoundly stressful life event, such as the Hanshin-Awaji earthquake, provides a clear and dramatic incident from which to assess subsequent health, the attribution of health change to life events experienced more commonly across a lifetime is less straightforward.

Measurement

Life event assessment techniques have evolved to include the use of checklists and interview methods and have been used in a wide variety of research designs to aid understanding of the risk of life events to health.

Checklists

During the late 1940s, Thomas Holmes and colleagues at the University of Washington started to investigate the relationship between adjustment to social stress and illness onset using a self-administered instrument, the Schedule of Recent Experience (SRE). The SRE included a list of 43 life change events intended to represent most circumstances experienced by the patient groups studied, and to which differing degrees of readjustment were required. A subsequent scaling study was designed to take account of both the intensity and the relative time judged to be needed to adjust to each life event on the list. This Social Readjustment Rating Scale (SRRS) included the life events ranked according to these degrees of readjustment – subsequently termed life change units (LCUs). The event of highest rank was death of spouse (with a mean value score of 100), relative to marriage, with a mean value score of 50, and, for example, death of close friend, which scored 37. Typically the LCUs for all events reported on the checklist to have been experienced during a given time period (e.g., the past year) were summed to give a measure of the cumulative social stress experienced. With varying degrees of modification, the SRRS has served as a model of a questionnaire format for assessing life event experience in relation to health. For example, in psychiatry, scaling studies focused on the capacity of life events to induce distress and were scaled in terms of their associated upset or undesirability. While the checklist approach provided a powerful impetus to study the association between life events and illness, these techniques attracted criticism. This stemmed from suggestions that the circumstances to be rated were defined vaguely, resulting in variability in item interpretation, that symptoms were included in the event lists, and that the assumption of additivity of event effects was untested. Despite these criticisms, the list techniques can provide a reliable assessment of the occurrence of specified adverse experiences, although they may be limited in their capacity to provide details of the context surrounding their occurrence.

Interviews

The Life Events and Difficulties Schedule (LEDS), an interview method for the assessment of stressful life events, was developed in the late 1960s and over the subsequent 30 years by George Brown and colleagues at London University. In contrast to the early respondent-based checklist assessment techniques, this approach was based on using the interviewer as the measuring instrument. Through the LEDS, ratings of adverse experience followed from consideration of both the context and meaning of the immediate circumstances associated with a stressful situation. Use of the LEDS was designed to provide measures of the long-term threat of life events experienced, to attempt to date their occurrence accurately, and to rate ongoing long-term difficulties. In addition, LEDS-based research drew attention to the importance of distinguishing the extent to which life events and long-term difficulties could be illness-related in order to help clarify their etiological significance for illness onset.

However, Bruce Dohrenwend and colleagues, at Columbia University, New York, raised fundamental criticisms of the LEDS core ratings of contextual threat. These criticisms were based upon their view that the contextual ratings represented a nonexplicit distillation of the event, the social circumstances surrounding its occurrence, and the personal history of the person who experienced the event, into one measure. Dohrenwend and colleagues argued that these situational and personal variables may themselves be important risk factors for illness, therefore creating ambiguity in understanding precisely which aspects of the stress process were associated with the illness outcomes of interest. They attempted to address these perceived problems with the LEDS approach through developing their own theoretical framework and measurement approach, using the Structured Event Probe and Narrative Rating method (SEPRATE) of life events measurement. The SEPRATE semistructured interview method was designed to provide measures that distinguished between the life event, the ongoing social situation present before event occurrence (for example, employment circumstances), and the personal dispositions and characteristics of the person who had experienced the life event. While the LEDS and SEPRATE share similarities in methodological approach, they differ markedly in their representation and rating of life event experience.

Health Associations

Efforts to synthesize research findings relating life events to health outcomes have been limited by the rarity of studies that meet stringent research design requirements. A commonly used set of criteria to help establish causality was proposed by the epidemiologist and statistician Sir Austin Bradford Hill. These criteria include consideration of the strength of the association, whether it is consistent (i.e., repeatedly demonstrated in different populations), whether there is evidence of temporality (i.e., the presence of the risk factor precedes onset of disease), and whether a dose–response relationship exists (i.e., disease risk increases monotonically with increasing exposure).

These criteria have not yet been fully met for any health outcome following from stressful life event experience. However, increasingly persuasive evidence is now accumulating in relation to the onset, and subsequent prognosis, of some health outcomes.

Life Events and Psychological Health

Evidence from both prospective cohort and record linkage studies has consistently shown an association between the experience of stressful life events and the subsequent onset of episodes of major depressive disorder. The strength of this association has been shown to vary according to the way in which life events were assessed: generally stronger associations were reported when events were assessed using the LEDS approach, rather than through use of the list techniques such as the SRE. These studies have also suggested evidence of a dose–response relationship, with the risk of depressive disorder onset increasing broadly in step with the severity of the events experienced. A dose–response association between the number of recently reported stressful life events and the annual prevalence of depressive disorder is illustrated in **Figure 1**.

Record linkage studies, through their use of very large populations, provide a potentially powerful research design with which to investigate the relationship between severely stressful events and psychiatric health. For example, one study linked records from the Danish Civil Registration System with the Danish Psychiatric Central Register to investigate the association between death of a child and subsequent parental admission to psychiatric hospital. Based on over a million persons identified in the registers and almost 12 000 deaths of children aged under 18 years, the study revealed a 67% increased risk of hospital admission for any psychiatric condition among the parents who had lost a child, with the risk being greatest for mothers and most pronounced for admission with a depressive condition.

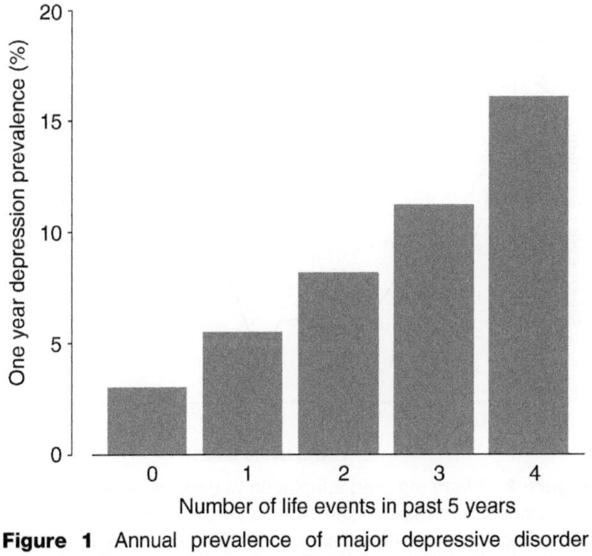

Figure 1 Annual prevalence of major depressive disorder according to the number of moderately or extremely upsetting (non-health-related) life events reported during the previous 5 years. Based upon 20 921 participants in the European Prospective Investigation into Cancer (EPIC)-Norfolk study in the United Kingdom.

The relationship between chronic enduring or progressively deteriorating stressful circumstances and psychiatric health is complex and difficult to study. For example, changes in the Japanese economy during the late 1980s, subsequently associated with escalating bankruptcy rates, has been interpreted as a significant contributory cause of increases in the male suicide rate, stemming from the high proportion of suicide notes in which economic circumstances were the stated reason for suicide. The Japanese male suicide rate increased from around 25 per 100 000 during the mid 1990s to over 35 per 100 000 at the beginning of the twenty-first century, when over 30 000 Japanese per year committed suicide, by then around twice the rate observed in the United States.

Life Events and Physical Health

Clinicians have long suspected stressful life events to be associated with the onset of physical disease (for example, this was noted by Sir James Paget, the surgeon and pathologist, in his *Clinical Lectures and Essays* in 1875). The assessment of stressful life event experience within chronic disease epidemiological study settings presents substantial methodological challenges related to cost, the need to limit participant burden, and the requirement of asking perhaps tens of thousands of study participants, ideally when they are all healthy, to recall their experience of stressful events over a particular time period. In consequence, within large-scale prospective cohort studies, the assessment of stressful life events has been largely restricted either to the use of short event lists or to specific events (e.g., bereavement). Record linkage research designs have investigated the risk of chronic disease and mortality associated with specific stressful events; for example, following the death or serious illness of a child or loss of a partner or twin. Both prospective cohort and record linkage studies have now provided evidence that under some circumstances such events may increase risk for congenital malformations, heart disease, and perhaps some cancers, just a few among many physical health outcomes studied.

Heart disease Sudden and particularly catastrophic life events, such as the 1995 Hanshin-Awaji earthquake in Japan, the 1999 Ji-Ji earthquake in

Taiwan, and the terrorist attacks on the World Trade Center in New York on September 11, 2001, have been associated with transient increases in blood pressure, increases in ventricular arrhythmias among patients with cardioverter defibrillators, and increases in the incidence of fatal and nonfatal cardiovascular events. Further, use of national registers in Denmark has shown that experiencing the unexpected death of a child (under 18 years) is associated with an increased subsequent risk of a heart attack (myocardial infarction) in the bereaved parents. The association between chronic stressful circumstances and cardiovascular events is less certain, but there is an increasing international consensus that a combination of high work demands and low job control is associated with cardiovascular events in certain occupational groups and that caregiving responsibilities for a disabled or ill partner for 9 or more h per week is associated with an increased risk of incident heart disease events in women.

Cancer Studies meeting stringent research design criteria that have been devoted to evaluating life events as possible determinants of cancer incidence and progression are rare. Evidence for the association between life events and cancer incidence is often contradictory, based on studies that often rely on imprecise case ascertainment methods, may be prone to recall bias in their assessment of life event histories, are able to include relatively few participants that develop cancer, and may be unable to include adjustment for factors known to be associated with cancer outcomes. Some of these limitations were overcome in a prospective study of a twin cohort of 10 808 women in Finland. During 15 years of follow-up, 180 incident breast cancers were diagnosed, and the results suggested that life events experienced during the 5 years before entry into the study were associated with an increased risk of breast cancer during follow-up. Three specific life events were found to be associated with an increase in breast cancer risk: divorce or separation, death of a husband, and death of a close relative or friend. The association between widowhood and divorce and subsequent cancer risk compared to married people has been investigated in a large Swedish study. A relatively consistent pattern of cancer risk was found in the divorced compared to the widowed (both with increases and decreases in risk, according to cancer site) that collectively may reflect changes in lifestyle following partner loss. Similar conclusions have been suggested to account for the evidence from record linkage studies that have found a slightly elevated overall cancer risk in mothers following death of a child.

Individual Differences

There are profound individual differences in the health consequences of stressful life events and difficult circumstances. These differences are most evident through studies of the health outcomes of people subsequent to their exposure to very stressful circumstances, including shipwreck, concentration camp experience, and terrorist attacks. Some people adapt to stressful circumstances more successfully than others. Not all people exposed to adverse or even traumatic circumstance experience health change. Identification of what distinguishes people in the way they are able to manage stressful life events can aid understanding of disease susceptibility and inform the design and delivery of effective care to reduce the long-term health impact of events. For example, a brief questionnaire designed to distinguish the extent to which people are optimistic about their lives and future expectations has shown that optimists have a reduced risk from dying due to cardiovascular causes over a 15-year period and after consideration of traditional risk factors. More direct evidence of individual differences in the capacity to adapt to stressful life events has followed from work originally inspired by Aaron Antonovsky's study of survivors of the Holocaust. This work has revealed how, despite their horrific experiences, some Holocaust survivors had subsequently been able to rebuild their lives successfully. Antonovsky defined sense of coherence (SOC), a theoretical construct based upon these observations, as a flexible and adaptive dispositional orientation enabling successful coping with adverse experience. **Figure 2** shows that individuals with a

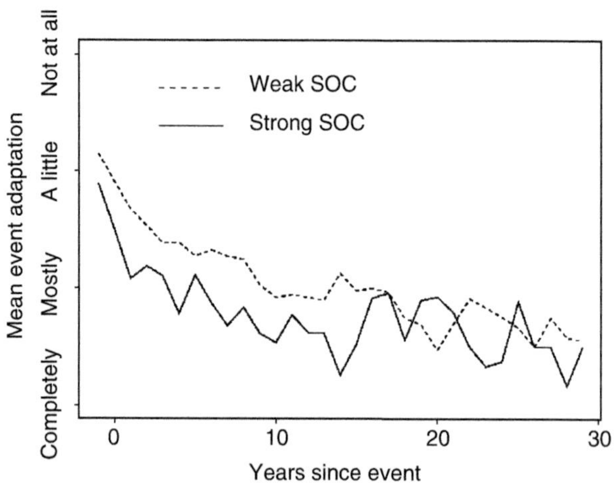

Figure 2 Mean reported adaptation to death of spouse or partner according to the elapsed time since the event occurred and according to sense of coherence (SOC). Based upon 20 921 participants in the European Prospective Investigation into Cancer (EPIC)-Norfolk study in the United Kingdom. Mean adaptation score was calculated from responses to the question "Do you feel that you have got over this now?" (1 = completely, 2 = mostly, 3 = a little, 4 = not at all).

weak SOC report that they take longer to get over the adverse effects of the death of their spouse or partner than those with a strong SOC and illustrates work that has provided support for the idea that SOC distinguishes adaptive capacity to adverse life event experience.

Further Reading

Antonovsky, A. (1987). *Unraveling the mystery of health.* San Francisco, CA: Jossey-Bass.

Cooper, C. L. (ed.) (2005). *Handbook of stress medicine and health* (2nd edn.) Boca Raton, FL: CRC Press.

Dohrenwend, B. P. (1998). *Adversity, stress and psychopathology.* New York: Oxford University Press.

Giltay, E. J., Kamphuis, M. J., Kalmijn, S., Zitman, F. G. and Kromhout, D. (2006). Dispositional optimism and the risk of cardiovascular death. The Zutphen Elderly Study. *Archives of Internal Medicine* **166**, 431–436.

Hansen, D., Lou, H. C. and Olsen, J. (2000). Serious life events and congenital malformations: a national study with complete follow-up. *Lancet* **356**, 875–880.

Harris, T. (2000). *Where inner and outer worlds meet. Psychosocial research in the tradition of George W. Brown.* London: Routledge.

Holmes, T. H. and Rahe, R. H. (1967). The social readjustment rating scale. *Journal of Psychosomatic Research* **11**, 213–218.

Kessler, R. C. (1997). The effects of stressful life events on depression. *Annual Review of Psychology* **48**, 191–214.

Li, J., Laursen, T. M., Precht, D. H., Olsen, J. and Mortensen, P. B. (2005). Hospitalization for mental illness among parents after the death of a child. *New England Journal of Medicine* **352**, 1190–1196.

Lillberg, K., Verkasalo, P. K., Kaprio, J., Teppo, L., Helenius, H. and Koskenvuo, M. (2003). Stressful life events and risk of breast cancer in 10,808 women: a cohort study. *American Journal of Epidemiology* **157**, 415–423.

Stansfeld, S. and Marmot, M. (2002). *Stress and the heart: psychosocial pathways to coronary heart disease.* London: BMJ Books.

Surtees, P. G., Wainwright, N. W. J. and Khaw, K.-T. (2006). Resilience, misfortune and mortality: evidence that sense of coherence is a marker of social stress adaptive capacity. *Journal of Psychosomatic Research* **61**, 221–227.

Sex Differences in Human Stress Response

B M Kudielka
University of Trier, Trier, Germany
D H Hellhammer
University of Trier, Trier, Germany
C Kirschbaum
Technical University of Dresden, Dresden, Germany

This is a revised version of the article by B M Kudielka, D H Hellhammer, C Kirschbaum, Encyclopedia of Stress First Edition, volume 3, pp 424–428, © 2000, Elsevier Inc.

Glossary

Cortisol — A glucocorticoid hormone produced by the adrenal cortex. Cortisol exhibits a pronounced circadian rhythm and responds to a wide range of stressors. It has many physiological effects and virtually every single nucleated cell in the body has cortisol receptors. It is predominantly (90–95%) bound to binding proteins in blood; only 5–10% of the total plasma cortisol circulates as biologically active, unbound, free cortisol.

Hypothalamic-pituitary-adrenal (HPA) axis — A central regulatory and control system of the organism that connects the central nervous system with the endocrine system. Under stress, the hypothalamus secretes corticotropin releasing hormone (CRH), which provokes the release of adrenocorticotropic hormone (ACTH) from the pituitary. ACTH triggers cortisol secretion from the adrenal cortex. The functioning of the axis is controlled by several negative feedback loops.

Lymphocytes — White blood cells responsible for the specific responses of the immune system to antigens. Based on the tissue where the stem cells mature to the specific lymphocyte, they are called B cells or T cells. B cells mature in the bone marrow and form the cellular basis for the humoral immunity (e.g., antibody production), whereas thymus-derived T lymphocytes (e.g., T helper cells and T suppressor cells) represent the effector cells of the specific cellular immunity.

Sex steroids Hormones produced in the gonads and, to a lesser degree, in the adrenal cortex. Estradiol and testosterone play major roles in the female and male reproductive system. In women, sex steroid concentrations show typical variations during the menstrual cycle. Sex steroids also influence the peripheral and central nervous system.

Sympathetic-adrenal-medullary (SAM) axis Sympathetic nerves, originating in the central nervous system, stimulate the adrenal medulla, which in turn secretes epinephrine and norepinephrine. These catecholamines mobilize energy-producing mechanisms quickly and downregulate less important organ functions.

Sex Differences in Health and Disease

Men and women are at differential risks for a number of illnesses. This observation is reflected in the sex-specific prevalence rates for several diseases. Women suffer more often from autoimmune illnesses such as lupus erythematosus, multiple sclerosis, and neurodermatitis, whereas men are more prone to develop coronary heart diseases or infectious diseases. Concerning psychiatric disorders, women more often develop anxiety, depression, phobias, panic disorders, or obsessive-compulsive disorder, whereas men more often are prone to antisocial behavior, substance abuse, or suicide. Although women consistently appear to report more physical and somatoform symptoms than men, the life expectancy for women is approximately 7 years longer than it is for men.

In addition to the clear sexual dimorphism with respect to certain diseases, sex differences exist in psychological and biological aspects of the human stress response. Investigation into sex-specific stress responses may help to reveal mechanisms that underlie somatic, psychosomatic, and psychiatric illnesses. Data showing that several diseases are associated with altered stress responses support this assumption.

On a behavioral level, psychiatric disorders such as depression and anxiety are interrelated with increased symptom reporting. On a physiological level, several of these disorders are accompanied by dysfunctional endocrine regulations. Major depression, susceptibility to infectious diseases, and cardiovascular problems seem to be associated with a hyperactive HPA axis, whereas autoimmune processes are associated more often with a hyporeactive HPA axis. The observation that (premenopausal) women (in contrast to men) seem to be protected from coronary heart disease parallels the finding that men show higher blood pressure changes and catecholamine increases under psychological stress. In addition to the described sex dimorphism with respect to disease and sex-specific stress responses in humans, it is generally accepted that exposure to stress can cause or intensify numerous diseases.

Thus, differences in health status may, at least in part, be related to sex differences in stress responses. Sex-specific stress responses do not seem to be epiphenomena of sex-specific prevalence rates of several disorders but, instead, appear to reflect causal links.

Sex Differences in Subjective Aspects of the Human Stress Response

Following Lazarus and Folkman, the extent of experienced stress is not determined by a situation or an event itself but is, instead, mediated by a three-phasic appraisal process. The importance or threat of the characteristics of a situation or an event is assessed in a primary appraisal loop. Simultaneously, in a secondary appraisal the amount of available coping capacity or resources is estimated. A final reappraisal determines the extent of experienced stress.

Several studies, ranging from everyday hassles to posttraumatic stress reactions, conclude that women subjectively experience more stress than men. A sociocultural approach focusing on external environmental factors emphasizes that women's lives are characterized more often by multiple social roles and lower socioeconomic status, which are both positively correlated with stressful life events. In addition to the finding that women experience more stress in everyday life, stress vulnerability and worry disposition also appear to be higher in women compared to men. This leads to the assumption that sex differences exist in people's readiness to perceive and appraise situations as stressful. This suggestion is supported by the finding that self-descriptions concerning self-esteem or self-confidence, self-efficacy, and sense of competence are slightly but consistently lower in women than in men. Although men repeatedly showed a more favorable locus of control and attribution style in questionnaire-derived studies, Miller and Kirsch concluded that data about sex differences in attributions, locus of control, and perceptions of control during stressful episodes remain inconsistent. Recent findings by Schulz and co-workers revealed that women's higher average scores in perceived stress, chance control orientation, stress-susceptibility, depressivity, and bodily complaints, as well as their lower scores in self-esteem and self-concept of ability, may be attributed to sex differences in worry disposition.

A higher sensitivity and attention to nonspecific stress symptoms appear to bring about more episodes of perceived stress in women. In contrast to women, men seem to be less sensitive in their perception of subtle bodily symptoms, and they are less prone to appraise bodily or emotional changes as significant. Concerning physical and somatoform symptoms, higher symptom reporting in women is described as a general phenomenon rather than one restricted to certain types of symptoms. This effect persists even after adjusting for psychiatric comorbidity such as depression and anxiety, disorders that are more prevalent in women and associated with increased reports of physical symptoms. The suggestion that women are more perceptive about emotions is supported by the finding that women outperform men at all ages in the encoding and decoding of emotions.

The differences in coping styles between men and women are small. Whereas women appear to prefer emotion-focused solutions including the greater use of social support and supportive networks, men focus more often on instrumental or problem-oriented coping. Reports on sex-specific effectiveness of coping strategies contradict the former notion that women's coping strategies could be inadequate or less effective for alleviating distress.

Investigations of perceived stressfulness after confrontation with various standardized laboratory stressors repeatedly led to similar reports of feelings of distress in men and women. Whereas performance in laboratory stress tests was not associated with sex, women tend to judge their own efforts and performances as poorer than men do.

The assessment of subjective aspects of the human stress response is always based on self-reports measured by standardized questionnaires, interviews (structured or half-structured), and open (unstructured) reports. Therefore, it should be considered that sex-related response differences to stress could also reflect sex-specific biases in the willingness (or capability) to report distress.

Sex Differences in Physiological Aspects of the Human Stress Response

Different regulatory systems of the human body are activated by stress. Endocrine stress-responsive systems such as the HPA and SAM axes help the organism adapt to increased demands and maintain homeostasis after challenge. In addition to hormonal responses, stress also provokes changes in cardiovascular and immunological parameters.

Hypothalamic-Pituitary-Adrenal Axis

Investigation of HPA axis responses to different types of stressors revealed that physical exercise (>70% VO_{2max}) and psychological challenges are potent activators of the HPA axis. Whereas the majority of studies did not reveal any sex differences in response to physical exercise, confrontation with psychosocial stimuli leads to higher adrenocorticotropic hormone (ACTH) and free cortisol levels in adult men than in women. This sex difference is conserved after menopause and in elderly individuals. Total cortisol secretion, however, does not differ between sexes in young adults. Although men and women show similar total cortisol responses after stress, a sexual dimorphism exists in the amount of bioavailable free cortisol, an observation calling for simultaneous measurements of total and free cortisol levels. These findings can, at least in part, be explained by greater ACTH pulses in men as well as by the higher sensitivity to ACTH of the adrenal cortex in women.

Observed sex differences in HPA axis stress responses may be due to sexual dimorphisms in brain functions and circulating sex steroid and corticosteroid-binding globulin (CGB) levels. Prime candidates for explaining sex differences in HPA axis stress responsiveness are the gonadal steroids. Among them, estradiol seems to exert modulating effects on HPA axis functioning, including HPA axis responsiveness and sensitivity to glucocorticoid negative feedback. Animal studies consistently revealed that estradiol has a strong stimulatory influence on HPA axis functioning with modulatory effects on mineralocorticoid and glucocorticoid receptors.

Although human data are more contradictory than evidence from animal literature, gonadal steroids also seem to exert important modulatory effects on HPA axis functioning in humans. In a series of studies from our laboratory, free cortisol responses systematically varied as a function of menstrual-cycle phase. Women in the luteal phase show free cortisol stress responses comparable to men, whereas women in the follicular phase and women taking oral contraceptives have significantly lower free cortisol responses. Although the total plasma cortisol net stress responses differ neither between men and women nor between different menstrual-cycle phases, the absolute levels are elevated in women with oral contraceptive use. A short-term estradiol treatment potentiated HPA axis responses to acute psychosocial stress in young men. Furthermore, a 2-week estradiol substitution seemed to diminish the endocrine response of postmenopausal women to exogenous corticotropin releasing hormone (CRH) after dexamethasone premedication, as observed in women with and without short-term estradiol treatment. In addition, a comparison with a third group of premenopausal women indicates that the feedback sensitivity of elderly estradiol-treated women approximates the endocrine response of premenopausal (untreated) women. However, this treatment did not change the acute HPA axis stress responses to psychosocial stress (Trier Social Stress Test). In sum, it should be acknowledged that there is still a paucity of data on the effects of gonadal steroids on the regulation of the human HPA (and SAM) axis. There is a definite need for future in-depth studies on these issues.

Sympathetic-Adrenal-Medullary Axis

Studies investigating SAM axis responses to stress showed that stress-induced epinephrine increases are higher in men than in women, suggesting that men are more sensitive to sympathetic stimulation via emotional arousal. In contrast, no sex effects are reported for norepinephrine concentrations. However, contradictory results also exist.

Reproductive hormones appear to have a significant impact on catecholamine stress responses. This assumption is confirmed first by findings of altered catecholamine levels throughout the menstrual cycle with enhanced epinephrine levels during the luteal phase. Second, comparisons between pre- and postmenopausal women revealed that stress-related epinephrine responses are increased in postmenopausal women and that estradiol treatment reduced catecholamine reactivity to stress. Third, short-time estradiol administration modulates catecholamine reactivity in healthy young men, although the direction of the effect remains contradictory. Although the majority of studies point to an estradiol-mediated reduction in SAM axis responses to laboratory stressors, a few carefully conducted studies show sex steroids to have no or a stimulating effect.

Cardiovascular Responses

In a meta-analysis, Stoney and coworkers summarized sex differences in stress-related heart-rate and blood pressure changes. They concluded that women have higher heart rates at rest as well as slightly larger increases during challenge, whereas men exhibit higher systolic blood pressure changes. Allen and colleagues also showed higher heart-rate increases in women and higher blood pressure changes in men after confrontation with various laboratory stress tasks, supporting the conclusion that women are more likely to be cardiac reactors and men are more prone to be vascular reactors. We aggregated heart-rate responses across five different studies in healthy children and in younger and elderly adults. Accordingly, enhanced heart-rate stress reactivity can be observed in girls and young adult females compared to boys and young adult men. However, in older men and women peak heart-rate responses are comparable, with only men returning to prestressor baselines during recovery.

Although the data are inconsistent, reports of blood pressure changes as a function of menstrual-cycle phase point to sex steroids having an impact on cardiovascular functioning. The fact that coronary heart disease morbidity and mortality rates increase in women after menopause, a time characterized by the marked decrease of reproductive hormones, confirms the protective role of sex steroids. In line with this idea, reports show that postmenopausal women have a higher cardiovascular responsiveness than premenopausal women.

Whereas postmenopausal estrogen use predominantly reduces the risk of coronary heart disease in women, exogenous estrogen use in clinical trials or hormonal replacement therapy studies do not consistently confirm the protective role of estrogens. The apparently conflicting results of exogenous estrogen use on cardiovascular functioning could be explained by a dual action of estrogens. Estrogens may increase the risk of thrombo-embolic events due to an adverse influence on coagulation, and simultaneously they may help to prevent atherogenic events through favorably changed lipid and lipoprotein levels.

Immunological Responses

In general, immunological activity appears to be higher in women than in men. Whereas levels of circulating immunoglobulins are higher and antibody responses to a variety of pathogens are larger in females, sex differences in cell-mediated immunity can vary depending on the immunological parameter studied. Sex differences in basal immunological functioning may result from the stimulation of lymphoid tissues by sex steroids. In general, estrogens appear to suppress T-cell-dependent immune function, but can increase antibody reactivity to antigens. Testosterone (and other androgens) has an immunosuppressive effect and increases susceptibility to infection, although it may help to prevent the development of autoimmune processes. In sum, sex hormones have been shown to modulate a large variety of mechanisms involved in the immune response. Evidence is accumulating that shows that estrogenic and androgenic actions on cells can be mediated not only through classical intracellular receptors but also through membrane receptors on cell surfaces of compounds of the immune system. Wunderlich and coworkers investigated possible cross-talk of nongenomic testosterone signaling with other genotropic signaling pathways in the rat. Furthermore, in addition to direct receptor-mediated influences, indirect effects on immunological functioning and disease processes may be exerted by sex-steroid-induced changes in other biological systems that are interrelated with the regulation of the immune system. For example, the androgenic steroid hormone dehydroepiandrosterone sulfate (DHEAS) was recently shown to inhibit apoptosis in human peripheral blood lymphocytes through a mechanism independent of either androgen or estrogen receptors.

Although there is a voluminous literature showing the impact of acute laboratory stress on rapid immune cell changes, sexual dimorphisms in immune responses to stress in humans have not been extensively examined and the reported results remain contradictory. Whereas Kiecolt-Glaser and colleagues found that women are more likely to elicit immunological changes after controversial discussions with their husbands, as reflected by a summary immune change score (based on killer cell lysis, blastogenic responses to two mitogens, the proliferative response to a monoclonal antibody to the T_3 receptor, percentage of macrophages, and number of T lymphocytes), Scanlan and coworkers concluded that immunological parameters appear to be more affected by psychosocial stressors (hassles and caregiving) in men than in women. Recently, Pehlivanoglu and colleagues observed a shift from cellular to humoral immunity (only) in men and showed evidence that acute stress may cause different immunological changes across the female menstrual cycle. In addition to these sexual dimorphisms, the use of oral contraceptives (OC) can also alter stress-induced immune responses in women. Furthermore, sex and OC intake may exert differential effects on the immune system by modulating glucocorticoid sensitivity of pro-inflammatory cytokine production.

In sum, immune functions at rest and under stress differ significantly between men and women, apparently due to sex-related differences in sex steroid levels.

Further Reading

Allen, M. T., Stoney, C. M., Owens, J. F., et al. (1993). Hemodynamic adjustments to laboratory stress: the influence of gender and personality. *Psychosomatic Medicine* 55, 505–517.

Cleary, P. D. (1987). Gender differences in stress-related disorders. In: Barnett, R. S., Biener, L. & Baruch, G. K. (eds.) *Gender and stress*, pp. 39–72. New York: Free Press.

Kiecolt-Glaser, J. K., Malarkey, W. B., Chee, M., et al. (1993). Negative behavior during marital conflict is associated with immunological down-regulation. *Psychosomatic Medicine* 55, 395–409.

Kirschbaum, C., Schommer, N., Federenko, I., et al. (1996). Short term estradiol treatment enhances pituitary-adrenal axis and sympathetic responses to psychosocial stress in healthy young men. *Journal of Clinical Endocrinology and Metabolism* **81**, 3639–3643.

Kroenke, K. and Spitzer, R. L. (1998). Gender differences in the reporting of physical and somatoform symptoms. *Psychosomatic Medicine* **60**, 150–155.

Kudielka, B. M., Buske-Kirschbaum, A., Hellhammer, D. H., et al. (2004). Differential heart rate reactivity and recovery after psychosocial stress (TSST) in healthy children, younger adults, and elderly adults: the impact of age and gender. *International Journal of Behavioral Medicine* **11**, 116–121.

Kudielka, B. M., Buske-Kirschbaum, A., Hellhammer, D. H., et al. (2004). HPA axis responses to laboratory psychosocial stress in healthy elderly adults, younger adults, and children: impact of age and gender. *Psychoneuroendocrinology* **29**, 83–98.

Kudielka, B. M. and Kirschbaum, C. (2005). Sex differences in HPA axis responses to stress: a review. *Biological Psychology* **69**, 113–132.

Kudielka, B. M., Schmidt-Reinwald, A. K., Hellhammer, D. H., et al. (1999). Psychological and endocrine responses to psychosocial stress and dexamethasone/corticotropin-releasing hormone in healthy postmenopausal women and young controls: the impact of age and a two-week estradiol treatment. *Neuroendocrinology* **70**, 422–430.

Lazarus, R. S. and Folkman, S. (1984). *Stress, appraisal and coping*. New York: Springer.

Lutzky, S. M. and Knight, B. G. (1994). Explaining gender differences in caregiver distress: the roles of emotional attentiveness and coping styles. *Psychology and Aging* **9**, 513–519.

McCruden, A. B. and Stimson, W. H. (1991). Sex hormones and immune function. In: Ader, R., Felten, D. L. & Cohen, N. (eds.) *Psychoneuroimmunology*, pp. 475–793. San Diego, CA: Academic Press.

Miller, S. M. and Kirsch, N. (1987). Sex differences in cognitive coping with stress. In: Barnett, R. S., Biener, L. & Baruch, G. K. (eds.) *Gender and stress*, pp. 278–307. New York: Free Press.

Pehlivanoglu, B., Balkanci, Z. D., Ridvanagaoglu, A. Y., et al. (2001). Impact of stress, gender and menstrual cycle on immune system: possible role of nitric oxide. *Archives of Physiology and Biochemistry* **109**, 383–387.

Polefrone, J. M. and Manuck, S. B. (1987). Gender differences in cardiovascular and neuroendocrine response to stress. In: Barnett, R. S., Biener, L. & Baruch, G. K. (eds.) *Gender and stress*, pp. 13–37. New York: Free Press.

Raison, C. L. and Miller, A. H. (2003). When not enough is too much: the role of insufficient glucocorticoid signaling in the pathophysiology of stress-related disorders. *American Journal of Psychiatry* **160**, 1554–1565.

Rohleder, N., Wolf, J. M. and Kirschbaum, C. (2003). Glucocorticoid sensitivity in humans – interindividual differences and acute stress effects. *Stress* **6**, 207–222.

Scanlan, J. M., Vitaliano, P. P., Ochs, H., et al. (1998). CD4 and CD8 counts are associated with interactions of

gender and psychosocial stress. *Psychosomatic Medicine* **60**, 644–653.
Schulz, P., Schlotz, W., Wolf, J., et al. (2002). [Gender differences in stress-related variables: the influence of worry-disposition]. *Zeitschrift für Differentielle und Diagnostische Psychologie* **23**, 305–326.
Stoney, C. M., Davis, M. C. and Matthews, K. A. (1987). Sex differences in physiological responses to stress and in coronary heart disease: a causal link? *Psychophysiology* **24**, 127–131.
Takahashi, H., Nakajima, A. and Sekihara, H. (2004). Dehydroepiandrosterone (DHEA) and its sulfate (DHEAS) inhibit the apoptosis in human peripheral blood lymphocytes. *Journal of Steroid Biochemistry and Molecular Biology* **88**, 261–264.
Whitacre, C. C. (2001). Sex differences in autoimmune disease. *Nature Immunology* **2**, 777–780.
Wunderlich, F., Benten, W. P., Lieberherr, M., et al. (2002). Testosterone signaling in T cells and macrophages. *Steroids* **67**, 535–538.
Young, E. A. (1995). The role of gonadal steroids in hypothalamic-pituitary-adrenal axis regulation. *Critical Reviews in Neurobiology* **9**, 371–381.

Ethnicity, Mental Health

K Iley
Canterbury Christ Church University, Canterbury, UK
J Y Nazroo
University of Manchester, Manchester, UK

Glossary

Census — A census is a count or survey of all households and people within a particular location. In the United Kingdom a census has been carried out every 10 years since 1841. The 1991 Census was the first one to ask individuals to define their ethnicity.

Ethnicity — The identification, by self or others, with a social group and or social collectivity on the basis of shared values, beliefs, customs, traditions, language, or lifestyle.

Patriarchy — Traditionally means rule of the father and used to describe the dominance of men over women.

Race — A contentious concept within British sociology, which is normally associated with a group connected by a common biological/genetic origin, typically associated with skin color.

Introduction

In this article we consider the key findings that have emerged on ethnic differences in mental health, with particular reference to the United Kingdom. This will be followed by a brief discussion of ethnic minority people's experiences of mental health services and the implications this has for healthcare provision and practice. We will conclude with a discussion of the conclusions we can draw on ethnic inequalities in mental health and the implications this has for our wider understanding of the experiences of ethnic minority people in United Kingdom and how these relate to stress and mental health. But we begin by introducing the concept of ethnicity.

Ethnicity

Approaches to ethnicity have been concerned with understanding how ethnicity relates both to social structures and how it relates to social relationships and identities, allowing us to provide a sensitive and contextual understanding of ethnicity, rather than resort to explanations based on stereotypes. So, research in the United Kingdom has demonstrated the social and economic inequalities faced by ethnic minority people and how economic inequalities and racism relate to ethnic inequalities in physical and mental health. In addition, importance is placed on the notion of ethnicity as an identity that reflects self-identification with cultural traditions, and which provide both meaning and boundaries between groups. So, although there is strong evidence to show that socioeconomic disadvantage contributes to ethnic inequalities in health, it is suggested that there remains a cultural component to ethnicity that could play a defining role.

When considering the relationship between culture, ethnicity, and mental health, however, it is vital to avoid reducing ethnic differences in mental health to stereotyped notions of fixed cultural or biological difference. Ethnicity is considered to reflect identification with sets of shared values, beliefs, customs, and lifestyles and has to be understood dynamically, as an active social process. In particular, the influence of an ethnic identity on individuals and their health depends on the wider context in which that identity is lived.

Ethnicity and Mental Health in the United Kingdom

The difference in rates of mental illness among different ethnic groups in the United Kingdom is probably one of the most controversial issues in the health inequalities field. Given the topic, which potentially allows the alignment of mental disorder with ethnic minority status, the controversial nature of the field is not surprising. And this controversy is aggravated by the complexity of conducting research on ethnic differences in mental illness and the consequent disputed nature of research findings. Much of the controversy has focused on the high rates of hospital treatment for schizophrenia and other forms of psychosis among the African-Caribbean population, where the alignment of mental disorder with ethnicity is most apparent. Interestingly, these findings are reflected in research in the United States and the Netherlands, where black populations are also shown to have high rates of psychotic illness. In the United Kingdom, evidence suggesting low rates of mental illness among the South Asian population, but high rates of suicide and attempted suicide among young South Asian women has also caused controversy. The following provides a summary of key findings from the United Kingdom.

Psychotic Illness

Psychotic illnesses, which include schizophrenia, are relatively infrequent; they are thought to affect around one person in 250 in the United Kingdom, but often result in severe disability. Typically they involve a fundamental disruption of thought processes, where the individual suffers from a combination of distressing delusions and hallucinations.

Most research on ethnic differences in psychotic illnesses has been based on treatment rates, and over the past three decades such studies in the United Kingdom have consistently shown elevated rates of schizophrenia among African-Caribbean people compared with the white population. African-Caribbean people are typically reported to be three to five times more likely than whites to be admitted to hospital with a first diagnosis of schizophrenia. These findings have been repeated in studies that have looked at first contact with all forms of treatment, rather than just hospital services, although the rates in one such study were only twice those of the white population. Some of the more recent of these studies have also looked at those of African ethnicity and have reported similarly raised rates of psychotic illness in this group. Explorations of the demographic characteristics of black people admitted to hospital with a psychotic illness suggest that these illnesses are particularly common among young men, and some studies have suggested that the rates are very high among young African-Caribbean people who were born in the United Kingdom, reporting that rates of first contact with psychiatric services for psychotic illness among this group are 18 times the general population rate.

Given the consistency of the evidence based on treatment statistics, it is somewhat surprising that the only national community based studies of mental illness among ethnic minority groups, the Fourth National Survey of Ethnic Minorities (FNS) and the Ethnic Minority Psychiatric Illness Rates in the Community (EMPIRIC) study, produced rather different findings. Overall, they found that Caribbean people had rates of psychotic illness that were at most twice as high as those in the general population. And when differences were considered across gender, age, and migrant/nonmigrant groups it was found that the prevalence of psychotic illness among: men; young men; and nonmigrant men; was no greater than that for equivalent white people. For example, in the FNS the annual prevalence of psychotic disorder among Caribbean men was estimated as 10 per 1000, while among white British men it was estimated as eight per 1000.

Findings on rates of psychotic illness among South Asian people are even more mixed. Studies of hospital-based treatment suggest that rates of admission for psychotic illness among South Asian people are similar to those among white people. This has been confirmed by a more comprehensive prospective study of first contact for schizophrenia with *all* treatment services in one area of London, but an earlier study using the same methods in another London district suggested that rates of psychotic illness among South Asian people were raised to similar levels to those found among black Caribbean people. Indeed, there is evidence suggesting that rates of psychotic illness among each of the ethnic minority groups defined by the 1991 Census categories are similarly raised in comparison with a white group. This, of course, suggests that it is misleading to maintain an exclusive focus on those of African-Caribbean origin when examining ethnic differences in psychotic illness in the United Kingdom.

In contrast to the findings for contact with treatment services, the community based FNS and

EMPIRIC prevalence studies suggested that rates of psychotic illness might not be raised for South Asian people, and may be lower for Bangladeshi people, than those for white British people. In support of the conclusions drawn by some researchers, these community surveys also suggested a high rate of psychosis among white people who were not of British origin.

Depression

Neurotic disorders, which include depression, are much more common than psychotic disorders. A national survey in the United Kingdom suggested that in the week before interview about one person in 16 was affected by such a disorder. They are usefully separated into two categories, anxiety and depression that, although common, do involve considerably more than a sense of anxiety or sadness. Here we will focus on depression, because of the lack of data on ethnic differences in anxiety.

According to treatment statistics, rates of depression among African-Caribbean people appear to be markedly lower than those for white people, and rates of depression among South Asian people appear to be a little lower than those for white people. For South Asian people, these findings have been confirmed in community studies, including the FNS. However, the more recently conducted, and more thorough, EMPIRIC study suggested few differences between South Asian groups and white people, with higher rates of depression among the Pakistani population.

In comparison with the high rates of treatment for psychotic illness among African-Caribbean people, the low rates of treatment for depression are a puzzle. Most factors that might be implicated in the higher rates of psychotic disorders should also lead to a higher rate for other mental illnesses. In addition, in contrast to the low treatment rates, evidence from the FNS suggests that the prevalence of depression among Caribbean people in the community is, in fact, more than 50% higher than that among whites. Moreover, that study also suggested that despite this higher prevalence, rates of treatment for depression among Caribbean people were very low.

In contrast to the low rates of hospital admission for depression among those born in the Caribbean and South Asia, it has been reported that rates of admission for depression among those living in England but born in Northern Ireland and Ireland were markedly higher than for those born and living in England. The high rate of depression among white people who were not of British origin was confirmed in the community based FNS, which reported that this group had rates that were two-thirds higher than the white British group, and was confirmed for Irish men in EMPIRIC.

Suicide

In contradiction to the apparent lower overall relative rates of mental illness among South Asian people, analyses of immigrant mortality statistics show that mortality from suicide are higher for young women born in South Asia, and this is particularly the case for very young women (aged 15–24 years), where the rate is two to three times the national average. In contrast to the findings for young South Asian women, these studies also showed that men and older women (aged 35 years or more) born in South Asia had lower rates of suicide. Analysis of the most recent data on immigrant mortality has been more detailed, because it could be coupled with the 1991 Census, which included a question on ethnicity as well as country of birth. This confirmed the overall pattern just described, but showed that the high rates appear to be restricted to those born in India and East Africa, rather than Pakistan or Bangladesh.

In terms of morbidity, rather than mortality, again the picture is mixed with studies of treatment suggesting very high rates of suicidal ideation, attempted suicide, and suicide among both male and female South Asians. In contrast, the only studies to look at suicidal thought among national community populations (the FNS and EMPIRIC) found that the rates of suicidal ideation were not raised among South Asian groups and, if anything, lower among South Asian women than white women regardless of age.

Problems with Existing Sources of Data

Although mental illness is a relatively common condition, it is difficult to measure and the defining characteristics are contested. Both the definition and the measurement of mental illness depend on the presence of clusters of psychological symptoms that indicate a degree of personal distress, or that lead to behaviors that cause such distress to others. The clusters of symptoms associated with particular forms of mental illness are clearly defined by psychiatrists, although the elicitation of these symptoms for diagnostic or research purposes can be difficult, particularly in cross-cultural studies.

One of the central problems arises from the reliance of most work on data based on contact with treatment services. Contact with treatment services, even when access is universal as in the United Kingdom's National Health Service, reflects illness behavior (i.e., the way that symptoms are perceived, evaluated, and acted upon), rather than illness *per se*. This raises a number of linked problems, particularly as illness behavior is likely to be affected by a number of factors that vary by ethnicity, such as socioeconomic position, health beliefs, expectations of the sick role, and lay referral systems. And these problems become particularly important for work on rates of psychosis, where contact with services might be against the patient's wishes. So, despite the consistency of research findings showing that African-Caribbean people have higher rates of treatment for psychosis, some commentators have not accepted the validity of the interpretation of these data and continue to suggest that a higher incidence (rather than a higher treatment rate) remains unproven, because of the serious methodological flaws with the research that has been carried out.

Briefly, the kind of problems that are focused on include: underestimation of census-based denominators for African-Caribbean people, leading to overestimation of admission rates (although not to the extent that could explain the many times higher rates of admission); overestimation of first onsets of psychosis, because of under-identification of previous episodes for African-Caribbean people (because of high geographical mobility leading to records of previous admissions being missed and a reluctance to disclose previous diagnoses because of a concern about the impact of these on how they might be managed); variations in the routes of admission and treatment by ethnicity, with African-Caribbean people over-represented among patients compulsorily detained, more likely to have been in contact with the police or forensic services prior to admission (despite them being both less likely than whites to display evidence of self-harm and no more likely to be aggressive to others prior to admission), and more likely to have been referred to these services by a stranger rather than by a relative or neighbor. Taken together, these comments suggested that there are a variety of potential problems with existing work and, consequently, that there must remain some doubt about the higher rates of psychosis reported among the African-Caribbean group.

It is equally possible that the reported differences between white and South Asian groups and the inconsistencies found in these could, as for the African-Caribbean group, be a result of the methodological limitations of studies in this area. In addition to the difficulties of relying on treatment data, outlined above, the lower rates of mental illness among South Asian people could reflect language and communication difficulties, or a general reluctance among South Asian people to consult with doctors over mental health problems. More fundamentally, they may reflect a difference in the symptomatic experience of South Asian people with a mental illness compared with white people. In particular, it has been suggested that South Asian people may experience particular culture-bound syndromes, that is a cluster of symptoms which is restricted to a particular culture, such as sinking heart, and consequently not be identified as mentally ill.

Explaining Key Findings and Contradictions

There a number of explanations considered for ethnic differences in mental health and these are similar to those considered for other ethnic inequalities in health in the epidemiological literature. These include migration, genetic differences, culture, racism, and socioeconomic position.

Migration

First, different rates of mental health across migrant and nonmigrant groups could be a consequence of factors related to the actual process of migration. Social selection into a migrant group could have favored those with a higher or lower risk of developing illness, or the stresses associated with migration might have increased risks. There is evidence to both support and counter these suggestions. In the case of the apparently higher rates of schizophrenia among African-Caribbean people in the United Kingdom, investigations of the rates of schizophrenia in Jamaica and Trinidad suggest that they are much lower than those for African-Caribbean people in the United Kingdom and, in fact, similar to those of the white population of the United Kingdom. This would suggest that the higher rates are either a consequence of factors related to the migration process, or of the greater stresses surrounding the lives of ethnic minority people in the United Kingdom.

However, there is evidence that shows that rates of schizophrenia for African-Caribbean people born in the United Kingdom are even higher than for those who migrated, suggesting that factors relating directly to the process of migration may not be involved, although these data (like most work in this area) are dependent on a very small number of identified cases.

Genetic Differences

As with all work on ethnicity and health, there has been discussion of the possibility that differences may be a consequence of a genetic factor that correlates with ethnic background, but little supporting evidence has been marshaled. Evidence suggests large differences in risk within ethnic categories, implying that any genetic basis for mental illness does not correlate closely with ethnic background. For example, the evidence on schizophrenia cited in the previous section, which shows that there are important differences between African-Caribbean people who stayed in Jamaica or Trinidad (who do not have raised rates), those who migrated to the United Kingdom (who appear to have raised rates), and those who were born in the United Kingdom (who appear to have markedly raised rates), suggests that the higher rates cannot be straightforward consequence of ethnic differences in genetic risk.

Culture

Not surprisingly, most research that has focused on cultural explanations for ethnic differences in mental health has based the cultural argument on speculative and stereotyped characterizations of the cultures of ethnic minority groups, which do not acknowledge the dynamic nature of culture.

It has been suggested that overall lower rates of mental illness among South Asian people could be a consequence of a strong and protective Asian culture, which provides extended and strong communities with protective social support networks. In contrast, in the attempt to explain the high mortality rates of suicide among young women born in South Asia and living in the United Kingdom, South Asian communities are portrayed as constraining, demanding, and conflictual, rather than supportive and cohesive, and so contributing to the high suicide rates.

Of course, such stereotypes will not hold when closely examined. For example, despite the focus on patriarchal South Asian families, there are, in fact, great similarities between the motives of white and South Asian patients for their suicidal actions. So, although it is worthy of considering how culture informs our understanding of ethnic minority people and their experiences of illness, it is necessary to question the stereotypes we use and to understand ethnic identities as dynamic and dependent on context.

Racism and Socioeconomic Position

Different rates in mental health across different ethnic groups might be a consequence of stress resulting from the different forms of discrimination and racism that ethnic minority people face in the United Kingdom. This could be a direct result of the experience of discrimination and harassment, or a result of the social disadvantages that racism leads to. It would not be surprising if the poor run-down, inner city environments and poor housing that many ethnic minority people live in, and their poorer employment prospects and standards of living, led to greater mental distress. As elsewhere in the ethnicity and health field, there has been considerable criticism of the failure to take into account explanatory variables related to social disadvantage in research that links ethnicity to poor mental health, as there is a strong possibility that these underlie the relationship. And there is a growing body of evidence linking racism and discrimination directly, and indirectly, to adverse mental health outcomes.

Conclusions

This article suggests that many basic questions concerning the relationship between ethnicity and mental health remain controversial. There remains a question of whether the use of western psychiatric instruments for the cross-cultural measurement of psychiatric disorder is valid and produces a genuine reflection of the differences between different ethnic groups. This has been raised particularly in relation to the low detection and treatment rates for depressive disorders among South Asians, but may apply to other disorders and other ethnic minority groups. It is also likely that treatment-based statistics do not accurately reflect the experiences of the populations from which those in treatment are drawn.

Perhaps, as other writers have pointed out, the most important conclusion to draw is that it is vital to avoid reducing ethnic differences in mental health to stereotyped notions of fixed cultural or biological difference, there is a need to explore the factors associated with ethnicity that may explain any relationship between ethnicity and mental health, such as the various forms of social disadvantage and consequent stressors that ethnic minority people face. And it remains important to explore how racism and the social disadvantages that this leads to structure the experiences of ethnic minority people when they come into contact with mental health services. Despite this, the focus on biological rather than social explanations for ethnic differences in mental illness continues in both the United States and the United Kingdom.

Further Reading

Adebimpe, V. R. (1995). Race, racism, and epidemiological surveys. *Hospital and Community Psychiatry* **45**, 27–31.

American Psychiatric, Association (1995). *Diagnostic and statistical manual IV.* Washington DC: American Psychiatric Association.

Crawford, M. J., Nur, N., McKenzie, K., et al. (2005). Suicidal ideation and suicide attempts among ethnic minority groups in England: results of a national household survey. *Psychological Medicine* **9**, 1369–1377.

Harrison, G., Owens, D., Holton, A., et al. (1988). A prospective study of severe mental disorder in Afro-Caribbean patients. *Psychological Medicine* **18**, 643–657.

Iley, K. and Nazroo, J. Y. (2001). Ethnic inequalities in mental health: a critical examination of the evidence. In: Culley, L. & Dyson, S. (eds.) *Sociology, ethnicity and nursing practice*, pp. 67–89. Basingstoke: Palgrave.

Iley, K. and Nazroo, J. (In press). Sociology of mental health and illness. In: Bhui, K. & Bhugra, D. (eds.) *Textbook of culture and mental health disorder.* London: Hodder Arnold.

Karlsen, S., Nazroo, J. Y., McKenzie, K., et al. (2005). Racism, psychosis and common mental disorder among ethnic minority groups in England. *Psychological Medicine* **35**, 1795–1803.

King, M., Coker, E., Leavey, G., et al. (1994). Incidence of psychotic illness in London: comparison of ethnic groups. *British Medical Journal* **309**, 1115–1119.

King, M., Nazroo, J., Weich, S., et al. (2005). Psychotic symptoms in the general population of England: a comparison of ethnic groups (The EMPIRIC study). *Social Psychiatry and Psychiatric Epidemiology* **40**, 375–381.

Kleinman, A. (1987). Anthropology and psychiatry: the role of culture in cross-cultural research on illness. *British Journal of Psychiatry* **151**, 447–454.

McGovern, D. and Cope, R. (1987). First psychiatric admission rates of first and second generation Afro-Caribbeans. *Social Psychiatry* **22**, 139–149.

Nazroo, J. Y. (2001). *Ethnicity, class and health.* London: Policy Studies Institute.

Sashidharan, S. and Francis, E. (1993). Epidemiology, ethnicity and schizophrenia. In: Ahmad, W. I. U. (ed.) *Race and health in contemporary Britain.* Buckingham, UK: Open University Press.

Selten, J. P., Slaets, J. P. and Kahn, R. S. (1997). Schizophrenia in Surinamese and Dutch Antillean immigrants to the Netherlands: evidence of increased incidence. *Psychological Medicine* **27**, 807–811.

Weich, S., Nazroo, J., Sproston, K., et al. (2004). Common mental disorders and ethnicity in England: the EMPIRIC study. *Psychological Medicine* **34**, 1543–1551.

II. GENETICS AND GENOMICS – SUSCEPTIBILITY TO STRESS

Neuroticism, Genetic Mapping of

M W Nash
King's College London, London, UK

Glossary

Complex traits Phenotypes governed by variation in many genes; often continuously and/or normally distributed. The trait does not segregate in the population following any obvious patterns. Environmental influences often account for as much as, or more than, genetic influences.

Genome The set of all genes for a particular organism. In humans this includes both nuclear and mitochondrial DNA sequences.

5-HTTLPR Gene polymorphism in the 5′-promoter region of the gene encoding the serotonin (5-hydroxytryptamine; 5-HT) transporter (5-HTT) that has been implicated in susceptibility to life events/stressors.

LOD score Logarithm of the odds score favoring linkage. The higher the score, the greater the evidence for linkage.

Mendelian or simple traits Phenotypes governed by a single major locus or gene and hence the traits can be seen to segregate in the population following obvious additive, dominant, or recessive patterns.

Phenotype Any observable and measurable characteristic of an organism produced by genetic and/or environmental influences.

Quantitative trait locus (QTL) A locus implicated in genetic variation that causes a change in a continuous phenotype.

What Is Neuroticism, and Is It Genetic?

Neuroticism is a unique dimensional measure of personality thought to capture emotional stability and a temperamental sensitivity to negative stimuli. Indeed, it is a widely agreed upon higher order factor in many different personality constructs. Currently, three measures of personality are commonly used in genetic research: Eysenck's Personality Questionnaire, Cloninger's Temperament and Character Inventory, and the Neuroticism Extraversion Openness (NEO) personality inventory. For Cloninger's measure of harm avoidance (HA) and Eysenck's measure of neuroticism (EPQ-N), there is some evidence that these different personality constructs are influenced by similar genetic and environmental variables. In the case of the EPQ-N, high scorers are conceived to be overly emotional, react strongly to stimuli, and find it difficult to recover after an emotionally stimulating experience, while low scorers are conceived to be calm, even tempered, and emotionally controlled. The genetic influence on neuroticism and harm avoidance has been widely assessed, and the estimates of heritability are 40–60% of the phenotypic variance. The EPQ-N is known to overlap genetically with many internalizing disorders, such as major depression, panic disorder, and generalized anxiety disorder, and because of this, neuroticism has been used in psychiatric genetic research to identify the genetic variation causing individual differences in the susceptibility to both depression and anxiety.

Which Regions of the Genome Are Linked to Neuroticism?

Traditionally, there have been two statistical approaches to relate variation of the genome to a phenotype of interest, known as linkage mapping and association mapping. Linkage mapping has played a huge historical role in the gene mapping of Mendelian traits. In essence, the method relies on the phenomenon of allele sharing among relatives. For example, monozygotic twins share 100% of their genome, while siblings and dizygotic twins should share only 50% – on average – of their genome. To illustrate this, if two siblings are both highly neurotic, then genetic variation at a region of the genome that is truly linked to neuroticism would be expected to be shared by the siblings. If such a phenomenon is observed in more siblings than would be expected by chance, this region of the genome is declared linked to neuroticism. Linkage is a useful approach for coarse mapping, as it identifies large regions of the genome as being linked to the phenotype, but this is also a disadvantage, as large regions can contain hundreds of candidate genes. As this analysis cannot distinguish which gene or genetic variant is responsible for the linkage, it is usual after the identification of a region to perform the finer association mapping approach to localize more precisely the disease gene (see next section).

To date, there have been seven linkage studies examining a neuroticism-like phenotype. The first reported study, undertaken by Cloninger and colleagues, examined HA and observed significant linkage to the long (p) arm of chromosome 8. Additive and nonadditive interaction of the chromosome 8 peak with other loci suggested significant interaction with chromosomes 11, 18, 20, and 21. A subsequent study assessed selected regions of the genome for linkage to HA and also found linkage in an overlapping region of chromosome 8. It is not possible, however, to deduce that the same sequence variant(s) is responsible for the linkage in both these studies. Further fine mapping of the chromosome 8p region in the same sample refined the region to one around the neuregulin gene (*NRG1*), which has been implicated in schizophrenia susceptibility. The NRG1 protein is involved in signaling based on the glutamate neurotransmitter and plays a central role in neural development. Interestingly, neuroticism and HA have been reported as elevated in first-degree relatives of schizophrenics and schizotypal individuals. A re-analysis of the original data set, using a novel method, reproduced the evidence for linkage to the chromosome 8p markers. As these four studies are derived from only two samples, it is difficult to decide if a true quantitative trait locus (QTL) actually resides on chromosome 8p. The possibility that *NRG1* is a candidate for harm avoidance is intriguing, but the gene needs to be extensively examined in multiple samples before any robust conclusion can be drawn.

The first published linkage analysis of the EPQ-N was carried out by Fullerton and colleagues in a UK selected sibling sample. The main findings were QTLs on chromosomes 1, 4, 7, 12, and 13. Further evidence was presented that these loci for neuroticism might be gender specific: the QTLs on chromosomes 1, 12, and 13 appeared to be female specific, while a QTL on chromosome 8, which was not found to be genome-wide significant in the complete sample analysis, appeared to be male specific. It is interesting to note that the chromosome 8 locus is in close proximity to the chromosome 8p locus identified in HA. The second published study used a composite index of four self-report measures of anxiety and depression, including Eysenck's measure of neuroticism in a large UK-based sibship sample. As opposed to only examining Eysenck's neuroticism measure, Nash and colleagues used structural equation modeling on the four self-report measures to derive a phenotypic composite index of the shared genetic liability to both depression and anxiety. While no significant findings were obtained, linkage peaks closely approaching significance were obtained on chromosomes 1p and 6p for both the composite index and neuroticism, with a high correspondence of results between the two phenotypes. Splitting the sample by gender led to the identification of a linkage peak for females on chromosome 12, while also indicating female specificity of the chromosome 1 peak and male specificity of the chromosome 6 peak. The most recent linkage publication on EPQ-N was performed in a New Zealand sample. While no peak reached statistical significance, a suggestive finding of linkage was obtained on chromosome 12, with nominal findings of linkages on chromosomes 1, 3, 6, 11, 15, and 17. Comparing the results from these three studies indicates a low correspondence between the results. There is possible overlap on chromosomes 1 and 12. The peak on chromosome 12 is potentially exciting, as this also overlaps with linkage peaks from both unipolar and bipolar depression. Indeed, as discussed later, variants of a gene within this peak have recently been observed to segregate with major depression and might also be associated with individual variation in neuroticism.

Similarly, comparisons between all the studies on neuroticism and harm avoidance show only slight correspondence. This is not unexpected, unless a major locus (responsible for >20% phenotypic variance) was involved. While linkage is a powerful method for simple traits with genes of major effect, its poor ability to reliably detect loci with a small phenotypic effect relegates the method to a preliminary tool providing genomic targets on which to focus fine mapping projects. Its contributions in this field at best provide suggestive evidence that chromosomes 1, 8, and 12 might harbor genetic variants that are associated with neuroticism/harm avoidance.

Have Association Studies Identified Any Genes Associated with Neuroticism?

Association mapping has historically been employed to evaluate the potential contribution of specified candidate genes, or as a follow-up, fine mapping tool to linkage analysis. Due to technological advances in speed and the reduction in expense in measuring differences in the genome, whole genome association mapping will eventually become the predominant mapping approach. The simplest version of association mapping is in case control studies of unrelated individuals and essentially examines whether or not there is a correlation between the genetic variation and the phenotype. This basic approach suffers from the fact that a much larger number of sequence variants need to be measured to capture adequately the effective genetic variation compared to linkage analysis. Nevertheless, the increased ability to detect small changes is the most attractive feature of this approach to gene mapping.

Function-Based Candidate Genes

Perhaps the biggest shift in thinking with respect to psychiatric and personality genetics has been the reduction in the expected effect size of a single genetic variant. While initial expectations were that a single genetic variant might account for around 10% of the phenotypic variance, it is now thought that 1%, or much less, is a more realistic expectation for single variants. Commonly, sample sizes are inadequate to detect such effects reliably. To tackle this problem, meta-analytic techniques can be implemented that use the results of multiple studies to estimate reliably the effect sizes and significance of genetic variants. In the only published meta-analysis of genetic polymorphisms in personality, Munafo and colleagues examined commonly researched genetic variants in the serotonin transporter (*SLC6A4*) and various dopamine genes (*DRD4, DRD2, DRD3*, and *DAT1*). Of all the results, the only significant meta-analytic association was between a polymorphism in *SLC6A4* and neurotic/avoidant traits.

Current evidence indicates that the serotonin transporter gene (*SLC6A4*), located on the long arm of chromosome 17 (17q), is probably the only gene that can be considered associated with neuroticism, albeit only weakly. The mature protein of this gene transports serotonin from the synaptic cleft back into the presynaptic neuron for reuse and is responsible for the quantity of serotonin in the synaptic cleft. A sequence variant, known as 5-HTTLPR, is present in either a short or long form in a region of the gene called the promoter, which regulates the rate at which the mRNA of the gene is made. The first study of this variant identified an association of the number of short variants with an increase in neuroticism. Subsequently, there have been many attempts at replicating this finding with varying degrees of success. To address this issue, there have been several meta-analyses of the many findings, with a general consensus supporting a small but positive association. Recently, Caspi and colleagues observed that the relationship of stressful life events and depression was mediated by 5-HTTLPR, such that individuals with two long alleles were unchanged in their risk to depression as life events increased, while the risk of depression was increased in those carrying one or more short alleles. This finding has subsequently been replicated for depression, but comprehensive studies looking only at neuroticism and 5-HTTLPR have found no mediation of the variant on the effect that life events have on neuroticism. It is highly probable that 5-HTTLPR and neuroticism are weakly associated; what is unknown, and a source of current interest, is the developmental mechanisms that 5-HTTLPR affects, which lead to its association with individual differences in neuroticism.

A more recent line of research has been driven by theories of aberrant neuronal apoptosis and neurogenesis in major depression. Based on such theories, some research has been carried out on genetic variants known to affect these mechanisms. The most studied of these is the brain-derived neurotrophic factor gene (*BDNF*), located on chromosome 11p. The BDNF protein has a well-documented role in neuronal development, survival, and plasticity, making it an attractive candidate for many psychiatric disorders. Indeed, variants in the gene have been associated with disorders such as obsessive-compulsive disorder, bipolar disorder, and major depressive disorder. Because neuroticism is genetically related to major depression and is a phenotypic marker for vulnerability to depression, genetic variants in the *BDNF* gene have been examined for their relationship with neuroticism. The original association with this gene examined a single nucleotide polymorphism that changes the 66th amino acid from a valine to a methionine and its association with neuroticism as measured by the NEO personality scale. This study found an apparently strong finding, with those individuals carrying the Met/Met genotype having substantially lower neuroticism scores than the rest of the sample. Subsequent follow-up studies using the NEO personality scale or HA have not found such strong evidence, and a recent comprehensive study examining the EPQ-N found no evidence for an association. It appears that although *BDNF* might be a plausible candidate gene for neuroticism, the data simply do not currently support this. As these studies have focused on only one variant in the gene, it is plausible that other variants in the gene are associated with neuroticism.

Position-Based Candidate Genes

Despite the promising leads from linkage studies, no positional candidates have emerged so far, but there have been some possible leads from related scientific fields. *RGS2*, or regulator of G-protein signaling 2, is a positional candidate gene from linkage studies that examined emotionality in mice. This gene is located on mouse chromosome 1 and corresponds to a region on human chromosome 1. Whether this gene is responsible for the linkage signal seen on this chromosome has not yet been established. Nevertheless, there have been reports that variants in the human version of this gene might be associated with agoraphobia. Another possible gene is *APAF1*, apoptosis protease activating factor 1, involved in the apoptosis pathway. This gene, located at 12q, was recently associated with major depression in Utah families. Functional studies indicated that only those variants that segregated with major depression had a functional effect on the apoptosis pathway. Given the genetic relationship between the EPQ-N and major depression, it is possible that *APAF1* also contributes to individual differences in neuroticism. This gene is located within the chromosome 12 linkage peak identified in two studies of neuroticism, as mentioned previously, lending weight to the suggestion that genetic variation in this gene might be associated with neuroticism.

Roles of Candidate Genes in Stress

There are a number of possible mechanisms that might explain the relationship of the aforementioned candidate genes with stress. Upon being stressed, the body enters into various response patterns, including at the molecular level an increase in firing from serotonergic neurons. As the role of the serotonin transporter is the reuptake of serotonin from the synaptic cleft, the rate at which new transporter can be made might affect the rate at which the biochemical system regains homeostasis. Because the short, low-activity 5-HTTLPR allele carriers produce less mRNA, these individuals might return to their biochemical baseline slower than long allele homozygotes. This delay might then leave these individuals more susceptible to the detrimental effects of stress. Another aspect of these detrimental effects is the neuronal toxicity of glucocorticoids, which are released as a negative feedback mechanism during response to a stressor, and it is known that glucocorticoids are capable of damaging hippocampal neurons. The rate and impact of this damage might be mediated by both BDNF and APAF1. BDNF is involved in neuronal survival, while APAF1 is involved in cell death. The functional variation that has been identified for these genes might cause some individuals to be more resilient to the toxic effects of stress, while making others more vulnerable. This model suggests that individuals who carry the S allele of 5-HTTLPR, who are homozygous for the *BDNF* Met allele, and who also have the apoptosis rate-increasing alleles of *APAF1* may be more vulnerable to the detrimental effects of stress.

See Also the Following Articles

Serotonin Transporter Genetic Modifications.

Further Reading

Caspi, A., Sugden, K., Moffitt, T. E., et al. (2003). Influence of life stress on depression: moderation by a polymorphism in the 5-HTT gene. *Science* **301**, 386–389.

Cloninger, C. R. (1986). A unified biosocial theory of personality and its role in the development of anxiety states. *Psychiatric Developments* **4**, 167–226.

Dina, C., Nemanov, L., Gritsenko, I., et al. (2005). Fine mapping of a region on chromosome 8p gives evidence for a QTL contributing to individual differences in an anxiety-related personality trait: TPQ harm avoidance. *American Journal of Medical Genetics, Part B: Neuropsychiatric Genetics* **132**, 104–108.

Fullerton, J., Cubin, M., Tiwari, H., et al. (2003). Linkage analysis of extremely discordant and concordant sibling pairs identifies quantitative-trait loci that influence variation in the human personality trait neuroticism. *American Journal of Human Genetics* **72**, 879–890.

Lake, R. I., Eaves, L. J., Maes, H. H., et al. (2000). Further evidence against the environmental transmission of individual differences in neuroticism from a collaborative study of 45,850 twins and relatives on two continents. *Behavior Genetics* **30**, 223–233.

Lesch, K. P., Bengel, D., Heils, A., et al. (1996). Association of anxiety-related traits with a polymorphism in the serotonin transporter gene regulatory region. *Science* **274**, 1527–1531.

Munafo, M. R., Clark, T. G., Moore, L. R., et al. (2003). Genetic polymorphisms and personality in healthy adults: a systematic review and meta-analysis. *Molecular Psychiatry* **8**, 471–484.

Nash, M. W., Huezo-Diaz, P., Williamson, R. J., et al. (2004). Genome-wide linkage analysis of a composite index of neuroticism and mood-related scales in extreme selected sibships. *Human Molecular Genetics* **13**, 2173–2182.

Neale, B. M., Sullivan, P. F. and Kendler, K. S. (2005). A genome scan of neuroticism in nicotine dependent smokers. *American Journal of Medical Genetics, Part B: Neuropsychiatric Genetics* **132**, 65–69.

Sen, S., Nesse, R. M., Stoltenberg, S. F., et al. (2003). A BDNF coding variant is associated with the NEO personality inventory domain neuroticism, a risk factor for depression. *Neuropsychopharmacology* **28**, 397–401.

Willis-Owen, S. A., Fullerton, J., Surtees, P. G., et al. (2005). The Val66Met coding variant of the brain-derived neurotrophic factor (BDNF) gene does not contribute toward variation in the personality trait neuroticism. *Biological Psychiatry* **58**, 738–742.

Willis-Owen, S. A., Turri, M. G., Munafo, M. R., et al. (2005). The serotonin transporter length polymorphism, neuroticism, and depression: a comprehensive assessment of association. *Biological Psychiatry* **58**, 451–456.

Zohar, A. H., Dina, C., Rosolio, N., et al. (2003). Tridimensional personality questionnaire trait of harm avoidance (anxiety proneness) is linked to a locus on chromosome 8p21. *American Journal of Medical Genetics, Part B: Neuropsychiatric Genetics* **117**, 66–69.

Genetic Predispositions to Stressful Conditions

D Blackwood and H Knight
University of Edinburgh, Edinburgh, UK

This is a revised version of the article by D Blackwood, Encyclopedia of Stress First Edition, volume 2, pp 212–217, © 2000, Elsevier Inc.

Glossary

Genes — It is estimated the human genome contains approximately 30,000 genes distributed on the 23 pairs of human chromosomes, and about one-third of genes are expressed in the brain. Each gene is the specific DNA code for a protein.

Genetic association studies — Studies designed to detect differences in the frequencies of DNA polymorphisms in a group of individuals with a particular phenotype contrasted with a group of control subjects from the same population.

Genetic polymorphism — The occurrence of two or more variants (alleles) of DNA sequence in a population. There are many types of sequence variation in the human genome, including single nucleotide polymorphisms (SNPs), microsatellites, deletions, and insertions that have proved valuable for locating genes in human disease using linkage and association strategies. A well-known example of genetic polymorphisms is those giving rise to the proteins of the ABO blood groups.

Genotype — The complete genetic composition of an organism.

Life events — Events usually measured by a trained interviewer using standardized interview schedules to obtain a record of events over a stated time. The inventory is likely to cover common and major events, including financial and marital problems, bereavement, ill health, employment change and infringements of the law. Some investigators separate the effects of different classes of life events, for example, an independent event such as a close friend being involved in an accident is contrasted with the subject him- or herself being in an accident, an event over which the subject may have some control or which directly threatened him or her.

Phenotype — The physical expression of the genotype.

twin studies — In genetic research, studies based on the fact that identical (monozygotic, or MZ) twins have exactly the same genes and nonidentical (dizygotic, or DZ) twins share on average 50% of their genes. Both types of twins share similar environments. In characteristics that are genetically determined, MZ twin pairs are more alike (concordant) than DZ pairs, whereas MZ and DZ concordance rates are similar in phenomena due solely to environmental influences.

It has often been taken for granted that anxiety and depression are the natural consequences of stressful events such as sudden bereavement, loss of a job, or marital disharmony and that stresses in childhood such as those related to poor parenting, physical or emotional abuse, or loss of a family member may have an impact on behavior well beyond childhood. However, many early studies of the effects of stressful situations on behavior have not taken into account the effects of genes. It is now abundantly clear that genetic factors play an important and sometimes major role in many human behaviors, personality dimensions, and the development of specific patterns of illness.

How Genes and Stressful Events Can Interact

Kendler and Eaves gave a detailed account of three models to explain how genes and the environment can interact to cause psychiatric illness. These models also help us understand how genetic influences and stressful events interact in everyday life not necessarily associated with psychiatric symptoms. They form a useful basis for discussing a number of recent empirical studies.

The first and simplest model hypothesizes that symptoms of anxiety and depression are the result of the addition of genetic and environmental contributions. This assumes that people, regardless of their genotype, will respond in the same way to an environmental stress, and the probability of being exposed to a stress is independent of genetic background. This model has been the basis of much research in social psychiatry and has, for example, highlighted the importance of early loss and poor social support as risk factors for the development of depression during adulthood in women. Such a direct causal link between environmental challenges and behavior is illustrated by the normal physiological and behavioral response to a life-threatening situation that is often termed the fight-or-flight response. However, the assumption that environmental stresses and genotype act independently does not explain the empirical observation that some individuals appear to be more sensitive than others to stressful life events.

A second model proposes that genes influence the individual's response to stressful events in the environment. The experience of life events differs widely between individuals and is related to personal characteristics including self-esteem, social support, mood, and personality traits. An example might be that individuals with high scores on neuroticism (a trait that is in part genetically determined) respond to loss or personal threat differently than those with low scores on neuroticism. Animal studies provide an example of how gender differences influence response to stress. Shors and colleagues have reported that the effect of acute stress on memory in rats differs between males and females; the degree of retrograde amnesia or enhanced memory depends on the sex of the animal. This suggests that the genetic differences between the sexes may underlie the expression of different stress response strategies.

Environmental control of the expression of genes is illustrated by animal studies showing that the stress of maternal separation during early development influences the growth of specific brain structures, leading to changes in adult behaviors. Different strains of animals respond differently to early stress, confirming a genetic background to the response. Under this model, however, genotype and environment are not correlated. The model accounts for the influence of genetic factors on the response of an individual to stressful events, but it does not include an effect of genes on the probability that a person will be exposed to stressful environmental situations.

A third, and in many ways the most interesting, model states that a person's genotype alters the probability that he or she will be exposed to a stressful environment. Genes and environment do not act independently, but are correlated. In effect, individuals throughout their lives select the level of environmental stress to which they are exposed. Specific stressful events such as road traffic accidents and injuries at work relate to a number of factors, including personality, drug and alcohol intake, and psychiatric illness. A common but indirect example is a person who is alcoholic and exposed to the consequences of heavy drinking. Since alcoholism is partly a heritable condition, as shown by family twin and adoption studies, one of the effects of the genes that increase risk of drinking behavior is also to increase exposure of the alcoholic to a range of stressful life events, including marital difficulties, assaults, road traffic accidents, and homelessness. Genes may also influence how a person recalls, perceives, and reports on their experiences of stressful life events.

Measuring Life Events

Over the past 30 years the concept of life events has been developed and refined as a means to study the effects of stressful conditions in the environment on human behavior and psychopathology. Scales such as the Social Readjustment Rating Scale of Holmes and Rahe were developed to be used as a measure of an individual's exposure to environmental stress and have become well-researched tools in social psychiatry. However, the reporting of life events may be influenced indirectly by genetic factors. One of the first studies to address the issue of how life event reporting is governed by social and other factors was carried out in New Zealand by Fergusson and Horwood, who obtained information on life events exposure including financial problems, marital problems, bereavement, ill health, and employment changes over a 6-year period for over 1000 women. The results made it clear that reporting stressful events was not random, and two major determinants of vulnerability to reporting life events were the level of social disadvantage of the woman and her level of trait neuroticism derived from the Eysenk Personality Inventory. Women of socially disadvantaged backgrounds and women with high neuroticism scores consistently reported high exposure to life events over the 6-year period.

Twin Studies of Exposure to Stress

Twin studies that include the comparison of monozygotic (identical) and dizygotic (nonidentical) twin pairs provide a powerful means to quantify the relative contributions to human behaviors of genetic and environmental factors. Rigorous statistical analysis including correlations between twin pairs permits calculation of variance due to genetic factors and shared and individual environments. If a twin experiences a life event that is entirely random and not influenced by his or her personal characteristics, we would not expect the co-twin to show increased likelihood of experiencing a similar event. The co-twin would have the same risk as the general population. If shared family environment was responsible for the life event, both MZ and DZ twins would share an equally increased exposure. If genetic factors contribute to the event, MZ twins will show greater concordance than DZ twins for that variable because they have more genes in common.

Kendler, in a study of more than 2000 twin pairs selected from the population in Virginia, found clear evidence that reported life events were influenced by both genetic and environmental factors. There was a significant familial resemblance for reported total life events: the correlations for MZ twins (0.43) and

DZ twins (0.31) both differed significantly from zero ($p < 0.001$), and the correlation for monozygotic twins consistently exceeded that for dizygotic twins. These results support the view that personality characteristics increase the probability of experiencing stressful life events. The genetic effect was observed only when life events were divided into those that affected the individual directly (personal events), for example, if the individual was in a car accident, as opposed to events involving someone else (network events), for example, if a close relative was in a car accident. Personal events included marital difficulties, being robbed or assaulted, interpersonal difficulties, financial problems, illness or injury, and legal problems, and these were all significantly influenced by genetic factors that explained nearly 20% of the variance. Shared environment had little effect on personal events. In contrast, network events affecting other people were not influenced by genetic factors, and the similarities between twins were entirely attributable to shared family environment. It is understandable that personal events should be under some degree of genetic control, since these events are dependent on the person's behavior whereas net work events are not.

This twin study confirmed that the occurrence of stressful life events is more than just bad luck. A combination of familial and genetic influences may predispose the individual to create for themselves a high-risk environment leading to a complex relationship between life events and stress-related disorders. In a further analysis of the female twins from the Virginia Twin Registry, Kendler and Karkowski-Shuman demonstrated that the genetic liability for depression in these twins was associated with an increased risk for stressful life events that included assault, marital problems, job loss, serious illness, financial problems, and social difficulties with relatives and friends. In the same twin sample, the genetic liability to alcoholism was related to the risk of being robbed and having trouble with the police. One of the ways that genes contribute to psychiatric illness is probably by causing individuals to select themselves into high-risk environments. Silberg, in a study of juveniles from the Virginia Twin Registry, proposed a model whereby depression in girls is partly influenced by genes that mediate adverse life events, and the influence of genes on life events is not stable but increases during adolescence.

Lyons specifically examined how genes influenced exposure to combat trauma in a study of more than 4000 male twin pairs who had served in the Vietnam War. A range of data was collected, including volunteering for service in Vietnam, actual service, a composite index of combat experiences, and the award of combat decorations. Correlations within twin pairs for actually serving in Vietnam were 0.41 (MZ) and 0.24 (DZ), and those for combat experiences were 0.53 (MZ) and 0.3 (DZ). These figures generated an estimate of heritability of 35 to 47%. The family environment had no significant effect on any of the variables, and the results are unlikely to be due to biases from self report because being awarded a combat medal gave similar correlations. The differences between MZ and DZ twin pairs show that exposure to combat is partly heritable and is not influenced by the socioeconomic status of the family of origin. A number of factors could influence combat experience, including the personality trait of novelty seeking, which is known to be genetically determined. Individuals scoring high on novelty seeking will be more likely to volunteer for active service. Similarly, genetic traits that increase the likelihood of a person suffering physical and psychiatric illnesses will act to decrease the likelihood that the person will seek out and experience exposure to trauma in combat.

A twin study by Stein extended these observations to noncombat situations in a study of 400 Canadian civilian twin pairs rated for exposure to trauma and symptoms of posttraumatic stress disorder (PTSD). Seventy-five percent of these twins reported experience of trauma that could be divided into assaultive (robbery or sexual assault) and nonassaultive (road traffic accident or natural disaster). Analysis of heritabilities showed that genetic effects contributed to risk of exposure to assaultive but not nonassaultive trauma, and there was a correlation between genetic effects and PTSD symptoms. It was concluded that many of the same genes that influence exposure to assaultive trauma appear to influence susceptibility to PTSD symptoms in their wake.

Studies of twins have provided important evidence that genetic predisposition has an important role in stress-related activity and the experience of stressful life events ranging from engagement in wartime combat to exposure to assault in civilian life. It is also clear that genetic factors influence how people respond to stress, explaining why some people and not others develop symptoms of PTSD. How these genetic influences are mediated is not known, but a variety of mechanisms have been proposed.

Molecular Genetic Approaches

We can now be fairly sure that a person's complement of genes strongly influences personality traits, but it is highly unlikely that in due course a gene for neuroticism or any other personality dimension will be uncovered. It is more probable that these traits are determined by a number of genes, and the inheritance of different variants of these genes will lead to the particular traits in a manner that has long been familiar to animal breeders.

Complex phenotypes including human personality characteristics are often termed quantitative traits because a number of different genes are thought to act additively in a quantitative manner to produce the phenotype. The genes contributing to the additive effect are termed quantitative trait loci (QTL). The terms polygenic (caused by many additive or interacting genes) and multifactorial (caused by many genes interacting with environmental factors) have also been used to describe the same situation in which a complex phenotype is under a variety of genetic influences. The completion of the sequencing of the human genome, followed by the Hapmap project, which catalogued hundreds of thousands of normal DNA sequence variants (polymorphisms) present at high-density across the genome, have given researchers unrivalled tools for detecting genes contributing to inherited human diseases and complex behavioral traits. Linkage studies use many markers on each of the 23 pairs of chromosomes to identify the small DNA region that is inherited along with a particular disease or trait within a particular family. Another approach for identifying genes contributing to monogenetic disease or complex disorders is to study very large cohorts of subjects rated for a particular quantitative trait and compare the frequency of selected DNA polymorphisms between cases and a matched sample of controls recruited from the same population. Association studies are used to study candidate genes or small selected regions of a chromosome previously identified by family linkage analysis. Candidate genes coding for proteins in neurotransmitter pathways, including the serotonin (5-HT) and dopamine systems, have been the focus of particular attention because these neurotransmitters are known from animal and clinical studies to play an important role in regulating mood and a variety of behaviors relevant to traits of impulsiveness, sensation seeking, and addictive behavior. The neurotransmitter 5-HT is an important regulator of early brain development, and 5-HT neurons play known roles in integrating emotion, cognition, and motor function. Genes related to 5-HT are good candidates for a role in human personality, and the 5-HT transporter gene apparently influences a constellation of traits related to anxiety and depression. Individuals who carry a common small deletion in the promoter region of the 5-HT transporter gene are more susceptible to depression. A possible role for the transporter gene as a mediator of the effects of environmental stress on moods was described by Caspi in a study of a New Zealand birth cohort of individuals. At the age of 26, these individuals were assessed for symptoms of depression and anxiety, and self-reported life events occurring in the previous 5 years were recorded. To address the question of why stressful experience leads to depression in some people and not in others, the 5-HT transporter gene was studied and a crucial difference was observed between individuals who became depressed after experiencing stress and those who were tolerant of stress. Those who became depressed were more likely than nondepressed individuals to carry a small deletion on the promoter region of the gene. This raises the possibility that different variants of the 5-HT promoter gene could moderate how a person is going to react to adverse life experiences.

The neurotransmitter dopamine, like 5-HT, is distributed widely in the nervous system and has a range of functions, including the modulation of mood. It is of considerable interest that a receptor in the dopamine family (DRD4) may influence novelty-seeking behavior. In a study described by Noble, a person who inherits one variety of the DRD4 receptor appears to be more likely to rate highly when assessed for novelty seeking. The same trait was also more common in boys with one particular set of variants in the DRD2 gene. However, the combined DRD4 and DRD2 polymorphisms contributed more markedly to novelty-seeking behavior than when these two gene variants were individually considered. Substantially more needs to be done to unravel the complex relations between stress and symptoms in populations, and it is likely that many more candidate genes will be examined by these methods in large populations to try to detect gene–environment interactions.

Neurotransmitter function is just one of many possible areas of gene–environment interaction providing a link between chronic stress and ill health. An entirely different approach was reported by Epel and colleagues, who investigated the effects on cellular aging of chronic psychological stress experienced by a group of mothers looking after a chronically ill child. They found a significant association between perceived stress and shorter telomere length in peripheral blood mononuclear cells. Telomeres are regions at the ends of each chromosome. It has been noted that telomere length becomes progressively shorter in cells as they age. In this study, the women who reported the highest levels of emotional stress had, on average, shorter chromosome telomeres than the women who looked after children without disability. Thus, reduced telomere length due to increased oxidative stress in the cell, a determinant of longevity of cells, was associated with perceived psychological stress. It was striking that telomere shortening in women presumed to be under the most stress was shorter on average by an amount equivalent to 10 years of aging compared to low-stress women.

Another area of current interest is how genetic factors during prenatal development and childhood may exert an influence on the way the adult responds to stress several decades later. Welberg and Seckl have extensively reviewed the role of steroids and the hypothalamic-pituitary-adrenocortical (HPA) axis as a system involved in prenatal programming in the brain. In animal studies, prenatal stress leads to long-lasting effects on the HPA axis function in adult offspring, in general programming a persistently hyperactive system and producing clear alterations in the animals' behavior and response to stressful situations. Adult rats exposed to prenatal stress show an increase in behaviors reminiscent of human anxiety. Extrapolation from animal studies to human situations requires extreme caution. However, in a number of clinical studies poor maternal nutritional status in pregnancy and low birth weight were correlated with increased blood pressure, obesity, and glucose intolerance later in life. A possible link between such early life stress and altered behavior or psychopathology in the offspring once they reach adulthood remains an interesting conjecture, and steroids in the HPA axis are the focus of considerable research as possible mediators of such a link.

Further Reading

Brown, G. V. and Harris, T. O. (1993). Aetiology of anxiety and depressive disorders in an inner-city population 1. Early adversity. *Psychological Medicine* **23**(1), 143–154.

Epei, E. S., Blackburn, E. H., Lin, J., et al. (2004). Accelerated telomere shortening in response to life stress. *Proceeding of the National Academy of Sciences USA* **101**(49), 17312–17315.

Caspi, A., Sugden, K., Moffitt, T. E., et al. (2003). Influence of life stress on depression: moderation by a polymorphism in the 5-HTT gene. *Science* **301**(5631), 386–389.

Kendler, K. S., Neale, M., Kessler, R., Heath, A. and Eaves, L. (1993). A twin study of recent life events and difficulties. *Archives of General Psychiatry* **50**(10), 789–796.

Kendler, K. S. and Karkowski-Shuman, L. (1997). Stressful life events and genetic liability to major depression: genetic control of exposure to the environment? *Psychological Medicine* **27**(3), 539–547.

Lvons, M. J., Goldberg, J., Eisen, S. A., et al. (1993). Do genes influence exposure to trauma? A twin study of combat. *American Journal of Medical Genetics* **48**(4), 22–27.

Mormede, P., Courvoisier, H., Ramos, A., et al. (2002). Molecular genetic approaches to investigate individual variations in behavioral and neuroendocrine stress responses. *Psychoneuroendocrinology* **27**(5), 563–583.

Noble, E. R., Ozkaragoz, T. Z. and Ritchie, T. L. (1998). D2 and D4 dopamine receptor polymorphisms and personality. *American Journal of Medical Genetics* **88**(3), 257–267.

Seedat, S., Niehaus, D. J. and Stein, D. J. (2001). The role of genes and family in trauma exposures and posttraumatic stress disorder. *Mol Psychiatry* **6**(4), 360–362.

Shors, T. J. (2004). Learning during stressful times. *Learning and Memory* **11**(2), 137–144.

Silberg, J., Pickles, A., Rutter, M., et al. (1999). The influence of genetic factors and life stress on depression among adolescent girls. *Archives of General Psychiatry* **56**(3), 225–232.

Stein, M. B., Jang, K. L., Taylor, S., Vernon, P. A. and Livesley, W. J. (2002). Genetic and environmental influences on trauma exposure and posttraumatic stress disorder symptoms, a twin study. *American Journal of Psychiatry* **159**(10), 1675–1681.

Veenema, A. H., Meijer, O. C., de Kloet, E. R. and Koolhaas, J. M. (2003). Genetic selection for coping style predicts stressor susceptibility. *Journal of Neuroendocrinology* **15**(3), 256–267.

Welberg, L. A. and Seckl, J. R. (2001). Prenatal stress, glucocorticoids and the programming of the brain. *Journal of Neuroendocrinology* **13**(2), 113–128.

Serotonin Transporter Genetic Modifications

K Sugden
Social, Genetic and Developmental Psychiatry Centre, London, UK

Glossary

Enhancer — A short region of DNA that can be bound with proteins (such as transcription factors) to enhance transcription levels of genes. An enhancer does not necessarily have to be located close to the genes it affects, although some enhancers are found within intronic sequences.

Messenger RNA (mRNA) — The primary sequence transcribed from the DNA template. mRNA has intronic sequences (i.e., sequences not represented in the transcript exiting the nucleus) removed by splicing and encodes the amino acid sequence of a protein.

Poly-adenylation	The cleavage of mRNA and addition of 50–200 adenosine residues, a poly-A tail. Polyadenylation is an important post-transcriptional modification that ensures the appropriate termination of the molecule at the 3′ end and helps in both the export of the mRNA from the nucleus and protection from exonucleases.
Polyadenylation site	The point of polyadenylation of newly transcribed mRNA.
Serotonin (5-hydroxy-tryptamine, 5-HT)	A protein present in many tissues, especially blood and nervous tissue; it stimulates a variety of smooth muscles and nerves and functions as a neurotransmitter.
Single nucleotide polymorphisms (SNPs)	Single-base changes in a DNA sequence, for example a C to T substitution. SNPs can be found in the coding (exonic) and noncoding region (e.g., untranslated region, promoter, or intron) of a gene, and coding SNPs can be synonymous (no change in resultant amino acid) or non-synonymous (change in resultant amino acid).
Transcription	The synthesis of an RNA copy from a sequence of DNA; the first step in gene expression.
Transcription factor binding site	A consensus sequence within a gene, promoter, or regulatory region that is recognized and bound by a transcription factor that then regulates the transcription of that gene.
Variable number of tandem repeats (VNTR)	A polymorphism within a DNA sequence that comprises varying numbers of repeating units. VNTRs can be microsatellites (usually repeat units of 2–8 bp) or minisatellites (more than 8 bp). VNTRs are hypermutable and often give rise to many alleles of different lengths.

The Serotonin Transporter

The serotonin transporter (5-HTT) is important in the termination and modulation of serotonergic neurotransmission by sodium-dependent reuptake of serotonin into the presynaptic neuron, which thus terminates the synaptic actions of serotonin and recycles it into the neurotransmitter pool. The transporter is the site of action of a number of commonly used antidepressants, such as selective serotonin reuptake inhibitors (SSRIs), fluoxetine (Prozac^{TM}), sertraline (Zoloft^{TM}), and paroxetine (Paxil^{TM}), and tricyclic antidepressants. A number of psychostimulants such as cocaine, methylphenidate, and MDMA (ecstasy) may also interact with 5-HTT. For this reason, *5-HTT* has become one of the most widely studied genes in the field of behavior, especially in the context of psychiatric disorders such as depression, neuroticism, and suicidal behavior.

The *5-HTT* Gene

The gene encoding the 5-HTT protein in humans has been mapped to the chromosomal location 17q11.2 and consists of 14 exons spanning approximately 38 kb. Several studies have focused on screening the genomic region for variation, and a number of polymorphisms have been characterized. Currently, at least 62 SNPs with frequency data within the gene, untranslated, or promoter region of *5-HTT* are listed in the Entrez SNP database (dbSNP). Most of these SNPs have not yet been investigated in the context of complex behavior, and any role they might have in regulation of the gene is still unknown.

Functional Polymorphisms of the *5-HTT* Gene

There are some regions within *5-HTT* that have been demonstrated to affect the expression of the gene. The most common of these are described next (see **Figure 1**).

The Serotonin Transporter-Linked Polymorphic Region

One of the most documented variants within *5-HTT* is the serotonin transporter-linked polymorphic region (*5-HTTLPR*; **Figure 1c**), a polymorphic GC-rich repetitive element within the proximal 5′ regulatory region. In humans (and indeed in primates), the *5-HTTLPR* is polymorphic, consisting of a variable number of 20- to 23-bp repeats. The *5-HTTLPR* exists as two common alleles: the short allele (S, 14 repeats) and the long allele (L, 16 repeats). There is evidence that this polymorphic region has functional significance; in JAR (human carcinoma) cells, the L allele confers higher activity than the S allele, whereas lymphoblastoid cells with the LL genotype have 1.4–1.7 times the amount of mRNA as SS or SL cells. Furthermore, the uptake of labeled serotonin in LL genotype cells is 1.9–2.2 times that in cells carrying one or two copies of the S variant. More recently, it has been shown that the *5-HTTLPR* gene actually exhibits a number of alleles of varying repeat numbers. Furthermore, the S and L alleles are themselves variable, so that, although their length is similar, SNPs occur within their repeating units. In total, at least 14 alleles of varying length and sequence have been identified, four different S alleles (14-A to 14-D), six different L alleles (16-A to 16-F), and alleles consisting of 13, 15, 18, 19, 20, and 22 repeats. The longer alleles appear to exhibit a silencer effect on the gene, having lower activity than 14- and 16-repeat variants; however, these alleles are extremely rare and appear to be found in specific populations only, such as the

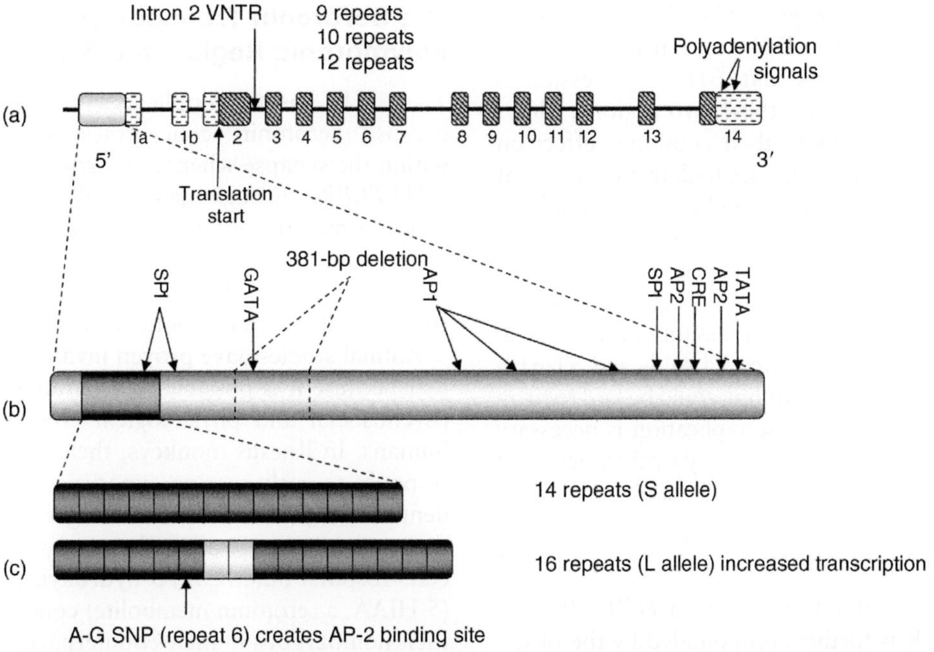

Figure 1 Serotonin transporter gene (not to scale). a, Organization of the gene; b, promoter region; c, *5-HTTLPR* as either the S or L allele. In a, the coding exons are represented by diagonally marked boxes; noncoding exons are represented by dashed boxes. The position of the promoter (light grey) and intron 2 VNTR are shown. In b, the position of some postulated transcription factor binding sites are shown by arrows; the region of the 381-bp deletion is demonstrated by dashed lines, as is the position of the *5-HTTLPR* (dark grey box). In c, the light boxes represent the position of the two repeat units that are inserted in the L allele; the position of the A-G SNP is also shown.

20-repeat allele in the Japanese population. Recently, it has been demonstrated that an A-G SNP (dbSNP reference number rs25531) within the sixth repeat of the *5-HTTLPR*, represented by the 14-D and 16-D alleles, creates a binding site for the transcription factor AP-2 that might affect the rate of transcription of the gene.

Recently however, the functional effect of the *5-HTTLPR* polymorphism has been called into question because *in vivo* experiments failed to find the same genotypic effect as that observed in cell lines. For example, the *5-HTTLPR* genotype has no effect on the 5-HTT binding of a serotonergic ligand, a measure of 5-HTT availability, in human brain. In other words, if the *5-HTTLPR* is driving differential transcription, it has no eventual effect on *5-HTT* availability. Similarly, some experiments suggest that 5-HTT binding in the brain does not differ by *5-HTTLPR* genotype. If these results are robust, then it may be that the expression patterns in cell-based assays do not accurately reflect the pattern of expression *in vivo*. Indeed, it has been shown that the regulation of the 5-HTT depends on the presence of the substrate (serotonin, 5-HT) rather than on any genetically driven effect. This might be an indication of the many levels of complex regulation that genes are subject to *in vivo* that may not be accurately modeled by cell-line *in vitro* approaches; the functional effect of the *5-HTTLPR* observed in cells might be adapted by the complex intra- and extracellular factors that brain neurons are exposed to.

Intron 2 Variable Number of Tandem Repeats

Along with the *5-HTTLPR*, there are other proposed transcriptional regulatory regions within the *5-HTT*. One example is a VNTR within intron 2 that has been shown to have differential enhancer activities in the mouse embryo and in human embryonic stem (ES) cells (**Figure 1a**). The VNTR consists of 9–12 copies of a 16- or 17-bp repeat, the 12-repeat allele (STin12) having greater enhancer activity than the 10-repeat allele (STin10) in both model systems. This ability to regulate expression is cell-specific in humans, in that it is observed in ES cells but not HeLa cells. However, as in the case of the *5-HTTLPR*, the regulation is much more complex than the effect of repeat length; the VNTR does not comprise a succession of perfect repeats, rather there are seven varying repeat sequences and the differences between alleles is described by the deletion of specific repeat elements. The functional effect of the VNTR is regulated by at least two transcription factors – CCTC-binding factor (CTCF) and Y box binding protein (YB-1) – that bind to a sequence that is deleted in the nine-repeat allele (STin9). YB-1 is inhibitory, so binding to the VNTR results in decreased expression. However, the addition of YB-1 results in a release from inhibition of the STin9 VNTR in COS-7 cells because the inhibitory site is deleted. This effect is antagonized by CTCF and is not observed with either the STin10 or STin12.

This evidence suggests that *5-HTT* expression is differentially regulated by these two regions. However, little is known about their combined effect on transcription. The only evidence to date indicates that the expression of the gene is highest in lymphoblastoid cells having both *5-HTTLPR* L/L and STin12/STin12 genotypes. The expression is lowest in cells with at least one S and one STin10 allele. Based on previous evidence of higher expression of 5-HTT with LL- and STin12/STin12-compared to S- and STin10-containing genotypes, this finding could be said to fit an *a priori* hypothesis; but some replication is necessary before any firm conclusions on the synergistic action of the *5-HTTLPR* and intron 2 VNTR can be made.

Other Regulatory Elements

The transcriptional effect of the *5-HTTLPR* and intron 2 VNTR is further compounded by the observation of splicing variation within the 5′ untranslated region, so that two alternative forms of *5-HTT* mRNA exist. Within the human brain and placenta, exon 1B is alternatively spliced and appears in transcripts to a varying degree, whereas exon 1A seems to be the principal transcription initiation point. This type of alternative splicing could help to specify cell-specific activity of the 5-HTT and ensure appropriate levels of neurotransmission in different tissues. This tissue-specific splicing of 5′ untranslated exons is also observed in the brain and gut in rats, indicating that it is a common mechanism of regulating protein expression. Furthermore, tissue-specific mRNA splicing might also be precipitated through multiple polyadenylation sites found in exon 14. This mechanism dictates alternate transcription stop sites that give rise to mRNA transcripts of varying length that, like alternative splicing of exons, might regulate tissue-specific expression. It has also been proposed that the structure of the *5-HTTLPR* is likely to result in a 381-bp deletion in the promoter region (**Figure 1b**) and that this deletion is present in 20–60% of genomic DNA derived from human brain and blood. Specific breakpoints suggest that the event is similar to V(D)J rearrangement often observed in antibody genes. This rearrangement results in looping out the 381-bp DNA sequence so that the two breakpoints are adjacent and are subsequently joined together, resulting in the deletion of the looped-out sequence.

The consequences of this deletion are not known, but it is suggested that the event is likely to be regulated by tissue- and *5-HTTLPR*-dependent mechanisms. However, this effect of mosaicism has yet to be consistently observed in multiple populations.

The Serotonin Transporter-Linked Polymorphic Region and Stress

The 5-HTT has been implicated in the stress response because serotonin concentrations are increased within the synapse when under stress. Given that the *5-HTTLPR*, through gene-regulatory mechanisms, might affect the efficiency by which serotonin is transported back in to presynaptic neuron, the *5-HTTLPR* is an ideal polymorphism candidate for studies of stress and its outcomes.

Animal studies have proven invaluable in this context because it is possible to accurately control both psychosocial and physiological effectors, unlike in humans. In Rhesus monkeys, there are variations in response to early rearing experience that are dependent on the primate *5-HTTLPR* genotype. Monkeys that possess an S allele have significantly lower cerebrospinal fluid (CSF) 5-hydroxyindoleacetic acid (5-HIAA, a serotonin metabolite) concentrations than their homozygous L-allele counterparts. This suggests that serotonin reuptake is lowered in monkeys with an S allele, but the effect is specific to those who were peer-reared (early stressful environment) rather than parent-reared. No differential effect of genotype is seen between parent-reared monkeys. This suggests that early experience has some effect on the functioning of the serotonin system within primates and that the *5-HTTLPR* genotype becomes important only when stressful events are experienced. There also exists a knockout mouse for the serotonin transporter, a genetically manipulated mouse that is deficient in the *5-Htt* gene. Stressed mice that are heterozygous or homozygous for the knockout mutation (i.e., mice that have lower or negligible levels of 5-HTT) have a greater response to stress (measured as increased levels of stress hormone adrenocorticotropic hormone, ACTH) than homozygous wild-type mice. The levels of ACTH are the same in knockout and wild-type mice when they are not stressed, again suggesting that it is the variability in 5-HTT density that participates in interindividual differences in stress response.

In humans, neuroimaging research suggests that individual differences in stress perception are mediated by genetic variations in the *5-HTTLPR*. Individuals with one or two copies of the S allele of the *5-HTTLPR* exhibit greater amygdala neuronal activity to fearful stimuli than individuals homozygous for the L allele. This suggests that the SS- and SL-genotype individuals respond to the same stressful event to a greater magnitude than the LL individuals. In addition, it has been demonstrated that there is a differential response to brain-derived neurotrophic factor (BDNF) by *5-HTTLPR* genotype. BDNF is involved in activating the stress response, so this suggests that variability in *5-HTT* may influence variability in other downstream molecular processes that 5-HTT is associated with. Some of the strongest evidence to date that the *5-HTTLPR* can modulate the human stress response comes from a longitudinal study of almost 1000 individuals from Dunedin, New Zealand, in which it was shown that variation in the *5-HTTLPR* can modify the effect of stress on the outcome of depression. Stressful life events, such as the breakdown of a marriage or unemployment can lead to depression; however, this is not true for all individuals who experience stress. It was found that individuals who had the LL genotype of the *5-HTTLPR* were protected against the effects of stress in that their rates of depression were much lower than SS- and SL-genotype individuals with similar levels of stressful life events. This effect was seen whether the stress was experienced proximally (within the previous 5 years) or earlier (in childhood). The rates of depression in individuals who had not experienced stress were similar regardless of genotype. Consequently, evidence from these diverse sources suggests that variation in the *5-HTTLPR* can influence psychopathological reactions to stress and that it can account for some of the variability in individual response.

Further Reading

Benjamin, A. B., Ebstein, R. P. and Belmaker, R. H. (eds.) (2002). *Molecular genetics and the human personality.* Washington, DC: American Psychiatric Publishers.

Bennett, A. J., Lesch, K. P., Heils, A., et al. (2002). Early experience and serotonin transporter gene variation interact to influence primate CNS function. *Molecular Psychiatry* 7, 118–122.

Caspi, A., Sugden, K., Moffitt, T. E., et al. (2003). Influence of life stress on depression: moderation by a polymorphism in the 5-HTT gene. *Science* **301**(5631), 386–389.

Hariri, A. R., Mattay, V. S., Tessitore, A., et al. (2002). Serotonin transporter genetic variation and the response of the human amygdala. *Science* **297**(5580), 400–403.

Heils, A., Teufel, A., Petri, S., et al. (1996). Allelic variation of human serotonin transporter gene expression. *Journal of Neurochemistry* **66**(6), 2621–2624.

Klenova, E., Scott, A. C., Roberts, J., et al. (2004). YB-1 and CTCF differentially regulate the 5-HTT polymorphic intron 2 enhancer which predisposes to a variety of neurological disorders. *Journal of Neuroscience* **24**(26), 5966–5973.

Kraft, J. B., Slager, S. L. and McGrath, P. J. (2005). Sequence analysis of the serotonin transporter and associations with antidepressant response. *Biological Psychiatry* **58**(5), 374–381.

Lesch, K. P. (1998). Serotonin transporter and psychiatric disorders: listening to the gene. *Neuroscientist* **4**(1), 25–34.

Lesch, K. P. (2001). Serotonin transporter: from genomics and knockouts to behavioral traits and psychiatric disorders. In: Briley, M. & Sulser, F. (eds.) *Molecular genetics of mental disorders*, pp. 221–267. London: Martin Dunitz.

Murphy, D. L., Li, Q., Engel, S., et al. (2001). Genetic perspectives on the serotonin transporter. *Brain Research Bulletin* **56**(5), 487–494.

Nakamura, M., Ueno, S., Sano, A., et al. (2000). The human serotonin transporter gene linked polymorphism (5-HTTLPR) shows ten novel allelic variants. *Molecular Psychiatry* **5**(1), 32–38.

Relevant Website

Entrez SNP database. http://www.ncbi.nlm.nih.gov/SNP/

Monoamine Oxidase

P Huezo-Diaz and I W Craig
King's College London, London, UK

Glossary

Allele — One of two or more possible forms of a gene. An individual may possess two identical, or two different, alleles, except for those of the genes on the X chromosome in males because they possess only a single copy of this chromosome.

Antisocial behavior (ASB) — A pervasive pattern of disregard for and violation of the rights of others occurring since age 15 years old.

Cycle of violence — The observed relationship between violent parenting and violence in the parents' offspring.

Major effect gene — A gene whose influence can be detected without the need to control for environmental factors.

Null mutation	A mutation that completely eliminates the function of the gene.
Promoter	The section of DNA that precedes a gene and controls its activity.

Stress and the Cycle of Violence

A common observation in studies of ASB and aggression in humans is the cycle of violence, in which there is a tendency for individuals who were exposed to abusive parents and/or difficult childhoods to manifest antisocial personalities in adulthood. Not all individuals exposed to abusive childhoods, however, develop antisocial and violent tendencies. The challenge is, therefore, to establish the extent to which genetic predispositions and the extent to which stressful environments are responsible for eliciting the violent behavior. Recent research suggests that there is an interaction between the two that may underpin this repeating pattern.

Genetic Factors in Aggression and Violence

Results from more than 50 behavioral genetic studies indicate that, on average, approximately 41% of the variance of ASB is due to genetic factors, approximately 16% is due to shared environmental factors and approximately 43% is due to nonshared environmental factors. The same overall pattern appears to hold for violence. Epidemiological studies have also consistently shown that the risk of aggression is greater in males than in females, and this raises the possibility that genetic and environmental influences contribute differentially to the risk of aggressive behavior depending on gender. Twin studies indicate that common environmental factors, sex-specific genes, and the interaction between the two play an important role in increasing liability toward aggressive behavior in males, even though females have a higher heritability and males a higher common environmental liability.

Evidence for a direct role of testosterone levels, which could be genetically determined, in promoting aggression in humans is not clear-cut. This leaves open the possible influence of other specific genetic factors that may contribute to increased aggression in males; recent interest has focused on the monoamine oxidase A gene, *MAOA*, in this regard.

MAOA as a Candidate Gene

The main role for the monoamine oxidase (MAOA) enzyme is thought to be in degrading serotonin following its reuptake from the synaptic cleft, although it is also capable of degrading both norepinephrine and dopamine. It therefore plays a key role in the regulation of nerve transmission, and alterations in its activity produced by pharmacological intervention or through genetic variants are likely to have profound effects on behavior. Indeed, drugs inhibiting its activity have long been employed in the treatment of behavioral disorders, particularly depression.

A wide range of genetic variants of the *MAOA* gene exists in the general population. One of the most significant is a DNA motif localized in the promoter 1.2 kb upstream from the *MAOA* coding region, comprising a 30-bp repeat existing in 3, 3.5, 4, or 5 copies (**Figure 1**). It has been shown that the copy number has a significant effect on the level of the gene's expression. The two predominant forms observed in the population are those with three or four repeats of the motif, with the three-copy version having reduced transcriptional activity compared to the four-copy allele. The gene is located on the X chromosome, which means that females have two copies but males have only one. Any defect in the gene in males is therefore exposed because they are unaffected by the status of a second copy.

A possible direct role for *MAOA* in predisposing violence, ASB, and conduct disorders was suggested by studies of males from a Dutch pedigree who exhibited a complex behavioral syndrome (including impulsive aggression). All affected individuals suffered from a mutation in the *MAOA* gene that resulted in zero activity of the enzyme. A role for *MAOA* deficiency in promoting aggression is further supported by studies on mutant mice that had deletions of portions of their monoamine oxidase gene, resulting in the lack of enzyme activity in the brain and liver. Behavioral studies on the adult male mice indicated heightened aggression in response to intruders and also increased inappropriate courtship behaviors. These have been the only reports to date of the phenotypic consequences of null mutations. The existence of high- and low-activity *MAOA* alleles in the human population, however, raises the intriguing possibility that lower levels of the enzyme may predispose male individuals to ASB and/or violent behavior.

There have been a variety of reports suggesting a role for variants at the *MAOA* locus in the context of violence and/or ASB, particularly in relation to subgroups of males with alcoholism and attention deficit and hyperactivity disorders. Generally, it appears that individuals with the low-activity allele are at risk, but there is no overall consensus concerning its possible status as a major effect gene. Nevertheless, a significant and intriguing interaction between stressful environments and low-activity variants of *MAOA* in promoting violence and ASB has recently emerged.

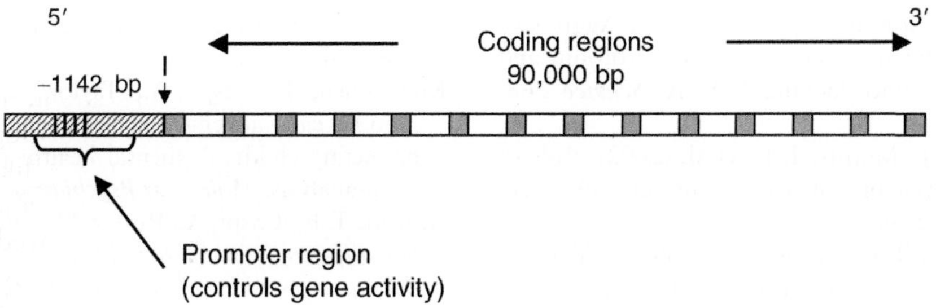

Figure 1 Representation of the monoamine oxidase gene (*MAOA*). The promoter region (in diagonal lines) controls the levels of gene activity and contains a 30-bp repeat (often referred to as a variable-number tandem repeat, VNTR). Different copy numbers of the basic motif have different effects on transcription. Three- and four-copy motifs are the most common in the population, with the former conferring lower activity than the latter. Rare alleles with 2-, 3.5-, and 5-copy motifs are also observed. I indicates position of transcription initiation (RNA synthesis). Exons (coding regions) are in gray (not to scale).

The Role of Stress and Abusive Upbringing in Aggression and Violence

Given the observed relationship between abusive environments and antisocial outcomes, the *MAOA* gene became a candidate for a genetic predisposing factor that may interact with stress induced by adverse early rearing experiences to promote ASB. Caspi and associates, in 2002, were the first to study the interactions between environment and *MAOA* activity variants in the etiology of ASB in males by investigating the patterns of antisocial outcomes in a range of male children who had been maltreated. A broad range of measures for ASB was followed in the males from a longitudinal cohort of approximately 800 individuals who were age 26 at the time of data collection. The information available relevant to ASB included the commission of violent crimes, a personal disposition toward violence, and adolescent conduct disorder (assessed according to *Diagnostic and Statistical Manual,* 4th edn., criteria). Whichever measure of antisocial outcomes was examined, a significant association between maltreatment and ASB conditional on the individual's *MAOA* genotype was observed. Whereas maltreated males with low-activity alleles were significantly at risk of conviction for violent crime or of exhibiting other ASB, those with high-activity alleles were not. An increasing tendency to antisocial acts by those with more extreme childhood maltreatment was observed for males with the low-activity allele, but not for those protected by a high-activity allele.

Similar observations have since been reported in studies employing data from white male twins from the community-based longitudinal Virginia Twin Study for Adolescent Behavioural Development. Several other studies have been completed, and an analysis of all the information currently available is broadly supportive of an interaction between variants of this gene and stressful environments in predisposing ASB.

It is of interest that an analogous promoter variant system of this X chromosome gene has been discovered in rhesus macaque monkeys. A variable-repeat motif of 18 bp has been identified and shown to regulate the expression of *MAOA*. Of particular relevance to the putative role of functional *MAOA* variants in humans is that male macaques with the low-activity form were found to be more aggressive in competing for food.

The physiological relationship between the stress caused by abusive upbringing and the apparent protection provided by the high-activity allele for *MAOA* is not yet clear. Stress is known to elicit an increase in levels of transcription factors, such as c-Fos. These factors, in turn, may upregulate genes encoding components of neurotransmitter pathways, and it is possible that the apparent risk conferred by the low-activity allele of *MAOA* reflects a relative inability to respond to the effects of stress arising from maltreatment.

Conclusion

The lack of a functional copy of the *MAOA* gene in humans and mice results in ASB and aggression, and the less-functional fundamental variation of the gene appears to have related behavioral consequences. In particular, there is a complex interaction between the response to chronic stress and functional variants of the gene and the likelihood of individuals developing ASB or violent behavior. Longitudinal studies of the effects of childhood maltreatment and its interaction in males with high- or low-activity genetic variants of the *MAOA* gene suggest that the high-activity allele may confer protection in males because carriers are much less likely to develop ASB and aggressive behavior than are those with low-activity alleles.

Further Reading

Brunner, H. G., Nelen, M., Breakefield, X. O., et al. (1993). Abnormal behavior associated with a point mutation in the structural gene for monoamine oxidase A. *Science* 262, 578–580.

Cases, O., Seif, I., Grimsby, J., et al. (1995). Aggressive behaviour and altered amounts of brain serotonin and norepinephrine in mice lacking MAOA. *Science* **268**, 1763–1766.

Caspi, A., McClay, J., Moffitt, T. E., et al. (2002). Role of genotype in the cycle of violence in maltreated children. *Science* **297**, 851–854.

Craig, I. W. (2005). The role of monoamine oxidase A, MAOA, in the aetiology of antisocial behaviour: the importance of gene environment interactions. In: Bock, G. & Goode, J. (Eds.) *Molecular mechanisms influencing aggressive behaviours* (Novartis Foundation Symposium 268), pp. 227–237. New York: John Wiley & Sons.

Deckert, J., Catalano, M., Syagailo, Y. V., et al. (1999). Excess of high activity monoamine oxidase A gene promoter alleles in female patients with panic disorder. *Human Molecular Genetics* **8**, 621–624.

Denney, R. M., Koch, H. and Craig, I. W. (1999). Association between monoamine oxidase A activity in human male skin fibroblasts and the genotype of the MAO promoter-associated variable number tandem repeat. *Human Genetics* **105**, 541–551.

Foley, D. L., Eaves, L. J., Wormley, B., et al. (2004). Childhood adversity, monoamine oxidase A genotype, and risk for conduct disorder. *Archives of General Psychiatry* **61**, 738–744.

Kim-Cohen, J., Caspi, A., Taylor, A., et al. (in press). MAOA, early adversity, and gene-environment interaction predicting children's mental health: new evidence and a meta-analysis. *Molecular Psychiatry.*

Moffitt, T. E., Caspi, A., Rutter, M. and Silva, P. A. (2001). *Sex differences in antisocial behaviour: conduct disorder, delinquency and violence in the Dunedin Longitudinal Study.* Cambridge, UK: Cambridge University Press.

Newman, T. K., Syagailo, Y. V., Barr, C. S., et al. (2005). Monoamine oxidase A gene promoter variation and rearing experiences influences aggressive behaviour in rhesus monkeys. *Biological Psychiatry* **57**, 167–172.

Sabol, S. Z., Hu, S. and Hamer, D. (1998). A functional polymorphism in the monoamine oxidase A gene promoter. *Human Genetics* **103**, 273–279.

Vierikko, E., Pulkkinen, L., Kaprio, J., et al. (2003). Sex differences in genetic and environmental effects on aggression. *Aggressive Behaviour* **29**, 55–68.

Relevant Website

http://www.ojp.usdoj.gov/bis.

III. MENTAL DISORDERS

A. Personality and Personality Disorders

Stress of Self Esteem

J C Pruessner, S Wuethrich and M W Baldwin
McGill University, Montreal, Quebec, Canada

Glossary

Cortisol — A steroid hormone secreted by the human adrenal glands. It is often released in high amounts during periods of stress. High doses lead to interference with the proper functioning of the immune system.

Hippocampus — Seahorse-shaped structure that extends along the inferior horn of each lateral ventricle of the brain and consists of gray matter covered on the ventricular surface with white matter. A part of the limbic system, it is involved in the storage of memory for intermediate periods and the consolidation of those memories into permanent form.

Hypothalamic-pituitary-adrenal (HPA) axis — The major part of the neuroendocrine system that controls reactions to stress and has important functions in regulating various body processes such as digestion, the immune system, and energy usage. Most species (from humans to simple organisms) share components of the HPA axis. It regulates a set of interactions among glands, hormones, and parts of the midbrain that mediate the general adaptation syndrome proposed by Selye.

Locus of control — The perception of factors responsible for the outcome of an event. An individual with high internal locus of control believes that his or her own actions caused the outcome. Conversely, an individual with high external locus of control believes the outcome was determined by outside forces.

Personality — The complex of all attributes – behavioral, temperamental, emotional, and mental – that characterize an individual.

Self-esteem — The global value we place on ourselves.

Stressor — Any emotional or physical demand (positive or negative) that gives or results in stress.

The Role of Personality in the Perception of Stress

Lazarus, who has devoted much of his work to the study of stress, noted early on that stressful conditions per se fail to produce reliable effects on task performance. Keeping all situational variables constant, the same stressor can have minimal effect, lead to performance improvement, or result in significant performance impairment across subjects. This led him and others to suggest that individual differences in motivational and cognitive variables are likely to interact with situational components, and what is considered threatening for some, and thus stressful and performance impairing, might be considered as stimulating by others, and thus produce beneficial effects on performance.

Subsequent research identified the process of evaluation as crucial in explaining the impact of psychological variables on the stress response. Any internal or external stimulus is perceived as stressful only if it is evaluated as harmful or threatening. The early notion of the importance of the evaluation has received recent validation with the identification of social evaluative threat as the single most important factor in determining the stressfulness of a situation in laboratory stress studies.

The Importance of Self-esteem and Locus of Control in the Perception of Stress

A case can be made that the personality variables self-esteem and locus of control play a central role in the evaluation of many situations and thus contribute to the experience of stress. Self-esteem is broadly defined as the value we place on ourselves. Epidemiological studies have shown that low self-esteem is associated with negative life outcomes, including substance abuse, delinquency, unhappiness, depression, and worsened recovery after illnesses. On the other hand, high self-esteem has been linked to happiness and longevity. In studies of aging, a positive self-concept has been identified to play a key role in successful aging, predicting independence, cognitive stability, and general health in old age.

Internal locus of control can be defined as the perception that one's outcomes are determined by one's actions. Not surprisingly, internal locus of control and self-esteem are usually highly correlated. The key link of these variables to the experience of stress lies in their impact on the evaluation of any given situation. We postulate that in the evaluation of whether a given situation is threatening or benign, self-esteem and internal locus of control systematically interact with situational factors. If a person

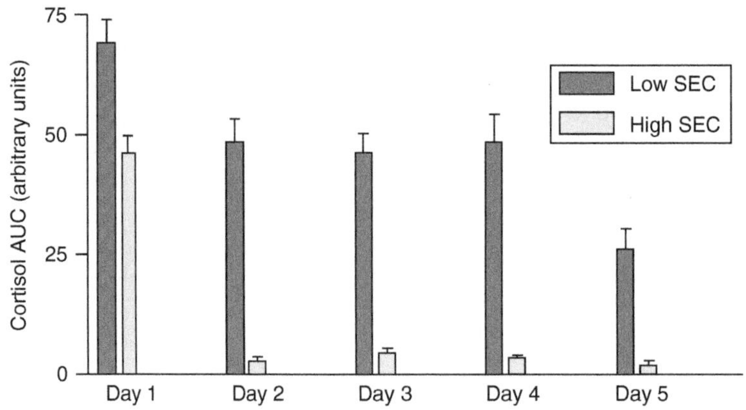

Figure 1 Cortisol responses (AUC, area under the curve) on repeated exposure to the Trier Social Stress Test (TSST) on 5 subsequent days in subjects with high self-esteem and high locus of control (high SEC; $n = 13$) and low self-esteem and low locus of control (low SEC; $n = 7$).

attributes little importance to him- or herself and thinks that he or she has little impact on the outcome of his or her own actions, this person will find more situations uncontrollable and unpredictable, and consequently will evaluate more situations as threatening and harmful.

Endocrinological Evidence for the Role of Self-esteem and Locus of Control in the Perception of Stress

Evidence for the impact of self-esteem and locus of control on stress perception emerged when subjects were exposed to repeated psychological stress, using the Trier Psychosocial Stress Test (TSST). In this paradigm, subjects have to give an impromptu speech and perform serial subtraction tasks in front of an audience, usually for about 10 min. The audience consists of two to three persons who are instructed to maintain a neutral expression, being neither explicitly rejecting nor confirmative in their facial expression or gestures. During the speech, the audience interacts with the subject only to indicate the amount of time that is left to talk or to ask specific questions. In the case that a subject stumbles, they encourage the subject to continue the speech. During the serial subtraction task, the subject is interrupted only when making a mistake. The subject is then corrected and instructed to start the task over. The task was designed to represent a significant social-evaluative threat and indeed has been shown to be a powerful stressor, stimulating the hypothalamic-pituitary-adrenal (HPA) axis and leading to significant free cortisol increases within 15 to 30 min following the onset of the task. This first study aimed to validate the long-standing hypothesis that in humans, repeated exposure to the same stressor would lead to quick habituation of the stress response. In order to test the habituation of the stress response, 20 young healthy male college students were exposed to the TSST on five subsequent days. For this purpose, the TSST was modified using different speech topics and serial subtraction tasks on each day. Interestingly, only 13 of the 20 subjects showed the typical habituation pattern, with a normal stress response on day one being significantly reduced on day two, and no longer present on the subsequent days. In the seven remaining subjects, however, the cortisol stress response continued to be present on all days and only showed a tendency to decline toward the end of the testing (**Figure 1**). When analyzing the available psychological variables, it became apparent that low internal locus of control and low self-esteem were the best predictors of failing habituation of the cortisol stress response to repeated stress exposure. This can be interpreted as a sign that these personality variables interact with the evaluation of a situation during repeated exposure. The absence of differences in the stress response between the two groups of subjects on day one was at the time attributed to the effect of novelty – the novelty of the situation might have made it unpredictable and uncontrollable for everybody on the first exposure and might thus have masked the impact of personality variables on stress perception and response. One conclusion at the time was that in order to reveal the effect of personality variables on the stress evaluation and response, one would likely need repeated exposures to the same stressor in order to reveal the influence of personality variables on stress.

However, it is known that personality variables tend to have relatively weaker effects when situational factors are very strong. In a second study, the threatening aspects of the situation were reduced, and self-esteem and locus of control had an impact on the perception of stress on the first exposure to a stimulus. Here, computerized mental arithmetic was combined with an induced failure design to invoke stress. In the setup used in this task, 52 students performed the task on computer terminals in front of them. Half of the students were exposed to a difficult version leading to low performance, compared to an easy version of the task with high performance for the other half. The students played the task in three 3-min segments and had to announce their performance score after each segment to the investigator, who wrote the scores down on a board for everybody to see. Saliva sampling before, throughout, and after the task allowed the assessment of the cortisol dynamics in relation to this paradigm. Interestingly, this task triggered a significant cortisol release only in the subjects who were in the low-performance group and had low self-esteem and low internal locus of control. Neither low performance alone nor low self-esteem and internal locus of control alone were significant predictors of cortisol release, supporting the notion that these personality variables produce effects only in interaction with a potentially stressful situation (**Figure 2**). The evaluation of the situation is suggested to be at the core of this interaction.

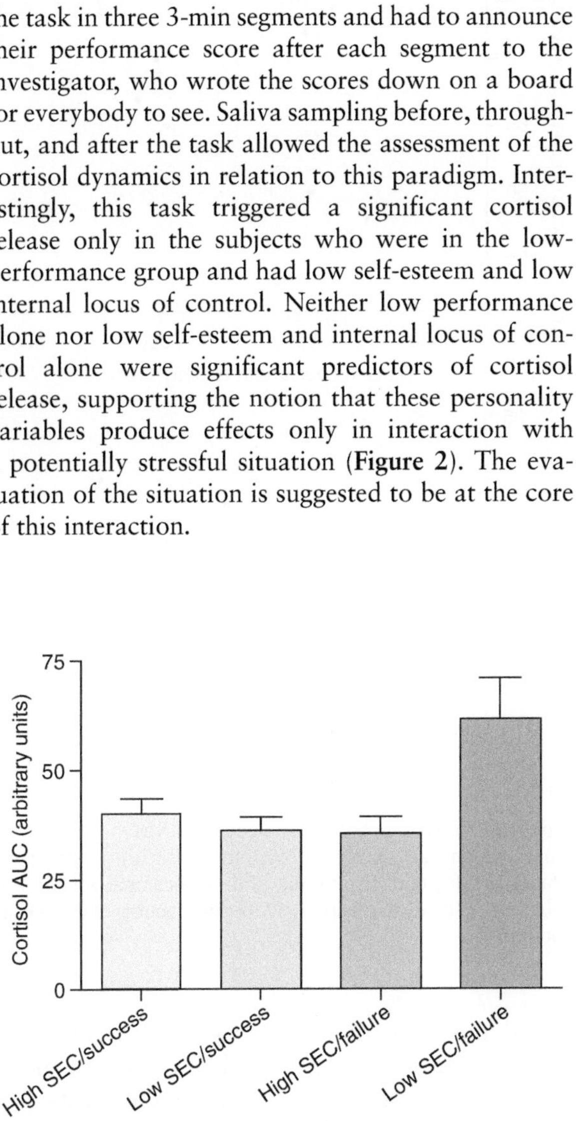

Figure 2 Cortisol stress responses to the Trier Mental Challenge Task (TMCT) in four groups of subjects, separated for high and low self-esteem and locus of control and high and low performance in the mental arithmetic. The performance was manipulated by the investigator.

The Hippocampus as a Possible Mediator of the Relationship between Self-esteem, Locus of Control, and Stress

Although studies on brain correlates of personality variables and endocrine function in humans are only starting to appear, a picture is emerging that puts the spotlight on the hippocampus as a likely mediator between the previously reported personality variations and stress responses. The hippocampus is one of the major limbic system structures involved in the regulation of the stress response, and variations in hippocampal volume (HCV) have been postulated and shown to be systematically linked to excessive HPA axis activity. Early models postulated that associations between HCV and HPA axis activity might represent the consequence of excessive exposure of the hippocampus to glucocorticoids, due to their powerful neurotoxic properties.

More recently, however, evidence for a link between naturally occurring variations in HCV and HPA function has surfaced. Functionally, the hippocampus is the primary structure for memory contextualization, and it is here that a link to self-esteem and locus of control could occur. When an individual is faced with a potentially threatening and harmful situation, he or she employs memories of past events to contribute to the evaluation of the current event. However, if specific situational and environmental characteristics associated with negative past events cannot be recalled, this lack of awareness of situational circumstance can lead to an overgeneralization of negative past events and thus an increased likelihood to consider the current situations as stressful as well. Thus, poor contextualization mediated by the hippocampus could be linked to higher stress responses, on the one hand, and lower self-esteem on the other.

This hypothesis of a link between HCV, personality variables, and stress responses was tested in 17 healthy young male college students. All subjects underwent extensive psychological assessment for assessment of personality variables, including self-esteem and locus of control. In addition, they underwent magnetic resonance imaging employing a structural T1-weighted acquisition protocol, which produces high-resolution images of the cerebrum. A recently developed manual segmentation protocol was then applied to all images that included nonuniformity correction, signal intensity normalization, and Tailarach-like transformation for standardization of brain size. This protocol allows for manual assessment of hippocampal volumes. Finally, all subjects were exposed to a computerized stress task, similar to the mental arithmetic task described earlier. Saliva samples before, during, and after the task accompanied the testing to capture the cortisol stress response. Results first replicated earlier findings of mental arithmetic stress: only the subjects with low self-esteem and low internal locus of control showed a significant release of cortisol. Extending earlier findings, however, a correlation emerged between the cortisol stress response and self-esteem ($r = -0.45$, $p < 0.05$). Furthermore, a significant correlation emerged between the cortisol stress response and the total hippocampal volume ($r = -0.53$, $p = 0.03$), suggesting that the size of the hippocampus is related to the regulation of the HPA (**Figure 3a**). Finally, supporting the initial hypothesis, a link was observed between internal locus of control and HCV ($r = 0.66$, $p = 0.006$; **Figure 3b**) and self-esteem and HCV ($r = 0.58$, $p = 0.02$; **Figure 3c**).

Testing for the specificity of the effect with regard to the hippocampus, total brain gray matter was employed as control structure in correlations with both personality variables and cortisol response. None of the tested correlations were significant, suggesting that the observed relationships were indeed specific to this medial temporal lobe area.

Conclusion: Personality Variables, Brain Structures, and Stress Responses in a Developmental Context

It will be a challenging task for future studies to ascertain the origin of the relationship observed between personality variables, hippocampal volume, and stress response. There are a number of possibilities as to how these associations could develop. One model puts naturally occurring variations in hippocampal volume at the origin of these functional relationships. It can be speculated that HCV is a consequence of multiple interacting factors during critical developmental stages, leading to the variation in HCV that follows a normal distribution pattern. If, however, the size of this structure determines memory contextualization capabilities, this variation would then have personality and stress-related consequences. The impaired source monitoring would lead to an overgeneralization of the experience of failure and rejection, and consequently to a self-perception of being a failure or being socially rejected in general, which might produce low self-esteem and low locus of control during childhood and adolescence. The observed higher cortisol responses would then not be a direct consequence of small HCV, but of the increased stress perception due to consistent unfavorable evaluations of ambiguous situations. Of course, the question arises why overgeneralization

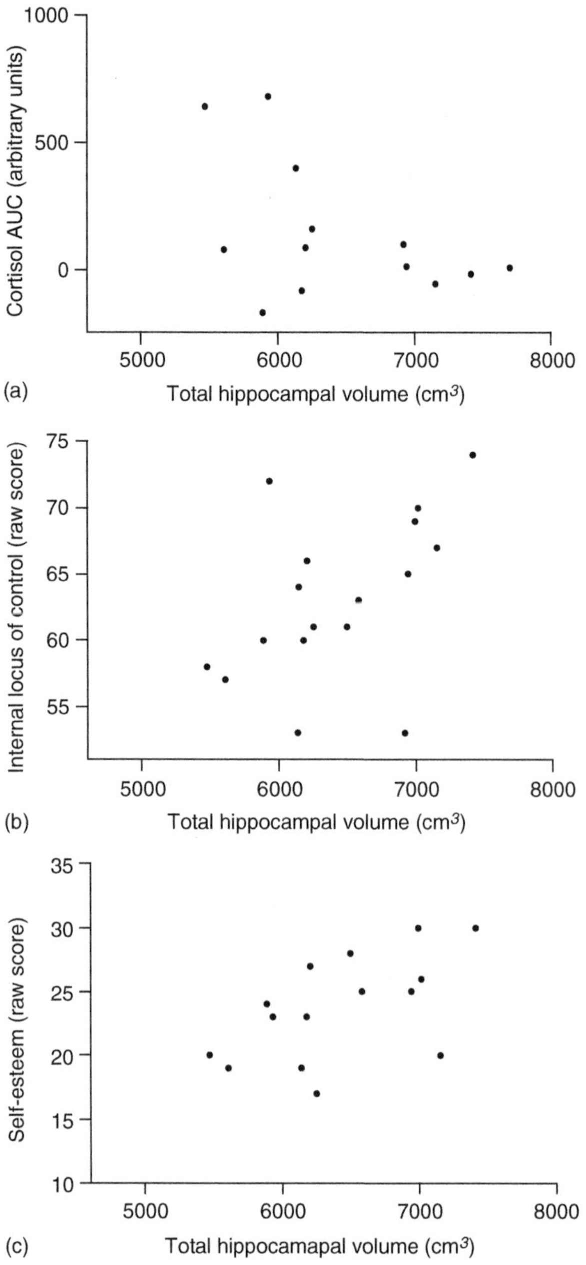

Figure 3 Correlation between hippocampal volume and cortisol stress responses to a mental arithmetic task (a), hippocampal volume and locus of control (b), and hippocampal volume and self-esteem (c) in a group of 17 healthy young male college students.

should then not also be an issue for positive life events, in other words, a general lack of source monitoring for both positive and negative life events with no consequences on self-perception. One possible explanation could be seen in the stress-specific function of the hippocampus within the limbic system. There is evidence that it is specifically the hippocampus together with the anterior cingulate that is involved in the stress response. It is also known that the anterior cingulate is particularly involved in error monitoring, which means that its involvement is restricted to situations in which a mismatch between expectations and reality occurs. These circumstances would make a specific role of the hippocampus in reaction to negative life events more probable.

Based on the findings to date, we suggest that reduced HCV might play a role in the development of low self-esteem. This may in turn produce a higher susceptibility of perceiving ambiguous situations as threatening, and thus stressful. The idea that HCV variation might be the cause for adverse functional and behavioral consequences, rather than their consequence, has recently been proposed in conjunction with risk factors for developing posttraumatic stress disorder (PTSD) in a study investigating hippocampal volume in twin brothers. Here, in subjects who developed PTSD as a consequence of participating in the Vietnam War, the researchers observed lower hippocampal volume compared to subjects who went to war but did not develop PTSD. Intriguingly, however, lower hippocampal volume could also be observed in the PTSD subjects' twin brothers – who never went to war – leading to the speculation that HCV might be a risk factor for, rather than a consequence of, developing PTSD.

As mentioned earlier, the possibility that HCV plays a causal role is supported by the fact that consistent results were found even among relatively young adults. Recently, variations in HCV in young populations have been reported, suggesting that there is a considerable range of hippocampal volumes already in young subjects. At the same time, self-esteem is known to be a stable trait, with considerable intra-individual stability throughout life. This supports a model in which variations in brain morphology could become a pathway to certain personality characteristics and behavioral phenotypes early in life, but longitudinal studies will be needed to examine these changes over time and provide validation for the assumed associations.

Further Reading

Baltes, M. M. and Baltes, P. B. (1990). *Successful aging.* Cambridge, UK: Cambridge University Press.

Baumeister, R. F., Campbell, J. K., Krueger, J. I. and Vohs, K. D. (2003). Does high self-esteem cause better performance, interpersonal success, happiness, or healthier lifestyles? *Psychological Science in the Public Interest* **4**, 1–44.

Dickerson, S. S. and Kemeny, M. E. (2004). Acute stressors and cortisol responses: a theoretical integration and synthesis of laboratory research. *Psychological Bulletin* **130**(3), 355–391.

Fuchs, E. and Flugge, G. (2003). Chronic social stress: effects on limbic brain structures. *Physiology and Behavior* **79**(3), 417–427.

Gilbertson, M. W., Shenton, M. E., Ciszewski, A., Kasai, K., Lasko, N. B., Orr, S. P., et al. (2002). Smaller hippocampal volume predicts pathologic vulnerability to psychological trauma. *Nature Neuroscience* **5**(11), 1242–1247.

Hoyle, R., Kernis, M. H., Leary, M. R. and Baldwin, M. W. (1999). *Selfhood: identity, esteem, control.* Boulder, CO: Westwood.

Kirschbaum, C., Bartussek, D. and Strasburger, C. J. (1992). Cortisol responses to psychological stress and correlations with personality traits. *Personality and Individual Differences* **13**(12), 1353–1357.

Lazarus, R. S. (1999). *Stress and emotion: a new synthesis.* New York: Springer.

Leary, M. R. and McDonald, G. (2003). Individual differences in self-esteem: a review and theoretical integration. In: Leary, M. R. & Tangney, J. P. (eds.) *Handbook of self and identity,* pp. 401–420. New York: Guilford Press.

Petrie, K. and Rotheram, M. J. (1982). Insulators against stress: self-esteem and assertiveness. *Psychological Report* **50**(3 Pt 1), 963–966.

Pruessner, J. C., Hellhammer, D. H. and Kirschbaum, C. (1999). Low self-esteem, induced failure and the adrenocortical stress response. *Personality and Individual Differences* **27**(3), 477–489.

Pruessner, J. C., Collins, D. L., Pruessner, M. and Evans, A. C. (2001). Age and gender predict volume decline in the anterior and posterior hippocampus in early adulthood. *Journal of Neuroscience* **21**(1), 194–200.

Pruessner, J. C., Baldwin, M. W., Dedovic, K., et al. (2005). Self-esteem, locus of control, hippocampal volume, and cortisol regulation in young and old adulthood. *Neuroimage* **28**, 815–826.

Sapolsky, R. M. (1999). Glucocorticoids, stress, and their adverse neurological effects: relevance to aging. *Experimental Gerontology* **34**(6), 721–732.

Sinha, R., Lacadie, C., Skudlarski, P. and Wexler, B. E. (2004). Neural circuits underlying emotional distress in humans. *Annals of the New York Academy of Sciences* **1032**, 254–257.

Borderline Personality Disorder

H W Koenigsberg and L J Siever
Bronx VA Medical Center, Bronx, NY, USA

This is a revised version of the article by L J Siever and H W Koenigsberg, Encyclopedia of Stress First Edition, volume 1, pp 339–341, © 2000, Elsevier Inc.

Glossary

Neurotransmitter — One of a number of chemical substances which, when released at the terminal of one neuron and captured by a specialized receptor on the surface of another neuron, transmit a signal from one neuron to another.

Personality — Enduring patterns of perceiving, relating to, and thinking about the environment and oneself.

Personality disorder — The disturbance resulting from maladaptive personality traits which cause functional impairment or substantial distress.

Phenomenology and Epidemiology of Borderline Personality Disorder

Borderline personality disorder (BPD), a disorder characterized by emotional instability and impulsivity, is one of the more serious personality disorders. It is associated with high levels of distress, significant impairments in social and occupational functioning, and a risk of suicide approaching 10%. As a personality disorder, BPD reflects an enduring and inflexible maladaptation in an individual's characteristic pattern of perceiving, relating to, and thinking about the environment and self. In BPD, the individual is highly reactive to psychosocial events such as losses, separations, and frustrations. The individual with BPD may show intense but shifting extremes of emotion, often involving anger and depression. He or she may engage in impulsively self-destructive acts, or may recurrently threaten or attempt suicide. His or her relationships with others are typically intense and unstable, often oscillating between idealization and devaluation of others. By the same token, his/her own sense of identity is unstable and people with BPD are unsure of their goals, values, or sense of self. They may be terrified of real or imagined abandonment and may frantically attempt to control others to prevent this. Under the stress of losses, frustrations, or intense interpersonal relationships, individuals with BPD may regress, becoming more infantile or experiencing transient lapses in reality testing, which can take the form of hallucinations or delusional ideas. They often experience a sense of boredom and inner emptiness. It is estimated that about 2% of the population meets criteria for BPD. It is more often diagnosed in women and is more common among first degree relatives of those with the disorder.

Role of Neurobiology

BPD appears to be the result of converging biological predispositions and early-life experience. Two biologically mediated dimensions of personality are particularly prominent in BPD, impulsive-aggression and affective instability. In borderline patients, the impulsive-aggression is most often self-directed, but it can also be directed to others. Impulsive-aggression has been shown to be associated with dysregulation in the serotonin neurotransmitter system. Cerebrospinal fluid levels of 5-hydroxyindoleacetic acid (5-HIAA), a breakdown product of serotonin, are inversely correlated with the degree of impulsive-aggressive and suicidal behavior in depressed patients and in patients with personality disorders. Borderline patients show a blunted response to the ingestion of fenfluramine, a serotonin-releasing and potentiating agent which triggers release of the hormone prolactin, and the degree of blunting in prolactin response to fenfluramine correlates with the level of impulsive-aggression manifest in the patient's life history. Studies, which use positron emission tomography (PET) scanning to show regional metabolic activity in the brain, have demonstrated that in BPD patients the response to the fenfluramine is diminished specifically in those brain regions responsible for inhibiting impulsive behaviors. Similar results were found using other serotonergic challenge agents.

The noradrenergic (norepinephrine) neurotransmitter system is also implicated in aggression in patients with personality disorders. Cerebrospinal fluid levels of 3-methoxy-4-hydrophenylglycol (MHPG), a norepinephrine breakdown product, have been shown to correlate positively with impulsive-aggressive behavior. The responsivity of the noradrenergic system can be assayed by measuring the growth hormone response to clonidine. Growth hormone release in response to clonidine directly correlates with irritability. Since norepinephrine activity is associated with alertness, attention to external stimuli, and extraversion, it may be connected with outward-directed aggression. The interaction between serotonin and noradrenergic systems may determine the nature of aggression in BPD. Low serotonergic activity may predispose to impulsive aggression, which appears to be outward directed when noradrenergic activity is high and inward directed when noradrenergic activity is low. Studies have suggested that the activity of another neurotransmitter, arginine vasopressin, may directly correlate with levels of aggression in personality disorders.

Affective instability may be associated with dysregulation of the neurotransmitter, acetylcholine. When borderline patients were given an acetylcholine-potentiating agent, physostigmine, they responded by becoming transiently more dysphoric for several minutes to 1 hour, whereas nonBDP patients did not show this reaction. The affective effect of physostigmine was associated with the patients' degree of affective instability, identity confusion, unstable relationships and feelings of emptiness and boredom, suggesting that these symptoms may all be related to affective instability.

Role of Life Experience

Early-life experience also appears to contribute to the development of BPD. Histories of repeated childhood physical or sexual abuse are commonly found among borderline patients, although such abuse experiences are also associated with a variety of other psychiatric disorders as well. Severe physical or emotional neglect may also predispose to BPD. Intense levels of aggressive drive, either resulting from an inborn predisposition or exceptionally powerful anger-inducing life experiences such as abuse, painful illness, or devastating losses, are also believed to contribute to borderline pathology. Some researchers have suggested that individuals who go on to develop borderline personalities have had impairments in their ability to evoke memories of their caretakers for use in soothing themselves in the absence of the caretaker. Other researchers emphasize the interaction of the affectively unstable child with a caretaking environment in which strong feelings are disavowed and the child is made to feel that his or her feelings are invalid.

Psychological Structures in the Borderline Patient

Psychoanalytic investigators have postulated that borderline individuals protect themselves from recognizing the consequences of their unacceptable feelings by developing inflexible and maladaptive defense mechanisms, such as splitting. Splitting is a defense in which the individual partitions his or her psychic experience into compartments which keep aggressive feelings away from images of loved and needed others. The partitioning of memory, which is the essence of splitting, may itself be a consequence of the impact of affective instability upon emotion-state-dependent memory processes. Thus the use of splitting, with its associated anxiety-controlling effects, may derive from a psychobiological vulnerability to affective dysregulation. The extensive use of the splitting defense fragments the individual's internal images of self and others. This produces a confused sense of self and identity and contradictory pictures of others.

Treatment of Borderline Personality Disorder

Because of their ingrained nature, personality disorders are slow to change, and the impulsiveness and affective instability characteristic of BPD makes this disorder often difficult to treat. While no single treatment has been identified as the treatment of choice for BPD, patients have responded well to a number of psychotherapeutic approaches and to medications. Recent work has extended earlier observations that such anticonvulsant/mood-stabilizing medications as topirimate, divalproex sodium, lamotrigine, and carbamezepine can reduce anger, aggression, irritability, and impulsivity in borderline patients. Borderline patients also show a global positive response to the mood stabilizer, lithium carbonate. Monoamine oxidase (MAO) inhibitors, which affect several neurotransmitter systems, reduce depression, anxiety, hostility, self-destructiveness, and interpersonal sensitivity in BPD. Selective serotonin-reuptake inhibitor (SSRI) antidepressants have been shown to diminish hostility in borderline patients and may also reduce impulsive-aggression and depression. Low doses of antipsychotic medications have reduced the transient psychotic symptoms, hostility, impulsiveness, and, in some studies, depression in BPD. The newer atypical antipsychotic medications have been shown to reduce hostility, suspiciousness, paranoia, anxiety, and depressive symptoms in the disorder. At present, it remains an open question whether the beneficial effects of medication last beyond the 6–12-week periods examined in most studies. For patients with severe self-destructiveness and those who tend to be more action-oriented than introspective, a form of cognitive behavioral therapy, dialectical behavior therapy (DBT), has been shown to diminish self-destructive behavior and reduce the need for inpatient treatment. One recent study demonstrated that DBT in combination with the atypical antipsychotic medication, olanzepine, was more effective than DBT alone. Psychodynamic psychotherapies, which have helped borderline patients develop an integrated sense of themselves and others and have led to enhanced interpersonal and career functioning, are suitable for patients who can contain dangerous behavior with the structure of an outpatient treatment contract and who are interested in identifying, understanding the origins of, and changing maladaptive interpersonal patterns. For some patients, sequential treatment with medication, DBT, and psychodynamic psychotherapy may be the optimal approach.

See Also the Following Articles

Multiple Personality Disorder.

Further Reading

Coccaro, E. F., Kavoussi, R. J., Hauger, R. L., et al. (1998). Cerebrospinal fluid vasopressin levels correlates with aggression and serotonin function in personality-disordered subject. *Archives of General Psychiatry* **55**, 708–714.

Cowdry, R. W. and Gardner, D. L. (1988). Pharmacotherapy of borderline personality disorder: alprazolam, carbamezepine, triflupoperazine, and tranylcypromine. *Archives in General Psychology* **45**, 111–119.

Kernberg, O. F. (1975). *Borderline conditions and pathological narcissism.* New York: Aaronson.

Koenigsberg, H. W. (1993). Combining psychotherapy and pharmacotherapy in the treatment of borderline patients. In: Oldham, J. M., Riba, M. B. & Tasman, A. (eds.) *American Psychiatric Press Review of Psychiatry,* Vol 12. Washington DC: American Psychiatric Press.

Koenigsberg, H. W., Harvey, P. D., Mitropoulou, V., et al. (2002). Characterizing affective instability in borderline personality disorder. *American Journal of Psychiatry* **159**, 784–788.

Koenigsberg, H. W., Woo-Ming, A. M., and Siever, L. J. (In press). Psychopharmacological treatment of personality disorders. In: Nathan, P. R. & Gorman, J. M. (eds.) *A guide to treatments that work*, 3rd edn., New York: Oxford University Press.

Linehan, M. M. (1993). *Cognitive-behavioral treatment of borderline personality disorder.* New York: Guilford.

New, A. S., Hazlett, E. A., Buchsbaum, M. S., et al. (2002). Blunted prefrontal cortical 18fluorodeoxyglucose positron emission tomography response to meta-chlorophenylpiperazine in impulsive aggression. *Archives in General Psychiatry* **59**, 621–629.

Siever, L. J. and Davis, K. L. (1991). A psychobiological perspective on the personality disorders. *American Journal of Psychiatry* **148**, 1647–1658.

Skodol, A. E., Siever, L. J., Livesley, W. J., et al. (2002). The borderline diagnosis ii: biology, genetics, and clinical course. *Biological Psychiatry* **51**, 951–963.

Multiple Personality Disorder

R P Kluft
Temple University, Philadelphia, PA, USA

This is a revised version of the article by R P Kluft, Encyclopedia of Stress First Edition, volume 2, pp 786–790, © 2000, Elsevier Inc.

Glossary

Alter — A distinct identity or personality state with its own characteristic and relatively enduring pattern of perceiving, relating to, and thinking about the environment and self. An alter has its own identity, self-representation, autobiographic memory, and sense of ownership of its own thoughts, feelings, and actions. Some synonyms are personality, personality state, subpersonality, alter personality, and disaggregate self-state.

Dissociation — "Disruption in the usually integrated functions of consciousness, memory, identity, or perception" (American Psychiatric Association, 2000: 519); the segregation of some subsets of information from other subsets of information in a relatively rule-bound manner (Spiegel, 1986: 123).

Ego state — "An organized system of behavior and experience whose elements are bound together by some common principle but that is separated from other such states by boundaries that are more or less permeable" (Watkins and Watkins, 1993: 278).

Iatrogenesis — The creation (or worsening) of a problematic condition as a result of the interventions of a helping professional.

Integration — The unification of all personalities into a single coherent identity; the cessation of separateness of a particular personality or group of personalities; the interventions made by a therapist to bring together two or more personalities at a particular point in time.

Personality — An enduring pattern of behavior, adaptation, and inner experience that is pervasive over time and across situations (in general psychology); synonym for alter (in dissociative disorders).

Resolution An outcome in which a multiple personality patient has achieved smooth function, continuity of contemporary memory, and the relief of distressing symptoms due to the more facile cooperation and collaboration of the remaining personalities. Some personalities may have integrated.

Shift A change in the personality system such that while the personality or alter in apparent executive control has not changed or been replaced, it is being influenced by different alters behind the scenes than it had been, leading to minor changes in the appearance, actions, and speech of the alter in apparent executive control.

Switch A transition from one personality being in apparent executive control to another personality being in apparent executive control.

Introduction

Multiple personality (dissociative identity disorder in the United States) has been described as difficult to understand, difficult to diagnose, difficult to treat, and difficult to discuss objectively not only because of its complexity, but also because of the controversies that often surround it. Its study draws upon the literatures of dissociation, hypnosis, memory, cognitive psychology, social psychology, development, trauma, attachment and psychoanalysis, among others, requiring researchers and clinicians to grapple with concerns and issues that often appear remote and obscure.

History

Conditions in which an individual's customary personality or way of being is replaced by an alternative (and often very different) personality or way of being, whose activities are unknown to the customary personality, were virtually worldwide and commonplace prior to the modern scientific era. Possession states were attributed to the intrusion of various forces, spirits, angels, demons, gods, or ancestors. Judeo-Christian possession states included forms in which the intruding entity took over completely, leaving the possessed person without memory for the intruding entity's actions, and forms in which both customary personality and intruding entity were aware of one another and contended for control (somnambulistic and lucid possession, respectively).

As possession was discredited (circa 1775–1800), cases with these phenomena were reported and described in secular terms (e.g., exchanged identity, doubling of the personality). By the 1830s, French physician Antoine Despine and his physician son and nephew had observed and treated series of such patients. Utilizing contemporary methods and magnetism, a precursor of hypnosis, successful treatments and integrations were achieved. Throughout the nineteenth century there was considerable interest in multiple personality.

However, rising forces in psychiatry and psychology eclipsed its study. Bleuler subsumed multiple personality under schizophrenia. Freud abandoned dissociation for repression. Janet was marginalized by psychoanalysis and the discrediting of his mentor, Charcot. Behaviorism disregarded multiple personality. Within a generation, multiple personality was largely forgotten except as a historical curiosity.

Two books, *The Three Faces of Eve* and *Sybil,* brought multiple personality to the attention of North American readers. A small but increasing number of North American clinicians began to report numbers of such patients (1970s–80s). Sensitized by feminism and the plight of Viet Nam veterans to the sequelae of abuse for women, children and combat veterans, they understood multiple personality as a chronic posttraumatic dissociative condition. Cases were recognized with increasing frequency. This experience was duplicated in The Netherlands and elsewhere.

In the 1990s there were highly polarized debates about whether multiple personality was iatrogenic, instigated and sustained by clinicians' interest in motivating patients to demonstrate the condition's phenomena, and whether the abuses alleged by patients, often recalled after years of apparent amnesia, were false, suggested by leading questions or subtle expressions of interest.

It remains unclear whether multiple personality can be created by iatrogenic factors alone. Some reports indicate that efforts to create conditions similar to multiple personality have been undertaken by various intelligence agencies. Some social psychology manipulations can cause subjects to demonstrate some characteristics of multiple personality under experimental conditions. However, no evidence demonstrates that clinicians exert influences similar to the interventions of either covert agencies or laboratory experiments. While some individuals are subject to develop false memories, many memories that became available after long absence from awareness have proven accurate.

Definition and Characteristic Findings

Criteria

The American Psychiatric Association's *Diagnostic and Statistical Manual of Mental Disorders,* 4th edition, text revision (DSM-IV-TR) offers four

Table 1 DSM-IV diagnostic criteria for dissociative identity disorder[a]

A. The presence of one or more distinct identities or personality states (each with its own relatively enduring pattern of perceiving, relating to, and thinking about the environment and self).
B. At least two of these identities or personality states recurrently take control of the person's behavior.
C. Inability to recall important personal information that is too extensive to be explained by ordinary forgetfulness.
D. The disturbance is not due to the direct physiological effects of a substance (e.g., blackouts or chaotic behavior during alcohol intoxication) or a general medical condition (e.g., complex partial seizures). Note: in children, the symptoms are not attributable to imaginary playmates or other fantasy play.

[a]From the American Psychiatric Association (2000), p. 529. Reprinted with permission from the Diagnostic and Statistical Manual of Mental Disorders, Copyright 2000. American Psychiatric Association.

diagnostic criteria for dissociative identity disorder (multiple personality) (**Table 1**).

Phenomena

Multiple personality involves problems with identity, memory, thinking, containment, cohesive conation, and the switch process. Problems of identity may include the presence of other identities (alters), depersonalization, an absence of or confusion about identity, alters' impingements on one another, and the combined presence of two or more alters. Problems of memory may include amnesia for past events, losing blocks of contemporary time, uncertainty about whether events did or did not occur, fragmentary recall, and experiencing events as dream-like, unreal, or of uncertain reality. There are often amnesia barriers across the alters, which may be aware or unaware of one another or display directional amnesia. In directional amnesia, alter A may know about alter B and be aware of B's thoughts and activities, while B knows little or nothing about A, is unaware of A's thoughts, and has no recall of what happens when A is in control.

Problems of thinking include cognitive errors, magical thinking, and the toleration of mutually incompatible ideas and perceptions without appreciating the impossibility of their coexisting (trance logic). They stem from distortions of reality made to accommodate to intolerable childhood circumstances.

Problems of containment include the intrusions of alters into one another and leakage of the memories, feelings, and sensations of one alter into the awareness and experience of another.

Problems of cohesive conation (will and intentionality) refer to difficulties in the distribution of executive control across the alters. Patients' sense of control of themselves and their actions may be compromised, along with their sense of ownership, responsibility, and voluntary control of themselves and their actions.

Problems of the switch process refer to changes of executive control that are jarring, incomplete, or so frequent that the person cannot concentrate or pay attention consistently enough to accomplish necessary functions and tasks.

Personalities

Personalities, personality states, subpersonalities, personifications, self-states, and alters are synonyms. They are relatively stable and enduring entities with fairly consistent ways of perceiving, relating to, and thinking about the environment and self. They are experienced as having their own identities, self-images, personal histories, and senses of ownership of their own activities and mental contents. Personalities usually but not inevitably have names. Some names may refer to attributes or emotions or humiliating insults. Usually a rather passive, guilt-ridden, dependent, masochistic, and depressed personality in apparent control most of the time bears the legal name. Alternate personalities may differ in name, age, race, gender, sexual orientation, areas of knowledge, predominant affect, vocabulary, and apparent intelligence. Alters may or may not be aware of one another. Alters may relate to one another in a potentially complex inner world. They constitute ongoing sets of parallel processes; that is, as one alter is dealing with the outside world, another may be making comments on or to the first, while others are interacting with one another, oblivious to external events. Neuropsychophysiological studies often demonstrate significant differences in different types of personality.

Personalities arise as desperate coping strategies, initially serving adaptive and defensive purposes. Achieving a degree of autonomy and persisting beyond the situations to which they were responses, they may become increasingly problematic and disruptive. Alters are formed by repudiating a sense of self and a representation of self in interactions with others that have become intolerable, severing empathic connection and erecting boundaries between the self that has become intolerable and a more adaptive identity created to manage the adaptation believed to be required. This new alter, envisioned and experienced as real, is accepted and interpreted as real. Its alternate autobiographic memories are endorsed as real.

For example: Lois, a 5-year-old girl, is molested by her previously warm and loving Uncle Ben. She is deeply attached to her uncle and does not want to lose him, afraid of the consequences of telling her

Table 2 Coping strategies and alter formation of 'Lois'[a]

Cognitive coping strategy	*Alter created*
This did not happen	A Lois who knows, and a Lois who does not
I must have deserved it	Bad Lois, whose behavior would explain trauma as punishment
I must have wanted it	A sexual alter, Sherrie
I can control it better if I take charge	An aggressively sexual alter, Vickie
I would be safe if I were a boy	Louis, Lois' male twin
I wish I were a big man	Big Jack, based on some person of power who could prevent this
I wish I were the one who could hurt someone and not be hurt	Uncle Ben, or a more disguised identification with the aggressor
I wish I could feel nothing	Jessie, who endures all yet feels nothing
I wish someone could replace me	The Girls, who encapsulate specific experiences of trauma unknown to Lois
I wish someone would comfort me	Angel, with whom Lois imagines herself to be while the body is being exploited and the Girls are experiencing the trauma

[a]From Kluft (1999), p. 5.

parents, confused about the feelings and sensations arising in her, wishing this molestation had never occurred, and wanting someone to rescue her. **Table 2** illustrates numerous coping strategies and alters that might be created to embody them. Strategies strongly influence the transformations of identity and autobiographic memory that alters will embody. For example, Bad Lois must repudiate knowledge that would demonstrate that Lois is an innocent victim. Louis not only must disregard attributes and experiences that would compel him to acknowledge he is a little girl, but also may need to hallucinate having a male body with appropriate musculature, facial hair, and genitalia.

Alters often experience themselves as having relationships with one another in an inner world that may be experienced as possessing reality and importance that is equally or more compelling than the external world. Inner world events may be reported as if they had occurred in external reality, and vice versa.

Comorbidity

Multiple personalities commonly suffer additional mental disorders. It may be difficult to be sure whether the diagnostic criteria for some of these other disorders are satisfied by symptoms emerging from multiple personality or whether they indicate co-occurring diagnoses that require treatments of their own. Posttraumatic stress disorder, major depression, various substance abuses, borderline personality disorder, other anxiety and affective disorders, somatoform disorders, sexual dysfunctions, eating disorders, and other personality disorders commonly co-occur. Symptoms of another disorder may be found in all or most of the personalities, but sometimes only in particular personalities. Distinguishing between comorbidities and look-alike epiphenomena can prove challenging.

Prognosis may be determined more by the treatability of comorbid conditions than by the multiple personality. For example, a multiple personality with posttraumatic stress disorder and a depression that responds well to medication has a much better prognosis than one with posttraumatic stress disorder, anorexia nervosa, rapid-cycling bipolar disorder, and borderline personality disorder.

Etiology

The predominant theory of the etiology of multiple personality holds that this condition comes into being when a child with high hypnotic potential and problematic support from caretakers and/or attachment issues experiences overwhelming traumatic stress, usually on a repeated basis, and is not protected, comforted, and supported in a way that alleviates the child's distress. The iatrogenesis hypothesis was noted previously. Many scholars consider both alternatives plausible and do not assume that either precludes the possibility of the other.

Data consistent with the predominant theory include the high hypnotizability of this patient group, documentation of abuse in 95% of two cohorts of young dissociative patients, and epidemiological studies in many nations using reliable and valid screening and diagnostic instruments finding a similar incidence of multiple personality (4–6% of psychiatric inpatients) in many nations with very different degrees of awareness of and sympathy toward the diagnosis of multiple personality. If clinicians with special interest in multiple personality act in such a way as to create it, an assumption of the iatrogenesis hypothesis, significantly higher percentages should be encountered in countries in which clinicians are accused of applying such pressures.

Observations consistent with the iatrogenesis hypothesis are the development of transient multiple personality-like phenomena in laboratory settings, reports of the creation of artificial multiple personality by intelligence agencies, and the fact that multiple personality patients have been known to create additional personalities in response to therapists' suggestions. Those most experienced with multiple personality hold that multiple personality cannot be created by therapists under normal clinical circumstances, but that additional personalities can be created in response to perceived pressures from a therapist.

Diagnosis

It was long thought that multiple personality was rare and sufficiently flamboyant to make its presence self-evident. Multiple personality has proven to be far from rare, usually covert, and commonly misdiagnosed for an average of 6.8 years. With the demonstration of widespread false negative diagnoses, diagnostic efforts were accorded greater importance.

The Natural History of Multiple Personality

While a small percentage (6%) of adult multiple personalities are florid and overt most of the time, the vast majority either take pains to avoid drawing attention to their situations and/or have only windows of overtness, usually in the context of psychosocial stress or encountering situations that in some way are analogous to overwhelming childhood events or that force them to contend with an abusive figure from their childhood (or someone who is perceived as similar to such a figure). Usually personalities either are relatively quiescent or exert their influence from behind the scenes by shifting or intruding into or otherwise influencing (by persuasion or threat) the personality in apparent executive control. They may contrive to pass as the usually apparent personality.

Multiple personality usually is clandestine in children and difficult to distinguish from various turmoils and early manifestations of psychotic disorders in adolescents. Young adults often work to avoid detection and deny manifestations of the condition. As individuals mature, they usually enter a complex matrix of work, family, and relationships and are less closely connected with important figures of their childhood. Less immediately pressured to keep childhood issues out of awareness and increasingly experiencing situations that are related to or analogous to childhood experiences (including intercurrent adult trauma), they often become symptomatic and seek treatment for what appears to be anxiety or depression. Treating clinicians may recognize or suspect dissociative phenomena.

Diagnostic Approaches

Considering the usually covert nature of multiple personality, it cannot be assumed that it will declare itself in typical clinical interviews or mental status examinations, or even in therapy sessions. Clinicians have derived lists of suggestive signs of multiple personality. Experience-derived suggestive signs include common findings in multiple personalities' histories and indications of dissociated behavior (i.e., having been given many different diagnoses, being told by others of disremembered out-of-character behavior, finding objects, productions, or writing in one's possession that one cannot recall acquiring or creating). Loewenstein developed a mental status that studies six relevant symptom clusters: (1) indications of multiple personality processes at work (e.g., differences in behavior, linguistic indications, switching/shifting); (2) signs of the patient's high hypnotic potential (e.g., enthrallment, trance logic, out-of-body experiences); (3) amnesia; (4) somatoform symptoms; (5) posttraumatic stress disorder symptoms; and (6) affective symptoms.

Instruments have been developed to screen patients for dissociative phenomena; high scores or particular patterns of response suggest that further evaluation is needed. Structured diagnostic interviews have enabled actual diagnostic assessment. The most well-known of these are the Dissociative Experiences Scale (Bernstein and Putnam) for screening and the Structured Clinical Interview for the Diagnosis of DSM-IV Dissociative Disorders – Revised (Steinberg) for diagnostic purposes.

Differential Diagnosis

The differential diagnosis includes other dissociative disorders, psychotic disorders, affective disorders, borderline personality disorder, partial complex seizures, factitious disorders, and malingering. Evaluators knowledgeable about all of these disorders usually find differential diagnosis to be straightforward. Evaluators unfamiliar with dissociative disorders commonly encounter difficulties because phenomena of many of these conditions overlap.

Treatment

Approaches and Modalities

Treatment resembles a stage-oriented trauma therapy, modified to include work with alters. However, work with some alters and issues may be quite advanced and work with others may be just beginning while still others have not yet been discovered. The treatment may be understood as a series of short-term therapies imbricated within the process of a long-term psychotherapy. Virtually every therapeutic model and modality has been applied to multiple personality. In practice, advocates of different theoretical models and treatment approaches find themselves making many similar interventions. In successful treatments, the pragmatic realities of dealing with multiple personality tend to determine what is done.

Treatment Stages

In the three-stage model of modern trauma therapy outlined by Herman, a phase of safety, in which the patient receives sanctuary and support and is strengthened, is followed by a phase of remembrance and mourning, in which the mind's representation of its traumatic experiences is explored, processed, and mastered and in which the losses and consequences associated with traumatization are grieved. The mind is reintegrated, and roles and functions are resumed in a phase of reconnection.

In the nine-stage treatment of multiple personality (Kluft, 1999a,b) with multiple personality (1) the psychotherapy is established and (2) preliminary interventions are made to establish safety, develop a therapeutic alliance that includes the alters, and enhance the patient's coping capacities. Then follows (3) history gathering and mapping to learn more about the alters, their concerns, and how the system of alters functions. Then is it possible to begin (4) the metabolism of trauma within and across the alters. As the alters share more, work through more, communicate more effectively with one another, and achieve more mutual awareness, identification, and empathy, their conflicts are reduced, as is contemporary amnesia. They increasingly cooperate and experience some reduction of their differences and senses of separateness. This is called (5) moving toward integration/resolution. More solidified stances toward one's self and the world are reached in (6) integration/resolution. Smooth and functional collaboration among the alters, usually including the blending of several personalities, is called a resolution. Blending all alters into a subjective sense of smooth unity is an integration. Then the patient focuses on (7) learning new coping skills, working out alternatives to dissociative functioning, and resolving other previously unaddressed concerns. Issues continue to be processed, and mastery without resort to dysfunctional dissociation is pursued in (8) solidification of gains and working through. Finally, treatment tapers, and the patient is seen at increasingly infrequent intervals in a stage of (9) follow-up.

Typical Issues

Treatment may prove arduous and challenging to patient and therapist alike. Work with traumatic material can be upsetting and destabilizing. Worse than the material itself is the pain of integrating what patients learn into their perceptions of their relationships with significant others who may appear to have been perpetrators of previously unremembered mistreatment. This is complicated by the fact that it is usually not possible to either validate or invalidate most of the traumatic memories that emerge. Patients should be informed about the possibility that material that emerges and may be useful for treatment may not prove to be accurate.

Processing traumatic memories has been controversial because the accuracy of initially unavailable memories has been challenged and the affects experienced in association with this processing may cause upset and trigger self-destructive impulses. Occasionally decompensation occurs. Some multiple personalities cannot tolerate such work. However, thus far, reported successful recoveries to the point of integration have involved processing traumatic memories. Studies have demonstrated that many recovered memories of multiple personality patients have been confirmed, and some have been proven inaccurate. Current opinion suggests that deliberate processing of traumatic memories should not proceed unless patients have demonstrated adequate strength and stability for such work. All others should be treated supportively, addressing traumatic memories only when they are intrusive, are disruptive, and cannot be put aside.

Patients typically have periods of wanting to disavow everything said in therapy, trying to banish painful memories of trauma, betrayal, and loss associated with important people in their lives in order to retain relationships and a sense of safety within those valued relationships. Tact, containment, and circumspection are required from therapist and patient alike. The patient should be protected from becoming overwhelmed by and lost in the traumatic material, and treatment should be paced to safeguard the patient's safety and stability. All pressures to get everything out and over with must be resisted.

The alter system is designed to facilitate escape from pain and difficulty or, failing that, to reframe or disguise it. Alters often reenact scenarios that (in their perceptions) are tried and true methods of keeping pain at bay, even if they disrupt the patient's treatment, life, and relationships. Containing and/or minimizing such events is an ongoing challenge to the treatment, rarely completely successful until therapy is well advanced.

Some have advised against working with alters lest separateness be reified and reinforced by their being addressed directly and individually, and recommend speaking in ways that always convey that the patient is a single person. In practice, working directly with alters often may make them more prominent transiently, but as they are worked with, empathized with, and helped to communicate with other alters, their separateness is eroded. All published series of successful integrations have been contributed by authors who work directly with alters.

The therapist should treat all of the personalities with respect, simultaneously appreciating the immediacy, forcefulness, and defensive aspects of their entrenched and subjectively compelling senses of separateness, and that all express aspects of a single individual, whose personality structure is to have multiple personalities. Interventions to contain alters' dysfunctional behaviors, aggressiveness toward other personalities, self-destructiveness, and irresponsible autonomy (e.g., failing to care for children, who may be seen as belonging to another personality) may prove necessary. The therapist may call upon personalities to work on their particular issues in the treatment and to facilitate their cooperation with the treatment and one another.

Treatment must respect the entirety of the patient's concerns. Specific multiple personality treatment may be deferred repeatedly to address pressing concerns and other mental health issues. For example, a woman with multiple personality whose child develops cancer is not in a position to pursue trauma work.

Patient Subgroups

Some multiple personality patients cannot achieve the goals of the early stages of treatment and move on to process traumatic events and bring personalities together. Those with severe comorbidity and maladaptive character issues may never achieve enough stability to follow that path. Their treatment will involve ongoing efforts to enhance safety and strength and will defer trauma work unless material is intrusive and unavoidable. Therapy prioritizes better coping strategies and enhanced cooperation among alters. An intermediate group will go through phases in which trauma work can be done and phases in which it cannot be tolerated. Therapists should be flexible and err on the side of caution whenever uncertain about the safety of trauma work.

Hypnosis

Multiple personality is associated with high hypnotizability, a stable trait. Hypnosis may occur because a clinician performs an induction procedure, because an individual induces self-hypnosis, or because spontaneous trance is triggered by some stimulus or activity, such as strong emotion or meditation. Therefore, therapists cannot control whether hypnosis occurs in the course of a therapy. Bearing this in mind, therapists should avoid making remarks that might suggest that particular events have taken place or that particular persons were involved in doing harmful things, because they may be heard as powerful hypnotic suggestions.

Notwithstanding such concerns, hypnotic interventions can play a major role in stabilizing multiple personality patients, managing abreactions, containing powerful emotions, accessing alters for therapeutic work, and promoting integration.

Miscellaneous Concerns

Forensic Aspects of Multiple Personality

The relevance of multiple personality as a defense varies tremendously depending upon (1) diverse requirements for the insanity defense in different jurisdictions and (2) the phenomenology in particular multiple personalities. Criminal acts may have taken place because of the impact of multiple personality upon a person's capacity to know his or her own mind and control its various aspects, without thereby satisfying legal definitions of insanity.

The assessment of defendants claiming to have or thought to have multiple personality should proceed with a keen eye toward discerning both factitious and malingered presentations, informed by a state-of-the-art knowledge of multiple personality drawn from the modern clinical literature.

The Impact of Controversy

Controversy magnifies the burden of having, treating, or researching multiple personality. Multiple personality patients must contend with the impact of efforts to deny the reality of their condition and the credibility of what they believe to be their autobiographic memories, attacks on the competence and credibility of those who treat them, and criticism and rejection from those who believe, either accurately or inaccurately, that the multiple personality patient is revealing their secrets or making scandalous accusations against them or those they love in treatment. Therapists treating such patients must contend with ongoing questioning of their efforts, methods, and intentions and accusations that they are encouraging iatrogenesis and confabulated false memories. Researchers have difficulty obtaining funds to expand our knowledge of this condition and may be endangering the trajectory of their careers by working in this area.

Concluding Remarks

Notwithstanding the complexity and difficulty associated with multiple personality, this disorder often proves treatable to a satisfactory outcome and offers unique insights into the impact of overwhelming stressors upon human memory and identity and into the neuropsychophysiology of mental structures and functions. It is moving into the mainstream of the mental health professions and should be of concern to all mental health professionals.

Further Reading

Bernstein, E. and Putnam, F. W. (1986). Development, reliability, and validity of a dissociation scale. *Journal of Nervous and Mental Disease* **174**, 727–734.

Boon, S. and Draijer, N. (1993). *Multiple personality in the Netherlands: a study on reliability and validity of the diagnosis.* Amsterdam: Swets & Zeitlinger.

Coons, P. M. (1980). Multiple personality: diagnostic considerations. *Journal of Clinical Psychiatry* **141**, 330–336.

Kluft, R. P. (1999a). Current issues in dissociative identity disorder. *Journal of Practical Psychiatry and Behavioral Health* **5**, 3–19.

Kluft, R. P. (1999b). An overview of the psychotherapy of dissociative identity disorder. *American Journal of Psychotherapy* **55**, 289–319.

Kluft, R. P. (2005). Diagnosing dissociative identity disorder. *Psychiatric Annals* **35**, 633–643.

Kluft, R. P. and Fine, C. G. (eds.) (1993). *Clinical perspectives on multiple personality disorder.* Washington, D.C.: American Psychiatric Press.

Loewenstein, R. J. (1991). An office mental status examination for complex chronic dissociative symptoms and multiple personality disorder. *Psychiatric Clinics of North America* **14**, 567–604.

Putnam, F. W. (1989). *Diagnosis and treatment of multiple personality disorder.* New York: Guilford.

Putnam, F. W. (1997). *Dissociation in children and adolescents: a developmental perspective.* New York: Guilford.

Ross, C. A. (1997). *Dissociative identity disorder: diagnosis, clinical features, and treatment of multiple personality.* New York: Wiley.

Spiegel, D. (1986). Dissociating damage. *American Journal of Clinical Hypnosis* **29**, 123–131.

Steinberg, M. (1994). *Structured clinical interview for DSM-IV dissociative disorders, revised.* Washington, D.C.: American Psychiatric Press.

Tutkun, H., Sar, V., Yargiuc, I., Ozpulat, T., Yanik, M. and Kiziltan, E. (1998). Frequency of dissociative disorders among psychiatric inpatients in a Turkish university clinic. *American Journal of Psychiatry* **155**, 800–805.

Watkins, H. and Watkins, J. (1993). Ego-state therapy in the treatment of dissociative disorders. In: Kluft, R. P. & Fine, C. G. (eds.) *Clinical perspectives on multiple personality disorder,* pp. 277–299. Washington, D.C.: American Psychiatric Press.

Trans-sexualism

R A Allison
American Medical Association, Phoenix, AZ, USA

Glossary

Assignment The process society follows to designate a person as a male or a female.

Crossdresser A person who wears the clothing of the opposite sex, but does not self-identify as a transsexual.

Female-to-male (FTM) A person born biologically female, whose gender identity is male, who may undergo medical and surgical changes to confirm her male identity.

Gender dysphoria A person's persistent feeling of discomfort with the gender assigned at birth.

Gender identity A person's inner feeling of self-identification as male or female. Gender identity in some people may be intermediate, neither fully male nor fully female. Some people experience changes in their understanding and acceptance of gender identity with the passing of time.

Gender identity disorder (GID) A medical term, used as a synonym for transsexualism. GID is listed in the *Diagnostic and Statistical Manual of Mental Disorders.*

Gender role The category (male, female, or ambiguous) in which society places a person, based on physical characteristics and behavior.

Male-to-female (MTF) A person born biologically male, whose gender identity is female, who may undergo medical and surgical changes to confirm her female identity.

Reassignment Actions taken to change society's designation of a person as a male or a female.

Transgender people Transsexual people, crossdressers, and people of less-fixed gender identity; sometimes used to describe people who live in their desired gender role but do not seek surgical reassignment.

Transition The process a person follows to live in his or her preferred gender; encompasses the physical changes brought about by hormones and surgical procedures, as well as the social changes of experiencing life and relationships in the new gender.

Transsexual A person who experiences persistent and severe discomfort in the gender assigned

	at birth and who wishes to permanently live in the opposite gender role, with all the physical and social changes that role implies.
Transvestite	A crossdresser. This is an older term, used in the mid-twentieth century, and is not currently preferred by most people because it has been associated with a strictly sexual motivation.

Introduction and Definitions

We humans choose certain characteristics by which we define ourselves. The earliest and most essential definition is whether an individual is a man or woman, boy baby or girl baby. The distinction is established at birth, and nurseries are furnished in pink or blue. The basis for the distinction is our external appearance. Our genitalia determine the life we are expected to lead. All humankind is divided distinctly into these two groups: except when it is not.

In fewer than 1/1000 children – the true incidence is still not known – a persistent discomfort exists with the individual's physical sex. This discomfort is present from earliest memory. There is no identifiable behavioral influence to produce it. The child grows and matures unremarkably, to all external appearances; but the child's thought patterns and behavioral instincts are those of the opposite gender.

Such people live their childhood in frustration, knowing something is wrong but being unaware of the specific issue. Finally, due to logical reasoning or reading of someone else's experiences, the child or young adult awakens to the truth. The inner conflict is unrelated to behavior (lifestyle) or preference of sexual partner; rather, it is a conflict involving one's core identity. Medical terms such as gender dysphoria or gender identity disorder (GID) are sometimes used to describe the condition, but it is perhaps best known by the popular name, transsexualism.

Childhood Experiences of Transsexual People

Most adult transsexual people can remember feeling different from their same-sex peers. Before they knew the physical differences between boys and girls, and long before they began to experience feelings of sexual attraction, they knew they belonged in the opposite camp. Such knowledge can be terrifying in an environment where conformity is demanded and diversity is rejected.

Gender-variant behavior in children is not uncommon. Tomboy behavior in girls is usually tolerated better than effeminate behavior in boys. Many boys who play with dolls and other girls' toys grow up to become heterosexual men; some grow up to be gay men; and a few never consider themselves men at all, but they may fear for their safety if other children regard them as sissies. Childhood conformity and peer pressure are the first obstacles transgender people encounter in their journey toward transition.

Factors that Discourage Transition

Even stronger than a child's peer relationships are the bonds of family. Parents, brothers, and sisters are the most influential people in any child's life. In contrast to the previously held views of some mental health professionals, who theorized that transsexualism results from family dysfunction in early childhood, many transsexual people report normal and loving family relationships. Even so, it is rare for a transsexual child to feel comfortable discussing gender feelings with family. Perhaps the child loves his or her parents and fears hurting them with so startling a revelation; or perhaps the fear of punishment creates a determination to hide the truth. Such fears are not without merit – it is true that many parents are ill prepared to deal with such a revelation by a child.

Psychological stress is a natural result of the child's practice of denial, which many continue well into adulthood. Some children are so affected by the stress that their school progress is impaired. Others find temporary escape in retreat into books and studies. Music or other hobbies may serve as a welcome distraction from their worries. Some even practice denial so strongly that they seek the other extreme; for example, a boy may strive to excel at sports or to engage in high-risk behavior, placing himself in physical danger, to deny his feeling of being a girl. Indeed, some teens and young adults enlist in the military services in an effort to cure such feelings.

Even in childhood, religion may play a large role in the stress a transsexual child faces. Most religions teach absolute truths, and do not tolerate departures from those absolutes. The child is taught that his or her feelings are sinful or evil but that they can be overcome through the faith process. Most children are eager to believe such doctrine, hoping that they can be made normal so their parents and peers will accept them. When the religious experience fails to change a child's gender identity, the child is left with feelings of failure and self-doubt. A significant number of transsexual adults report so much despair as children or teenagers that they considered suicide.

The onset of puberty is a very stressful time for transsexual children. Their dreams of becoming normal members of their desired gender are severely challenged as female-to-male (FTM) people develop breasts and menstrual activity and male-to-female (MTF) youth experience growing to tall stature, beard growth, and a deepening voice. These physical changes require years of treatment through surgery, hormones, and electrolysis to correct – if they can be corrected at all.

The ultimate denial of an individuals' transsexualism focuses on their attempt to live a normal life through marriage and parenthood. In years past, transsexual young adults lacked the information and resources available today. Believing themselves doomed to a life of quiet unhappiness, they pinned their last hopes on marriage and family to cure them of their dysphoria. However, within a few years, they realized this too could not cure their sense of identity. Unfortunately, at this point other people have entered their lives in intimate roles, and any ultimate disclosure and transition will be disruptive to the entire family. Because of this, some people make the decision to delay transition until their children are older; this is the reason we see so many people begin transition after age 40. A decision to delay carries its own dangers; a child who reaches puberty before learning of a parent's transsexualism usually will react more negatively than a child who is made aware at a younger age.

The Transition Process

Eventually the transsexual person reaches a point of understanding – this is the way my life is going to be. Denial, family pressure, religious fervor, and even marriage have all failed to change the person's gender identity. The incredible pressure can be relieved only through acceptance and transition. The process of disclosure and beginning transition is sometimes called coming out.

This is perhaps the time of the most intense stress a transsexual person experiences. Every aspect of life is at risk: family, friends, status, job, and finances. The importance of advance planning becomes crucial. People who felt they would be warmly accepted may be devastated by the rejection they experience. Job loss, although not universal, is still very common. Income is gone, at a time when it is needed more than ever. The expenses of transition can be enormous; the psychological counseling alone is more than some people can afford, and the various surgical procedures may cost tens of thousands of dollars and very few are covered by insurance. Efforts to find a new job during transition, in the new gender role, are made more difficult because a lifetime of documentation – birth certificate, Social Security records, passport, diplomas, credit ratings – are all on record under the old name. Furthermore, a person in early transition still has behavior patterns from a lifetime of socialization in the birth gender. Such behavior may be overcome quickly for some people as they find the freedom to behave naturally as a member of their desired gender, but others struggle for years to shed male mannerisms. When added to a physical appearance that still reflects the birth gender, the new mannerisms make it difficult for some to blend into society without attracting unwelcome attention.

For some, the stresses of transition prove too great. As a result of economic demand, family pressure, or the hope of a religious cure, some people abandon transition and return to their original gender role. For most, this return is temporary, and the transition process resumes once they are better prepared to cope with the stress.

Hormonal and Surgical Changes

During and after transition, the effects of cross-gender hormone therapy produce results that often are dramatic. FTM people experience a deepening of the voice and the growth of facial hair. The most obvious early effect of hormones for MTF people is breast enlargement. These effects are obvious to friends, family, and coworkers. At this point, transsexual people may feel a sense of relief because they no longer have to hide their identity or their plan to transition.

Of course, hormones do not produce a complete transformation to the new gender. Other physical differences, including skull and jaw structure, cannot be reversed by hormone treatment. Surgical procedures to eliminate prominent male jaw and chin shape, as well as the exaggerated prominence of the brows, can be of great help in allowing MTF people live normal lives without constant exposure. FTM people often seek mastectomy to make life less stressful.

Ultimately, the transition process culminates in sex reassignment surgery (SRS). In this operation, the surgeon removes some of the old sex organs and creates an appearance as close as possible to the desired gender. Most surgeons who perform SRS follow rather strict guidelines of patient selection to minimize the risk of postoperative regret.

Health Effects of Stress for Transsexual People

A number of physical and psychological effects may result from a transsexual person's decisions related to transition. Many effects occur prior to coming out. The stress of keeping hidden a life-changing truth may be a factor in all types of stress-related illness, including high blood pressure, migraine or other headaches, peptic ulcer disease, and inflammatory bowel disease.

The psychological impact of stress often manifests as chronic anxiety or depression. The degree of psychological distress may be so severe that the person cannot function normally in a work or school environment. Anxiolytic medications, especially benzodiazepines, are often prescribed; even more commonly given are antidepressants. Some degree of depression is extremely common in transsexual people who have experienced rejection or loss.

Suicide, or suicidal gesture, is a continuing concern for many transsexual people. There are three periods when transsexuals are at greatest risk for suicide. The first occurs early in life, when the young person experiences despair from being unlike his or her peers; the stress of keeping such knowledge undisclosed is magnified by the failure of attempts to eliminate the dysphoria. The second period of high suicide risk occurs just prior to the person's acceptance of his or her transsexualism and decision to proceed with transition and is associated with the last attempt to avoid disclosure and to have, to outward appearances, a normal life. As already mentioned, acceptance and transition may relieve this stress and the associated depression.

The third period of high suicide risk occurs after the completion of transition. The person may have high expectations of success in the chosen gender, and some expectations are more likely to be realized than others. Most people find acceptance by society and may continue their careers or begin new ones. Some, however, lose their jobs and are unable to find employment sufficient to pay expenses. Family and friends may continue to reject the transsexual to the point of shunning the person. Perhaps most devastating, the transsexual may be unable to find a life partner whose love and acceptance is unconditional.

The psychological counseling included in a well-planned transition process should address these expectations so that transsexuals can consider how to deal with failure to meet them. Some people, unfortunately, view the counseling process as simply another obstacle to be overcome in order to obtain their desired surgery. The lack of attention to good counseling during transition may increase the likelihood of regret, depression, and even suicide in the years that follow.

Religion and the Transsexual Person

It is accurate to generalize that people whose religious heritage is liberal, or who have no religious affiliation, experience less stress with transition than people who come from a conservative religious background. This generalization can apply to conservative Christianity, and also to Judaism and Islam. Some churches, particularly the Roman Catholic church, have made specific doctrinal statements describing transsexualism as unacceptable. Other Protestant churches may include transsexualism with homosexuality and issue a general condemnation of all gender and sexual diversity.

People who have been raised in such denominations experience a high degree of stress. Their religion tells them it is a sin to change from one gender to the other, and it threatens them with eternal punishment if they disobey. The church maintains that a person can, through faith, turn away from transsexualism and live a normal life. For many, the church is their major support network; the thought of being cast out is unbearable. Yet their life experience tells them otherwise – they have already experienced failure of their faith to bring about this change to normalcy.

These people are forced to choose between two difficult paths. Either they must continue to live in denial, experiencing the stress of secrecy and eventually reaching the point of having to face the truth, or they must face the truth early, risking probable rejection and becoming disillusioned with their faith. Many such people do find their way to more liberal, accepting churches, but others abandon their faith altogether and may become quite hostile to any form of religion.

Violence and Fear

It is not coincidence that transsexual people are more likely to be the victims of violent crime. Several factors explain this increased risk. Young, aggressive males, the group most likely to show violent behavior, have a high incidence of homophobia. If a homophobic male encounters someone who is visibly gender variant, he may feel his own masculinity is threatened; he may even feel the need to prove his manhood by attacking the queer.

In addition, when a person is not initially perceived as transsexual but is discovered to be so later, there may be anger because of the perception of having been deceived. Well-publicized cases of people such as Gwen Araujo and Brandon Teena, both of whom were murdered under these circumstances, illustrate the dangers of antitranssexual violence.

Such is the reality faced by transsexual people in our society. Most people take a healthy approach to such risks by avoiding situations in which the danger is apparent. Others may avoid all social occasions and relationships; their excessive fear of violent reactions prevents their having a normal social life.

Intimacy and the Transsexual Person

Many transsexual people find themselves alone at the beginning of transition. Either they have not been in a relationship or their spouse has refused to be a part of their future plans. These people can benefit from the transition counseling process if they are willing to take the time to explore their future intimacy needs. Such exploration can be stressful in itself, however. People in transition learn that gender identity is independent of sexual orientation. An MTF transsexual person, for example, who was attracted to women prior to transition may ultimately seek intimacy with a man or with a woman. The problem comes when the desired partner has to deal with the reality of the transsexual person's past. A relationship with a man is often jeopardized by the man's feelings of homophobia and inability to get past the idea that his partner is not a real woman. Less likely, but also possible, is the failure of a lesbian relationship due to the female partner's similar feelings. It is possible to find love posttransition, but the increased difficulty of doing so is a great source of stress.

A different dynamic occurs when the spouse of a transsexual person chooses to remain in the relationship posttransition. What was initially a heterosexual relationship now is seen by the world as a homosexual one, with all the associated societal stress such couples encounter. The continued relationship becomes quite a strain on the spouse; for example, the wife of a MTF transsexual soon realizes that she cannot change her sexual orientation to lesbian, just as a gay person cannot decide to become straight. Couples who stay together after transition are the rare exception, and in general the two people involved are very mature and are strong and secure in their commitment to one another despite the stress of daily confrontation.

Aging and Death and the Transsexual Person

The subject of aging has only recently been discussed in depth among transsexual people because the number of people completing transition remained small until the 1980s. Now some people from that era are entering their 60s and 70s, and aging and health issues have begun to assume a prominence in their priorities and present unique stress situations.

Many elderly people count on their children or grandchildren for physical support, to attend to their medical needs, and to take them for doctor visits or hospital emergencies. Transsexual people may lack that support because of family rejection. They face the stress of finding other support among friends, and sometimes a network of elder transsexuals may form for mutual support. The idea of loss of independence is stressful for everyone, but especially so for people who may wear breast binders or hair-replacement systems.

The medical needs of the aging transsexual people are often unique. Physicians called to see a transsexual patient in an emergency may not possess the knowledge or the desire to provide appropriate treatment for these unique needs. It may be difficult to find a doctor willing to continue hormone therapy in an older individual or to screen for diseases associated with the person's birth gender.

A case was reported of an FTM person who developed ovarian cancer. He was rejected for treatment by several physicians, who could not accept a person who presented as a male but had ovaries. The patient eventually died from his disease, which had gone untreated unnecessarily. It is also possible (unlikely, but reported) for an MTF person to develop cancer of the prostate, and it is very rare for such people to submit to the usual screening blood tests.

End of life issues need to be addressed in transsexual people with special concern. It is very important that transsexual people have a partner or sympathetic friend to serve as health-care power of attorney. Likewise, it is important for them to have a will specifying how they wish to be buried or cremated. This will avoid the situation in which family members disregard the individual's stated wishes and bury him or her as the birth gender, even many years posttransition.

Conclusion

Transsexualism, more common than once thought, affects thousands of people who are subject to increased stress due to rejection or confrontation from family, friends, employers, religious institutions, and even total strangers. Coping with these stresses on a daily basis may make the transsexual person mature and strong, or it may be devastating. Understanding and acceptance may reduce the constant stress and enable the transsexual person to make valuable contributions to society.

Further Reading

Boylan, J. F. (2003). *She's not there: a life in two genders.* New York: Broadway Books.

Brown, M. L. and Rounsley, C. A. (1996). *True selves: understanding transsexualism for families, friends, coworkers, and helping professionals.* San Francisco, CA: Jossey-Bass.

Cromwell, J. (1999). *Transmen and FTMs: identities, bodies, genders, and sexualities.* Urbana, IL: University of Illinois Press.

Ettner, R. (1996). *Confessions of a gender defender: a psychologist's reflections on life among the transgendered.* Chicago, IL: Spectrum Press.

Ettner, R. (1999). *Gender loving care: a guide to counseling gender-variant clients.* New York: W. W. Norton.

Green, J. (2004). *Becoming a visible man.* Nashville, TN: Vanderbilt University Press.

Israel, G. E. and Tarver, D. E., II (1997). *Transgender care: recommended guidelines, practical information and personal accounts.* Philadelphia, PA: Temple University Press.

Kaiser Permanente National Diversity Council (2004). *A provider's handbook on culturally competent care: lesbian, gay, bisexual, and transgender population* (2nd edn.). Oakland, CA: Kaiser Permanente National Diversity Council.

Lev, A. I. (2004). *Transgender emergence: therapeutic guidelines for working with gender-variant people and their families.* New York: Haworth Press.

Stryker, S. and Whittle, S. (2006). *The transgender studies reader.* New York: Routledge.

Type A Personality, Type B Personality

W S Shaw
University of Massachusetts, Worcester, MA, USA
J E Dimsdale
University of California, San Diego, CA, USA

This is a revised version of the article by W S Shaw and J E Dimsdale, Encyclopedia of Stress First Edition, volume 3, pp 624–630, © 2000, Elsevier Inc.

Glossary

Free-floating hostility — Behavior characterized by hostile vocal inflection and facial expression, ill temper, cynicism, sleeplessness, irritability, and interpersonal conflict.

Structured interview — An assessment technique involving a series of questions meant to elicit impatience, hostility, and competitiveness among those believed to have type A-defining characteristics.

Time urgency — Behavior characterized by extreme haste, punctuality, time monitoring, and tendencies to engage in polyphasic activities with poor recall of events.

Type A behavior — "An action-emotion complex that can be observed in any person who is aggressively involved in a chronic, incessant struggle to achieve more and more in less and less time, and if required to do so against the opposing efforts of other things and other persons" (Friedman and Rosenman, 1974: 67).

Type B behavior — A relative absence of the behavioral characteristics defined as type A.

Introduction

For centuries, observers have suggested that certain personality patterns are toxic to the heart. Early reports were based on clinical observations and, as is typical in the history of medicine, such reports were either case reports or pronouncements (in lieu of data) by respected authorities. From 1930 to 1950, such reports were typically framed from a psychoanalytic perspective. However, shortly afterward, a new conceptualization emerged. The investigators claimed to have recognized a coronary-prone personality pattern but chose to label it in a value-neutral fashion as type A behavior pattern.

Historical Perspective

Few health-related psychological constructs have received the scientific interest and widespread public recognition of the type A personality classification. Scientific interest in type A and its relation to coronary heart disease began in the 1960s with a research team at the Mount Zion Hospital in San Francisco, California. Meyer Friedman, Ray Rosenman, and colleagues identified a constellation of personality traits that were observed disproportionately among their patients presenting with coronary heart disease (CHD). These traits (labeled type A or coronary-prone) included excessive drive, time urgency, ambition, impatience, aggressiveness, hostility, and competitiveness. When confronted with stressful situations, type A individuals were believed to react with rapid, explosive retorts and increased muscle tension. These behaviors were thought to cause heightened or excessive wear on the cardiovascular system and thereby increase the risk of CHD. The relative absence of these traits defined type B or non-coronary-prone behavior.

Clinical reports suggesting a coronary-prone behavior pattern led to a multitude of epidemiological and experimental studies in the 1970s and 1980s to examine these relationships in the general population and to elucidate biological mechanisms. Assessment techniques were developed, including structured interviews, self-report questionnaires, and behavioral observations. Studies examined the relationship of type A to CHD incidence, angina, myocardial infarction (MI), atherosclerosis, and cardiovascular reactivity. Early epidemiologic studies supported an association between type A and CHD, and this led to a 1981 consensus statement by the Review Panel on Coronary-Prone Behavior and Coronary Heart Disease (organized by the National Heart, Lung, and Blood Institute) listing type A as a viable risk factor for heart disease.

Despite the early support for type A, a proliferation of research in the 1980s failed to replicate earlier findings, and several related psychological constructs (hostility, anger, and aggression) emerged as stronger predictors of CHD. As a result, interest in type A has waned in recent years. By the late 1980s, two meta-analyses concluded that the accumulated empirical studies were inconsistent and that prospective evidence linking type A to CHD was weak. Since that time, behavioral CHD research has emphasized hostility and other related constructs over the global type A characterization. However, originators of the type A concept continue to defend its role as a CHD risk factor, blaming poor assessment techniques and a substantial drift from its original conceptualization for the discrepant research findings.

As late as the 1990s, interest in the health implications of type A behavior continued, albeit in a more limited scope. Meyer Friedman and his colleagues at the University of California, San Francisco, continued to refine clinical assessment techniques and develop interventions for reducing type A behavior. Others sought to examine type A behavior with respect to other psychosomatic health problems. Today, there is declining research interest in type A as a behavioral health risk. **Figure 1** illustrates the rapid rise and fall of this construct as a title word in psychological research publications over the past 40 years. Nevertheless, type A has served as an important catalyst for the explosion of scientific and public interest in behavioral factors associated with health, especially cardiovascular disease.

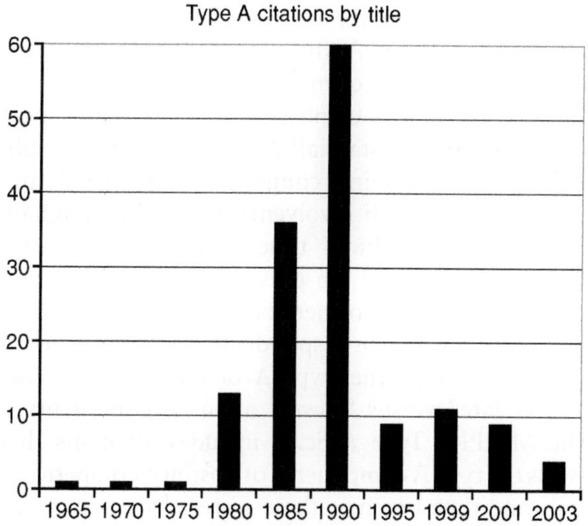

Figure 1 Type A journal title citations.

Conceptualization and Assessment

Considerable conceptual confusion has surrounded the type A construct. Type A behavior has been variously described as a medical disorder, an inappropriate coping mechanism, a strong need for productivity, or a pattern of physiological reactivity. Although most research has presumed type A behavior constitutes an enduring personality trait, other studies have attributed type A behavior to specific cognitions that can be modified through therapeutic interventions. Much of the accumulated discrepancy in results between studies of type A may be attributable to poor agreement in construct definition and assessment.

Type A behavior was first assessed through clinical ratings applied to structured interviews or videotaped structured interviews, and these interview techniques have been further updated and expanded by Meyer Friedman and colleagues. The current technique combines both observations and subjective reporting of patients using eliciting remarks. The interview consists of multiple queries that are designed to elicit manifestation of time urgency and free-floating hostility that emerge for type A, but not for type B, individuals. Questions include "Do you mind very much waiting in grocery checkout, bank, or theater lines or waiting to be seated in a restaurant?" (time urgency) and "Do you often find it difficult to fall asleep or to continue to sleep because you are upset about something a person has done?" (hostility). Scoring is based on both endorsements of items and the presence of psychomotor signs. For time urgency, signs include aspects of facial tension, posture, speech, breathing, and perspiration. For free-floating hostility, these include facial expression, eyelid movement, vocal orientation, and hand clenching. For each item, scores are clinical ratings varying in assigned weights and ranges. Total scores range from 0 to 480, and a total score greater than 45 indicates the presence of type A traits.

As an alternative to the interview technique, self-report measures of type A were developed to simplify data collection for use in large-scale epidemiological studies of CHD. One of the earliest and most frequently used questionnaires is the Jenkins Activity Scale (JAS). Other pen-and-paper measures of type A behavior include the Framingham Type A Scale, the Bortner Scale, the MMPI-2 Type A Scale, the Gough

Adjective Checklist, the Thurstone Activity Checklist, the Coronary Prone Attitudes Scale, and the Ketterer Stress Symptoms Frequency Checklist.

The content and emphasis of type A self-report measures vary substantially. The JAS includes subscales of hard-driving competitiveness, speed and impatience, and job involvement. The Framingham Type A Scale includes time urgency, competitive drive, and perceived job pressures, but does not include hostility. The Bortner scale contains 14 adjective pairs between which respondents mark the level of agreement with either type A or type B traits (e.g., "Never late" versus "Casual about appointments"). The MMPI-2 Type A Scale includes 19 items that assess the type A components of hostility, competitiveness, and time urgency; these were selected from the total pool of MMPI-2 questions by expert consensus and verified using empirical tests of item-to-type A group classification. The Ketterer Scale compares self-ratings of type A characteristics with parallel ratings of a friend or family member.

The reliability of the various interview and self-report measures is quite good. For example, interrater correspondence for discriminating type A and B individuals using the videotaped structured interview has ranged from 75 to 90%. For the MMPI-2 Type A Scale, test–retest reliability is high ($r = 0.82$), and internal consistency is moderately high ($\alpha = 0.72$), at least for male respondents. Other self-report measures of type A show similar levels of reliability. Prevalence estimates of type A behavior have varied from 50 to 75% depending on the populations studied and assessment techniques employed.

The validity of self-report measures of type A were originally documented by comparing scores between type A and type B individuals already categorized using the gold-standard interview technique. Although both interview and self-report assessment techniques have good reliability, the two approaches are only modestly interrelated. For example, the JAS showed a 73% agreement with the type A interviews in a cross-validation sample of 419 men participating in the Western Collaborative Group Study. Similarly, the Bortner scale was shown to explain only 53% of the variability in type A clinical interview ratings. This has led to considerable debate as to whether self-report questionnaires of type A are a valid means of describing the same constellation of features identified by the structured interview. Studies using self-report measures have generally provided less association with cardiovascular health outcomes than have interview techniques. As a result, self-report measures of type A have been criticized for relying on the insight of respondents, restricting the range of type A traits, and being influenced by the social undesirability of many items. Because self-report measures do not involve a live interaction with the individual, these scales may not accurately assess the action–emotion complex described by the creators of the interview technique.

Empirical Support

Data on the association between type A and CHD have been inconsistent. Three early large-scale epidemiological studies supported an association between type A and CHD incidence: the Western Collaborative Group in 1975, the Framingham Heart Study in 1980, and the French-Belgian Cooperative Study Group in 1982. All three investigations found that type A individuals had a significantly increased risk of CHD in individuals followed closely for 5–8 years. In the Western Collaborative Group study, 3200 employed men with no heart disease were followed for 8 years. Type A individuals (by structured interview) were found to have a 2.2 relative risk of CHD relative to type B individuals. The Framingham Heart Study, which included a more representative sampling of both men and women, showed relative risk ratios for white-collar men of 2.9 for total CHD, 7.3 for MI, and 1.8 for angina without MI; however, risks were substantially less for women and for blue-collar men. The French-Belgian Cooperative Heart Study followed 2811 male civil servants and factory workers for an average of 5 years. The relative risk ratio for type A men was 1.8 for total CHD. The latter two studies used self-report measures of type A.

Other subsequent epidemiological studies showed little or no relationship. For example, in the Normative Aging Study, correlations of the JAS type A score with CHD risk were not statistically significant. In a 40-year follow-up of 280 men from the 1947 Cardiovascular Disease Project at the University of Minnesota, no statistically significant association was found between the MMPI Type A Scale and CHD. In a large-scale 7-year prospective study (Multiple Risk Factor Intervention Trial, MRFIT), there was no association between type A and risk of coronary events, and this applied to both interview and self-report methods of type A classification. The type A–CHD relation has been much smaller in prospective versus cross-sectional studies, in meta-analyses synthesizing results from multiple studies, and among more diverse groups. Although many plausible explanations have been offered for differences among study results, meta-analyses and other attempts to synthesize results across studies have failed to provide consistent support for type A as a unique and valid predictor of CHD.

The generalizability of initial research linking type A to CHD has also been criticized because early studies were limited to middle-aged, working, White American males. Among more diverse populations, associations between type A and CHD have been weaker or nonexistent. Studies of both type A and hostility in Japan, for example, have shown little association with CHD. Instead, a type C behavior pattern, characterized by a job-centered lifestyle and social dominance at work, was predictive of CHD in working Japanese men. The type A construct may not apply for women due to the greater social unacceptability of type A traits for women.

Intervening biological mechanisms to explain the type A–CHD association have focused primarily on the hyperreactivity of the cardiovascular and neuroendocrine systems; however, results have been inconsistent. Quantitative reviews have suggested some heightened reactivity in systolic blood pressure response and catecholamine response, but results vary by gender, type A-assessment technique, and the nature of laboratory stressors. Ambulatory blood pressure studies have also indicated some relationship between type A and cardiovascular reactivity. Type A scores have been related to the actual extent of coronary artery atherosclerosis, as judged from cardiac catheterization. Here again, initial studies were positive, but subsequent studies failed to reveal such links.

Other studies have included type A as a potential mediator of health behavior. For example, type A individuals underestimate their degree of physical exertion in response to exercise. They also work longer and at greater intensity when given a self-selected work-pace task. This may explain some of the relationships between type A and cardiovascular health outcomes such as recurrent MI or unexplained cases of sudden death.

Despite the huge accumulated literature on type A, hostility, and CHD, interventions targeting type A behavior are rare. One exception is a 14-month type A counseling approach developed at Mount Zion Hospital purportedly to change belief systems, engage in exercises to modify a sense of time urgency or free-floating hostility, and increase perceptions of personal security. This intervention has been reported to reduce the frequency of silent myocardial ischemia; however, the studies have been performed on small nonrepresentative samples of post-MI coronary patients. It is not known which therapeutic techniques included in this broad-based intervention were most effective.

Component Factors

Because the interview assessment of type A included a number of signs and symptoms, researchers became interested in the specific component factors that might contribute to CHD risk and whether type A was unique in this respect compared with other personality variables. These investigations ultimately led to a shift in the focus of CHD behavioral studies away from the type A global constellation of symptoms. When the total score and subscale scores of the JAS were contrasted, the hard-driving competitiveness factor was more strongly associated with cardiovascular disease than was speed and impatience, job involvement, or the overall type A score. Other studies showed support for hostility as the key underlying component. For example, of 12 behavioral characteristics extracted from the structured interview, a reanalysis of the Western Collaborative Group Study data showed that the hostility component alone accounted for all of the variance explained by type A.

In their 1987 meta-analysis, Booth-Kewley and Friedman identified 18 overlapping personality variables from various assessment measures for the purposes of comparing relative strengths of association. These included global type A scores; subscale measures of speed and impatience, job involvement, hard-driving competitiveness, and time urgency; and non-type A measures of anger, hostility, aggression, depression, extraversion, and anxiety. These analyses showed that depression was more strongly associated with CHD than was type A, and CHD correlations with hostility, aggression, and extraversion were of a similar magnitude to type A. This meta-analysis and subsequent studies ultimately led to the conclusion that only the type A components related to anger, hostility, and aggression were responsible for increased CHD risk. In particular, hostility, which had long been suspected as a risk factor for CHD, was found to explain nearly all the shared variance between type A and CHD.

Today, the expanding interest in hostility as a predictor of CHD has eclipsed the original global type A as a potential risk factor. However, conceptual and assessment controversies continue as various components of hostility are hypothesized to underlie associations with CHD. Cynical hostility, as measured by the Cook–Medley scale of the MMPI, was shown to predict a fivefold increase in CHD risk in a 25-year follow-up of 255 medical students. Suppressed anger was associated with a twofold increase in mortality among 696 Michigan residents followed over 12 years. Studies linking hostility to CHD have shown associations with angiographically documented CHD. However, their cross-sectional nature precludes definitive conclusions regarding cause and effect. Prospective studies with 5- to 25-year follow-ups have shown associations between hostility and later CHD development, but similar associations exist with all-cause mortality. Therefore, the specificity of hostility with regard to CHD remains unclear.

Beyond Coronary Heart Disease

Although the focus of type A research has been primarily on CHD, hypertension, and related cardiovascular health outcomes, several studies have examined the impacts of type A behaviors in the context of entirely different medical conditions. These have included chronic fatigue syndrome, irritable bowel syndrome, and other health problems thought to involve psychological risk factors. These studies have generated no consistent pattern of findings that implicate type A as a central causal factor, although it periodically emerges as a significant predictor of various health outcomes. The most common explanation for this finding is that type A behavior may play a mediating role in health behaviors (exercise, diet, smoking, etc.).

Despite the popular use of the type A label to describe the overachieving efforts of co-workers and family members, there have been relatively few studies of the interpersonal and occupational consequences of type A behavior. In cross-sectional studies, type A overlaps with other measures of personality and temperament (e.g., narcissism, optimism, and aggression), yet type A has not emerged as an independent mental health risk factor. In relation to perceptions of stress and satisfaction at work and home, the impacts of type A behavior have been inconsistent. Based on the available evidence, the type A constellation of personality traits is an uncertain predictor of social and emotional well-being.

Conclusion

Any fair-minded observer would be immediately impressed by the numerous links between behavior and coronary disease. The impact of various risk-enhancing and risk-reducing behaviors is unchallenged. Similarly, the impact of unusual life stressors in provoking a deterioration in already-existing CHD is reasonably established. It is less clear that a habitual personality or behavior pattern leads to the development of CHD. Ambiguities in recognizing that personality and defining its central features have plagued this area. Nonetheless, data do suggest some links between type A behavior and CHD. Current work focuses less on type A itself than on the quest for its toxic core, its mechanism of action, and the possibilities of intervention.

Further Reading

Booth-Kewley, S. and Friedman, H. (1987). Psychological predictors of heart disease: a quantitative review. *Psychological Bulletin* **101**, 343–362.

Dimsdale, J. (1988). A perspective on type A behavior and coronary disease. *New England Journal of Medicine* **318**, 110–112.

Friedman, M. and Ghandour, G. (1993). Medical diagnosis of type A behavior. *American Heart Journal* **126**, 607–618.

Friedman, M. and Powell, L. H. (1984). The diagnosis and quantitative assessment of type A behavior: introduction and description of the videotaped structured interview. *Integrated Psychiatry* **2**, 123–129.

Friedman, M. and Rosenman, R. (1974). *Type A behavior and your heart.* New York: Knopf.

Gallacher, J. E. J., Sweetnam, P. M., Yarnell, J. W. G., et al. (2003). Is type A behavior really a trigger for coronary heart disease events? *Psychosomatic Medicine* **65**, 339–346.

Grunbaum, J., Vernon, S. W. and Clasen, C. M. (1997). The association between anger and hostility and risk factors for coronary heart disease in children and adolescents: a review. *Annals of Behavioral Medicine* **19**, 179–189.

Harbin, T. J. (1989). The relationship between the type A behavior pattern and physiological responsivity: a quantitative review. *Psychophysiology* **26**, 110–119.

Haynes, S. G., Feinleib, M. and Kannel, W. B. (1980). The relationship of psychosocial factors to coronary heart disease in the Framingham Study. III: Eight-year incidence of coronary heart disease. *American Journal of Epidemiology* **111**, 37–58.

King, K. B. (1997). Psychologic and social aspects of cardiovascular disease. *Annals of Behavioral Medicine* **19**, 264–270.

Matthews, K. and Hanes, S. (1986). The type A behavior patterns and coronary disease risk: update and critical evaluation. *Journal of Epidemiology* **123**, 923–960.

Melamed, S., Harari, G. and Green, M. S. (1993). Type A behavior, tension, and ambulatory cardiovascular reactivity in workers exposed to noise stress. *Psychosomatic Medicine* **55**, 185–192.

Review Panel on Coronary-Prone Behavior and Coronary Heart Disease (1981). Coronary prone behavior and coronary heart disease: a critical review. *Circulation* **63**, 1199–1215.

Thoreson, C. E. and Powell, L. H. (1992). Type A behavior pattern: new perspectives on theory, assessment, and intervention. *Journal of Consulting & Clinical Psychology* **60**, 595–604.

B. Anxiety and Fear

Anxiety

A Öhman
Karolinska Institutet, Stockholm, Sweden

This is a revised version of the article by A Öhman, Encyclopedia of Stress First Edition, volume 1, pp 226–230, © 2000, Elsevier Inc.

Glossary

Anxiety — Apprehensive anticipation of uncertain, often ill-defined dangers.

Fear — Emotional state associated with attempts to cope with threatening events.

Panic attack — A sudden surge of anxiety associated with physiological symptoms (e.g., heart-rate increases) and catastrophic feelings (e.g., fear of dying) that come suddenly and seemingly unprovoked.

State anxiety — The level of anxiety at a defined point in time.

Trait anxiety — An individual's habitual level of anxiety.

Anxiety is an aversive emotional state associated with the apprehensive anticipation of more or less likely future dangers. It incorporates the somatic symptoms of tension and dysphoric feelings.

Anxiety and Fear

Anxiety is closely related to fear (see **Fear**). The traditional distinction has been that anxiety, in contrast to fear, lacks an obvious eliciting stimulus. According to the definitions given here, anxiety and fear occupy different temporal locations in relation to threatening events, anxiety typically being anticipatory to, and fear elicited by, threatening stimuli. Furthermore, whereas the threat in anxiety often is imagined, in fear it is typically real. These differences promote different phenomenologies in the two states, with anxiety dominated by an unpleasant feeling of foreboding and fear by an urge to escape. However, the perhaps most fruitful distinction can be derived from the controllability of the threat. Fear is predicated on the hope that the situation can be coped with, that it is controllable. Fear, therefore, is a source of motivation because it supports active attempts to deal with the threat by, for example, escape or avoidance. Anxiety, on the other hand, results when the coping attempt fails, that is, when the situation is perceived as uncertain or uncontrollable. With few or inefficient means to cope with the threat, the option that is left is the apprehensive anticipation of the more or less likely expected disaster.

This analysis gives anxiety and fear a joint origin in an evolved defense system that has served through eons of time to protect organisms from survival threats. The primary emotional counterpart is fear, which supports adaptive coping with threat. However, depending on restrictions in the controllability of the situation, there is a dynamic interplay between the closely related emotional qualities of fear and anxiety. Because fear is the prototype reflected in anxiety, the two emotional states have many similarities, for example., in terms of components (aversive feelings, physiological responses, and behavior; see **Fear**). Thus, the two states may often be hard to distinguish, but this is due to the fact that they are fused in the real world rather than to conceptual obscurity.

Placing anxiety and fear at different regions of a controllability dimension has the added virtue of relating both these states to another related concept dominated by dysphoric feelings – depression. Thus, whereas fear is the emotional concomitant in situations of somewhat controllable threat, anxiety takes over when the uncontrollability of the situation undermines active coping attempts. With further and more lasting uncontrollability, coping becomes fruitless, which makes the organism helpless and replaces anxiety with depression. Thus, the conceptual view advanced here is compatible with the emerging notion of negative affect as a pervasive higher order factor behind both anxiety and mood disorders.

Different Types of Anxiety

Situational versus Free-Floating Anxiety

There are several more or less interdependent bases for distinguishing between different types of anxiety. The controllability analysis puts anxiety on a continuum between fear and depression. There are other related continua that are often invoked in this context. One is that of situational versus free-floating (generalized) anxiety. Situational anxiety is bound to a particular stimulus, such as the stimulus in phobic anxiety. Whether anxiety of this type should be called anxiety or fear depends on the controllability of the fear stimuli in the situation. In situationally unfocused or free-floating anxiety, the intensity of the anxiety does not vary with the situation, but is always present at a noticeable level.

Panic Attacks versus Generalized Anxiety

Free-floating (generalized) anxiety is correlated with worries (e.g., about finances or academic performance). It is often contrasted with panic attacks, which have been claimed to represent a distinct subtype of anxiety. A panic attack is a sudden surge of often overwhelming anxiety dominated by physical symptoms such as shortness of breath, dizziness, palpitations, trembling, sweating, nausea, hot flashes, and chest pain. It may also involve feelings of depersonalization and fears of dying or going crazy. A panic attack may appear to be spontaneous, coming out of the blue, or to be situationally provoked. For example, a social phobic may experience panic when forced to face a threatening social context.

Some people have occasional panic attacks with no or only little residual anxiety between the attacks. However, because a panic attack is such an overwhelmingly aversive experience, the person may start to develop anticipatory anxiety about further attacks. As a result, occasional attacks will now appear against a fluctuating background of anticipatory anxiety, and the distinction between panic and generalized anxiety will become somewhat blurred.

Factor Analytically Derived Varieties of Anxiety

Factor-analytic work on observed and self-reported anxiety symptoms in normals and patients confirms clinical observations in delineating two clusters of anxiety. Thus, there is one cluster of somatic overreactivity composed of symptoms such as sweating, flushing, shallow breathing, and reports of heart palpitations, intestinal discomforts, and aches and pains. The other cluster may be called cognitive or psychic anxiety and is composed of intrusive and unwanted thoughts, worrying, ruminations, restlessness, and feelings of muscle tension.

Trait versus State Anxiety

The distinction between panic and generalized (free-floating) anxiety is related to another important distinction. A particular person may suffer from habitually elevated anxiety, never feeling completely free of apprehension and worry. This habitually elevated anxiety is called trait anxiety. Nevertheless, the level of anxiety may still vary somewhat across time and situations. The momentary level of anxiety at a particular time (e.g., during a panic attack), on the other hand, is called state anxiety. Even though people with high trait anxiety tend also to have high state anxiety in most situations, there may be situations in which the state anxiety of low-trait-anxious people is still higher because of stressful circumstances.

Clinical versus Normal Anxiety

Anxiety is both a phenomenon of everyday life and an important sign of psychopathology. Thus, there is a need to distinguish between normal and clinical anxiety. In general, clinical anxiety is more intense, recurrent, and persistent than normal anxiety. Furthermore, whereas normal anxiety is proportional to the real danger of the situation, the intensity of clinical anxiety is clearly above what is reasonable, given the objective danger involved, tending to paralyze individuals and undermine their coping efforts. Consequently, it results in impeded psychosocial or physiological functioning, which may promote contact with treatment facilities.

Anxiety and Cognition

To be anxious implies a preoccupation with threat and danger. For example, people with high anxiety tend specifically to overestimate the likelihood that they will experience negative events, but they do not differ from people with low anxiety in judging the likelihood that they will experience positive events. Anxiety and cognition, in fact, are intimately related to one another in a two-way communication in which anxiety determines cognition and cognition determines anxiety.

Attentional Bias for Threat

The immobility exhibited by animals that freeze in the face of danger is associated with hypervigilance to the environment. Similarly, there is a large research literature documenting that anxiety is associated with hypervigilance and an attentional bias for threat. For example, when simultaneously exposed to two visual stimuli, one threatening and the other nonthreatening, anxiety patients tend systematically to attend to the threatening stimulus, as revealed by their shortened reaction times to probe stimuli occurring at the location of the threatening stimulus. Low-anxiety people, on the other hand, tend to shy away from threat; their reaction times are faster for probe stimuli at the location of nonthreatening stimuli. This general finding is valid regardless of the threat conveyed by the pictorial (e.g., angry faces) or word (e.g., cancer) stimuli. Similarly, if people high or low in anxiety are asked to name the color in which words are printed (the Stroop paradigm), the color-naming latency is longer for threatening than for nonthreatening words in anxious (but not in nonanxious) people. This implies that high-anxiety people are distracted by attention to the threatening word content.

The attentional bias for threatening stimuli in highly anxious research participants does not require conscious recognition of the stimuli. Several studies have shown that similar results are obtained when the threatening stimuli are presented masked by other stimuli, thus precluding their conscious recognition. For example, using the Stroop color word paradigm, longer color-naming latencies to threatening words are observed in highly anxious people, even if the word is shown only for 20 ms and immediately masked by illegible letter fragments of the same color. This finding implies that the attentional bias operates at an automatic, preattentive level of information processing. Thus, outside the conscious awareness of individuals, this attentional bias determines that they preferentially attend to threatening events in their surroundings. This preference for focusing attention on threat no doubt helps maintain the anxiety.

Expectancy and Interpretational Bias

Attentional bias provides a case in which anxiety drives cognition. However, it is also abundantly clear that cognition drives anxiety. This is particularly well documented for panic. A compelling argument can be advanced to the effect that catastrophic interpretations provide a necessary condition for the elicitation of panic. According to the dominating model, stress or anxiety results in an autonomic arousal that is perceived by the person. The perception of this bodily change prompts more anxiety and further autonomic arousal in a vicious circle. But it is only when the interpretation of the bodily symptoms becomes catastrophic (e.g., when the person feels that they signal serious illness or imminent death) that the full-blown panic attack emerges.

Several lines of evidence support this model. For example, when panic attacks are pharmacologically promoted in panic patients (e.g., through lactate infusion or CO_2 inhalation), panic is unlikely if patients are informed about the expected effects of the manipulation. If they are not informed, or misinformed, on the other hand, panic patients (but not social phobics) are likely to experience panic. Similarly, if panic patients inhaling CO_2 are led to believe that they can manipulate the CO_2 saturation in the inhaled air by pressing a panic button, this induced sense of illusory control protects them from panic attacks and decreases their self-rated anxiety. Conversely, if panic patients are led to believe through false physiological feedback that their heart is racing, they become more anxious and show more psychophysiological arousal than control subjects.

Anxiety Disorders

Disorders of anxiety are common in the population, afflicting about one-quarter of adult individuals. One group of the anxiety disorders, phobias, is more closely related to fear than to anxiety (see **Fear**).

Panic Disorder

Recurrent panic attacks have a key position in the diagnosis of anxiety disorders, and they are what the diagnostician first looks for. Panic disorder is a condition characterized by recurring and crippling panic, typically associated with distressing worries about future panic attacks. As a result, the normal social life of the individual is compromised. Typically panic disorder occur in the context of agoraphobia (see **Fear**), in which the person starts to avoid situations in which he or she will be left helpless and vulnerable in the event of a panic attack.

Generalized Anxiety Disorder

If the anxiety is manifested as uncontrollable and excessive anxiety and worry about events or activities (e.g., finances or school performance), generalized anxiety disorder may be diagnosed. Patients with this disorder worry more or less constantly and their worries are less controllable and more self-driven and ruminative than normal worries. Typically the worry is combined with somatic symptoms or other anxiety symptoms such as restlessness, fatigue, irritability, muscle tension, and concentration and sleep difficulties.

Posttraumatic Stress Disorder

Posttraumatic stress disorder has its origin in intense traumas, that is, in situations whose danger and aversiveness are outside the range of usual human experience, such as in natural disasters, war, violent crime, or severe accidents. In this disorder, the traumatic event is persistently reexperienced (e.g., in the form of flashbacks), stimuli or events associated with the trauma elicit intense anxiety and are avoided, and the person feels generally numbed with regard to emotions. Common anxiety symptoms experienced by people suffering from posttraumatic stress disorder include difficulties sleeping and concentrating, irritability or outbursts of anger, hypervigilance, and exaggerated startle.

Obsessive-Compulsive Disorder

Obsessions are persistent thoughts, impulses, or images; compulsions are repetitive behaviors such as hand washing and checking or mental activities such as praying or silently repeating words. The essential features of obsessive-compulsive disorder are recurrent, uncontrollable obsessions or compulsions that are performed with the ostensible purpose of reducing anxiety. The obsessions and compulsions are associated with marked distress, and they interfere with the normal routines, even though the victim, at least at some point, has recognized that they are excessive or unreasonable.

The Genetics of Anxiety Disorders

Statistical modeling based on comorbidity data in twins suggests that there are two independent genetic factors involved in the anxiety disorders. The anxious-misery factor is related to panic disorder, agoraphobia, posttraumatic stress disorder, generalized anxiety disorder, and depression, whereas the fear factor predisposes for specific phobias. The model suggests only a limited role for shared (within-family) environmental factors, but it suggests a substantial role for unique environmental factors (i.e., factors affecting one family member but not others) for all disorders. This genetic difference between the disorders may explain why those related to the anxious-misery factor all respond to the same medication (selective serotonin-uptake inhibitors), which is ineffective in specific phobias. It may also be reflected in psychophysiological data showing a distinct fear response in specific phobics who are exposed to their fear object or situation but normal psychophysiological resting levels. The disorders relating to the anxious-misery factors, on the other hand, show elevated resting levels and little psychophysiological mobilization during stress.

The Neuroanatomy of Anxiety

From the perspective taken here, in which anxiety is seen as a sibling of fear, it is a natural assumption that their neural substrate shows considerable overlap. A neural network for fear activation is centered on the amygdala (see **Fear**). It is an attractive notion that this circuit is sensitized and hyperreactive in anxiety states. Furthermore, there are data suggesting that a brain area closely related to the amygdala, the bed nucleus of the stria terminalis, has a downstream connection, similar to that of the amygdala, to hyhpothalamic and brain-stem nuclei controlling different components of fear and anxiety, such as autonomic responses and fear behavior. However, whereas the amygdala mediates short-term fear responses to specific stimuli, the bed nucleus of the stria terminalis is more dependent on long-term contextual stimuli for its activation. This effect appears to be mediated by an abundance of receptors for the corticotropin releasing hormone (CRH) in the bed nucleus of the stria terminalis, which mediates the activation of the hypothalamic-pituitary-adrenal axis. Thus, this opens the possibility of separable but closely related anatomical loci for fear and anxiety. Fear may be primarily dependent on the effects of specific stimuli on the amygdala, and anxiety may be primarily dependent on the effect of contextual stimuli and CRH in the bed nucleus of the stria terminalis.

See Also the Following Articles

Fear.

Further Reading

American Psychiatric Association. (1994). *Diagnostic and statistical manual of mental disorders* (4th edn.). Washington, DC: American Psychiatric Association.

Barlow, D. H. (2002). *Anxiety and its disorders: the nature and treatment of anxiety and panic* (2nd edn.). New York: Guilford Press.

Hettema, J. M., Prescott, C. A., Myers, J. M., et al. (2005). The structure of genetic and environmental risk factors for anxiety disorders in men and women. Archives of General Psychiatry **62**, 182–189.

LeDoux, J. E. (1996). *The emotional brain.* New York: Simon & Schuster.

Mineka, S. and Zinbarg, R. (1996). Conditioning and ethological models of anxiety disorder: stress-in-dynamic-context anxiety models. In: Hope, D. A. (ed.) *Nebraska symposium of motivation. Vol. 43: Perspectives on anxiety, panic, and fear*, pp. 135–210. Lincoln, NE: University of Nebraska Press.

Mogg, K. and Bradley, B. P. (1998). A cognitive-motivational analysis of anxiety. *Behaviour Research and Therapy* **36**, 809–848.

Öhman, A. (2000). Fear and anxiety: evolutionary, cognitive, and clinical perspectives. In: Lewis, M. & Haviland, J. M. (eds.) *Handbook of emotions* (2nd edn., pp. 573–593). New York: Guilford.

Walker, D. L., Toufexis, D. J. and Davis, M. (2003). Role of the bed nucleus of the stria terminalis versus the amygdala in fear, stress, and anxiety. *European Journal of Pharmacology* **463**, 199–216.

Fear

A Öhman
Karolinska Institutet, Stockholm, Sweden

This is a revised version of the article by A Öhman, Encyclopedia of Stress First Edition, volume 2, pp 111–115, © 2000, Elsevier Inc.

Glossary

Agoraphobia	An intense fear and avoidance of situations in which one would be helplessly exposed in case of a panic attack.
Amygdala	A collection of interconnected nuclei in the anterior medial temporal lobe, which is the hub of the brain network controlling the activation of fear responses.
Autonomic nervous system	A part of the peripheral nervous system concerned with the metabolic housekeeping of organisms. In general, the activation of its sympathetic branch results in the expenditure of energy and the activation of the parasympathetic branch results in the restoration of energy.
Fear	The emotional state associated with attempts to cope with threatening events.
Social phobia	An intense fear and avoidance of being socially evaluated or scrutinized.
Specific phobia	An intense fear and avoidance of specific objects or situations.

Fear is an activated, aversive emotional state that serves to motivate attempts to cope with events that provide threats to the survival or well-being of organisms. The coping attempts are typically centered on defensive behaviors such as immobility (freezing), escape, and attack.

Components of Fear

A fear response comprises several partially independent components, such as subjective feelings (accessible through verbal reports), peripheral physiological responses, and overt behavior. In humans, the phenomenological quality of fear is best described as an aversive urge to get out of the situation. This is a familiar feeling for every human being and a frequent target for artistic representation.

Fear is closely associated with the activation of the autonomic nervous system. Depending on situational constraints, the direction of this activation may differ. If the threat is not imminent and appears stationary, the typical response is one of freezing or immobility. This is associated with enhanced attentiveness toward the environment and the potential threat stimulus and with a vagally mediated deceleration of the heart. If the threat is imminent or approaching, there is a pervasive mobilization of the sympathetic branch of the autonomic nervous system, including heart rate acceleration and increases in blood pressure and circulating catecholamines (primarily epinephrine) from the adrenal medulla. These responses lay a metabolic foundation for taxing overt reactions of flight or fight.

In terms of behavior, there is an important distinction between expressive and instrumental overt acts. Expressive behavior includes automatic tendencies to withdraw from the threat and a typical facial expression of fear. The latter is composed of elevated eyebrows, wide open eyes, and a mouth that is either slightly opened or shut with depressed mouth corners. Instrumental behavior primarily concerns escape from and avoidance of the fear stimulus.

Measures of Fear

Measures of fear can be readily derived from the various components of fear. The intensity of the subjective component of fear can be directly assessed through ratings that may be anchored, for example, at a zero level of no fear at all, with a maximal level of fear corresponding to the most intense fear ever experienced by the subject.

Many fear indices have been derived from effectors innervated by the autonomic nervous system. Some of these measures, such as heart rate deceleration and skin conductance responses, are primarily related to the increased attentiveness associated with the initial stages of fear. Other measures, such as increases in heart rate or blood pressure, reflect the sympathetic mobilization that supports active coping attempts. Endocrine indices are available from the adrenal medulla and the adrenal cortical hormones. Measures among the former, such as circulating epinephrine, are often assumed to index successful coping, whereas measures from the latter, such as cortisol, are regarded as related to failing coping attempts.

Many behavioral measures have been used to assess fear. Typically they focus on avoidance behavior. For example, in a standard behavioral avoidance test to assess specific human fears, subjects are encouraged to approach their feared object as close as they dare, and the minimal achieved distance (touching included) is taken as inversely related to avoidance. In animals, the strength of escape behavior or the duration of freezing responses can be measured, depending on the experimental situation. In rodents, who typically freeze when fearful, the effect of a fear stimulus can be assessed by its interfering effect on a regular background behavior, such as operant lever pressing for food rewards on a variable interval schedule.

On the premise that defensive reflexes are primed by an induced fear state, the modulation of such reflexes by fear stimuli can provide accurate information about fear both in animals and humans. Typically, the startle reflex is studied using whole-body startle in rodents and the eyeblink component of startle in humans. The typical result is an enhancement of the startle reflex to a standard startle probe stimulus (e.g., a white noise with abrupt onset) when it is presented against a background of a fear stimulus compared to when the probe is presented alone.

It is important to realize that different measures of fear are not necessarily highly intercorrelated, even when assessing the effects of a common fear stimulus. This is because the fear response is better conceptualized as a loosely coupled ensemble of partially independent response components, sensitive to various modulating parameters, than as a unitary internal state mechanically elicited by the appropriate fear stimulus.

Fear Stimuli

There are innumerable events and situations that are feared by humans. Loosely speaking, they have in common that they provide a threat to the integrity of the individual, either in a physical or in a psychological sense. Many of the stimuli that are feared by humans are feared by other mammals as well. They include, for instance, loud noises, predators, and dominating conspecifics.

Classification of Fear Stimuli

In general, behaviors can be classified as communicative or noncommunicative depending on whether they elicit an active response from the environment. Communicative behavior is directed toward other living creatures, whereas noncommunicative behavior is directed toward the physical environment. Communicative behavior can be further subdivided into behavior directed toward members of another species, such as in predator–prey relationships, and members of the own species in what is commonly regarded as social behavior. Applied to fear, this classification system distinguishes among fear of physical stimuli, fear of animals, and social fears.

Physical stimuli Humans and other animals fear many types of physical stimuli, particularly those that may inflict tissue damage, thus inducing pain. A primary stimulus dimension is that of intensity. Highly intense stimuli of any modality may induce pain, and certainly they elicit fear and associated attempts to escape in most animals. Complex events that incorporate high-intensity stimulation, such as lightning and thunder, often evoke intense fright. But there are other complex events or situations whose fear-eliciting power is less directly dependent on simple stimulus dimensions. The effectiveness of such situations can be understood only in relation to the recurrent threat they have provided throughout evolution. Examples that come to mind include heights, small enclosures, wide-open spaces, and darkness or light (for species primarily active in daylight or at night, respectively).

Animal stimuli Species typically share ecological niches, and thus the presence of other animals has been a shaping force in evolution. Species compete for similar food supplies, and in predation, one species provides the food supply for another. In this latter case, avoiding capture as prey is a prerequisite for reproduction; therefore, potential prey species fear their predators. There is also a widespread fear of potentially poisonous animals, such as snakes, spiders, and insects, and these fears may be better represented as fear of (and disgust for) contamination rather than as fear of the animal itself.

Social stimuli No animal is more dangerous to humans than other humans; the most dangerous predators are humans who are ready to use violence to exploit the resources of other humans. Conflicts with fellow humans, however, are not restricted to fights about tangible resources. Typically they deal with something more abstract, but also more pervasive – power. Like other primates, human groups are structured in terms of dominance, that is, some members dominate others. Fear is part of the submissiveness shown by the dominated group members when confronting a dominant conspecific. This fear is not automatically connected to escape or (least of all) to attack, but it is shown in a readiness to emit signals of submissiveness and in refraining from competition. In humans (and other primates), it denotes a fear of being negatively evaluated, of losing face in front of the group, rather than of physical harm.

Moderating Factors

Several general dimensions modify the fear elicited by these types of fear stimuli. One of them is closeness. In general, the closer the fear stimulus, the stronger the fear response. This may, in fact, provide an explanation for the effect of stimulus intensity on fear – an intense stimulus is likely to be very close. Prey animals (e.g., gazelles) show a minimal reactive distance before they overtly take notice of a predator (e.g., a lion). If the predator is far away or appears to be resting, it is monitored only by increased attention. If it gets closer or appears to be hunting, the attention enhancement is accompanied by defenses such as immobility. When the predator gets dangerously close, finally, there is active defense such as flight.

A second moderating factor is movement of the stimulus and the direction of the movement. Approaching objects, in general, elicit more fear than stationary objects or objects moving away. For example, more fear is generated by a fearsome authority figure who is heading in our direction than by one who is heading in another direction.

A third class of moderating factors involves predictability and/or controllability of the fear stimulus. An abruptly occurring stimulus is, by definition, not predicted and elicits immediate fear. Fear stimuli that are predictable may also be behaviorally controlled, for example, through avoidance. Less predictable or controllable stimuli elicit more fear. However, it is only reasonable to talk about increasing fear as long as the uncontrollability does not completely undermine the coping attempts. When the situation is too uncontrollable to support active attempts to cope, fear is replaced by anxiety, and when the organism eventually gives up and becomes helpless, anxiety is replaced by depression (see **Anxiety**).

Fear Learning

Events such as obstructed breathing, physical constraints, and rapidly approaching large objects can be regarded as innate fear stimuli and may be called natural fear triggers. However, even though evolution has equipped us with defenses for a number of events that have threatened our survival in the long past of our species, modern humans, for good reason, fear many stimuli that simply were not around during our evolution. Thus, these stimuli must have acquired their fear-eliciting power through learning. They may be called learned fear triggers.

Pavlovian conditioning is the central mechanism for associative fear learning. Through Pavlovian conditioning, a natural fear trigger may transfer its potential to a new, previously neutral stimulus, thus turning it into a learned trigger. The procedure for achieving this is simply to present the two stimuli together, so that the to-be-learned trigger serves as a signal for the natural trigger. This is direct Pavlovian conditioning, but the procedure also works in a social arrangement in which one individual sees another individual express intense fear of the to-be-learned trigger. In this way, fear may transfer to new stimuli and circumstances, and, particularly for a species that has access to language, with its associative structure, this means that fear may come to be elicited from large classes of new stimuli only remotely associated with the original natural trigger.

An interesting possibility is that fear is more easily transferred to some stimuli that by themselves do not elicit fear, even though throughout evolution they have occurred in threat-related contexts. However, because of this long historic association with threats to survival, they may be evolutionarily prepared to enter easily into association with fear after only minimal aversive experience. For example, even though rhesus monkeys do not show an innate fear of snakes, they easily learn such fear after seeing conspecifics in fearful interactions with snake-related stimuli. Similar easy fear learning to neutral stimuli such as flowers is not obvious.

Pathological Fear: Phobias

Fear may sometimes be excessive to the extent that it interferes with normal adaptive functioning. Intense, involuntary, and rationally unfounded fear of a specific object or situation that provokes maladaptive avoidance is called a phobia. Phobias are classified into three categories depending on the feared object or situation.

Specific Phobias

Specific phobias concern circumscribed objects or situations, such as knives, other sharp objects, and dental treatments. One subgroup of specific phobias involves nature fears, such as fears of water or thunderstorms. Another important category centers on fear of animals; snakes, spiders, dogs, cats, and birds are typical examples. A third category involves fear of blood, taking injections, and mutilated bodies. Contrary to other anxiety disorders, which often incorporate a fear of fainting, this type of phobia is the only one actually associated with fainting as a result of a pronounced vasovagal response to exposure to the phobic situation.

Social phobias Some people tremble at the mere thought of meeting new people or having to formally address a group. In general, they fear social situations that involve being scrutinized or evaluated by others and the associated risk of being socially humiliated. Social phobia is more debilitating than specific phobia because social situations are central to human adjustment. For example, consistently avoiding such situations or enduring them only with intense dread may be detrimental both to academic and vocational careers.

Agoraphobia Agoraphobia (from the Greek *agora*, which means marketplace) denotes an intense fear of being out among people in crowded places such as in supermarkets or on public transportation vehicles. However, the fear is less concerned with this particular situation than with an intense fright of being overwhelmed by fear or anxiety in a situation in which no help or assistance is available; the common denominator is that the person would be left helpless without any escape route back to safety in the event of a sudden fear attack. Safety typically is defined as being at home, and thus many agoraphobics become captives in their homes, only able to leave if accompanied by a trusted companion.

Preparedness and Phobias

It is reasonable to assume that phobias derive primarily from learned fear triggers. Even though phobias are fairly common in the population, the overwhelming majority does not show a phobia-level fear of, say, snakes, knives, blood, underground trains, or airplanes. Thus, the assumption that phobics somehow have associated fear to the phobic situation is readily invoked. If this were the case, we would expect a correlation between common ecological traumas and phobias. However, there is an obvious discrepancy between the distribution of phobic situations and the distribution of traumas in our environment. For example, many people have aversive experiences with broken electrical equipment, but there are few bread-toaster phobics needing clinical assistance. On the other hand, clinicians encounter many spider and bird phobics, even in environments completely lacking poisonous spiders or threatening birds. This discrepancy between traumas and phobias can be accounted for by the preparedness hypothesis because phobic objects and situations appear more obviously related to threats in an evolutionary than in a contemporary perspective. In fact, most phobic situations (animals, heights, enclosures, dominant conspecifics, lack of escape routes, etc.) have provided recurrent threats to humans and our predecessors throughout evolution. As a result, humans may have become biologically predisposed easily to associate such situations with fear even after only minimal trauma. Nonprepared situations, such as cars, on the other hand, may not come to elicit fear even after having been paired with excessive traumas.

The Neurophysiology of Fear

Research during the last 2 decades has delineated a neural network in the brain that controls fear responses and fear learning. This network is centered on the amygdala, a small set of nuclei in the anterior temporal lobe that has long been identified as a limbic structure associated with emotion.

A primary role for the amygdala appears to be the evaluation of input to the brain in terms of its potential threat. This purpose is achieved by the lateral nucleus, which receives fully processed sensory information from the cortex as well as only preliminarily processed information from subcortical structures such as the thalamus. These two routes to the amygdala have been described as the high and the low routes, respectively. Because the low route depends on monosynaptic linkage between the thalamus and the amygdala, the incompletely processed information conveyed by this route reaches the amygdala faster than the polysynaptically wired information conveyed by the high route. As a consequence, the amygdala can start recruiting defense responses even before the veridicality of the threat stimulus is confirmed by the full cortical analysis.

The high route, therefore, is not necessary for eliciting fear, but the low route may be necessary both for fear elicitation and fear learning. Fear may be elicited and learned in animals even after the ablation of the relevant sensory cortices, and in humans, fear responses can be elicited and learned via stimuli that are prevented from conscious recognition through backward masking. Thus, fear responses are recruited after a quick and nonconscious analysis of the stimulus, which explains the automatic, nonvoluntary character of intense fear, such as in phobias.

After threat evaluation in the lateral and basolateral nuclei of the amygdala, the information is conveyed to the central nucleus, which controls various efferent aspects of the fear response. Neural pathways to the lateral hypothalamus activate sympathetically controlled responses, such as heart-rate acceleration and skin conductance responses, and parasympathetically dominated responses, such heart-rate decelerations, are influenced through the vagal motor nucleus and the nucleus ambiguus of the brain stem, which also can be controlled from the amygdala. Through connections between the central nucleus and the paraventricular nucleus in the hypothalamus, corticotropin releasing hormone can be released, which, via adrenocorticotropic hormone from the anterior pituitary, activates corticosteroid stress hormones from the adrenal cortex. Paths to the tegmentum, including the locus coeruleus, activate the dopaminergic, noradrenergic, and cholinergic arousal systems of the forebrain, resulting in electroencephalogram (EEG) activation and increased vigilance. Overt motor responses associated with fear such as freezing, fight, and flight are activated by connections between the central nucleus of the amygdala and the dorsal and ventral periaqueductal gray of the brain stem. The facial expressions of fear are activated through the facial motor nucleus and the seventh cranial nerve, the nervus facialis. The modulation of the startle reflex, finally, is accomplished through neurons connecting the central nucleus of the amygdala with the central nexus for the startle reflex, the nucleus reticularis pontis caudalis in the brain stem. This circuit accounts both for peculiarities of fear activation such as its independence of conscious recognition of the fear stimulus and the complex efferent organization of the fear response. Furthermore, its sensitization through various procedures may contribute to the understanding of pathological fear and anxiety.

See Also the Following Articles

Anxiety; Fear and the Amygdala.

Further Reading

Davis, M. and Whalen, P. J. (2001). The amygdala: vigilance and emotion. *Molecular Psychiatry* **6**, 13–34.
Lang, P. J., Bradley, M. M. and Cuthbert, B. N. (1997). Motivated attention: affect, activation, and action. In: Lang, P. J., Simons, R. F. & Balaban, M. T. (eds.) *Attention and orienting: sensory and motivational processes*, pp. 97–135. Mahwah, NJ: Lawrence Erlbaum.
LeDoux, J. E. (1996). *The emotional brain.* New York: Simon & Schuster.
Öhman, A. and Mineka, S. (2001). Fears, phobias, and preparedness: toward and evolved module of fear and fear learning. *Psychological Review* **108**, 483–522.
Rosen, J. B. and Schulkin, J. (1998). From normal fear to pathological anxiety. *Psychological Review* **105**, 325–350.

Fear and the Amygdala

R Norbury
Warneford Hospital and University of Oxford, Oxford, UK
G M Goodwin
University of Oxford, Oxford, UK

Glossary

Amygdala	A complex brain structure with numerous subnuclei located deep within the temporal lobe of the brain.
Backward masking paradigm	A paradigm in which an initial emotional face (e.g., fear) is presented for a very short duration (17–33 ms) and then immediately replaced by a neutral face presented for a longer duration (~200 ms). In this situation, the initial image is subliminal; subjects report that they have seen only the neutral expression.
Excitatory postsynaptic potential (EPSP)	A depolarization of the postsynaptic membrane.
Fear	An unpleasant, powerful emotion caused by anticipation or awareness of potential or actual danger.
Fear conditioning	A form of emotional learning in which an emotionally neutral or conditioned stimulus acquires the ability to elicit behavioral and physiological responses associated with fear after being associated with an aversive unconditioned stimulus.
Long-term potentiation (LTP)	The long-lasting strengthening of the connection between two neurons.
Neuroimaging	A number of powerful noninvasive techniques, including positron emission tomography (PET) and functional magnetic resonance imaging (fMRI), that allow the examination of regional patterns of brain activation in the living human brain with considerable spatial resolution, but limited temporal resolution, in the order of seconds as determined by vascular responses associated with neural activity.
Startle response	An innate reflex observed in nearly all animals, including humans, that manifests as an involuntary motor response to any unexpected noise, touch, or sight. In studies of emotion, it has been used to measure the aversiveness of emotive stimuli.

Amygdala Anatomy

The amygdala is an almond-shaped structure located deep within the temporal lobe of higher animals. It was first identified by Burdach in the early nineteenth century, who described a group of cells, or nuclei, now referred to as the basolateral complex. Subsequently, however, the amygdala was shown to be both more complex and more extended, comprising more than twelve subnuclei. In rats, current nomenclature divides the amygdala nuclei into three main groups: (1) the basolateral complex, which includes the lateral nucleus, the basal nucleus, and accessory basal nucleus; (2) the cortical nucleus, which includes the cortical nuclei and the lateral olfactory tract; and (3) the centromedial nucleus, comprising the medial and central nuclei.

Afferent and Efferent Connections

The amygdala receives input from all sensory systems: olfactory, somatosensory, gustatory, visceral, auditory, and visual. Olfactory inputs arise at the olfactory bulb and project to the lateral olfactory tract. Somatosensory inputs pass via the parietal insular cortex in the parietal lobe and via thalamic nuclei to the lateral, basal, and central nuclei. Primary gustatory and visceral sensory areas project to the basal nucleus and central nucleus. In contrast, auditory and visual information, thought to be important in fear conditioning, arise from association areas rather than from the primary sensory cortex.

The amygdala has widespread efferent connections to cortical, hypothalamic, and brain-stem regions. The basolateral complex projects to the medial temporal lobe memory system (e.g., the hippocampus and perirhinal cortex), and the basal nucleus has a major projection to prefrontal cortex, nucleus accumbens, and the thalamus. Thus, the anatomy of the amygdala is consistent with its role in fear processing. The amygdaloid complex receives inputs from all sensory modalities and activates brain regions important to measurable neurobehavioral correlates of fear. How it works offers an insight into the nature of emotion in humans and animals.

The Amygdala and Fear Conditioning in Animals

Much of the scientific interest in the amygdala stems from its established role in fear conditioning, research that has been carried out mostly in rats. Classical Pavlovian fear conditioning is a type of emotional learning in which an emotionally neutral conditioned stimulus (CS), often a tone, is presented in conjunction with an aversive unconditioned stimulus (US), typically a small electric shock to the foot of the animal. After one or more pairings, the emotionally neutral stimulus (CS) is able to elicit a constellation of species-specific conditioned responses (CRs) that are characteristic of fear, such as freezing or escape behavior, autonomic responses (elevated heart rate and blood pressure), potentiated acoustic startle to aversive acoustic stimuli, and increased neuroendocrine responses (release of stress hormones). Fear conditioning therefore allows new or learned threats to activate ways of responding to threat that have been long established in evolution.

Numerous studies have demonstrated that lesions to the amygdala impair the acquisition and expression of conditioned fear in rats. The basolateral complex of the amygdala is a substrate for sensory convergence from both the cortical and subcortical areas, and it is considered a putative locus for CS–US association during fear conditioning. Thus, its cells encode this emotional learning. By contrast, the central nucleus of the amygdala projects to brain regions implicated in the generation of fear responses, such as the hypothalamus; it may therefore act as a common output pathway for the generation of fear-conditioned responses. Consistent with this hypothesis, lesions to either the basolateral or central nucleus of the amygdala impair the both the acquisition and expression of conditioned fear.

The amygdala pathways involved in fear conditioning have also been studied using electrophysiological studies (see **Figure 1**). During fear conditioning, the convergence of CS and US inputs to the basolateral complex results in sustained enhancement, or long-term potentiation, of EPSPs evoked by the CS (**Figure 1**). Thus, the amygdala is able to both integrate and associate sensory information and influence the motor and physiological responses associated with fear conditioning.

The Amygdala and Fear in Humans

Evidence from Lesion Studies

Damage to the amygdala, or areas of the temporal lobe that include the amygdala, also produces deficits in fear processing in humans. In a recent study, a patient with Urbach–Wiethe disease (S.M.), a rare congenital lipoid storage disease that results in the bilateral degeneration of the amygdala, underwent fear conditioning with either visual or auditory CSs and a loud noise as the US. Compared to normal control subjects, S.M. showed no evidence of fear conditioning (as measured by galvanic skin response). Notably, S.M.'s recall of events associated with fear conditioning was intact. These data support the hypothesis that the amygdaloid complex plays a key role in the acquisition of Pavlovian fear conditioning, whereas the hippocampus is important in acquiring declarative knowledge of the conditioning contingencies. In a further study with the same patient, it was demonstrated that bilateral amygdala damage impaired the recognition of fearful facial expressions. Other patients with Urbach–Wiethe disease have also been shown to be impaired in

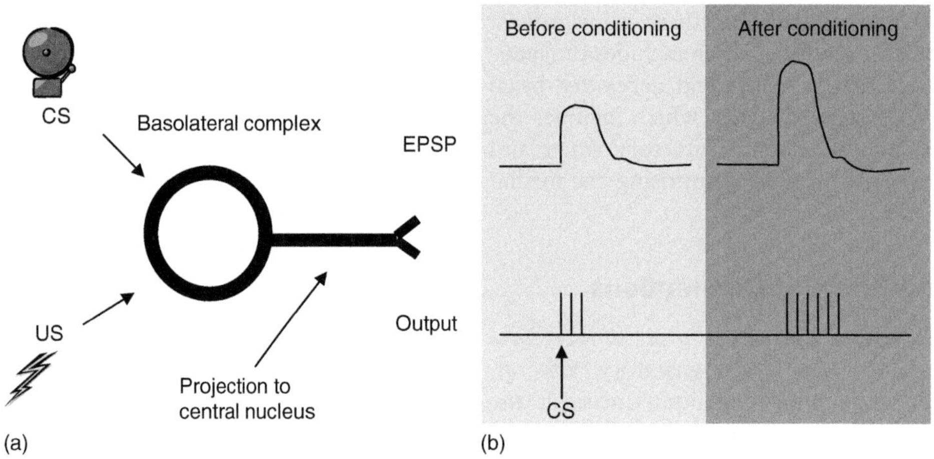

Figure 1 During fear conditioning convergence of inputs (CS and US) induce long-term potentiation of EPSPs evoked by the CS. a, Schematic; b, graphs. CS, conditioned stimulus; EPSPs, excitatory postsynaptic potentials; US, unconditioned stimulus.

recognizing fearful facial expressions. S.M., however, had no difficulty in recognizing people by their faces or in learning the identity of new faces. These results suggest that the human amygdala is directly involved in the processing of emotion but not in recognizing aspects of facial appearance. There is also evidence to suggest that the impairment of the perception of expressive signs of fear in patients with amygdala damage extends beyond facial expressions; bilateral amygdala damage has also been associated with impairment in the recognition of vocalic expressions of threat.

The effect of amygdala damage on the startle response has also been studied in humans. A recent study compared the startle response in a 32-year-old male with a localized legion in the right amygdala with that of eight age-matched controls. The control subjects displayed the well-documented effect of aversive stimuli potentiating startle magnitude. In the patient with the right-amygdala lesion, no startle potentiation was observed in response to aversive versus neutral stimuli. Together, studies of patients with amygdala damage suggest that this structure plays a key role in the perception and production of negative emotions, particularly fear.

Evidence from Neuroimaging Studies

During the early 1990s, researchers began to explore the role of the amygdala in fear processing using neuroimaging (e.g., positron emission tomography, PET; and functional magnetic resonance imaging, fMRI) and continue to do so today. So far, amygdala activity has been assessed predominantly using two basic paradigms: fear conditioning and presentation of emotional facial expressions.

Functional MRI experiments have demonstrated increased amygdala activity during both the early acquisition and early extinction of fear conditioning to a visual stimulus. Indeed, it has been suggested that the amygdala's role is limited to early conditioning or early extinction, when response contingencies change. That is, the amygdala is particularly important for forming new associations as relationships – emotional learning and unlearning.

The amygdala may also be responsible for generating coordinated reflexive behavioral responses to highly aversive stimuli. The animal literature shows that the amygdala, specifically the central nucleus, generates conditioned autonomic, behavioral, and endocrine responses in acute stress paradigms. CSs, which may be interpreted as changing the animal's emotional set, increase the response in startle paradigms, for example. Clearly, this kind of response may be quite primitive, but lesioning experiments demonstrated definite mediation by the amygdala. It is usually assumed the amygdala may be involved in the selection of more purposive motor-behavioral responses in response to more subtle aversive conditions.

The second major neuroimaging protocol for assaying amygdala activity is the presentation of faces expressing different emotions. It is difficult to overemphasize the importance of facial expressions in social communication. Facial expressions act at a number of levels to signal important information; expressions of disgust enable the avoidance of the ingestion of harmful substances, and fearful facial expressions rapidly communicate the presence of imminent threat. More subtly, cues from the faces of others are continuously informing us of our social impact and acceptability, and we, in turn, communicate our feelings and intentions through our own facial gestures and expressions.

It is no surprise, therefore, that facial expressions have provided a useful experimental tool to measure fear-related amygdala activity. Many studies have demonstrated that the amygdala is preferentially activated during the presentation of fearful facial expressions. Moreover, even when subjects are unaware of seeing a fearful face, by the use of a masking protocol or when attention is directed away from the fearful face, the amygdala is still activated. Such findings suggest that the extraction of potentially threatening information within the amygdala may not be sufficient for conscious face perception but it may well be necessary. The amygdala may act to direct attention toward emotionally salient events that are ambiguous or require further processing. Indeed, anatomical studies in rats suggest that sensory information travels to the amygdala via two distinct pathways: a short, rapid thalamic route, and a longer cortical pathway. It is proposed that the short thalamic pathway rapidly prepares the animal for a potentially aversive encounter independent of conscious processing, which occurs later via the slower cortical route. A similar two-way route to the amygdala has yet to be anatomically defined in humans; however, evidence from a number of well-designed fMRI experiments point to the existence of these two pathways (**Figure 2**). First, as already described, the amygdala responds to fearful faces even when presented outside conscious awareness. Second, in an extension of the masking paradigm, Whalen and colleagues presented degraded versions of fearful and happy expressions by displaying only the eye whites immediately masked by a complete image of a neutral expression. Fearful faces are typically associated with the enlarged exposure of the sclera, and it was observed that the crude information provided by the wide eyes of fearful expressions was sufficient to stimulate the amygdala. Analogously, Vuilleumier and coworkers used fMRI to compare amygdala and cortical responses to rapidly presented (200 ms) fearful and neutral faces that had been filtered to extract either low-spatial-frequency information (giving a blurry image) or high-spatial-frequency information (giving a finely detailed, sharp image) (**Figure 3**). As detected by fMRI, the finely detailed images elicited a greater response in a region of the cortex called the fusiform face area, a brain region widely implicated in the conscious recognition of faces and facial expressions. The amygdala was relatively unresponsive to these images even if they were fearful in nature. Low-spatial-frequency fearful faces, however, produced a robust response in the amygdala. Although these findings could imply the existence of a two-pathway route to the amygdala in humans, with dissociation between neural responses in amygdala and fusiform gyrus across different spatial frequency ranges for face stimuli, they do not prove it. However, they suggest that the amygdala does not require very complex configural stimuli, such as presented by the complete image of a face, in order to respond to emotion. It is obviously possible that crude fragmentary information related to emotionally salient signals could be rapidly communicated via a subcortical route. Extreme facial expressions of emotion may be well adapted to attract immediate attention via this mechanism.

Given the involvement of the amygdala in fear processing, there is increased interest in the role of this structure in anxiety disorders, such as post-traumatic stress disorder (PTSD), and obsessive-compulsive disorder (OCD), and in depression. For example, patients with PTSD show increased blood

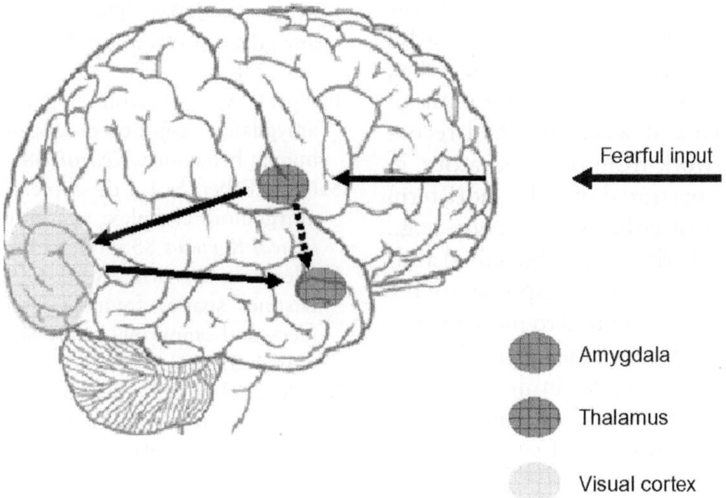

Figure 2 Two-pathway hypothesis for amygdala activation to fear. The short, rapid thalamic route is shown by the dashed arrow; the longer cortical pathway is shown by bold arrows. (For clarity, subcortical structures are shown overlaid on brain surface.)

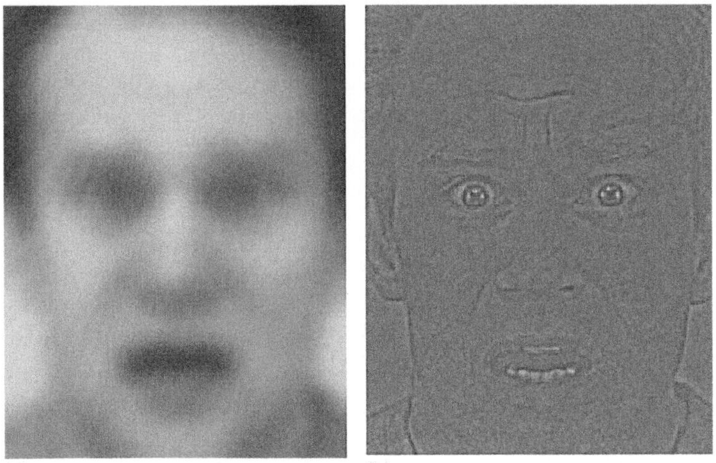

Figure 3 Processing of images by the amygdala and cortical regions. a, Low-frequency image; b, finely detailed image. The rapid subcortical pathway may allow low-frequency inputs to reach the amygdala rapidly, whereas finely detailed images are further processed in cortical regions (e.g., fusiform gyrus).

flow in the right amygdala (as measured by PET) in response to the presentation of images designed to activate traumatic memories, compared to neutral images. Using fMRI, it has also been demonstrated that individuals with OCD have significantly increased activity bilaterally in the amygdala in response to ideographically tailored stimuli designed to provoke their symptoms.

Functional MRI can also be used to investigate how pharmacological treatment for anxiety and depression modulates amygdala activity. A number of studies have demonstrated that the increased amygdala response to negative facial expressions seen in depression is reduced following effective treatment with serotonergic antidepressants. Although these results suggest an important role for the amygdala in the recovery from depression, it remains unclear if this normalization of amygdala response to fearful faces with time is a direct action of the drug or, rather, a reflection of the current symptom state (the scans of patients when depressed and when they had recovered were compared). Work from our laboratory, in healthy volunteers, demonstrated that the short-term administration (7 days) of either serotonergic (e.g., citalopram) or norepinepherine (e.g., reboxetine) antidepressants reduces the amygdala response to the masked expressions of fear compared to placebo controls. Significantly, these effects on the amygdala were observed in the absence of changes in mood. These results suggest that antidepressants have rapid, direct effects on the amygdala. Moreover, if similar effects are seen in clinical populations, drug modulation of amygdala activity in response to negative stimuli may be a key component in patients' recovery from depression and anxiety.

See Also the Following Articles

Anxiety; Fear; Posttraumatic Stress Disorder, Delayed; Posttraumatic Stress Disorder – Clinical; Posttraumatic Stress Disorder – Neurobiological basis for.

Further Reading

Harmer, C. J., Mackay, C. E., Reid, C. B., et al. (2006). Antidepressant drug treatment modifies the neural processing of nonconscious threat cues. *Biological Psychiatry* **59**, 816–820.

Ledoux, J. (2003). The emotional brain, fear, and the amygdala. *Cellular and Molecular Neurobiology* **23**, 727–738.

Phelps, E. A. and LeDoux, J. E. (2005). Contributions of the amygdala to emotion processing: from animal models to human behaviour. *Neuron* **48**, 175–187.

Sah, P., Faber, S. L., de Armentia, L., et al. (2003). The amygdaloid complex: anatomy and physiology. *Physiological Reviews* **83**, 803–834.

Vuilleumier, P., Armony, J. L., Driver, J., et al. (2003). Distinct spatial frequency sensitivities for processing faces and emotional expressions. *Nature Neuroscience* **6**, 624–631.

Whalen, P. J., Kagen, J., Cook, R. G., et al. (2004). Human amygdala responsivity to masked fearful eye whites. *Science* **306**(5704), 2061.

Defensive Behaviors

D C Blanchard, M Yang, M Hebert and R J Blanchard
University of Hawaii, Honolulu, HI, USA

This is a revised version of the article by D C Blanchard, M Hebert and R J Blanchard, Encyclopedia of Stress First Edition, volume 1, pp 652–656, © 2000, Elsevier Inc.

Glossary

Chronic mild stress (CMS) A pattern of anhedonia involving reduced positive response toward normally rewarding items, such as a sweetened liquid or intracranial stimulation in reward sites, following intermittent exposure to a variety of mildly stressing stimuli or events. These behavioral outcomes, like those of both learned helplessness and subordination, have been shown to be responsive to antidepressant drugs.

Defensive behavior An array of evolved behavioral responses (e.g., flight or freezing) to threat stimuli such as predators or attacking conspecifics. Individual defensive behaviors are modulated by features of both the threat stimulus and the situation in which they are encountered. Many defensive behaviors are relatively consistent across mammalian species and may be a component of stress- or defense-related psychopathologies.

Defensive threat/attack Display of weapons (e.g., teeth and claws) and strength (e.g., through loud vocalization) in response to close contact by an attacker, followed by bites or blows to particularly vulnerable sites on the attacker's body (typically, face and eyes).

Dominance/subordination A pattern of relationships between a consistent winner (dominant) and a consistent loser (subordinate) in agonistic encounters. Both dominant and subordinate often show behavioral and physiological signs of stress, but these may be modulated by compensatory mechanisms in the dominant that are not available to the subordinate. Subordination has been used as a model of chronic social stress.

Learned helplessness (LH) A pattern of reduced learning, particularly in active avoidance situations and of reduced activity in a threat context, following exposure to uncontrollable aversive events. This, like the chronic mild stress paradigm, has been proposed as a model of depression.

Offensive attack An attack, typically (but not always) toward conspecifics, in the context of a dispute over important resources such as territory, access to mates, or food. An offensive attack is aimed toward species-typical sites on the opponent, often areas in which bites or blows do little serious damage. In contrast to defensive threat/attack, fear reduces offensive attack.

Risk assessment A pattern of orientation, attention, and exploration with regard to potential threat stimuli, enabling an animal to gather information about their location, identity, and threat status. This information facilitates an optimally adaptive response to a genuine threat or promotes a return to nondefensive behavior if no threat is present.

Defensive behaviors are those activities that occur in response to the host of life-threatening dangers encountered in every natural environment, from predators, from conspecific attack, and from threatening features of the environment. They constitute the behavioral component of the stress response and have evolved on the basis that, to particular types of threat stimuli and in particular situations, each such behavior has proved to be optimally adaptive in terms of enhancing the extended reproductive success of the individual. These behaviors range from active investigation of threat stimuli to actions facilitating escape from or termination of threat. Because the extended reproductive success of females may, in an important way reflect the survival of offspring in their care, the optimal defensive behaviors for males and females may differ: The magnitude and mechanisms of gender difference in defense are poorly understood, but there is speculation that these may be related to the substantial and consistent differences in vulnerability to particular psychiatric disorders for men and women.

Defensive Behaviors and the Stimuli That Elicit Them

Much recent work on defensive behaviors has focused on response to predators or attacking conspecifics, threat stimuli (especially the former) that elicit a number of defensive behaviors in rodents without the necessity of pain or prior experience. Although the defensive behaviors of higher primates are undoubtedly more complex than those of rodents and may involve some specific learning components, there appears to be an essential continuity of defense patterns across mammals such that research on the behavioral, neural, and neurochemical aspects of the defense systems may be very relevant to analysis of defense-related behaviors, including psychopathologies, in people.

Defensive behaviors are modulated by features of both the threat stimulus and the situation in which it is presented). The major (self-)defensive behaviors are:

1. *Flight* from the threatening stimulus, and avoidance of that stimulus if it is at a distance. These behaviors are facilitated by the presence of an escape route or a place of concealment and are dominant responses to high-level threat when such features are available.
2. *Freezing* when no escape route or place of concealment is available. Freezing involves orientation toward the threat source and immobility in a species-typical posture. Like flight, it increases in intensity as the threat approaches, up to a level of proximity that elicits defensive threat/attack.
3. *Defensive threat* occurs as the threat stimulus nears the subject. It consists of a weapons display (teeth bared, claws unsheathed) and loud sonic vocalizations such as screams.
4. *Defensive attack* occurs at even shorter threat-subject distances. This attack is often oriented toward particularly vulnerable sites such as the predator/attacker's face and eyes.
5. *Risk assessment* occurs when the threat is potential rather than present (e.g., predator odor or novel situation) or of low intensity and includes sensory sampling (visual/auditory scanning, sniffing) and approach and investigation of the threat source, alternating with rapid retreat. Risk assessment is associated with low-profile postures and rapid movement interspersed with periods of immobility; these reduce the likelihood of detection as the animal approaches and investigates the threat stimulus. These activities enable the gathering of information, facilitating identification and localization of the threat source. If it proves to be a real danger, defenses such as flight or defensive threat/attack ensue. Alternatively, if risk assessment permits a determination that the situation is safe, then the animal can resume its normal activities (food gathering, self-care, or offspring care, etc.).
6. *Alarm vocalizations* occur in many (perhaps most) mammalian species with a colonial lifestyle. Such cries warn other group members of the appearance of a predator. In some primate species, different types of predator (e.g., terrestrial vs. aerial) elicit different alarm cries, permitting the listener to take defensive action appropriate to that predator.

These defensive behaviors all occur in the context of physical threat. Threat to resources elicits a very different behavior, offensive attack or aggression, which has a much weaker association with fearfulness or psychological stress. Both offensive and defensive (i.e., self-defensive) attack toward conspecifics in mammals tend to be oriented toward specific areas on the body of the opponent, and these target sites may provide an additional means of differentiating offensive and defensive attack modes. The former tends to be aimed at sites where bites or blows will produce pain without a high risk of damage to vital organs, whereas the latter is typically targeted toward the face of the threatener. This, for both conspecific and predator attackers, is both the site of particularly vulnerable and important organs, such as the eyes, and of the major offensive weapons of many animals, that is, the teeth. Because conspecific attack is so precisely targeted, an additional group of defenses against conspecific threat involves concealment of these especially likely targets of attack. These target-protection defenses, in combination with attacker behaviors that seek to thwart the defender (target concealment) strategy and reach the preferred attack target, may give fighting among conspecific mammals a dancelike quality in which the actions of one animal are immediately countered by appropriate actions of the other.

All of these defensive behaviors involve a strong component of orientation toward (or, in the case of flight, away from) the threat stimulus. In contrast, analyses of chronic internal pain (a stressful event not involving an external stimulus) suggest that the behavioral defense to this may be quiescence, involving reduced activity and inattention to external stimuli.

Across-Species Generality

These defensive behaviors and their specific associations with particular elements of the threat stimulus and the environment in which it is encountered show a high degree of cross-species generality in mammals. The generality is probably not limited to mammals, but mammals do appear to rely more strongly on this range of behavioral defenses than do other animals. Structural defenses (e.g., armor, venom, and poisonous tissues) and cryptic coloration are emphasized in lower vertebrates and invertebrates, whereas birds show an obvious specialization toward flight.

The behavioral repertory, including defensive behavior, of higher primates is more varied and sophisticated than that of more primitive mammals (e.g., rodents). However, the same defensive behaviors noted for rodents also occur in primates, albeit with greater elaboration of cognitive and communicatory elements. Examples are threat-differentiated alarm vocalizations, social or observational learning of threat stimuli (based on the defensive behaviors of conspecifics to these stimuli), and the formation of conspecific coalitions involving mutual defense and protection. Studies of defensive behaviors in humans are necessarily more indirect. However, choices of responses to scenarios designed to focus on features of the threat stimulus and the situation in which it is encountered strongly suggest that the relationship between stimulus/situational features and particular defenses in humans are broadly similar to those described in nonhuman animals.

Defensive Behaviors as Independent Biobehavioral Systems

Much classic research on defensive behavior had an initial "site" focus, in that it involved attempts to describe the immediate response of an animal to electrical or chemical stimulation of particular brain structures. Although a number of forebrain sites yield behaviors (e.g., vocalizations) that appear to be related to defensiveness, the most thoroughly investigated area has been the periaqueductal gray (PAG) region of the midbrain. This contains a number of longitudinally coursing columns in which stimulation can produce defensive threat/attack, flight, and freezing or quiescence. Some controversy surrounds the interpretation of stimulation of the ventral PAG column in terms of the last two alternatives. Responses related to defensive threat appear to be more common in the anterior components of these systems, whereas flight and freezing occur with stimulation in more posterior sites. It is particularly interesting that the PAG has been mapped in both cats and rats and that the specific areas where particular behaviors are elicited by stimulation appear to be very consistent.

Typically such studies did not provide a strong threat stimulus, or even an opponent to which the animal could orient and react, making interpretations of behavior more difficult. More recent attempts to determine the neural systems of defense have involved specific stimuli, notably presentation of a cat or cat odor to the subject rat. These studies indicate that cat stimuli elicit a strong c-Fos expression in specific areas of the amygdala, lateral septum, and specific nuclei of the hypothalamus, notably the dorsal premammillary nucleus. Lesions of the last of these strongly reduce responsivity to a cat or cat odor, but do not have a major impact on freezing following foot shock, suggesting considerable stimulus or stimulus modality specificity of control of defense in some forebrain structures. In addition to anatomical differences, there appear to be differences in the neurochemistry of the biobehavioral defensive systems, providing a basis for findings of differential response of these systems to psychoactive drugs.

Acute versus Chronic Behavioral Defenses

In addition to acute exposure paradigms, a number of models of chronic social or predator threat have been devised and used to evaluate behavioral and physiological effects of longer-term stress. In a particularly desirable habitat, with females and a burrow system, male rodents quickly create a strong dominance hierarchy based on victory and defeat. Defeated subordinate male rats spend most of their time within a particular chamber or tunnel, from which they attempt to exclude the victorious male (dominant); defensive threat/attack is a particularly effective defense in a tunnel. From these sites, subordinates also consistently monitor the dominant's location, avoiding the surface area when it is present and fleeing when they are in the open area and the dominant appears. Subordinates spend most of their waking time in defensive behavior and lose weight even when food and water are freely available.

Much of the defensive behavior of a subordinate rat to a dominant is very similar to that seen on initial exposure to a threat stimulus, except that it is more protracted. However, prolonged exposure to threat/stress may produce deleterious behavioral changes such as reduced activity, a shift away from active defense toward more passive defenses, and possibly a shift to a quiescent state in which the animal becomes less, or less effectively, attentive to possible environmental dangers. In learning situations, particularly those involving an active avoidance response, deficits in responding by animals chronically exposed to an uncontrollable stressor are characterized as indicating LH. A potentially similar phenomenon in subordinate rats involves greatly prolonged risk assessment without transition to nondefensive behavior. This may also reflect a learning deficit and it, like the active avoidance deficit of LH rats, may be quite maladaptive. The prolonged (and often inadequately cautious) risk assessment behavior exposes the animal to danger if a threat is present, whereas the failure to resume normal behavior patterns is maladaptive if there is no threat present.

Another behavior associated with chronic stress (in a CMS model) is anhedonia, typically indexed by reduced consumption of sweetened liquids. In fact, the CMS animals may actually show heightened preference for more intensely sweetened liquids.

Defensive Behaviors, Stress, and Psychopathology

Defensive behaviors – both those seen in response to acute threat and the altered patterns expressed after chronic threat/stress – have many parallels to the behavioral components of a range of human psychopathologies. In particular, risk-assessment behaviors appear to be very similar to the increased vigilance and scanning characteristic of generalized anxiety disorder, whereas reduced activity, anhedonia, and deficits in active avoidance learning have parallels in depression.

An additional parallel between the chronic stress models and depression is through alterations in the functioning of the hypothalamic-pituitary-adrenal (HPA) axis and changes in brain neurotransmitter systems. Different physiological systems have often been emphasized in investigations of the various chronic stress models (LH, CMS, and subordination), and so a consensus on their commonality of effects is difficult to obtain. HPA axis changes appear to be most severe for subordinates, many of whom show greatly decreased levels of corticosterone binding globulin, reduced corticosterone (CORT) response to acute stress, and reduced corticotropin-releasing factor (CRF) in the paraventricular nuclei of the hypothalamus, indicating the involvement of brain mechanisms in this deficit. Subordinates also show sharply reduced levels of testosterone, reflecting both peripheral and central effects of stress, with the former appearing prior to the latter. For the most part, LH is not associated with these hormonal effects, particularly when the criterion of experiencing uncontrollable versus controllable shock is applied. This very stringent criterion, using chronic but controllable shock as a control condition, may obscure some important changes in stress-linked physiological systems. As befits the term chronic mild stress, the CMS model also fails to produce notable hormonal changes. However, all three models have been associated with brain neurochemical changes, particularly involving biogenic amines, and a number of these brain changes, as well as the behaviors with which the models are associated, have been shown to be reversible after treatment with antidepressants. These hormonal and brain effects, in addition to the changes in defense and other behaviors after chronic stress, suggest that animal models of chronic stress may provide some very relevant analogs to depression and further emphasize the potential value of use of these behaviors as preclinical models for research on the pharmacology of emotion-linked disorders.

This approach has produced many interesting results. Risk-assessment behaviors show a selective response to anxiolytic drugs such as classic benzodiazepines. Antipanic drugs (e.g., alprazolam, imipramine, fluoxetine, and phenelzine) decrease flight behaviors, whereas the panicogenic agent yohimbine increases flight. As with clinical findings, the effects of these antipanic drugs on flight require chronic administration, whereas the initial injection of imipramine and fluoxetine may actually exacerbate defense. Both CMS and LH models have proved to be responsive to a variety of antidepressant drugs. However, the various behavioral effects of the latter model, such as reduced activity and disrupted learning of an active avoidance response, may show differential patterns of response to antidepressant and anxiolytic drugs. Both acute and chronic social defeat produce behavior changes that are normalized by fluoxetine, a selective serotonin reuptake inhibitor that has antidepressant as well as antipanic effects. In general, these findings suggest that, although acute and chronic stress may produce a wide pattern of changes in defensive and other behaviors, it is the behavioral response itself, rather than the stress paradigm, that may provide the clearest and most direct relationship to particular stress-linked psychopathologies.

See Also the Following Articles

Anxiety.

Further Reading

Bandler, R. and Keay, K. A. (1996). Columnar organization in the midbrain periaqueductal gray and the integration of emotional expression. *Progress in Brain Research* **107**, 285–300.

Blanchard, D. C., Griebel, G. and Blanchard, R. J. (2003). The mouse defense test battery: pharmacological and behavioral assays for anxiety and panic. *European Journal of Psychology* **463**, 97–116.

Blanchard, D. C., Hynd, A. L., Minke, K. A., et al. (2001). Human defensive behaviors to threat scenarios show parallels to fear- and anxiety-related defense patterns of nonhuman mammals. *Neuroscience and Biobehavioral Reviews* **25**, 761–770.

Blanchard, D. C., Spencer, R., Weiss, S. M., et al. (1995). The visible burrow system as a model of chronic social stress: behavioral and neuroendocrine correlates. *Psychoendocrinology* **20**, 117–134.

Canteras, N. S., Ribeiro-Barbosa, E. R. and Comoli, E. (2001). Tracing from the dorsal premammillary nucleus prosencephalic systems involved in the organization of innate fear responses. *Neuroscience and Biobehavioral Reviews* **25**, 661–668.

Davis, M. (1997). Neurobiology of fear responses: the role of the amygdala. *Journal of Neuropsychiatry and Clinical Neuroscience* **9**, 382–402.

Dielenberg, R. A., Hunt, G. E. and McGregor, I. S. (2001). "When a rat smells a cat": the distribution of Fos immunoreactivity in rat brain following exposure to a predatory odor. *Neuroscience* **104**, 1085–1097.

Gray, J. A. and McNaughton, N. (2000). *The neuropsychology of anxiety: an enquiry into the functions of the septo-hippocampal system* (2nd edn.). Oxford: Oxford University Press.

Maier, S. F., Ryan, S. M., Barksdale, C. M., et al. (1986). Stressor controllability and the pituitary-adrenal system. *Behavioral Neuroscience* **100**, 669–674.

Willner, P., Muscat, R. and Papp, M. (1992). Chronic mild stress-induced anhedonia: a realistic animal model of depression. *Neuroscience and Biobehavioral Reviews* **16**, 525–534.

Panic Disorder and Agoraphobia

J C Ballenger
Medical University of South Carolina, Charleston, SC, USA

This is a revised version of the article by J C Ballenger, Encyclopedia of Stress First Edition, volume 3, pp 119–123, © 2000, Elsevier Inc.

Glossary

Panic attacks (PA)	The name used currently for unexpected attacks of fear.
Panic disorder (PD)	Originates from the Greek god of flocks, Pan, who would frighten animals and humans out of the blue.
Spontaneous panic attacks	The main characteristic of PD that is central to its recognition and diagnosis.

Symptoms

One of the main characteristics of panic disorder (PD) is spontaneous out of the blue panic attacks (PAs). PAs usually occur immediately upon exposure or in anticipation of exposure to particular situations, often ones in which panic attacks have previously occurred.

Symptoms of PAs in order of their frequency are palpitations, pounding heart, tachycardia, sweating, trembling or shaking, shortness of breath or smothering, feeling of choking, chest pain or discomfort, nausea or abdominal distress, feeling dizzy, unsteady, lightheaded or faint, derealization or depersonalization, fear of losing control or going crazy, fear of dying, chills, and hot flashes.

Panic attacks usually last for several minutes, but they can also last for hours. In one of the largest modern PD clinical trials, patients averaged one to two PAs per week. However, the frequency and severity of PAs vary greatly between individuals and, at times, in individuals. Some may have only one to three PAs per year, whereas others may have multiple PAs on a daily basis. Some individuals will even have bursts of PAs and then not experience attacks for a long period of time.

Because PAs are extremely frightening, patients will often develop a logical fear that they will reoccur. This anticipatory anxiety increases prior to exposure to situations in which patients have experienced previous PAs. Because of this, PD patients often develop agoraphobia, which is avoidance of certain places or situations. Agoraphobics often avoid situations in which they have had PAs because they are afraid that escape would be difficult or embarrassing or that help might not be available during these attacks. In community samples, one-third to one-half of patients who meet criteria for PD also have significant agoraphobia avoidance.

There are typical situations that are avoided most frequently. These include taking buses, trains, or planes; riding in or driving a car; being in large crowds; standing in lines; shopping; and being in spaces where they might feel trapped (e.g., bridges, tunnels, elevators). Patients experiencing a PA will often have an overwhelming need to escape or return to a place of safety, like home. These patients do not actually fear the situation itself but are afraid of the feelings of panic that might happen while in that situation.

Many patients even have PAs that begin during sleep. These nocturnal panic attacks are quite common, and the majority of PD patients experience them. These PAs occur during the beginning states of the sleep cycle and are essentially identical to daytime PAs.

There also is a close relationship between depression and PD. In various samples, comorbid or secondary depression ranged from 22 to 68%. Proper recognition of comorbid depression is especially important because of the marked increase in suicide attempts (23.6–50%) in patients with both PD and depression.

Diagnosis

The diagnosis of PD has several requirements.

1. Recurrent, unexpected PAs (situational PAs could also occur, but there would need to be at least two unexpected PAs by history).
2. Panic attacks need to be followed by at least 1 month of (1) persistent anxiety about the potential recurrence of further PAs, (2) persistent anxiety about the implications of these attacks (e.g., going crazy, something wrong medically), or (3) a significant behavioral change because of these attacks.

PD in the General Medical Setting

There is poor recognition of PD in the general medical setting. It is often undiagnosed, because physical symptoms of PD can be mistakenly linked to other medical conditions. However, panic-like symptoms can occur in a few medical conditions (e.g., hyperthyroidism, pheochromocytoma, seizures, cardiac arrhythmias, and chronic obstructive pulmonary disease).

Conservative estimates of PD in primary care have ranged from 3 to 8%, with at least 50% of patients with PD being unrecognized. The average length of time for a patient in the general medicine setting to be diagnosed correctly with PD is 10 years, with an escalation of the use of health-care services over this 10-year period. Overall, PD patients are three times more likely to utilize general medical services than the traditional patient in a primary care setting. The percentage of PD patients is also markedly higher in certain medical groups (e.g., cardiology and gastroenterology).

A study sponsored by the World Health Organization (WHO) studied primary care patients in 14 different countries. Ninety-nine percent of patients with one PA in the previous month had an anxiety disorder or depression or a subthreshold anxiety disorder or depressive disorder. If replicated, it would appear that the occurrence of even a single PA should serve as a signal for increased scrutiny for anxiety and depressive syndromes.

Epidemiology

There is a striking uniformity worldwide for the observed prevalence of PD, generally averaging between 1 and 2% in multiple studies. In the WHO Primary Care Survey of 14 countries mentioned previously, the prevalence for PD ranged from a low of 1.4% to a high of 16.5% for PAs and 0–03.5% for PD itself. The average for PD was 1.1% (current) and 3.5% (lifetime), which was similar to community samples. As mentioned, rates are much higher in certain medical settings, ranging from 15% in dizziness clinics to 16–65% in cardiology practices and 35% in hyperventilation clinics.

Risk Factors

In treatment samples, PD has been observed to be at least two times more prevalent in females than in males. Males tend to have a longer duration of illness but are less likely to seek help or develop agoraphobia and depression. The onset of PD for both genders usually occurs between 15 and 24 years of age, with a second peak at 45–54 years of age. The onset of PD after the age of 65 is rare (0.1%).

As mentioned previously, agoraphobia is also more prevalent in females, with the highest rates of PD and agoraphobia occurring in widowed, divorced, or separated individuals living in cities. Early parental loss, limited education, and physical or sexual abuse are also risk factors for PD.

Genetic factors can even be associated with PD. Heightened anxiety, known as behavioral inhibition, is higher in children of anxiety-disordered parents and in children of adults with PD. As these children have aged, they have been observed to have higher rates of anxiety and phobic disorders.

Precipitating events have been reported in 60–96% of PD cases. Multiple studies also suggest that traumatic early events may figure into the vulnerability leading to PD.

Course and Prognosis

Available evidence suggests that PD is a chronic condition, once criteria for the disorder are met. It is common for patients to report symptoms that they have had for 10–15 years prior to diagnosis. As mentioned previously, the Klein model suggests that spontaneous PAs are the first manifestation of the illness, followed by anticipatory anxiety and then agoraphobia in some individuals.

In fact, most PD patients do not have PAs as their first symptoms. Over 90% have had mild phobic or hypochondriac symptoms prior to the onset of their first PA. The first PA is usually experienced in a phobogenic situation, such as a public place, street, public transportation, crowd, elevator, tunnel, bridge, or open space. Despite this, the Klein model remains largely correct and helpful in conceptualizing the development of the condition and its treatments.

After diagnosis and some sort of treatment, functional recovery occurs in the majority of patients. Poor responses to treatment were associated most consistently with initial high symptom severity and high agoraphobic avoidance at baseline. A poor response is also associated with a low socioeconomic status, less education, longer duration, limited social networks, death of a parent, divorce or unmarried status, and personality disorders.

Treatment

Since the early 1960s, effective psychological and pharmacological treatments for PD have been developed.

Tricyclic Antidepressants (TCAs)

In the 1960s, the TCA imipramine was one of the first effective drug treatments. Important advantages of imipramine include its once-a-day dose, its low cost, and the extensive research that has been conducted on its effectiveness. Its principal difficulties are initial hyperstimulation reactions, significant weight gain with long-term use, and the dangers involved with an overdose. The highly serotonergic clomipramine became the most popular treatment in Europe during the 1970s, 1980s, and 1990s.

Monoamine Oxidase Inhibitors (MAOIs)

During the 1960s, MAOIs were also proven to be effective in the treatment of PD. The most definitive trial was an early comparison of phenelzine and imipramine in the mid-1970s. This was the first trial to suggest that MAOIs might be the most effective medication class, especially if the PD patient is depressed. The biggest drawbacks of MAOIs are the need for a patient to be on a restricted diet and the danger of hypertensive crisis if the diet is not followed. There are also dangers if certain other medications are used, especially certain analgesics and other antidepressants. The principal side effects are insomnia, weight gain, postural hypotension, anticholinergic side effects, and sexual dysfunction.

The reversible MAOIs, brofaramine and meclobemide, have stimulated interest because they require no restrictive diet. However, trials with meclobemide were unable to distinguish medication from placebo, and despite promising early results with brofaramine, its development has been discontinued. There is still active research in this area.

Benzodiazepines (BZs)

High potency BZs (e.g., alprazolam, clonazepam) were developed in the 1980s and are also used in the treatment of PD. In fact, BZs remain the most frequently utilized treatment for PD worldwide, probably because of their quick onset of action, increased efficacy against anticipatory anxiety, low cost, and tolerability. They are frequently utilized in conjunction with the antidepressants. The principal drawback to BZs is the general concern with their abuse potential, although it is alcoholics and opiate or pill addicts that abuse the drug. Abuse in uncomplicated PD patients is extremely rare. Other side effects include the high rate of withdrawal symptoms and relapse that can occur after discontinuing BZ treatment.

Selective Serotonin Reuptake Inhibitors (SSRIs)

More recent studies in the 1990s have demonstrated that the SSRIs are effective, and they are now frequently recommended as the first treatment of choice. This is largely based on the many controlled trials documenting the high tolerability of SSRIs and the decreased rate of jitteriness and hyperstimulation responses often associated with tricyclic antidepressants. They are preferred over benzodiazepines in patients with significant difficulty with depression. Most (70–85%) patients retain their benefit when SSRIs are tapered and discontinued after 12 months of successful treatment.

Psychological Treatments: Psychodynamic Psychotherapy

Although psychodynamic psychotherapy remains a popular treatment for many psychiatric disorders, including PD, there is limited research demonstrating its efficacy in PD. An emotion-focused treatment for PD has been developed that explores typical fears of being abandoned or trapped as stimuli for panic attacks. This often involves a 12-session acute treatment with 6 sessions of monthly maintenance. Patients are encouraged to identify, reflect upon, and attempt to change problematic feelings and their responses.

Behavioral Treatments

There is a rapidly increasing body of evidence for combinations of exposure-based treatments and cognitive-behavioral therapy (CBT) that are effective in the treatment of PD.

Exposure Treatments

Behavioral treatments, involving *in vivo* exposure, require patients to gradually systematically re-expose themselves to their phobic situations. A large number of studies have documented that 58–83% of patients improve after exposure treatments.

One consistent observation of exposure-based treatments is its long-lasting effects. In one trial with 110 individuals treated with 12 weeks of exposure-based treatment, 74% of the sample achieved panic-free status, and this improvement was maintained in almost all patients throughout a 7-year follow-up. Studies that have compared the use of exposure to CBT have found them to be essentially equal in efficacy. There appears to be little benefit from the combination, although the dropout rate was lower.

Evidence supporting the importance of exposure-based treatments is very clear, but many patients remain symptomatic. In addition, many studies report that between 10 and 25% of patients drop out of the therapy because it is an anxiety-provoking treatment method.

Cognitive-Behavioral Therapy

Cognitive-behavioral therapy is based on the theory that patients with PD interpret physical symptoms in a catastrophic way and that these cognitive distortions need to be challenged and corrected. CBT of PD evolved from early work of Aaron Beck but has been applied to PD primarily by Barlow and colleagues and is called panic control therapy (PCT).

Treatment generally involves an initial education component, which is followed by the identification of critical misinterpretations of panic symptoms. Patients are then taught ways in which they can challenge and correct these misinterpretations. This includes evaluating how likely (or unlikely) the imagined consequences are and how catastrophic it would be even if their worse fears did happen. Most CBT is also combined with interoceptive exposure to the physical symptoms that frighten them. For instance, a patient fearful of dizziness might be spun in a chair.

Although applied relaxation has been shown to be somewhat effective in PD, other studies have demonstrated that CBT, especially combined with interoceptive exposure (i.e., PCT), is more effective than medication.

Most experts would agree that the treatment of PD with pharmacotherapy and a CBT approach – employing a combination of exposure and cognitive therapy – are roughly comparable in efficacy. The most carefully performed trial demonstrating this was a multicenter, 11-week acute trial comparing imipramine to CBT. Both CBT and imipramine performed equally well, but the combination of CBT and imipramine was not proven to be any more effective in the treatment of PD. This trial provided evidence that CBT applied early in treatment did not offer protective effects against imipramine relapse. However, other data suggest that it is protective if given during the discontinuation period.

Selection of Treatments

Pharmacotherapy (BZs or antidepressants) and CBT/exposure treatments appear to be equally effective, although response is perhaps faster with medication treatment and longer term response is better in some patients with CBT/exposure-based treatments. Most often, selection of treatment is determined by patient choice or individual characteristics.

One important issue in the treatment of PD is that the majority of patients do not fully recover with either pharmacotherapy or psychotherapy. For both types of treatment, only 25–45% of patients could be considered fully recovered, despite the excellent progress that has been made since the 1980s. This has led to ongoing research attempts to find more effective treatment methods for PD.

See Also the Following Articles

Anxiety.

Further Reading

Ballenger, J. C. (1998). Treatment of panic disorder in the general medical setting. *Journal of Psychosomatic Research* **44**, 5–15.

Ballenger, J. C. (1998). Comorbidity of panic and depression: Implications for clinical management. *International Journal of Clinical Psychopharmacology* **13**(Supplement), 513–517.

Ballenger, J. C. (2003). Selective serotonin reuptake inhibitors in the treatment of the anxiety disorders. In: Nutt, D. & Ballenger, J. C. (eds.) *Anxiety disorders*, pp. 339–361. Oxford, UK: Blackwell Science.

Ballenger, J. C., Burrows, G. and DuPont, R. L., Jr., et al. (1988). Alprazolam in panic disorder and agoraphobia. Results from a multicenter trial. I. Efficacy in short-term treatment. *Archives of General Psychiatry* **455**, 413–422.

Ballenger, J. C., Lydiard, R. B. and Turner, S. M. (1997). Panic disorder and agoraphobia. In: Gabbard, G. O. (ed.) *Treatments of psychiatric disorders* (2nd edn., vol. 2), pp. 1421–1452. Washington, D.C.: American Psychiatric Press.

Ballenger, J. C., Davidson, J. R. T., Lecrubier, Y. and Nutt, D. J. (International Consensus Group on Depression and Anxiety), et al. (1998). Consensus statement on panic disorder from the International Consensus Group on Depression and Anxiety. *Journal of Clinical Psychiatry* **59**, 47–54.

Klein, D. F. (1964). Delineation of two drug responsive anxiety syndromes. *Psychopharmacology* **5**, 397–408.

Klerman, G. L., Weissman, M., Ovellette, R., Johnson, J. and Greenwald, S. (1991). Panic attacks in the community: social morbidity and health care utilization. *Journal of the American Medical Association* **265**, 742–746.

Margraf, G., Barlow, D. H., Clark, D. M. and Telch, M. J. (1993). Psychological treatment of panic: work in

progress in outcome, active ingredients, and follow-up. *Behavioral Research Therapy* **31**, 1–8.
Marks, I. M. (1969). *Fears and phobias.* London: Heinemann.
Mavissakalian, M. R. and Prien, R. F. (eds.) (1996). *Long-term treatments of anxiety disorders.* Washington, D.C.: American Psychiatric Press.
Rosenbaum, J. F., Biederman, J., Gersten, M., et al. (1988). Behavioral inhibition in children of parents with panic disorder and agoraphobia: a controlled study. *Archives of General Psychiatry* **45**, 463–470.
Roy-Byrne, P. P. and Cowley, D. S. (1995). Course and outcome in panic disorder. A review of recent follow-up studies. *Anxiety* **1**, 151–160.
Sartorius, N., Ustun, T. B., Jorges-Alberto, C., et al. (1993). An international study of psychological problems in primary care. *Archives of General Psychiatry* **50**, 819–824.

Death Anxiety

R Kastenbaum
Arizona State University, Tempe, AZ, USA

This is a revised version of the article by R Kastenbaum, Encyclopedia of Stress First Edition, volume 1, pp 645–651, © 2000, Elsevier Inc.

Glossary

Existentialism	A philosophical position that emphasizes the individual as alone in the world and responsible for his or her own life and values.
Hospice	A programmatic approach to providing comfort to terminally ill people and their families.
Ontological confrontation	An experience that forces one to acknowledge the reality and salience of death.
Near-death experience (NDE)	An altered state of consciousness usually occurring after traumatic injury that is often recalled as a comforting and revelatory episode.
Palliative care	Medical and nursing procedures designed to relieve pain and suffering rather than extend life by all possible means.
Thanatophobia	Fear of death and of whatever has become associated with death.

Empirical and Clinical Studies of Death Anxiety

The experience of anxiety is much the same whatever its source: a sense of danger and foreboding accompanied by physical manifestations such as changes in heart rate and respiration. Precisely how death anxiety differs from other forms of anxiety – if at all – is a question that has received little attention. Instead, most academic studies have relied on self-report questionnaires. Respondents usually respond by agreeing or disagreeing with direct questions such as "I fear dying a painful death." Fortunately, there have also been multilevel and interview studies that enhance our understanding.

Self-Reported Death Anxiety in Everyday Life

Most studies have been conducted with healthy adults, with attention given to their level of anxiety and gender, age, and other demographic variables.

The general population: How anxious about death? Most adults in the United States report themselves as having moderately low levels of death anxiety. This consistent finding often has been interpreted to mean that we labor to keep our anxieties hidden both from ourselves and others. Supporting this interpretation are studies that have detected physiological indications of stress at the same time that subjects report feeling no death-related anxiety at all. It is therefore argued that we are all anxious about death on the gut level, though are reluctant to admit so. An alternative interpretation is that we usually have a low walking-around level of death anxiety that only surges up when a threat is detected. There is a readiness for emergency response, but from moment to moment life is not an emergency. This issue is revisited in the section on theoretical approaches.

Is there a gender difference in death anxiety? Women in the United States usually report higher levels of death anxiety than men. The few studies conducted in other nations find the same pattern. We can choose among several interpretations:

- Women are too anxious about death.
- Men are not anxious enough about death.
- There is no actual difference in level of death anxiety between the sexes, but women are more willing to acknowledge and express their concerns.

In weighing these alternative interpretations, it is useful to recognize the exceptional contribution made by women in providing care and comfort to dying people and their families. Much of the leadership and manpower in the international hospice movement has come from women, who also are far more likely than men to enroll in death education courses. Women have generally been more responsive to the needs of people with life-threatening conditions and more cognizant and accepting of their own feelings about death. Men generally seem more guarded and uncomfortable when circumstances remind them of their vulnerability. These gender differences have been related to childhood socialization patterns in which the expression of feelings, especially those of vulnerability, is encouraged in girls but discouraged in boys.

Women may be too anxious about death if the criterion is subjective comfort, but men may be not anxious enough if the criterion is the readiness to respond to the mortal jeopardy of self and others. Research also suggests gender differences in the type of situations that arouse the most anxiety. Men express more fear of extinction and the way their post-death self will be remembered. Women express more fear of the dying process and of being unable to make adequate arrangements for the well-being of their families. These differences should not be overestimated. There are marked individual differences in personality within each gender.

Is there an age difference in death anxiety? Do we become more anxious as we grow older because of the decreasing distance from death? Or do we become less anxious because we develop a more mature outlook on life and death?

Age differences, when found, indicate less fear of death among elderly people. Concerns are more likely to center around the challenges and stresses of daily life, such as protecting relationships and self-esteem. However, it should be kept in mind that each generation passes through unique historical circumstances with distinctive configurations of social attitudes, economic up- and downturns, technological innovations, and threats to life. The fact that most elders have been reporting low or moderate levels of death anxiety probably represents the interaction of their distinctive life histories and current health and socioeconomic status, as well as their personal accommodations to the aging process. Qualitative studies have identified specific concerns that are most salient for people at different points in their life course. Young people seem most apprehensive about the possible loss of loved ones, death as punishment, and the finality of death. Midlife adults express most concern about premature death and fear of pain in dying. Older adults do not fear death as much as they do the prospect of becoming helpless and dependent on others during their final phase of life.

There is little support for the hypothesis that people become more anxious as the distance from death decreases with advanced age. Self-actualization and existential theories propose that acceptance of death is a mark of maturity. This is an attractive proposition, but not an established fact. It might be overreaching to insist that philosophical acceptance of death is the only way a mature person can come to terms with mortality. Furthermore, other explanations might account for the relatively low death anxiety found among elderly adults. Some people experiencing social isolation, financial concern, and age-related physical problems express a readiness to have their lives come to an end – an attitude that is also reflected in the high completed suicide rates for elderly white men. Low death anxiety might then be related to dissatisfaction with a life that is no longer considered worth living.

What are the demographics of death anxiety? People in favorable socioeconomic circumstances tend to report lower levels of death anxiety. Education, affluence, and status serve as buffers against death anxiety (though not impenetrable buffers). Growing up in an intact family and having a secure interpersonal environment also offer some protection against high death anxiety. Married people generally live longer and are less likely to commit suicide. We might therefore expect that married people would experience less anxiety than those who are single or divorced, but, surprisingly, this proposition has not been systematically examined.

Religious beliefs and practices have a complex relationship with death anxiety. Anthropologists and historians have argued that religion originated as a response to the fear of death. A particular religion operating within a particular cultural context might be effective in controlling death anxiety with comforting rites of passage and images of blessings in the afterlife. The opposite effect is also possible, however. Presenting death in frightening images is an effective way of keeping anxiety bubbling and therefore motivating people to seek protection by obedience to the establishment. In today's mass and heterogeneous societies, religion offers a broad array of beliefs and practices, some of which seem likely to reduce and others to increase death anxiety. Some people of faith might have less fear of death because they expect a joyful afterlife, while others are beset by anxiety about damnation. Surveys continue to indicate that most people in the United States do believe in an afterlife. Studies of terminally ill people suggest that there is more anxiety about suffering and dependency during the dying process than fear of death as such. Religious faith and belief in an afterlife seem to help many people face the prospect of death, but they are still vulnerable to anxiety about the dying process and the effects of their death on others. It has become clear, however, that many people feel more secure during their final illnesses when they know that they will be given full benefit of the religious and social customs that are meaningful within their group.

What are the personality and lifestyle correlates of death anxiety? People who are afflicted with many other fears are likely to have relatively high death anxiety as well. People with humorless authoritarian personalities are the least likely to sign the organ donation forms attached to their drivers' licenses, suggesting a higher level of death-related anxiety. A dominating need to control situations and to win at all costs has been related to a feeling of vulnerability: catastrophic anxiety and death must be warded off by exercising power over the course of events. Similarly, some people who seem to live outside of themselves through causes and cults do so to achieve a sense of participatory immortality and thereby escape the sting of death anxiety. By contrast, people with deep interpersonal attachments who have a strong sense of purpose in life tend to have a lower level of death anxiety.

Death Anxiety in Particular Situations

Our focus now shifts from characteristics of the individual to the types of situations in which individuals may find themselves. We draw now upon a wide range of observations beyond self-report questionnaires.

Transitional situations We often experience heightened death anxiety in transitional situations. Starting or losing a job and moving to a new community are common examples of transitions that have no evident relationship with death but that can engage feelings of uncertainty and threat. Separation, divorce, and other significant changes in relationships can also arouse a sense of vulnerability, which, on the emotional map, is not far from fear of mortality. Even detection of the first gray hair can trigger the recognition that one is no longer young, thereby arousing the lurking fears of aging and death. Determined attempts to look young often express a convergence of fears: "I will be less attractive, less valued, less useful – and I will become the sort of person who is most likely to die – the old-timer."

The community at large can also experience heightened stress during periods of transition and uncertainty. Apprehension about unemployment, inflation, inadequate health-care benefits, and difficulties in coping with bureaucracy and technology can all contribute to a sense of helplessness, which, in turn, increases permeability to awareness of mortality. A society that has lost confidence in its purpose and competence may contribute to heightened death anxiety throughout all ages, ranks, and echelons.

Touched by death Exposure to death does not always make us anxious. Sometimes we seal off such episodes quickly before they can penetrate our awareness. At the extreme, we may deny the significance of the event, as when the victim of a heart attack insists that he is just fine and does not need medical attention. More often, though, we use subtle defensive strategies to avoid the impact of an exposure to death. For example, at a funeral we may not permit ourselves to acknowledge a possible resonance between the neighbor who died of pulmonary disease and our own habit of smoking. "It's too bad about the neighbor, but I don't smoke the same brand of cigarettes." Many of us are gifted in the ability to shed exposures to death in order to preserve the comforting routines of everyday life. Nevertheless, some exposures to death do get through to us. Usually these exposures take one of two forms: a personal brush with death or the death of another person.

It is not uncommon for the stress reaction to develop after a life-threatening emergency. A competent driver or pilot, for example, is likely to respond to an emergency with quick and skillful actions. Only when the danger has passed will the emotional reaction seize its opportunity, perhaps taking the form of a transient posttraumatic stress episode. Anxiety aroused due to a close call with death usually dissipates quickly, although there may be heightened sensitivity to future risk situations. What has become known as a near-death experience (NDE) is a different case. These episodes almost invariably involve risk to life that the individual could not deal with through personal initiative and action (e.g., the passenger in a car hit in a broadside collision). The NDE is an episode split off from the person's usual life and marked by unusual, dream-like events. Instead of intense anxiety, however, many reports depict a remarkable feeling of serenity and liberation. Some people believe that they not only have been touched by death but also were actually in death for a short period of time. There are varying interpretations of the actual state of being during a NDE, but a great many reports that anxiety about death completely dissipated after the experience.

By contrast, the death of another person is often mentioned as the wake-up call that leads to anxious realization of one's own mortality. Most often it is the death of a parent that produces an increased sense of personal vulnerability. "Death is coming after me, now!" as a 50-ish woman exclaimed after the death of her mother. The death of a long-lived cultural icon can also lead to feelings of vulnerability and abandonment. In addition, we are likely to experience an upsurge of death-related anxiety when a person seen as much like ourselves passes away. Our behavior toward others when they are terminally ill and during the funeral process can be markedly influenced by anxieties aroused by our feeling that "this could be happening to me."

Facing death: Life-threatening illness The prospect of our own death may flash before us in a quickly developing episode as already noted. It is a different matter, however, when the threat is persistent, as in the case of life-threatening illness. Coping with a threat to life varies with both the individual and the medical condition (e.g., a cardiac disorder that might end one's life at any time or advanced pulmonary disease in which every breath is a struggle as the disease continually progresses). Nevertheless, there are also some common issues that often intensify anxiety. These include (a) uncertainty about diagnosis and prognosis, (b) learning that one has a life-threatening condition, (c) progression of symptoms and dysfunctions that suggest that treatment efforts are failing, (d) interpersonal cues that others also recognize the end is approaching, along with concern about losing one's most valued relationships, (e) concern about practical end-of-life matters, (f) concern about the overall meaning of one's life, and (g) anxiety about experiencing helplessness and pain in the end phase of the dying process. Patients often are aware of the anxiety that exists in others around them: it has been found that physicians often experience intense discomfort in the terminal-care situation and therefore try to limit their contacts with the patients. It is not unusual for death anxiety to be reinforced and multiplied throughout the entire terminal-care interpersonal network.

There is some evidence to suggest that episodes of intense anxiety can trigger sudden death in people with coronary heart disease. These findings support earlier observations that a person literally can be scared to death. However, a moderate level of anxiety might be more protective than a denial reaction. It has often been suggested, but not yet firmly established, that high levels of anxiety can also increase the risk of death in other life-threatening conditions.

Anxiety peaks most often at two points. The first jolt usually occurs when the person discovers that his or her illness is terminal. Suicidal ideation can develop during this chaotic period of panic and depression. Trustworthy and sensitive communication on the part of family and health-care providers can prevent a plunge into the depths of despair or an anxious leap into self-destruction. The second anxiety peak, again accompanied by depression, arises as a result of continued physical deterioration, fatigue, and apprehension regarding progressive loss of function. "I'm just so tired of dying" is how more than one person has expressed it. Here anxiety is focused less on death than on the fear of being abandoned and isolated while continuing to suffer for no good reason that the person can see. Euthanasia is not sought by all people in the end-phase of their terminal illnesses, however. Many continue to experience life as meaningful and to be protected from disabling anxiety by positive belief systems and loving support from the people most important to them.

Anxiety and depression associated with terminal illness have often been the result of social isolation and inadequate control of pain and other symptoms. The pioneering contributions of Elisabeth Kubler-Ross and Dame Cicely Saunders have done much to improve this situation. Kubler-Ross, a psychiatrist, encouraged professional and family caregivers to overcome their own anxieties about interacting with terminally ill people. Saunders, a nurse and physician, launched and guided the international hospice movement that provides a broad spectrum of symptom relief with a combination of compassionate care and palliative expertise. As their own lives neared the end, Kubler-Ross and Saunders both received the benefits of the hospice care they had helped make possible for people around the world. Recently, the medical establishment has shown signs of agreeing with the hospice premise that pain should be regarded as one of the vital signs to be assessed and effectively treated in all physician–patient interactions. Team approaches to the comfort of terminally ill people and their families with priorities given to the dying person's own lifestyle and values have also contributed to reducing anxiety throughout the final phase of life.

Major mental health problems People who feel that their worlds are exploding or collapsing often express intense anxiety about death. Some of the most striking expressions of death anxiety are found during psychotic episodes, whether functional or triggered by a drug-altered state of mind. Whatever the specific cause, it is usually the sense of losing total control over one's life that has precipitated the episode. Dying and death become metaphorical expressions of this panic. Severely depressed people may even present themselves as dead, thereby having passed beyond the reach of death anxiety. Helpful interventions include providing a higher degree of stability and simplicity in the sociophysical environment and creating situations in which the individual can begin to experience again a sense of competence and control. Approaches as different as expressive and drug therapies can also be useful.

Theories of Death Anxiety

General theories of stress and anxiety have potential for contributing to the understanding of death-related concerns. Here we focus on theories that were intended specifically for comprehension of death anxiety.

Freud and Becker: Rival Theories

Two theories may be considered classic for their bold positions and widespread influence. These views could not be more opposed in their fundamental propositions, although there are commonalities as well.

Sigmund Freud held that we cannot truly have a fear of death because we cannot believe in our own death. Notice that person who is standing off to the side and viewing your death – it is you, the spectator self who is still very much alive. Personal death is not comprehended by the foundational logic of our unconscious processes, while on the conscious level, we have not actually experienced death. An expressed fear of death (thanatophobia), then, is a phobic symptom that conceals the actual, deeper source of anxiety lodged in childhood experiences and stimulated by current life developments. This influential view relegated death anxiety to a derived, secondary status and thereby not of much interest in its own right. Later in his own pained and stressful life, Freud came to see dying and death as issues very much deserving of attention, but it was his earlier formulation that continued to prevail.

Ernest Becker challenged Freud's interpretation from an existential standpoint. For Becker, all anxiety is an expression of death anxiety. Our core fear of nonbeing attaches itself to an almost infinite variety of situations and symbols. This is where society comes in – it exists largely to protect us from being consumed by death anxiety. Becker charges that our language and customs are designed to disconnect us from ontological encounters with mortality. Even our technologically resplendent civilization remains basically a theatrical performance piece to which we all contribute our talents and suspension of disbelief. We agree not to notice that we all happen to be mortal. The person who really believes in death – and is therefore really anxious about it – is often the person we call schizophrenic. Being normal means being fairly successful in protecting ourselves against facing up to reality.

Both the Freudian/psychoanalytic and the Becker/existential theories have served as useful guides to observation and reflection. Different as they are, however, both share the premise of universal application and the flaw of unverifiability. There are situations in which one theory or the other seems applicable, but also situations in which neither seem sufficient.

Emerging Theories

Several new theories have emerged, each offering a distinctive perspective and drawing upon a distinctive realm of empirical research. Terror management theory is an empirically oriented offshoot of Becker's position. Its core proposition is that self-esteem and a positive worldview serve as effective barriers to death anxiety. When we feel ourselves imperiled, we can call upon our sense of self-worth and confidence as well as our belief that our society is basically sound and the universe a friendly place in which to dwell. Whatever contributes to growth of self-esteem and confidence and whatever contributes to the moral character and resilience of society can stand between ourselves and mortal terror.

Developmental learning theory places death anxiety within the mainstream of sociobehavioral research. We learn to fear, avoid, or cope with death-related phenomena just as we learn to deal with all other life challenges: through a long process of maturation and social interaction. It is not necessary to assert either that all anxiety or no anxiety is related to death or that we all have some kind of fixed response to death-linked situations and symbols. As a society and as individuals, the shape and intensity of our anxieties and coping strategies are pretty much in our own hands, and are likely to vary from generation to generation.

Edge theory shifts the emphasis from fear of death to the readiness to respond to threats to life. Two frequently held assumptions are set aside. First, the question of whether or not we can truly comprehend death is not as important as it once seemed. The point is that we do recognize threats to survival, whether of ourselves or of others. A vigilance function is with us from birth. Like other living creatures, we are equipped with the ability to detect serious threats and go on alert. The second assumption set aside is that we try desperately to hide our intense anxieties about death from ourselves and others. According to edge theory, however, we do not carry about a burden of repressed death anxiety. Instead, our moderate everyday approach to life is occasionally challenged by a potentially dangerous situation. We have a momentary sense of being on the edge of nonbeing. In such situations we go on alert and try to identify the source of the danger. If we can then either dismiss or take action to overcome the threat we experience only a sense of heightened activation. It is when we feel on the edge and cannot respond to the threat that are likely to be flooded by death anxiety.

Points of difference aside, current research and theory suggest that the understanding of stress management throughout life requires attention to the ways in which we come to terms with our mortality.

See Also the Following Articles

Anxiety; Fear; Suicide, Psychology of.

Further Reading

Becker, E. (1973). *The denial of death*. New York: Free Press.

Clark, D. (2003). Saunders, Cicely. In: Kastenbaum, R. (ed.) *Macmillan encyclopedia of death and dying,* (vol. 2)), pp. 743–745. New York: Macmillan Reference USA.

Freud, S. (1951). Thoughts for the times on war and death. In: *Collected works,* (vol. IV)), pp. 288–317. London: Hogarth Press.

Hayslip, B., Jr. (2003). Death denial. Hiding and camouflaging death. In: Bryant, C. (ed.) *Handbook of death and dying*, pp. 34–42. Thousand Oaks, CA: Sage.

Kastenbaum, R. (2004). *Death, society, and human experience* (8th edn.). Boston, MA: Allyn & Bacon.

Kastenbaum, R. (2004). *On our way. The final passage through life and death.* Berkeley, CA: University of California Press.

Kaufmann, W. (1976). *Existentialism, religion and death.* New York: New American Library.

Kubler-Ross, E. (1969). *On death and dying.* New York: Macmillan.

Tomer, A. (2003). Terror management theory. In: Kastenbaum, R. (ed.) *Macmillan encyclopedia of death and dying,* (vol. 2)), pp. 885–887. New York: Macmillan Reference USA.

C. Obsessive–Compulsive Disorder

Obsessive–Compulsive Disorder

R T Rubin
VA Greater Los Angeles Healthcare System, Los Angeles, CA, USA
B J Carroll
Pacific Behavioral Research Foundation, Carmel, CA, USA

This is a revised version of the article by R T Rubin, Encyclopedia of Stress First Edition, volume 3, pp 77–82, © 2000, Elsevier Inc.

Glossary

Anti-depressants	Drugs that are used in the treatment of depression and other psychiatric disorders, including obsessive–compulsive disorder (OCD).
Basal ganglia	Groups of neurons deep in the brain that serve as integrative way stations for brain circuits.
Cerebral cortex	The outer layer of the brain, composed mainly of nerve cells (neurons).
Compulsions	Repetitive behaviors or mental acts that reduce anxiety or distress.
Neuro-transmitters	Chemicals that carry messages from one nerve cell to another.
Obsessions	Intrusive and inappropriate recurrent and persistent thoughts.

Introduction

Psychiatric disorders are considered functional when there is no clearly understood central nervous system (CNS) pathophysiology underlying them. Thus, schizophrenia, the major affective illnesses, and anxiety disorders have been and are still considered functional psychiatric illnesses. This is an evolving nomenclature, however – as our knowledge about the pathophysiology of the brain in these disorders increases, the adjective functional conveys less and less meaning.

The brain substrates of the major psychiatric disorders are being examined in several ways. Complex genetic underpinnings are slowly being defined. Structural and functional imaging studies of the brain are providing some anatomical localization, limited by the resolution of the imaging techniques and the particular methodology of each study. Specific classes of drugs are known to be therapeutic for specific disorders, but the balance among chemical systems in the brain makes inferences about disturbance of a specific system in a particular psychiatric disorder difficult. Furthermore, no drug is curative of any psychiatric disorder. Obsessive–compulsive disorder (OCD) is one of the functional psychiatric illnesses that is giving way to an understanding of its pathophysiology in the brain. Stress can play a major role in the severity of OCD, and the illness itself can be very stressful to afflicted persons.

Clinical Characteristics of OCD

OCD is classified among the anxiety disorders. Its hallmarks are recurrent obsessions and/or compulsions severe enough to be time consuming (more than 1 h/day) or to interfere with occupational or social functioning. At some point, the individual must recognize that these symptoms are excessive or unreasonable (this does not apply to children), and, if another major psychiatric disorder is present, the content of the obsessions or compulsions must be unrelated to it. Finally, the OCD must not be a direct result of a drug or an underlying medical condition.

Obsessions are recurrent and persistent thoughts, impulses, or mental images that are experienced as intrusive and inappropriate, that cause marked anxiety and distress, and that are not simply excessive worries about real-life problems. The individual recognizes that the mental intrusions are a product of his or her own mind (this distinguishes them from psychotic symptoms such as thought insertion) and attempts to neutralize them with other thoughts or actions (for example, compulsive rituals). The content of obsessions is most often violent (for example, the murder of one's child), sexual, contaminative (for example, touching unclean objects), or doubting (for example, worrying repeatedly about having performed a particular act).

Compulsions are repetitive behaviors or mental acts engaged in to reduce anxiety or distress. Common compulsive behaviors are hand washing, ordering of objects, and repetitive checking (for example, a locked door); common mental acts are repetitive counting, praying, and saying words silently. The frequency and severity of these obsessions and compulsions as necessary for a diagnosis are a minimum for these activities; not infrequently, many hours each day are spent in the throes of OCD, and compulsions may be physically damaging (for example, washing one's hands until the skin is raw). As mentioned, the individual knows these are alien thoughts and behaviors and is distressed by them, but is powerless to moderate them.

There appear to be different OCD symptom profiles across subjects. An analysis of scores on the Yale-Brown Obsessive-Compulsive Scale in more than 300

OCD patients showed that there were four relatively independent clusters of symptoms: obsessions and checking, symmetry and order, cleaning and washing, and hoarding. Other recognized clinical variants include obsessional slowness (for example, taking several hours to perform routine bathing, grooming, and dressing each day) and obsessional rumination, commonly with a hypochondriacal theme. The background personality of individuals with OCD tends to be rigid and perfectionistic. The end result of severe OCD can be impressively bizarre behavior: the housewife who must purchase new china whenever guests are invited; the adult son who cannot join his parents for the weekend because he spends 12 hours checking that his house has been properly locked; the hoarder whose house is stuffed with trash and newspapers to the point that it is declared a fire hazard. At present, there are no laboratory tests that are diagnostic of OCD.

The lifetime prevalence of OCD is 2–3%; thus, it is not rare. OCD occurs equally in men and women and usually begins in early adulthood, although childhood OCD is not uncommon. It may co-occur with other psychiatric illnesses such as major depression, other anxiety disorders, and eating disorders. There is a high incidence of OCD (30–50%) in patients with Gilles de la Tourette syndrome, which consists of severe tics (sudden, involuntary muscle movements) and involuntary utterances, occasionally vulgar in nature. Tourette syndrome is quite rare, but approximately 5% of OCD patients may have some form of it, and 20–30% of OCD patients have a history of tics. Indeed, one formulation considers that an obsession is a psychic tic. OCD affects both twins more often in monozygotic (single-egg) twins than in dizygotic twins, and there is a higher incidence of OCD in first-degree relatives (parents, siblings, and children) of both OCD and Tourette syndrome patients than in the general population. OCD patients in stressful life situations often have a worsening of their symptoms, for example, more frequent intrusive obsessional thoughts or more frequent compulsive behaviors such as repetitive hand washing.

Biological Characteristics of OCD

Neurotransmitters (for example, serotonin, norepinephrine, and dopamine) are chemicals in the brain that are released by neurons and carry a chemical message across a short space (synapse) to activate receptors on downstream neurons. An interesting treatment finding is that OCD responds best to drugs that are serotonin uptake inhibitors (SUIs) in the brain. These drugs (for example, clomipramine, fluoxetine, paroxetine, sertraline, and fluvoxamine), block the serotonin transporter, which recycles the neurotransmitter serotonin from the synapse back into the nerve cell that released it. By blocking transporter uptake, these drugs increase synaptic serotonin concentrations, at least in the short term. This implies that reduced serotonin neurotransmission may be a neurochemical basis for OCD, but clear evidence of this, by measurement of serotonin or its metabolites, transport mechanisms, or receptors, has not yet been forthcoming.

Complicating this perspective is recent evidence that chronic treatment with an SUI completely blocks the rise of extracellular brain serotonin that occurs in response to stress. Serotonin is mainly an inhibitory neurotransmitter in the brain, especially in areas that are implicated in OCD, such as orbital prefrontal cortex and hippocampus. In these sites, serotonin reduces the firing of cortical pyramidal cells that are essential components of the cortico-striato-thalamo-cortical circuits now implicated in OCD and major depression. SUIs are most often used as antidepressants, and it is interesting that OCD and major depression, two illnesses with different symptom patterns (although occurring together in some patients), respond to treatment with the same drugs. The common factor is now considered to be that these disorders have a similar neuropathology that is expressed in functionally segregated neuronal circuits in the brain. Relief of OCD symptoms by SUIs is not complete (about 35% on average), and only about 50% of patients respond, suggesting that more than one brain neurotransmitter system may be involved. The addition of antipsychotic drugs (for example, haloperidol) that block dopamine receptors on neurons, thereby reducing dopamine neurotransmission, can be effective, certainly when there is a tic disorder associated with the OCD, and perhaps in cases refractory to SUI treatment. Other drugs useful in selected cases as adjuncts to treatment with SUIs are lithium (used most commonly to treat manic-depressive illness) and fenfluramine, a direct stimulator of serotonin receptors. Interestingly, dextroamphetamine, a dopamine and norepinephrine neurotransmission-potentiating drug, can reduce OCD symptoms in some patients.

Another aspect of OCD that supports an underlying brain abnormality is the presence of OCD-like disorders in other mammalian species, including subhuman primates, dogs, cats, horses, pigs, cows, sheep, bears, and parrots. Compulsive behaviors in these species include repetitive grooming to the point of skin damage; hair and feather pulling; tail chasing, pacing, whirling, bouncing, and somersaulting; sucking, bar biting, and lip flapping; compulsive sexual behaviors; aggression; checking; and territorial marking. Some equine and canine compulsive behaviors are familial and breed-specific, providing support for genetic factors in these conditions.

It cannot be determined which of these behaviors animals engage in to reduce anxiety or distress vs. which are distressing to the animal, but the animal is powerless to control them, the latter being a necessary criterion for the diagnosis of OCD in humans, as indicated previously. Some behaviors, such as pacing, whirling, and compulsive sexual activity, may be engaged in because a captive animal is deprived of necessary physical exercise and environmental stimulation, and these behaviors provide some degree of pleasure and relief from boredom. Nevertheless, some compulsive behaviors are pathological, such as acral lick in dogs, resulting in dermatitis, and avian compulsive feather picking. Several of these animal behaviors have been treated successfully with SUIs as well as with dopamine-blocking drugs.

The pharmacology of drugs useful in treating OCD points to which brain areas might be involved. Both the cerebral cortex of the frontal lobes (frontal cortex), which receives prominent serotonin connections from brain stem nuclei, and the basal ganglia, which receive dopamine connections from the substantia nigra, have been considered in OCD pathology. However, it should be noted that psychological treatments such as behavior therapy also can have a significant therapeutic effect, and brain imaging studies have shown that behavior therapy can induce changes in brain metabolism in OCD similar to those induced by drug therapy. Whether psychological therapy induces changes in neurotransmitter activity similar to those induced by pharmacotherapy is as yet unknown. In some instances of severe, incapacitating OCD that was unresponsive to all other treatments, stereotaxic cingulotomy (surgery that interrupts connections between the thalamus and the prefrontal cortex) has been effective. A significant minority of such patients experience gratifying clinical remission, but a partial response is equally common. Some 30–50% of patients, however, have little improvement from surgery.

Brain Circuit Theories of OCD

Brain circuit theories of OCD represent variations on the postulated involvement of certain areas of the frontal parts of the brain (frontal lobes) and their functional connections with deeper parts of the brain – the basal ganglia, thalamus, and other structures, including hippocampus and amygdala. There also are connections from these structures back to the cortex itself. In a general sense, the frontal lobes of the brain mediate executive functions, that is, an individual's decision-making and behavioral actions based on detailed evaluation of environmental demands, along with an appreciation of their historical context and a coordinated affective/emotional component. Particular areas of the frontal cortex mediate executive behavior, social behavior, and motivation.

The underlying theme of the brain circuit theories of OCD is that the lower, or orbital, frontal cortex is a generator of afferent impulses to the caudate nucleus, which is a part of the basal ganglia, and the caudate in turn serves as a filter or gating area. The caudate nucleus is considered to normally suppress extraneous thoughts, sensations, and actions, with little need for control by the frontal cortex. Some investigators have hypothesized a primary defect in caudate function in OCD, which leads to an increased requirement for the frontal cortex to suppress and emotionally neutralize intrusive neuronal activity. Other investigators have viewed overactivity of the orbital frontal–thalamic circuit as the cause of compulsions in OCD, since compulsions represent unmodulated behavioral drive. The functional result is that the caudate nucleus cannot reasonably filter all the neuronal impulses sent to it from frontal cortical areas; some inappropriate or otherwise innocuous stimuli therefore are passed on to other structures, where they acquire excessive emotional meaning that results in inappropriate thoughts and actions.

Electroencephalographic (brain wave) studies of OCD subjects undergoing cognitive neuropsychological testing also support involvement of the frontal lobes, and functional neuroimaging studies suggest increased blood flow and metabolic overactivity of the orbital frontal cortex. Imaging studies of the caudate nucleus are less consistent in their findings. Thus, it is not possible at present to determine from imaging studies where in the frontal cortical/caudate nucleus/thalamus/frontal cortical circuit the primary defect resides. Structural lesions (for example, strokes and tumors) of both the frontal cortex and the basal ganglia have been associated with obsessions and stereotyped behaviors resembling compulsions. And, as mentioned, drug treatments of OCD do not particularly clarify the matter, since alteration of cortical serotonergic systems with SUIs often results in only partial relief of symptoms, and dopamine-enhancing drugs, which act on caudate nucleus dopamine systems, have some role in the management of OCD symptoms, especially when there is associated tic disorder.

Current theories emphasize hyperactivation of the lateral orbitofrontal loop in OCD, with overactivity of the orbital frontal cortex, the anterior cingulate cortex (ACC), and the caudate nucleus. As indicated previously, these brain structures also have been implicated in major depression and anxiety disorders. The ACC has been further implicated in OCD through correlative functional magnetic resonance imaging (MRI) studies of ACC activity and error checking. Compared to normal control subjects, patients with OCD have excessive error-related activation of the rostral ACC, which is correlated with the severity of OCD symptoms. One of the primary executive functions of the ACC is error detection or mismatch recognition; dysfunction in this brain region might well be associated with the inability of OCD patients to achieve cognitive closure. Failure to achieve cognitive closure is precisely what they demonstrate in their inability to terminate rituals and obsessions despite intellectual awareness that these behaviors are not justified. For the OCD patient, it is never okay: there is always the possibility that he or she has failed to rule out some contingency. This cognitive style is also apparent in formal testing of, for example, deductive and inductive reasoning: Patients with OCD have no problem with deductive reasoning, but they are significantly impaired on inductive reasoning tasks.

Neuropsychological Testing in OCD

Neuropsychological tests can tap some of the components of frontal lobe function, but it is difficult to implicate the involvement of a particular area of the frontal lobes in OCD from impaired performance on a specific neuropsychological test. Studies indicate deficits in OCD patients' ability to shift task set. This is consistent with theories of disrupted response feedback, in which repeated compulsive acts are required to determine their adequacy. An inherent need for high accuracy in a given individual may aggravate the tendency to lose response feedback, setting up the repetitive behavioral pattern.

Another issue is whether neuropsychological deficits or changes in brain metabolic activity appears first. Altered metabolic activity may result in the behavioral and neuropsychological test changes found in OCD, but it also may be true that the anxiety and need for absolute mastery caused by the illness itself underlie the increased cerebral metabolic activity noted on electroencephalogram (EEG) and functional neuroimaging studies.

Neuroimaging Studies in OCD

With the advent of neuroimaging techniques, it now is possible to probe the structure and function of the living human brain. Brain structure can be viewed with x-ray computed tomography (CT) and MRI. Nuclear medicine techniques such as single-photon and positron-emission computed tomography (SPECT and PET) allow the visualization and quantitation of regional cerebral blood flow, glucose metabolic rate, and neurotransmitter receptor occupancy, which are indirect probes of regional neuronal function. SPECT and PET use radiolabeled compounds as tracers; as these compounds decay, high-energy photons are emitted that are counted by external detectors. The distribution of the tracer molecules is computed, and cross-sectional images of the brain are created in which image brightness is proportional to the underlying physiological process being measured.

Studies of brain structure with CT and MRI in OCD patients have not demonstrated consistent abnormalities. Most of these studies, however, focused on the caudate nucleus or lateral cerebral ventricles; less attention has been paid to the frontal lobes. Taken together, the findings suggest that structural abnormalities may be more associated with subtle neurological deficits accompanying OCD in some patients than with the disorder itself.

In contrast to the contradictory data from structural imaging studies, a consistent finding in SPECT and PET functional neuroimaging studies of OCD has been increased frontal cortical blood flow and glucose metabolism (hyperfrontality), although the precise cortical location has varied. The hyperfrontality does not seem to be a reflection of heightened anxiety in OCD patients. On the other hand, a relationship may exist between OCD hyperfrontality and serotonin neurotransmitter dysfunction. SUIs not only reduce OCD symptoms, but also alleviate the hyperfrontality, as shown by SPECT and PET.

A tendency toward lateralized right frontal hyperactivity in OCD also has been noted. Right frontal hypermetabolism in OCD is consistent with theories of frontal emotional lateralization. The right frontal cortex is considered to play a greater role in perception of and reaction to negative primary emotions and stimuli, whereas the left frontal cortex may be more active in response to positive stimuli and positive social emotions. The inability of OCD patients to suppress negative primary emotions and thoughts occurs along with their right frontal hyperactivity. A similar formulation of predominantly right prefrontal activity has been advanced for major depression. Suppression of right hemisphere cerebral activity, either with the Wada test (transient suppression of a cerebral hemisphere by barbiturate injection into the same-sided carotid artery) or as a result of lesions, is associated with decreased apprehension, euphoric mood, and minimization of negative emotions, while left hemisphere suppression produces feelings of depression, guilt, and worries about the future. With regard to basal ganglia function, neither structural nor functional neuroimaging studies strongly substantiate the hypothesis of a caudate abnormality in OCD. They do not rule out this possibility, but rather indicate that whatever abnormality might exist has not been consistently seen with current functional neuroimaging technology.

Conclusions

There is considerable variation in obsessive and compulsive symptoms, ranging from normal time-limited worry, through obsessive–compulsive personality disorder, to self-consuming OCD. The criteria for OCD represent a consensus statement among mental health professionals, based not only on the nature of the OCD symptoms but also on their frequency and interference with social and occupational functioning. OCD thus remains an arbitrarily defined syndrome, no matter how much expertise underlies the definition, so long as there are insufficient empirical data to validate its qualitative difference from obsessive–compulsive personality disorder, as well as from other major anxiety syndromes.

While animal models of OCD provide an interesting theoretical perspective, as noted earlier, this analogy also suffers from a certain nonspecificity. Repetitive behaviors such as pacing, whirling, hitting oneself, toe walking, and rocking, as well as increased anxiety, also are common symptoms of autism, a pervasive developmental disorder that begins in early childhood and persists into adult life. In autistic adults, dietary tryptophan depletion, which depletes brain serotonin, increases these repetitive behaviors, and treatment with SUIs decreases them. This suggests an involvement of brain serotonin neurotransmitter systems in autism similar to that in OCD.

It is interesting to speculate on the opposite of OCD, that is, excessive neglect in conducting one's activities of daily living. A large segment of society fails to adequately check their surroundings and to protect themselves from even known threats. Preventable accidents are a leading cause of mortality and morbidity, and epidemics of avoidable diseases such as AIDS are only too well known. This can be considered inappropriate denial of dangerous situations that have the potential to cause real harm to the individual. However, we approach inappropriate denial and risk taking only from a cognitive, educational standpoint, for example, trying to convince persons at risk to just say no. Perhaps our relative failure to make headway with such an approach suggests that we should take a fresh, psychobiological look at this aspect of behavior. For example, how is compulsive risk taking psychobiologically similar to or different from compulsive checking and hand washing? Psychologically they could be viewed as opposite ends of a spectrum, the former representing pathological self-neglect and the latter pathological self-protection. These and other issues remain the exciting areas of future research into OCD.

Acknowledgment

This work was supported by NIH grant MH28380.

See Also the Following Articles

Depression and Manic–Depressive Illness.

Further Reading

American Psychiatric Association. (1994). *Diagnostic and statistical manual of mental disorders* (4th edn.). (DSM-IV). Washington, D.C.: American Psychiatric Association.

Barr, L. C., Goodman, W. K., Price, L. H., McDougle, C. J. and Charney, D. S. (1992). The serotonin hypothesis of obsessive compulsive disorder: implications of pharmacologic challenge studies. *Journal of Clinical Psychiatry* **53**(Supplement), 17–28.

Chamberlain, S. R., Blackwell, A. D., Fineberg, N. A., Robbins, T. W. and Sahakian, B. J. (2005). The neuropsychology of obsessive compulsive disorder: the importance of failures in cognitive and behavioral inhibition as candidate endophenotypic markers. *Neuroscience and Biobehavioral Reviews* **29**, 399–419.

Cummings, J. L. (1995). Anatomic and behavioral aspects of frontal-subcortical circuits. *Annals of the New York Academy of Science* **769**, 1–13.

Denys, D., Zohar, J. and Westenberg, H. G. M. (2004). The role of dopamine in obsessive-compulsive disorder: preclinical and clinical evidence. *Journal of Clinical Psychiatry* (Supplement 14), 11–17.

Dodman, N. H., Moon-Fanelli, A., Mertens, P. A., Pflueger, S. and Stein, D. J. (1997). Veterinary models of OCD. In: Hollander, E. & & Stein, D. J. (eds.) *Obsessive-compulsive disorder*, pp. 99–144. New York: Mrcel Dekker.

Fitzgerald, K. D., Welsh, R. C., Gehring, W. J., et al. (2005). Error-related hyperactivity in the anterior cingulate cortex in obsessive-compulsive disorder. *Biological Psychiatry* **57**, 287–294.

Hoehn-Saric, R. and Benkelfat, C. (1994). Structural and functional brain imaging in obsessive-compulsive disorder. In: Hollander, E., Zohar, J., Marazziti, D. & & Olivier, B. (eds.) *Current insights in obsessive-compulsive disorder*, pp. 183–211. New York: Wiley.

Jenike, M. A. (1995). Obsessive-compulsive disorder. In: Kaplan, H. I. & & Sdock, B. J. (eds.) *Comprehesive textbook of psychiatry* (6th en.,pp. 1218–1227). Williams & Wilkins: Baltimore, MD.

Jenike, M. A. (2004). Obsessive-compulsive disorder. *New England Journal of Medicine* **350**, 259–265.

McGuire, P. K., Bench, C. J., Frith, C. D., et al. (1994). Functional anatomy of obsessive-compulsive phenomena. *British Journal of Psychiatry* **164**, 459–468.

Otto, M. W. (1992). Normal and abnormal information processing: a neuropsychological perspective on obsessive-compulsive disorder. *Psychiatry Clinics of North America* **15**, 825–848.

Pelissier, M. C. and O'Connor, K. P. (2002). Deductive and inductive reasoning in obsessive-compulsive disorder. *British Journal of Clinical Psychology* **41**(Part 1), 15–27.

Rubin, R. T. and Harris, G. J. (1999). Obsessive-compulsive disorder and the frontal lobes. In: Miller, B. L. & & Cummings, J. L. (eds.) *The hum frontal lobes: functions andisorders*, pp. 522–536. New York: Guilford.

Rubin, R. T., Villanueva-Meyer, J., Ananth, J., Trajmar, P. G. and Mena, I. (1992). Regional xenon 133 cerebral blood flow and cerebral technetium 99m HMPAO uptake in unmedicated patients with obsessive-compulsive disorder and matched control subjects. *Archives of General Psychiatry* **49**, 695–702.

Saxena, S., Brody, A. L., Schwartz, J. M. and Baxter, L. R. (1998). Neuroimaging and frontal-subcortical circuitry in obsessive-compulsive disorder. *British Journal of Psychiatry* **173**(Supplement 35), 26–37.

Zielinski, C. M., Taylor, M. A. and Juzwin, K. R. (1991). Neuropsychological deficits in obsessive-compulsive disorder. *Neuropsychiatry, Neuropsychology, and Behavioral Neurology* **4**, 110–126.

D. Posttraumatic Stress Disorder

Acute Stress Disorder and Posttraumatic Stress Disorder

R Yehuda and C M Wong
Mt. Sinai School of Medicine and Bronx Veterans Affairs, New York, NY, USA

This article is reproduced from Encyclopedia of Stress First Edition, Volume 1, pp 1–7, © 2000, Elsevier Inc.

Glossary

Acute stress disorder A mental condition that can occur following exposure to extreme stress or trauma but by definition does not last longer than 1 month [i.e., after 1 month, if the symptoms persist, it is appropriate to consider the diagnosis of posttraumatic stress disorder (PTSD)].

Avoidant symptoms Experiences that represent measures taken by the individual to avoid feeling, thinking, or coming into contact with reminders of the trauma; these experiences can also include having difficulty recalling important events of the trauma, avoiding people and places associated with the trauma, and generally feelings of emotional numbness, detachment from others, and feeling like there is no future.

Depersonalization An alteration in the perception or experience of the self so that one feels detached from, and, as if one is an outside observer of, one's mental processes or body (e.g., feeling like one is in a dream).

Derealization An alteration in the perception or experience of the external world so that it seems strange or unreal (e.g., people may seem unfamiliar or mechanical).

Dissociation A disruption in the usually integrated functions of consciousness, memory, identity, or perception of the environment. The disturbance may be sudden or gradual, transient, or chronic.

Dysphoria An unpleasant mood such as sadness, anxiety, or irritability.

Flashback A recurrence of a memory, feeling, or perceptual experience from the past.

Hyperarousal symptoms Experiences that involve more physical reactions to trauma, including difficulty with sleep and concentration, irritability, and anger, needing to be on guard overly much, and having an exaggerated startle response to unexpected noises.

Intrusive symptoms Experiences in which trauma survivors relive the trauma or become distressed by reminders of the trauma. These include unwanted thoughts and images, nightmares and bad dreams, extreme distress when exposed to a trigger or reminder, and a physiological response to triggers, including palpitations, sweating, and shortness of breath.

Posttraumatic stress disorder A mental condition that can occur following exposure to extreme stress or trauma and lasts for 1 month or longer. Acute PTSD lasts from 1 to 3 months according to current formulations in the DSM-IV. Chronic PTSD lasts 3 or more months according to current formulations in the DSM-IV. In delayed onset PTSD, the onset of symptoms begins 6 or more months after the traumatic event(s) according to current formulations in the DSM-IV.

Stressor In this context, it is a life event or life change that is so challenging as to potentially be associated with the onset, occurrence, or exacerbation of a psychological symptom or a mental disorder.

Traumatic event According to DSM-IV, an experience that involves death or serious injury or another threat to one's physical integrity. A person does not need to actually experience the physical injury to be traumatized – just the knowledge that a person could have been severely injured or had a serious threat of injury and the feelings that accompany this realization are enough to produce a posttraumatic reaction.

Both acute stress disorder (ASD) and posttraumatic stress disorder (PTSD) are conditions that can occur in people who have been exposed to a traumatic life event. Traumatic events are thought to occur in at least 50% of the population. A traumatic event is defined in the *American Psychiatric Association's Diagnostic and Statistical Manual for Mental Disorders*, 4th edn (DSM-IV) as an experience in which a person underwent, witnessed, or was confronted with "an event that involved actual or threatened death or serious injury, or a threat to the physical integrity of self or others" and a subjective response of "intense fear, helplessness, or horror." The definition of trauma is purposely identical for both ASD and PTSD because what differentiates the two conditions is the point in time following the event at which the symptoms are experienced. Not all people who have experienced trauma will develop ASD and/or PTSD. ASD defines the immediate response to trauma for up to 4 weeks posttrauma, whereas PTSD encompasses a more chronic response to trauma beginning 1 month after the trauma and lasting at least 1 month after that. Recent estimates suggest that as much as 14% of persons in the United States will develop these conditions at some point during their lives. Given the chronic nature of PTSD and the extreme disability that can be associated with this condition, this statistic is alarming and points to PTSD as a major public health problem.

Introduction

Posttraumatic stress disorder was originally defined in 1980 to describe long-lasting symptoms that occur in response to trauma. The diagnosis revived psychiatry's long-standing interest in how stress can result in behavioral and biological changes that ultimately lead to disorder. At the time the formal diagnosis of PTSD was being conceptualized, the field was focused heavily on describing the psychological consequences of combat Vietnam veterans and others who had chronic symptoms following exposure to events that had occurred years and even decades earlier. It was widely assumed that the symptoms that persisted in these survivors were extensions of those that were present in the earlier aftermath of a traumatic event. Indeed, some data from recently traumatized burn victims supported the idea that symptoms such as intrusive thoughts were present in the early aftermath of a trauma. However, at the time the diagnosis was established, there were no longitudinal data – either retrospective or prospective – that formally established the relationship between acute vs chronic posttraumatic symptoms.

Chronic PTSD was not initially conceptualized as being qualitatively different from what might have been observable in trauma survivors in the acute aftermath of the trauma. Rather, chronic PTSD suggested a failure of restitution of the stress response. The implicit assumption behind the diagnosis was that most trauma survivors initially developed symptoms as a direct result from exposure to the event.

As the awareness of the longterm effects of trauma became more widespread, investigators began to explore the reaction of trauma survivors in the immediate aftermath of the event. Studies of the acutely traumatized revealed that survivors do experience symptoms in the immediate aftermath. Clinicians felt it important to provide mental health interventions as early as possible so as to perhaps prevent the development of more chronic conditions. ASD first appeared as a diagnosis in the DSM-IV in 1994 in order to provide a diagnosis for people before they were eligible to receive the diagnosis of PTSD (i.e., having symptoms for less than 1 month's duration). Thus, ASD arose in part out of the need for justification for acute intervention. However, as described later, the syndrome of ASD has features that are not directly associated with the more chronic response of PTSD.

One of the important findings to be generated from research in the last two decades is that PTSD does not occur in everyone exposed to trauma, nor is PTSD the only possible response to trauma. Prospective longitudinal studies have now demonstrated that mood and other anxiety disorders can also occur following a traumatic event, and these may be present even in the absence of PTSD. The question of why some people develop PTSD and others do not has not been fully resolved and is the subject of current investigation in the field. However, insofar as this condition no longer serves to characterize a universal stress response, it has been important to redefine the nature of traumatic stress responses and determine the risk factors for developing these conditions. It has also been important to consider the relationship between acute and chronic stress response.

Relationship between Acute Stress Disorder (ASD) and Posttraumatic Stress Disorder (PTSD)

Figure 1 shows a time continuum that describes the onsets of ASD and acute, chronic, and delayed PTSD. In ASD, symptoms must last for at least 2 days up to 4 weeks. In PTSD, the symptoms last for a period of at least a month following the traumatic event(s) and can be either acute (symptom duration of 3 months or less) or chronic (symptom duration of more than 3 months). The onset of PTSD can be delayed for months and even years.

Proponents of ASD hoped the diagnosis would help survivors mobilize acute intervention, thereby preventing more chronic disability. The idea of an acute stress disorder was initially considered to be superfluous with the diagnosis of adjustment disorder, which was defined in 1980 to describe early symptoms after any stressful event. The proponents of ASD, however, were interested in emphasizing that, unlike adjustment disorders that were expected to resolve even without treatment, ASD was expected to develop into PTSD. Furthermore, ASD focused on a different set of symptoms that were precursors of PTSD such as dissociation.

Indeed, the symptom of dissociation is a prominent difference between ASD and adjustment disorder. Interestingly, dissociation per se is not a symptom of PTSD. However, there is much support for the idea that if people dissociate at the time of trauma, they are at an increased risk to develop PTSD (**Table 1**).

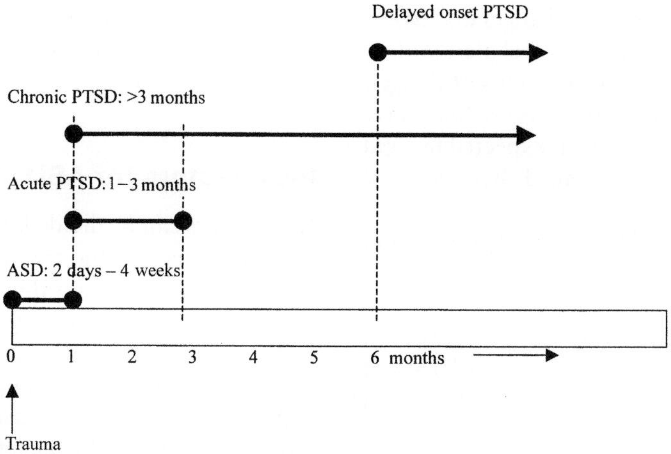

Figure 1 Time line comparing ASD and PTSD.

Table 1 Comparison of symptoms of adjustment disorder, ASD, and PTSD

Adjustment disorder	*ASD*	*PTSD*
With anxiety	Intrusive reexperiencing	Intrusive reexperiencing
With depression	Avoidance	Avoidance
With mixed anxiety and depression	Hyperarousal	Hyperarousal
With disturbance of conduct		
With mixed disturbance of emotions and conduct	Dissociation	
	Subjective sense of numbing, detachment, or absence of emotional responsiveness	
	A reduction in awareness of his or her surroundings (e.g., being in a daze)	
	Derealization	
	Depersonalization	
	Dissociative amnesia (i.e., inability to recall an important aspect of the trauma)	

Most studies examining the relationship between dissociation at the time of a trauma and development of PTSD have been retrospective, in some studies, assessing the dissociation 25 years after the traumatic experiences. This means that assessment of dissociation is based largely on subjective recollections of victims. However, in studies that have been prospective, peritraumatic dissociation was still found to be one of the best predictors of PTSD 6 months and 1 year following the trauma in a group of mixed civilian trauma. Posttraumatic depression was also a good predictor for the occurrence of PTSD at 1 year. This would perhaps support the idea of including dissociation as a criterion for ASD given its predictive property for the future development of PTSD.

ASD and PTSD are both characterized by the development of intrusive, avoidant, and hyperarousal symptomatology following a traumatic event. These three symptom clusters represent different expressions of the response to trauma.

Intrusive symptoms describe experiences in which the survivor relives the event in their mind. After a traumatic event, it is common for the survivor to have thoughts of the event appear in one's mind and to think about the event despite not wanting to. Frightening thoughts or nightmares about the event are also common, and the person may feel very distressed. Sometimes a survivor may even have physical symptoms such as heart palpitations, sweating, and an increased breathing rate in response to being reminded of the event.

In addition to experiencing one or more of the just-mentioned intrusive symptoms, the survivor may make one or more attempts to avoid being reminded of the traumatic experience. The individual may go out of her way to avoid being in situations that remind her of the event. The individual may forget details about the traumatic event. The survivor may also experience a more generalized feeling of wanting to shut out the world, which is manifested by a feeling of emotional numbness and an inability to connect with others.

Finally, the trauma survivor may experience a range of more physiological symptoms, such as an inability to sleep, inability to concentrate, and anger and irritability. The individual may constantly feel alert and on guard, scanning the environment for signs of danger. The survivor may be very sensitive to noises and have an exaggerated startle response to unexpected or loud sounds. These symptoms are called hyperarousal symptoms.

The conceptualization of ASD remains in evolution at the writing of this volume. The salient question is whether ASD is really a disorder that indicates a deviation from a normative response to stress. To the extent that ASD is a good predictor of PTSD, it may be that this syndrome captures elements of a maladaptive response.

Epidemiology

In considering the prevalence rates of ASD and PTSD, the main observation is that neither are inevitable responses to stress.

The range of prevalence rates of ASD for various types of trauma, including traumatic brain injury (TBI), disasters, and shootings, ranges from 7.2 to 33%, which interestingly are about the same as those for PTSD (see later).

The range of prevalence rates of PTSD in trauma survivors in DSM-IV is 3–58%. This great variation is thought to reflect mostly a difference in the type and quality of the trauma experienced. However, it may also reflect study methodology (i.e., whether people were evaluated in person or on the phone; whether they were selected randomly or from a convenience sample, and/or whether the study was conducted in the immediate aftermath of the trauma or years later). Studies have found that there were differences in the rates of PTSD depending on the type of trauma experienced. For example, 65% of men and 45.9% of women with PTSD reported rape as their most upsetting trauma. Other types of trauma associated with high probabilities of PTSD development include combat exposure (38.8%), childhood neglect (23.9%) and childhood physical abuse (22.3%) in men, and sexual molestation (26.5%), physical attack (21.3%), being threatened by a weapon (32.6%), and childhood physical abuse (48.5%) in women.

In the aggregate, PTSD is estimated to occur on average in 25% of individuals who have been exposed to traumatic events with rates considerably higher for life-threatening events than for those with lower impact. Lifetime prevalence of exposure to at least one traumatic event was also found to range from 40 to 55% in various studies. In the National Comorbidity Survey (NCS), it was found that about 8% of the population were exposed to four or more types of trauma, some of which involved multiple occurrences. The lifetime prevalence of PTSD has consistently been demonstrated to be twice as high in women as in men.

Risk Factors for ASD and PTSD

Risk factors can be divided into two broad categories: those pertinent to the traumatic event (e.g., severity or type of trauma) and those relevant to individuals who experience the event (e.g., gender, prior experiences, personality characteristics). Although some risk factors for PTSD appear to be related to prior experiences, data have also emerged implicating biological and possibly genetic risk factors for PTSD.

Risk factors for the development of ASD include female gender, high depression scores in the immediate aftermath of the event, an avoidant coping style, and the severity of the traumatic event. These are similar to the risk factors that have been associated with the development of chronic PTSD. However, it should be noted that this has not been an area of extensive study.

Risk factors for PTSD also include female gender, posttraumatic depression, an avoidant coping style, and the severity of trauma. However, additional risk factors have also been noted, such as a history of stress, abuse, or trauma, a history of behavioral or psychological problems, preexisting psychiatric disorders, a family history of psychopathology, genetic factors, subsequent exposure to reactivating environmental factors, initial psychological reaction to trauma such as emotional numbing, early separation, preexisting anxiety and depressive disorders, and depression at the time of trauma. Parental PTSD has also been found to be a risk factor for the development of PTSD.

Comorbid Disorders

PTSD rarely occurs in the absence of other conditions. Approximately 50–90% of individuals with chronic PTSD have a psychiatric comorbidity. This reinforces the idea that PTSD is not distributed randomly throughout the population, but rather that there are subgroups of people that are more vulnerable to the development of PTSD and other psychiatric disorders. This also raises the question of whether PTSD develops as a separate disorder from other psychiatric comorbidities seen in association from it or whether people who have these constellations of disorders are more likely to get PTSD.

Common comorbidities in PTSD patients include major depressive disorder, alcoholism, drug abuse, personality disorders, anxiety disorders such as panic disorder, and generalized anxiety disorder and dissociative disorder.

Symptoms of depression are observed frequently in trauma survivors with PTSD. A significant correlation between early PTSD symptoms and the occurrence of depression seems to predict the chronicity of PTSD. The sequence in which PTSD and major depressive disorder (MDD) occurs following trauma is of particular interest. Some studies proposed that depression is "secondary" to PTSD because its onset followed that of PTSD. In the NCA, patients with comorbid PTSD and MDD reported that the onset of the mood disorder followed that of PTSD in 78.4% of the sample. Vietnam veterans also reported that the onset of their phobias, MDD, and panic disorder followed that of the PTSD. Retrospective studies were flawed in that patients may not recall accurately which symptom came first after being symptomatic for decades. In contrast, Israeli combat veterans reported a simultaneous onset of PTSD and MDD in 65% of the sample, with 16% reported having the MDD precede the PTSD.

In a groundbreaking prospective, longitudinal study, it was demonstrated that the presence of depression in the early aftermath of a trauma was associated with the subsequent development of PTSD. These data contradict the notion that comorbid conditions in PTSD reflect secondary consequences of the PTSD symptoms and suggest instead that other psychiatric symptoms influence the presence of PTSD symptoms. Indeed, a history of previous psychiatric symptoms is a predictor of PTSD, but posttraumatic symptoms may also be strong predictors.

Biological Findings in ASD and PTSD

One of the most provocative observations in both ASD and PTSD that has emerged is that the biological findings do not conform to classic patterns of biological stress responses that have been described in animal and human models of the stress response. This is particularly true in the area of neuroendocrinology of PTSD. The distinctness in the biology of PTSD and stress further supports the idea that PTSD represents a circumscribed and specific response to a traumatic event that may be different from a normative response in which the reaction does not reach a certain magnitude or, if it does, becomes attenuated quickly.

There have been only a few studies of the biology of ASD; however, the biological alterations in ASD seem to resemble those in PTSD. First and foremost, there has been a demonstration of the enhanced negative feedback inhibition of the hypothalamic-pituitary-adrenal (HPA) axis, similar to findings in PTSD (see later). At 2 weeks posttrauma, rape victims who subsequently recovered from ASD at 3 months showed a "normal" response to dexamethasone administration, whereas rape victims who failed to recover from ASD at 3 months showed a hypersuppression of cortisol on the dexamethasone suppression test (DST).

In another study, women with a prior history of rape or assault had significantly lower cortisol levels in the immediate aftermath of rape compared to those who did not. A past history of rape or assault is generally considered to be a potent predictor for the development of PTSD. In a study of motor vehicle accident victims, a lower cortisol response in the immediate aftermath of the trauma was associated with the presence of PTSD at 6 months, whereas higher cortisol levels at the time of the trauma were associated with the development of depression at 6 months. These data indicate that it might be possible to identify high-risk ASD patients through biological means.

In PTSD, there have been far more studies that have yielded fairly consistent results. The studies demonstrate a different profile of HPA alterations in PTSD compared to that in other psychiatric disorders such as major depression. In the aggregate, these studies have demonstrated a hypersensitization of the HPA axis to stress that is manifested by a decreased cortisol release and an increased negative feedback inhibition. Hypersecretion of the corticotropin-releasing hormone (CRH) has also been described in PTSD, as has blunting of the adrenocorticotropic hormone (ACTH) response to CRH. Other studies have demonstrated lower 24-h urinary cortisol excretion levels in PTSD patients compared to other psychiatric groups and normal controls. PTSD subjects have also been shown to have lower plasma cortisol levels in the morning and at several time points throughout the circadian cycle and to have a greater circadian signal-to-noise ratio compared to normal controls.

In addition, studies support the notion that the enhanced negative feedback regulation of cortisol is an important feature of PTSD. PTSD subjects have an increased number of lymphocyte glucocorticoid receptors (which are needed for cortisol to exert its effects) compared to psychiatric and nonpsychiatric control groups and show an enhanced suppression of cortisol in response to dexamethasone. This response is distinctly different from that found in depression and other psychiatric disorders.

There have been numerous other systems studies in PTSD such as the sympathetic nervous system, the serotonergic system, and the immune system. Psychophysiological, neuroanatomical, cognitive, and behavioral alterations have also been noted; however, it is beyond the scope of this volume to encompass and discuss all these findings.

Treatment of ASD and PTSD

There are several types of specialized treatments that have been developed in recent years to address the specific needs of trauma survivors who suffer from both ASD and PTSD. These treatments include cognitive behavioral therapy, psychotherapy, group therapy, and medication therapy. Chronic PTSD appears to be more resistant to treatment than acute PTSD. It is usually necessary to employ a combination of therapies in the treatment for PTSD, but the success rate of specialized trauma-focused treatment is quite encouraging.

Summary

ASD and PTSD represent responses that can occur following exposure to traumatic events. To date, it is useful to conceptualize ASD and PTSD as two distinct conditions that are very much related. ASD often but not always leads to a development of PTSD. ASD and PTSD seem to share similar symptoms, prevalence, risk factors, and neurobiological alterations. ASD appears to be easier to treat than chronic PTSD, which suggests that it is probably useful to treat traumatic stress symptoms earlier rather than later in the course of adaptation to trauma.

Acknowledgments

This work was supported by NIMH R-02 MH 49555 (RY), Merit Review Funding (RY), and APA/PMRTP 5T32-MH-19126-09/10 (CMW), and VA-Research Career Development award (CMW).

See Also the Following Articles

Posttraumatic Stress Disorder in Children; Posttraumatic Stress Disorder, Delayed.

Further Reading

Andreasen, N. C. (1980). Posttraumatic stress disorder. In: Kaplan, J. L., Freedman, A. M. & Saddock, B. J. (eds.) *Comprehensive Textbook of Psychiatry* (3rd edn. Vol. 2), pp. 1517–1525. Baltimore: Williams & Wilkins.

Breslau, N., Davis, G. C., Andreski, P., Peterson, E. L. and Schultz, L. R. (1997). Sex differences in posttraumatic stress disorder. *Archives of General Psychiatry* **54**, 1044–1048.

Foa, E. B. (ed.) (1993). *Posttraumatic Stress Disorder. DSM-IV and Beyond.* Washington, DC: American Psychiatric Press.

Friedman, M. J., Charney, D. S. and Deutch, A. Y. (eds.) (1995). *Neurobiological and Clinical Consequences of Stress: From Normal Adaptation to Post-traumatic Stress Disorder.* Hagerstown, MD: Lippincott-Raven.

Kessler, R. C., Sonnega, A., Bromet, E. and Nelson, C. B. (1995). Posttraumatic stress disorder in the National Comorbidity Survey. *Archives of General Psychiatry* **52**, 1048–1060.

Shalev, A. Y., Freeman, S., Peri, T., Brandes, D., Shahar, T., Orr, S. P. and Pitman, R. I. K. (1998). Prospective study of posttraumatic stress disorder and depression following trauma. *American Journal of Psychiatry* **155**, 630–637.

Yehuda, R. (ed.) (1998). *Psychological Trauma.* Washington, DC: American Psychiatric Press.

Yehuda, R. (ed.) (1999). *Risk Factors for Posttraumatic Stress Disorder. Progress in Psychiatry Series.* Washington, DC: American Psychiatric Press.

Yehuda, R. and McFarlane, A. C. (eds.) (1997). *Psychobiology of Posttraumatic Stress Disorder.* New York: New York Academy of Sciences.

Posttraumatic Stress Disorder in Children

A M La Greca
University of Miami, Coral Gables, FL, USA

This is a revised version of the article by A M La Greca, Encyclopedia of Stress First Edition, volume 3, pp 181–185, © 2000, Elsevier Inc.

Glossary

Avoidance or numbing — Refers to symptoms of posttraumatic stress syndrome (PTSD), such as avoiding thoughts, feelings, or conversations about the traumatic event, avoiding reminders of the event, diminished interest in normal activities, or feeling detached or removed from others.

Hyperarousal — Refers to symptoms of PTSD, such as difficulty sleeping or concentrating, irritability, angry outbursts, hypervigilance, and an exaggerated startle response.

Life threat — The perception that one's life is in danger; it is a key aspect of exposure to traumatic events, and is believed to be critical for the emergence of PTSD and related symptoms.

Loss and disruption — Loss (of family and friends, of personal property and possessions) and disruption of everyday life (displacement from home, school, or community); it is also an aspect of exposure to traumatic events and can contribute to PTSD in children.

Re-experiencing — Refers to symptoms of PTSD, such as recurrent or intrusive thoughts or dreams about the event, or intense distress at cues or reminders of the event.

Posttraumatic stress disorder (PTSD) refers to a set of symptoms that develop following exposure to an unusually severe stressor or event. Typically, the event is one that causes or is capable of causing death, injury, or threat to the physical integrity of oneself or another person. In order to meet criteria for a diagnosis of PTSD, a child's reaction to the traumatic event must include intense fear, helplessness, or disorganized behavior. In addition, specific criteria for three additional symptom clusters must be met: re-experiencing, avoidance/numbing, and hyperarousal. Re-experiencing includes symptoms such as recurrent or intrusive thoughts or dreams about the event and intense distress at cues or reminders of the event; for young children, re-experiencing also may be reflected in repetitive play with traumatic themes or by a re-enactment of traumatic events in play, drawings, or verbalizations. Avoidance or numbing includes symptoms such as efforts to avoid thoughts, feelings, or conversations about the traumatic event, avoiding reminders of the event, diminished interest in normal activities, and feeling detached or removed from others. Hyperarousal symptoms include difficulty sleeping or concentrating, irritability, angry outbursts, hypervigilance, and an exaggerated startle response; these behaviors must be newly occurring since the event. For a diagnosis of PTSD, the above symptoms must be manifest for at least 1 month, and be accompanied by significant impairment in the child's functioning (e.g., problems in school, friendships, or family relations). In addition, acute PTSD is specified if the duration of the symptoms is less than 3 months; chronic PTSD is specified if the duration of symptoms is 3 months or longer.

Traumatic Events

In recent years, media coverage of devastating natural disasters, bombings, and terrorist activities has drawn attention to the significant trauma that children and adults experience following such events. It has become increasingly apparent that exposure of children to such traumatic events may lead to reactions that interfere substantially with their day-to-day functioning and cause them significant distress. Specifically, exposure to natural disasters (e.g., hurricanes, tsunamis, tornadoes, fires, earthquakes, or floods) and to human-made disasters and acts of violence (e.g., plane crashes, sinking of ferrys, war, terrorist attacks, bombings, sniper shootings) represent traumatic events that may result in the emergence of PTSD. Although considerable attention has been devoted to the effects of terrorism and community-wide disasters, it is also the case that children who experience motor vehicle accidents, life-threatening illnesses or medical procedures, or violence of a personal nature (e.g., physical and sexual abuse, rape, kidnapping, and community violence) also are vulnerable to developing PTSD. This article describes common symptoms of PTSD in children and factors that contribute to the development and course of this disorder.

Posttraumatic Stress Disorder in Children: Clinical Picture

The diagnostic category of PTSD was introduced in the third edition of the American Psychiatric Association's *Diagnostic and Statistical Manual of Mental Disorders* (DSM-III). At that time, PTSD was primarily considered to be an adult disorder. More recently, there has been a growing awareness that children and adolescents also experience PTSD, which is reflected in the current edition of the DSM (DSM-IV). (See previous description of the criteria for the disorder.)

Community studies of children following traumatic events suggest that the most commonly reported PTSD symptoms are those of re-experiencing the event. For example, up to 90% of children exposed to a catastrophic hurricane reported symptoms of re-experiencing 3 months after the disaster. In contrast, symptoms of avoidance and numbing are far less common in children and, in fact, their presence may be a good indicator of PTSD.

Due to their limited verbal capacity, the diagnosis of PTSD is especially difficult in very young children, such as infants, toddlers, and early preschoolers. In such cases, generalized anxiety, fears, avoidance of certain situations that may be linked to the traumatic event, and sleep disturbances may be useful indicators of PTSD.

PTSD may also be present (i.e., co-morbid) with other psychological difficulties. In particular, PTSD often is co-morbid with anxiety disorders (i.e., separation anxiety disorder, specific phobias, generalized anxiety disorder, panic, and agoraphobia) and with affective disorders (e.g., major depressive disorder and dysthymia). Traumatic events that involve the loss of loved ones (e.g., earthquakes and bombings) are especially likely to lead to depressive reactions in children.

Prevalence and Developmental Course

Prevalence

It is difficult to estimate the prevalence of PTSD in children and adolescents because studies have been extremely diverse with respect to the type of trauma evaluated, assessment methods used, and the length of time that passed since the traumatic event occurred. Community studies suggest that approximately 24–39% of children and adolescents exposed to trauma (e.g., community violence or a natural disaster) meet criteria for PTSD. Rates of PTSD have been reported to be even higher among children and adolescents who witness death or physical injury in conjunction with acts of violence or following disasters associated with mass casualties.

When subclinical levels of PTSD are considered, up to 55% of the children in large community samples have reported at least moderate levels of PTSD symptoms during the first 3 months following a traumatic event, such as a hurricane. Thus, symptoms of PTSD appear to be common among children exposed to trauma, although fewer children and youth will meet criteria for a PTSD diagnosis.

Developmental Course

Little is known about the course of PTSD symptoms in children over time. However, it does appear that PTSD symptoms may emerge in the days or weeks following a traumatic event, and can take months or years to dissipate in some children. In the absence of re-exposure to trauma or of the occurrence of other traumatic events, the typical developmental course of symptoms appears to be one of lessening frequency and intensity over time. For example, 3 months after a highly destructive natural disaster (Hurricane Andrew: a Category 5 hurricane, that struck South Florida in 1992), 39% of the children informally met criteria for PTSD disorder, but this was reduced to 24% at 7-months postdisaster, and to 18% by 10-months postdisaster. A subgroup of children who reported moderate-to-severe PTSD symptoms was followed 42 months postdisaster, revealing that 40% continued to report moderate-to-severe PTSD symptoms as well as impairment in their functioning; yet, almost none of the children who had mild or no symptoms at 10-months postdisaster reported any symptoms later on. Similarly, 51.5% of the adolescents who survived the sinking of the cruise ship Jupiter in 1988 (with 400 British school children on board) developed PTSD after the disaster, but 5–8 years later, only 17.5% still had PTSD.

These data suggest a steady reduction in the frequency and severity of PTSD and its symptoms over time (with no further exposure to similar trauma), although a significant minority of children and adolescents do not recover and continue to report substantial difficulties years later. The findings also indicate that it is highly unusual for children and adolescents to report significant symptoms of PTSD 1 year or more after a traumatic event, if they did not experience such symptoms closer to the event. Although there may be a brief period of shock or numbing, or sometimes elation and relief at still being alive, most children who develop PTSD will evidence stress symptoms within the first few months of the traumatic event.

Persistence of Symptoms

Overall, findings confirm that children's reactions to disasters and other traumatic events are not merely transitory feelings that dissipate quickly. On the contrary, they appear to linger and persist and are likely to cause distress to children and their families for some time. One factor that contributes to the persistence of PTSD symptoms in children over time is the occurrence of other significant life stressors. Children who encounter major life stressors (e.g., a death or illness in the family or parental divorce) in the months following a traumatic event, do not recover quickly, and report persistently high levels of PTSD symptoms over time.

Demographic Trends

Gender and Age

Some studies indicate that PTSD appears more frequently among girls than boys, but this has not consistently been the case. Preadolescent children may be more vulnerable to PTSD than older youths, although it is difficult to draw generalizations regarding children's vulnerability to PTSD at different ages, as findings on age-related differences have been inconsistent and may be influenced by diverse developmental manifestations of PTSD.

Ethnicity

PTSD appears to occur across diverse ethnic and cultural groups. Community studies suggests that minority youths exposed to severe natural disasters report more symptoms of PTSD and have a more difficult time recovering from such events than nonminority youths. It is possible that socioeconomic factors might account for such findings, in that children and families from minority backgrounds may have less financial resources or less adequate insurance to deal effectively and efficiently with the postdisaster rebuilding process.

This could prolong the period of life disruption and loss of possessions that ensues after destructive natural disasters.

Factors that Precipitate Posttraumatic Stress Disorder in Children

Exposure to Trauma

A wide range of traumatic events have been linked to the emergence of PTSD in children and adolescents. However, two key aspects of exposure to these traumatic events are thought to contribute to children's reactions: the presence or perception of life threat, and personal loss and disruption of everyday events.

The presence or perception of life threat is considered to be essential for the emergence of PTSD. It is easy to understand why children who witness or are exposed to acts of violence, such as sniper shootings or severe physical abuse by a caretaker, feel that their life is in danger. It is also the case, however, that catastrophic natural disasters or personal disasters (such as residential fires) can elicit perceptions of life threat in children, even if no one is injured or hurt. For example, although very few lives were lost in South Florida as a result of Hurricane Andrew, the extensive destruction of homes and property that occurred during the storm was terrifying to many children and adults. In one study, 60% of the children interviewed "thought that they were going to die" during the storm. Thus, perceptions of life threat can occur in the absence of actual loss of life or serious injury.

Evidence also underscores the importance of loss (of family and friends or personal property and possessions) and disruption of everyday life (displacement from home, school, or community) as contributing to PTSD in children. The life changes that result from this aspect of exposure to a traumatic event also predicts PTSD symptoms in children and adolescents.

The duration and intensity of life-threatening events are additional aspects of traumatic exposure associated with children's PTSD symptom severity. The prolonged nature of certain traumatic events (e.g., floods or child abuse) is very distressing to children when no immediate relief is in sight.

Role of Prior Psychological Functioning

Children with pre-existing psychological problems, especially anxiety, may be more vulnerable to developing PTSD following traumatic events. For example, children's anxiety levels 15 months before a traumatic event have been found to predict their levels of PTSD symptoms 3 and 7 months postdisaster, even when controlling for children's exposure to the event. This suggests that anxious children may have a vulnerability to PTSD, even if their degree of exposure to a trauma is relatively low. In addition, children who had greater levels of exposure to the disaster (i.e., more life threat or more loss/disruption) showed an increase in anxiety symptoms following the disaster relative to children with less disaster exposure. Other studies have shown predisaster levels of depression predicted postdisaster PTSD among adolescents exposed to a destructive natural disaster (earthquake).

Aspects of the Recovery Environment

Certain aspects of the posttrauma recovery environment may either contribute to the development and persistent of symptoms of PTSD, or may help to alleviate or mitigate such symptoms. Intervening life events/stressors and re-exposure to the traumatic event have been linked with greater persistence of PTSD and its symptoms among children and adolescents. In addition, parents' psychosocial functioning, including their levels of psychopathology and their own reactions to the disaster, are likely to affect children's postdisaster functioning. For example, mothers' distress in the aftermath of Hurricane Hugo, which struck Charleston South Carolina in 1989, was associated with the persistence of their children's postdisaster emotional difficulties. Other research has supported a linkage between children's symptoms of PTSD and parents' trauma-related symptoms. Finally, children with more negative coping strategies for dealing with stress (e.g., anger or blaming others) show greater persistence in their symptoms of PTSD over time.

In contrast, the availability of social support has been found to mitigate the impact of trauma on children. Following traumatic events, such as severe abuse or catastrophic disasters, children with higher levels of social support from significant others (parents, teachers, friends, and classmates) report fewer symptoms of PTSD than those with low levels of social support. Because of these findings, efforts to enhance the social support of children exposed to trauma, and to encourage adaptive coping skills, may be useful for strategies for interventions with children following traumatic events.

Assessing Posttraumatic Stress Disorder Symptoms in Children

Evaluating the presence of PTSD symptoms in children and adolescents can be challenging and will depend, to some extent, on the age or developmental level of the child. For children of elementary school age and older (i.e., 7 years and above), the child or adolescent is likely to be the best informant; parents often underestimate symptoms of PTSD in their children.

The use of child-oriented structured interviews that contain items pertinent to the PTSD diagnosis, such as the Anxiety Disorders Interview Schedule for Children or the Diagnostic Interview Schedule for Children represent the most desirable way to assess such reactions. For screening purposes, when a large number of children are being evaluated, or when personnel constraints preclude the use of individual interviews, child-oriented self-report measures, such as the PTSD Reaction Index, have been found to be extremely useful.

Assessing symptoms of PTSD in children of preschool age and younger typically requires the input of the parent or primary carer. Parent-versions of structured interviews would be the desired format to use, or parent-competed questionnaires reporting on children's PTSD symptoms. For young children, behavioral observations can be especially important in evaluating their reactions. Behaviors to evaluate include signs of distress, arousal, or fear, and behavioral avoidance of trauma-related objects, events, or situations.

See Also the Following Articles

Acute Stress Disorder and Posttraumatic Stress Disorder; Posttraumatic Stress Disorder, Delayed; Posttraumatic Stress Disorder – Clinical; Posttraumatic Stress Disorder – Neurobiological basis for.

Further Reading

American Psychiatric Association (1994). *Diagnostic and statistical manual of mental disorders* (4th edn.). (DSM-IV) Washington, DC: American Psychiatric Association.

American Academy of Child Adolescent Psychiatry (1998). AACAP Official Action: Practice parameters for the assessment and treatment of children and adolescents with posttraumatic stress disorder. *Journal of the American Academy of Child and Adolescent Psychiatry* **37**, 4S–26S.

Applied Research & Consulting LLC and the Columbia University Mailman School of Public Health. (2002). *Effects of the World Trade Center attack on NYC public school students: initial report to the New York City Board of Education.* Available online at:. http://eric.ed.gov/ERICDocs/data/ericdocs2/content_storage_01/0000000b/80/27/ce/00.pdf. Last accessed 11 October 2006.

Asarnow, J. (1999). When the earth stops shaking: earthquake sequelae among children diagnosed for pre-earthquake psychopathology. *Journal of the American Academy of Child and Adolescent Psychiatry* **38**, 1016–1023.

Drell, M. J., Siegel, C. H. and Gaensbauer, T. J. (1993). Posttraumatic stress disorder. In: Zeanah, C. H. (ed.) *Handbook of infant mental health*, pp. 369–381. New York: Guilford Press.

Goenjian, A. K., Pynoos, R. S., Steinberg, A. M., et al. (1995). Psychiatric comorbidity in children after the 1988 earthquake in Armenia. *Journal of the American Academy of Child and Adolescent Psychiatry* **34**, 1174–1184.

Green, B. L., Korol, M. S., Grace, M. C., et al. (1991). Children and disaster: gender and parental effects on PTSD symptoms. *Journal of the American Academy of Child and Adolescent Psychiatry* **30**, 945–951.

Gurwitch, R. H., Sitterle, K. A., Young, B. H., et al. (2002). The aftermath of terrorism. In: La Greca, A. M., Silverman, W. K., Vernberg, E. M., et al. (eds.) *Helping children cope with disasters and terrorism*, pp. 327–358. Washington, DC: American Psychological Association.

La Greca, A. M., Silverman, W. K., Vernberg, E. M., et al. (1996). Symptoms of posttraumatic stress after Hurricane Andrew: a prospective study. *Journal of Consulting and Clinical Psychology* **64**, 712–723.

La Greca, A. M., Silverman, W. K., Vernberg, E. M., et al. (eds.) *Helping children cope with disasters and terrorism.* Washington, DC: American Psychological Association.

La Greca, A. M., Silverman, W. K. and Wasserstein, S. B. (1998). Children's predisaster functioning as a predictor of posttraumatic stress following Hurricane Andrew. *Journal of Consulting and Clinical Psychology* **66**, 883–892.

Nolen-Hoeksema, S. and Morrow, J. (1991). A prospective study of depression and posttraumatic stress symptoms after a natural disaster: the 1989 Loma Prieta Earthquake. *Journal of Personality and Social Psychology* **61**, 115–121.

Vernberg, E. M., La Greca, A. M., Silverman, W. K., et al. (1996). Predictors of children's post-disaster functioning following Hurricane Andrew. *Journal of Abnormal Psychology* **105**, 237–248.

Vogel, J. and Vernberg, E. M. (1993). Children's psychological responses to disaster. *Journal of Clinical Child Psychology* **22**, 464–484.

Yule, W., Udwin, O. and Bolton, D. (2002). Mass transportation disasters. In: La Greca, A. M., Silverman, W. K., Vernberg, E. M., et al. (eds.) *Helping children cope with disasters and terrorism*, pp. 327–358. Washington, DC: American Psychological Association.

Posttraumatic Stress Disorder, Delayed

A Holen
Norwegian University of Science and Technology, Trondheim, Norway

This is a revised version of the article by A Holen, Encyclopedia of Stress First Edition, volume 3, pp 179–180, © 2000, Elsevier Inc.

Glossary

Delayed posttraumatic stress disorder (D-PTSD)	Posttraumatic stress disorder when the onset of symptoms occurs at least 6 months after the stressor.
Stressor	A traumatic event that gives rise to major stress responses.

Diagnostic Systems and Delayed Posttraumatic Stress Disorder

Posttraumatic stress disorder (PTSD) can be found in both the *Diagnostic and Statistical Manual of Mental Disorders,* 4th edition (DSM-IV) of the American Psychiatric Association and the *International Classification of Diseases* (ICD-10) of the World Health Organization. The stressor criterion and the three symptom cluster criteria (intrusion, avoidance, and psychophysiological arousal), as well as the time frames, are fairly similar, though some differences exist.

In DSM-III through DSM-IV, PTSD is subsumed under anxiety disorders. When the disorder lasts at least 1 month and persists for less than 3 months after the stressful event, PTSD is considered acute. If the duration is more than 3 months, then PTSD is regarded as chronic.

In ICD-10, PTSD is placed under the heading F43, "Reaction to severe stress and adjustment disorders." The ICD-10 defines "Post-traumatic stress disorder" (F43.1) when the diagnostic criteria are met within 6 months of a major stressful event or of a period of stress. The ICD-10 gives yet another option: when patients have a chronic course, which involves major and lasting personality changes, the diagnosis of "Enduring personality changes, not attributable to brain damage and disease" (F62) may be used. So far, there has been limited research into long-term personality changes.

Both DSM-IV and ICD-10 concur that delayed PTSD (D-PTSD) is diagnosed when at least 6 months have passed between the exposure of a major stressor and the full onset of PTSD.

Nature of the Delay Period

D-PTSD occurs when a person is reasonably well adapted for the initial 6 months or more after experiencing a major stressor but develops PTSD symptoms, such as intrusion, avoidance, and increased arousal related to the initial event, at some later stage. None of the diagnostic systems, however, characterize the nature of the delay period. Still, there is a limited body of research available to shed light on the subject. North et al., in a study published in 1997, found no cases of delayed-onset PTSD in 136 survivors 1 year after a mass shooting incident. Considerable discrepancy of identified PTSD cases was apparent between index and follow-up. The authors argued that inconsistency in reporting rather than true delayed onset was responsible for PTSD cases identified 1 year after the trauma. After the Oklahoma City bombing, survivors were studied 6 and 17 months postdisaster by the same author. Again, no delayed-onset cases were verified. At a 5-year follow-up, Holen found only one case of D-PTSD in the 72 survivors from the North Sea oil rig disaster.

A prospective study by Bryant et al. of 103 motor vehicle accident survivors studied within 1 month of the stressor and again at 6 months and 2 years post-accident identified five patients with PTSD at 2 years; they had not met the PTSD criteria at 6 months. Additionally, the authors reported that delayed-onset cases suffered subsyndromal levels of PTSD, with elevated resting heart rate levels prior to diagnosis. Buckley et al. also found delayed-onset survivors from motor vehicle accidents to be more symptomatic initially than those who did not develop PTSD. In addition, the delayed-onset survivors tended to have poorer social support systems than controls both prior to and after the stressor. Furthermore, the delayed-onset survivors had lower global assessment of function (GAF) scores than controls in the month prior to the motor vehicle accident. Schnurr et al. found that women were more likely to be in the delayed-onset cluster. In a prospective study of traffic accident victims by Koren et al., only 2 of 39 survivors without PTSD at 1 year posttrauma demonstrated delayed-onset PTSD 4 years later. In discussing compensation issues, Eitinger and Holen argued that bridge symptoms, i.e., subclinical symptoms that persist from the time of the trauma to the manifestations of full-blown PTSD, may serve as precursors to delayed responses. In follow-up studies of the population from the collapse of the Buffalo

Creek dam, Green et al. reported that 11% of the cases not identified with PTSD in 1974 met the criteria in 1986.

In a study published in 1989, Solomon et al. reviewed 150 randomly selected files of veterans who sought treatment for combat-related disorders; all the veterans were from the 1982 Lebanon war. Four reasons were given for why they asked for health services. In 10% of the sample, the delayed-onset PTSD was preceded by an initial asymptomatic period. After the war, some other veterans uninterruptedly suffered mild PTSD-associated symptoms until accumulated tension or exposure to subsequent adversity, either military or civilian in nature, resulted in full-blown PTSD. Such exacerbations of PTSD were seen in 33% of the veterans. Reactivation of an earlier combat stress reaction was found in 13% of the cases. The reactivation started only after an asymptomatic period and in connection with threatening military stimuli. Some veterans had no single trigger; they seemed to build up tensions over time with various exposures. Finally, one group of veterans was characterized by delayed treatment seeking for chronic PTSD; this accounted for as much as 40% of the cases. In the absence of proper definitions, the first three groups, i.e., those with an initial asymptomatic period, those with exacerbations, and those with reactivated responses, may qualify as varieties of D-PTSD or they may represent different kinds of posttraumatic processing. The veterans from the 1982 Lebanon war with delayed-onset PTSD used significantly more emotion-focused and distraction coping on the Ways of Coping Checklist than control subjects. Furthermore, they used coping skills significantly less than those with immediate-onset PTSD.

From 1968 to 1973, decades before PTSD was invented, Eitinger and Stroem studied the health of Norwegian concentration camp survivors. They reported a high occurrence of late-onset somatic and psychiatric manifestations associated with concentration camp syndrome, or the KZ syndrome.

In a study of aging Resistance veterans from Holland, Aarts et al. found that the period between the end of the war and when the first symptoms of PTSD appeared varied considerably. First onset of PTSD symptoms appeared in 26% of the cases during the first 5 years after World War II. However, in about 50% of the veterans, PTSD manifested after more than 20 years.

Discussing Delayed Posttraumatic Stress Disorder

There are many uncertainties and controversies in the current conceptualizations of D-PTSD. Some authors report no cases of D-PTSD and raise doubts about the legitimacy of the concept. Others bring up the question of whether D-PTSD represents a latent disorder or simply is unrecognized PTSD. In recent years, a growing number of studies involving both motor vehicle accidents and combat-related stressors have demonstrated occurrence rates of D-PTSD around 10% when manifestation of the disorder is preceded by an asymptomatic period. Moreover, several studies point toward vulnerability factors in both the survivors and their environments. Persons who tend to have subsyndromal symptom levels in the delay period are more likely to have poorer social networks, poorer coping skills, and lower GAF scores.

Some researchers, such as Horowitz, argue that posttraumatic symptoms may wax and wane with triggers or life events. According to the diagnostic criteria of PTSD in the DSM-IV, the triggers are internal or external cues that symbolize or resemble aspects of the primary stressor. When a person is exposed to triggers, his or her state may change from asymptomatic or subthreshold to symptomatic, or from prodromal mild to severe, and thus meet the diagnostic criteria of D-PTSD. Most researchers and clinicians would probably regard triggers as idiosyncratic, low-grade events with no or only a minimal impact on most people, which, in contrast, lead to major responses in survivors. On the contrary, events leading to reactivation may be regarded as having more impact and being traumatic in a general sense. The notion of reactivation implies that past traumas lower the threshold for certain stressors that may symbolize or resemble the primary stressor, and entail far stronger responses than would be seen in most people. The boundaries between episodes of reactivation as part of D-PTSD and episodes of a new PTSD are rather blurred.

In discussing D-PTSD and concepts such as triggers, reactivating events, and primary stressors, the need for clearer definitions becomes quite apparent. Furthermore, gradients and/or classifications of events may be relevant. More studies are needed to shed light on these issues as well as on the course of the posttraumatic processing. What roles do the primary stressor, the subsequent triggers and aversive events, personality, and the social environment play when full-blown PTSD occurs after a completely asymptomatic period, or after a time dominated by subthreshold levels of PTSD symptoms? If the subthreshold symptoms affect the life of the person to a maladaptive degree yet do not meet the criteria of PTSD, the person might within certain time limits be diagnosed as having an adjustment disorder.

Many central questions regarding D-PTSD are still unanswered. We do not know much about possible links to aging. More research is needed to expand our current knowledge about the vicissitudes of delayed posttraumatic stress.

See Also the Following Articles

Acute Stress Disorder and Posttraumatic Stress Disorder; Anxiety; Depression and Manic–Depressive Illness.

Further Reading

Arts, P. G. H., Op den Velde, W., Falger, P. R. J., et al. (1996). Late onset of posttraumatic stress disorder in aging resistance veterans in the Netherlands. In: Ruskin, P. E. & Talbott, J. A. (eds.) *Aging and the posttraumatic stress disorder*, pp. 53–76. Washington, D.C.: American Psychiatric Press.

Bryant, R. A. and Harvey, A. G. (2002). Delayed-onset posttraumatic stress disorder: a prospective evaluation. *Australian and New Zealand Journal of Psychiatry* **36**, 2005–2009.

Buckley, T. C., Blanchard, E. B. and Hickling, E. J. (1996). A prospective examination of delayed onset PTSD secondary to motor vehicle accidents. *Journal of Abnormal Psychology* **105**, 617–625.

Eitinger, L. and Strøm, A. (1973). *Mortality and morbidity after excessive stress.* Norway: Universitetsforlaget.

Green, B. L., Lindy, J. D., Grace, M. C., et al. (1990). Buffalo Creek survivors in a second decade: stability of stress symptoms. *American Journal of Orthopsychiatry* **60**, 43–54.

Holen, A. (1990). *A long-term outcome study of survivors from a disaster: the Alexander L. Kielland disaster in perspective.* Oslo, Norway: University of Oslo.

Horowitz, M. J. (1986). *Stress response syndromes.* Northvale: Aronson.

Koren, D., Arnon, I. and Klein, E. (2001). Long term course of chronic posttraumatic stress disorder in traffic accident victims: a three-year prospective follow-up study. *Behavior Research and Therapy* **39**, 1449–1458.

North, C. S., Smith, E. M. and Spitznagel, E. L. (1997). One year follow-up of survivors of a mass shooting. *American Journal of Psychiatry* **154**, 1696–1702.

North, C. S., Pfefferbaum, B., Tivis, L., et al. (2004). The course of posttraumatic stress disorder in a follow-up study of survivors of the Oklahoma City bombing. *Annals of Clinical Psychiatry* **16**, 209–215.

Pomerantz, A. (1991). Delayed onset of PTSD: delayed recognition or latent disorder? *American Journal of Psychiatry* **148**, 1609.

Schnurr, P. P., Lunney, C. A., Sengupta, A. and Waelde, L. C. (2003). A descriptive analysis of PTSD chronicity in Vietnam veterans. *Journal of Trauma and Stress* **16**, 545–553.

Solomon, Z., Kotler, M., Shalev, A. and Lin, R. (1989). Delayed onset PTSD among Israeli veterans of the 1892 Lebanon war. *Psychiatry* **52**, 428–436.

Solomon, Z., Mikulincer, M. and Waysman, M. (1991). Delayed and immediate onset posttraumatic stress disorder. II. The role of battle experiences and personal resources. *Social Psychiatry and Psychiatric Epidemiology* **26**, 8–13.

Stroem, A. (ed.) (1968). *Norwegian concentration camp survivors.* Norway: Universitetsforlaget.

HPA Alterations in PTSD

R Yehuda
Mount Sinai School of Medicine, New York, NY, USA

Glossary

Hypothalamic-pituitary-adrenal (HPA) — The HPA system is one of the major two neuroendocrine stress response systems of the body. Stress stimulates the release of the hypothalamic neurohormonal peptides, corticotropin releasing hormone and arginine vasopressin, that stimulate secretion of the pituitary adrenocorticotropic hormone (ACTH), which in turn stimulates the secretion of adrenal corticosteriods. In addition to its role in the stress response, the HPA system plays a role in and serves as a biomarker of mental disorders and especially depression and posttraumatic stress disorder (PTSD).

Introduction

The study of the neuroendocrinology of posttraumatic stress disorder (PTSD) has presented an interesting paradox – some of the alterations described have not historically been associated with pathological processes. In particular, initial observations of low cortisol levels in a disorder precipitated by extreme stress directly contradicted the emerging and popular formulation of hormonal responses to stress, the glucocorticoid cascade hypothesis, which posited that stress-related psychopathology involves hypercortisolism as either a cause or consequence of disorder. It is now clear that insufficient glucocorticoid signaling may produce detrimental consequences as robust as those associated with glucocorticoid toxicity.

With respect to PTSD, the majority of studies demonstrate alterations consistent with an enhanced negative feedback inhibition of cortisol on the pituitary and/or an overall hyperreactivity of other target tissues (adrenal gland and hypothalamus). Findings of low cortisol and increased reactivity of the pituitary in PTSD are also consistent with reduced adrenal output, although it is more difficult to fully explain cortisol elevations in response to stress and neuroendocrine challenge with this model.

Insofar as there have been discrepancies in the literature with regard to basal hormone levels, investigators more recently theorized that models of enhanced negative feedback, increased hypothalamic-pituitary-adrenal (HPA) reactivity, and reduced adrenal capacity may explain different facets of the neuroendocrinology of PTSD, including preexisting risk factors that may be related to certain types of early experiences, at least in certain people who develop PTSD. Notwithstanding that some aspects of HPA alterations may predate exposure to a traumatic event that precipitates PTSD, alterations associated with enhanced negative feedback inhibition also appear to develop over time in response to the complex biological demands of extreme trauma and its aftermath. Moreover, the findings of increased HPA reactivity may sometimes reflect a more nonspecific response to ongoing environmental challenges associated with having chronic PTSD. Certainly the absence of cortisol alterations in some studies imply that the alterations associated with low cortisol and enhanced negative feedback are present only in a biological subtype of PTSD. The observations in the aggregate, and the alternative models of pathology or adaptation suggested by them, must be clearly understood when using neuroendocrine data in PTSD to identify targets for drug development.

Basal Cortisol Levels in Posttraumatic Stress Disorder

The majority of the evidence supports the conclusion that cortisol levels in PTSD are different from those observed in acute and chronic stress and in major depression; that is, they are lower, rather than higher, compared to normal. However, it should be noted that there have been many reports that failed to observe low cortisol levels and (although fewer) that have reported cortisol increases in PTSD. This discrepancy may be due to the fact that basal alterations of cortisol in PTSD are subtle. That is, even when cortisol is reported to be significantly lower in PTSD, levels fall within the normal endocrinological range. There are numerous other sources of potential variability in such studies related to the selection of subjects and comparison groups, adequate sample size, and inclusion/exclusion criteria, as well as considerations that are specific to the methods of collecting and assaying cortisol levels, that can explain the discrepancies in the findings. However, the simplest explanation for the disparate observations is that cortisol levels may not represent stable trait markers and are likely to fluctuate, making it difficult to consistently observe group differences.

There is better agreement in studies of circadian rhymicity of cortisol in PTSD, although these are fewer in numbers. The advantage of these studies is that plasma samples can be obtained continuously throughout the 24-h cycle under controlled conditions. Thus, not only is it possible to confirm overall mean cortisol release but also to determine the times of day at which alterations are most likely to be present and note changes in circadian rhythm parameters. Indeed, it appears that the major difference between PTSD and non-PTSD groups is that cortisol levels are lower in the late night and remain lower for a longer period of time in PTSD during hours when subjects are normally sleeping.

Even in cases in which there is failure to find group differences in cortisol levels, there are often correlations within the PTSD group with indices of PTSD symptom severity or trauma exposure. Most often, investigators have reported negative correlations between cortisol levels (particularly integrated mean 24-h cortisol levels) and PTSD symptoms in combat veterans. Low cortisol levels have also been negatively correlated with duration since trauma, implying that low cortisol is associated with early traumatization. In fact, in some recent studies, cortisol levels were inversely related to childhood traumatic experiences, including emotional abuse, even in the absence of PTSD.

Cortisol levels have also been correlated with findings from brain imaging studies in PTSD. In one report, there was a positive relationship between cortisol levels and hippocampal acetylaspartate (NAA), a marker of cell atrophy presumed to reflect changes in neuronal density or metabolism, in subjects with PTSD, suggesting that, rather than having neurotoxic effects, cortisol levels in PTSD may have a trophic effect on the hippocampus. Similarly, cortisol levels in PTSD were negatively correlated with medial temporal lobe perfusion, whereas anterior cingulate perfusion and cortisol levels were positively correlated in PTSD but negatively correlated in trauma survivors without PTSD. These inverse correlations may result from an augmented negative hippocampal effect secondary to increased sensitivity of brain glucocorticoid receptors, which would account for the inverse correlation in PTSD despite equal cortisol levels in both the PTSD and non-PTSD groups. On the other hand, the positive correlation between regional cerebral blood flow in the frontocingulate transitional cortex and cortisol levels in PTSD may reflect unsuccessful attempts of the frontocingulate transitional cortex to terminate the stress response, which has also been linked with low cortisol.

Cortisol may be related to specific or state-dependent features of the disorder, such as comorbid depression or the time course of the disorder. There is a long and rich tradition in psychosomatic medicine underscoring the importance of examining intrapsychic correlates of individual differences in cortisol levels in PTSD, reflecting emotional arousal and opposing antiarousal disengagement defense mechanisms or other coping styles. Finally, recent evidence also suggests that cortisol levels further decrease over time and in old age in trauma survivors.

Cortisol Levels in Response to Stress

Although cortisol levels may be lower at baseline, they may actually be elevated in PTSD relative to comparison subjects when challenged by physiological or psychological stressors. In particular, subjects with PTSD appear to show more anticipatory anxiety to laboratory stressors, which is reflected by increased cortisol levels. These studies provide at least some evidence that the adrenal is capable of producing ample cortisol levels at baseline and in response to stress. In fact, transient increases in cortisol levels are consistent with the notion of a more generalized HPA axis reactivity in PTSD, as reflected by enhanced negative feedback inhibition.

Basal Corticotropin Releasing Hormone and Adrenocorticotropic Hormone Levels in Posttraumatic Stress Disorder

Interestingly, all published reports examining the concentration of corticotropin releasing hormone (CRH) in cerebrospinal fluid (CSF) in PTSD have concluded that levels of this peptide are increased in PTSD. The assessment of CSF CRH does not necessarily provide a good estimate of hypothalamic CRH release but, rather, an estimate of both the hypothalamic and extrahypothalamic release of this neuropeptide. Nonetheless, that there is increased CRH release is somewhat of a paradox considering the lower cortisol levels. With respect to adrenocorticotropic hormone (ACTH), the majority of studies have reported no detectable differences in ACTH levels between PTSD and comparison subjects even when cortisol levels obtained from the same sample were found to be significantly lower.

Lower cortisol levels in the face of normal ACTH levels can reflect a relatively decreased adrenal output. Yet, under circumstances of classic adrenal insufficiency, there is usually increased ACTH release compared to normal levels. Thus, in PTSD, there may be an additional component of feedback on the pituitary acting to depress ACTH levels so that they appear normal rather than elevated. Indeed, elevations in ACTH are expected not only from a reduced adrenal output but also from increased CRH stimulation. On the other hand, the adrenal output in PTSD may be relatively decreased but not enough to substantially affect ACTH levels. In any event, the normal ACTH levels in PTSD in the context of the other findings suggest a more complex model of the regulatory influences on the pituitary in this disorder than reduced adrenal insufficiency.

Glucocorticoid Receptors in Posttraumatic Stress Disorder

Type II glucocorticoid receptors (GRs) are expressed in ACTH- and CRH-producing neurons of the pituitary, hypothalamus, and hippocampus and mediate most systemic glucocorticoid effects, particularly those related to stress responsiveness. Low circulating levels of a hormone or neurotransmitter can result in increased numbers of available GRs to improve response capacity and facilitate homeostasis. However, alterations in the number and sensitivity of both type I (mineralocorticoid) and type II GRs can also significantly influence HPA axis activity and, in particular, can regulate hormone levels by mediating the strength of negative feedback. In PTSD, there is evidence for both an increased number of GRs (measured in lymphocytes) and increased responsiveness of the GR.

Observations regarding the cellular immune response in PTSD are also consistent with enhanced GR responsiveness in the periphery, as indicated by increased beclomethasone-induced vasoconstriction and enhanced delayed-type hypersensitivity of skin test responses. Because immune responses, like endocrine ones, can be multiply regulated, these studies provide only indirect evidence of GR responsiveness. However, when considered in the context of the observation that PTSD patients showed an increased expression of the receptors in all lymphocyte subpopulations, despite a relatively lower quantity of intracellular GRs, as determined by flow cytometry, and in the face of lower ambient cortisol levels, the findings more convincingly support an enhanced sensitivity of the GRs to glucocorticoids. Furthermore, there appears to be an absence of alterations of the mineralocorticoid receptor in PTSD, as investigated by examining the cortisol and ACTH response to spironolactone following CRH stimulation.

With respect to increased glucocorticoid responsiveness, this was recently determined using an *in vitro* paradigm in which mononuclear leukocytes were incubated with a series of concentrations of dexamethasone (DEX) to determine the rate of inhibition of lysozyme activity. Subjects with PTSD showed evidence of a greater sensitivity to glucocorticoids as reflected by a significantly lower mean lysozyme median inhibitory concentration of DEX ($IC_{50\text{-}DEX}$; in nanomoles per liter). The lysozyme $IC_{50\text{-}DEX}$ was significantly correlated with age at exposure to the first traumatic event in subjects with PTSD. The number of cytosolic GRs was correlated with age at exposure to the focal traumatic event.

The Dexamethasone Suppression Test in Posttraumatic Stress Disorder

In contrast to observations regarding ambient cortisol levels, results using the dexamethasone suppression test (DST) present a more consistent view of reduced cortisol suppression in response to DEX administration. The DST provides a direct test of the effects of GR activation in the pituitary on ACTH secretion, and cortisol levels following DEX administration are thus interpreted as an estimate of the strength of negative feedback inhibition, provided that the adrenal response to ACTH is not altered. Using 0.50 mg DEX, most investigators have found a more dramatic reduction in plasma cortisol levels. This exaggerated cortisol suppression in response to DEX has been observed in PTSD related to people with combat exposure, survivors of childhood sexual abuse, Holocaust survivors, children exposed to disaster, women exposed to domestic violence, and mixed groups of trauma survivors.

The Metyrapone Stimulation Test

Metyrapone prevents adrenal steroidogenesis by blocking the conversion of 11-deoxycortisol to cortisol, thereby unmasking the pituitary gland from the influences of negative feedback inhibition. If a sufficiently high dose of metyrapone is used, such that an almost complete suppression of cortisol is achieved, this allows a direct examination of pituitary release of ACTH without the potentially confounding effects of differing ambient cortisol levels. When metyrapone is administered in the morning when HPA axis activity is relatively high, maximal pituitary activity can be achieved, facilitating an evaluation of group differences in pituitary capability. The administration of 2.5 mg metyrapone in the morning resulted in a similar and almost complete reduction in cortisol levels in both PTSD and normal subjects (i.e., removal of negative feedback inhibition) but in a higher increase in ACTH and 11-deoxycortisol in combat Vietnam veterans with PTSD, compared to nonexposed subjects. In the context of low cortisol levels and increased CSF CRH levels, the findings supported the hypothesis of a stronger negative feedback inhibition in PTSD. Both pituitary and adrenal insufficiency are not likely to result in an increased ACTH response to the removal of negative feedback inhibition because the former is associated with an attenuated ACTH response and reduced adrenal output would not necessarily affect the ACTH response. To the extent that ambient cortisol levels are lower than normal, an increased ACTH response following the removal of negative feedback inhibition implies that, when negative feedback is intact, it is strong enough to inhibit ACTH and cortisol. The increased ACTH response is most easily explained by increased suprapituitary activation; however, a sufficiently strong negative feedback inhibition would account for the augmented ACTH response even in the absence of hypothalamic CRH hypersecretion.

Evidence of increased ACTH was not observed when a lower dose of metyrapone was used, administered over a 3-h period at night (750 mg at 7:00 a.m. and 10:00 a.m.). However, interestingly, the manipulation produced a more robust suppression of cortisol in comparison subjects. Using a similar methodology, the effects of metyrapone was used to evaluate CRH effects on sleep. ACTH and cortisol levels were increased in the PTSD group relative to the controls the next morning, suggesting that the same dose of metyrapone did not produce the same degree of adrenal suppression of cortisol synthesis. Under these conditions, it is difficult to evaluate the true effect on ACTH and 11-deoxycortisol, which depends on achieving complete cortisol suppression, or at least the same degree of cortisol suppression, in the two groups. The endocrine response to metyrapone in this study do not support the model of reduced adrenal capacity because this would have yielded a large ratio of ACTH-to-cortisol release, yet the mean ACTH/cortisol ratio prior to metyrapone was no different in the PTSD subjects and the controls. On the other hand, the mean ACTH/cortisol ratio postmetyrapone was lower, although not significantly, suggesting, if anything, an exaggerated negative feedback rather than reduced adrenal capacity.

The Corticotropin Releasing Hormone Challenge Test and Adrenocorticotropic Hormone Stimulation Test in Posttraumatic Stress Disorder

The infusion of exogenous CRH increases ACTH levels and provides a test of pituitary sensitivity. A blunted ACTH is classically thought to reflect a reduced sensitivity of the pituitary to CRH, reflecting a downregulation of pituitary CRH receptors secondary to CRH hypersecretion. The results of studies in PTSD subjects using this challenge have also been mixed. Some studies have demonstrated a blunted ACTH response to PTSD; however, insofar as this blunting did not occur in the presence of hypercortisolism, as in depression, the attenuated ACTH response may reflect an increased negative feedback inhibition of the pituitary secondary to increased GR number or sensitivity. This explanation supports the idea of CRH hypersecretion in PTSD and explains the pituitary desensitization and resultant lack of hypercortisolism as arising from a stronger negative feedback inhibition. An augmented ACTH response to CRH has also been reported, which the authors interpreted as reflecting increased reactivity of the pituitary, although here too there was no evidence for increased cortisol levels.

Findings of Cortisol in the Acute Aftermath of Trauma

Recent data provided some support for the idea that low cortisol levels may be an early predictor of PTSD rather than a consequence of this condition. Low cortisol levels in the immediate aftermath of a motor vehicle accident predicted the development of PTSD in a group of accident victims consecutively presenting in an emergency room in two studies. In a sample of people who survived a natural disaster, cortisol levels were similarly found to be lowest in those with highest PTSD scores at 1 month posttrauma; however cortisol levels were not predictive of symptoms at 1 year. In the acute aftermath of rape, low cortisol levels were associated with prior rape or assault, themselves risk factors for PTSD, but not with the development of PTSD *per se*.

These findings imply that cortisol levels might have been lower in trauma survivors who subsequently developed PTSD even before their exposure to trauma and might therefore represent a preexisting risk factor. Consistent with this, low 24-h urinary cortisol levels in adult children of Holocaust survivors were specifically associated with the risk factor of parental PTSD. Interestingly, the risk factor of parental PTSD in offspring of Holocaust survivors was also associated with an increased incidence of traumatic childhood antecedents. In this study, both the presence of subject-rated parental PTSD and scores reflecting childhood emotional abuse were associated with low cortisol levels in offspring. Thus, it may be that low cortisol levels occur in those who have experienced an adverse event early in life and then remain different from those not exposed to early adversity. Although there might reasonably be HPA axis fluctuations in the aftermath of stress, and even differences in the magnitude of such responses compared to those not exposed to trauma early in life, HPA parameters would subsequently recover to their (abnormal) prestress baseline.

Low cortisol levels may impede the process of biological recovery from stress, resulting in a cascade of alterations that lead to intrusive recollections of the event, avoidance of reminders of the event, and symptoms of hyperarousal. This failure may represent an alternative trajectory to the normal process of adaptation and recovery after a traumatic event.

One of the most compelling lines of evidence supporting the hypothesis that lower cortisol levels may be an important pathway to the development of PTSD symptoms are the results of studies showing that the administration of stress doses of hydrocortisone prevents the development of PTSD and traumatic memories and attenuate these symptoms once present. These findings support the idea that low cortisol levels may facilitate the development of PTSD in response to an overwhelming biological demand, at least in some circumstances.

Conclusion

Cortisol levels are most often found to be lower than normal in PTSD subjects, but can also be similar to or greater than those in comparison subjects. Findings of changes in circadian rhythm suggest that there may be regulatory influences that result in a greater dynamic range of cortisol release over the diurnal cycle in PTSD. Thus, although cortisol levels may be generally lower, the adrenal gland is certainly capable of producing adequate amounts of cortisol in response to challenge.

The model of enhanced negative feedback inhibition is compatible with the idea that there may be transient elevations in cortisol, but suggests that, when present, these increases are shorter-lived due to a more efficient containment of ACTH release as a result of enhanced GR activation. An increased negative feedback inhibition results in reduced cortisol levels under ambient conditions. In contrast to other models of endocrinopathy, which identify specific and usually singular primary alterations in endocrine organs and/or regulation, the model of enhanced negative feedback inhibition in PTSD is in large part descriptive and currently offers little explanation of why some individuals show such alterations of the HPA axis following exposure to traumatic experiences and others do not.

The wide range of observations observed in the neuroendocrinology of PTSD underscores the important observation that HPA response patterns in PTSD are fundamentally in the normal range and do not reflect endocrinopathy. In endocrinological disorders, in which there is usually a lesion in one or more target tissue or biosynthetic pathway, endocrine methods can usually isolate the problem with the appropriate tests and then obtain rather consistent results. In psychiatric disorders, neuroendocrine alterations may be subtle, and therefore, when using standard endocrine tools to examine these alterations, there is a high probability of failing to observe all the alterations consistent with a neuroendocrine explanation of the pathology in tandem or of obtaining disparate results within the same patient group owing to a stronger compensation or reregulation of the HPA axis following challenge.

The next generation studies should aim to apply more rigorous tests of neuroendocrinology of PTSD based on the appropriate developmental issues and in consideration of the longitudinal course of the disorder and the individual differences that affect these processes. No doubt such studies will require a closer examination of a wide range of biological responses, including the cellular and molecular mechanisms involved in adaptation to stress, and an understanding of the relationship between the endocrine findings and other identified biological alterations in PTSD.

Acknowledgments

This work was supported by MH 49555, MH 55-7531, and MERIT review funding.

See Also the Following Articles

Depression and Manic–Depressive Illness; Depression, Immunological Aspects.

Further Reading

Baker, D. G., West, S. A., Nicholson, W. E., et al. (1999). Serial CSF corticotropin-releasing hormone levels and adrenocortical activity in combat veterans with posttraumatic stress disorder. *American Journal of Psychiatry* **156**, 585–588[errata] 986.

Bremner, J. D., Vythilingma, M., Vermetten, E., et al. (2003). Cortisol response to a cognitive stress challenge in posttraumatic stress disorder related to childhood abuse. *Psychoneuyroendocrinology* **28**, 733–750.

Boscarino, J. A. (1996). Posttraumatic stress disorder, exposure to combat, and lower plasma cortisol among Vietnam veterans: findings and clinical implications. *Journal of Consulting and Clinical Psychology* **64**, 191–201.

Delahanty, D. L., Raimonde, A. J. and Spoonster, E. (2000). Initial posttraumatic urinary cortisol levels predict subsequent PTSD symptoms in motor vehicle accident victims [in process citation]. *Biological Psychiatry* **48**, 940–947.

Holsboer, F. (2000). The corticosteroid receptor hypothesis of depression. *Neuropsychopharmacology* **23**, 477–501.

Raison, C. L. and Miller, A. H. (2003). When not enough is too much: the role of insufficient glucocorticoid signaling in the pathophysiology of stress related disorders. *American Journal of Psychiatry* **160**, 1554–1565.

Schelling, G., Briegel, J., Roozendaal, B., et al. (2001). The effect of stress doses of hydrocortisone during septic shock on posttraumatic stress disorder in survivors. *Biological Psychiatry* **50**, 978–985.

Yehuda, R. (2002). Status of cortisol findings in PTSD. *Psychiatric Clinics of North America* **25**, 341–368.

Yehuda, R., Boisoneau, D., Lowy, M. T., et al. (1995). Dose-response changes in plasma cortisol and lymphocyte glucocorticoid receptors following dexamethasone administration in combat veterans with and without posttraumatic stress disorder. *Archives of General Psychiatry* **52**, 583–593.

Yehuda, R., Halligan, S. L. and Grossman, R. (2001). Childhood trauma and risk for PTSD: relationship to intergenerational effects of trauma, parental PTSD and cortisol excretion. *Development and Psychopathology* **2001**, 733–753.

Yehuda, R., Levengood, R. A., Schmeidler, J., et al. (1996). Increased pituitary activation following metyrapone administration in post-traumatic stress disorder. *Psychoneuroendocrinology* **21**, 1–16.

Yehuda, R., Shalev, A. Y. and McFarlane, A. C. (1998). Predicting the development of posttraumatic stress disorder from the acute response to a traumatic event. *Biological Psychiatry* **44**, 1305–1313.

Yehuda, R., Teicher, M. H., Trestman, R. L., et al. (1996). Cortisol regulation in posttraumatic stress disorder and major depression: a chronobiological analysis. *Biological Psychiatry* **40**, 79–88.

Posttraumatic Stress Disorder – Neurobiological basis for

M Barad
University of Los Angeles, Los Angeles, CA, USA

Glossary

α_2-Adrenergic receptor A receptor for the neurotransmitter norepinephrine; largely expressed presynaptically and acts to inhibit further release of norepinephrine.

Adrenergic system The cells and pathways in the brain that use the neurotransmitter norepinephrine, either by releasing it or by expressing receptors that respond to it.

Corticotropin releasing hormone (CRH) A peptide neurotransmitter released by the median eminence of the hypothalamus to stimulate the hypothalamic-pituitary-adrenal axis. It also acts widely in the brain as a neurotransmitter.

Cortisol The primary glucocorticoid hormone.

Denditic pruning Reductions in the branching dendrites of neurons, the part of the neuron that receives signals from other neurons.

Functional imaging The examination of the brain by magnetic resonance imaging or positron emission tomography, yielding cross-sectional images of the brain and highlighting areas of increased or decreased blood flow that reflect localized brain activity.

Glucocorticoids Steroid hormones, especially cortisol, that regulate metabolism and the stress response.

Hippocampus A brain structure crucially involved in complex memories (those available to consciousness).

Hypothalamic-pituitary-adrenal (HPA) axis The regulatory pathway from the brain to the adrenal cortex that regulates the release of cortisol.

Longitudinal studies Studies that follow the development of a disease in an individual over time, along with its biological correlates. By comparing variables before and after the development of a disease, these studies allow a stronger identification of the pathological effects of the disease process than other types of studies.

Metachlorophenylpiperazine (m-CPP) A serotonin agonist.

Naltrexone An antagonist of opioids receptors.

Opioid system The cells and pathways in the brain that use endorphins, or endogenous opioids, as neurotransmitters, either by releasing them or expressing receptors that respond to them. These are the same receptors that bind opium and other opioid drugs.

Provocation studies Studies that use drugs or environmental stimuli (e.g., stories, images, or tasks) to provoke a specific brain response.

Serotonin system The cells and pathways in the brain that use the neurotransmitter serotonin, either by releasing it or by expressing receptors that respond to it.

Structural imaging The examination of the brain using high-resolution magnetic resonance imaging (or, in the past, computed tomography) to carefully quantify the size of identifiable structures.

Twin studies Research comparing identical twins, one of whom suffers a pathology, such as posttraumatic stress disorder. Because the healthy twin is genetically identically and shares much the same environment as the patient, the similarities in his brain structure or function to that of the patient, which differ from the average population and are similar to the patient population, suggest a preexisting condition or vulnerability to disease.

Yohimbine A pharmacological antagonist of α_2-adrenergic receptor.

General Considerations

In general, two approaches have been used to examine the neurobiological basis of posttraumatic stress disorder (PTSD): imaging and biological measures. Imaging has been used to examine the anatomy of the brain and its activity both at rest and during a number of symptom provocation and cognitive challenges. Biological measures have been used to measure a number of candidate hormonal and neurotransmitter systems, again, both at rest and after symptom provocation. We consider some of the findings of these studies here.

It is important to remember that most studies of PTSD compare PTSD patients to normal controls. Such studies cannot differentiate between a finding in the PTSD patient that is the result of the disease process of PTSD and follows the traumatic event and a finding that preceded the trauma and thus may indicate a source of vulnerability to PTSD. Only longitudinal and twin or family studies can effectively differentiate between those possibilities, and there have been few such studies to date.

It is likely that preexisting factors, whether genetic or acquired from previous experience, are crucial to the development of PTSD. Exposure to trauma is not enough, no matter how severe. Only a small proportion of people exposed to trauma, even horrific trauma, develop PTSD. In the United States, approximately 90% of the population is exposed to at least one traumatic event serious enough to satisfy the trauma criterion for PTSD. However, only approximately 8% of the population develops PTSD. This means that it is particularly important to understand the neurobiological factors that contribute to vulnerability to PTSD or to its inverse, resiliency.

One obvious biological factor that seems to play a role in vulnerability to PTSD is sex. Women are twice as likely to develop PTSD after a trauma than men, although the interaction between biology and type of trauma is a complicated one. Women are much more likely to develop PTSD after an assault and men are much more likely to develop PTSD after being raped (even though their risk of rape is lower); both sexes have an equal risk of PTSD after natural disaster. These patterns suggest that the differences in rates of PTSD between men and women overall have something to do with the meaning of the type of trauma to each sex. Both sexes suffer equally from natural disasters, which affect everyone in the area, whereas physical or sexual assault emphasizes the relative weakness of the victim.

PTSD is, by definition, a chronic condition in which symptoms persist for at least 1 month. However, in the immediate aftermath of a trauma, almost everyone experiences symptoms of PTSD. Thus, the symptoms of PTSD are almost certainly part of the normal human response to stress. It is the failure of recovery that is characteristic of PTSD, so it may be that the right place to look for vulnerability is in the mechanisms of recovery. Such mechanisms may include biological mechanisms, such as the glucocorticoid response to stress, or psychological mechanisms, such as the ability of people to suppress fearful responding in the short term through inhibition by prefrontal cortex or in the long term through behavioral extinction or desensitization of fearful responses to the reminders of the trauma.

Physiological Measures

Frightening experiences elicit a characteristic stress response. The faster response to a frightening stimulus is the adrenergic stress response, which orchestrates the readiness of an animal or a human to protect itself, the fight-or-flight response originally described by Walter Cannon. Simultaneously, a second, slower stress system is activated, the hypothalamic-pituitary-adrenal (HPA) axis, which results in the production of the effector glucocorticoid cortisol, as first described by Hans Selye. One important action of the slower cortisol response is to shut down or limit the adrenergic response.

Disruptions in stress hormone regulation stand out prominently in the neurobiology of PTSD. Some of the first studies of PTSD patients indicated not only that PTSD patients show increased excretion of epinephrine and norepinephrine at baseline but also that adrenergic system is hyperreactive. The administration of yohimbine to PTSD patients provided the most striking demonstration of the increase of adrenergic tone and its relation to PTSD symptoms. Yohimbine blocks the α_2 receptors for norepinephrine. These receptors are presynaptic on adrenergic terminals and act like a thermostat to inhibit the release of norepinephrine into the synapse. The administration of yohimbine is mildly anxiogenic in normal controls, but in PTSD patients it caused great distress, precipitating flashbacks in 40% and panic attacks in 70%, whereas none of the controls experienced either. These data indicate a profound dysregulation of the adrenergic system. Interestingly, yohimbine also provokes panic attacks in patients with panic disorder but not in patients with schizophrenia, depression, obsessive-compulsive disorder, or generalized anxiety disorder and also not in normals. Thus, PTSD may share some part of its pathophysiology with panic disorder.

Increases of adrenergic tone and reactivity may be of great importance in the symptomatology of PTSD. It is clear from the experiment that increases of adrenergic neurotransmission may be precipitating some of the most troubling symptoms of PTSD, including not only flashbacks and the physiological hyperreactivity characteristic of panic attacks but also intrusive thoughts, emotional numbing, difficulty concentrating, and increased startle. However, it has also been extensively demonstrated in preclinical studies that the adrenergic system is crucial to memory strength, and particularly to the establishment of fearful or distressing memories. This explains in part why memories of frightening events are so vivid. Thus, high levels of norepinephrine during traumatic experiences may well strengthen the formation of distressing memories and make them more vivid for PTSD patients.

When challenged with yohimbine, the family members of PTSD patients do not have more panic attacks than normal subjects, whereas the healthy family members of panic disorder patients do have high rates of panic attacks upon yohimbine challenge. This suggests that a hyperreactive adrenergic system may be a predisposing factor for panic disorder, whereas the adrenergic hyperreactivity of PTSD patients may be acquired.

What might account for that hyperreactivity? One hypothesis is an insufficient regulation by an inadequate glucocorticoid response. We might expect from the strong response to trauma in PTSD patients that cortisol levels, as part of the stress response, should be high. In fact, most studies have found that glucocorticoid levels are low at baseline in PTSD patients and that the feedback inhibition of glucorticoid synthesis is overly strong. Thus, when injected with an exogenous glucocorticoid, dexamethasone, patients with PTSD suppress the production of endogenous cortisol for a significantly longer time than normal controls. This is true even though the levels of the hypothalamic hormone that drives cortisol synthesis and release, corticotropin releasing hormone (CRH), are high in PTSD patients.

By contrast, in depression, high CRH levels drive high levels of circulating cortisol. The contrasting pattern in PTSD suggests that feedback inhibition of the HPA axis is dominant over CRH drive. Low circulating levels of cortisol may well allow the adrenergic response to stress to run out of control. But are these low levels in PTSD patients the result of a burnout of the cortisol system by sustained high cortisol during and after the trauma?

Two longitudinal studies of motor vehicle-accident victims have addressed this question. In one study, 15-h urinary cortisol excretion was measured after accidents; in the other, cortisol levels were measured in blood samples drawn on the way to the emergency room. In both studies, the victims who went on to develop PTSD had significantly lower cortisol after their accidents than those who did not. Thus, even just after their trauma, the cortisol levels of those who later went on to PTSD were lower. This begins to hint that lower cortisol in PTSD patients may not be the result of burnout after prolonged elevations around the time of trauma but rather a preexisting state that contributes to a vulnerability to PTSD.

This preexisting state is almost certainly not entirely genetic. For example, in rape victims, cortisol levels after the rape were lower in those who had sustained a previous assault, and the victims of previous assaults were three times as likely to go on to develop PTSD. Women who had no previous trauma had cortisol levels that averaged three times higher than those who did and had higher cortisol levels when the index rape was more severe. Women with previous trauma showed no increase in cortisol levels in response to increased severity of rape.

However, the question remains whether low cortisol levels existed even before the rape. By comparing the children of Holocaust survivors to children of European Jews who escaped the Holocaust, Rachel Yehuda and her colleagues have examined this question. The children of holocaust survivors are almost four times as likely to develop PTSD as the controls. The children of Holocaust survivors show lower cortisol excretion than do the controls, which argues for a preexisting defect in the cortisol system. However, this group was not homogeneous. When neither parent nor child had PTSD, cortisol excretion was the same as that of controls. However, when the parent had PTSD, the cortisol excretion was lower in the offspring; it was lowest when both parent and child had PTSD. Thus, it is clear that low PTSD levels are a preexisting risk factor that may not only be due to previous trauma. It is tempting to think that this risk factor is due to the transmitted anxiety of parents with PTSD, acting like a previous assault in rape victims to lower cortisol. However, there remains a potential for a genetic explanation. It might be that the Holocaust survivors with PTSD also had low cortisol as a risk factor for their PTSD and transmitted that risk genetically rather than behaviorally.

All of these data on endocrine stress responses outline one potential chain of causation in generating the clinical picture of PTSD. A hypoactive cortisol response may lead to the dysregulation of the adrenergic stress response. An ungoverned adrenergic system may increase the intensity of traumatic memories, the strength of association of those memories with a wide range of stimuli in the environment, and the physiological and psychological arousal when those memories are recalled.

Beyond the alterations in the endocrine stress responses, other physiological abnormalities have been identified in PTSD patients. Endogenous opioids are low in PTSD sufferers, who also show a reduced pain threshold. However, when exposed to traumatic reminders, Vietnam veterans with PTSD showed a higher pain threshold that could be reversed by naltrexone (which blocks opioids receptors). Thus, PTSD patients appear to have both decreased resting levels of endogenous opioids and a more reactive opioid system. This may lead to cycles of trauma reminders inducing numbing, followed by opioid withdrawal (and PTSD) symptoms such as irritability and disturbed sleep. Because these hyperarousal symptoms of opioid withdrawal may be mediated by adrenergic activity, low tonic opioid levels may act in concert with low cortisol to increase adrenergic reactivity.

One study examined the effect of a serotonin agonist metachlorophenylpiperazine (m-CPP) on PTSD patients compared with the effect of yohimbine and placebo. As in the studies of yohimbine, m-CPP caused panic attacks in a substantial number of the patients, along with exacerbations of other PTSD symptoms. A similar number of patients experienced panic attacks and worsened PTSD symptoms after m-CPP injections. Interestingly, different subsets of patients tended to get panic attacks with the two agents. Another study showed that PTSD patients had a higher frequency of being homozygous for the short allele of the serotonin promoter, a genotype associated with depression after life stressors. Thus, although fewer data indicate a role for serotonergic than for noradrenergic mechanisms, serotonergic mechanisms may make a second and possibly independent contribution to PTSD vulnerability or pathophysiology.

Brain Imaging

Three areas of the brain have received particular attention in imaging studies of PTSD, because there are *a priori* reasons to suspect their involvement. The hippocampus has been examined in detail because a wealth of preclinical studies indicate that chronic stress has profound effects on this structure. The amygdala has been examined because this brain structure has an orchestrating role in all fear learning. Finally, the prefrontal cortex has been examined because of its role in suppressing amygdaloid activation.

Structural Imaging

A variety of studies in animals indicate that elevated levels of the stress hormone cortisol is damaging to the hippocampus. Long-term exposure to exogenous glucocorticoid steroids and prolonged stress (which presumably elevates endogenous levels of these steroids) both damage the CA3 region of the hippocampus and cause dendritic pruning of neurons there, with the net effect of decreasing hippocampal volume. Although lower levels of cortisol are usually observed in PTSD patients, it is reasonable to hypothesize that cortisol levels might have been extremely high at the time of traumatic exposure.

Consistent with this hypothesis, hippocampal volumes in PTSD patients are decreased compared to controls in a number of structural imaging studies of combat veterans and of adult victims of childhood sexual abuse that compared PTSD patients to others exposed to combat or sexual abuse without PTSD. However, results have been less consistent with other patient populations and have not been observed in Holocaust survivors or patients with personality disorders who suffer from PTSD.

These studies are cross-sectional, comparing PTSD patients to controls, and do not address whether the hippocampal volume deficits might predate the trauma and development of PTSD. One study of identical twins in which one twin was a Vietnam combat veteran addressed this question indirectly. This study found that smaller hippocampal volume in the combat-exposed twin correlated to the severity of his PTSD symptoms. However, the hippocampal volume of the non-combat-exposed twin correlated just as closely with the severity of his brother's symptoms. These data suggest strongly that small hippocampi are a risk factor for, rather than a result of, combat exposure. Two longitudinal studies have also addressed this question, and neither found decreases of hippocampal volume associated with the development of PTSD or with ongoing PTSD pathology. Similarly, no changes in amygdala volume have been seen in PTSD patients.

Functional Imaging

Brain structure may be of less importance than brain function in psychiatric disease, including in PTSD. Functional imaging, looking at brain activity as reflected by blood flow, may thus be a better indicator of pathological brain function, especially when performed using biological or psychological probes designed to stimulate functional systems. Functional studies have focused attention on the amygdala, a brain region important for orchestrating the fear response, as well as in related paralimbic and frontal structures. This approach remains in its early stages, and a clear anatomical pattern has not yet emerged, perhaps because of the wide variation in patient populations and provocation protocols in use.

One interesting approach has been to use pharmacological provocation with yohimbine, the antagonist of inhibitory presynaptic α_2 autoreceptors. As previously described, yohimbine, when injected into PTSD patients, exacerbates symptoms and causes panic attacks and flashbacks. In a positron emission tomography (PET) imaging study, yohimbine injections tended to increase metabolism in a variety of cortical regions including the prefrontal, temporal, parietal, and orbitofrontal cortices in control subjects, but tended to decrease metabolism in those regions in PTSD patients. These data indicate that the adrenergic dysregulation observed in PTSD patients profoundly changes brain activation patterns and suggests a role for those brain structures with changed activity in suppressing the set of symptoms evoked by yohimbine, specifically panic attacks and flashbacks.

Psychologically driven provocation studies have generally shown differences in brain activation between PTSD patients and controls, although these have not always been consistent. Left amygdala activity was increased by combat sounds, compared to white noise, in Vietnam veterans with PTSD but not in combat-exposed veterans without PTSD or in normal controls. In another similar study with combat sound, veterans with PTSD showed activation of the right amygdala as well as in other regions. In another comparison of veterans with and without PTSD who were asked to visualize combat, the veterans showed activation in the right amygdala as well as in the ventral anterior cingulate gyrus. However, when actually viewing combat images, no such activation was seen; however, PTSD patients showed decreased activity in Broca's area, an area important for language generation.

Trauma scripts and viewing of traumatic images have generally not yielded amygdala activation, whereas visualization and simple stimuli, such as combat sounds, which bypass the cortex, effectively activate that structure. Interestingly, masked presentations of fearful faces, too brief to register consciously, caused exaggerated amygdala responses in veterans with PTSD compared to healthy veterans.

On the other hand, script-driven provocation has effectively activated the posterior cingulate and motor cortex in women with a history of childhood sexual abuse with PTSD compared to those without PTSD. Women with PTSD also failed to activate Broca's area and the anterior cingulate compared to controls, who did.

In summary, the functional imaging data so far do support changes in the function of the amygdala and of the limbic and prefrontal cortices in PTSD. However, the exact nature of those changes and their significance in the symptomatology and pathophysiology of PTSD remain to be defined.

See Also the Following Articles

Acute Stress Disorder and Posttraumatic Stress Disorder; Fear and the Amygdala; Posttraumatic Stress Disorder in Children; Posttraumatic Stress Disorder, Delayed; Posttraumatic Stress Disorder – Clinical.

Further Reading

Bremner, J. D. (2002). Neuroimaging studies in post-traumatic stress disorder. *Current Psychiatry Reports* **4**, 254–263.

Bremner, J. D. (2005). Effects of traumatic stress on brain structure and function: relevance to early responses to trauma. *Journal of Trauma and Dissociation* **6**, 51–68.

Foa, E. B. and Street, G. P. (2001). Women and traumatic events. *Journal of Clinical Psychiatry* **62**(supplement 17), 29–34.

Gilbertson, M. W., Shenton, M. E., Ciszewski, A., et al. (2002). Smaller hippocampal volume predicts pathologic vulnerability to psychological trauma. *Nature Neuroscience* **5**, 1242–1247.

Grossman, R., Buchsbaum, M. S. and Yehuda, R. (2002). Neuroimaging studies in post-traumatic stress disorder. *Psychiatric Clinics of North America* **25**, 317–340.

Resnick, H. S., Yehuda, R., Pitman, R. K., et al. (1995). Effect of previous trauma on acute plasma cortisol level following rape. *American Journal of Psychiatry* **152**, 1675–1677.

Rinne, T., Westenberg, H. G., den Boer, J. A., et al. (2000). Serotonergic blunting to meta-chlorophenylpiperazine (m-CPP) highly correlates with sustained childhood abuse in impulsive and autoaggressive female borderline patients. *Biological Psychiatry* **47**, 548–556.

Southwick, S. M., Bremner, J. D., Rasmusson, A., et al. (1999). Role of norepinephrine in the pathophysiology and treatment of posttraumatic stress disorder. *Biological Psychiatry* **46**, 1192–1204.

Vermetten, E. and Bremner, J. D. (2002). Circuits and systems in stress. II: Applications to neurobiology and treatment in posttraumatic stress disorder. *Depression and Anxiety* **16**, 14–38.

Yehuda, R. (2002). Current status of cortisol findings in post-traumatic stress disorder. *Psychiatric Clinics of North America* **25**, 341–368.

Yehuda, R. (2004). Risk and resilience in posttraumatic stress disorder. *Journal of Clinical Psychiatry* **65**(supplement 1), 29–36.

Yehuda, R., Schmeidler, J., Wainberg, M., et al. (1998). Vulnerability to posttraumatic stress disorder in adult offspring of Holocaust survivors. *American Journal of Psychiatry* **155**, 1163–1171.

Posttraumatic Stress Disorder – Clinical

N C Feeny and L R Stines
Case Western Reserve University, Cleveland, OH, USA
E B Foa
University of Pennsylvania, Philadelphia, PA, USA

Glossary

Arousal A cluster of PTSD symptoms that includes difficulty concentrating, sleep disturbance, irritability and anger, exaggerated startle response, and overalertness.

Avoidance A cluster of PTSD symptoms that includes behavioral and cognitive avoidance (i.e., avoidance of thoughts, feelings, and reminders of the trauma), emotional numbing, loss of interest in activities, feeling disconnected from others, psychogenic amnesia, and a sense of foreshortened future.

Cognitive-behavioral treatments A class of psychosocial treatment approaches focused on the interrelationships among thoughts, behaviors, and emotions.

Posttraumatic stress disorder (PTSD) An anxiety disorder that develops in response to a traumatic event and is characterized by three clusters of symptoms: reexperiencing, avoidance, and physiological hyperarousal. PTSD is diagnosed after a 1-month period of sustained problems following the traumatic event.

Reexperiencing A cluster of PTSD symptoms that includes reexperiencing the traumatic event through intrusive distressing thoughts, nightmares, flashbacks, and intense emotional upset and physiological arousal on exposure to reminders of the trauma.

Trauma An event that a person experiences, witnesses, or learns about that involves actual or threatened physical injury or death and to which the person responds with feelings of fear, helplessness, or horror.

Overview of Posttraumatic Stress Disorder

Prevalence of Traumatic Events

According to the *Diagnostic and Statistical Manual of Mental Disorders* (4th edn.; DSM-IV) a trauma is an event that involves actual or perceived physical threat or injury, to which a person responds with fear, helplessness, or horror. Although in the past, trauma was conceptualized as unusual and outside the realm of human experience, large epidemiological studies have demonstrated high rates of trauma exposure among adults. In a nationally representative sample of 6000 U.S. adults, Kessler and colleagues found that 60% of men and 51% of women reported experiencing at least one traumatic event in their lifetime. Similar findings emerged from Norris's 1992 study using a large, racially diverse sample – 74% of men and 65% of women reported experiencing at least one traumatic event. A lower prevalence of trauma was found in a sample of members of a health maintenance organization – 43% of men and 39% of women experienced a trauma in their lifetime. Taken together, these studies suggest that trauma is very common among adults in the United States.

Diagnostic Criteria of Posttraumatic Stress Disorder

The constellation of psychological difficulties that is observed most often following a trauma is called posttraumatic stress disorder (PTSD). PTSD is an anxiety disorder, and its symptoms fall into three clusters: reexperiencing the traumatic event (e.g., intrusive and distressing thoughts, flashbacks, and nightmares), avoidance of trauma-related reminders (e.g., avoiding thoughts or situations related to the trauma, emotional numbing, sense of foreshortened future), and hyperarousal (e.g., sleep disturbance, difficulty concentrating, irritability, and hypervigilance). In order to meet diagnostic criteria for PTSD, these difficulties must last for more than 1 month and cause substantial impairment in social or occupational functioning.

Prevalence and Course of Posttraumatic Stress Disorder

In the general population, the lifetime prevalence of PTSD is estimated to be around 9%. Estimates suggest that women are two times more likely to develop PTSD than men (e.g., 10% of women vs. 5% of men in the general population). Because a diagnosis of PTSD requires an exposure to a traumatic event, rates of PTSD are inherently higher among those who have experienced such an event, with lifetime prevalence estimated at 25%. Among trauma survivors, the prevalence of current PTSD varies quite widely. For example, 15% of Vietnam combat veterans, 12–65% of female assault survivors, and up to 40% of survivors of serious motor vehicle accidents have been reported to meet diagnostic criteria for PTSD. Thus, although trauma exposure is quite common, persistent psychological difficulties in the aftermath of a traumatic event are less so and vary in frequency, in part, as a function of the traumatic experience.

In the initial days and weeks following a trauma, it is common to experience difficulties such as fear, disrupted sleep, and difficulty concentrating. Although most people experience such difficulties shortly after a traumatic event, the majority also experience a natural reduction in these difficulties over the following several months. Some trauma survivors, however, continue to experience significant PTSD symptoms for months and even years after exposure to the traumatic event. After 1 year, chronic PTSD is unlikely to remit without treatment; thus there is a critical need for effective treatments.

Cognitive-Behavioral Treatments for Posttraumatic Stress Disorder

Several cognitive-behavioral therapies for PTSD have been developed and tested in prospective randomized studies. These treatments include prolonged exposure therapy (PE), stress inoculation training (SIT), cognitive therapy (CT), cognitive processing therapy (CPT), and eye movement desensitization and reprocessing (EMDR). In this section, these treatments are reviewed and selected outcome studies that evaluate the efficacy of these treatments are presented.

Prolonged Exposure Therapy

Exposure therapy has been extensively evaluated as a treatment for persistent, pathological anxiety. The chief aim of this form of treatment is to help patients confront feared and avoided objects, situations, memories, and images until anxiety declines. PE for trauma survivors with PTSD is a treatment program that is based on the notion that avoidance of trauma-related memories and external reminders interferes with recovery from the traumatic event. Specifically, avoidance prevents opportunities to emotionally process the trauma memory, to learn to distinguish safe from unsafe situations, and to disconfirm erroneous trauma-related cognitions, thus maintaining the unrealistic cognitions underlying PTSD that the world is utterly dangerous and that the trauma survivor is extremely incompetent in coping with stress. This view of the mechanisms involved in exposure therapy is central to emotional processing theory.

PE includes two forms of exposure: imaginal exposure and *in vivo* exposure. Imaginal exposure involves repeatedly recounting the traumatic memory. Specifically, the patient is instructed to vividly imagine the traumatic event and to describe it in detail aloud, along with the thoughts and feelings that occurred during the event. Imaginal exposure is typically conducted during several treatment sessions and via homework of listening to audiotapes of the in-session recounting of the memory. *In vivo*, or real-life, exposure involves systematic and repeated confrontation with safe or low-risk trauma-related reminders that evoke excessive or unrealistic anxiety. *In vivo* exposure is typically conducted outside of the treatment sessions as homework, during which the patient confronts situations, places, objects, or activities that are realistically safe but that trigger trauma-related fear and anxiety because they are related to the trauma. With *in vivo* exposure, the patient is encouraged to remain in the anxiety-provoking situation until his or her fear decreases by a significant amount. Other components of PE include psychoeducation about common reactions to traumatic events and breathing retraining.

Across several studies in different centers, PE has consistently been found to be highly effective. PE has demonstrated outcomes superior to supportive counseling (SC) and a wait-list control (WL). Most patients who receive PE experience a significant reduction in PTSD, depression, anxiety, anger, and guilt and experience improvements in overall functioning. In fact, in the treatment guidelines developed by experts in the field in conjunction with International Society for Traumatic Stress Studies (ISTSS), PE was identified as the most empirically supported intervention for PTSD.

Stress Inoculation Training

SIT was among the first of the cognitive-behavioral treatments to be applied to PTSD. According to the theory underlying SIT, stress occurs when people experience environmental events as exceeding their coping resources and thereby as threatening to their safety or welfare. Anxiety is a normal response to stress and signals people to increase efforts to cope with or somehow manage the stress-eliciting situation. In the case of individuals with PTSD, the anxiety evoked by trauma-related reminders is excessive and disruptive. Thus, SIT involves the learning and repeated practice of specific coping skills, with the goal of helping patients to develop or enhance their ability to manage stress effectively and to reduce anxiety. Coping skills typically include tools such as breathing and relaxation training, guided self-dialog, assertiveness training, role-playing, covert modeling, and cognitive restructuring.

The efficacy of PE, SIT, SC, and WL were compared for female sexual-assault survivors with chronic PTSD. PE and SIT showed significant pre- to posttreatment reductions in reexperiencing and avoidance symptoms, whereas SC and WL did not. Also, at the end of treatment, 50% of patients who had SIT and 40% who had PE no longer met the criteria for PTSD; in contrast, only 10% of patients who had SC and none who had WL lost their diagnosis. At follow-up, there was a tendency for patients in the PE group to show further improvement in PTSD symptoms, whereas patients in the SIT and SC groups did not.

In a second study, the efficacy of PE and SIT was compared to the efficacy of a combination of both treatments (PE/SIT) and WL. All three active treatments resulted in considerable symptom reduction and were more effective than WL. However, PE appeared superior to the other treatments, leading to greater reductions of anxiety and depression, with fewer dropouts than both SIT and PE/SIT. At the end of treatment, 70% of patients who had PE, 58% who had SIT, and 54% who had PE/SIT lost their PTSD diagnosis compared to none in the WL group. At follow-up, women who received PE exhibited better social functioning than did those who received SIT or PE/SIT.

Cognitive Therapy

The aims of CT or cognitive restructuring (CR) for PTSD patients are to help patients to understand the role of their beliefs and appraisals of situations in influencing their emotional reactions, to identify trauma-related irrational thoughts or beliefs that trigger avoidance and/or excessive negative emotions (e.g., fear, shame, and rage), and to learn to challenge unrealistic beliefs and expectations in a rational evidence-based manner. In challenging these beliefs, evidence is weighed and alternative ways of viewing the situation are evaluated. In treatment sessions, and in daily life, patients practice responding to automatic thoughts and interpretations by reviewing the facts, considering alternative explanations, and sometimes experimenting with different ways of behaving in response to situations or events that elicit anxiety and other negative emotions. As a consequence, patients learn to evaluate whether their trauma-related beliefs and expectations accurately reflect reality and are appropriate or helpful and modify them accordingly.

In a 2005 randomized trial, PE was compared with a program that included PE and CR (PE/CR) in female victims of sexual and nonsexual assault. The results suggest that both PE and PE/CR produce substantial improvements on multiple outcomes, including evaluator ratings of PTSD severity, depression, and social functioning. Similar to the PE/SIT findings, combining PE with CR did not improve the efficacy of PE. In an examination of PE in a sample of mixed trauma victims with chronic PTSD, Marks et al. compared PE to CR, PE/CR, and a relaxation control condition (R). The results suggest that PE, CR, and PE/CR are all quite effective and superior to R. Again, both PE and CR were effective, and combining them did not improve efficacy.

Cognitive Processing Therapy

Another cognitive behavioral therapy program for PTSD is CPT. CPT was originally developed for use with sexual assault victims and comprises elements of both CT and PE. Specifically, CPT includes CR around beliefs in five core areas – safety, power and control, esteem, trust, and intimacy – written exposure (i.e., writing about the traumatic memories and reading the account aloud to the therapist).

Resick et al. compared the efficacy of 12 sessions of CPT, 9 sessions of PE, and WL in rape victims with chronic PTSD. Results indicated that after 9 weeks of PE and 12 weeks of CPT, both treatments were highly effective in reducing PTSD; posttreatment only 19.5% of completers of CPT and 17.5% of PE met the criteria for PTSD. Among the completers, 76% of patients who had CPT and 58% of patients who had PE met the criteria for good end-state functioning (i.e., low PTSD and depression). Gains were maintained over time as well. At a 3-month follow-up, only 16.2% of those who received CPT and 29.7% of those who received PE were PTSD positive. Finally, at a 9-month follow-up, 80.8% of CPT and 84.6% of PE patients remained in sustained remission from PTSD symptoms. In sum, CPT appears to be an efficacious intervention for the short- and long-term treatment of PTSD. This study also provides further evidence for the efficacy of PE.

Eye Movement Desensitization and Reprocessing

EMDR emerged as a treatment for PTSD in the early 1990s, and since that time, a number of studies have investigated its efficacy. A core component of this intervention is theorized to be the therapist's repeated elicitation of rapid, saccadic eye movements (or other bilateral stimulation) from the patient during the processing of traumatic memories. Shapiro theorized that rapid eye movements in some way override or reverse neural blockage or obstruction induced by the traumatic event. During EMDR treatment sessions, patients are asked to generate an image of the trauma and to focus on trauma-related thoughts, feelings, and/or sensations. Simultaneously, the therapist elicits the saccadic eye movements by having patients visually track a finger rapidly waved back and forth in front of their face. Other forms of laterally alternating stimuli (e.g., tapping or alternating sounds) are sometimes used rather than the original finger tracking. Patients are asked to evaluate the cognitions associated with these images and experiences and to generate alternative cognitive appraisals of the trauma or their behavior during the event. As patients focus on the distressing images and thoughts, and later focus on the alternative cognition, the saccadic eye movement (or another form of bilateral stimulation) is intermittently generated.

EMDR has been the focus of considerable controversy due to early claims regarding remarkable success in only a single session. Of the studies evaluating the efficacy of EMDR, more recent studies have typically used well-controlled designs and thus yielded clearly interpretable results. One well-controlled 1997 study evaluated the efficacy of EMDR relative to WL for PTSD in female rape victims. Three sessions of EMDR resulted in greater improvement of PTSD symptoms (57% reduction in PTSD at posttreatment) than WL (10% reduction at posttreatment). However, in contrast to other controlled studies, one therapist conducted all the treatments, and therefore the contribution of therapist and treatment effects are confounded. A direct comparison between EMDR and a combined treatment of PE plus stress inoculation training (called trauma treatment protocol, TTP) was conducted by DeVilly and Spence. Both TTP and EMDR reduced PTSD severity (63 and 46%, respectively), but TTP patients maintained their gains at follow-up, whereas EMDR patients showed higher rates of relapse (symptom reduction at follow-up of 61 and 12%, respectively). Rothbaum, Astin, and Marsteller compared PE, EMDR, and WL in female sexual assault victims. Compared to WL, both treatments resulted in a significant reduction in PTSD severity and related psychopathology. Immediately after treatment, only 5% of PE participants and 25% of EMDR participants continued to meet PTSD diagnostic criteria, compared to 90% of WL participants. The active treatments were significantly different from WL but did not differ from one another. At follow-up, however, significantly more participants receiving PE (78%) achieved good end-state functioning than did participants receiving EMDR (35%). Taylor and colleagues compared PE, EMDR, and R and found that PE produced significantly greater reductions in reexperiencing and avoidance symptoms than EMDR and R, which did not differ from one another. Indeed, a 2001 meta-analysis found EMDR to be no more effective than exposure therapy programs and, moreover, suggested that the eye movements integral to the treatment and its underlying theory are unnecessary.

In summary, several cognitive-behavioral therapy programs have received empirical support for their efficacy in reducing PTSD severity and diagnosis in controlled studies: PE, SIT, CT, CPT, and EMDR. Studies that have attempted to combine these empirically supported approaches into new treatment packages to improve outcome have failed to demonstrate superior outcomes compared to the single-treatment protocols in these clinical trials.

Real-World Treatment Considerations

Treatment Tolerability and Preference

It also important to explore the tolerability and acceptability of empirically supported treatments for PTSD. Notably, although concerns have been raised by some clinicians and researchers that PE is too difficult to tolerate and may lead to symptom worsening and treatment drop-out, there is evidence that PE is tolerable. For example, Foa and colleagues examined self-reported symptom exacerbation in a sample of women with chronic assault-related PTSD who were receiving PE. After the first imaginal exposure, only a minority of participants in the study exhibited reliable symptom exacerbation during treatment: 10.5% reported an increase in PTSD symptoms, 21.1% reported an increase in anxiety, and 9.2% reported an increase in depression. Significantly, patients who reported such symptom exacerbation benefited from PE as much as those who did not report such exacerbation and were not more likely to drop out of treatment. Thus, although some patients experienced a brief period of exacerbation of symptoms during PE, this exacerbation decreased within 2 weeks and was unrelated to treatment outcome or completion. With respect to the completion of treatment, additional evidence supports that PE is tolerable. A 2003 review of dropout rates from various cognitive-behavioral therapy treatments for PTSD across 25 controlled studies indicated no significant differences in dropout rates among trials of PE, CT, SIT, EMDR, and combined treatments. PE did not produce a higher rate of treatment dropouts than other PTSD treatments; thus, concerns about excessive treatment dropout from PE appear to be unwarranted.

In fact, recent data demonstrate that treatments including PE are actually preferred over other psychosocial and psychopharmacological treatments. In a forced-choice comparison of treatment preference between PE and sertraline (an antidepressant medication) for PTSD, approximately 87% of female college students chose PE compared to only 7% who chose medication (6% chose no treatment). Consistent with these data, Tarrier and colleagues found that adults strongly prefer PE for PTSD compared to other psychosocial interventions, including EMDR, group therapy, and psychodynamic psychotherapy.

Treatment Dissemination

Disseminating empirically supported treatments such as PE to community-based clinicians is an important step in bridging the critical gap between research and practice for trauma survivors with PTSD. In one of the first studies to evaluate such dissemination, Foa and colleagues trained clinicians at a community-based rape crisis center in the delivery of PE for assault survivors with PTSD. These community clinicians provided treatment to a subset of participants in a randomized controlled trial, and their outcomes were compared to participants treated by those with expertise in PE at an academic medical center. After an initial training with follow-up consultation and supervision, results showed that the community mental health counselors obtained outcomes comparable to the university-based providers. This provides good evidence that empirically supported treatments such as PE can be successfully disseminated.

Childhood Sexual Abuse-Related Posttraumatic Stress Disorder

Despite the documented efficacy of PE for PTSD, there is some concern reported in the clinical literature that adults who have PTSD secondary to maltreatment during childhood, specifically child sexual abuse, may be a particularly vulnerable population for whom PE may be too difficult to tolerate. In response to this concern, a new treatment protocol, skills training affect and interpersonal regulation plus modified prolonged exposure (STAIR/MPE), was designed as a two-phase treatment, with phase 1 consisting of skills training in affect and interpersonal regulation and phase 2 consisting of modified PE (imaginal exposure plus coping skills training, with no *in vivo* exposure). Data suggested that STAIR/MPE resulted in significant reductions in PTSD and depression compared to WL. However, a critical weakness of this study is that this combination treatment was not compared to the usual PE. It is of note that two recent clinical trials demonstrated that cognitive-behavioral treatments are effective for reducing PTSD among child sexual abuse survivors without a skills-building component. Moreover, a subanalysis of the data from Foa et al.'s 2005 study demonstrated that patients whose PTSD was related to child sexual abuse benefited from PE and PE/CR as much as did those whose PTSD was related to adult trauma. Thus, it seems that the skills-building component, which extends the number of treatment sessions and may delay recovery time, is unnecessary above the brief treatments that have empirical support.

Conclusion

Although exposure to potentially traumatic events is quite common, only a small minority of people develop persistent psychological difficulties such as PTSD in response to a trauma. The most validated types of treatment for PTSD are cognitive-behavioral therapies, and among the cognitive-behavioral therapy approaches available, PE has the strongest empirical support. Further, recent data suggest that PE is a preferred treatment among those who are given various treatment descriptions for PTSD. Concerns over the tolerability of PE, specifically that PE may lead to symptom exacerbation or premature dropout, are not supported by data. STAIR/MPE, a modified version of PE, has been shown to be helpful for childhood sexual abuse survivors with PTSD. However, this modified treatment has not been compared directly to already validated treatments for PTSD such as PE. Thus, at this point, we cannot determine whether it offers incremental benefit above such treatments. Future research should continue to evaluate ways to enhance treatment outcome and to disseminate efficacious treatments to a larger number of those who suffer with PTSD.

See Also the Following Articles

Acute Stress Disorder and Posttraumatic Stress Disorder; Posttraumatic Stress Disorder in Children; Posttraumatic Stress Disorder, Delayed; Posttraumatic Stress Disorder – Neurobiological basis for.

Further Reading

American Psychiatric, Association (1994). *Diagnostic and statistical manual of mental health disorders* (4th edn.). Washington, DC: American Psychiatric Association.

Cloitre, M., Koenen, K. C., Cohen, L. R., et al. (2002). Skills training in affective and interpersonal regulation followed by exposure: a phase-based treatment for PTSD related to childhood abuse. *Journal of Consulting and Clinical Psychology* **70**(5), 1067–1074.

Foa, E. B., Dancu, C. V., Hembree, E. A., et al. (1999). A comparison of exposure therapy, stress inoculation training, and their combination for reducing posttraumatic stress disorder in female assault victims. *Journal of Consulting and Clinical Psychology* **67**(2), 194–200.

Foa, E. B. and Rothbaum, B. O. (1998). *Treating the trauma of rape*. New York: Guildford Press.

Kessler, R. C., Sonnega, A., Bromet, E., et al. (1995). Posttraumatic stress disorder in the national comorbidity survey. *Archives of General Psychiatry* **52**, 1048–1060.

Zoellner, L. A., Feeny, N. C., Cochran, B., et al. (2003). Treatment choice for PTSD. *Behaviour Research & Therapy* **41**(8), 879–886.

Nightmares

M Hirshkowitz and A Sharafkhaneh
Baylor College of Medicine and Michael E. DeBakey Veteran Affairs Medical Center, Houston, TX, USA

This is a revised version of the article by M Hirshkowitz and C A Moore, Encyclopedia of Stress First Edition, volume 3, pp 49–52, © 2000, Elsevier Inc.

Glossary

Hypnagogic and hypnopompic hallucinations — Vivid sensory images occurring at the transition between sleep and wakefulness. Hypnagogic refers to hallucinations occurring as a person falls asleep while hypnopompic images occur as a person awakens. Hypnagogic imagery may be particularly vivid during rapid eye movement (REM) sleep occurring at sleep onset (as in narcolepsy). Similarly, dreamlike hypnopompic images may continue during wakefulness upon sudden or partial awakening from REM sleep. Hypnagogic and hypnopompic hallucinations may be accompanied by a complete inability to move (sleep paralysis).

Nachtmare — Nacht (night) + mare (spirit or monster). Mythologies throughout the world describe devils, demons, evil spirits, ogres, ghosts, vampires, old hags, and witches that attack individuals while they sleep. The *mare* usually sits on or crushes the sleeper's chest causing a smothering sensation and an inability to breathe. Additionally, the individual is usually unable to move. Sometimes there are sexual overtones as well with the spirit raping or assaulting the person while they lay paralyzed. This description suggests the occurrence of the parasomnia sleep paralysis accompanied by a hypnagogic or hypnopompic hallucination.

Night terror (also known as sleep terror) — A sleep disorder usually arising from slow-wave sleep that involves a sudden awakening with intense fear. The afflicted individual usually emits a sharp piercing scream. Autonomic nervous system activation accompanies the awakening and the individual will often have tachycardia, tachypnea, sweating, and increased muscle tone. The individual typically acts confused, disoriented, and inconsolable during the episode; however, there may be complete amnesia about the episode upon awakening the next morning.

Parasomnia — A disorder of arousal, partial arousal, or sleep stage transition. Parasomnias occur episodically during sleep and may interfere with sleep, sometimes producing insomnia or daytime sleepiness.

Rapid eye movement (REM) sleep — REM sleep is one of the five sleep stages defined in humans. REM sleep was discovered by Eugene Aserinsky who noted eye movements occurring every 90–100 minutes during sleep. In initial studies, dream recall was better correlated with awakenings from REM than other sleep stages. Consequently, REM sleep came to be considered the biological substrate of dreams.

Sleep paralysis — The inability to perform voluntary movements upon awakening from sleep or just before sleep onset. The individual is fully conscious, usually feels acutely anxious, typically is unable to vocalize, and may have hallucinatory activity accompanying the paralysis episode.

Nightmares, according to current terminology, are unpleasant, distressing, or frightening dreams that usually occur during rapid eye movement (REM) sleep. The International Classification of Sleep Disorders–Second Edition (ICSD-2) formally classifies the nightmare disorder as a parasomnia usually associated with REM sleep. Nightmares, as currently defined are "coherent dream sequences that seem real and become increasingly more disturbing as they unfold. Emotions usually involve anxiety, fear, or terror but frequently also anger, rage, embarrassment, disgust, and other negative feelings. Dream content most often focuses on imminent physical danger to the individual but can also involve distressing themes." The fears produced by the dream usually dissipate rapidly after awakening and clear sensorium returns.

Phenomenology of Frightening Awakenings

Although nightmares are currently conceptualized as frightening dreams that usually produce an awakening from REM sleep, the term derives from *nachtmare* which refers to a quite different phenomenon. The nachtmare (or night spirit) has taken many forms in folk lore and superstition, ranging from vampires (in Medieval Eastern Europe) to witch riders (among preAmerican Civil War slaves). Contemporary alien attacks are likely an offshoot of the same disorder.

The nachtmare accompanies sleep paralysis with frightening hypnagogic or hypnopompic hallucinations and characteristically arise during the transition from wakefulness to sleep. The sleeper has difficulty breathing due to the creature sitting on his or her chest, there may also be a sense of sexual molestation, the sleeper may feel that their life force is being sucked out of them. To complicate things further, the mythical nachtmares Incubus and Succubus are commonly associated with yet as distinctly different phenomenon: the sleep terrors (*Pavor nocturnus*). Sleep terrors usually occur in slow-wave sleep, are not dreamlike, and are poorly recalled. The person may remember a frightening image; however, narrative and plot are rare.

By contrast, the nightmare in modern parlance explicitly arises from a dream, implying imagery, narrative, and plot. Individuals awakened from a dream typically recollect its content. Nightmares may afflict 10–50% of children and 50–85% of adults have at least an occasional nightmare. Overall estimates for the prevalence of nightmares range from 2–8% in the general population. Nightmares arising from either acute or posttraumatic stress disorders (PTSDs) may occur in stage 2 sleep as well as during REM sleep. However, there are other widely recognized types of awakenings associated with subjective reports of panic, dysphoria, or anxiety. These included sleep-related panic attacks, sleep terrors, and sleep paralysis with hypnagogic or hypnopompic hallucinations. These paroxysmal events arise from different stages of sleep. Like REM sleep nightmares, sleep-related panic attacks are characterized by awakening with fear. Polysomnography reveals that these episodes customarily occur during sleep stage 2, often during transition to slow-wave sleep. However, sleep-related panic attacks may occur, although rarely, at the wake-to-sleep transition.

Nightmares and Posttraumatic Stress Disorder

Nightmare frequency increases during periods of stress and after an individual experiences a distressing event (e.g., an automobile accident, burglary, rape, or death of a friend or relative). Stress and sleep deprivation are also thought to exacerbate sleep paralysis, sleep terrors, and sleep-related panic attacks. One approach to exploring the relationship between stress and these phenomena is to study the sleep in individuals with PTSD.

Silva and colleagues reported on symptoms in 131 physically or sexually abused women interviewed in a primary care setting. They found that 65% reported bad dreams, flashbacks, and/or terror attacks. These women had higher intrusion and avoidance scores. Nightmares are also reported in school age children after being involved as passengers in traffic accidents. Psychological consequences were common and persisted in 33% of children after 4–7 months. Eleven percent were thought to be severely afflicted on follow up with 17% reporting nightmares and other sleep difficulties. Nightmares related to trauma are known to persist for prolonged periods. A study of Dutch war veterans found nightmares and anxiety dreams 40 years after the traumatizing event. In a large survey of Vietnam War veterans, using a careful sampling technique, nightmare frequency strongly correlated with combat exposure. Insomnia also was associated with combat exposure but not to the same degree as nightmares. By contrast, neither chronic medical illnesses nor psychiatric disorders (panic disorder, major depression, mania, and alcohol abuse) could predict nightmare frequency.

Although recurrent distressing dreams are a key PTSD diagnostic feature according to DSM-IV, the nature of these nightmares is in question. Many clinicians assume that PTSD nightmares represent a REM sleep phenomenon; however, PTSD nightmares are poorly understood. In many respects their features conform to those present in REM sleep nightmares. They typically contain imagery, narrative, and plot. However, the repetitive, recurring nature of these nocturnal frightening phantasms makes them unusual. Another uncommon characteristic of chronic PTSD nightmares is that they narrate traumatic events, often without elaboration or symbolism. Several published descriptions of PTSD nightmares include the adrenergic concomitants tachycardia and sweating that are atypical of REM sleep. These features more commonly accompany sleep terrors. Thus, it is not surprising that some sleep experts contend that PTSD nightmares can arise from any stage of sleep. Hartmann in his extensive monograph on nightmares flatly states that PTSD nightmares "... are not typical REM nightmares; they occur sometimes in stage 2 and sometimes in all stages of sleep and even at sleep onset..." Kramer and Kinney also emphasize that PTSD nightmares can arise from both REM and stage 2 sleep.

Ross and associates argue strongly that REM sleep disturbance is closely involved in the pathogenesis of PTSD. This disturbance may be either "inappropriate recruitment of essentially normal REM sleep processes" or involvement of "inherently dysfunctional REM sleep mechanisms". They correctly contend that the vividness and recallability of PTSD nightmare content has more in common with REM than non-REM mentation. REM sleep is comprised of an array of individual features, including: low amplitude, mixed frequency electroencephalograph (EEG) activity; rapid eye movements; muscle atonia; pontine geniculate occipital (PGO) discharges; small muscle twitches; periorbital integrated potentials (PIPs); and middle ear muscle activity (MEMA). Although these activities usually occur in concert, they sometimes dissociate, as in REM sleep behavior disorder (RBD). In RBD, the atonia that characteristically accompanies REM sleep is absent. In fact, Ross and colleagues suggest RBD as a possible model for the pathophysiological mechanism underlying PTSD nightmares. In their overnight polysomnographic studies, these researchers showed that combat veterans with PTSD had elevated REM sleep percentage, longer average REM cycle duration, and increased REM density (number of eye movements per minute of REM sleep) compared to controls. These same investigators also report more phasic leg muscle activity during REM sleep in veterans with PTSD than in those without PTSD. Admittedly, the sample was small; however, these studies provide a foundation for further research.

Neuropharmacology of REM sleep clearly demonstrates involvement of cholinergic mechanisms. It is also widely accepted that acetylcholine plays an important role in the formation of memories. It has also been postulated that REM sleep mediates memory consolidation. When high adrenergic arousal accompanies a remembered experience (as occurs with acute trauma or re-experiencing a distant trauma), it appears that the memory process functions differently. Memories can be triggered by adrenergic arousal. The relationship between this arousal, flashbacks, and nightmares underlie current neuropsychiatric conceptualization of the consequences of traumatic stress. REM sleep has been characterized as a parasympathetic state with bursts of sympathetic activity (associated with phasic events). Nightmares and recurrent dreams may be considered a failure of dreamwork to handle emotionally laden, presumably adrenergically coupled experiences.

PTSD nightmares are reported in 92% of patients with flashbacks and 57% of patients without flashbacks, they seldom occur during laboratory sleep studies. This is the case even among patients who indicate having nightmares four or more times per week. Nonetheless, on several occasions during our 30 years of clinical polysomnography experience, patients had nightmares while sleeping in the laboratory. On those rare occasions, we noticed increased REM density just before awakenings associated with nightmares. Consultation with several sleep disorder medicine colleagues revealed that this is a widely held impression (e.g., Drs. Hartmann (Boston, MA), Roffwarg (Jackson, MS), Mendelson (Chicago, IL), and Mahowald (Minneapolis, MN). To the best of our collective knowledge and according to thorough search using medical databases, little systematic data exists beyond description of the phenomenon. Ross and associates mention exceedingly high REM density preceding a nightmare that fortuitously occurred during their study. We also have observed vastly increased phasic activity in combat veterans with PTSD referred to our Sleep Diagnostic Clinic for evaluation of insomnia, nightmares, or daytime sleepiness.

A phasic activity threshold likely exists that is necessary but not sufficient to produce nightmares. The level of phasic activity is elevated in patients with PTSD compared to control subjects. This conceptualization is analogous to the relationship between hypersynchronous slow-wave activity and parasomnias of arousal (confused awakening, sleepwalking, and sleep terror). Another perspective is suggested by the well-established relationship between sleep and some forms of epilepsy. Abnormal spike activity is enhanced by sleep deprivation. Interestingly, some neurophysiologically oriented researchers have posited a kindling model for flashbacks and nightmares. More research is needed to illuminate the biological substrate underlying the dysphoric mentation and paroxysmal awakenings that we call nightmares.

Treatment Approaches

Nightmares are experienced acutely (at some period during the lifetime) in many individuals. Furthermore, they typically resolve without intervention. However, persistent nightmares, particularly if the dream content is recurrent, can be a marker for significant psychopathology. In such cases, treatment is advised especially when the nightmare produces serious distress, insomnia, or interferes with daily activities. Similarly, nightmares in early childhood (preschool and early school years) are of less concern (assuming they are outgrown) than those beginning or persisting in late childhood and adolescence. In adults, the frequency of psychopathology is higher among patients suffering from chronic nightmares than in control subjects. Hartmann posits that nightmare sufferers have thin boundaries, are more vulnerable, and have weaker psychological defenses. He also suggests that these individuals are at risk for schizophrenia. In addition to this profile for patients with nightmares, traumatic events apparently can induce nightmares. The nightmares may be immediate or delayed. They may afflict the individual acutely or persist for many years. Finally, drug abuse, drug or alcohol withdrawal, and specific medications are associated with nightmares. Thus, treatment must start with a careful history emphasizing current stressors, possible traumatic experiences, psychopathology (in patient and family), alcohol and drug abuse, and medication regimen.

Several medications have been associated with increased chance of nightmares. Some of them act by potentiating REM sleep and others by producing REM sleep rebound on withdrawal. Such drugs include L-DOPA, reserpine, thiothixene, alpha methyldopa, metoprolol, propranalol, simvastatin, and atorvastatin. Interestingly, in addition to several statins appearing to induce nightmares, there is also a report by Arargun and associates (2005: 361–364) that nightmares are associated with low serum lipid levels.

Altering dose or substituting other pharmacological agents would be the first step in such cases. Alcohol or stimulant withdrawal also potentiates nightmares via presumed REM sleep mechanisms. In such cases, nightmares should be time-limited and resolve when sleep normalizes. If nightmares persist, intervention should be considered.

When psychopathology is found, it should be treated directly. Psychotherapy is thought to be beneficial. It is worth emphasizing that insomnia resulting from fear of sleep can pose a serious treatment obstacle. Sleep deprivation exacerbates nightmares, sleep terrors, and sleep paralysis attacks. Thus, the nightmare may perpetuate insomnia and thereby produce a vicious cycle. Behavioral interventions for insomnia are safe and effective in both the short and long term. Improved sleep hygiene, stimulus control therapy, sleep restriction therapy, and/or cognitive therapy are recommended. Krakow and Zadra (2006: 45–70) directly target the nightmare with imagery rehearsal therapy (IRT) with good results using four, 2-hour sessions. Another reportedly successful behavioral approach is lucid dream therapy. A lucid dream is one in which the dreamer becomes aware that he or she is dreaming. In an uncontrolled case series of five individuals that could be trained to recognize their dream state, nightmare frequency declined. Whether the decline related to increased lucidity or volitional alteration of dream content is unknown. In some cases, medications may be needed. Several medications reportedly provide some relief from nightmares when administered to patients with PTSD. Davidson and colleagues report decreased nightmare and general sleep disturbance scores in response to the atypical antidepressant nefazodone in a group of 17 patients treated with up to 600 mg day^{-1} for 12 weeks. Other antidepressants have been tried. Cavaljuga and co-workers (2003: 12–16) found fluoxetine more effective at reducing nightmares than amitriptyline; however, amitriptyline was more effective overall in acute PTSD. In another study by Gupta and co-workers, cyproheptadine (4–12 mg at bedtime) was found to be beneficial on retrospective review of nine patient charts. Response to this histamine-1 blocking, serotonin antagonist ranged from decreases in nightmare frequency (or intensity) to complete remission.

At present, the most systematic work on pharmacological treatment of nightmares is with prazosin. Peskind and colleagues (2003: 165–171) treated nine older men with posttraumatic nightmares with 2–4 mg prazosin 1 hour before bedtime. The drug substantially reduced nightmares in eight of the patients and was well tolerated. Furthermore, a 20-week, double-blind, crossover trial was conducted by Raskind and associates (2003: 371–373) in 10 Vietnam theatre combat veterans. A mean dose of 9.5 mg of prazosin was given at bedtime. Drug, compared to placebo, significantly reduced scores on recurrent distressing dreams.

In a review article concerning nightmare treatments, van Liempt (2006: 193–202) concludes that open-label reports suggest efficacy for some antidepressants, anticonvulsants, and atypical antipsychotic drugs. Placebo-controlled studies show possible efficacy with olanzapine and prazosin. We find these preliminary results are encouraging; however, more double-blind, placebo-controlled trials are needed. Finally, assorted benzodiazepines can provide relief from dream anxiety and help improve sleep. However, few randomized, placebo-controlled, clinical trials have been conducted and they had small sample sizes. Furthermore, the withdrawal effects from pharmacotherapeutic interventions have not been systematically studied.

Further Reading

Arargun, M. Y., Gulec, M., Cilli, A. S., et al. (2005). Nightmares and serum cholesterol level: a preliminary report. *Canadian Journal of Psychiatry* **50**, 361–364.

Bell, C. C., Shakoor, B., Thompson, B., et al. (1984). Prevalence of isolated sleep paralysis in black subjects. *Journal National Medical Association* **76**, 501–508.

Boriani, G., Biffi, M., Strocchi, E., et al. (2001). Nightmares and sleep disturbances with simvastatin and metoprolol. *Annals of Pharmacotherapy* **35**, 1292.

Cavaljuga, S., Licanin, I., Mulabegovic, N., et al. (2003). Therapeutic effects of two antidepressant agents in the treatment of posttraumatic stress disorder (PTSD). *Bosnian Journal of Basic Medical Sciences* **3**, 12–16.

Davidson, J. R., Weisler, R. H., Malik, M. L., et al. Treatment of posttraumatic stress disorder with nefazodone. *International Clinical Psychopharmacology* **13**, 111–113.

Diagnostic Classification Steering Committee. (1990). *International classification of sleep disorders – 2nd edition: diagnostic and coding manual.* Westchester, IL, USA: American Academy of Sleep Medicine.

Ermin, M. K. (1987). Dream anxiety attacks (nightmares). *Psychiatric Clinics of North America* **10**, 667–674.

Firestone, M. (1985). The "old hag" sleep paralysis in Newfoundland. *Journal of Psychoanalytic Anthropology* **8**, 47–66.

Gupta, S., Popli, A., Bathurst, E., et al. (1998). Efficacy of cyproheptadine for nightmares associated with post-traumatic stress disorder. *Comprehensive Psychiatry* **39**, 160–164.

Hartmann, E. (1984). *The nightmare: the psychology and biology of terrifying dreams*. New York: Basic Books.

Hauri, P. J., Friedman, M. and Ravaris, C. L. (1989). Sleep in patients with spontaneous panic attack. *Sleep* **12**, 323–337.

Kales, A., Soldatos, C., Caldwell, A., et al. (1980). Nightmares: clinical characteristics and personality patterns. *American Journal of Psychiatry* **137**, 1197–1201.

Krakow, B. and Zadra, A. (2006). Clinical management of chronic nightmares: imagery rehersal therapy. *Behavioral Sleep Medicine* **4**, 45–70.

Kramer, M. and Kinney, L. (1988). Sleep patterns in trauma victims with disturbed dreaming. *Psychiatric Journal of the University of Ottawa* **13**, 12–16.

Morin, C. M., Colecchi, C., Stone, J., et al. (1999). Behavioral and pharmacological therapies for late-life insomnia: a randomized controlled trial. *JAMA* **17**, 991–999.

Neylan, T. C., Marmar, C. R., Metzler, T. J., et al. (1998). Sleep disturbance in the Vietnam generation: findings from a nationally representative sample of male Vietnam veterans. *American Journal of Psychiatry* **155**, 929–933.

Peskind, E. R., Bonner, L. T., Hoff, D. J., et al. (2003). Prazosin reduces trauma-related nightmares in older men with chronic posttraumatic stress disorder. *Journal of Geriatric Psychiatry and Neurology* **16**, 165–171.

Raskind, M. A., Peskind, E. R., Kanter, E. D., et al. (2003). Reduction of nightmares and other PTSD symptoms in combat veterans by prazosin: a placebo-controlled study. *American Journal of Psychiatry* **160**, 371–373.

Ross, R. J., Ball, W. A., Sullivan, K. A., et al. (1989). Sleep disturbance as the hallmark of PTSD. *American Journal of Psychiatry* **146**, 697–707.

Silva, C., McFarlane, J., Soeken, K., et al. (1997). Symptoms of post-traumatic stress disorder in abused women in a primary care setting. *Journal of Womens Health* **6**, 543–552.

van Liempt, S., Vermetten, E., Geuze, E., et al. (2006). Pharmacotherapy for disordered sleep in post-traumatic stress disorder: a systematic review. *International Clinical Psychopharmacology* **21**, 193–202.

Woodward, S. H., Arsenault, N. J., Murray, C., et al. (2000). Laboratory sleep correlates of nightmare complaint in PTSD inpatients. *Biological Psychiatry* **48**, 1081–1087.

E. Mood Disorders: Depression

Affective Disorders

D F MacKinnon
Johns Hopkins University School of Medicine,
Baltimore, MD, USA

This is a revised version of the article by D F MacKinnon, Encyclopedia of Stress First Edition, volume 1, pp 87–94, © 2000, Elsevier Inc.

Glossary

Affect	Objective manifestations of emotional state, including facial expression, demeanor, neurovegetative functioning, and behavior, but also verbal statements reflecting mood, self-attitude, and vital sense.
Disease	A clinical syndrome with characteristic signs and symptoms, related to dysfunction in a bodily organ, caused at least in part by biological forces.
Mood	Sustained subjective emotional state.
Neuro-vegetative functioning	Motivated behavior essential to biological functioning, including sleep, appetite, and libido.
Psychosis	Severe symptoms of mental illness involving dysfunction in rational thought and reality testing, including hallucinations and delusions.
Self-attitude	Feelings of personal worth, ranging from grandiosity to self-loathing.
Vital sense	Feelings of physical well-being, including energy, clarity and speed of thought.

Affective disorders are psychiatric syndromes characterized by significant disturbances in mood, the sense of self-worth, and the feelings and functions of physical well-being. Affective disorders can lead to occupational and interpersonal impairment and often (perhaps not often enough) the pursuit of treatment. Suicide is an all-too-common outcome of a severe affective disorder. Major depression, according to the United Nations World Health Organization, is the second leading cause worldwide of lost years of health and productivity. Mood swings routinely wreck marriages and careers and trigger and sustain substance abuse. The clinical features, management, and biology of mania and major depression are described elsewhere in this work; therefore, the present article examines the concept of affective disorders from the multiple perspectives of phenomenology, meaning, behavior, and temperament to complement the growing biological understanding of these disorders.

Phenomenology of Affective Disorders

The clinical syndrome of all affective disorders is a persistent and pervasive disturbance in mood, self-attitude, vital sense, and neurovegetative functioning. In depression, the varieties of mood disturbance include not only melancholia or sadness, but also apathy, anxiety, and irritability. Some patients describe depression as the absence of any feeling. The mood of a manic patient may be elated, but also irascible to the point of belligerence, expansive without a sense of euphoria, or simply excitable.

Self-attitude, the feeling of personal worth, is insidiously disturbed in affective disorders. The disturbance in self-valuation often impedes treatment. Depressed patients may delay treatment because the suffering they experience seems somehow deserved; ultimately suicide may be desired because the patient feels that he or she is such a burden on others. Manic patients may feel smarter than the doctor and others, and may feel misunderstood or insulted by the suggestion they are ill.

Affectively ill patients have a disturbance in the sense of physical well-being, or vital sense. In depressed patients, physical well-being is lacking; patients feel tired, weak, slow, and inept; cognition is halting or uncertain. Manic patients tend to feel energized, quick, tireless, and powerful. Thoughts move swiftly; the patient may have the sense that he or she is thinking circles around others, while others may find the patient's ideas loose, connected by the thinnest of associations – clanging speech, riddled with puns and rhymes, is seen in severe cases – or at the most severe, incomprehensible. Neurovegetative functioning – the body's internal regulation of activity and metabolism – is typically disturbed in both syndromes. Depressed patients may have insomnia or may sleep to excess without feeling rested. Manic patients may feel little to no need to sleep and may arise rested after a few hours and carry on in this manner to the marvel (or annoyance) of others. Appetites tend to diminish with depression (though some will overeat or binge); in mania the drive for food is less often disturbed, but the drives for sex, acquisition, and excitement are enhanced.

Affective disorders are diagnosed from clinical history and observation of the patient's demeanor and behavior. The clinician is more certain of the diagnosis upon hearing the patient's own description of troubling mental phenomena and personally observing signs (e.g., emaciation, lethargy, agitation, rapid speech) consistent with the clinical syndrome. There are no laboratory tests to reveal affective disorder.

The Experience of Affective Disorders

Literature abounds with poignant and gritty descriptions of what it is like to be manic or depressed. A pervasive theme in these descriptions is the relative inability of a person in the grip of a severe mania or depression to perceive that the accompanying attitudes, responsiveness, and emotional states are pathologically disconnected from or disproportionate to the true circumstances. A depressed mood, sleepless nights, lack of appetite, feelings of worthlessness, and wishes for death often seem to a depressed patient to follow inevitably an unwanted change in life such as a divorce or job loss. A profound sense of meaninglessness is attributed to the world, rather than to the patient's altered perception of the world. The elated mood in mania seems to the inexperienced patient to be the natural consequence of possessing superhuman energy and confidence. The heightened sense that everything is possible seems a quality of the world, in the eyes of the manic patient, and not a distortion driven by an abnormal mood.

Insofar as depressive and some manic states are unpleasant, patients generally understand them to be a response to stress, with the implied assumption that they have had a nervous breakdown because they were unable to handle the stress. On being diagnosed with an affective disorder, many patients are relieved to hear their distress attributed to a medical illness or chemical imbalance in the brain, especially when told of the successful record of biological treatment. Patients with repeated episodes of mania and depression eventually come to see the disease as a primary problem, rather than a secondary result of life circumstances. It begins to seem more plausible that, while some episodes may certainly have followed a significant change in life circumstances, others were unprovoked, or even preceded a change in circumstances; indeed, it may occur to the experienced patient that the changes were in some cases caused by the affective disorder. Was a patient's emotional state so inconstant that romantic partners found the relationship intolerable? Did a drop in energy and motivation result in an unfavorable change in job status, which heralded a suicidal episode? Did a patient feel elated because of a vacation in the tropics, or did the motivation to travel stem from a markedly heightened capacity for excitement, pleasure, and financial largesse?

Thus, the general question of whether stress causes affective instability or affective instability causes stress cannot be answered definitively by asking the patient, as the illness distorts the patient's ability to tell the difference. This is one fundamental difference between an affective disorder and a disorder of the visceral or peripheral organs: in the latter case, the intact mind, seated in the brain, receives unambiguous information from another organ about a disease process, e.g., pain, shortness of breath, weakness. With affective disorders, the major symptoms are in the mind, where they impede perceptions and judgments.

Behavior in Affective Disorders

From the perspective of a family member or treating clinician, the most salient features of an affective disorder are the behavioral difficulties it drives. Most alarmingly, affective disorders often drive self-destructive behavior. The vast majority of suicide victims can be diagnosed, in retrospect, with affective disorder. When the suicidal behavior does not result in death, it nevertheless may permanently strain relationships with those the patient intended to leave behind.

Suicide is the direst behavioral outcome of affective disorder, but not the only significant maladaptive behavior. At the core of maladaptive, affectively driven behaviors is the change in hedonic capacity that typically accompanies them. Where reward is absent, as in the anhedonic, depressed patient, experiences may seem flat and meaningless, and in many cases painful and enervating. A depressed patient may withdraw to bed, avoid family, friends, and work, and seek solace in alcohol or drugs. When reward comes too easily or powerfully, as in mania, the impulse to spend, drive, and love recklessly, to flout the law and social mores, and to abuse alcohol and drugs is nearly irresistible. For the manic patient there is an indiscriminate sense of excitement over a world of newly perceived opportunities for enjoyment, resulting in costly, uninhibited, social and financial decisions.

It is important to note that affective disorders are not essential in such behaviors. Many people who attempt suicide, avoid work, spend recklessly, or drink heavily lack the signs and symptoms of affective disorders. Many patients with affective disorders (perhaps most) manage, somehow, to constrain their behavior. Patients who change their behavior in the midst of an episode of affective disorder may benefit from confrontation and counseling about the consequences of their behavior. Some therapists think of the self-defeating and self-deprecating thoughts and attitudes that arise during depression as behaviors amenable to confrontation and redirection; this idea is the basis of cognitive therapy.

The degree of behavioral impairment associated with affective disorder can be a function not only of the severity of the symptoms, but also of the vulnerability of the patient to behavioral excess or instability. A libertine when stable is more likely than a saint to engage in reckless acts when affectively ill, if only because the means to such acts are more familiar. An academically and economically marginal college student knocked out of school by affective illness may have a harder time getting back on track than a middle-class mid-career middle manager in a solid marriage. A student not only lacks the benefit of a structured life upon which to recover, but may also have the option unavailable to the older person of re-entering a state of dependency on parents, a state that may reinforce functional debilitation. Patients and families are wisely counseled not to make major changes in career, family, or housing in the midst of an episode of mania or depression. The fewer the changes, the less the risk of serious impairment, and the easier the rehabilitation once the episode clears.

Affective Disorders and Personality

Greater symptom severity may drive one patient's behavior to go awry while a less afflicted patient remains relatively steady, but personality and life circumstances also contribute. Some affectively ill patients prone to dysfunctional behavior may have personality disorders at baseline. Personality disorder refers, in diagnostic nomenclature, to enduring patterns of temperamental vulnerability and problematic behavior. These disorders may themselves be defined by their affective components, e.g., the labile affect of the borderline patient or the constricted affect of the schizoid patient. Thus, it can be hard to tell if a patient who seems to meet diagnostic criteria for a personality disorder really has an affective disorder. Patients in a manic state often display labile affect and indifference to the feelings of others (and other borderline or narcissistic traits), and depressed patients often appear cold and constricted. Thus, it is generally prudent to wait to assign a definitive personality disorder diagnosis to an affectively ill patient until after the affective syndrome clears up and the patient can be observed in the well state.

The concept of affective disorder also becomes salient when considering individuals who seem characterologically gloomy, moody, or excitable. Although they are counted as having mild forms of affective disorder, the existence of chronically gloomy (dysthymic) and chronically moody (cyclothymic) individuals illustrates the permeable boundaries between entities considered as medical disorders versus those understood as features of character or temperament. Indeed, affective and personality disorders may not be fully independent in their origins. It seems plausible to assume that childhood or adolescent onset of affective disorder is likely to result in persistent – even permanent – changes in the direction of personality development. Whereas affectively stable individuals learn through experience to properly associate their behaviors with desired social and interpersonal consequences, the experience of affective disorder, which warps these affective connections during critical stages of adult development, may lead to the sort of immature emotionality and self-defeating behavior that characterize the personality disorders.

Varieties of Affective Disorder

There are many ways to categorize affective disorders. The most salient clinical distinction is between manic-depressive and melancholic (depressive) disorders. Modern nosology refers to these disorders as bipolar disorder and major depressive disorder. Beyond the differentiation by polarity, affective disorders are classified according to severity and chronicity. **Figure 1** illustrates the spectrum of affective disorders, ranging from mild, transient normal mood fluctuations to severe, rapid-cycling bipolar disorder type I.

In clinical reality, the differentiation of mania from depression is not always so clear. Many patients experience either a mixture or the rapid alternation of manic and depressive symptoms. One way to understand these mixed states (following Kraepelin) is to postulate that there are different components of affect (we might call them mood, cognition, and energy) that tend to cycle in synchrony during typical manic (high mood, rapid and copious thoughts, high energy) and depressive (low mood, sluggish and paltry thoughts, diminished energy) episodes, but that synchrony is lost in mixed states (**Figure 2**). A patient in a common presentation of mixed state will tend to have a dysphoric (irritable, nihilistic) mood but such racing thoughts and restless energy that the patient will appear irascible and feel highly uncomfortable. In practice, the mixed state is seen as a high-risk state for suicide. In contrast, a patient with agitated depression combines dysphoric mood with restless energy and a poverty of thought, generally manifested as a tendency to ruminate on a single, depressive theme. Other combinations, in particular those involving euphoric mood without high energy, seem more rare, though it may be that these patients are rarely brought to treatment.

History of the Concept of Affective Disorders

Descriptions of melancholia and mania date back to Hippocrates, and many medical writers throughout

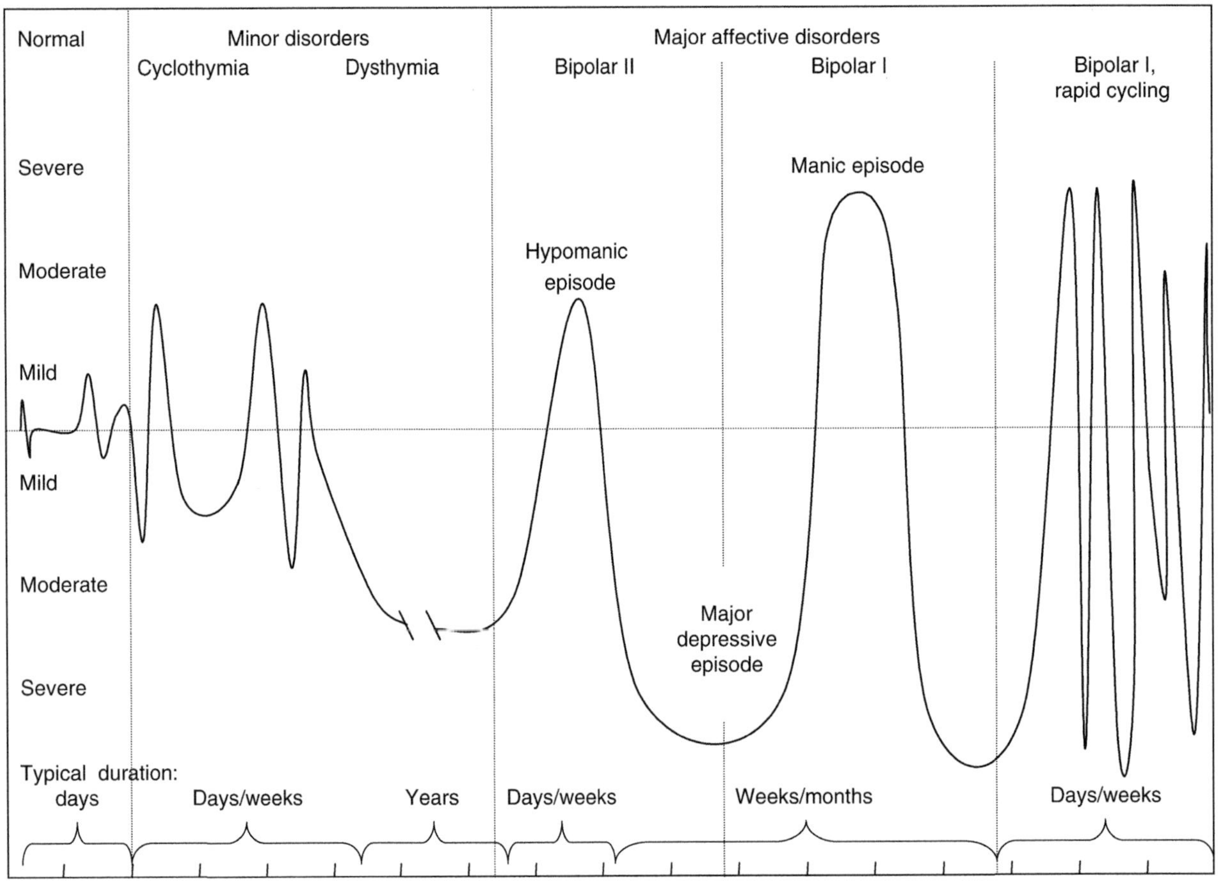

Figure 1 Affective disorder diagnoses as a function of the frequency and amplitude of mood variability. Note that normal mood changes may be frequent but are mild and transient, while the more severe mood swings tend to last weeks, months, and in the case of dysthymia, years.

history were able to describe the manic-depressive syndrome in a way familiar to modern psychiatrists. Until the nineteenth century, the prevailing explanations for affective disorders relied on the humoral theory. Abnormal balances of bodily fluids such as black bile (the roots for the term melancholia) or yellow bile (an excess of which was associated with the choleric, or irritable, temperament) were felt to be the cause of affective imbalance.

By the nineteenth century, ideas about the organic basis of disease had become more sophisticated, and observations of psychopathology were made systematically with the view that affective disorders had their basis in an as-yet-unknown disease of the brain. An exemplar of this trend was Emil Kraepelin, who delineated the patterns of symptoms and course in the institutionalized severely mentally ill under his care. Kraepelin noted a general difference in the course and affective symptomatology in the two groups of patients: those having a remitting/relapsing forms of psychosis marked by prominent signs of affective disturbance, and those having a chronic psychosis with affective flattening. Kraepelin called the remitting/relapsing disorder manic-depressive insanity and the chronic psychotic conditions paranoia (including dementia praecox, now better known as schizophrenia).

Psychiatric epidemiologists have established that affective disorders are not only found in the severely, institutionalized mentally ill, but also are fairly common in the general population. About 1 in 100 individuals in population surveys meet diagnostic criteria for bipolar disorder, and 5–10% have a major depressive episode at some time in life. Many patients with affective disorders do not develop psychosis or require hospitalization; a rather large percentage never enters treatment.

Historical accounts of the obviously manic and melancholic are not too hard to find; it is harder to account for the large number of those who, it is supposed, experienced milder forms of mania and depression but understood these experiences in nonmedical terms. Traces of these experiences perhaps are found in the annals of art, literature, politics, business, philosophy, exploration, science, and religion, where a mild depression in a receptive mind may produce enduring insights about the fragility of existence or tenderness to the suffering of others.

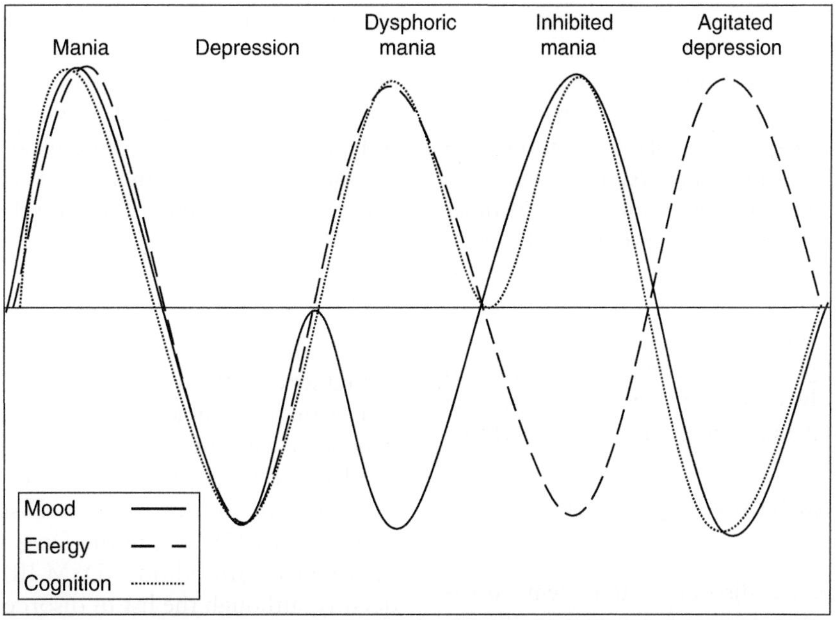

Figure 2 Kraepelin's schema of mixed affective states. The coexistence of a morose mood (low emotion) with physical restlessness or agitation (high volition) and racing thoughts (high intellect) creates a typical mixed state.

Mild manic states may have contributed to expansive works of art or ambitious, risky exploration and entrepreneurship. Affectively colored cultural contributions are not necessarily pathological, though the experience of the passionate, creative, or daring historical figure might resemble in detail the experience of a typical patient with an affective disorder. It is just as possible that the availability of effective antidepressive and antimanic treatments in times past might have robbed the world of some works of genius as it is possible that the geniuses themselves might have been spared much suffering and contributed even more had treatment been available.

Affective Disorders as Diseases

Efforts to link affective disorders to external circumstances have yielded distinctions between mourning and melancholia (Freud), and reactive versus endogenous depression. But if it is unclear whether stress causes depression or vice versa, then a simpler, assumption-free explanatory model is required if we are to understand the normal dejection that results from, say, a romantic setback, versus the prolonged sadness that accompanies the grieving process, versus a pathological affective disorder. Unlike emotional reactions, affective disorders are clinical syndromes with stereotypical patterns of sign, symptoms, course, and treatment response. Unlike grieving, affective disorders are associated in some cases with known brain disease. Affective disorders are best understood as medical diseases, i.e., as syndromal entities emerging from biological dysfunction in the brain and body.

Like other medical diseases, affective disorders are not limited by culture, intelligence, education, socioeconomic status, or experience. Nor do the symptoms of affective disorder vary much across cultures, although one might expect to see culturally and individually specific manifestations of these symptoms. The typical symptoms of affective disorder cluster over a similar course and respond to the same biological treatments anywhere in the world. Affective disorders, moreover, may arise from known medical causes. Huntington's disease, a genetic disorder of progressive dementia and abnormal movement, carries a high risk for manic-depressive disorder. Some patients develop their first depression after a stroke (particularly a stroke in the left frontal part of the brain). Certain medications can cause a clear depressive syndrome; knowledge of the pharmacology of such drugs spawned research into medications to reverse the depressive syndrome. Cortisol-like drugs (e.g., prednisone) frequently induce manic symptoms in people with no history of affective disorder. If such known changes to the anatomy and biochemistry of the brain can trigger the characteristic signs and symptoms of affective disorder, then it seems reasonable to conclude that the commonly observed affective disorders arise from biological mechanisms as yet unknown, but knowable.

In contrast, clinical problems related to mood alone are strongly culture bound and uniquely expressed, generally have few if any symptoms other than a bad mood, and cannot be mimicked by drugs or other medical diseases. Unpleasant or unmanageably intense mood reactions of this sort are best viewed primarily as discouragement, demoralization, the blues, or in the official nomenclature, adjustment disorders. Grief, on the other hand, has a syndromal quality to it, with characteristic sensations: the welling-up feeling, the false recognition of the departed in a crowd. Uncomplicated grief is not a disease, of course, but a normal part of human experience: painful, but rich with personal meaning. In real clinical situations, it is not always simple to distinguish grieving from moping from depression, but it is essential to try.

Affective versus Other Psychiatric Disorders

Patients with affective disorder often seem superficially to have other sorts of psychiatric illness, and vice versa. While affectively ill patients may demonstrate cognitive dysfunction (poor attention and concentration in depression, disorganization and distractibility in mania), mania and depression are not a cognitive disorder, like dementia, since the cognitive difficulties tend to clear up with normalization of the mood. In contrast to a chronic psychotic disorder such as schizophrenia, psychotic symptoms in patients with affective disorder tend to occur only when the patient is in the grip of severe mania or depression. In practice, however, the boundaries of affective and psychotic disorders are not always well defined. Some believe that schizophrenia and bipolar disorder have the same cause, with schizoaffective disorder as an intermediate type; it seems more likely that both disorders have complex causes and that some of these causes affect the presentation and course of illness in either disorder. Anxiety disorders, too, may be related to affective disorders; indeed, anxious moods, phobic avoidance, panic disorder, and obsessive–compulsive disorder are seen frequently in patients with affective disorder. Anxiety disorders share some of the characteristic symptoms of affective disorders: disturbances of mood and physical well-being, but miss the typical affective disturbances in self-worth, sleep, and appetite.

In summary, affective disorders are fairly common and often severe medical diseases afflicting mood, self-attitude, vital sense, and the bodily functions of sleep, appetite, and libido. Some patients exhibit marked changes in behavior, while others maintain the appearance of normality despite their symptoms. Although a patient with an affective disorder (and loved ones and caregivers) will often search for a meaningful explanation for the symptoms, the source of the problem is likely to be in the functioning of the brain. Stress may trigger the onset of an affective disorder in a vulnerable individual; affective disorders certainly cause stress. Patients with affective disorders require not only biological treatment of the disease, but also management of self-destructive behavior and rehabilitation once the episode clears.

A Note on Nomenclature

Strictly speaking, there is no longer a universally accepted set of "affective disorders". Earlier generations of psychiatrists spoke of manic-depressive reactions, depressive neuroses, and affective psychoses, which melded into the category of affective disorders in the *International Classification of Diseases,* 9th edition (ICD-9), in 1975, and in the *Diagnostic and Statistical Manual,* 3rd edition (DSM-III) in 1983. Subsequently, although the list of disorders included in the category remained more or less constant, the labeling in both classification schemes changed from "affective" to "mood" disorders in their next editions. The significance of this change in terminology is hard to estimate, as the definitions of affect and mood vary from source to source. Taking the prevailing view that affect encompasses mood along with its various associated qualities, the term affective disorders is preferred in a discussion of the conceptual foundations of these disorders, as it seems more descriptive. All of the disorders counted as mood disorders in current diagnostic schemes are disorders of much more than the prevailing emotional state, while in any given patient, change in the mood itself may be a minor problem compared to changes in energy, motivation, and neurovegetative functioning.

See Also the Following Articles

Depression and Manic–Depressive Illness; Suicide, Psychology of; Suicide, Sociology of.

Further Reading

DePaulo, J. R. and Horvitz, L. A. (2002). *Understanding depression: what we know and what you can do about it.* Hoboken, NJ: John Wiley & Sons.

Goodwin, F. K. and Jamison, K. R. (1990). *Manic depressive illness.* New York: Oxford University Press.

Jamison, K. R. (1993). *Touched with fire: manic-depressive illness and the artistic temperament.* New York: Free Press.

Jamison, K. R. (1995). *An unquiet mind.* New York: Vintage Books.

Kraepelin, E. (1990). *Manic depressive insanity and paranoia* (reprint edn.). Salem, NH: Ayer Company.

McHugh, P. R. and Slavney, P. R. (1998). *The perspectives of psychiatry* (2nd edn.). Baltimore, MD: Johns Hopkins University Press.
Mondimore, F. M. (1999). *Bipolar disorder: a guide for patients and families.* Baltimore, MD: Johns Hopkins University Press.
Robins, L. N. and Regier, D. A. (1991). *Psychiatric disorders in America: the epidemiologic catchment area study.* New York: Free Press.
Styron, W. (1992). *Darkness visible.* New York: Vintage Books.

Depression and Manic–Depressive Illness

R T Rubin and B J Carroll
VA Greater Los Angeles Healthcare System, Los Angeles, CA, and Pacific Behavioral Research Foundation, Carmel, CA, USA

This is a revised version of the article by R T Rubin, Encyclopedia of Stress First Edition, volume 1, pp 666–674, © 2000, Elsevier Inc.

Glossary

Affect	The objective (observable) component of emotions (appearing depressed, angry, elated, etc.), in contrast to mood.
Antidepressants	Drugs that are used in the treatment of depression.
Bipolar illness (disorder)	Manic-depressive illness (disorder).
Cerebral cortex	The outer layer of the brain, composed mainly of nerve cells (neurons).
Cerebral ventricles	Cerebrospinal fluid-filled spaces within the brain.
Electroconvulsive therapy (ECT)	A treatment for severe depression or bipolar disorder; a brief electric current is passed through the brain to induce a grand mal convulsive seizure.
Mood	The prevailing subjective (experienced) emotional tone (sadness, happiness, elation, anger, etc.), in contrast to affect. (Mood is to affect as climate is to weather.)
Neurotransmitters	Chemicals that carry messages from one nerve cell to another.

Introduction

The term depression covers a spectrum of disorders. These range from temporarily feeling down about something that has gone wrong in one's life to long and severe depressions that have a genetic and biological basis and that often are incapacitating to the afflicted person in his or her occupational and social life. The term manic-depression likewise covers a spectrum of disorders from temperamental instability of mood (i.e., cyclothymia) to a severe psychotic disorder with recurrent episodes of mania and depression. These are inappropriate swings of mood and behavior in opposite directions – excessive elation as well as significant depression.

Depression and manic-depression are psychiatric disorders that currently are considered functional, in that there is no clearly understood central nervous system (CNS) pathophysiology underlying them. This is a nomenclature in transition, however – as knowledge about the pathology of the brain in these and otherpsychiatric illnesses increases, the adjective "functional" conveys less and less meaning. Furthermore, when these mood disorders are so severe that they impair the daily life of the individual, somatic (physical) treatments are almost always required, including antidepressants, mood-stabilizing drugs such as lithium, and, when drug therapy fails, electroconvulsive therapy (ECT).

This article focuses on the more severe disorders of mood, in particular major depression (also called unipolar depression) and bipolar disorder. The CNS substrates of these illnesses are being examined in several ways, and their genetic underpinnings are slowly being defined. Structural and functional imaging studies of the brain are providing some anatomical localization, limited by the resolution of the imaging techniques and the particular imaging method used.

Several classes of antidepressant drugs are useful for treating major depression, but the interactions among chemical systems (neurotransmitters) in the brain make it difficult to predict which antidepressant will work best for a particular patient. Lithium is the most broadly effective treatment for bipolar illness, but a number of anticonvulsant and antipsychotic drugs, as well as antidepressants, also may be helpful in various clinical circumstances. Stress can play a major role in the severity and duration of both major depression and bipolar disorder. Moreover, the illnesses themselves, given the incapacitating nature of their symptoms, can be very stressful to afflicted people. In both disorders, one's psychological pain and despair can be so severe that suicide may be contemplated and even attempted.

Clinical Characteristics of Major Depression and Manic-Depression

Major depression and manic-depression are classified among the mood disorders. Major depression (unipolar depression) consists of one or more depressive episodes, defined as 2 weeks or more of depressed mood or loss of interest or pleasure in nearly all activities, with at least four additional symptoms from the following: increased or decreased appetite and/or weight; increased or decreased sleep; change in psychomotor activity (retardation or agitation); decreased energy; feelings of worthlessness or guilt; difficulty thinking, concentrating, or making decisions; and repeated thoughts of death, including suicidal thoughts, plans, or attempts. The symptoms must be severe enough to cause significant distress or to interfere with the person's occupational or social functioning. Finally, the major depressive episode must not be a direct result of a drug or an underlying medical condition.

Based on these criteria for the diagnosis of major depression, we can see that it is a very broad category of mental illness. The diagnostic criteria are disjunctive in that there are few mandatory symptoms, and individual patients may have few symptoms in common. To address this concern about heterogeneity, subtypes of major depressive disorder have been defined that require a more restricted list of symptoms. In particular, melancholic major depression focuses on physiological symptoms. Its diagnosis requires having the criteria for major depression plus either loss of pleasure in all (or almost all) activities or lack or reactivity to usually pleasurable stimuli, along with at least three additional symptoms from the following: a distinct quality to the depressed mood (different from a feeling of grief), the depressive symptoms being regularly worse in the morning, early morning awakening (at least 2 hours earlier than usual), marked psychomotor retardation or agitation, significant loss of appetite and/or weight, and excessive or inappropriate guilt. These also are disjunctive criteria, associated with significant heterogeneity. Melancholic major depression usually requires antidepressant medication, and sometimes ECT, for effective treatment.

Another feature of major depression may be the presence of psychotic features (delusions that are usually mood-congruent, or hallucinations). This form of depression may require treatment with antipsychotic as well as antidepressant drugs. The timing of major depressive episodes also may be linked to the season of the year, particularly to the light-dark cycle – seasonal affective disorder, as this condition is known, usually occurs in the winter when the days are short. Exposure to very bright light for several hours each morning may be useful as an adjunct to antidepressant drugs in the treatment of seasonal affective disorder.

A manic episode consists of a period of abnormally and persistently elevated, expansive, or irritable mood lasting for at least 1 week (less if the person is hospitalized), with at least three of the following additional symptoms: inflated self-esteem or grandiosity, decreased need for sleep, pressure of speech, flight of ideas or subjective feeling that his or her thoughts are racing, being easily distracted, increased activities (work, social, sexual) or psychomotor agitation, and excessive involvement in pleasurable activities that are potentially harmful (e.g., excessive alcohol intake, buying sprees, sexual indiscretions, or foolish business decisions).

Although these diagnostic criteria also are disjunctive, the heterogeneity of manic patients is generally much less than that of depressed patients. As with major depression, the symptoms must be severe enough to cause significant distress or to interfere with the person's occupational or social functioning, and the manic episode must not be a direct result of a drug or an underlying medical condition. And, as with major depression, psychotic features also may be part of the clinical picture. Finally, although mania and depression are conceptualized as polar opposite forms of mood disorder (hence the term bipolar disorder), coexisting manic and depressive symptoms are very common. When depressive and/or anxiety symptoms are prominent in a manic episode, the term mixed bipolar disorder is applied. Analyses of symptoms in mania have consistently revealed dimensions of depression and anxiety, elation-grandiosity, pressured behavior, psychosis, and irritable hostility. These separate components may display differential responsiveness to treatments; for example, elation-grandiosity may respond to lithium, irritable hostility to anticonvulsant mood stabilizers, and psychosis to antipsychotic drugs.

Bipolar I disorder is defined as a clinical course of one or more manic or mixed episodes, the latter being defined as criteria for both manic episode and major depression when they have been met nearly every day for at least 1 week. The most common form of bipolar illness is manic episodes alternating with major depressive episodes, which may or may not be separated by intervals of normal mood. Mixed episodes are less common, and the rarest pattern is to have manic episodes only, with no depressive features. Occasionally, several major depressive episodes may occur before the first manic episode becomes evident. Bipolar II disorder is defined as recurrent major depressive episodes with hypomanic episodes. Hypomanic episodes must meet the criteria for manic episodes, except they can be of shorter duration and lesser severity.

Epidemiologic studies indicate that the lifetime prevalence of major depression is about 10–25% for women and about half that for men; thus, it is one of the commonest psychiatric disorders. Fewer than half these survey-defined cases come to clinical attention, however. About twice as many adolescent and adult females are affected as males. In children, the prevalence of major depression is about equal between boys and girls. Thus, the hormonal changes of puberty may play a role in its greater incidence in adolescent and adult females. In contrast to widespread clinical belief a few decades ago, there is no increase in major depression in women at the time of menopause.

Approximately one-third of clinical major depressions improve with treatment and do not recur; approximately one-third show remission with treatment but do recur a number of times throughout the life of the individual; and approximately one-third may improve with treatment, but there remains a chronic, underlying depression of lesser severity. This chronic depression may meet the criteria for dysthymic disorder, which requires, among other criteria, depressed mood for more days than not, for at least 2 years. Major depressive episodes occurring against a background of dysthymia has been called double depression. The term refractory depression is applied to patients who fail to respond to at least two adequate trials of treatment; these make up approximately 15% of clinical major depressive episodes.

Major depression can co-occur with many other psychiatric illnesses such as anxiety disorders, eating disorders, drug abuse and alcoholism, dementias, and psychotic disorders, as well as in the context of many medical illnesses. In these instances, it is referred to as secondary major depression, in contrast to primary major depression, in which the depressive illness itself predominates. Primary major depression also may have some of these illnesses as secondary diagnoses; the determining factor is which came first. For example, anxiety symptoms sufficient to meet a diagnosis of generalized anxiety disorder occur with some frequency in major depression and are considered secondary because the depressive illness preceded them. Regardless of whether the depression is primary or secondary, these comorbid conditions have significant adverse effects on the clinical course of patients with major depression.

Although the classical descriptions of major depression and mania do not focus on cognitive function, it is now clear that pervasive, subtle impairments of executive function and declarative memory do occur during episodes of mood disturbance and that these features sometimes persist between episodes, especially in bipolar subjects. In elderly patients, more striking cognitive impairment may occur as part of a depressive episode. In particular, depressive pseudo-dementia (false dementia) should be considered in elderly depressed patients who have significant impairment of cognitive function and who might otherwise be diagnosed as having a dementia such as Alzheimer's disease. The distinction between depressive pseudo-dementia and true dementia is extremely important, because pseudo-dementia resolves with successful treatment of the underlying depression, whereas true dementia generally does not respond to currently available treatments.

Not only is major depression an important illness today, but within 15 years it is predicted to become the second most incapacitating illness throughout the world, just a small percentage behind cardiovascular disease. Thus, major depression is fast becoming a significant public health problem. As global populations age, a newly recognized form of major depression in the elderly, termed vascular depression, is increasing in prevalence. This condition results from disease of the small arteries supplying the brain. It has an unusually late age of onset for unipolar depression (after age 50), and it is recognized by the magnetic resonance imaging (MRI) features of deep white-matter hyperintensities; subcortical gray matter hyperintensities, especially in the caudate nuclei; and micro-infarcts (tissue death from blocked blood supply). All these features occur as well in vascular dementia, which is a significant long-term outcome of vascular depression. Risk factors for vascular depression include hypertension, diabetes mellitus, and abnormal plasma lipid profiles.

The lifetime prevalence for bipolar I illness is about 1% and for bipolar II illness about 0.5%. These illnesses usually begin in adolescence or young adulthood and are equally prevalent in males and females. As mentioned, recurrent alternating manic and depressive episodes represent the most common form; if four or more manic or depressive episodes occur within a year, the illness is considered rapidly cycling and may require frequent hospitalizations and certain medication combinations for its control.

As with the other severe psychiatric disorders, both major depression and manic-depression can be made worse by stressful life situations. Major depression not uncommonly is preceded, if not precipitated, by a significant loss in a person's life, be it death of a significant other, job loss, or financial reversal. As mentioned, the psychological pain and turmoil of a severe depression, coupled with additional physical factors such as insomnia, can in turn be extremely stressful to the sufferer, and, on occasion, suicide may be considered the only way out. Fortunately, almost every major depression is treatable, and suicidal thoughts that are present in the depths of the depressive episode almost always disappear with treatment.

Bipolar disorder is more internally driven (less affected by external stressors), but the illness itself can have extremely stressful consequences for the individual. It is a challenging condition for family members as well, as evidenced by the fact that the rate of marital failure in bipolar disorder exceeds that in any other psychiatric condition. During a manic episode the person may run afoul of the law and be arrested; may spend his or her life savings foolishly and be reduced to poverty; or may behave recklessly and suffer physical injury, for example by reckless or drunken driving with involvement in an auto accident or sexual promiscuity with the contraction of a disease such as AIDS. Bipolar disorder, being a recurrent disorder, can result in many psychiatric hospitalizations over an individual's lifetime.

Biological Characteristics of Depression and Manic-Depression

There appears to be a genetic contribution to both major depression and bipolar disorder. Both illnesses more frequently coexist in monozygotic (single-egg) than in dizygotic twins, but the difference is much more pronounced for bipolar disorder. Similarly, there is a higher incidence of these disorders in the first-degree relatives of patients with both major depression and bipolar disorder; again, the relationship is stronger for bipolar disorder. A consistent observation is that the most common psychiatric disorder in the relatives of subjects with bipolar disorder is unipolar depression. This has led to suggestions of a two-gene vulnerability in bipolar cases. For both of these illnesses, however, as for all the major psychiatric disorders, the modes of inheritance have not been established. Except for a few bipolar disorder families, the modes of inheritance do not appear to fit either an autosomal or an X-linked pattern but most likely are multifactorial, involving several genes of varying influence. Nongenetic contributing factors, as well as different genetic loadings in different families, may interact to produce the same phenotypic outcome.

A particularly intriguing area of research is the interaction of gene polymorphisms and life stresses in the onset of major depressive episodes. A particular polymorphism in the serotonin transporter gene, the presence of two short alleles, appears to confer a greater vulnerability to depressive episodes following mild stressful life events than the presence of either one or two long alleles. There is only a weak overall relationship between the serotonin transporter polymorphism and occurrence of major depression, so life stresses apparently are the precipitating factors. The genetic polymorphism confers vulnerability to developing depression following less severe stresses.

There are several neurochemical theories of the etiology of depression and bipolar disorder, all of which involve abnormal function of CNS neurotransmitters and/or the chemical changes they activate in nerve cells (neurons). Neurotransmitters (for example serotonin, norepinephrine, and dopamine) are chemicals in the brain that are released by neurons and carry a chemical message across a short space (synapse) to neighboring neurons that have receptors for that neurotransmitter. Deficiencies of norepinephrine and serotonin neurotransmission and excessive acetylcholine neurotransmission are among the oldest theories of depression and best supported by research studies.

In both unipolar major depression and the depressive phase of bipolar disorder, reductions in the metabolic products of norepinephrine and serotonin have been found in blood, urine, and cerebrospinal fluid, suggesting that both these neurotransmitter systems may be underactive, but the reductions in metabolites have been relatively small. In manic patients, the administration of physostigmine, a drug that inhibits the breakdown of acetylcholine, immediately stops the mania and produces a depressionlike state. Physostigmine also produces a depressionlike state in normal subjects. These findings suggest an overactivity of cholinergic neurotransmission in depression, and other studies have shown depressed patients to be supersensitive to cholinergic drugs in their sleep patterns, constriction of the pupils of their eyes, and so forth.

The most compelling evidence for the neurotransmitter theories of depression comes from the effects of drugs used to treat major depression and bipolar disorder. There are several classes of antidepressant drugs, and many of them block the cell membrane transporters for norepinephrine and/or serotonin, which recycle the neurotransmitters from the synapse back into the nerve cells that released them. By blocking transporter uptake, antidepressants increase synaptic neurotransmitter concentrations. Studies have shown that, in the intact human being, even very specific neurotransmitter uptake inhibitors eventually influence multiple neurotransmitter systems because of the physiological interactions among them. If one neurotransmitter system is perturbed by a drug acting on it specifically, the other systems tend to change to come back into balance with it.

More recent theories of antidepressant drug action emphasize follow-on actions of the drugs beyond inhibiting neurotransmitter reuptake by monoaminergic neurons. For example, an intracellular cascade occurs involving the activation of intracellular messengers (adenylyl cyclase and tyrosine protein kinases, the transcription factor cAMP response element binding protein (CREB), and increased mRNA for neurotrophins such as brain-derived neurotrophic factor (BDNF)).

The time course for full clinical response to all antidepressant drugs is 3–6 weeks, even though their specific pharmacological effects occur within 12–24 h. What is common to almost all antidepressants is that downregulation of postsynaptic noradrenergic receptors in the CNS occurs over the same number of weeks as required for the clinical response. Noradrenergic receptor downregulation may be an ultimate result of the increased availability of norepinephrine as a synaptic neurotransmitter, signaling that noradrenergic neurotransmission has increased to such an extent that the number and sensitivity of postsynaptic receptors need to be reduced in compensation. This finding suggests that a common neurochemical pathology in depressed patients may be a relative underactivity of noradrenergic neurotransmission, which is rectified by drug treatment. The restoration of noradrenergic transmission by antidepressant treatments, including ECT, may be linked to the trophic action of BDNF in restoring functional synapses between noradrenergic neurons and their target neurons in prefrontal cortex and limbic system sites.

There are disturbances in several physiological systems that occur as part of depression and the depressive phase of bipolar disorder. Sleep disturbance has been mentioned as part of the diagnostic criteria. Electrophysiological studies of sleep (polysomnography) have revealed typical changes, including less total sleep time, fragmentation of the orderly cycling of sleep stages with more frequent awakenings throughout the night, and early occurrence of rapid eye movement sleep (REM or dreaming sleep). In normal people, the first REM episode occurs about 60–90 min after sleep is established (REM latency). This interval may be severely shortened in major depression, so much so that the person may go directly into REM sleep when sleep is first established (sleep-onset REM). The occurrence of REM sleep is influenced by CNS cholinergic neurotransmission; as mentioned, the administration of cholinergic neurotransmission-stimulating drugs to depressed people and control subjects while asleep produces a significantly shorter REM latency in the depressives than in the controls. This is one of the findings supporting the cholinergic overdrive hypothesis of major depression.

Another important physiological disturbance in major depression and bipolar disorder is increased activity of the hypothalamic-pituitary-adrenal cortical (HPA) axis. This endocrine axis consists of cells in the hypothalamus of the brain that secrete corticotropin-releasing hormone (CRH) and vasopressin (AVP), which are carried to the anterior pituitary gland and stimulate the secretion of adrenocorticotropic hormone (ACTH) from the anterior pituitary into the blood stream. In turn, ACTH stimulates the adrenal cortex to secrete glucocorticoids, mineralocorticoids, and adrenal androgens into the bloodstream. Glucocorticoid hormones increase glucose production in the liver and promote lipid breakdown in fat tissue, thereby increasing circulating glucose available for muscle and other tissue use. The principal glucocorticoid in humans is cortisol (hydrocortisone). Mineralocorticoid hormones reduce the excretion of sodium and enhance the excretion of potassium and hydrogen ions by the kidney; the principal mineralocorticoid in humans is aldosterone. Adrenal androgenic hormones have weak male sex hormonelike effects.

The HPA axis is very responsive to both physical and psychological stressors. The secretion of CRH is regulated by several of the CNS neurotransmitters considered important in depressive illness, including norepinephrine, serotonin, and acetylcholine. The increased activity of this endocrine axis that occurs in 30–50% of patients with major depression and in the depressive phase of bipolar disorder is likely caused by an underlying neurotransmitter dysfunction in the brain. Increased HPA axis activity can be documented by the finding of increased ACTH and cortisol in blood, urine, and cerebrospinal fluid and by ACTH and cortisol resistance to suppression with the potent, synthetic adrenal glucocorticoid, dexamethasone. Dexamethasone acts primarily at the pituitary gland to suppress the secretion of ACTH, which, in turn, suppresses the secretion of hormones from the adrenal cortex. Resistance to dexamethasone suppression in depressed patients originally was interpreted as evidence of overdrive from the brain on the pituitary. However, it is now known that dexamethasone may be cleared from the body more rapidly in the nonsuppressing subjects, with resulting lower plasma dexamethasone concentrations. This factor has to be considered when the test is being used.

When stimulated for a period of time, endocrine glands often hypertrophy (grow in size), and both increased pituitary size and increased adrenal gland size have been reported in major depression. Adrenal size reverted to control values following successful antidepressant treatment. These adrenal gland changes are similar to those occurring during and after chronic stress in animals. The long-term effects of chronic exposure to high cortisol levels in depressed patients include loss of bone density, impairment of immune function, increased incidence of adult-onset diabetes mellitus and cardiovascular disease, and premature mortality. Collectively, these are termed indicators of high allostatic load in depression.

Neuroimaging Studies in Depression and Manic-Depression

With the advent of neuroimaging techniques, it now is possible to probe the structure and function of the living human brain. Brain structure can be viewed with X-ray computed tomography (CT) and MRI. Magnetic resonance spectroscopy (MRS) can determine the concentrations of certain chemical substances in the CNS. Nuclear medicine techniques such as single-photon computed tomography (SPECT) and positron-emission computed tomography (PET) allow the visualization and quantitation of regional cerebral blood flow, glucose metabolic rate, and neurotransmitter receptor occupancy, which are indirect probes of regional neuronal function. SPECT and PET use radiolabeled compounds as tracers; as these compounds decay, high-energy photons are emitted, which are counted by external detectors. The distribution of the tracer molecules is computed, and cross-sectional images of the brain are created in which image brightness is proportional to the underlying physiological process being measured. The newest technique, functional MRI (fMRI), also indicates blood flow in different areas of the brain.

Studies of brain structure with CT and MRI in patients with major depression and bipolar disorder have demonstrated a number of abnormalities, but it is not clear how specific these changes are. Enlarged cerebral ventricles in relation to overall brain size have been reported in a number of studies, but similar findings have been reported in patients with other psychiatric illnesses, such as schizophrenia. Different groups of patients (unipolar and bipolar), different ways of measuring and reporting ventricular volume, and different control groups have been used, but meta-analysis of many studies has pointed toward a significant enlargement of the ventricles in unipolar and bipolar patients compared to controls. The difference is more marked in elderly subjects. There appears to be no consistent relationship between structural changes in the brain and severity of the illness. Reduced volume of the subgenual anterior cingulate gyrus has been found in familial, pure, primary, unipolar depression, and this feature has been correlated with glial cell loss in the same region.

Reduced volume of the hippocampus also has been reported inconsistently in major depression. Initial suggestions that this feature is related to elevated cortisol exposure have not been confirmed. Moreover, hippocampal volume reduction also has been reported in nondepressed patients with cardiovascular disease. The finding of reduced hippocampal volume in depression, therefore, may simply reflect the high load of cardiovascular disease in these patients.

Elderly patients with vascular depression may show subcortical hyperintensities. These are areas within the white matter (neuron fiber tracts) and the subcortical grey-matter nuclei (neuron cell bodies) that are bright on T2-weighted MRI scans. They are associated with risk factors for cerebrovascular disease and may be areas of demyelination, local brain swelling, and small, old strokes. Elderly patients with major depression and bipolar patients of all ages have more extensive (in total area) subcortical white-matter hyperintensities than do age-matched healthy controls. The presence of subcortical hyperintensities in elderly depressed patients correlates with a greater sensitivity to the side effects of antidepressant medications, including delirium, a greater risk of developing tardive dyskinesia (a movement disorder) from neuroleptic (antipsychotic) medication, and a longer recovery time from ECT.

MRS has been used to study several compounds in the brain in major depression and bipolar disorder. Phosphomonoesters, a component of cell membranes, have been found to be both elevated and decreased. Phosphocreatine, a high-energy phosphate, has been more consistently decreased. MRS of fluorine-containing drugs, such as some antidepressants, and of lithium provides brain concentrations of these compounds in patients under treatment and may eventually be helpful in guiding dosage adjustments to achieve maximum therapeutic response. SPECT and PET functional neuroimaging studies of major depression and bipolar disorder have shown decreased prefrontal cortical and anterior cingulate gyrus blood flow and glucose metabolism, although these findings have not been consistent. In addition, there have been inconsistent reversals of these abnormalities in treated patients; however, it does appear that successful antidepressant pharmacotherapy is associated with increased blood flow and/or metabolism in the prefrontal cortex, cingulate cortex, and/or the basal ganglia (caudate nucleus, globus pallidus, and putamen).

Brain Circuit Theories of Depression and Manic-Depression

Brain circuit theories of major depression and bipolar disorder all represent variations on the postulated involvement of certain areas of the frontal parts of the brain (frontal lobes) and their functional interconnections with deeper parts of the brain – the cingulate gyrus, basal ganglia, thalamus, and other structures, including hippocampus and amygdala. Several of these structures make up the limbic system, a phylogenetically older part of the brain that influences emotional coloration and behavioral reactivity. In a general sense, the frontal lobes of the brain mediate executive functions; that is, an individual's decision-making and behavioral actions based on a detailed evaluation of environmental demands, along with an appreciation of their historical context, and a coordinated affective/emotional component. Particular areas of the frontal cortex mediate executive behavior, social behavior, and motivation.

The underlying theme of the brain circuit theories of major depression and the depressive phase of bipolar disorder is that the cognitive dorsal prefrontal cortex cannot effectively modulate the ventral orbitofrontal and medial prefrontal cortex and the limbic system components of emotions, so that what in a normal individual would be an expression of sadness becomes magnified and prolonged into a major depression when the interactive circuitry is not functioning properly. Ascending monoamine projections from the brainstem involving dopamine, norepinephrine, and serotonin set the tone in the emotional circuits comprising the prefrontal cortex, ventral striatum, mediodorsal thalamus, and projections back to the prefrontal cortex. When these delicate, unmyelinated, slow-conducting monoamine projections are damaged or rendered dysfunctional, monoamine control of the emotional circuits becomes abnormal.

Several distinct pathologic processes may cause such disconnection of the monoaminergic projections from their target neurons in prefrontal cortex and subcortical sites. These include loss-of-function polymorphisms of the BDNF gene, with resultant vulnerability to stress or glucocorticoids through reduced terminal arborization of monoaminergic axons; vascular lesions of the monoaminergic fibers in their passage through the midbrain and internal capsule; degenerative changes in brainstem monoaminergic cell nuclei as happens in Parkinson disease, Huntington disease, and Alzheimer disease; and functional impairment of the monoaminergic neurons by drugs such as reserpine, which prevent vesicular storage of the monoamine neurotransmitters, with resultant depletion of tissue monoamine concentrations. No matter which of these processes is operative, the final effect is loss of monoamine control over activity in the prefrontal-subcortical emotion circuits and the appearance of a primary or secondary depressive syndrome. In these syndromes, the expressed symptoms are very similar, regardless of the underlying pathology. The aforementioned reductions in resting prefrontal cortical blood flow and glucose metabolism, as determined by functional neuroimaging with SPECT, PET, and fMRI support this brain circuit theory. Likewise, increased activity in these same regions is seen when negative emotional processing tasks are performed by depressed patients.

Psychological Testing in Depression and Manic-Depression

Many general psychological tests contain questions pertaining to mood, and these tests usually give a score that indicates the degree of depression. Because depression and manic-depression are often recognizable clinically, however, psychological testing is usually not done unless there are ancillary questions, such the possibility of associated dementia or psychosis. Psychological testing also may be helpful in differentiating depressive pseudo-dementia from primary dementia. In a patient presenting with dementia, an indication of depressive features by psychological testing, which may not have been apparent clinically, usually signals the need for antidepressant treatment. In such cases, following successful treatment of the depression, the dementia also should have improved, which can be determined by repeat psychological testing.

There also are some rating scales designed specifically to quantitate depression. The Hamilton Rating Scale for Depression (HAM-D), which is scored by the person examining the patient, is the gold standard for clinical trials of antidepressant efficacy. Self-rated scales such as the Beck Depression Inventory (BDI) and the Carroll Depression Scale (CDS) also are used. The HAM-D tends to emphasize the physiological aspects of depression, such as sleep and appetite disturbance and physical symptoms of anxiety. The BDI emphasizes the cognitive component of depression; that is, how the person thinks about him- or herself when depressed. Short, self-rated depression screening scales also are used in epidemiologic studies and in primary medical care settings.

Treatment of Major Depression and Manic-Depression

The first issue in the treatment of patients with major depressive and bipolar disorder is to assess their immediate personal safety in light of the severity of their illness. For depressed patients, this always includes an assessment of their suicide potential. For manic patients, it includes not only an assessment of their suicide potential, especially in mixed bipolar disorder, but also whether their behavior is harmful (e.g., excessive alcohol intake, buying sprees, sexual indiscretions, or foolish business decisions, as mentioned earlier). The most certain way to interrupt behavioral indiscretions and protect the individual from suicide attempts is hospitalization in a specialized psychiatric unit whose staff is trained in the care of such patients. If the patient resists hospitalization, an involuntary hold may be medically and legally justified. A locked psychiatric unit, which prevents the patient from leaving, may be necessary until the illness is sufficiently under control that the patient's better judgment returns.

The treatment of major depression and bipolar disorder almost always requires drug therapy with antidepressants and/or mood-stabilizing drugs. There are several chemical classes of antidepressant drugs, and they have specific pharmacological activities in the CNS. As previously mentioned, many of them block the transporters for norepinephrine and/or serotonin, which recycle the neurotransmitters from the synapse back into the nerve cells that released them. By blocking transporter uptake, antidepressants increase synaptic neurotransmitter concentrations.

The time course for a full clinical response to antidepressant drugs is 3–6 weeks, even though their pharmacological effects occur within 12–24 h. Often, improved sleep may be an early sign of response to medication, especially with antidepressants that have sedative side effects. Objective signs of improvement usually precede the patient's feeling better; for example, the person may be sleeping and eating better, may have more energy and a higher level of activities, and may be speaking more cheerfully, but he or she still may be complaining about feeling as depressed as before. The subjective depressed mood is often the last aspect of the illness to improve. Because the subjective experience of depression is so psychologically painful and stressful, it is very important that a patient with suicide potential not be released from the hospital until he or she is in sufficient behavioral control to no longer be a suicide risk after discharge.

As mentioned, some antidepressants are specific uptake inhibitors of norepinephrine and others of serotonin, but it is not possible to predict which depressed patient will respond to which antidepressant. This is most likely on the basis of the physiological interactions of neurotransmitter systems and, as previously indicated, the fact that almost all antidepressants result in downregulation of postsynaptic noradrenergic receptors and induction of BDNF over the same time course as clinical improvement occurs. Antidepressants therefore are usually chosen on the basis of their side effects and cost, those under patent being more expensive than those available in generic form. Many of the older antidepressants have prominent side effects, such as causing dry mouth, blurred vision, and especially changes in the electrical conduction system of the heart. This last side effect can be particularly dangerous in accidental or deliberate drug overdose.

The class of antidepressant drugs currently in greatest use is the serotonin uptake inhibitors (SUIs). The first SUI accepted for clinical use in the United States was fluoxetine (Prozac). The SUIs may not be quite as effective as the original tricyclic and monoamine oxidase inhibitor antidepressant drugs, especially in severe depression, but they have fewer side effects, especially cardiac, which makes them generally safer drugs to use. They do have other side effects that must be considered, including weight gain, decreased sexual drive, akathisia (inner restlessness), and some increased risk of suicidal thinking or gestures. Although it has not been established that antidepressant drugs provoke completed suicides, regulatory warnings emphasize that patients must be followed closely for this risk during the early weeks of treatment.

Recent studies have shown that the efficacy of the SUIs in the broad, heterogeneous group of patients diagnosed with major depression is modest at best. The Number Needed to Treat (NNT) is a standard therapeutics measure that denotes the number of patients who must receive a drug for one drug-attributable therapeutic outcome to be achieved, that is; over and above the placebo response rate. For the SUIs, the NNT ranges from five to twelve, whereas the NNT for the early tricyclic antidepressant drugs in severe, hospitalized depressed patients was three. Recent studies also confirm that there is no significant difference in response or remission rates between SUIs and some other newer antidepressants vs. placebo in mild depression. The National Institute for Clinical Excellence (NICE) in Britain therefore has recommended that nondrug treatments be used first in mild depression.

A new class of antidepressant drugs that block synaptic reuptake of both norepinephrine and serotonin (e.g., venlafaxine and duloxetine) has recently appeared. The dual action of these drugs recapitulates the pharmacodynamic profile of original antidepressant agents such as imipramine, amitryptiline, and phenelzine, but with a greatly reduced side-effect profile. These dual-action drugs appear to be more effective than the SUIs in treating major depression. For example, in direct comparisons, the NNT for venlafaxine to produce remission is five, compared with ten for the SUIs.

The other major class of drugs used in mood disorders, especially in bipolar disorder, is the mood stabilizers. For manic patients, lithium is the most effective. Lithium is a metal ion, in the same class in the periodic table of elements as sodium and potassium. Lithium has a number of effects on neurotransmission in the CNS. It has a relatively narrow therapeutic index; that is, the blood concentrations at which lithium exerts toxicity are not very far above the concentrations required for its therapeutic effect. Therefore, patients taking lithium require frequent measurement of their circulating lithium concentrations, especially at the outset of treatment, to determine the daily dose necessary to achieve a therapeutic blood level. Lithium takes several weeks to achieve its full antimanic effect. It is a mood stabilizer rather than a pure antimanic compound, so bipolar patients who switch from mania into depression are usually continued on their lithium if an antidepressant is added.

For major depressive and bipolar patients, additional dimensions of their illnesses may suggest the need for other medications in addition to antidepressants and lithium. For example, prominent psychotic features in either illness may call for an antipsychotic medication to be used concomitantly. For the treatment of depression, hormone supplements such as estrogens in women and thyroid hormone may be helpful. For the treatment of bipolar disorder, a number of anticonvulsant medications have been shown to be effective, often as augmentation of lithium treatment. Compounds such as carbamazepine, valproate, and lamotrigine are currently in use, and several newer anticonvulsants are being tested for their mood-stabilizing properties.

After the successful drug treatment of a first lifetime episode of major depression, continuation treatment at full dosage is advised for 9 to 12 months to prevent relapse. The slow reduction of the medication then is attempted. Patients who experience recurrent depression, particularly those who have had three or more lifetime episodes, require long-term antidepressant maintenance treatment at full dosage to prevent recurrences. Controlled trials have established that, even after 3 years of successful preventive drug treatment, 50% of such patients will have a recurrence within 6 months of stopping their medication.

Bipolar patients need to have medication adjustments made according to the frequency of their manic and depressive mood swings; it may take years for the timing of these cycles to be clearly understood. Both disorders should be viewed as chronic illnesses, often relapsing over a person's lifetime. If strenuous attempts at drug treatment of either disorder fail, ECT often will provide definitive relief of symptoms. Usually, 10 treatments are given, three per week. The patient may suffer some memory loss during and following the treatments, but this is short-lived, whereas the therapeutic effect can be remarkable, especially in patients resistant to drug therapy. Unilateral, brief pulse application of electrical current to the nondominant hemisphere can reduce these memory changes significantly. Maintenance ECT, often one treatment every month or so, can be useful to keep the person in remission from his or her illness.

In addition to pharmacotherapy and ECT, psychotherapies of different types, such as cognitive-behavioral therapy, often are useful to help the person change his or her lifestyle and manner of thinking about adversity. An improvement in self-esteem often results, which may protect against future episodes of depression or at least may reduce their severity.

Conclusion

Major depression and manic-depression (bipolar disorder) represent serious psychiatric illnesses. In addition to interfering with occupational and social functioning, these illnesses put the sufferer at personal risk – a potential for suicide attempts in the case of depression and impulsive behaviors such as excessive alcohol intake, buying sprees, sexual indiscretions, and foolish business decisions in the case of a manic episode. Severe life stressors often precede a depressive episode, and both illnesses create their own stresses in the sufferer, including the psychological pain of depression and the untoward consequences of unrestrained manic behavior. Fortunately, there are effective pharmacological treatments that can produce remission in the majority of patients, and for those who do not respond to drug treatment, ECT is an excellent therapeutic modality. The neurological circuitry involved in mood disorders is being revealed, with the result that new treatment approaches are emerging.

Acknowledgments

This research is supported by NIH grant MH28380. Dr. Rubin has received no commercial company support. Dr. Carroll has had past consulting, speaking, or research support from the following companies: Abbott, Astra Zeneca, Becton-Dickinson, Cyberonics, Glaxo Smith Kline, Janssen, Johnson and Johnson, Lilly, Novartis, Pfizer, Roche, Warner Lambert-Parke Davis, and Wyeth.

Further Reading

Akiskal, H. S. (2000). Mood disorders: introduction and overview. In: Sadock, B. J. & Sdock, V. A. (eds.) *Kapla an& Sadock's comprehensive textbook of psychiatry* (7th edn., pp. 1284–1298). Philadelphia: Lippincott Williams & Wilkins.

Akiskal, H. S. (2000). Mood disorders: clinical features. In: Sadock, B. J. & Sdock, V. A. (eds.) *Kapla an& Sadock's comprehensive textbook of psychiatry* (7th edn., pp. 1338–1377). Philadelphia: Lippincott Williams & Wilkins.

American Psychiatric Association (1994). *Diagnostic and statistical manual of mental disorders* (4th edn.). Washington, DC: American Psychiatric Association.

Baldessarini, R. J. (2001). Drugs and the treatment of psychiatric disorders: depression and anxiety disorders. In: Hardman, J. G. & Limbird, L. E. (eds.) *Goodm & Gilman's the pharmacological basis of therapeutics* (10th e&n., pp. 447–483). New York: McGraw-Hill.

Baldessarini, R. J. and Tarazi, F. I. (2001). Drugs and the treatment of psychiatric disorders: psychosis and mania. In: Hardman, J. G. & Limbird, L. E. (eds.) *Goodm & Gilman's the pharmacological basis of therapeutics* (10th e&n., pp. 485–520). New York: McGraw-Hill.

Blazer, D. (2000). Mood disorders: epidemiology. In: Sadock, B. J. & Sdock, V. A. (eds.) *Kapla an& Sadock's comprehensive textbook of psychiatry* (7th edn., pp. 1298–1308). Philadelphia: Lippincott Williams & Wilkins.

Bloom, F. E. (2001). Neurotransmission and the central nervous system. In: Hardman, J. G. & Limbird, L. E. (eds.) *Goodm & Gilman's the pharmacological basis of therapeutics* (10th e&n., pp. 293–320). New York: McGraw-Hill.

Davis, K. L., Charney, D., Coyle, J. T. and Nemeroff, C. (eds.) (2002). *Psychopharmacology: the fifth generation of progress.* Philadelphia: Lippincott Williams & Wilkins.

Cummings, J. L. (1995). Anatomic and behavioral aspects of frontal-subcortical circuits. *Annals of the New York Academy of Sciences* **769**, 1–13.

Gabbard, G. O. (2000). Mood disorders: psychodynamic aspects. In: Sadock, B. J. & Sdock, V. A. (eds.) *Kapla an& Sadock's comprehensive textbook of psychiatry* (7th edn., pp. 1328–1338). Philadelphia: Lippincott Williams & Wilkins.

Hirschfeld, R. M. A. and Shea, M. T. (2000). Mood disorders: psychotherapy. In: Sadock, B. J. & Sdock, V. A. (eds.) *Kapla an& Sadock's comprehensive textbook of psychiatry* (7th edn., pp. 1431–1440). Philadelphia: Lippincott Williams & Wilkins.

Kelsoe, J. R. (2000). Mood disorders: genetics. In: Sadock, B. J. & Sdock, V. A. (eds.) *Kapla an& Sadock's comprehensive textbook of psychiatry* (7th edn., pp. 1308–1318). Philadelphia: Lippincott Williams & Wilkins.

Kitayama, I., Yaga, T., Kayahara, T., et al. (1997). Long-term stress degenerates but imipramine regenerates noradrenergic axons in the rat cerebral cortex. *Biological Psychiatry* **42**, 687–696.

Koschack, J. and Irle, E. (2005). Small hippocampal size in cognitively normal subjects with coronary artery disease. *Neurobiology of Aging* **26**, 865–871.

Krishnan, K. R. R. and Doraiswamy, P. M. (eds.) (1997). *Brain imaging in clinical psychiatry.* New York: Marcel Dekker.

Kupfer, D. J., Frank, E., Perel, J. M., et al. (1992). Five-year outcome for maintenance therapies in recurrent depression. *Archives of General Psychiatry* **49**, 769–773.

Nibuya, M., Morinobu, S. and Duman, R. S. (1995). Regulation of BDNF and trkB mRNA in rat brain by chronic electroconvulsive seizure and antidepressant drug treatments. *Journal of Neuroscience* **15**, 7539–7547.

Post, R. M. (2000). Mood disorders: treatment of bipolar disorders. In: Sadock, B. J. & Sdock, V. A. (eds.) *Kapla an& Sadock's comprehensive textbook of psychiatry* (7th edn., pp. 1385–1430). Philadelphia: Lippincott Williams & Wilkins.

Rush, A. J. (2000). Mood disorders: treatment of depression. In: Sadock, B. J. & Sdock, V. A. (eds.) *Kapla an& Sadock's comprehensive textbook of psychiatry* (7th edn., pp. 1377–1385). Philadelphia: Lippincott Williams & Wilkins.

Singh, V., Muzina, D. J. and Calabrese, J. R. (2005). Anticonvulsants in bipolar disorder. *Psychiatric Clinics of North America* **28**, 301–323.

Thase, M. E. (2000). Mood disorders: neurobiology. In: Sadock, B. J. & Sdock, V. A. (eds.) *Kapla an& Sadock's comprehensive textbook of psychiatry* (7th edn., pp. 1318–1328). Philadelphia: Lippincott Williams & Wilkins.

Thase, M. E., Entsuah, A. R. and Rudolph, R. L. (2001). Remission rates during treatment with venlafaxine or selective serotonin reuptake inhibitors. *British Journal of Psychiatry* **178**, 234–241.

Corticotropin-Releasing Factor Circuitry in the Brain – Relevance for Affective Disorders and Anxiety

D A Gutman and C B Nemeroff
Emory University School of Medicine, Atlanta, GA, USA

Glucocorticoids in Affective Disorders: Early Evidence

Evidence linking the hypothalamic-pituitary-adrenal (HPA) axis abnormalities with psychiatric symptoms dates back over 100 years. The occurrence of depression, anxiety, and in extreme cases psychosis, in both Cushing and Addison diseases, which are associated with excessive or markedly reduced levels of circulating glucocorticoids, respectively, served as an initial impetus for researchers to scrutinize HPA-axis function in psychiatric disorders. Some of the first direct evidence that posited a role between glucocorticoids and mood stemmed from studies that were carried out in the 1950s.

The concatenation of several lines of evidence revealed abnormalities in glucocorticoid (i.e., cortisol) function in depressed patients. These include elevated plasma cortisol concentrations, increased 24-h urinary free cortisol concentrations, and increased levels of cortisol metabolites in urine. Although not observed in every patient with major depression, elevated cortisol secretion in depression is among the most reproducible findings in all of biologic psychiatry.

Structural changes in the components of the HPA axis have also been documented in depressed patients. These include pituitary gland enlargement as demonstrated by magnetic resonance imaging (MRI) and moreover, the adrenal glands have also shown to be enlarged in depression as assessed by both imaging studies, as well as postmortem analysis of the adrenals, presumably due to the effects of adrenocorticotropic hormone (ACTH) hypersecretion.

Corticotropin-Releasing Factor

Although Saffran and Schally identified a crude extract that promoted the release of ACTH from the pituitary in 1955, the ultimate regulator of ACTH and cortisol release, corticotropin-releasing factor (CRF), was not isolated and chemically characterized until 1981. Working with extracts derived from 500 000 sheep hypothalami, Vale and colleagues at the Salk Institute elucidated the structure of CRF. This discovery led to the availability of synthetic CRF, which allowed for a comprehensive assessment of the HPA axis. Based on finding from numerous studies it is clear that CRF coordinates the endocrine, immune, autonomic, and behavioral responses of mammals to stress.

The hypothalamus serves as a regulatory point for a number of key functions including body temperature, hunger, thirst, and circadian cycles. Within the hypothalamus, CRF is synthesized primarily in the parvocellular neurons of the paraventricular nucleus (PVN). These PVN CRF neurons receive input from a variety of brain regions, including the amygdala, the bed nucleus of the stria terminalis (BNST), and the brain stem. CRF-containing neurons within the hypothalamus then project to the median eminence. The median eminence serves as a bridge between the hypothalamus and the anterior lobe of the pituitary gland. Within the median eminence, the release and release-inhibiting hypothalamic hypophysiotropic hormones are released from nerve terminals and enter the portal blood system which supplies the anterior pituitary gland.

In response to a variety of stressors, this neural circuit becomes activated, thereby releasing CRF into the hypothalamo-hypophysial portal system, where it activates CRF receptors on corticotrophs in the adenohypophysis to promote the synthesis of pro-opiomelanocortin and the release of its major posttranslation products, ACTH and β-endorphin. ACTH, released from the anterior pituitary, stimulates the production and release of cortisol from the adrenal cortex. These same hypothalamic CRF neurons also project to the spinal cord and brainstem nuclei, including the locus coeruleus (LC), the site of the noradrenergic neurons that project to the forebrain. Magnocellular neurons (literally large cells) in the PVN also produce vasopressin and oxytocin. Vasopressin has been regarded to potentiate the action of CRF on ACTH secretion.

Corticotropin-Releasing Factor Receptors

Two CRF receptor subtypes, CRF_1 and CRF_2, with distinct anatomic localization and receptor pharmacology, have been identified in rats and humans. Both receptors are members of the large G-protein receptor superfamily. The CRF_1 receptor is predominantly expressed in the pituitary, cerebellum, and neocortex in rats. Considerable evidence from laboratory animal studies has shown that CRF_1 receptors may specifically mediate some of the anxiogenic-like behaviors observed after administration of CRF.

In agreement with these findings, mice that have had their CRF_1 receptor knocked out were found to exhibit an impaired stress response. The CRF_1 receptor knockout mice were less anxious than their wild-type litter mates when tested in the elevated plus maze, a commonly used animal model of anxiety. This paradigm consists of an elevated maze in which two of the arms contain walls, whereas the other two arms are open. Rodents that spend more time on the open arms, where they are potentially exposed to predators or more likely could fall, are generally interpreted to be less anxious than animals that spend the preponderance of time in the closed arms. In addition, data in these transgenic mice showed a significant reduction in stress-induced release of ACTH and corticosterone (the primary glucocorticoid in rodents).

CRF_2 receptor knockout mice have also been generated. Deletion of the CRF_2 receptor gene during development has provided conflicting results, with increased anxiety observed in some but not all paradigms tested. These studies suggest that CRF_2 receptor blockade may lead to states of increased anxiety, though it is likely that both the environment and the genetic background on which the knockouts were bred contribute to the behavioral phenotype of these animals.

Research using selective CRF_2 receptor agonists and antagonists have also provided inconsistent results. Several studies have used the selective CRF_2 receptor antagonist antisauvagine-30 (ASV-30), which has been reported to be between 100- and 1000-fold selective for the CRF_2 receptor, depending upon whether the radiolabeled ligand is sauvagine or ASV-30, respectively. Direct administration of ASV-30 into the lateral septum was shown to reduce anxious behavior induced by immobilization stress in the elevated plus maze paradigm or by previous association with foot shock in mice. These behavioral data were corroborated in rats, where direct injection of ASV-30 into the cerebral ventricles reduced anxious behavior in the plus maze, defensive withdrawal, and a conditioned anxiety paradigm.

Compounds which selectively activate (i.e., agonists) the CRF_2 receptor have also been discovered. The peptides urocortin 2 and urocortin 3 are structurally and ancestrally related to CRF but show between 100- and 1000-fold selectivity at the CRF_2 receptor versus the CRF_1 receptor. Urocortin 3 has been shown to mildly suppress locomotion and has an anxiolytic-like profile in mice. However, another study from the same group of researchers demonstrated that urocortin 2 was inactive in the plus maze after acute administration but did increase exploratory behavior in the plus maze 4 h later. Thus, compounds reported to be both selective agonists and antagonists at the CRF_2 receptor have been shown to possess anxiolytic effects; clearly the precise role of this receptor in modulating stress-induced behaviors remains obscure.

Extrahypothalamic Corticotropin-Releasing Factor Circuits and Depression

Although initially investigated for its role as one of the key modulators of the HPA axis, further research has revealed that CRF controls not only the neuroendocrine, but also the autonomic (e.g., heart rate, blood pressure, etc.), immune, and behavioral responses to stress in mammals. Results from both clinical studies and a rich body of literature conducted primarily in rodents and nonhuman primates have highlighted the importance of extrahypothalamic CRF neurons. In rodents, primates, and humans, CRF and its receptors are heterogeneously localized with high concentrations in a variety of regions, including the amygdala, thalamus, hippocampus, and prefrontal cortex, among others. These brain regions serve as key regulators of the mammalian stress response and emotion.

The presence of CRF receptors in both the dorsal raphe and LC, the origin of the major serotonergic- and noradrenergic-containing perikarya, respectively, also deserves comment because most available antidepressants, including the tricyclic antidepressants and selective serotonin-releasing inhibitors (SSRIs), are believed to act via modulation of the serotonergic and/or noradrenergic systems. The neuroanatomic proximity of CRF and monoaminergic systems provides evidence for an interaction between CRF systems and certain antidepressants, thereby suggesting a mechanism by which antidepressants may affect the CRF system.

Corticotropin-Releasing Factor in Depression

Among the affective disorders, the role of CRF in major depression has been the most thoroughly investigated. Shortly after the isolation and characterization of CRF, a standardized intravenous CRF stimulation test was developed to assess HPA-axis activity. In this paradigm, CRF is administered intravenously (usually at a dose of 1 $\mu g\ kg^{-1}$ or a fixed dose of 100 μg), and the ACTH and cortisol responses are measured at 30-min intervals over a 2–3-h period. Numerous studies have now documented a blunted ACTH and β-endorphin response to intravenously administered ovine or human CRF in depressed patients compared with nondepressed people; the cortisol response in depressed patients and nondepressed control subjects did not consistently differ. This was one piece of evidence that contributed to the initial hypothesis that CRF may be hypersecreted in a subset of depressed patients.

More specifically, the attenuated ACTH response to CRF has been hypothesized to be due to chronic hypersecretion of CRF from nerve terminals in the median eminence, which results in downregulation of CRF receptors in the anterior pituitary, and/or to chronic hypercortisolemia and its associated negative feedback. CRF receptor downregulation results in reduced responsivity of the anterior pituitary to CRF, as has been repeatedly demonstrated in laboratory animals.

In support of the involvement of extrahypothalamic CRF systems in the pathophysiology of depression, numerous studies have demonstrated elevated CRF concentrations in the cerebrospinal fluid (CSF) of depressed patients, though some discrepant results have also been reported. It is likely that this increased CSF CRF is due to hypersecretion not only from hypothalamic CRF nerve terminals, but from extrahypothalamic sites as well.

Elevated CSF CRF concentrations have also been detected in depressed suicide victims. A reduction in concentrations of CRF in CSF has been reported in healthy volunteers treated with the tricyclic antidepressant desipramine and in depressed patients following treatment with fluoxetine or amitriptyline, providing further evidence of an interconnection between antidepressants, monoamine neurons, and CRF systems. Similar effects have also been reported after electroconvulsive therapy (ECT) in depressed patients.

The alterations in CSF CRF concentrations appear to represent a state, rather than a trait, marker of depression (i.e., a marker of current depression rather than a marker of vulnerability to depression). Furthermore, high and/or increasing CSF CRF concentrations despite symptomatic improvement of major depression during antidepressant treatment may be the harbinger of early relapse.

Consistent with altered concentrations of CRF found in clinical studies of depression, CRF binding site density and messenger ribonucleic acid (mRNA) expression have shown alterations in both preclinical and clinical studies, presumably in response to changes in CRF availability. Our group has previously reported a marked (23%) reduction in the number of CRF binding sites in the frontal cortex of suicide victims compared with controls; we have now replicated this finding in a second study. Raadsheer and colleagues demonstrated an increase in CRF mRNA expression in the PVN of depressed patients compared with controls.

Increased CRF mRNA and decreased CRF_1 mRNA have also been detected in the brains of suicide victims in subregions of the frontal cortex. Although conducted in different laboratories and on different tissue, and keeping in mind the relative difficulty in obtaining and analyzing human tissue, the general pattern of increased CRF concentrations and/or CRF mRNA and the relative decrease in CRF binding sites is consistent with the well-documented phenomenon of receptor up- and downregulation and the CRF hypersecretion hypothesis of depression.

While the exact mechanism contributing to CRF hyperactivity remains obscure, studies from our group and others have documented long-term persistent increases in HPA-axis activity and extrahypothalamic CRF neuronal activity after exposure to early untoward life events, e.g., neglect and child abuse, respectively, in both laboratory animals (rats and nonhuman primates), and patients. Early life stress apparently permanently sensitizes the HPA axis and extrahypothalamic CRF neurons and leads to a greater risk of depression developing later in life.

To measure HPA-axis responsivity to stress in humans, the Trier Social Stress Test (TSST) was developed. This laboratory paradigm involves a simulated 10-min public speech followed by a difficult mental arithmetic task. The TSST has been validated as a potent activator of the HPA axis in humans. Our group reported increased HPA-axis responsivity, presumably due to hypersecretion of CRF, after exposure to the TSST in both depressed and nondepressed women who were exposed to severe physical and emotional trauma as children. These data strongly suggest that CRF systems are particularly sensitive to the effects of early adverse life events.

Corticotropin-Releasing Factor and Anxiety Disorders

Involvement of CRF in anxiety disorders has been well documented in both animal and human studies. Best studied among this diverse group of disorders is posttraumatic stress disorder (PTSD), which has been most commonly studied in Vietnam combat veterans, though it is now widely recognized to occur after other life-threatening situations including victims of rape, natural disasters, and physical and sexual abuse as children. Combat veterans with PTSD exhibit significantly elevated CSF CRF concentrations, as well as alterations in the ACTH response to CRF challenge. In contrast to studies from depressed patients, low serum cortisol and urinary free cortisol levels have been repeatedly, yet unexpectedly, detected in PTSD, especially after dexamethasone administration. One possible mechanism that has been proposed by Yehuda and colleagues to explain these findings is heightened negative glucocorticoid feedback within the HPA axis in chronic PTSD patients.

Elevated CSF CRF concentrations have not been detected in patients with panic disorder, though a blunted ACTH response after CRF administration has been observed. Increased or normal concentrations of CSF CRF have been observed in patients with obsessive–compulsive disorder (OCD), though significant decreases in CSF CRF concentrations have been noted following a therapeutic response to clomipramine. Patients with generalized anxiety disorder (GAD), however, exhibit similar CSF CRF concentrations in comparison to normal controls.

Not surprisingly, increased concentrations of CSF CRF occur in alcohol withdrawal, a condition of sympathetic nervous system arousal and increased anxiety. In contrast, CSF CRF concentrations are reduced or are normal in abstinent chronic alcoholics with normal plasma cortisol concentrations. Although human data are limited in other addictive states, there is also a burgeoning laboratory animal literature which suggests that CRF may play a role in both the withdrawal and/or stress-induced drug relapse of a number of addictive compounds including nicotine, alcohol, cocaine, and benzodiazepines. To understand the exact role of CRF in anxiety will require considerable additional study.

Small-Molecule Corticotropin-Releasing Factor Antagonists

Although space constraints do not permit an extensive review of the entire preclinical literature, several additional points are worth noting. Findings from numerous studies have shown that when CRF is directly injected into the central nervous system (CNS) of laboratory animals it produces effects reminiscent of the cardinal symptoms of depression, including decreased libido, reduced appetite and weight loss, sleep disturbances, and neophobia. Certainly, by the late 1980s, a number of research groups, including our own, had hypothesized that a lipophilic, small-molecule CRF receptor antagonist that readily penetrates the blood–brain barrier after oral administration would represent a novel class of antidepressant and/or anxiolytic agents.

CRF_1 receptor antagonists possess activity in both animal models of anxiety and depression. CRF receptor antagonists have been tested in many different paradigms, including the elevated plus maze, foot shock, restraint stress, and defensive withdrawal. Pretreatment with CRF receptor antagonists decreases measures of anxiety induced by stressors. There is also some evidence that CRF receptor antagonists may reduce the effects of drug withdrawal and stress-induced relapse to drug seeking in rats. Based on this premise, newly developed CRF_1 receptor antagonists represent a novel putative class of antidepressants. Such compounds show activity in nearly every preclinical screening test for antidepressant and anxiolytic drugs.

Despite the rich preclinical and clinical literature supporting a potential role for CRF_1 receptor antagonists, there has only been one published study investigating the effects of a CRF_1 receptor antagonist in humans. A small open-label study examining the effectiveness of R121919, a CRF_1 receptor antagonist, in major depression was completed more than 5 years ago. This study of 20 patients showed that R121919 (5–40 mg day^{-1} or 40–80 mg day^{-1} for 30 days) was well tolerated and did not significantly affect plasma ACTH or cortisol concentrations at baseline or following CRF challenge. It is important that any potential CRF antagonist not lead to adrenal insufficiency, which can, of course, have grave medical consequences. Hamilton Depression Rating Scale and Hamilton Anxiety Scale severity scores were both significantly reduced following 30-day treatment with this drug. Although this small, pilot study does not provide unequivocal proof, it does provide further evidence that a selective CRF-receptor antagonist may possess antidepressant and antianxiety properties in humans. Although this drug is no longer in clinical development because of hepatotoxicity, several novel CRF_1 antagonists are currently under investigation.

Conclusions and Future Directions

Since the discovery of CRF more than 25 years ago, evidence has accumulated that it plays a preeminent role in the physiology of the stress response. Moreover the evidence of its involvement in pathophysiologic states such as major depression and anxiety disorders is compelling. The recent introduction of small-molecule CRF receptor antagonists as a putative novel class of antidepressant and anxiolytic drugs remains very promising. These compounds block the actions of exogenous and endogenous CRF in a variety of *in vivo* models, supporting a putative role for these agents in the treatment of stress and/or anxiety and affective disorders. The promising clinical results in patients with depression in the completed open trial of R121919 is of great interest and the results of controlled studies are eagerly awaited.

Acknowledgments

This work was supported in part by MH-58922 (Sylvio O. Conte Center for the Neuroscience of Mental Disorders) and MH-42088.

Further Reading

Bremner, J. D., Licinio, J., Darnell, A., et al. (1997). Elevated CSF corticotropin-releasing factor concentrations in posttraumatic stress disorder. *American Journal of Psychiatry* **154**, 624–629.

Gutman, D. A., Owens, M. J. and Nemeroff, C. B. (2005). Corticotropin-releasing factor receptor and glucocorticoid receptor antagonists: new approaches to antidepressant treatment. In: denBoer, J. A., George, M. S. & terHorst, G. J. (eds.) *Current and future developments in psychopharmacology*, pp. 133–158. Amsterdam: Benecke NI.

Heim, C., Newport, D. J., Miller, A. H., et al. (2000). Long term neuroendocrine effects of childhood maltreatment. *JAMA* **284**, 2321.

Sanchez, M. M., Young, L. J., Plotsky, P. M., et al. (1999). Autoradiographic and *in situ* hybridization localization of corticotropin-releasing factor 1 and 2 receptors in nonhuman primate brain. *Journal of Comparative Neurology* **408**, 365–774.

Steckler, T. and Holsboer, F. (1999). Corticotropin-releasing hormone receptor subtypes and emotion. *Biological Psychiatry* **46**, 1480–1508.

VanPett, K., Viau, V., Bittencourt, J. C., et al. (2000). Distribution of mRNAs encoding CRF receptors in brain and pituitary of rat and mouse. *Journal of Comparative Neurology* **428**, 191–212.

Depression, Immunological Aspects

M R Irwin
UCLA Semel Institute for Neuroscience, Los Angeles, CA, USA

Glossary

Cytokine A soluble protein that is produced by lymphocytes, monocytes, and macrophages, as well as by tissue cells and cells of the central nervous system; cytokines are released from a cell to influence the activity of other cells by binding a specific receptor and activating cell function.

Immune system A variety of interactive cells and soluble molecules that provide for the body's defense against invading external pathogens; the immune system is composed of two components: humoral or antibody responses and cell-mediated responses.

Inflammation A immune response that occurs to rid the body of an infectious agent or to remove and repair damaged tissue.

Major depressive disorder A disorder characterized by a period of at least 2 weeks of depressed mood or loss of interest in nearly all activities with the presence of at least four other symptoms drawn from a list that includes changes in appetite or weight, sleep, or activity; decreased energy; feelings of worthlessness or guilt; difficulty thinking or concentrating; and recurrent thoughts of death or suicidal ideation.

Psychoneuroimmunology A research field that investigates the physiological systems that integrate behavioral and immunological responses and examines the interactions between the nervous system and the immune system in the relationship between behavior and health.

Introduction

Many immunological changes reliably occur in patients with major depressive disorder, as recently described in comprehensive meta-analyses of over 180 studies with more than 40 immune measures. This article provides a brief overview of the immune system and the pathways that mediate connections between the central nervous system (CNS) and the immune system. A detailed review of the various immune findings that occur in major depression is presented with consideration of the behavioral correlates and biological mechanisms that might contribute to immune changes in major depression. Finally, the clinical implications of immune alterations in depression for infectious disease risk and inflammatory disorders are addressed.

Immune System

The immune system is the body's defense against invading external pathogens such as viruses and bacteria and from abnormal internal cells such as tumors.

Innate immunity refers to the body's resistance to pathogens that operates in a nonspecific way without recognition of the different nature of various pathogens, whereas specific immunity is acquired in response to the identification of non-self molecules called antigens. Macrophages and granulocytes are examples of nonspecific immune cells that react to tissue damage by consuming debris and invading organisms. Natural killer (NK) cells are another example of nonspecific immunity that acts to kill virally infected cells in a nonspecific way without need for prior exposure or recognition. In contrast, each T cell or B cell is genetically programmed to attack a specific target by secreting antibodies (B cell) or by killing cells of the body that harbor a virus (T cell). Both innate and specific immunity are orchestrated by the release of interleukins or cytokines from immune cells; cytokines are protein messengers that regulate the immune cells. This cytokine network aids in the differentiation of the immune response and in the coordination of its magnitude and duration. For example, there are two main classes of cytokines secreted by the T cells. One class of cytokines, T helper type 1 (Th1) cytokines, supports T cell responses (e.g., the ability of T cells to kill virally infected cells), whereas another class of cytokines, T helper type 2 (Th2), supports an antibody-mediated humoral immune response. However, these immunoregulatory processes cannot be fully understood without taking into account the organism and the internal and external milieu in which innate and specific immune responses occur.

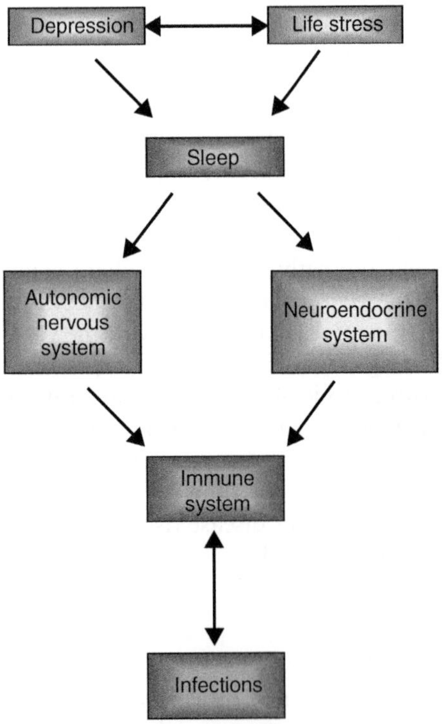

Figure 1 Hypothesized mediators of the effects of major depression on immunity and infectious disease risk in humans.

Biological Connections between the CNS and Immune System

Autonomic Nervous System

The CNS and the immune system are linked by two major physiological pathways: the hypothalamic-pituitary-adrenal (HPA) axis and the autonomic nervous system, composed of sympathetic and parasympathetic branches. The sympathetic nervous system (SNS) is a network of nerve cells running from the brain stem down the spinal cord and out into the body to contact a wide variety of organs, including the eyes, heart, lungs, stomach and intestines, joints, and skin. In organs where the immune system cells develop and respond to pathogens (e.g., bone marrow, thymus, spleen, and lymph nodes), sympathetic nerve terminals make contact with immune cells. Thus, sympathetic release of norepinephrine and neuropeptide Y, together with receptor binding of these neurotransmitters by immune cells, serve as the signal in this hard-wire connection between the brain and the immune system. In addition, sympathetic nerves penetrate into the adrenal gland and cause the release of epinephrine into the bloodstream, which circulates to immune cells as another sympathetic regulatory signal.

Many immune system cells change their behavior in the presence of neurotransmitters. Under both laboratory and naturalistic conditions, sympathetic activation has been shown to suppress the activity of diverse populations of immune cells including NK cells and T lymphocytes. In contrast, other aspects of the immune response can be enhanced. For example, catecholamines can increase the production of antibodies by B cells and the ability of macrophages to release cytokines and thereby signal the presence of a pathogen. Additional studies indicate that sympathetic activation can also shunt some immune system cells out of circulating blood and into the lymphoid organs (e.g., spleen, lymph nodes, thymus) while recruiting other types of immune cell into circulation (e.g., NK cells). In general, SNS activation can reduce the immune system's ability to destroy pathogens that live inside cells (e.g., viruses) via decreases of the cellular immune response, while sparing or enhancing the humoral immune response to pathogens that live outside cells (e.g., bacteria). Together, these observations are a cornerstone for understanding fundamental, neuroanatomic signaling between the autonomic nervous and immune systems.

Neuroendocrine Axis

The other way in which the brain can communicate with the immune system is the HPA system. This process begins in the hypothalamus, an area of the brain that governs basic bodily processes such as temperature, thirst, and hunger. Following the release of neuroendocrine factors from the brain, the endocrine glands secrete hormones into the circulation, which reach various organs and bind to hormone receptors on the organs. Under conditions of psychological or physical stress, for example, the hypothalamus increases its release of corticotropin-releasing hormone (CRH) into a small network of blood vessels that descends into the pituitary gland. In response to CRH, the pituitary gland synthesizes adrenocorticotropic hormone (ACTH), which travels through the bloodstream down to the adrenal glands and triggers the release of a steroid hormone called cortisol from the outer portion of the adrenal glands. Cortisol exerts diverse effects on a wide variety of physiological systems and also coordinates the actions of various cells involved in an immune response by altering the production of cytokines or immune messengers. Similar to sympathetic catecholamines and neuropeptide Y, cortisol can suppress the cellular immune response critical to defending the body against viral infections. Indeed, a synthetic analog of cortisol is often used to suppress excessive immune system responses (e.g., in autoimmune diseases such as arthritis or in allergic reactions such as the rash produced by poison oak). Cortisol can also prompt some immune cells to move out from circulating blood into lymphoid organs or peripheral tissues such as the skin. What is even more remarkable about the interactions between the neuroendocrine and immune system is that immune cells can also produce neuroendocrine peptides (e.g., endorphin, ACTH), which suggests that the brain, neuroendocrine axis, and immune system use the same molecular signals to communicate with each other.

Central Modulation of Immunity

Together, this converging evidence of brain–immune system interactions legitimizes the possibility that the brain has a physiological role in the regulation of immunity. Indeed, one key peptide involved in integrating neural and neuroendocrine control of visceral processes is CRH. Release of this peptide in the brain alters a variety of immune processes, including aspects of innate immunity, cellular immunity, and *in vivo* measures of antibody production. Relevant to immune alterations in depression, CRH is elevated in the cerebrospinal fluid of depressed patients. Hence, the brain through the endogenous release of CRH controls immune cells in lymphoid tissue in the same manner it controls other visceral organs, namely, by coordinating autonomic and neuroendocrine pathways; when these pathways are blocked by specific factors that bind to sympathetic or hormone receptors, the effects of CRH or brain stimulation on immune function are also blocked.

Depression Influences on Immunity

Enumerative Measures

Evidence for increases in the total number of white blood cells and in the numbers and percentages of neutrophils and lymphocytes was among the first immunological changes identified in depressed persons. Further evaluation of lymphocyte numbers in depression has used phenotype-specific cell surface markers to enumerate lymphocyte subsets and found that depression is negatively related to the number and percentage of lymphocytes (B cells, T cells, T helper cells, and T suppressor/cytotoxic cells) as well as the NK cell phenotype.

Functional Measures

For the evaluation of the function of the immune system in depressed patients, a majority of studies have relied on results from assays of nonspecific mitogen-induced lymphocyte proliferation, mitogen-stimulated cytokine production, and NK cytotoxicity. More than a dozen studies have been conducted on lymphocyte proliferation in depression, and there is a reliable association between depression and lower proliferative responses to the three nonspecific mitogens, including phytohaemagglutinin (PHA), concanavalin-A (Con A), and pokeweed (PWM). In addition, a number of independent laboratories have confirmed the finding of reduced NK activity in major depression.

Stimulated Cytokine Production

Studies of stimulated cytokine production have not yielded consistent findings. For example, increased lipopolysaccharide stimulated production of interleukin-1β (IL-1β) and IL-6 in depressed patients, but resulted in no change in the expression of another pro-inflammatory cytokine, tumor necrosis factor α (TNF-α). There are also reports of a shift in the relative balance of Th1 vs. Th2 cytokine production with increases in the capacity of lymphocytes to produce interferon in depression. However, no difference in the stimulated production of IL-2 has been found. These negative findings cannot be ascribed to differences in depressed samples, as depressed patients who show declines in NK activity show no difference in IL-2 production.

Inflammation and Circulating Levels of Inflammatory Markers

The presence of immune activation in major depression has also been evaluated by examining circulating levels of inflammatory markers, as well as Th1 cytokines; one study reported increases of plasma levels of IL-12 in a large cohort of depressed patients. Meta-analyses indicate that depression is associated with an increase in circulating levels of the pro-inflammatory cytokine IL-6. It is hypothesized that increases in circulating levels of pro-inflammatory cytokines are due to activation of monocyte populations, and increases in circulating levels of other pro-inflammatory cytokines such as TNF-α and IL-1β have also been reported in depressed patients. Additional studies have extended these observations and assayed markers of systemic inflammation such as acute phase proteins and/or levels of soluble interleukin-2 receptor (sIL-2R), although findings are mixed. Nevertheless, increases in C-reactive protein have been found in association with depression with elevated levels in healthy depressed adults, as well as in those depressed patients with acute coronary syndrome. In turn, systemic immune activation is thought to lead to endothelial activation in depression with increases in the expression of soluble intercellular adhesion molecule.

Dissociation between Declines of Innate Immunity and Inflammatory Markers

Little attention has been given to the potential relationship between measures of innate immunity, such as NK activity, and levels of inflammatory markers in the context of major depression. In a recent study, levels of NK activity, circulating levels of IL-6, sIL-2R, and acute phase proteins were measured in patients with current major depressive disorder. Whereas patients with major depressive disorder showed lower NK activity and higher circulating levels of IL-6, levels of NK activity were not correlated with IL-6 or with other markers of immune activation including acute phase proteins or sIL-2R. Such findings have implications for understanding individual differences in the adverse health effects of major depressive disorder. Some depressed persons show reductions of cellular and innate immune responses that are associated with infectious disease susceptibility, whereas other studies report that depression is linked to immune activation that is associated with risk of inflammatory disorders such as rheumatoid arthritis and cardiovascular disease.

Viral-Specific Immune Measures

Extension of these nonspecific measures of immunity to viral-specific immune response has suggested a functional decline in memory T cells that respond to at least one virus, namely, the varicella zoster virus, which is thought to be a surrogate marker for herpes zoster risk. Psychological stress is also associated with decline in specific immune responses to immunization against viral infections, although extension of this work to major depression has not yet been conducted.

Assays of *in Vivo* Responses

Basic observations in animals have raised the possibility that depression can alter *in vivo* immune responses, as administration of chronic stress suppresses the delayed type hypersensitivity (DTH) response. Translation of these findings suggests that suppression of the DTH response to a panel of antigenic challenges occurs in depression.

Clinical Moderating Variables

Heterogeneity in the effects of depression on immunity can be accounted for by a number of factors such as age, gender, ethnicity, adiposity, and health behaviors (e.g., smoking, alcohol consumption). Older adults show declines in cellular immunity, and the presence of comorbid depression appears to magnify further age-related immune alterations. Gender of the subject exerts differential effects on pituitary-adrenal and immune systems by modulating the sensitivity of target tissues, and women undergoing laboratory stress show exaggerated expression of cytokines that lead to inflammation as compared to men. Such inflammatory responses to stress may place depressed women at increased risk for autoimmune disorders. In contrast, declines of T cell and NK cell response appear to be more prominent in depressed men than in depressed women. Regarding ethnicity, African American ethnicity interacts with a history of alcohol consumption to exacerbate immune abnormalities, but the effects of ethnicity on depression-related immune alterations are not known. Increases in body mass index and the presence of obesity are associated with increases in markers of inflammation such as circulating levels of C-reactive protein and IL-6. It has been suggested that adiposity and greater body mass partially mediate the increase of inflammatory markers in depression, although other data indicate that elevated levels of inflammatory markers may occur only above a threshold of adiposity or in those with obesity. Finally, depressed patients who are comorbid for alcohol abuse or tobacco smoking show exaggerated declines of NK activity.

Behavioral Mechanisms: Role of Insomnia

Insomnia is one of the most common complaints of depressed subjects, with potential mediating effects on immune alterations in depression. Disordered sleep and loss of sleep are thought to adversely affect resistance to infectious disease, increase cancer risk, and alter inflammatory disease progression. Recent epidemiological data show that self-reported difficulty initiating sleep is a predictor of cardiovascular disease mortality, and objective measures of difficulty initiating sleep (i.e., prolonged sleep latency) yield a twofold elevated risk of death in a healthy older adult population. Animal studies further show that sleep deprivation impairs influenza viral clearance and increases rates of bacteremia, with translational data showing that acute sleep loss reduces immune response to immunization against influenza and hepatitis B.

In humans, normal sleep is associated with a redistribution of circulating lymphocyte subsets, increases of NK activity, increases of certain cytokines (e.g., IL-2, IL-6), and a relative shift toward Th1 cytokine expression that is independent of circadian processes. Conversely, sleep deprivation suppresses NK activity and IL-2 production, although prolonged sleep loss has been found to enhance measures of innate immunity and pro-inflammatory cytokine expression.

In depressed patients, subjective insomnia correlates with NK activity in depression, but not with other depressive symptoms. Recent studies in bereaved persons show that insomnia mediates the relationship between severe life stress and a decline of NK responses. Furthermore, in patients with primary insomnia, prolonged sleep latency and fragmentation of sleep are associated with nocturnal elevations of sympathetic catecholamines and declines in daytime levels of NK cell responses, similar to the abnormalities found in depression. Finally, EEG sleep measures in depressed patients showed that prolonged sleep latency and increases of REM density correlated with elevated levels of IL-6 and sICAM and fully accounted for the association between depression and IL-6.

Depression Treatment: Effects of Antidepressant Medications

Only a limited number of studies have investigated the clinical course of depression and changes of immunity in relation to antidepressant medication treatment and symptom resolution. In a longitudinal case-control study, depressed patients showed increases in NK activity during a 6-month course of tricyclic antidepressant medication treatment, although improvements in NK activity correlated with declines in symptom severity and not medication treatment status at the follow-up. However, both *in vivo* and *in vitro* treatment with fluoxetine, a selective serotonin reuptake inhibitor, results in enhanced NK activity along with changes in depressive symptoms, consistent with the effects of a number of other selective serotonin reuptake inhibitors on NK responses. Other studies have focused on pro-inflammatory cytokine expression and inflammation and concluded that antidepressants decrease pro-inflammatory cytokine (e.g., IL-1β, TNF-α, and IL-6) and induce a shift toward Th2 cytokine expression. However, such alterations in the production of cytokines appear to be confined to medication responders, suggesting that symptom resolution is a relatively more important predictor of the cytokine changes than antidepressant medication status.

Cytokines Influences on the CNS and Behavior: Implications for Depression

Not only does the brain participate in the regulation of immune responses, but also the CNS receives information from the periphery that an immune response is occurring with consequent changes in both electrical and neurochemical activity of the brain. During immunization to a novel protein antigen, the firing rate of neurons within the brain (e.g., ventromedial hypothalamus) increases at the time of peak production of antibody; this part of the brain controls autonomic activity. Cytokines released by immune cells are increasingly implicated as messengers in this bidirectional interaction, and the release of IL-1 following activation of macrophages with virus or other stimuli induces alterations of brain activity and changes in the metabolism of central brain chemicals and neurotransmitters such as norepinephrine, serotonin, and dopamine in discrete brain areas. Much recent data have focused on how these cytokines signal the brain given their large molecular size and inability to cross readily the blood–brain barrier. It is now known that IL-1 and possibly other inflammatory cytokines communicate with the brain by stimulating peripheral nerves such as the vagus that provide information to the brain. In sum, the immune system acts in many ways like a sensory organ, conveying information to the brain, which ultimately regulates neuroendocrine and autonomic outflow and the course of the immune response.

Immune activation also leads to changes of peripheral physiology and behaviors that are similar to a stress response. With peripheral immune activation, pro-inflammatory cytokines are expressed in the CNS, CRH is released by the hypothalamus, and there is an induction of a pituitary adrenal response and autonomic activity. Coincident with these physiological changes, animals show reductions in activity, exploration of novel objects, social interactions, food and water intake, and a willingness to engage in sexual behaviors. Taken together, this pattern of behavioral changes (i.e., sickness behaviors) is similar to that found in animals exposed to fear or anxiety-arousing stimuli and can be reproduced by the central or peripheral administration of IL-1. In contrast, central administration of factors that block IL-1 antagonizes these effects. These cytokine-brain processes are also implicated in increased sensitivity to pain stimuli that is found following nerve or tissue injury.

Translation of these data to clinical samples suggest that physiological activation of the immune system by bacterial products with the release of pro-inflammatory cytokines leads to increases of depressed mood and anxiety, and decreases of verbal and non-verbal memory function. Moreover, large doses of cytokines, given as immunotherapy for cancer or hepatitis C commonly induce depression-like symptoms such as depressed mood, inability to experience pleasure, fatigue, poor concentration, and disordered sleep, which can be effectively treated by giving antidepressant medications. Cytokines can also alter sleep in humans. Expression of the Th2 or anti-inflammatory cytokine IL-10 prior to sleep predicts amounts of delta sleep during the nocturnal period, whereas levels of pro-inflammatory cytokine IL-6 are associated with declines of delta sleep and increases of REM sleep. Likewise, pro-inflammatory cytokine activation is implicated in daytime fatigue, with links identified in cancer survivors as well as healthy older adults.

Clinical Implications of Psychoneuroimmunology

The factors that account for individual differences in the rate and severity of disease progression are not fully understood, although increasing evidence suggests that behavioral and multisystem physiological changes that occur during depression or stress come together to exacerbate the course of many chronic diseases. In the following sections, several pertinent diseases examples are discussed.

Cardiovascular Disease

Atherosclerosis is now thought to be an inflammatory process that involves a series of steps, each of which appears to be impacted by depression. Activated macrophages within the vascular space secrete pro-inflammatory cytokines, which in turn leads to expression of adhesion molecules. With recruitment of immune cells to the vascular cell wall or endothelium and the release of inflammatory cytokines, the vascular endothelium expresses adhesion molecules that facilitate further binding of immune cells. Importantly, psychological and physical stressors increase both release of pro-inflammatory cytokines and expression of adhesion molecules that tether (slow down) and bind immune cells to the vascular endothelium. Moreover, it appears that depression is associated with activation of the endothelium. Acute coronary patients who are depressed show an increased expression of an adhesion molecule that is released following activation of the vascular endothelium (i.e., soluble intracellular adhesion molecule). Importantly, this molecular marker of endothelial activation, as well as IL-6, predicts risk of future myocardial infarction, independent of cholesterol levels, smoking status, and obesity. In prospective studies, both depressed mood and inflammatory markers contribute independently to the risk for coronary heart disease, particularly in men.

HIV

HIV infection shows a highly variable course, and depression, bereavement, and maladaptive coping responses to stress (including the stress of HIV infection itself) have all been shown to predict the rate of immune system decay in HIV patients. For example, major depression in women with HIV infection was associated with lower NK activity, as well as increases in the numbers of activated CD8 lymphocytes and viral load, which suggested that declines of killer lymphocytes in association with depression may increase risk of HIV disease progression in women. Immune system decline and HIV replication are particularly rapid in patients living under chronic stress (e.g., gay men who conceal their homosexuality by living in the closet) and in patients with high levels of SNS activity (e.g., socially inhibited introverts). Tissue culture studies have shown that SNS neurotransmitters and glucocorticoids can accelerate HIV replication by rendering T lymphocytes more vulnerable to infection and by suppressing production of the antiviral cytokines that help cells limit viral replication.

Depression and Rheumatoid Arthritis: Neuroimmune Mechanisms

In a negative feedback loop, pro-inflammatory cytokines stimulate the HPA axis that results in the secretion of glucocorticoids, which in turn suppresses the immune response. However, in autoimmune disorders such as rheumatoid arthritis, it is thought that the counterregulatory glucocorticoid response is not fully achieved. In animals that are susceptible to arthritis, there is a central hypothalamic defect in the biosynthesis of CRH, blunted induction of ACTH and adrenal steroids, and decreased adrenal steroid receptor activation in immune target tissues that together contribute to weak HPA response, one that is not sufficient to suppress the progression of an autoimmune response. Rheumatoid arthritis patients also show a relative hypofunctioning of the HPA axis despite the degree of inflammation. Stress and depression can lead to HPA axis activation and to increases of pro-inflammatory cytokines, and recent data suggest that stressful events, particularly those of an interpersonal nature, provoke symptoms of disease such as greater pain and functional limitations. Moreover, the presence of depression in rheumatoid arthritis patients undergoing stress is associated with exaggerated increases of IL-6, a biomarker predictive of disease progression. Conversely, administration of a psychological intervention that decreases emotional distress produced improvements in clinician-rated disease activity in rheumatoid arthritis patients, although immunological mediators were not measured. Likewise, in the case of another autoimmune disorder, psoriasis, a stress reduction intervention, mindfulness meditation, was found to induce a more rapid clearing of the psoriatic lesions.

Cancer

Experimental studies conducted in animal models have shown that exposure to acute stress leads to decreases in NK cell function and facilitates the metastatic spread of NK-sensitive tumors. However, translation of these data has been challenging; clinical findings supporting a link between depression and cancer have been mixed, with limited evidence to support the contribution of immune mechanisms. Immunogenic tumors have rarely been investigated in the context of depression and psychoneuroimmunology. In addition, other physiological systems, such as the endocrine system, may also play a role; for example, dysregulated cortisol rhythm is associated with both reduced NK activity and increased mortality in metastatic breast cancer patients. Behavioral interventions in the setting of cancer recovery appear to impact disease outcomes such as recurrence and survival. In metastatic breast cancer patients, group psychotherapy led to improvements in mood and increased survival time, controlling for initial staging and medical care during the follow-up period. Among patients with malignant melanoma, group psychotherapy was associated with decreases in distress, increases in active coping, and increases in NK cytotoxicity, as well as a higher rate of survival. Both baseline NK cytotoxicity and improvements in coping behavior were associated with disease outcomes in this study.

Acknowledgments

This work was supported in part by grants A13239, DA16541, MH55253, AG18367, T32-MH19925, M01-RR00865, M01 RR00827, General Clinical Research Centers Program, and the Cousins Center for Psychoneuroimmunology.

See Also the Following Articles

Depression and Manic–Depressive Illness.

Further Reading

Ader, R., Felten, D. and Cohen, N. (eds.) (2001). *Psychoneuroimmunology.* San Diego, CA: Academic Press.

Capuron, L. and Dantzer, R. (2003). Cytokines and depression: the need for a new paradigm. *Brain, Behavior, and Immunity* **17**, S119–S124.

Empana, J. P., Sykes, D. H., Luc, G., et al. (2005). Contributions of depressive mood and circulating inflammatory markers to coronary heart disease in healthy European men: the Prospective Epidemiological Study of Myocardial Infarction (PRIME). *Circulation* **111**, 2299–2305.

Evans, D. L., Ten Have, T. R., Douglas, S. D., et al. (2002). Association of depression with viral load, CD8 T lymphocytes, and natural killer cells in women with HIV infection. *American Journal of Psychiatry* **159**, 1752–1759.

Friedman, E. M. and Irwin, M. (1997). Modulation of immune cell function by the autonomic nervous system. *Pharmacology Therapy* **74**, 27–38.

Irwin, M. (2002). Psychoneuroimmunology of depression: clinical implications (Presidential Address). *Brain, Behavior, and Immunity* **16**, 1–16.

Irwin, M., Pike, J. and Oxman, M. (2004). Shingles immunity and health functioning in the elderly. *Evidence Based Complementary and Alternative Medicine* **1**, 223–232.

Jung, W. and Irwin, M. (1999). Reduction of natural killer cytotoxic activity in major depression: Interaction between depression and cigarette smoking. *Psychosomatic Medicine* **61**, 263–270.

Kronfol, Z. and Remick, D. G. (2000). Cytokines and the brain: implications for clinical psychiatry. *American Journal of Psychiatry* **157**, 683–694.

Lesperance, F., Frasure-Smith, N., Theroux, P. and Irwin, M. (2004). The association between major depression and

levels of soluble intercellular adhesion molecule 1, interleukin-6, and C-reactive protein in patients with recent acute coronary syndromes. *American Journal of Psychiatry* **161**, 271–277.
Miller, G. E., Cohen, S. and Herbert, T. B. (1999). Pathways linking major depression and immunity in ambulatory female patients. *Psychosomatic Medicine* **61**, 850–860.
Miller, G. E., Freedland, K. E., Duntley, S. and Carney, R. M. (2005). Relation of depressive symptoms to C-reactive protein and pathogen burden (cytomegalovirus, herpes simplex virus, Epstein-Barr virus) in patients with earlier acute coronary syndromes. *American Journal of Cardiology* **95**, 317–321.
Motivala, S. J., Sarfatti, A., Olmos, L. and Irwin, M. R. (2005). Inflammatory markers and sleep disturbance in major depression. *Psychosomatic Medicine* **67**, 187–194.
Raison, C. and Miller, A. H. (2003). When not enough is too much: the role of insufficient glucocorticoid signaling in the pathophysiology of stress-related disorders. *American Journal of Psychiatry* **160**, 1554–1565.
Schleifer, S. J., Keller, S. E. and Bartlett, J. A. (1999). Depression and immunity: clinical factors and therapeutic course. *Psychiatry Research* **85**, 63–69.
Segerstrom, S. C. and Miller, G. E. (2004). Psychological stress and the human immune system: a meta-analytic study of 30 years of inquiry. *Psychological Bulletin* **130**, 601–630.
Vedhara, K. and Irwin, M. R. (2005). *Human psychoneuroimmunology.* Oxford, UK: Oxford University Press.
Zautra, A. J., Yocum, D. C., Villanueva, I., et al. (2004). Immune activation and depression in women with rheumatoid arthritis. *Journal of Rheumatology* **31**, 457–463.
Zorrilla, E. P., Luborsky, L. and McKay, J. R., et al. (2001). The relationship of depression and stressors to immunological assays: a meta-analytic review. *Brain, Behavior, and Immunity* **15**, 199–226.

Depression and Coronary Heart Disease

F Lespérance
Centre Hospitalier de l'Université de Montréal Research Center, University of Montreal, and Montreal Heart Institute Research Center, Montreal, Canada
N Frasure-Smith
Centre Hospitalier de l'Université de Montréal Research Center, University of Montreal, McGill University, and Montreal Heart Institute Research Center, Montreal, Canada

Glossary

Autonomic nervous system — The system that controls internal organs without a person being consciously aware. There are two parts to this system: the sympathetic nervous system and the parasympathetic (or vagal) nervous system.

Cognitive-behavior therapy (CBT) — A structured, usually time-limited, form of psychotherapy with active therapist involvement involving exercises and homework to alter dysfunctional thought patterns that are believed to underlie and perpetuate depression.

Endothelial dysfunction — One of the earliest signs of the development of coronary heart disease.

Endothelium — The lining of the arteries; responsible for arterial dilation and constriction in response to systemic demands and chemical stimuli.

Heart-rate variability — The degree to which the length of time between heart beats differs from beat to beat. Low heart-rate variability is a sign of inadequate vagal protection in the autonomic nervous system and predicts cardiac death in individuals with coronary heart disease.

Parasympathetic nervous system — Part of the autonomic nervous system that controls relaxation and promotes digestion; also called the vagal nervous system.

Sympathetic nervous system — Part of the autonomic nervous system that directs the fight-or-flight response to stress.

Sympathetic-vagal balance — The balance between the sympathetic nervous system and the parasympathetic (or vagal) nervous system; this balance is altered in depression.

Ventricular function — A measure of the heart's ability to pump blood; it is often reduced following myocardial infarction because of the damage that occurs to the heart muscle.

Introduction

Depression and coronary heart disease (CHD) are among the most prevalent disabling medical conditions worldwide. The Global Burden of Disease Study predicted that, by 2020, depression and CHD will be the two leading causes of early death and disability in the world. The term depression most frequently refers to a mental state with sustained sadness or loss of interest lasting at least several weeks, coupled with other symptoms such as fatigue, reduced sleep, and appetite and leading to significant occupational or interpersonal impairment. CHD includes all clinical manifestations associated with damage to the myocardium due to acute or chronic ischemia, which itself is most commonly caused by atherosclerotic narrowing of the coronary arteries. Interestingly, psychological stress, such as interpersonal conflicts, perceived or real losses, and work stress, are thought to contribute to the acute exacerbation of depression as well as of CHD.

Definitions of Depression

The *Diagnostic and Statistical Manual of Mental Disorders* (4th edn.; DSM-IV) of the American Psychiatric Association defines major depression as at least 2 weeks of daily (lasting most of the day) sadness or loss of interest plus at least five of the following symptoms: changes in appetite, changes in sleep patterns, psychomotor agitation or retardation, loss of energy or fatigue, feelings of worthlessness, inability to concentrate or make decisions, and thoughts of suicide or death.

Studies conducted in hospitalized cardiac patients have found that about one in six patients meet the criteria for a major depressive episode. This high peak prevalence during the hospitalization subsides, with approximately 10% of CHD patients depressed at 3 months after discharge. However, many patients do not meet the full criteria for major depression, but nevertheless present elevated levels of depressive symptoms. These patients may have a variety of clinical diagnoses. Some may suffer from a major depression in partial remission or dysthymia (chronic low-level depression); others may suffer from an adjustment disorder. There are many different self-report scales available to measure the overall intensity of depressive symptoms. The Beck Depression Inventory (BDI) is the most commonly used in research with CHD patients.

Even if major depression is not present, however, having high levels of depressive symptoms increases a patient's risk of cardiovascular events. Although major depression and elevated depressive symptoms are approximately three times as common in CHD patients as in the general community, the prevalence of depression in CHD patients is similar to that in patients with other chronic medical conditions.

The Course and Consequences of Depression in Coronary Heart Disease Patients

As for depressed patients without medical illnesses, the course of depression in CHD patients is frequently chronic. More than half of those who experience major depression during hospitalization after a myocardial infarction (MI, or heart attack) remain depressed or have elevated symptoms of depression 1 year later.

However, as important as its chronicity is the fact that depression is associated with a worse cardiac prognosis. Several reviews and meta-analyses have concluded that both major depression and high levels of depressive symptoms predict cardiac mortality in patients with established CHD, as well as the incidence of CHD among previously healthy subjects. The impact of depression is independent of other prognostic variables; that is, it is not explained by other possible confounding factors. This means, for example, that depression predicts cardiac mortality even after statistical control for other predictors of mortality such as age, ventricular function, hypertension, and diabetes. In addition to its independent impact on prognosis, the size of the impact of depression on CHD events is as large as that of these other important prognostic factors. Depression at least doubles the risk of cardiac mortality over time, and the risk increases with the severity of depressive symptoms.

INTERHEART, a very large case-control study conducted in 52 countries across all continents compared levels of modifiable risk factors in more than 11,000 survivors of a first MI and more than 13,000 control subjects. The study found that the population attributable risk (PAR) for depression is 9%, a risk as large as that of diabetes. The PAR takes into account the prevalence and degree of risk associated with a particular risk factor and is interpreted to mean that, if depression could be eliminated at the population level, we would observe a worldwide reduction of 9% in the incidence of first MIs.

The INTERHEART study also evaluated the contribution of different dimensions of stress to the incidence of MI. It found that all four dimensions of stress measured in the study (stress at work, stress at home, financial stress, and general stress) predicted the incidence of MI, with the PARs for stress ranging between 8 and 12%. In addition, the study found that a measure of locus of control, evaluating how much a person feels that he or she can control life circumstances, also predicted the incidence of MI, with a PAR of 16%. Finally, the occurrence of stressful life events in the last year, such as the death of a spouse or other family member, marital separation or divorce, or major familial conflict, was also more frequent among first MI patients than controls. In summary, this landmark study found that, on a worldwide basis, the contribution of psychosocial stress and depression to the incidence of MI was just behind that of smoking and was greater than that of abdominal obesity. INTERHEART also confirmed that the impact of depression and other psychosocial stresses is independent of age, smoking status, and other cardiovascular risk factors. It underscores the importance of the emotional and behavioral factors in physical health, and it should stimulate research to reduce depression, stress, and their consequences.

Mechanisms

Many biological pathways may be involved in the link between depression and CHD. Depression is similar to a state of chronic, severe psychological stress, and many of the biological systems involved in the stress response are dysregulated in depressed patients regardless of whether or not they have CHD. The sympathetic-vagal balance is tipped toward more noradrenergic activity, heart-rate variability is reduced, and there is an increased risk of ventricular arrhythmias. There is also an augmentation of the innate inflammatory response with more pro-inflammatory cytokines. Platelet activation is increased, facilitating blood-clot formation. There is hyperactivity of the hypothalamic-pituitary-adrenal (HPA) axis, which influences lipid and carbohydrate metabolism. In addition, it has been recently shown that depressed young adult patients without CHD have endothelial dysfunction, one of the early markers of atherosclerotic burden.

Because of the obvious role of the selective serotonin reuptake inhibitor (SSRI) antidepressants in mood regulation, there has been a great deal of interest in their potential cardiovascular benefits. Platelets contain serotonin granules that are secreted during the platelet activation phase, a process that facilitates blood-clot formation through the activation of the platelet's own serotonin receptors. In addition, platelets have a specific serotonin transporter, which acts to move (reuptake) the secreted serotonin back inside the platelet. SSRIs block this transporter, therefore gradually depleting serotonin in the platelets. Consequently, after several weeks of treatment, SSRIs seem to have blood-thinning effects. However, it is unknown whether this effect is of enough clinical relevance to prevent thrombotic cardiovascular events.

It is also possible that some environmental or genetic factors contribute to the physiopathology of CHD and depression at the same time. For example, a lower dietary intake of long-chain omega-3 fatty acids has been shown to predict the incidence of CHD and a wide variety of mood disorders. There is hope to identify common genetic predispositions for mood disorders and CHD. Specifically, the genes involved in the regulation of the biological systems mentioned thus far (i.e., the sympathetic-parasympathetic system, the inflammatory response, the HPA axis, platelet activation, and thrombus formation) can be profiled and used to evaluate whether specific genetic variations predict the development of CHD, depression, or both. For example, the genes regulating serotonin synthesis, metabolism, and reuptake, such as the serotonin transporter-linked polymorphic region (5-HTTLPR), may be associated with an increased risk of depression because of its role in the brain and with an increased risk of cardiovascular events because of its role in platelet aggregation.

Depression Treatment Trials in Coronary Heart Disease Patients

With the current deluge of mega-trials in cardiology testing new drugs and devices to prevent cardiovascular events among CHD patients, it is very disappointing that only one trial was specifically designed to evaluate whether an intervention for depression has an impact on CHD events. This is, at least partially, because of lack of funding resources; a depression treatment–CHD trial would necessarily depend on peer-reviewed public funding, whereas most of the large phase III drug trials in cardiology are currently supported by the pharmaceutical industry.

ENRICHD (Enhancing Recovery in Coronary Heart Disease) is the only trial carried out to date to evaluate the impact of depression treatment on cardiac events. ENRICHD was a National Heart, Lung, and Blood Institute (NHLBI)-sponsored, multicenter trial that assessed the potential benefit of 6 months of CBT in some 2400 depressed post-MI patients. Although patients receiving CBT experienced a significantly greater improvement in depression than those in the usual-care group, this study was unable to demonstrate that CBT prevented the recurrence of cardiac events. The physicians of patients in the usual-care group were informed that their patients were depressed, and there was a high rate of prescription of antidepressant medications in the usual-care group, reducing the contrast between the groups. Other earlier controlled clinical trials designed to treat psychological distress, rather than depression *per se*, were also not successful in demonstrating that treating distress reduces cardiac events.

Conclusion

Despite the extensive epidemiological data showing that an increased risk of cardiac events is associated with depression and considerable animal and human research suggesting that various physiopathological changes, similar to those observed in chronic severe stress, accompany depression, the data from controlled clinical trials do not support the use of any specific interventions for depression or psychological distress to prevent cardiac events in CHD patients.

Further Reading

Carney, R. M., Blumenthal, J. A., Freedland, K. E., et al. (2005). Low heart rate variability and the effect of depression on post-myocardial infarction mortality. *Archives of Internal Medicine* **165**, 1486–1491.

ENRICHD Investigators. (2003). Effects of treating depression and low perceived social support on clinical events after myocardial infarction. *Journal of the American Medical Association* **289**, 3106–3116.

Frasure-Smith, N. and Lesperance, F. (2005). Reflections on depression as a cardiac risk factor. *Psychosomatic Medicine* **67**(supplement 1), S19–S25.

Frasure-Smith, N., Lespérance, F. and Julien, P. (2004). Major depression is associated with lower omega-3 fatty acid levels in patients with recent acute coronary syndromes. *Biological Psychiatry* **55**, 891–896.

Hibbeln, J. R. and Makino, K. K. (2002). Omega-3 fats in depressive disorders and violence: the context of evolution and cardiovascular health. In: Skinner, E. R. (ed.) *Brain lipids and disorders in biological psychiatry*, pp. 67–111. Amsterdam: Elsevier Science.

Joynt, K. E., Whellan, D. J. and O'Connor, C. M. (2003). Depression and cardiovascular disease: mechanisms of interaction. *Biological Psychiatry* **54**, 248–261.

Kuper, H., Marmot, M. and Hemingway, H. (2002). Systematic review of prospective cohort studies of psychosocial factors in the etiology and prognosis of coronary heart disease. *Seminars in Vascular Medicine* **2**, 267–314.

Lespérance, F., Frasure-Smith, N., Theroux, P., et al. (2004). The association between major depression and levels of soluble intercellular adhesion molecule 1, interleukin-6, and C-reactive protein in patients with recent acute coronary syndromes. *American Journal of Psychiatry* **161**, 271–277.

Murray, C. J. L. and Lopez, A. D. (1997). Global mortality, disability, and the contribution of risk factors: Global Burden of Disease Study. *Lancet* **49**, 1436–1442.

Musselman, D. L., Evans, D. L. and Nemeroff, C. B. (1998). The relationship of depression to cardiovascular disease: epidemiology, biology and treatment. *Archives of General Psychiatry* **55**, 580–592.

Rosengren, A., Hawken, S., Ounpuu, S., et al. (2004). Association of psychosocial risk factors with risk of acute myocardial infarction in 11,119 cases and 13,648 controls from 52 countries (the INTERHEART study): case-control study. *Lancet* **364**, 953–962.

Schiepers, O. J., Wichers, M. C. and Maes, M. (2005). Cytokines and major depression. *Progress in Neuropsychopharmacology and Biological Psychiatry* **29**, 201–217.

Serebruany, V. L. (2006). Selective serotonin reuptake inhibitors and increased bleeding risk: are we missing something? *American Journal of Medicine* **119**, 113–116.

Suls, J. and Bunde, J. (2005). Anger, anxiety, and depression as risk factors for cardiovascular disease: the problems and implications of overlapping affective dispositions. *Psychological Bulletin* **131**, 260–300.

Vale, S. (2005). Psychosocial stress and cardiovascular diseases. *Postgraduate Medical Journal* **81**, 429–435.

Adjustment Disorders

M Dascalu and D Svrakic
Washington University School of Medicine, St. Louis, MO, USA

This article is reproduced from Encyclopedia of Stress First Edition, volume 1, pp 27–31, © 2000, Elsevier Inc.

Glossary

Bereavement	Loss through death.
Bereavement process	The umbrella term for bereavement reactions over time.
Bereavement reactions	Psychological, physiological, or behavioral responses to bereavement.
Crisis	A self-limited response to hazardous events and experienced as a painful state. It can last from a few hours to weeks.
Diagnostic and Statistical Manual of Mental Disorders DSM-IV	The latest and most up-to-date classification of mental disorders. It was published in 1994.
Temperament and character inventory (TCI)	A self-report questionnaire that allows diagnosis of personality disorders using a quantitative rating of seven factors, four dimensions of temperament (harm avoidance, novelty seeking, reward dependence, and persistence) and three dimensions of character (self-directedness, cooperativeness, and self-trancendence).

Definition

Adjustment disorder is characterized in DSM-IV by the development of emotional or behavioral symptoms in response to one or more identifiable psychosocial stressors. The symptoms are considered clinically significant because they either impair the individual's functioning or are subjectively perceived to cause distress in excess of what would be expected from exposure to the stressor(s). These symptoms neither fulfill criteria for an Axis I diagnosis nor represent the exacerbation of a preexisting Axis I or Axis II disorder. They are not caused by normal bereavement. The symptoms occur within 3 months of the onset of a stressor and in response to it and do not last longer than 6 months after the end of the stressor or its consequences. The nature and severity of the stressors is not specified in DSM-IV. They include interpersonal, occupational, or medical problems. The stress may be single or multiple, such as loss of job associated with divorce and physical illness. The stress may happen once or it may be chronic, lasting more than 6 months (such as living in poverty), or recurrent (such as seasonal business difficulties). It can affect only one person or many (as in a flood or an earthquake). Whatever the nature of the stressor the person is overwhelmed by it. The individuals may experience anxiety, depression or behavioral symptoms (e.g., erratic actions) or various combinations. If the symptoms progress to meet criteria for another Axis 1 disorder (e.g., major depression), a diagnosis of adjustment disorder can no longer be used.

Historically a diagnosis similar to adjustment disorder first appeared in DSM-II. Transient situational disorder was understood in a developmental context and its subtypes were defined accordingly; for example, "adjustment reaction" of childhood, adolescence, or adulthood. It required an unusually severe stress. The term adjustment disorder first appeared in DSM-III. A link to severe and unusual stress was no longer required, and the subtypes were recategorized according to their symptomatic presentation. In DSM-II and DSM-III the duration of adjustment disorder was not specified. In DSM-III-R, the duration of the illness was restricted to 6 months after the cessation of the stressor, and the subtype adjustment disorder with physical complaints was added.

Epidemiology

The adjustment disorders are considered to be very common. One epidemiological study conducted in children and adolescents found a prevalence rate of 7.6%. Precise data are not available for adults because the structured interviews used in general population do not include adjustment disorder. Several studies of the prevalence of adjustment disorders were done in clinical samples including patients admitted in the hospital for medical or surgical problems. The reported rates were between 5 and 13% in adults and up to 42% in children and adolescents. In a recent study of 1039 consecutive referrals to consultation–liaison psychiatry services, a diagnosis of adjustment disorder was made in 125 patients (12.0%). It was the sole diagnosis in 81 patients (7.8%) and in 44 (4.2%) it was diagnosed comorbidly with other Axis I and II diagnoses, most frequently with personality disorders and organic mental disorders. It had been considered as a rule-out diagnosis in a further 110 patients (10.6%).

Several studies found that this disorder is more common in women (sex ratio, 2:1).

Etiology

Adjustment disorder is caused by one or more stressors. There is a significant individual variation in response to stress so the severity of the stressors is not always predictive of the development of the illness.

Individual Factors

It is not clear why there is so much individual variation in the development of psychopathology in persons who experience similar stressors and also why when a reaction occurs the symptoms are so variable. Psychoanalytic researchers have highlighted the importance of development of adequate defense mechanisms as a child. Those who were able to develop mature defense mechanisms seem to be less vulnerable to and recover more quickly from the stressor. In this context, the roles of the mother and the rearing environment in a person's capability to respond adequately to stress are critical.

More recently, it has been shown that immature defense mechanisms correlate highly with poor character development as defined by the TCI (Temperament and Character Inventory). Poor character development is considered to be the common feature for the whole group of personality disorders as defined by DSM-IV. This implies that people who have a personality disorder are at a high risk for developing abnormal reaction to stress and then adjustment disorder. Conform to the definition both disorders can be diagnosed in the same time.

Several studies showed that children and adolescents are at a higher risk of developing an adjustment disorder than adults and that the illness is more frequent in females than in males.

Other Factors

The stressor severity is a complex function of multiple factors; for example, degree, quantity, duration, reversibility, environment, and timing. The severity of the stressors is not always predictive of the occurrence and severity of adjustment disorder, but without a doubt, serious and//or chronic stressors are more likely to cause an adjustment reaction. It is not clear if all persons are likely to develop symptoms if stress levels are increased enough. The nosological and phenomenological distinction between crisis and stress is critical for the understanding of individual variability in response to stress.

Diagnosis

Diagnostic Clues

The chief complaint may be a nervous breakdown, inability to manage problems of life, or anxiety or depression associated with a specific stressor; the patient's history reveals normal functioning before the onset of the stressor; and the patient's mental status examination shows symptoms of anxiety, depression, or disturbed conduct.

Clinical Features

Several studies reported that between 50 and 87% of patients present with depressed mood. Other common symptoms encountered in more than 25% of the patients include insomnia, other vegetative symptoms (e.g., palpitations), behavioral problems, social withdrawal, and suicidal ideation or gesture.

The development of depressive symptoms alone is less characteristic of children and adolescents. Two recent studies found that among children and adolescents with adjustment disorder, the majority presented with mixed emotional or mixed emotional and behavioral syndromes. In one study, 77% of adolescents but only 25% of adults had behavioral symptoms (disturbance of conduct).

Studies of adjustment disorder that used structured diagnostic instruments have reported a high level of comorbidity. In a mixed group of children, adolescents, and adults, approximately 70% of patients with adjustment disorder had at least one additional Axis I diagnosis.

Several studies have reported a significant association of adjustment disorder with suicidal behavior in adolescents and young adults. A couple of studies done in patients hospitalized after a suicidal gesture showed that more than 50% of the patients met criteria for adjustment disorder with depressed mood. Three retrospective studies of suicide completers below age 30 found that between 9 and 19% of the cases met criteria for adjustment disorder. This data suggest the seriousness of the illness in a subset of persons.

Subtypes of Adjustment Disorder

The adjustment disorders are classified according to the predominant clinical symptoms. Six subtypes are identified and coded in DSM-IV. Three define discrete symptomatic presentations (depressed mood, anxious mood, disturbance of conduct) and two describe mixed clinical presentations (mixed disturbance of anxiety and depressed mood, mixed disturbance of emotions and conduct). The final subtype, adjustment disorder unspecified, is a residual category for presentations not accurately described by one of the other subtypes. One additional subtype, adjustment disorder with suicidal behavior, was proposed for inclusion in DSM-IV. It was ultimately rejected because of concerns that it would discourage a more systematic assessment of symptoms in patients presenting with suicidal behavior.

1. Adjustment Disorder with Depressed Mood: The predominant manifestations are depressed mood, tearfulness, and hopelessness. This type must be distinguished from major depressive disorder and uncomplicated bereavement.
2. Adjustment Disorder with Anxiety. Symptoms of anxiety – such as palpitations, jitteriness, and agitation – are present in adjustment disorder with anxiety, which must be differentiated from anxiety disorders. The patient is usually nervous, fearful, and worried.
3. Adjustment Disorder with Mixed Anxiety and Depressed Mood: Patients exhibit features of both anxiety and depression that do not meet the criteria for an already established anxiety disorder or depressive disorder.
4. Adjustment Disorder with Disturbance of Conduct: The predominant manifestation involves conduct in which the rights of others are violated or age-appropriate societal norms and rules are disregarded. Examples of behavior in this category are truancy, vandalism, reckless driving, and fighting. The category must be differentiated from conduct disorder and antisocial personality disorder.
5. Adjustment Disorder with Mixed Disturbance of Emotions and Conduct: The combination of disturbance of emotions (anxiety and//or depression) and conduct sometimes occurs.
6. Adjustment Disorder Unspecified: Adjustment disorder unspecified is a residual category for atypical maladaptive reactions to stress. Examples include inappropriate responses to the diagnosis of physical illness, such as massive denial and severe noncompliance with treatment and social withdrawal without significant depressed or anxious mood.

Adjustment disorders are also classified according to the clinical course. They are acute if the symptoms last less than 6 months and chronic if the symptoms last longer than 6 months.

Differential Diagnosis

Adjustment disorders must be differentiated from a normal reaction to stress or from other psychiatric disorders that occur following a stress.

1. In acute stress disorder and posttraumatic stress disorder, the stress needs to be severe and it is more clearly specified. The stressors are psychologically traumatizing events outside the range of normal human experience so they are expected to produce the syndromes in the average human being. Both acute stress disorder and posttraumatic stress disorder are characterized by a specific constellation of affective and autonomic symptoms, which is not encountered in adjustment disorders.

2. In normal bereavement, despite difficulties in social and occupational functioning, the person's impairment remains within the expectable bounds of a reaction to a loss of a loved one.

3. Other disorders include major depressive disorder, brief psychotic disorder, generalized anxiety disorder, somatization disorder, conduct disorder, drug abuse, academic problem, occupational problem, or identity problem.

4. If the criteria for any of the above disorders are met, that diagnosis should be used instead of adjustment disorder, even if a stressor was present.

Course and Prognosis

Course

Adjustment disorder begins shortly after a significant stressor. By definition, the symptoms have to commence within the first 3 months after the onset of the stressor. Usually they start in the first couple of weeks. In most cases when the stressor ceases the symptoms remit quickly.

Prognosis

By definition, adjustment disorder is not an enduring diagnosis. The symptoms either resolve or progress to a more serious illness. In most cases, the prognosis is favorable with appropriate treatment, and most patients return to their previous level of functioning within 3 months. It appears that children and adolescents have a poor prognosis. Several studies, which surveyed adolescents up to 10 years after a diagnosis of adjustment disorder, found that only 44 to 60% of the original sample were well at follow-up. Some of the patients developed major mental disorders, such as schizophrenia, bipolar disorder, major depressive disorder, or substance-related disorders. It is not clear whether the poor outcome is due to adjustment disorder itself or to the frequent existence of comorbidity. At least one study that matched two groups for comorbidity (one with adjustment disorder and the other one without) found that adjustment disorder added no additional risk for poor outcome.

Treatment

Little is known about the proper treatment of adjustment disorder. There are few, if any, treatment studies in patients with adjustment disorder, and systematic clinical trials are necessary because adjustment disorder is one of the most common psychiatric diagnoses. The typical pharmacological intervention is always symptomatic. When given, medication is aimed to alleviate a specific symptom, but should always be in addition to psychosocial strategies.

Stressors

Whenever possible the etiologic stressors should be removed or ameliorated. Interventions designed to minimize the impact of the stressors on daily functioning should be considered.

Psychotherapy

This remains the treatment of choice for adjustment disorder. It can help the patient adapt to the stressor if it is not reversible or time limited. It can also serve a preventive role if the stressor does remit.

1. Crisis intervention is a brief type of therapy that may be useful to decrease stress and facilitate the development of external support. It is designed to resolve the situation quickly by supportive techniques, suggestions, reassurance, and environmental manipulation. The frequency and length of encounters with the therapist is tailored to the patients needs, and sometimes even short-term hospitalization might be warranted.

2. Individual psychotherapy offers the patient the opportunity to understand the personal meaning of the stressor and to develop coping skills.

3. Group psychotherapy can be remarkably useful for patients who experienced similar stresses; for example, a group of renal dialysis patients.

4. Family therapy can sometimes help in some patients, especially those with adjustment disorder with disturbance of conduct who may have difficulties with the school, authorities, or the law.

Pharmacotherapy

This may be useful in some patients when prescribed for brief periods. Depending of the subtype of adjustment disorder, an antianxiety agent or an antidepressant may help. Some patients with severe symptoms may also benefit from short course psychostimulant or antipsychotic medication. There are no studies regarding the use of specific medical agents in adjustment disorder. Few, if any, patients can be adequately treated by medication alone, and psychotherapy should be added to the treatment.

Conclusions

Adjustment disorders are an important and prevalent cause of personal discomfort, absenteeism, addiction, and suicide. This diagnosis should not be used to avoid stigmatization of a patient. Short psychotherapy is the treatment of choice, but pharmacotherapy is often used as an acute way to stabilize the patient and to prevent potentially disruptive behavior.

See Also the Following Articles

Anxiety; Bereavement.

Further Reading

Cloninger, C. R. and Svrakic, D. M. (2000). Personality disorders. In: Kaplan, H. I. & Sadock, B. J. (eds.) *Comprehensive Textbook of Psychiatry* (7th ed.). Baltimore: Lippincott Williams & Wilkins.

Kaplan, H. I., Sadock, B. J. and Grebb, J. A. (1994). *Synopsis of Psychiatry* (7th ed.). Baltimore: Williams & Wilkins.

Morrison, J. (1995). *DSM-IV Made Easy.* New York: Guilford.

Newcorn, J. H. and Strain, J. (1995). Adjustment Disorders. In: Kaplan, H. I. & Sadock, B. J. (eds.) *Comprehensive Textbook of Psychiatry.* Baltimore: Williams & Wilkins.

Popkin, M. K., Callies, A. L., Colon, E. A. and Stiebel, V. (1990). Adjustment disorders in medically ill inpatients referred for consultation in a university hospital. *Psychosomatics* **31**(4), 410–414.

Snyder, S., Strain, J. J. and Wolf, D. (1990). Differentiating major depression from adjustment disorder with depressed mood in the medical setting. *General Hospital Psychiatry* **12**(3), 159–165.

Strain, J. J., Smith, G. C., Hammer, J. S., et al. (1998). Adjustment disorder: A multisite study of its utilization and interventions in the consultation-liaison psychiatry setting. *General Hospital Psychiatry* **20**(3), 139–149.

Bereavement

P J Clayton
American Foundation for Suicide Prevention,
New York, NY, USA

This is a revised version of the article by P J Clayton, Encyclopedia of Stress First Edition, volume 1, pp 304–311, © 2000, Elsevier Inc.

Glossary

Bereavement The state or fact of being bereaved, suffering the death of a loved one; the loss of a loved one by death.

Disorders So disturb the regular or normal functions of; an abnormal physical or mental condition: ailment.

Grief Deep and poignant distress caused by loss, a cause of such suffering.

Mourning The act of sorrowing; a period of time during which signs of grief are shown.

Outcome Something that follows as a result or consequence.

Complicated grief A disordered psychic or behavioral state resulting from a deep and poignant distress caused by or as if by bereavement.

Introduction

Although no-one would argue that the loss by death of someone close is a significant life event, the degree of adversity that the death brings to the individual is variable. The field is just beginning to identify and study people who are most severely affected. In studying bereavement, most investigators have used entry in widowhood as the model, although the response to the death of a child is probably more stressful. This article will concentrate on research on bereavement which by definition is a reaction of a person to loss by death. Other terms in the literature which should not be confused with bereavement are grief, which is the emotional and psychological reaction to any loss but not limited to death, and mourning, which is the social expression of bereavement or grief, frequently formalized by custom or religion.

At this point there have been numerous longitudinal follow-up studies of people who have been recently bereaved. The majority deal with the widowed although there are excellent studies of children who have lost a parent. Despite the fact that the mode of selection, response rate, gender, age group, time since the death to the first interview, comparison groups, and the selection of instruments and outcome measures differ greatly from study to study, the similarities of outcome outweigh the differences. Our own data highlight the major outcomes, although important additional findings have been identified and there are still areas of controversy.

Bereavement is the ideal condition to study the effect of stress on the organism. It is not species specific so it can be defined identically across species and generations of species. It is a real event, not artificial, imagined, or devised, it is datable, it occurs in present time so it can be studied immediately, not retrospectively, and even prospectively. Finally, the significance of the event would not be disputed. Before reviewing the morbidity and mortality associated with this clear-cut, easily defined stress, it is important to emphasize that by far the most usual outcome following this experience is numbness for a very brief period, depression for a variable time, and then recovery. Recovery is the return of the individual to the level of functioning that he or she had established before the death and/or a change in a positive direction. In some cases this takes months, in others, up to 2 years or more. This is described by Lund et al. (1993: 24) in older adults. Only 10–15% of individuals develop chronic depression, with even fewer experiencing complicated grief. In studying the biology of this particular stress, whole populations have to be studied so that we define the usual, natural outcomes as well as the abnormal responses.

Depressive Symptoms and Course

In studying relatives' reactions to the loss of a significant person, we collected data on three different samples. The first sample was a group of 40 bereaved relatives of people who had died at a general hospital in St. Louis, United States. The second was a sample of widows and widowers chosen from the death certificates and seen at 1, 4, and 13 months after the deaths of their spouses. The third sample was a consecutive series of young (<45 years old) widowed people also seen within 1 month after the death and again at 1 year. The last two samples were matched through the voter registry with married people of the same age and sex who had not had first degree relatives die, and who were also followed prospectively to ascertain their morbidity and mortality. The findings are exemplified in **Table 1** which displays the depressive symptoms that were endorsed at 1 and 13 months. In the first month, a large majority of the sample experienced depressed mood; anorexia and beginning weight loss; insomnia that was initial, middle, and terminal; marked crying; some fatigue and loss of interest in their surroundings, but not necessarily the people around them; restlessness; and guilt. The guilt that these people expressed was different to the guilt seen in depressed patients. For the most part it was guilt of omission surrounding either the terminal illness or the death. Irritability was common but overt anger was uncommon. Suicidal thoughts and ideas were rare. When they did occur they occurred in younger men after the death of a wife or in men and women after the death of a child. Hallucinations were not uncommon. Many widows and widowers, when asked, admitted that they had felt touched by their dead spouse or had heard his or her voice, had seen his or her vision or had smelled his or her presence. The misidentification of their dead spouses in a crowd was extremely common.

Table 1 Frequency of depressive symptoms 1 and 13 months after bereavement

Symptoms	*Frequency (%)*	
	1 Month (n = 149[a])	*13 Months (n = 149[a])*
Crying	89	33[d]
Sleep disturbance	76	48[d]
Low mood	75	42[d]
Loss of appetite	51	16[d]
Fatigue	44	30[c]
Poor memory	41	23[d]
Loss of interest	40	23[d]
Difficulty concentrating	36	16[d]
Weight loss of $\geq$ 2.25 kg	36	20[c]
Feeling guilty	31	12[d]
Restlessness (*n* = 89)	48	45
Reverse diurnal variation	26	22
Irritability	24	20
Feels someone to blame	22	22
Diurnal variation	17	10
Death wishes	16	12
Feeling hopeless	14	13
Hallucinations	12	9
Suicide thoughts	5	3
Fear of loosing mind	3	4
Suicide attempts	0	0
Feeling worthless	6	11
Feels angry about death	13	22[b]
Depressive	42	16[d]

[a]n varies from symptom to symptom mostly 148;
[b]significant by McNemar's chi-square, degrees of freedom (df) = 1, $P \leq 0.02$;
[c]significant by McNemar's chi-square, df = 1, $P \leq 0.01$;
[d]significant by McNemar's chi-square, df = 1, $P \leq 0.001$. Reproduced with permission from Clayton, P. J. (1982). Bereavement. In: Paykel, E. S. (ed.) *Handbook of affective disorders*. London: Churchill Livingstone.

We matched some of our subjects with well-studied hospitalized depressed patients and found, as Freud suggested, symptoms such as feeling hopeless, worthless, being a burden, psychomotor retardation, wishing to be dead, and thinking of suicide differentiated the depressed from the bereaved.

By the end of the first year the somatic symptoms of depression had remarkably improved. Low mood (usually associated with specific events or holidays), restlessness, and poor sleep continued. The few psychological symptoms of depression, although rare, resolved less easily. In our studies, the symptoms were as frequent in men as in women, in people who had lost a spouse suddenly or after a lingering death, in people who had good or bad marriages, and people who were religious or nonreligious. Young people were more likely to have a severer immediate reaction, but by 1 year their outcome was similar. There was no relationship between financial status and outcome.

As **Table 2** shows, when the frequency of depressive symptoms were compared to the community controls, all symptoms were more common among the bereaved.

When depressive symptoms reported at 13 months were examined by those with symptoms for the entire year and those who had just developed them, the percent who had new symptoms was similar to those reported by the controls who had had no deaths (**Table 3**). Those who were disturbed early were more likely to be disturbed later. Delayed grief, like delayed posttraumatic stress disorder (PTSD), may be an interesting ideologic concept but remains unproven. It is also counterintuitive since the usual recognized reaction to a physical or psychological insult is an immediate injury with a gradual resolution. This has been confirmed by others.

Physical Symptoms, Substance Use, and Medical Treatment

We systematically ask about physical symptoms, usually associated with major depression, in both the recently widowed and control subjects (**Table 4**). In general, physical symptoms were not more frequent in recently bereaved and controls subjects. Nor did they change much over the year. The largest difference was recorded in "other pains" which were mainly in the elderly bereaved and consisted of arthritic type pains. In our studies, there were no more physicians' visits or hospitalizations in the year following the bereavement. This is controversial.

The most striking finding of this research is illustrated in **Table 4**. After a significant stress such as bereavement the use of alcohol, tranquilizers, and hypnotics significantly increased. For the most part these were not new users but people who had used them before. Cigarette smoking also increased. The morbidity and mortality of bereavement may be

Table 2 Frequency of depressive symptoms at any time in the first year of bereavement and in controls

Symptoms	*Frequency (%)*	
	Bereaved (n = 149[a])	*Controls (n = 131[a])*
Crying	90	14[e]
Sleep disturbance	79	35[e]
Low mood	80	18[e]
Loss of appetite	53	4[e]
Fatigue	55	23[e]
Poor memory	50	22[e]
Loss of interest	48	11[e]
Difficulty concentrating	40	13[e]
Weight loss of ≥2.25 kg	47	24[e]
Feeling guilty	38	11[e]
Restlessness	63	27[e]
Irritability	35	21[b]
Diurnal variation	22	14
Death wishes	22	5[e]
Feeling hopeless	19	4[d]
Hallucinations	17	2[e]
Suicidal thoughts	8	1[c]
Fear of losing mind	7	5
Suicide attempts	0	0
Worthlessness	14	15
Depressive syndrome	47	8[d]

[a]n varies from symptom to symptom;
[b]significant by chi-square, degrees of freedom (df) = 1, $P \leq 0.05$;
[c]significant by chi-square, df = 1, $P \leq 0.01$;
[d]significant by chi-square, df = 1, $P \leq 0.0005$;
[e]significant by chi-square, df = 1, $P \leq 0.0001$. Reproduced with permission from Clayton, P. J. (1982). Bereavement. In: Paykel, E. S. (ed.) *Handbook of affective disorders*. London: Churchill Livingstone.

Table 3 Frequency of depressive symptoms at 1 month

Symptom	*Those with symptoms at 1 month*		*Those without symptoms at 1 month (new symptoms)*	
	%	*n*	*%*	*n*
Crying	36	132	6	16
Sleep disturbance	59	113	11	35
Low mood	49	111	22	37
Loss of appetite	28	76	4	72
Fatigue	45	65	19	83
Poor memory	34	61	15	88
Loss of interest	40	57	12	84
Difficulty concentrating	33	52	6	94
Weight loss of ≥2.25 kg	22	51	17	92
Feeling guilty	25	49	6	97
Restlessness	63	43	28	46
Reverse diurnal variation	39	38	17	109
Irritability	37	35	15	113
Feels someone to blame	63	32	11	111
Diurnal variation	24	25	7	122
Death wishes	33	24	7	124
Feeling hopeless	55	20	6	128
Hallucinations	29	17	6	131
Suicidal thoughts	0	8	3	139
Fear of losing mind	0	5	4	143
Suicide attempts	0	0	0	147
Feeling worthless	56	9	8	139
Feel angry about death	63	19	16	128
Depressive syndrome	27	63	8	86

Reproduced with permission from Clayton, P. J. (1982). Bereavement. In: Paykel, E. S. (ed.) *Handbook of affective disorders*. London: Churchill Livingstone.

Table 4 Frequency of physical symptoms in 1 year in bereaved and controls

Symptom	*Frequency (%)*	
	Probands (n = 149)	*Controls (n = 131)*
Headaches	36	27
Dysmenorrhea	38	20
Other pains	44	18[b]
Urinary frequency	30	23
Constipation	27	24
Dyspnea	27	16[a]
Abdominal pain	26	11[c]
Blurred vision	22	13
Anxiety attacks	15	8
Alcohol use	19	9[a]
Tranquilizers	46	8[d]
Hypnotics	32	2[d]
Physician visits	79	80
Physician visits ≥ 3	45	48
Physician visits ≥ 6	27	29
Hospitalizations	22	14
General poor health	10	7

[a]Significant by chi-square, degrees of freedom (df) = 1, $P \leq 0.05$;
[b]significant by chi-square, df = 1, $P \leq 0.005$;
[c]significant by chi-square, df = 1, $P \leq 0.001$;
[d]significant by chi-square, df = 1, $P \leq 0.0001$; n varies slightly from symptom to symptom. Reproduced with kind permission of Springer Sciences and Business Media. *New results in depression*, 1986, Bereavement and its relation to clinical depression, Clayton, P. J. Berlin-Heidelberg: Spring-Verlag.

related to these changes in behavior. It also highlights how people behave after significant stress.

In a separate study, we examined 249 psychiatric inpatients and similarly matched hospital controls and found that there were no significant differences between the groups for the loss of a first degree relative or spouse in the 6 months or 1 year prior to admission to the hospital. In each case only 2% reported such a loss in the 6 months and 3 or 4% in the 7–12 months prior to the hospitalization. In the psychiatric patients, the major diagnosis was a mood disorder. There were diagnoses of alcoholism in both the bereaved psychiatric patients and bereaved hospitalized controls which related to their increased drinking after the death.

Psychiatric Disorders – Depression, Anxiety, and Mania

In our first study of widowhood, 35% of the subjects had a depressive syndrome at 1 month, 25% at 4 months, and 17% at 1 year. Forty-five per cent were depressed at some point during the year and 11% were depressed for the entire year. Adding the second younger sample, 42% were depressed at 1 month and 16% met the criteria at 1 year. Forty-seven per cent were depressed at some time during the year compared to 8% of controls and again, 11% for the entire year. These findings are remarkably similar to those of a study extensively reported by Zisook and Shuchter (1991: 1346; 1993: 157). They identified a large sample of widows and widowers from death certificates and solicited volunteers to be interviewed. The demographics of the final sample were very similar to the first widowed sample reported here. They reported that 24% of their sample was depressed at 2 months, 23% at 7 months, 16% at 13 months, and 14% at 25 months. In all of these studies the best predictor of depression at 13 months was depression at 1 month. In the Zisook and Shuchter studies, a past history of depression also predicted depression at 1 year. In our own studies, because we did not have enough depressed patients, it was any psychiatric morbidity prior to the death that predicted depression at 1 year. The other common correlate of depression at 1 year was poor physical health prior to the death of the spouse. So, prior poor physical or mental health predicted poor outcome at 13 months. Although there are methodologic issues in defining both anticipation of a death (e.g., expected versus unexpected) and outcomes (depression, death, remarriage, etc) in our data, unexpected deaths produced more severe immediate responses but the differences disappeared by 13 months, again confirmed by others. The best definitions of unexpected death, is a death in a healthy individual which occurred in less than 2 hours. Using that and comparing it to those bereaved after longer terminal illnesses we found that it has been reported that there was more morbidity especially as measured in physician visits, and long lingering grief symptoms.

In more then one study, about 25% of recently bereaved subjects met criteria for some anxiety disorder immediately following bereavement. More then half, however, had generalized anxiety disorder and that correlated with the severity of the depressive disorder. Others have shown, without clarifying the nature of the anxiety disorder, the major disorders that affect recently bereaved people are depressive disorder alone or concurrent depression and anxiety. New episodes of any anxiety disorder were rare after bereavement. It may be wisest to conclude that these are anxiety symptoms embedded in a depression disorder.

An occasional person, with a bipolar disposition, develops mania following a significant death, probably secondary to the sleep deprivation that the stress induces.

Complicated or Traumatic Bereavement

Lindemann (1944: 24) probably wrote the first papers on bereavement that dealt with prospective observations of 13 bereaved subjects who were hospitalized at Massachusetts General Hospital after the Coconut Grove fire. He combined these observations with those of his own patients who lost a relative during treatment, with relatives whom he saw of patients who died at the hospital, and of relatives of members of the Armed Forces. Although he considered his observations to be of normal grief, many of them were probably related to a pathologic response. More recently, investigators have begun to quantify the abnormal response. Prigerson and colleagues (1995: 616) have developed an inventory of complicated grief and shown it to be related to the severity of depressive symptoms, but with distinct symptoms. Building on earlier inventories such as the Texas Grief Inventory and the Grief Measurement Scale, they took symptoms such as preoccupation with death, crying, searching and yearning for the deceased, disbelief about the death, being stunned, and not accepting the death and added questions about preoccupation with thoughts of the deceased, anger, distrust, detachment, avoidance, replication of symptoms that the deceased experienced, auditory and visual hallucinations, and guilt, loneliness, bitterness, and envy of others who had not lost someone close. Their instrument was shown to be reliable and have criterion validity. Whether it is just defining the most severe depression is not yet clear. Modifying the Grief Measurement Scale in accordance with the above symptoms, Prigerson et al. (1997: 616) looked at a previously ascertained sample that were followed from before the death to until 25 months after the death. They found that if they identified bereaved at 6 months who scored high on their inventory, at 13 months there was a correlation between high scores and change in smoking and eating, depression, and high systolic blood pressure. At 25 months, these people had an increased risk to develop heart trouble and cancer and more often expressed suicidal ideation as ascertained on a single item. If they tried to separate the sample on complicated grief at 2 months, they could not predict unfavorable outcomes. There are others working on similar instruments, especially in Australia. They measured bereavement phenomena and developed a scale for core bereavement items. This scale also measures images and thoughts around the death, yearning and pining about the death, and some grief symptoms such as sadness, loneliness, longing, tearfulness, and loss of enjoyment. Their inventory was developed using parents of deceased children, bereaved spouses, and bereaved adult children who scored high in descending order on the inventory. However they have not yet correlated the questionnaire with outcome.

Some of the symptoms in all of these inventories are similar to symptoms that occur in PTSD, and it is difficult to justify a new category where the major difference is that in the bereaved, the mood is sadness and loneliness focused on the loss compared to fear or horror in PTSD. It is still an unanswered question. Should we have a diagnosis of complicated bereavement or acknowledge that after certain deaths, most especially those that are sudden and violent, some individuals will develop PTSD which is usually comorbid with major depression? Clearly these investigators are defining an important bereavement response that identifies survivors with a poorer outcome. For other researchers who are studying human reactions to stress, symptoms such as those in the inventory of complicated grief should be identified and studied prospectively. The identification of such a syndrome also makes it possible to study, more specifically, various interventions.

Mortality

More recently the method of study (collecting health data on a large core of men and women and following them prospectively to ascertain point of widowhood and using the Cox hazards regression mode to estimate the effect of bereavement on mortality while controlling for the effects of other covariates), should have greatly improved the validity of the mortality data. Unfortunately, there still are controversies. Three studies have used these methods. De Leon et al. (1993: 519) reported that elderly, young–old (aged 65–74 years), and old–old men (aged > 74 years) showed an increased mortality in the first 6 months of widowhood. But, because there was an age difference between the future widowed and nonwidowed, when they were age adjusted, the death rate fell to a nonsignificant level. Among young–old women there was also an increased risk of death in the first 6 months which only decreased slightly after the age adjustment, but enough to make it of borderline significance. The authors suggested that the "true risk period" may be even shorter than 6 months. Schaefer et al. (1995: 1142) also reported that mortality following bereavement was significantly elevated in both men and women after adjusting for age, education, and other predictors of mortality. Here, the highest mortality occurred 7–12 months following the bereavement. Ebrahim et al. (1995: 834) studied 7735 middle-aged men (40–59 years) over 5 years. They included never married, divorced, separated, widowed, and married men and found that there was no increase in mortality in men who became widowed during the follow-up time. There were only 24 men who became widowed in that follow-up period which probably limited the findings. Lusyne et al. (2001: 281) confirmed an excess mortality in the first 6 months of widowhood which was higher for men than women. As others had found, it was highest in the youngest bereaved (<60 years) and dropped with each older group and almost disappeared for the oldest old. There is also a twin study of mortality after spousal bereavement. Without relating whether the twins were mono- or dizygotic, the authors found an increased mortality for young–old (under 70 years) men and women during the first year of bereavement. The death hazard diminished the longer the bereaved were followed. The data were analyzed for smoking status, excessive alcohol consumption, education, body mass, cardiovascular disease, respiratory disease, and other chronic illness and found that these did not affect the relative hazard estimates. Other studies show that remarriage, which is much more likely to occur in men, protects men from death either because the healthier remarry or the remarriage in itself is protective. The death rates of those who remarry are similar to married men of the same age. Taken as a whole, these studies support the fact that there is probably an increased mortality after bereavement in men and women under 70 years of age in the first year.

From these studies there does not seem to be an increased mortality from any one particular cause, such as cancer or cardiovascular disease. Other studies, however, have shown an increase in suicide after a bereavement, although when looking at smaller samples most of those who committed suicide were psychiatrically ill prior to their spouses' deaths. A case control study of 100 elderly suicides compared to well-matched deaths from other causes, found that the major independent risk factors in those who committed suicide were family discord and mental disorders (mainly depression and substance abuse). Recent bereavement did not distinguish the two groups.

Pathologic Outcomes and Predictors of Outcome

Before reviewing the predictors of pathologic outcomes it should be noted that all studies of widowhood, including those on mortality, emphasize that psychological stability predicts a good outcome, although unfortunately no-one has measured personality traits or variables prior to entry into widowhood. Good health predicts a better outcome. And not having sleep difficulty or having low scores on depression ratings in the first month of bereavement also predicts a better outcome.

There are many ways to assess outcome. Loneliness certainly is the most characteristic outcome following bereavement and this persists in many for years. Under psychological morbidity, chronic depression as measured 1 year after the death and complicated bereavement both lead to a significant morbidity. There is also physical morbidity. The mortality noted postbereavement still needs further study.

There are very few definitive predictors of chronic depression. A past history of psychiatric illness particularly depression predicts it, poor prior physical health may predict it, and depression at 1 month after the bereavement definitely predicts it. Perhaps a bereavement that follows an instantaneous and totally unexpected death predicts it, although it might not be that it is the unexpected aspect of it, but rather whether it is violent in nature. Studies will clarify the predictions as data collection improves. All the other variables, gender, young age, perceived lack of social supports and socioeconomic income do not predict it. Gender is important to note, because major depression is overwhelmingly more common in women then in men but chronic depression after bereavement is not. Stress-related depression affects both genders equally.

Treatment

The vast majority of people who experience a loss will recover gradually without any interventions. It is just that fact that probably contributes to the conclusion in a recent salient review of all qualifying grief counseling studies, which the effect of such counseling is quite weak and in some cases could even be harmful.

In those who become chronically depressed or have complicated grief, an intervention at 6 months after the bereavement is indicated. In a recent report, 95 volunteers with complicated grief of long duration (>2 years) were randomized to treatment with either interpersonal therapy (IPT) or complicated grief therapy (IPT modified to include cognitive therapy based on techniques for addressing trauma). The results showed, when looking at treatment completers, the complicated grief therapy was superior to IPT especially in those with losses through violent deaths. Still, the response rate was only 51%. Patients also had high rates of comorbid depression and PTSD and 45% were taking antidepressants. It may be the kind of therapy for a specific group of bereaved that Jordan and Neimeyer (2003: 765) were urging researchers to study. Most importantly, the elements of these therapies may be applicable to other stress-related disorders.

Antidepressants have also been used and been shown to be efficacious. For example, an older study of treatment of bereavement-related major depressive episodes in later life with nortriptyline, IPT, the combination, or neither showed that nortriptyline alone or with IPT significantly improved the depressive disorder. IPT alone was not significantly different to the placebo. The outcomes are notable because very few people relapsed when the treatments were stopped and the response rate was relatively high in both nortriptyline treatment groups and the placebo group. Thus it seems to be a good condition to treat with antidepressant medication. It is also important to remember that should the patient be psychotic or suicidal, electroconvulsive therapy (ECT) is probably indicated.

Further Reading

Clayton, P. J. (1982). Bereavement. In: Paykel, E. S. (ed.) *Handbook of affective disorders.* London: Churchill Livingstone.

Clayton, P. J. (1986). Bereavement and its relation to clinical depression. In: Hippius, H., Klerman, G. L. & Matussek, N. (eds.) *New results in depression.* Berlin-Heidelberg: Spring-Verlag.

Clayton, P. (2004). Bereavement and depression. In: Roose, S. & Sackeim, H. (eds.) *Late life depression.* Oxford: Oxford University Press.

Clayton, P., Demarais, L. and Winokur, G. (1968). A study of normal bereavement. *American Journal of Psychiatry* **125**, 168–178.

Clayton, P. J. and Darvish, H. S. (1979). Course of depressive symptoms following the stress of bereavement. In: Barrett, J. E. (ed.) *Stress and mental disorder,* pp. 121–136. New York: Raven Press.

Clayton, P. J., Halikas, J. A. and Maurice, W. L. (1971). The bereavement of the widowed. *Disease of the Nervous System* **32**, 597–604.

Clayton, P. J., Herjanic, M., Murphy, G. E., et al. (1974). Mourning and depression, their similarities and differences. *Canadian Psychiatric Association Journal* **19**, 309–312.

Clayton, P. J., Parilla, R. H. Jr., and Bieri, M. D. (1980). Methodological problems in assessing the relationship between acuteness of death and the bereavement outcome. In: Reiffel, J. (ed.) *The psychosocial aspects of cardiovascular disease: the patient, the family and the staff,* pp. 267–275. New York: Columbia University Press.

De Leon, C. F. M., Kasl, S. F. and Jacobs, S. (1993). Widowhood and mortality risk in a community sample of the elderly: a prospective study. *Journal of Clinical Epidemiology* **46**, 519–527.

Ebrahim, S., Wannamethee, G., McCallum, A., et al. (1995). Marital status, change in marital status, and mortality in middle-aged British men. *American Journal of Epidemiology* **142**, 834–842.

Frost, N. R. and Clayton, P. J. (1977). Bereavement and psychiatric hospitalization. *Archives of General Psychiatry* **34**, 1172–1175.

Jordan, J. R. and Neimeyer, R. A. (2003). Does grief counseling work? *Death Studies* **27**, 765–786.

Lindermann, E. (1944). Symptomalogy and management of acute grief. *American Journal of Psychiatry* **101**, 141–148.

Lund, D. A., Caserta, M. S. and Dimond, M. F. (1993). The course of spousal bereavement in later life. In: Stroebe, M. S., Stroebe, W. & Hansson, R. O. (eds.) *Handbook of bereavement,* pp. 24–254. Cambridge: Cambridge University Press.

Lusyne, P., Page, H. and Lievens, J. (2001). Mortality following conjugal bereavement, Belgium 1991–96: the unexpected effect of education. *Population Studies* **55**, 281–289.

Prigerson, H. G., Bierhals, A. J., Kasl, S. V., et al. (1997). Traumatic grief as a risk factor for mental and physical morbidity. *American Journal of Psychiatry* **154**, 616–623.

Prigerson, H. G., Maciejewski, P. K., Reynolds, III, C. F., et al. (1995). Inventory of Complicated Grief. A scale to measure maladaptive symptoms of loss. *Psychiatry Research* **59**, 65–79.

Rubenowitz, E., Waern, M., Wilhelmson, K., et al. (2001). Life events and psychosocial factors in elderly suicides – a case-control study. *Psychological Medicine* **31**, 1193–1202.

Schaefer, C., Quesenberry, J. C. P. Jr. and Wi, S. (1995). Mortality following conjugal bereavement and the effects of a shared environment. *American Journal of Epidemiology* **141**, 1142–1152.

Shear, K., Frank, E., Houck, P. R., et al. (2005). Treatment of complicated grief. *JAMA* **293**, 2601–2608.

Zisook, S. and Shuchter, S. R. (1991). Depression through the first year after the death of a spouse. *American Journal of Psychiatry* **148**, 1346–1352.

Zisook, S. and Shuchter, S. R. (1993). Uncomplicated bereavement. *Journal of Clinical Psychiatry* **54**, 365–372.

Zisook, S., Chentsova-Dutton, Y. and Schuchter, S. R. (1998). PTSD following bereavement. *Annals of Clinical Psychiatry* **10**, 157–163.

F. Schizophrenia/Psychoses

Psychotic Disorders

J Ventura
University of California, Los Angeles, CA, USA

This is a revised version of the article by J Ventura and R P Liberman, Encyclopedia of Stress First Edition, volume 3, pp 316–326, © 2000, Elsevier Inc.

Glossary

Brief psychiatric rating scale (BPRS) One of the most widely used rating scales, nationally and internationally, for measuring psychiatric symptoms at baseline and for assessment of change over time. The BPRS allows for the rapid assessment of symptoms such as depression, anxiety, delusions, and hallucinations.

Cognitive appraisal An individual's evaluative thought process that instills a life event or situation with a particular meaning.

Coping response Cognitive and behavioral efforts used to master, tolerate, and reduce the demands of stressful events that tax or exceed an individual's resources.

Expressed emotion (EE) Attitudes and feelings expressed by a relative during family interactions; an individual with a psychotic disorder would describe this as critical comments, overt or subtle hostility, or emotional overinvolvement in the individual's affairs.

Independent life event A life event or situation that is not related to an individual's psychotic symptoms and is beyond his or her personal influence, for example, the death of a relative, the loss of a job because the entire company went out of business, or becoming the victim of an unprovoked attack.

Mediator A variable that explains how, why, or when to expect a relationship between a predictor (e.g., life event) and the criterion (e.g., psychosis).

Prospective studies Research in which the data are collected on an ongoing regular basis about all study participants, whether they are considered at risk for an illness or not and before the event being studied occurs (e.g., psychotic relapse).

Protective factor Individual characteristics, which may be biological, intrapersonal, interpersonal, or learned, that reduce or eliminate the risk of developing a psychosis.

Stress An adverse biological, physiological, or psychological state that develops when the demands on an individual exceed his or her capacity for adaptation.

Vulnerability to psychosis The enduring characteristics of individuals, which might be genetic, social, behavioral, biochemical, cognitive, or related to brain structure, that increase their susceptibility to developing psychosis.

Stress is a concept on whose definition few scholars or researchers can agree. Yet there is little dispute that stressful events can influence the onset and course of major psychotic disorders. A 1977 vulnerability–stress model by Zubin and Spring proposes that a relationship exists among the level of inherited vulnerability, stress that exceeds a certain threshold, and the onset or relapse of psychotic illness. According to this vulnerability model, individuals with high biological vulnerability are susceptible to the exacerbation of psychotic symptoms even when they experience low levels of stress; however, if the biological vulnerability is low, then high levels of stress are required before symptoms emerge. Differences in the rates of psychotic disorders found in males versus females, urban versus rural areas, and high-stress versus low-stress households support the importance of environmental factors in understanding gene–environment interactions.

Several empirical tests of the vulnerability–stress model have shown that an increase in the frequency of life events occurs in the month before a psychotic exacerbation. However, not all studies have found a reliable association between stressful life events and psychosis. Some researchers believe that the relationship in schizophrenia is weak when compared to more striking findings in patients with mood disorders. Although there is a convergence of evidence that stressful life events are triggers of psychosis, stressful events alone are neither necessary nor sufficient to account for illness onset, nor are they necessary as precursors of relapse. Antipsychotic medication may provide protection against stress and raise the threshold of vulnerability. An interactive vulnerability–stress–protective factors model (**Figure 1**) hypothesizes the existence of mediators of stress, some of which are considered protective such as cognitive appraisal of life events, social competence, social and familial support, and premorbid intelligence.

Stress in Psychotic Disorders: Conceptual Framework

All biomedical disorders, including those that manifest themselves by psychotic symptoms, are

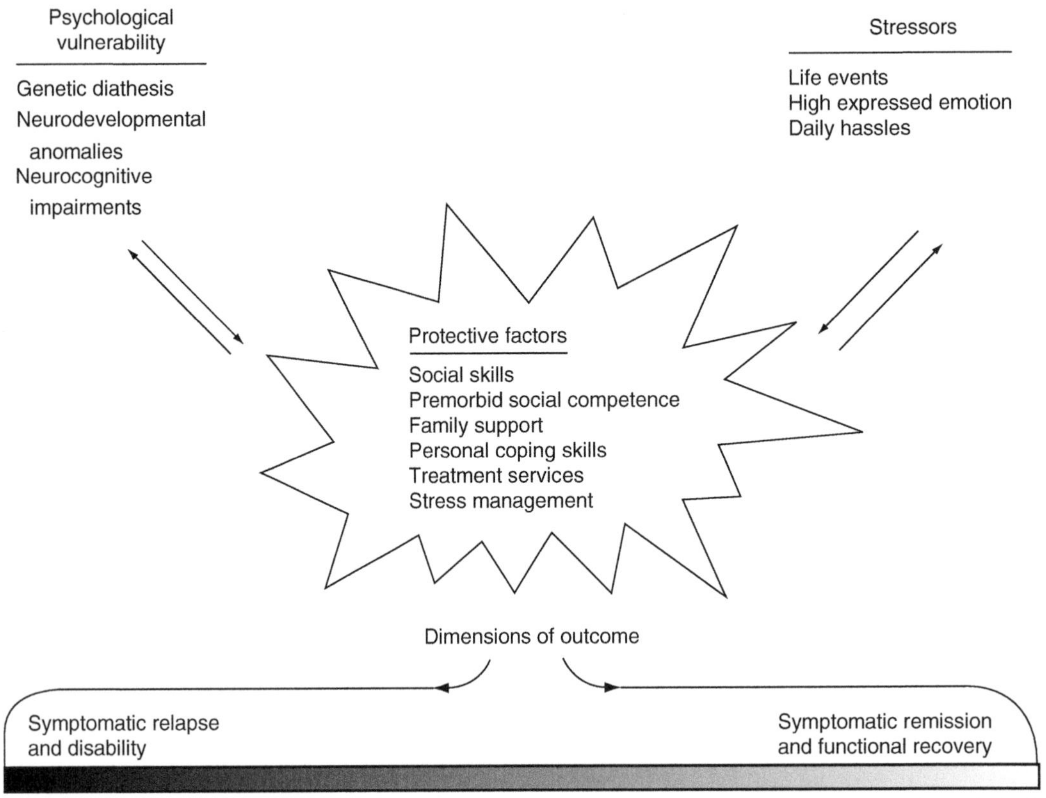

Figure 1 An interactive vulnerability–stress–protective factors model of risk factors for the onset and course of psychotic disorders.

stress-related biological illnesses. It doesn't matter whether it is the heart or the brain that is involved as the organ from which the illness arises, stressors impinge on the organ's genetic vulnerability to trigger episodes of symptoms, exacerbations, relapses, and disability. Moreover, protective factors in the individual or in the individual's environment can mitigate or buffer the noxious effects of stressors on vulnerable people. When protective factors – such as social competence, social and family support, intelligence, availability, and accessibility to preventive interventions and good quality treatment – outweigh stressors and vulnerability, health may be sustained and disability forestalled.

In this article, we identify some of the stressors that have been implicated in the induction of episodes of illness, relapse, and poor outcome in psychotic disorders. However, it is important to place the role of stressors within the framework of the vulnerability–stress–protective factors model so as to understand why an individual may experience an episode of illness when exposed to a stressor at one time but not when exposed to the same stressor at another time. In addition, the vulnerability–stress protective–factors framework permits clinical scientists to explain the enormous interindividual variability in susceptibility to stressors – in short, why some people, some of the time, do not experience stress and exacerbations of psychosis in response to certain stressors, but others do.

Stressful Life Events and Psychosis

The life charts of Adolf Meyer, published in 1951, were among the first records of clinical observations that emphasized the importance of psychosocial stressors and the development of pathological conditions. Over the past 3 decades, many researchers have attempted to empirically document the nature of the relationship between stressful life events and psychotic illness. Such studies are based on the notion that higher frequencies of events translate into higher levels of stress for patients. These studies can be grouped into those that compared schizophrenia patients and other psychiatric groups, those that compared schizophrenia patients with community controls, and those that examined the impact of stressful events on the onset and relapse of psychotic symptoms.

Most research has shown that, compared to schizophrenia patients, other psychiatric groups (usually depressed patients) reported either similar or significantly higher rates of stressful events prior to an episode. These differences were unexpected because there was an assumption that the rate of stressful life events in schizophrenia patients was higher than for patients with other psychiatric disorders. Schizophrenia patients are considered sensitive to even subtle changes in the environment. However, given that schizophrenia patients sometimes withdraw when stressed, their rate of life events may actually be lower than the rate for patients with other psychiatric disorders. Available evidence supports the conclusion that schizophrenia patients report fewer life events than other diagnostic groups. Furthermore, most studies have found that the strength of the relationship between stress and symptoms is more robust in patients with major depression than in patients with schizophrenia.

Most studies that used community controls as a comparison found that schizophrenia patients experienced a higher frequency of stressful events. However, some studies showed no difference. Interestingly, one prospective study found that normal controls actually had higher levels of stressful events than did schizophrenia patients. Several studies have shown an increased frequency of triggering life events in the month prior to the onset or relapse of schizophrenic symptoms. Even studies that did not find a sharp increase in the number of life events in the month prior to onset or relapse found that stressful life events had increased the risk of psychosis. There has been some investigation into whether life events play a more prominent role in the onset of psychosis than in relapse. Although there is no consistent evidence favoring a relationship between stress and onset (compared with stress and relapse), there is some indication that life events play a larger role in psychotic episodes that have a discrete (vs. insidious) onset.

Perhaps more relevant than the absolute frequency of events in patients or controls is the nature of the relationship between life events and psychotic illness. However, most of the studies of stress and psychosis focused on the frequency of events rather than the amount of threat posed. In fact, methods of measuring life event frequency (through open-ended interviews or life event inventories) are readily available. But, in some cases, events that were hoped for or expected (e.g., finding a suitable mate) but did not occur may also be perceived as stressful. Most researchers believe that the impact of a stressor is determined by an individual's cognitive appraisal and that the appraisal is altered in schizophrenia patients in a way that increases vulnerability to stress and psychosis; yet this important topic has received limited study. Perhaps the popular belief that most schizophrenia patients cannot accurately report their appraisal of life events dampens researchers' enthusiasm for comprehensive study.

Retrospective Studies of Life Events and Psychosis

In a classic and frequently cited 1968 British study, Brown and Birley interviewed schizophrenia patients and their families soon after a hospitalization regarding the 12-week period prior to the onset or relapse of psychosis. Schizophrenic patients reported an increased frequency of independent life events (independent of the insidious onset or occurrence of psychotic symptoms) in the 3-week period prior to the datable onset of their episode. Specifically, 46% of patients reported an independent life event in that 3-week period, compared with 14% for a sample of community controls during a comparable period. Except for the 3-week period prior to an episode, the life event rates between the two groups did not differ significantly. From these results, Brown and Birley concluded that life events play a role in triggering the onset or relapse of psychotic symptoms in schizophrenia.

The most ambitious attempt at a replication of the Brown and Birley findings was a 1987 multinational World Health Organization (WHO) study published by Richard Day and colleagues. The design of this WHO study was virtually identical to Brown and Birley's original work, including the use of retrospective reporting, although normal controls were not included. The life events data were collected in nine centers, five located in developed countries and four in developing countries. Day and colleagues replicated the finding that independent life events occur with increased frequency in the 3 weeks prior to psychotic episodes in schizophrenic patients. Although the lack of a comparison group is a serious concern, the consistency of these findings from different countries lends considerable support to the hypothesis that stressful life events may trigger episodes of schizophrenia.

Questions Concerning Retrospective Studies

Most of the classic research supporting the idea that stress triggers psychosis has been subject to criticism because the data was collected using retrospective methods, in which data regarding life events were collected after onset or relapse of psychosis. Because retrospective data gathering relies on the patient's memory of life events and the date of onset of psychotic symptoms, it is subject to considerable report distortion, particularly for events of smaller magnitude. Such distortion is likely to bias results when patients (or their families) are searching for an explanation for a known outcome, such as a psychotic episode. In addition, there is the issue of bias in the dating of the onset or relapse of psychosis in these studies. Such a bias favors finding a relationship between stress and psychosis even if there was none.

The prospective studies of the mid-1980s and 1990s, which used a follow-through design in the regular collection of life events data, were aimed at correcting the methodological flaws of the prior retrospective studies. In some studies, life events data were collected as often as biweekly, thereby minimizing errors associated with memory for stressors that preceded relapse. In addition, each patient's symptoms were assessed frequently, minimizing the distortion of an association between the presence of symptoms and certain events.

Prospective Studies of Life Events and Relapse

The first well-designed prospective study of schizophrenia outpatients addressed the question of whether a significant increase in symptoms occurs after independent life events rather than evaluating the frequency of life events in the month preceding symptom relapse. This study, which collected life events data on an ongoing regular basis, focused on the average effects of life events on illness. An increase in negative symptoms was found in response to stressful events but not an increase in positive psychotic symptoms. Based on this stringent test of the relationship between stress and psychosis, Jean Hardesty and colleagues concluded that independent life events have minimal bearing on florid psychotic symptoms in schizophrenia.

A 1989 prospective study by Ventura and colleagues introduced additional methodological improvements in data collection, including (1) careful monitoring of the amount of antipsychotic medication received, (2) the use of both an open-ended style of interviewing and a structured life events inventory, and (3) the classification of life events as independent only when they were both independent of the patient's illness and not within the patient's ability to influence them. Ventura et al. found, as had Brown and Birley, and Day and colleagues, an increase in the number of independent life events in the 4-week period before a relapse or significant exacerbation of positive symptoms; 5 of 11 (45%) patients had at least one independent life event in the month before relapsing, compared with 1 of 11 (9%) during a comparable period without relapse. Thus, a well-designed prospective study supported the conclusion that stressful life events play a role in triggering psychotic symptoms.

Stress Sensitivity

Researchers and clinicians alike have theorized that schizophrenia patients are sensitive to even very small negative changes in the environment. A series of studies using the Experience Sampling Method (ESM) has provided some evidence for the validity of this hypothesis. The ESM requires that patients wear a beeping watch that alerts them 10 times a day to record real-life activity and their emotional response over a 6-day period. Using the ESM, researchers in the Netherlands found that schizophrenia patients, compared to high-risk relatives and controls, are more likely to experience negative affect in response to minor life events. This negative affectivity is considered a vulnerability marker for future psychosis. In addition, using the ESM the researchers recorded life events in sets of twins, in which one twin scored high on a measure of psychosis proneness and the other scored low. The advantage of this method of research is that the well twin acts as a genetic control for the psychosis-prone twin. Twins who were prone to experiencing psychotic-like experiences were more likely to show sensitivity to minor stressful life events. These findings further support the hypothesis that stress sensitivity acts as a risk factor for psychosis.

General Conclusions on Life Events and Psychosis

Interestingly, similar conclusions about the relationship between stress and psychosis can be drawn from sophisticated prospective studies and the retrospective studies. There is strong evidence from both retrospective and prospective studies to support the triggering hypothesis, even though some studies were able to confirm only an increased risk of psychosis from stressful events. Although life events influence psychotic episodes, the occurrence of stressful life events is usually not sufficient to precipitate an increase in psychotic symptoms. Furthermore, life events are not always necessary for relapse to occur. Some studies found that more than one-half of relapsing patients did not experience a prior life event. Other factors, such as medication reduction/discontinuance or biological factors, may also contribute to the risk of relapse. These conclusions attest to the potential importance of mediators such as, cognitive appraisal and coping efforts, which produce differences in individual response to stress within groups of psychotic patients. The finding of increased negative symptoms in response to stressful events, instead of psychosis, indicates that not all patients respond to stress in the same way. Prospective research has also shown that life events do not have to be large in magnitude; both major and minor life events are predictors of symptom exacerbation and relapse in schizophrenia. Furthermore, stress sensitivity to daily hassles and minor life events has been associated with increased subjective distress and potential risk for future psychosis in schizophrenia.

Cognitive Appraisal of Stressful Events

Understanding the link between stressors and subsequent psychotic symptoms in schizophrenia may entail looking more closely at potential mediators such as patients' cognitive appraisal of life events. According to stress researchers, an individual's appraisal of an event always should be measured because appraisal determines the stressful nature of the event. In one stress–illness model, the perception of the stressor is schematically represented as a polarizing filter that can magnify or diminish the stressfulness of an event. Richard Lazarus and Susan Folkman hypothesized that appraisal is the first element of a two-phase cognitive-phenomenological process of coping and thereby is a factor in determining how much stress an individual experiences. After decades of research, Lazarus continued to assert that an individual's appraisal is necessary and sufficient in the generation of emotions in response to stressful events. Appraisal thus is relevant to understanding the relationship between stressful life events and subsequent illness.

Research suggests that schizophrenic patients, in particular, might respond in idiosyncratic ways to life events. Appraisal may play a larger mediating role in the relationship between life events and psychotic symptoms in schizophrenia patients than it does in other populations. Both psychoanalytic and cognitive information-processing theories suggest that schizophrenia patients rely on narrow and idiosyncratic meanings of events. Heightened sensitivity to environmental stimuli, coupled with cognitive distortions and psychotic thinking (e.g., persecutory ideas or referential thoughts to either perceived or existing threats) could result in increased stress. Research has shown that schizophrenia patients may overestimate the threatening nature of everyday events or situations and underestimate the effectiveness of their problem-solving ability. This tendency for altered appraisal may increase in patients as their condition worsens.

Can Stress Cause Psychotic Illness?

Although some investigators have argued that stressful life events can cause psychotic episodes in schizophrenia patients, others have argued that life events can only act as triggers of episodes. Central to this issue is whether psychosis can occur in individuals without inherited vulnerability and from stressful events that are definitely independent of the illness. Exposure to wartime combat, natural disasters, and other severe traumatic events that are clearly independent of the individual's influence have been shown to increase the risk of developing psychosis. According to one theory, psychosis can occur even in individuals without inherited vulnerability characteristics, especially if the stressor is severe. However, many individuals have been exposed to all types of stressful situations and catastrophic events and only a handful become psychotic. Some theorists believe that individuals who became psychotic must have some type of underlying vulnerability to illness and that therefore the stress merely acted as a trigger. The possibility also exists that the role of life events may be indirect and occur in conjunction with other risk factors.

Stressful Life Events and Depression in Psychosis

The presence of clinical depression in schizophrenia patients has generated a great deal of interest because of its significance as an early indicator of an impending psychotic relapse, association with an increased risk for suicide attempts, and relationship to psychiatric rehospitalization. Several theories have been put forward to explain the occurrence of depression in schizophrenia. Depression has been considered part of the postpsychotic phase when it occurs after a psychosis remits and as a reaction to the realization that the individual is in trouble or that his or her life has fallen far short of prior expectations. Other researchers view depressive symptoms as part of the acute psychotic process because it has been found to occur simultaneously with the exacerbations of positive symptoms. Depression may be a part of the patient's biological diathesis to schizophrenia and therefore an integral part of the disorder or an aspect of familial genetic liability to disturbances in mood. Some researchers view depression as an unwanted side effect of antipsychotic medication. However, observations by Eugen Bleuler and Emil Kraepelin of depression in schizophrenia during the preneuroleptic era suggest that depression is not simply secondary to antipsychotic medications. In any event, according to the vulnerability–stress–protective factors model, psychosocial stressors such as life events may be expected to increase the chances of an onset or exacerbation of depressive symptoms in psychotic patients.

Schizophrenia patients have reported a higher frequency of stressful life events during the 6 months before a depressive exacerbation and during the 12-month period prior to a postpsychotic depression. Early parental loss (before age 17) was also found to be more common in depressed than nondepressed chronic paranoid schizophrenia patients. In chronic schizophrenia patients, increased levels of depression have been found to be associated with psychosocial stressors, such as unemployment. Although much of this previous research had some methodological weaknesses, recent work with sound methods confirmed the earlier findings. A well-designed 2000 prospective study using survival analysis showed that stressful life events act as triggers of depressive exacerbation in recent-onset schizophrenia patients. These studies suggest that individuals with schizophrenia who experience undesirable life events may have a vulnerability to depression similar to mood disorder patients and individuals without psychiatric disorders. Thus, stressful events may play an even broader role in psychosis than is typically theorized by the vulnerability–stress–protective factors model.

Natural Disasters and Psychotic Disorders

There are various types of stressful life events that can have a negative impact on schizophrenia patients, ranging from minor daily hassles to major life events. These include catastrophic events such as natural disasters. One reliable predictor of psychiatric morbidity is the degree of exposure to the devastating physical consequences that follow natural disasters. Research on natural disasters showed consistently that the existence of a prior psychiatric disorder (or symptoms) is a risk factor for postdisaster psychopathology. Preexisting disorders such as major depression, posttraumatic stress disorder (PTSD), anxiety disorders, and alcohol dependence have been associated with postdisaster morbidity. One study found 98% of individuals with a prior psychiatric disorder had a diagnosable postdisaster psychiatric disorder, compared with 25% of postdisaster diagnosis in the group without a previous diagnosis. Most studies have been retrospective and therefore subject to recall bias, but these results have been supported in prospective research.

Contrary to what is predicted by the vulnerability–stress–protective factors model, most anecdotal accounts and a few studies indicated that psychiatric patients remain clinically stable or even improve during or after natural or human-made disasters (e.g., hurricanes, ice storms, nuclear power plant accidents, and missile attacks). During Hurricane Iniki, psychiatric inpatients in Hawaii responded with increased independence, defined as decreased requests for therapy. Similarly, during SCUD missile attacks on Israel throughout the Persian Gulf War, many psychiatric inpatients were described as having coped well, quietly entering sealed concrete bunkers and easily donning gas masks. During a state hospital fire, the patients assisted the hospital staff in the efforts to control the blaze.

In contrast to these prior reports, patients with psychotic disorders in some studies of disasters demonstrated evidence of heightened stress reactivity. On January 17, 1994, a 6.8-magnitude earthquake struck Northridge, California, and provided our research group with an unprecedented opportunity to study the impact of a natural disaster on psychotic patients. Our sample consisted of patients who were previously diagnosed as having a psychotic disorder and were active participants in research projects. As hypothesized, the degree of exposure to the earthquake was a statistically significant predictor of the amount of distress experienced. Schizophrenia patients reported higher levels of avoidance symptoms than did controls when assessed postearthquake. However, the groups did not significantly differ in their mean levels of intrusion symptoms. The specific elevation of avoidance symptoms is noteworthy because the early appearance of avoidance and emotional numbing has been found to be the strongest predictors of disaster-induced psychiatric morbidity, including PTSD. BPRS assessments were compared for patients for whom 1-week preearthquake and 1-week postearthquake ratings were available. We found a significant increase in postearthquake dysphoria but not in psychotic symptoms. In response to the September 11, 2001, terrorist attacks, there was no difference between inpatients in New York who did and inpatients who did not have the opportunity to directly view the disaster through downtown-facing windows. However, patients with a schizophrenia spectrum diagnosis showed evidence of worsening symptoms compared to those with affective disorder or other diagnoses. Although there is some evidence of confirmation of the stress reactivity hypothesis in response to disasters, the stress reactions of psychotic patients are not always consistent and might depend on the amount of exposure, type of disaster, and the setting.

Expressed Emotion as a Stressor

High expressed emotion (EE), the attitudes and feelings expressed by a family member to a patient with a psychotic disorder, is the most potent stressor precipitating relapses. EE is a misnomer because it does not refer to emotional expressiveness but, rather, to very specific and operationalized types of attitudes and feelings that are associated with stressful interactions within a family living with a severely mentally ill person. These attitudes and feelings take the form of critical comments, hostility, and emotional overinvolvement. Critical comments are complaints about specific behaviors or symptoms of the mentally ill family member, whereas hostility is generally directed at broader and more global personality characteristics. Emotional overinvolvement is overprotectiveness, intrusiveness, self-sacrificing behavior, and hovering over the patient by the family member. Conversely, low EE, which is associated with lower than average relapse rates, may subserve a protective function by insulating the individual from stressors with positive comments, positive reinforcement, and warmth.

Family members' levels of EE are reliably associated with patients' risks of relapse in the subsequent 9–12 months after a psychotic episode. Patients living with or having frequent contact with one or more high EE relatives have relapse rates 2–3 times greater than patients living with or having contact only with low EE relatives. This increased risk is present despite adequate treatment with antipsychotic medication. In a recent meta-analysis of 27 studies, the average rate of psychotic relapse in patients living with one or more high EE relatives was 52%, compared to 22% in patients coming from low EE families. The probability that this result was due to chance is virtually zero. This association of EE and relapse has been found for relapses in bipolar disorder, schizophrenia, and major depression.

Although there is no evidence whatsoever that EE or families have an etiological role in the first episode or development of psychosis, there is solid evidence that there is a causal link between EE and relapse. More than 15 treatment studies in several countries have shown that behavioral, social learning, and psychoeducational interventions that are well-organized, structured, and focused on teaching family members practical methods for understanding and coping with psychosis lead to reductions in EE and in relapses. Thus, the treatment research provides experimental evidence for the role of EE in stress-related relapse.

The association between EE and relapse in psychosis has been consistently found in developing countries (e.g., India) and developed countries (e.g., United States, United Kingdom, and Italy); however, cultural factors do play a role in the proportion of families from various cultures who are high versus low EE. For example, the proportion of high EE families is significantly lower in rural India than in urban India and is lower among unacculturated Mexican American families than among Anglo-American families. It is likely that cultural factors play a role in the way that families react to and cope with major mental illness in a relative, and this moves the understanding of EE into an interactional framework.

During direct observation of high EE family members interacting to solve a problem, the emergence of subclinical psychopathology in the patient triggered responses by the patient's relatives that might be viewed as incipient signs of high EE. Negative interactional cycles escalated, with efforts by the family to squelch the patient's deviant behavior, leading to more intense symptomatic behavior and greater negativity in the cycles. There is evidence also that enduring personality, attributional, and information processing factors in high EE relatives may contribute to the association between EE and relapses in psychotic disorders. For example, families who perceive the causes of the patients' problems or symptoms as being controllable by the patients (i.e., families with high internal locus of control) are more likely to be high EE. On the other hand, families that are rated as having higher tolerance, flexibility, empathy, and communication are more likely to be low EE.

The role of EE as a stressor in schizophrenia and other psychotic conditions is elucidated by the stress–vulnerability–protective factors model. Certain characteristics of relatives (e.g., attributional style) may predispose them to experience stress when they are faced with abnormal, unpredictable, and even dangerous behavior in their ill family member. They attempt to cope with this stress by using any means at hand – even criticism, hostility, or emotional overinvolvement – and this has counterproductive effects on the ill relative, causing that person stress and leading eventually to relapse after many cycles of stress superimposed on vulnerability in both the patient and relatives. The interactional nature of EE that develops in this synchronous fashion does indeed link stress, vulnerability, and protective factors in both the family members and patient.

Treatment as Protection against Stress and Psychosis

The Role of Antipsychotic Medication in Reducing Psychosis

In most, if not all studies, antipsychotic medications have repeatedly been shown to be effective for the treatment of psychosis and the prevention of relapse in schizophrenia. Brown and Birley reported that a larger percentage of patients who relapsed while taking an antipsychotic medication had experienced a life event compared to patients who relapsed while not on medication. Additional work by Brown and Birley in 1968 also suggested that "life events and reducing or stopping phenothiazines [antipsychotic medication] contribute as precipitants of acute schizophrenia." Similar results were published showing that a significantly greater proportion of the patients who relapsed on medication had experienced an independent life event, compared to nonrelapsing patients not on active medication. Leff proposed that regular antipsychotic maintenance medication produces a prophylactic effect against stress by raising a patient's threshold to relapse; this increased threshold makes the patient less likely to relapse unless exposed to major life stressors.

In a 1992 prospective study, Ventura et al. found that patients who had a psychotic exacerbation while on medication had more independent events in the prior month than did patients who had an exacerbation while off medication. As previously proposed by Leff, Ventura et al. concluded that taking an antipsychotic medication is protective and raises the threshold for relapse. However, another well-designed study did not completely support the hypothesis that life events are more relevant to relapse in patients on maintenance medication.

Behavioral Family Management for Reducing Stress Inherent in High Expressed Emotion

As shown in **Figure 2**, the daily hassles and challenging or stressful events of everyday life in a family with a relative who has a disabling psychosis can be dealt with in either of two ways. If the family is equipped with good coping and communication skills, these daily problems can be decompressed and solved without the emotional temperature in the family rising above the ill relative's vulnerability threshold, decreasing the risk of relapse. However, families that lack the know-how and skills to cope with the stressors of everyday life can, all too readily, succumb to a cycle of stress, poor communication, and mounting problems, leading to relapse. Given the large proportion of families that show high EE in the United States and most developed countries, an intervention program is essential to cool the family emotional temperature.

Behavioral family management, initially designed by Liberman, Falloon, and their colleagues at the UCLA Center for Research on Treatment and Rehabilitation of Psychosis, comprises education of the family and patient about the nature of the mental illness affecting the patient, information and advice about using community-based resources for treatment and rehabilitation, planned and structured training in communication skills, and training in problem solving. Research conducted and replicated on behavioral family management and related treatments has revealed that family-based stress management and skills training is a highly effective addition to the long-term clinical management of psychotic disorders. This modality of treatment has shown superiority in reducing relapse and rehospitalization rates, improving rates of remission of symptoms, enhancing social outcomes, and increasing family and economic benefits. Moreover, the technique can be adapted to be useful in a wide variety of settings, employed by many different disciplines of mental

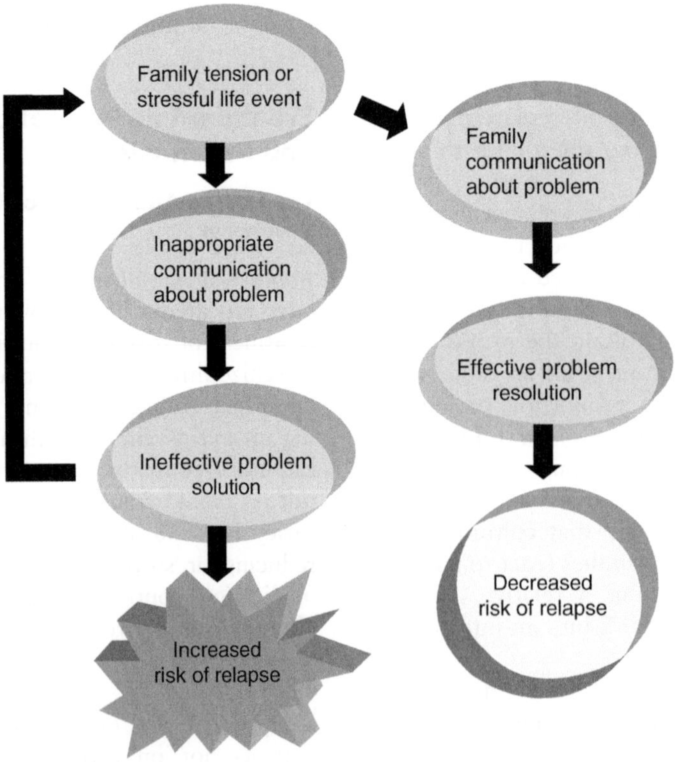

Figure 2 Role of the family in preventing relapse.

health workers, and effective in a spectrum of patient populations.

Coping with Stressful Life Events

Stressful life events occur often enough in the lives of schizophrenia patients to significantly increase the risk of psychotic relapse. Some research suggested that individuals who experience stress, but who do not relapse, possess psychological characteristics and cognitive functioning that may be associated with effective coping. In particular, the use of problem-focused coping strategies has been associated with good neurocognitive functioning and has been shown to lessen the impact of stressful life events by lowering the risk of relapse. High levels of self-esteem, hope, and insight and the perception of available social support were found in schizophrenia patients who reported using active problem-focused coping strategies. Protective mechanisms, such as effective coping behaviors, in patients and their families may have changed stressful situations into more minor events and reduced the risk of relapse. Positive symptoms have been reduced in patients who consistently applied coping strategies to stressful life events and used problem-solving techniques. These findings support the importance of coping behavior as a protective factor and mediator in the vulnerability–stress–protective factors model.

Despite good evidence for the value of using specific problem-focused coping strategies, schizophrenia patients may fail to use them. This differential use of coping strategies may explain the variability of schizophrenia patients' responses to stressful events. Even after training, they may continue to use ineffective strategies and report that the strategies they used most often were the least effective. Despite the fact that successful coping behaviors may be protective and can be learned, relatively few patients seem to avail themselves of the benefits of using coping strategies. In addition, because many schizophrenia patients have aversive reactions to stressful events, they may respond with avoidance and withdrawal to reduce their acute stress. Thus, further longitudinal research is needed to determine whether short-term or brief avoidance could in some way be adaptive or always leads to problems later.

Further Reading

Brown, G. W. and Birley, J. L. T. (1968). Crisis and life change and the onset of schizophrenia. *Journal of Health and Social Behavior* **9**, 203–214.

Bustillo, J., Lauriello, J., Horan, W., et al. (2001). The psychosocial treatment of schizophrenia: an update. *American Journal of Psychiatry* **158**(2), 163–175.

DeLisi, L., Cohen, T. and Maurizio, A. (2004). Hospitalized psychiatric patients view the World Trade Center disaster. *Psychiatry Research* **129**(2), 201–207.

Myin-Germeys, I., Krabbendam, L., Jolles, J., et al. (2002). Are cognitive impairments associated with sensitivity to stress in schizophrenia?: an experience sampling study. *American Journal of Psychiatry* **159**(3), 443–449.

Mylin-Germeys, I., van Os, J., Schwartz, J., et al. (2001). Emotional reactivity to daily life stress in psychosis. *Archives of General Psychiatry* **58**(12), 1137–1144.

Ventura, J., Nuechterlein, K. H., Subotnik, K. L., et al. (2000). Life events can trigger depressive symptoms in early schizophrenia. *Journal of Abnormal Psychology* **109**, 139–144.

Schizophrenia

M van den Buuse and D Copolov
The Mental Health Research Institute of Victoria, Parkville, Victoria, Australia

This is a revised version of the article by J M Crook and D L Copolov, Encyclopedia of Stress First Edition, volume 3, pp 393–397, © 2000, Elsevier Inc.

Glossary

Adrenocorticotropin (ACTH) — The pituitary hormone that stimulates the synthesis and secretion of adrenal corticosteroids and especially the glucocorticoids.

Corticotropin-releasing hormone (CRH) — The 41-amino-acid residue peptide released from hypothalamic neurons that mediates neural control of ACTH secretion. CRH has also been implicated in the central control of emotion and behavior.

Dexamethasone suppression test (DST) — A test designed to determine the responsiveness of the HPA axis to the negative feedback effects of the potent synthetic glucocorticoid dexamethasone. Major mental disorder is often associated with a blunted response to the DST.

Expressed emotion (EE) — Emotion expressed by close relatives toward family members with schizophrenia.

Hypothalamic-pituitary-adrenocortical (HPA) axis	The system that involves CRH-induced ACTH release, which in turn leads to adrenal glucocorticoid secretion. The latter moderates ACTH release by way of negative feedback regulation.
Magnetic resonance imaging (MRI)	An imaging technique commonly used primarily to produce high-quality images of brain.
Ultra-high risk (UHR)	A cohort of individuals identified as being at ultra-high risk to develop psychosis.

Introduction

Stress may have an impact on the course and severity of schizophrenia during a number of stages along the neurodevelopmental trajectory, including presymptomatic and early symptomatic phases as well as the phases associated with chronicity and relapse. Extensive neurobiological research has now identified molecular pathways and brain regions that are likely to be involved in the interplay between stress and schizophrenia. The interaction between these pathways has not, however, been the subject of pharmacological intervention studies. Most of the therapy-oriented research in this field has involved psychosocial approaches to reducing stress and minimizing the impact of life events in order to reduce symptom severity and the risk of relapse.

Schizophrenia: Definition and Etiology

Schizophrenia is an enigmatic illness of unknown cause, heterogeneous symptomatology, and unpredictable course, with a variable treatment response. While the precise definition of schizophrenia poses numerous difficulties, there is general agreement that the disorder involves a breakdown of integration among emotions, thoughts, and actions due to underlying neurobiological abnormalities. Common symptoms include disorganized thought processes, hallucinations, delusions, inappropriate or blunted affect, social withdrawal, and poverty of speech. Cognitive impairments, including deficits in working memory, attention, and executive functioning are also often found in the disorder. Because many of these symptoms occur in other disorders, they cannot be regarded as diagnostic when taken individually. According to most diagnostic systems, the diagnosis of schizophrenia requires specific psychopathologies to be present for at least 6 months.

The onset of schizophrenia is usually during late adolescence or early adulthood. Gender differences exist, with women on average having a later onset and a more benign course of the illness. The lifetime prevalence of schizophrenia is around 1% of the general population across all ethnic backgrounds, nationalities, and socioeconomic classes. Most people with the disorder are unemployed. Many live in substandard accommodation and experience drug or alcohol dependencies. Approximately 10% of people with schizophrenia commit suicide. Thus, schizophrenia represents a significant public health problem, from both an economic and a social point of view.

The Effects of External Stressors: Expressed Emotion and Life Events

Genetic factors play a major role in the development of schizophrenia; however, they alone do not explain the illness. First, multiple genes appear to be involved in the etiology of schizophrenia, collectively increasing susceptibility to the illness but each contributing only a small percentage to the risk. Furthermore, while family, twin, and adoption studies strongly support this genetic contribution, the finding of only 35–50% concordance for schizophrenia among monozygotic twins clearly supports the involvement of environmental factors. Epidemiological studies have identified several such adverse factors that may increase incidence of schizophrenia, such as pre- or perinatal obstetric complications, maternal influenza or rubella infection, or malnutrition and psychological trauma during pregnancy. For example, among both men and women conceived at the height of the Dutch famine in 1945, the risk of later developing schizophrenia was double that of individuals born before or after this period. Prenatal exposure to famine was also associated with decreased intracranial volume and white matter hyperintensities. These data have now been confirmed in a separate Chinese study, in which it was found that prenatal exposure to the 1959–61 famine more than doubled the risk of later developing schizophrenia. Both studies thus show that early stress caused by prenatal nutritional deficiency may play a role in the pathogenesis of schizophrenia. It should be noted that other nonstress factors could also play a role in the apparent link between famine and schizophrenia.

In addition to early environmental disturbances causing an increased risk, environmental factors later in life, such as drug abuse or psychosocial stress, may precipitate the disorder in predisposed individuals. For example, there is a significant relationship between the use of drugs of abuse, such as cannabis, and the exacerbation of psychosis and schizophrenia. The common denominator of all these early and late environmental factors is that they all induce stress, i.e., increased central and systemic release of stress hormones and disturbance of physiological and neurochemical homeostasis. The development of schizophrenia therefore may involve a disruption of early development, by either genetic or stress factors, which induces subtle changes along the neurodevelopmental trajectory. These changes could take place in synaptogenesis, synaptic pruning, axonal myelination, and neuronal proliferation in various brain regions, including cortex and hippocampus, but if they precede the onset of the disorder they either remain silent until the onset of the disorder or lead to very minor neuropsychiatric or behavioral changes in childhood and adolescence. Such changes have been reported and include a tendency for delayed neurological development, reduced social functioning, lower IQ, and neurological soft signs. However, while these associations are statistically significant, many individuals in the normal population also display such abnormalities. As a result, the presence of such mild abnormalities is not of clinical utility in the prediction of the development of schizophrenia. The emergence of psychotic symptoms may be triggered by additional stress, which may also be responsible for a later aggravation or reemergence of symptoms. One of the most influential versions of the neurodevelopmental hypothesis of schizophrenia thus comprises at least two principal components, highlighting postulated early changes in the brain, followed by later disturbances in psychological and physiological homeostasis – the so-called two-hit hypothesis of schizophrenia.

Early attempts to characterize the existence of stress-reactive schizophrenia were driven by the finding that attempts to overcome negative symptoms by social stimulation sometimes induced the reemergence of positive, psychotic symptoms of schizophrenia. This has since been tested through the study of expressed emotion (EE) – emotion expressed by close relatives toward family members with schizophrenia. Many, but not all, studies have shown that patients who experience a family environment with high EE, especially of a type that is chronic and critical in nature, have a greater propensity for psychotic relapse compared to patients from families with lower levels of EE.

Although EE studies have provided some of the strongest evidence for the stress reactivity of schizophrenia, the EE measure has been frequently misunderstood and misapplied. One of the most common mistakes is to conclude that critical and overinvolved caregivers are the major cause of poor clinical outcomes, with the result that family members are blamed for causing or exacerbating the illness. Such an approach fails to take into account the iterative relationship between high EE and patient relapse, which includes the impact of psychiatric illness on the patient's carers. In support of the iterative nature of this relationship is the established correlation between EE and family burden.

In comparison to EE, which is relatively ambient and consistent, thereby providing a probe for the impact of chronic stress on schizophrenia, life events are more discrete and less predictable, thereby providing a greater insight into the effect of acute stress on the condition. Although the majority of studies support an association between the propensity to experience episodes of schizophrenia and either the frequency of both major life events and daily hassles or their negative subjective appraisal, most of these studies have been retrospective and could therefore be affected by a search after meaning, which leads individuals to bias their recall in favor of giving undue importance to life events in order to explain their psychotic symptoms.

The anxiety associated with the psychotic experience itself may also contribute to relapse and symptom severity. Clearly, responses to delusions of persecution and danger or to hallucinations of a derogatory and intrusive nature may involve severe distress, which in turn may further exacerbate psychotic symptoms.

The Hypothalamic-Pituitary-Adrenocortical (HPA) Axis and Schizophrenia

There is good evidence that HPA axis dysfunction, as evidenced by nonsuppression in the dexamethasone suppression test (DST), occurs in approximately one in five subjects with schizophrenia, which is more than in normal subjects but less than in patients with depression. Post mortem studies have shown reduced glucocorticoid receptor expression in the hippocampus of subjects with schizophrenia, which might contribute to reduced negative feedback to the HPA axis and thus play a role in DST nonsuppression.

DST nonsuppression appears to be more common in patients who are in the acute or initial phases of their illness than in stable or chronic phases. This may explain some inconsistency in the literature, which could be attributable to differences between prodromal, first episode, and chronic patients. In addition, antipsychotic treatment has been shown to normalize at least some of the HPA axis disturbances, such as nonsuppression in the DST. The initial phase of psychosis has been shown to be associated with HPA axis hyperactivity, shown by elevated circulating cortisol cerebrospinal fluid CRH levels and impaired DST. First episode patients show enlarged pituitary volumes as measured by magnetic resonance imaging (MRI). This might reflect HPA axis hyperactivity, since enhanced CRH and adrenocorticotropin (ACTH) secretion leads to increased size and number of pituitary ACTH-producing cells. These effects could be the consequence of the previously mentioned distressing psychotic experience or, alternatively, could be involved in the induction of psychosis. To distinguish between these possibilities, pituitary volumes have been measured in a cohort of individuals identified as being at ultra-high risk (UHR) to develop psychosis. Importantly, these subjects were symptom-free and did not receive antipsychotic medication at the time of pituitary volume measurement. Within this UHR cohort, pituitary volume positively predicted future transition to psychosis, and subjects with the greatest increase in pituitary volume also showed the shortest time between being scanned and psychosis onset. Theoretically, UHR individuals with enlarged pituitary volumes might benefit from preventative treatments that target HPA axis overactivity, such as glucocorticoid receptor antagonists or CRH receptor antagonists.

While there is clear evidence for disturbances in HPA axis function in a subset of individuals with schizophrenia, the mechanism by which these disturbances mediate illness development and symptomatology is less clear. Chronically enhanced levels of glucocorticoid hormones are neurotoxic, for example, leading to macroscopic volume reduction and cell loss in the hippocampus as well as reduced neuronal volume and dendritic arborization. These effects could be associated with some of the cognitive impairments seen in patients with schizophrenia and could also explain some of the structural changes seen in the brains of patients with schizophrenia, such as reduced cortical and hippocampal volumes.

There appears to be a synergistic relationship between HPA axis activity and dopaminergic activity in the brain. Glucocorticoids increase dopamine metabolism in the striatum and dopamine release in the nucleus accumbens. If these effects apply to all areas of the brain, HPA axis disinhibition is likely to contribute to dopaminergic hyperactivity, which appears to be central to psychosis symptomatology. Positron emission tomography studies have shown that patients with schizophrenia display greater increases in central dopamine release in response to certain challenges, including low-dose amphetamine. All antipsychotic drugs share dopamine receptor antagonism as part of their pharmacological mode of action. Conversely, abnormalities in dopaminergic activity influence HPA axis activity and render an individual hyperresponsive to stress. The vulnerability-stress model of schizophrenia suggests that the illness is potentiated by stress due to this interplay with brain dopaminergic activity.

Stress, Early Development, and Schizophrenia: Neurobiological Findings

In an attempt to elucidate neurobiological mechanisms involved in the interaction of environmental factors and schizophrenia, animal model studies have simulated major life events during early stages of development. These animals, mostly rats, are then tested as adults in behavioral paradigms with relevance to schizophrenia. Developmental disruptions include neonatal stress induced by maternal deprivation, prenatal maternal stress, developmental stress induced by placental insufficiency, antimitotic treatment or vitamin D depletion, and prenatal or neonatal infection. Several studies have also used neonatal brain lesions, such as in the ventral hippocampus, frontal cortex, or amygdala. Such early interventions induce behavioral effects in the adult such as hyperlocomotion, enhanced sensitivity to psychotomimetic drugs (amphetamine, phencyclidine), disruptions of prepulse inhibition, and learning and memory deficits.

Another approach has been to study the influence of variations in maternal care. In these rat studies, dams were classified according to the level of maternal care, and behavioral and molecular changes in the offspring were examined. Offspring from mothers that displayed high levels of pup licking, grooming, and nursing differed in the level of DNA methylation from offspring from mothers that displayed low levels of these behaviors. These effects persisted into adulthood and resulted in specific changes in the regulation of glucocorticoid receptor expression. Offspring from mothers that displayed lower levels of maternal care showed lower levels of glucocorticoid receptor expression and greater plasma corticosterone increases to stress than offspring from mothers that displayed higher levels of maternal care. These studies show that early environmental factors, in this case the level of maternal care, induce long-term molecular and biochemical alterations leading to differences in glucocorticoid receptor expression and alterations in HPA axis activity. Such changes in stress responsiveness could be involved in the role of stress in schizophrenia.

Treatment Implications of the Vulnerability-Stress Model of Schizophrenia: Psychosocial Treatment Strategies

Psychosocial treatments are critical elements in the management of schizophrenia, provided that they are – as they need to be – in tandem with the keystone of treatment, antipsychotic medication. Stress management has received relatively little research attention in the treatment of the disorder, but there are suggestions that this form of treatment reduces the prevalence of hospitalization. Psychosocial treatment modalities that have received greater validation include family therapy, assertive community treatment, psychoeducation, social skills training, and cognitive-behavioral therapy. To the extent that these modalities improve coping skills, the positive outcomes they have been associated with in terms of relapse prevention and symptom amelioration might, in part, be a consequence of reduction in stress levels.

Conclusion

A variety of epidemiological, clinical, and neurobiological studies have suggested a nontrivial link between stress and schizophrenia, both during development and during the initial and established phases of the disease. These studies provide clues about brain mechanisms that could be the target of future new pharmacological treatments and about psychosocial strategies aimed at enhancing coping skills and reducing the impact of stress on the individual. However, as the available evidence is still controversial, further studies are clearly needed to better our understanding of the role of stress in schizophrenia.

See Also the Following Articles

Psychotic Disorders.

Further Reading

Bustillo, J., Lauriello, J., Horan, W. and Keith, S. (2001). The psychosocial treatment of schizophrenia: an update. *American Journal of Psychiatry* **158**, 163–175.

Corcoran, C., Walker, E., Huot, R., et al. (2003). The stress cascade and schizophrenia: etiology and onset. *Schizophrenia Bulletin* **29**, 671–692.

Cotter, D. and Pariante, C. M. (2002). Stress and the progression of the developmental hypothesis of schizophrenia. *British Journal of Psychiatry* **181**, 363–365.

Garner, B., Pariante, C. M., Wood, S. J., et al. (2005). Pituitary volume predicts future transition to psychosis in individuals at ultra-high risk of developing psychosis. *Biological Psychiatry* **58**, 417–423.

Gispen-de Wied, C. C. (2000). Stress in schizophrenia: an integrative view. *European Journal of Pharmacology* **405**, 375–384.

Hulshoff Pol, H. E., Hoek, H. W., Susser, E., et al. (2000). Prenatal exposure to famine and brain morphology in schizophrenia. *American Journal of Psychiatry* **157**, 1170–1172.

McGrath, J. J., Feron, F. P., Burne, T. H., Mackay-Sim, A. and Eyles, D. W. (2003). The neurodevelopmental hypothesis of schizophrenia: a review of recent developments. *Annals of Medicine* **35**, 86–93.

Miller, P., Lawrie, S. M., Hodges, A., et al. (2001). Genetic liability, illicit drug use, life stress and psychotic symptoms: preliminary findings from the Edinburgh study of people at high risk for schizophrenia. *Social Psychiatry and Psychiatric Epidemiology* **36**, 338–342.

Mueser, K. T. and McGurk, S. R. (2004). Schizophrenia. *The Lancet* **363**, 2063–2072.

Pantelis, C., Yucel, M., Wood, S. J., McGorry, P. D. and Velakoulis, D. (2003). Early and late neurodevelopmental disturbances in schizophrenia and their functional consequences. *Australia and New Zealand Journal of Psychiatry* **37**, 399–406.

Van den Buuse, M., Garner, B. and Koch, M. (2003). Neurodevelopmental models of schizophrenia: effects on prepulse inhibition. *Current Molecular Medicine* **3**, 459–471.

Van den Buuse, M., Garner, B., Gogos, A. and Kusljic, S. (2005). Importance of animal models in schizophrenia research. *Australia and New Zealand Journal of Psychiatry* **39**, 550–557.

Weaver, I. C., Cervoni, N., Champagne, F. A., et al. (2004). Epigenetic programming by maternal behavior. *Nature Neuroscience* Aug 7(8), 847–854.

G. Substance Related Disorders

Interactions Between Stress and Drugs of Abuse

P V Piazza and M Le Moal
Université de Bordeaux, Bordeaux, France

This article is reproduced from Encyclopedia of Stress First Edition, volume 2, pp 586–594, © 2000, Elsevier Inc.

Glossary

Dopamine — A neurotransmitter that, with norepinephrine and serotonin, belongs to the class of monoamines. In the central nervous system there are two principal groups of dopaminergic neurons, one in the mesencephalon projecting to a large number of brain structures and the other in the hypothalamus, controlling hormonal function in the hypophysis. Mesencephalic dopaminergic neurons are divided into two major subgroups: (1) The nigrostriatal neurons (A9) that have cell bodies in the substantia nigra-pars compacta (SNc) and that principally project to the dorsal striatum and the caudate nucleus and (2) the meso-limbic-cortical neurons (A10) with cell bodies in the ventral tegmental area (VTA) and that project to the ventral striatum, nucleus accumbens, and cortical and limbic structures, such as the amygdala and the hippocampus.

Drug self-administration — Intravenous drug self-administration is one of the most used models for studying drug abuse in animals. This test measures the learning of an operant response, such as pressing a lever, which stimulates drug infusion, i.e., this test measures the capacity of pharmacological substances to act as positive reinforcers.

Glucocorticoids — Consisting of cortisol in humans and corticosterone in rodents, this is the final step of the activation of the hypothalamo-pituitary-adrenal axis. These hormones have large effects in the periphery, where they modify energy metabolism and the activity of the immune system. Glucocorticoids also act at the level of the central nervous system. These hormones cross the blood–brain barrier easily and bind to two types of specific intracellular receptors, which are hormone-activated transcription factors. Glucocorticoids also seem to have direct membrane effects, although the mechanism of this action remains unclear.

Negative reinforcer — A stimulus that induces a subject to respond in a manner that interrupts the response. Foot shock is the most common negative reinforcer used in animals. Stressors are usually stimuli that can also act as negative reinforcers.

Positive reinforcer — A stimulus that increases the probability of a response. For example, positive reinforcers are food, a receptive sexual partner, and drugs of abuse.

Introduction

This article analyzes the interactions between stress and the responses to drugs of abuse. In particular, it focuses on intravenous drug self-administration, one of the principal experimental models of drug abuse. Much of our information on the interaction between stress and drugs of abuse is based on experimental studies and in particular from research in rats. Although several authors have proposed that stress is related positively to abuse of both opioid and psychostimulant drugs, a firm causal link between stress and drug abuse cannot be established on the basis of studies in humans. There are two main reasons for this. First, the variables under investigation, i.e., the history and the experiences of the subject, in humans cannot be manipulated directly under controlled experimental conditions, but only assessed indirectly on the basis of retrospective self-reports of stress. Second, a reliable measure of the outcome of stress on drug abuse implies that all individuals have equal access to drugs under identical environmental conditions. Again, this experimental setting is impossible to achieve in humans. As will be reviewed, this type of experimental investigation has revealed some of the biological factors that mediate stress-induced propensity to self-administer drugs of abuse.

Influence of Stressors on Drug Self-Administration

Definition of Stress

Stress is a very vague concept often used with different meanings that principally refer to a subjective state with a strong negative connotation. Because subjective states cannot be investigated directly in animals, experimental research on stress has focused principally on the behavioral and biological responses to the forced exposure to stimuli or situations that are normally avoided by the individual. This is why stimuli used as experimental stressors are very often identical to aversive stimuli used as negative reinforcers in learning tasks. Consequently, stress, as studied in animals, probably corresponds to "the internal status induced by the exposure to threatening and aversive stimuli." However, what is principally studied in stress research is a panoply of responses induced by aversive stimuli.

Model of Intravenous Drug Self-Administration

The experimental study of drug abuse has been made possible by the discovery that animals self-administer drugs intravenously. This behavior shares many similarities with drug use in humans. First, animals self-administer practically all the drugs that induce addiction in humans. Second, the patterns of self-administration of the different drugs in humans and animals are similar. Finally, the large individual differences in the response to drugs of abuse that characterize humans are also found in animals.

Self-administration measures positive reinforcing effect of drugs, i.e., the learning of an operant response, such as pressing a lever, that has as a consequence the delivery of a drug infusion. In general, changes in the rate of the response reinforced by the drug are considered to reflect changes in the sensitivity to its addictive properties.

Self-administration is usually studied using three different and complementary approaches: acquisition, retention, and reinstatement. The influence of different forms of stress on the three aspects of self-administration will be analyzed separately.

Influence of Stress on the Acquisition of Self-Administration

Acquisition studies evaluate the propensity of an individual to develop drug self-administration. For this purpose, the effects of first contact with low doses of the drug are studied, and parameters such as threshold or rate of acquisition are taken into account.

In adult animals, artificial and physical stressors, such as repeated tailpinch (**Figure 1**, top) and electric foot shock, facilitate the acquisition of the self-administration of psychostimulants, such as cocaine and amphetamine. Food restriction is another physical stressor that facilitates the acquisition of psychostimulant, opiate, and alcohol self-administration.

The acquisition of psychostimulant self-administration is also enhanced in male and female rats exposed to an aggressive biological 'congener' and in male rats raised in colonies in which there is a high level of social competition, i.e., colonies in

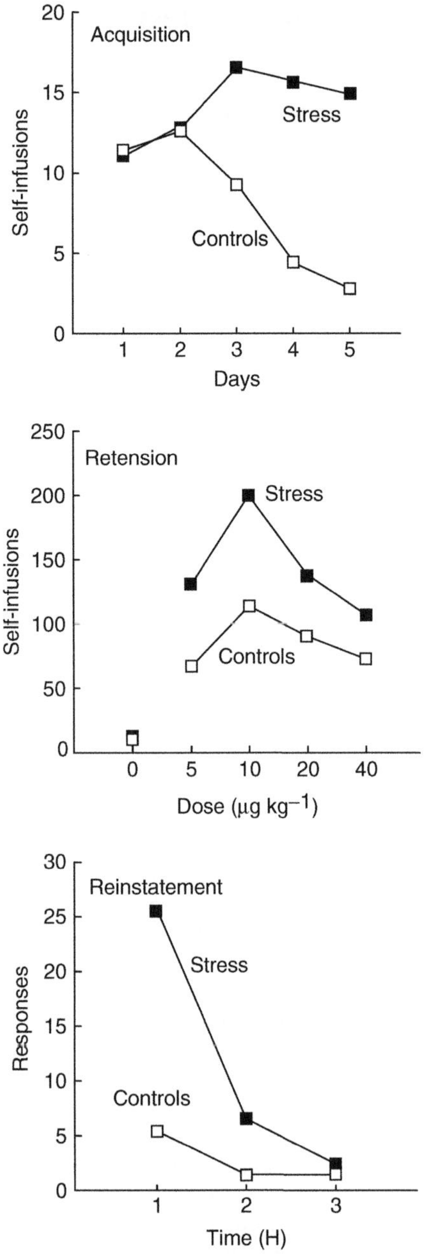

Figure 1 Examples of the effects of stress on intravenous self-administration. Top: effects of tail pinch on the acquisition of the self-administration of amphetamine (10 μg/infusion). Center: effects of food restriction on the dose–response curves of etonitazene self-administration. Bottom: influence of electric foot shock on the reinstatement of heroin self-administration. Stress facilitates the acquisition of self-administration, induces an upward shift of the dose–response function, and triggers the reinstatement of drug-seeking behavior. Redrawn with permission from, respectively, Piazza, P. V., Deminiere, J. M., Le Moal, M., et al. (1990). Stress- and pharmacologically-induced behavioral sensitization increases vulnerability to acquisition of amphetamine self-administration. *Brain Research* **514**, 22–26; Carrol, M. E. and Meich, R. A. (1984). Increased drug-reinforced behavior due to food deprivation. *Advances in Behavioral Pharmacology* **4**, 47–88; and Shaham, Y. and Stewart J. (1995). Stress reinstates heroin-seeking in drug-free animals: an effect mimicking heroin, not withdrawal. *Psychopharmacology* **111**, 334–341.

which male rats fight to establish and maintain the social hierarchy that will determine access to females. Facilitation of the acquisition of morphine and alcohol oral self-administration, as well as of heroin intravenous self-administration is also induced by social isolation.

Early life events, such as prenatal stress, also increase the propensity to develop amphetamine self-administration. Such an effect has been observed in adult rats whose mothers had been submitted to a restraint procedure during the third and fourth weeks of gestation.

Influence of Stress on Retention

Retention studies are performed after prolonged training with high doses of drug and allow estimation of changes in (i) the sensitivity to the reinforcing effects of drugs and (ii) the motivation to self-administer drugs. The sensitivity to drugs is assessed by performing dose–response curves. In this case, the dose of the drug per infusion is varied, usually between sessions, and the rate of responding is recorded. Motivation for drugs is evaluated principally by means of progressive ratio schedules. In this case, the dose is maintained constant and the ratio requirement (number of responses necessary to obtain one infusion) is increased progressively. The highest ratio reached by the subjects (breaking point) is considered an index of its motivation to self-administer drugs.

Changes in dose–response functions for psychostimulant and/or opiate self-administration have been observed after social stress, social isolation, and food restriction (**Figure 1**, center). In all these cases, the stressors induce an increase in the rate of response over a large range of doses, resulting in a vertical upward shift of the dose–response function. This type of shift in dose–response curves suggests an increase in the reinforcing efficacy of drugs in stressed animals. This idea is confirmed by progressive ratio studies. Thus, over a large range of doses, the breaking point for heroin self-administration has been consistently higher for animals subjected to repeated electric foot shock than for control rats.

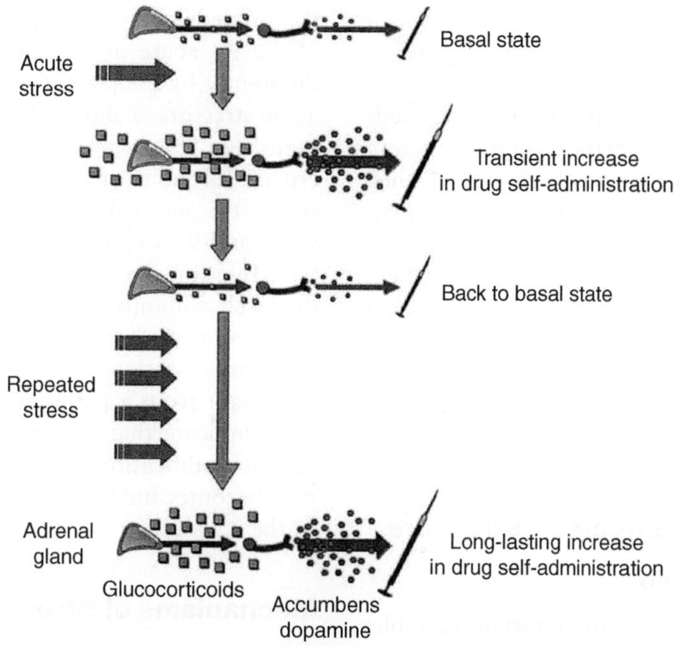

Figure 2 Possible pathophysiological mechanisms of the increase in drug self-administration induced by acute and repeated stress. The concentrations of glucocorticoids (large squares) determine the level of dopamine release in the nucleus accumbens (small squares). In basal conditions (basal state), glucocorticoid secretion and dopamine release are low, as is sensitivity to drugs of abuse. Acute stress increases glucocorticoid secretion, which, by enhancing the release of dopamine, results in an increase in the sensitivity to the reinforcing effects of drugs of abuse. However, activation of the negative feedback that controls the secretion of these hormones brings the system back to basal levels within 2 h. The increase in the concentrations of glucocorticoids induced by repeated exposure to stress will progressively result in a long-lasting increase in the secretion of these hormones and in the release of dopamine in the nucleus accumbens. These changes will, in turn, determine a long-lasting increase in the sensitivity to the reinforcing effects of drugs of abuse. The transient increase in glucocorticoids and dopamine observed after acute stress may explain why, in this case, an increase in drug self-administration is found only if the exposure to drugs closely follows the stressor. The long-lasting increase in the activity of these two biological factors could explain why, after repeated stress, an increase in the sensitivity to drugs is also found long (weeks) after the end of the stressor.

A large variability has been observed in the effect of social isolation. Indeed, higher, slightly higher, equal, or lower sensitivities to cocaine have all been described in socially isolated rats as compared to grouped rats. The conditions that were considered as controls could also contribute to such variability. In fact, the rate of self-administration of control animals, and not the one of isolated rats, is what really differentiates some of these reports. Not surprisingly, the effects of social isolation appeared weaker when other conditions that facilitate self-administration, such as priming injections of the drug and pretest periods of food restriction, were used concomitantly.

Influence of Stress on Reinstatement

Reinstatement studies are considered a measure of relapse in drug intake. In this case, the behavior is studied after the extinction of previously acquired self-administration. Extinction is usually obtained by substituting the drug with a vehicle solution. Following extinction, the administration of stimuli known to induce craving for the drug in abstinent human addicts, such as low doses of the drug, will reinstate responses to the stimulus that elicited the infusion of the drug during acquisition. The rate of response to this stimulus is the principal measure of reinstatement.

Stressors increase reinstatement of drug self-administration. In rats in which the response to heroin (**Figure 1**, bottom) or cocaine has been extinguished by substituting the drug with a saline solution, repetitive electric foot shock induces the reinstatement of response to the drug. Stress-induced reinstatement seems to be a very robust and well-documented phenomenon, and it is of comparable intensity to the one induced by other experimental manipulations known to induce reinstatement, such as the infusion of low doses of the self-administered drugs.

Factors Influencing Effects of Stressors

Predictability and Intensity

Predictability and intensity seem important variables in mediating the effects of stress on drug self-administration. Unpredictable stressors have higher effects than predictable ones. Furthermore, stressors, especially when acute, need to be of a certain intensity in order to increase self-administration. The relationship between the intensity of the stressor and its outcome on drug seeking is also shown by reinstatement studies. Thus, the rate of reinstatement has been found to be a function of the duration of the shocks. However, in the case of prolonged exposure to stress, the duration of the stress seems less important. Similar facilitory effects on self-administration have been found for stressors that are continuous and for those that are of short duration and administered repeatedly.

Physical Versus Psychological Threats

Although 'physical' stressors involving a noxious stimulus such as electric foot shock and tail pinch increase self-administration, physical aggression per se does not seem to be a necessary condition for mediating stress effects. In fact, pure psychological stress is also able to increase drug self-administration. For example, it has been shown that witnessing another rat receiving foot shocks facilitates the acquisition of cocaine self-administration. Similarly, in social aggression experiments, the facilitation of self-administration is also found when the intruder is always protected by a screen grid and consequently never submitted to physical attacks.

Time Contingencies

Both acute and repeated exposure to stress can increase the propensity to develop drug self-administration. However, acute and chronic stress are influenced differently by temporal contingencies. In the case of acute stressors, a short interval between the stressful event and the exposure to the drug appears to be crucial. In contrast, after a prolonged exposure to stress, the interval between the termination of the stress and the exposure to the drug does not seem to be a relevant variable. In this case a facilitation of drug self-administration has also been found when the stress is terminated weeks before the start of the self-administration session. These observations are important from a pathophysiological point of view. They indicate that repeated stress can induce long-lasting modifications that result in a drug-prone state that becomes independent from the actual presence of the stressor.

Mechanisms of Stress Action

Different mechanisms could mediate the effects of stress on drug self-administration and much remains to be done on this field of research. We will focus principally on the possibility that stressors sensitize the endogenous system of reward by an action on dopaminergic neurons and glucocorticoid hormones. Mesencephalic dopaminergic neurons, particularly their projection to the nucleus accumbens, are considered one of the principal substrates of drug-reinforcing effects. Glucocorticoid hormones are the final step of the activation of the hypothalamic-pituitary-adrenal axis. The secretion of glucocorticoids by the adrenal gland is considered one of the principal biological adaptations to external aggression.

Clearly, an interaction between glucocorticoids and dopamine should not be considered as the only possible mechanism mediating stress effects, but as the best studied of only one of the likely possibilities. **Figure 2** shows schematically the interactions among stress, glucocorticoids, and dopaminergic neurons.

Sensitization of the Reward System

One of the mechanisms by which stress could modify the sensitivity of an individual to drugs of abuse is by modifying the activity of those neurobiological systems that mediate the addictive properties of drugs.

Role of mesencephalic dopaminergic neurons Mesencephalic dopaminergic neurons seem to be a likely candidate for such a neurobiological system. The role of these neurons in drug abuse has been emphasized in several good reviews. In particular, the release of dopamine in the nucleus accumbens is considered one of the major mechanisms of the addictive properties of drugs. Practically all drugs of abuse increase dopamine release in this brain area, and an increase or a decrease in dopaminergic activity in the nucleus accumbens corresponds, respectively, to an increase or a decrease in the reinforcing properties of drugs. Several types of acute stress transiently increase dopamine release in the nucleus accumbens. In parallel, repeated stress induces a long-lasting increase in the release of this neurotransmitter, particularly of drug-induced dopamine release.

Role of glucocorticoid hormones Glucocorticoid hormones seem to be the link between environmental experiences and mesencephalic dopaminergic neurons. In basal conditions, the administration of glucocorticoids at levels that are in the stress range can increase dopamine release in the nucleus accumbens, whereas the suppression of glucocorticoid secretion has the opposite effect. During stress, a selective blockade of stress-induced secretion of glucocorticoids reduces dopamine release by around 50%. Finally, the development of the long-lasting sensitization of the dopaminergic response to psychostimulants and opioids induced by stress is suppressed by the blockade of corticosterone secretion.

That glucocorticoids hormones, through their action on dopamine release, could increase the behavioral responses to drugs is supported by a supplementary set of data. First, administration of glucocorticoids, at levels that are in the stress range, increases the propensity to self-administer amphetamine. Second, the blockade of stress-induced corticosterone secretion induces a downward shift in the dose–response curve for cocaine self-administration, i.e., changes opposite to those observed after stress. Third, the blockade of corticosterone secretion can reverse the stress-induced sensitization of the dopaminergic and behavioral responses to cocaine.

Mechanisms of reinstatement The hypothalamic-pituitary-adrenal axis and dopaminergic neurons also seem to play a role in reinstatement, but in a way that differs from the one described for drug self-administration.

For example, a concomitant blockade of D1 and D2 dopaminergic receptors is needed to block stress-induced reinstatement, whereas selective antagonists of either receptor suffice to decrease the positive reinforcing effects of drugs. In parallel, although the injection of glucocorticoids alone can induce reinstatement, blockade of the secretion of these hormones does not prevent the stress-induced reinstatement of heroin self-administration. In contrast, the blockade of glucocorticoid secretion seems to block the stress-induced reinstatement of cocaine self-administration.

Stress-Induced Impulsivity

Changes in impulsivity could be an alternative mechanism by which stress modifies drug self-administration. A deficit in the inhibitory processes that normally operate to control the reward effect of a stimulus is considered an important dimension of impulsivity. This type of impairment could contribute to the increase in drug self-administration induced by stress. This idea is prompted by the effects of social aggression on the rate of responding during time-out periods, i.e., fixed time periods that follow each drug infusion and during which responses are not expected. During time-out, control animals learn quickly to reduce response rates and to wait for the next period of drug availability, whereas stressed rats maintain high rates of response during these time periods. The possibility that an inhibitory deficit is involved in excessive drug consumption is also backed by the finding that the inability to delay gratification predicts alcohol self-administration.

Although stress-induced impulsivity seems an interesting mechanism, further experiments should specifically test the actual occurrence of such a change in behavior. At the neurochemical level it will be important to correlate such potential changes in behaviors with neurobiological modifications involved in impulsivity, such as a decrease in serotoninergic activity.

Does Stress Induce a Drug-Prone Phenotype?

The Individual-Centered Vision of Addiction

It is a common observation that although a large number of people take drugs for variable periods of time, only few of them develop a true addiction, i.e., a compulsive drug use that becomes the main goal-directed activity of the subject. One of the theories that has been used to explain such individual differences in the development of addiction postulates the existence of a drug-prone phenotype, i.e., drug abuse is a pre-existing pathological condition revealed by the drug. Addiction would appear only in certain individuals because their biological phenotype will generate a 'pathological response' to drugs. This pathological response would make the addictive properties of drugs much greater in some subjects, increasing their likeliness to develop drug abuse.

Knowledge about Drug-Prone Phenotypes

Research in rodents has identified some of the biological factors that could determine a drug-prone phenotype. As indicated earlier, large individual differences in the propensity to develop drug self-administration have been described in laboratory rats, and the propensity of an individual animal to develop self-administration correlates with its behavior in other experimental situations. For example, animals that show the highest locomotor activity when exposed to a novel environment, a procedure that can be seen as a model of mild stress, also show the highest propensity to self-administer amphetamine.

Animals predisposed to drug addiction show a faster acquisition of drug self-administration, an upward shift of the dose–response function, and reach higher ratio requirements. They also show a higher release of dopamine into the nucleus accumbens in response to a drug challenge and a longer glucocorticoid secretion in response to stress. Finally, the higher dopaminergic activity of animals that are spontaneously drug prone seems to be glucocorticoid dependent. These rats are more sensitive to the dopaminergic effect of glucocorticoids, and blockade of glucocorticoid reduces their dopaminergic hyperactivity.

Stress-Induced Phenotype

Data presented in this article suggest that stressful experiences are one of the determinants of a drug-prone phenotype. Indeed, stressors can induce a long-lasting increase in drug self-administration, and such an effect occur place at an early stage of life, as exemplified by prenatal stress. Further support for this idea arises from the comparison of the characteristics of individuals who are spontaneously drug prone with those of subjects in which such a predisposition has been induced by stress. Indeed, dopaminergic hyperactivity and a dysregulation of glucocorticoid hormone activity, similar to that observed in subjects susceptible to drug addiction, have also been found in individuals made vulnerable by stress.

Conclusions

In conclusion, stress experiences increase the propensity of an individual to develop drug self-administration, inducing a drug-prone phenotype. Stress-induced increases in the secretion of glucocorticoids, which in turn enhance the drug-induced release of dopamine in the nucleus accumbens, seem to be an important substrate of such an effect of stress.

These observations highlight the importance of environmental experiences in the etiology of drug abuse. This confirms the hypothetical role of stress suggested by correlative studies in humans. Second, the observations support the idea that drug abuse is not simply induced by chronic drug intake, but that the phenotype of the individual plays an important role in determining the development of such a pathological behavior.

See Also the Following Article

Drug Use and Abuse.

Further Reading

Carrol, M. E. and Meich, R. A. (1984). Increased drug-reinforced behavior due to food deprivation. *Advances in Behavioral Pharmacology* **4**, 47–88.

de Kloet, E. R. (1992). Brain corticosteroid receptors balance and homeostatic control. *Frontiers of Neuroendocrinology* **12**, 95–164.

Kalivas, P. W. and Stewart, J. (1991). Dopamine transmission in the initiation and expression of drug- and stress-induced sensitization of motor activity. *Brain Research Reviews* **16**, 223–244.

Piazza, P. V. and Le Moal, M. (1996). Pathophysiological basis of vulnerability to drug abuse: Role of an interaction between stress, glucocorticoids and dopaminergic neurons. *Annual Review of Pharmacology and Toxicology* **36**, 359–378.

Piazza, P. V. and Le Moal, M. (1997). Glucocorticoids as an endogenous substrate of reward. *Brain Research Reviews* **25**, 359–372.

Piazza, P. V. and Le Moal, M. (1998). The role of stress in drug self-administration. *Trends in Pharmacological Sciences* **19**, 7–74.

Schuster, C. R. and Thompson, T. (1969). Self-administration and behavioral dependence on drugs. *Annual Review of Pharmacology* **9**, 483–502.

Shaham, Y. (1996). Effect of stress an opioid-seeking behavior: Evidences from studies with rats. *Annals of Behavioral Medicine* **18**, 255–263.

Wise, R. A. (1996). Neurobiology of addiction. *Current Opinion in Neurobiology* **6**, 243–251.

Alcohol, Alcoholism, and Stress: A Psychobiological Perspective

A N Taylor and P Prolo
University of California, Los Angeles, and Veterans Administration Greater Los Angeles Health Care System, Los Angeles, CA, USA
M L Pilati
Rio Hondo College, Whittier, CA, USA

This is a revised version of the article by A N Taylor and M L Pilati, Encyclopedia of Stress First Edition, volume 1, pp 131–135, © 2000, Elsevier Inc.

Glossary

Alcohol abuse — The use of alcohol in a manner harmful to the individual and/or others, such as contributing to the failure to fulfill familial or work obligations but not a severe enough problem to meet criteria for alcohol dependence. *Diagnostic and Statistical Manual of Mental Disorders*, 4th edition (DSM-IV-TR), makes a distinction between substance abuse and dependence; once the criteria for dependence have been met, a diagnosis of substance abuse is not possible.

Alcohol dependence — According to DSM IV-TR criteria, a failure to control alcohol use despite repeated attempts, continued use despite the knowledge of adverse consequences, and, in general, compulsive use of alcohol. Alcohol dependence may or may not be accompanied by physiological dependence.

Alcoholism — Excessive alcohol use. Although there is no formally accepted definition of alcoholism, the criteria for alcohol dependence are most frequently used by researchers.

Circadian rhythms — Biological rhythms that have a cycle of about 24 h; derived from the Latin *circa diem* "about a day."

Endorphin compensation hypothesis — A hypothesis that proposes that the use of alcohol following stress is an attempt to compensate for a decrease in the levels of β-endorphin resulting from the termination of the stressor.

Relapse prevention model — A model that proposes that the goal of treatment for addictive behaviors is to develop the means for coping with stressful situations that put the addict at risk for relapse.

Stress-response-dampening model — A model that proposes that alcohol use is reinforced by its ability to ameliorate responses to stress.

Introduction

The effects of alcohol on the mind, brain, and body are as diverse as the effects of stress. However conceptualized, stress is consistently associated with psychological manifestations, including anxiety, irritability and anger, sad and depressed moods, tension, fatigue, and with certain bodily manifestations, including perspiration, blushing or blanching of the face, increased heart rate, decreased blood pressure, and intestinal cramps and discomfort. Sleep duration and quality are also severely impaired by stress. In the field of substance addiction, both acute and chronic alcohol intake have a disruptive effect on a variety of stressors, both at physiological and psychosocial levels. Three fundamental issues arise: (1) the consequences of stress on normal subjects and alcoholics are not uniform, and the psychopathological and physiopathological impact of stress may be significantly greater in some people than in others; (2) the impact of stress is dynamic and multifaceted, such that the same person may exhibit a variety of manifestations of the psychoneuroendocrine-immune stress response with varying degrees of severity in different situations; and (3) the outcome of stress can be variable in the sense that normal subjects and alcohol abusers may position themselves along the spectrum of allostatic regulation, somewhere between the allostatic state (i.e., toward regaining physiological balance) and allostatic overload (i.e., toward physiological collapse, with associated potential onset of varied pathologies). In brief, subjects with different levels of chronic stress (i.e., major life events or minor hassles) may be expected to respond dramatically differently. Finally, inherited changes in response to alcohol, such as an increase in the ability of alcohol to lessen the impact of stressful events, may themselves confer susceptibility to alcohol abuse. Our understanding of the relationships between alcohol and stress is based on different lines of research both on animal and human subjects.

Alcohol and the Stress Response

Alcohol and the Neuroendocrine-Immune Response to Stress

Acute alcohol administration has a stimulatory action on the hypothalamic-pituitary-adrenal (HPA) axis and related brain systems in humans and rodents, that is, the brain and pituitary β-endorphin (β-EP) systems and the sympathetic nervous system. Alcohol-induced neuroendocrine effects are characterized by dose-dependent elevations in plasma glucocorticoids, adrenocorticotropic hormone (ACTH), β-EP, and catecholamines. Ethanol activation of the HPA axis is abolished by hypophysectomy or treatment with corticotropin-releasing hormone (CRH) antiserum in rodents, suggesting that it is primarily modulated by ACTH secretion and that CRH is an essential intermediate in the stimulation of ACTH by ethanol. Acute ethanol exposure generally activates the HPA axis when blood alcohol concentrations (BACs) exceed intoxicating levels of 100 mg dl−1, although HPA activation can also occur at lower BACs. In contrast, the ethanol-induced HPA response of some individuals may be either unaffected or blunted. There are also contributions from environmental and genetic factors to this variability.

Chronic exposure to ethanol has a more variable effect on the HPA axis and the β-EP system, ranging from stimulation to either response attenuation or tolerance. For example, a small percentage of alcoholic individuals (<5%) develop clinical features of hypercortisolism or Cushing's syndrome. However, animal studies suggest that chronic ethanol exposure can result in tolerance to the stimulatory effect of ethanol on CRH release in vitro and can impair the ability of the HPA axis to respond to stress. Indeed, alcoholic men have been reported to show blunted ACTH and cortisol responses to CRH and ACTH challenges, as well as other signs of HPA axis dysfunction (i.e., impaired feedback regulation).

Alcohol consumption acts on the autonomic nervous system as well as the neuroendocrine system, in particular the HPA axis. The latter plays a pivotal role in regulating immune surveillance mechanisms, including the production of cytokines that control the inflammatory process as well as events responsible for healing. Given the multidirectional communication among the neuroendocrine, immune, and nervous systems, alcohol can be expected to impact all three interacting systems, in both feed-forward and feedback directions.

Alcohol and the Cardiovascular Response to Stress

The impact of alcohol on cardiovascular responses varies with the state of the subject at the time of alcohol exposure (i.e., baseline or post-stress) and with the cardiovascular measures employed. Although alcohol has been shown to increase resting heart rate, it also is known to produce a paradoxical decrease in blood pressure in both humans and animals. Thus, alcohol's effect on heart rate is comparable to that of stress, whereas its impact on blood pressure is inconsistent. Heart rate, as a psychophysiological measure of the stress response, has provided evidence for the general assumption that alcohol is often used as a means of relief from the physical and psychological effects of stress. However, human research designed to assess the stress-response-dampening model of alcohol use has had mixed results. There is some indication that contradictions in experimental findings may be due to varying alcohol doses, differences in the subjects employed, and differences in the timing of the stress exposure and the alcohol presentation. Making the issue even more complex is the evidence indicating that altered responses to alcohol may have a genetic basis, possibly even conferring susceptibility to alcohol abuse on those with a family history of such substance-abuse problems. Studies failing to see a stress-response dampening effect of alcohol have often employed rather low doses, providing a logical explanation for differing results; it has also been established that alcohol increases baseline levels of physiological arousal. Thus, when looking at the effects of alcohol on the response to a given stressor and calculating change from baseline, results will differ depending on whether the baseline used is a pre- or postethanol measurement.

Effects of Stress on Alcohol Consumption

Stress and Alcohol Use

Animal studies indicate that stress increases alcohol consumption when the stress, whether physical or social, is chronic, unavoidable, and uncontrollable. Evidence from human and animal studies indicates that alcohol has profound anxiolytic effects. In rodents, tolerance to the anxiolytic effects of low or moderate doses of ethanol was shown to develop rapidly and, as such, may explain the augmented consumption of alcohol required to maintain its tension-reducing effects. In addition, adverse experiences early in life, such as maternal separation, have been found to be associated with excessive alcohol consumption in monkeys as well as in humans. Furthermore, prenatal factors, such as maternal stress and drugs or alcohol consumption during pregnancy, can dysregulate physiological and behavioral stress responses in adulthood. Such findings suggest that early life experiences can result in long-lasting psychobiological changes that may manifest as enhanced alcohol consumption in order to achieve tension reduction.

Consistent with the stress-response dampening model, it is a common and long-held assumption that alcohol is often used as a means of coping with stress. Recently, however, with the observation that alcohol may or may not dampen physiological responses to stress, new theories have evolved. One that is consistent with many observations and the effectiveness of new pharmacological treatments for alcoholism is the endorphin compensation hypothesis. This hypothesis proposes that alcohol is consumed following the termination of stress because the presence of stress increases levels of the endogenous opioid β-EP. Alcohol is sought for its ability to increase β-EP levels and compensate for the deficit that results when the stress has been removed. Consistent with this hypothesis is the use of naltrexone, an opiate antagonist, in the treatment of alcoholism.

Sleep and Alcohol Use

Sleep disturbance is a common complaint of alcohol-dependent patients. Various studies have demonstrated a strong association between poor sleep and psychological factors, especially in relation to perceived stress and associated increases in CRH and cortisol, the hypothalamic and adrenal products of the HPA axis. Both hormones are known to lead to arousal and sleeplessness in human subjects and experimental animals.

The daily sleep–wakefulness cycle is synchronous with circadian patterns of body temperature in humans and animals such that maximum body temperatures occur during the active portion of each day and minimum body temperatures occur during the inactive or sleep portion. In rodents, the daily active period corresponds with the dark phase of the daily light–dark cycle while sleep occurs during the light phase. Acute administration of ethanol was found to alter the rodent's circadian body temperature and activity rhythms in a dose- and time-dependent manner. Chronic exposure to ethanol has also been shown to alter the amplitude of the rat's circadian body temperature and activity rhythms. Confirmation of these findings in translational studies on human subjects could provide a further basis for alcohol-induced sleep disturbances.

Trauma and Alcohol Use

Despite the controversy as to whether or not alcohol is used to minimize the impact of stress or to compensate for some post-stress condition, there is an abundance of correlational data linking increases in alcohol use with exposure to or the experience of traumatic or uncontrollable stressful events. For example, studies have demonstrated that there is an increase in social indices of alcohol use (such as arrests for driving while intoxicated) following disasters.

Not only are changes in a population's alcohol consumption associated with traumatic events that affect a community (e.g., natural disasters), but a high percentage of those seeking treatment for alcoholism are survivors of abuse or suffering from post-traumatic stress disorder or other anxiety disorders. Although it may be difficult to determine a direct relationship between victimization and alcohol misuse, attempts to define whether or not alcohol abuse preceded, coincided with, or followed trauma have consistently found that trauma did, in fact, precede alcohol misuse. Furthermore, trauma severity is positively correlated with alcohol consumption and the severity of alcohol-related problems. There is reason to believe that, whereas stress plays a role in the etiology of all drug dependence, the drug selected by men is more likely to be alcohol. Thus, there appears to be a gender difference in the drug of choice for the individual struggling with the aftermath or presence of stressful life conditions.

Traumatic Brain Injury and Alcohol Use

Traumatic brain injury (TBI) and its sequelae are of pivotal importance in the young generation (e.g., in victims of car accidents and in deployed soldiers and war veterans) with consequences ranging from physical disabilities to long-term behavioral and social deficits. Close to 25% of TBI cases are associated with alcohol abuse, and alcoholism may, in and of itself, complicate long-term TBI recovery. A growing body of evidence raises the possibility that alcohol intoxication or dependence in combination with TBI may lead to increased deleterious effects on cognitive functioning. Moreover, serious alterations in neuroendocrine and immune regulation have been noted following chronic alcohol use and TBI in animal models and humans that can impair recovery and rehabilitation efforts after brain injury. However, the role of alcohol as an interactive or additive agent in these findings has not been fully assessed.

Alcoholism, Stress, and Relapse

Stressful life events have long been thought to play a role in the return to alcohol use following cessation of problematic drinking behavior. The role of stress in relapse has received much attention, with more recent reviews concluding that less severe psychosocial stress may not increase the likelihood of relapse, whereas severe acute stressors and chronic stressors perceived as highly threatening may contribute to an increased risk of relapse. In considering the role of stress in relapse, however, the capabilities of the individual must be considered. The impact of even severe stress and whether this leads to relapse are mediated by both protective and risk factors that render the individual more or less likely to return to problematic alcohol use. Risk factors that may increase the likelihood of relapse to substance abuse include the persisting physiological symptoms of abstinence (e.g., HPA axis dysfunction, characterized by a blunted ACTH response to a challenge with CRH).

The role of stress has been the focus of many alcoholism treatments. Most notably, the relapse prevention model introduced by Marlatt and George in 1984 proposes that the goal of treatment for addictive behaviors must be to develop the means for coping with stressful situations. In order to change addictive patterns, situations that are high-risk for relapse need to be identified and methods for coping with such situations developed. According to the model, cessation of addictive behavioral patterns can be achieved through the mastery of handling such high-risk situations. The relapse prevention model has been the focus of much research, although empirical support for its effectiveness is difficult to obtain. Despite research suggesting that relapse does occur in situations identified as being high-risk, the subjective nature of such retrospective reports calls any definitive conclusions into question.

Modifiers of the Stress–Alcohol Interaction

Genetics

Various inbred murine and rodent strains differ in their sensitivities to alcohol at the endocrine and behavioral levels. In the past 2 decades, with the application of selective breeding techniques, rodent models of alcoholism have been derived with high and low oral alcohol preference. Such animal models are particularly useful in the identification of genetic traits associated with the physiological and behavioral bases of alcohol drinking. For example, results indicate that the β-EP system of alcohol-preferring rats is hyperresponsive to alcohol. Thus, the activation of the endogenous opioid system may either enhance the reinforcing effects of low-dose alcohol or attenuate the aversive effects of high-dose alcohol and thereby affect alcohol consumption, consistent with the previously noted endorphin compensation hypothesis.

The genetic basis for susceptibility to alcohol abuse and dependence has long been accepted, and numerous studies have been conducted to determine how those with a family history of alcoholism (family history positive, FHP) might differ from those without such an inherited risk (family history negative, FHN). There is increasing support that altered neuroendocrine responses to alcohol in the sons of alcoholic men provide a possible basis for the genetic component in the development of alcoholism. For example, nonalcoholic male offspring of alcoholic fathers (known to be at three- or fourfold higher risk for alcoholism than sons of nonalcoholics) demonstrate, in comparison to the sons of non-alcoholics, lower cortisol responses to alcohol, an impaired ACTH response to CRH, increased alcohol-induced plasma β-EP levels, and an enhanced ACTH response to the opioid receptor antagonist, naloxone. These findings indicate that FHP men have altered hypothalamic CRH neuronal activity. Although it is not clear how these alterations may contribute to the development of abusive patterns of alcohol use, these studies suggest that the CRH-mediated response of the HPA axis or the β-EP system to alcohol may serve as a marker to distinguish individuals at risk for alcoholism. Interestingly, these markers do not effectively distinguish FHP women, supporting the notion that there are gender differences in the role of genetic factors in the etiology of alcoholism.

Expectancy

Adding an additional level of complexity to the determination of the effects of alcohol on the human stress response is the vast literature demonstrating that expectancies have a significant impact on the response to alcohol ingestion. It may be that many reported differences in the literature are created by the influence of cognition on reactivity to alcohol and are due to the timing of stress presentation with respect to alcohol use. Indeed, it appears that intoxication prior to stress exposure may alter the cognitive reaction to the stimulus and, as a result, the response to the stressful stimulus may be minimized. Thus, it may be that alcohol does not merely dampen the stress response but that alcohol may also act to reduce the physiological response to a stressor by altering the appraisal of the stressful stimulus. Such a conclusion is supported by studies that find that more complex paradigms are more likely to result in alcohol stress-response dampening.

Conclusion

There is clearly a relationship between alcohol and stress, although the nature of this association is complex and not easily described. A brief look at the relevant literature demonstrates that the interaction of alcohol and stress varies with characteristics of the subject studied, the environment, the alcohol dose, the nature of the stressor imposed, and the timing of the exposure to alcohol and the stressor. Thus, stress, alcohol, and alcoholism are interrelated, but the nature of this relationship is highly variable. The ineffectiveness of many strategies for prevention and treatment of alcohol abuse and the variation in clinical history represent a challenge and an opportunity to better understand the relationship between alcohol and stress.

See Also the Following Articles

Drug Use and Abuse.

Further Reading

Aston-Jones, G. and Harris, G. C. (2004). Brain substrates for increased drug seeking during protracted withdrawal. *Neuropharmacology* **47**(supplement 1), 167–179.

Besedovsky, H. O. and Del Rey, A. (2001). Cytokines as mediators of central and peripheral immune-neuroendocrine interactions. In: Ader, R., Felten, D. L. & Cohen, N. (eds.) *Psychoneuroimmunology,* (3rd edn. Vol. 1), pp. 1–17. San Diego, CA: Academic Press.

Cloninger, C. R. (1987). Neurogenetic adaptive mechanisms in alcoholism. *Science* **236**, 410–416.

Corrigan, J. D., Whitneck, G. and Mellick, D. (2004). Perceived needs following traumatic brain injury. *Journal of Head and Trauma Rehabilitation* **19**, 205–216.

Crum, R. M., Ford, D. E., Storr, C. L., et al. (2004). Association of sleep disturbance with chronicity and remission of alcohol dependence: data from a population-based prospective study. *Alcoholism: Clinical and Experimental Research* **10**, 1533–1540.

Froelich, J. C. (1993). Interactions between alcohol and the endogenous opioid system. In: Zakhari, S. (ed.) *Alcohol and the endocine system,* NIAAA research monograph, **23**, pp. 21–36. Bethesda, MD: National Institutes of Health.

Higley, J. D., Hasert, M. F., Suomi, B. J., et al. (1991). Nonhuman primate model of alcohol abuse: effects of early experience, personality, and stress on alcohol consumption. *Proceedings of the National Academy of Sciences USA* **88**, 7261–7265.

Marlatt, G. A. and George, F. R. (1984). Relapse prevention: introduction and overview of the model. *British Journal of Addiction* **79**, 261–273.

Pohorecky, L. A. (1991). Stress and alcohol interaction: an update of human research. *Alcoholism: Clinical and Experimental Research* **15**, 438–459.

Schuckit, M. (1998). Biological, psychological and environmental predictors of the alcoholism risk: a longitudinal study. *Journal of Studies on Alcohol* **59**, 485–494.

Stewart, S. H. (1996). Alcohol abuse in individuals exposed to trauma: a critical review. *Psychology Bulletin* **120**, 83–112.

Taylor, A. N., Chiappelli, F. and Yirmiya, R. (2001). Fetal alcohol syndrome and immunity. In: Ader, R., Felten, D. L. & Cohen, N. (eds.) *Psychoneuroimmunology* (3rd edn. Vol. 2), pp. 49–71. San Diego, CA: Academic Press.

Taylor, A. N., Tio, D. L., Heng, N. S., et al. (2002). Alcohol consumption attenuates febrile responses to lipopolysaccharide and interleukin-1β in male rats. *Alcoholism: Clinical and Experiment Research* **26**, 44–52.

Vgontzas, A. N., Zoumakis, M., Bixler, E. O., et al. (2003). Impaired nighttime sleep in healthy old vs. young adults is associated with elevated plasma IL-6 and cortisol levels: physiologic and therapeutic implications. *Journal of Clinical Endocrinology and Metabolism* **88**, 2087–2095.

Volpicelli, J. R., Tiven, J. and Kimmel, S. C. (1987). Uncontrollable events and alcohol drinking. *British Journal of Addiction* **82**, 381–392.

Waltman, C., McCaul, M. E. and Wand, G. S. (1994). Adrenocorticotropin responses following administration of ethanol and ovine corticotropin-releasing hormone in the sons of alcoholics and control subjects. *Alcoholism: Clinical and Experimental Research* **18**, 826–830.

Wand, G. S., Mangold, D. and Mahmood, M. (1999). Adrenocorticotropin responses to naloxone in sons of alcohol-dependent men. *Journal of Clinical Endocrinology and Metabolism* **84**, 64–68.

Zimmermann, U., Spring, K., Kunz-Ebrecht, S. R., et al. (2004). Effect of ethanol on hypothalamic-pituitary-adrenal system response to psychosocial stress in sons of alcohol-dependent fathers. *Neuropsychopharmacology* **29**, 1156–1165.

Smoking and Stress

F J McClernon
Duke University Medical Center, Durham, NC, USA
D G Gilbert
Southern Illinois University-Carbondale, Carbondale, IL, USA

This is a revised version of the article by D G Gilbert and F J McClernon, Encyclopedia of Stress First Edition, volume 3, pp 458–465, © 2000, Elsevier Inc.

Glossary

Acetylcholine — A neurotransmitter in the brain that has receptors on nerve cells that nicotine stimulates and promotes the firing of.

Affect — Moods, emotions, and feelings, including negative affect (e.g., anxiety, depressive mood, and anger) and positive affect (e.g., euphoria, vigor, and pleasant feelings).

Cognitive dysfunction — The impairment or biasing of information processes such as perceptual, attentional, and memorial functions that can be caused by temporary physiological and mood states, as well as by longer-lasting forms of psychopathology, neurological abnormality, or temperamental bias.

Dopamine — A neurotransmitter in the brain having a number of functions, including the enhancement of attention and signaling of reward in response to appetitive stimuli.

Neuro-transmitter — A chemical released at the synapse (junction) between nerves that promotes the conduction of nerves impulses from one nerve to another.

Nicotine — The primary psychoactive component of tobacco smoke; it binds to endogenous nicotinic acetylcholine receptors, which results in a variety of neuronal actions.

Situation x trait adaptive response (STAR) model — An integrative model that emphasizes the interaction of situational factors with genetic and personality factors in determining who is likely to become a smoker, how rewarding smoking will be, and when and how often smoking is likely to be rewarding to the individual as a coping tool.

Tar — The mass of some 5000 components of tobacco smoke, excluding nicotine and gases (e.g., carbon monoxide).

Introduction

Smoking remains the number one preventable cause of death and disability in the United States and is a burden on people, economies, and health-care systems worldwide. Knowledge about the relation of smoking and stress has expanded exponentially in the last 3 decades as a result of new findings in the fields of genetics, neuroscience, and clinical research. This research has revolutionized thinking about who smokes and why it is so difficult for many to quit. Genes have been found to play a significant role in determining who becomes and remains a smoker. Some of the genes that predispose some people to smoke predispose the same individuals to experience higher than normal levels of stress and negative mood states. These and related findings indicate that there are many clinically and theoretically important relations among smoking, stress, and coping.

Personality Traits, Genetic, and Biological Predictors of Smoking and Stress

Evidence shows clear and substantial relations among smoking, stress-related personality traits, and psychopathology. Further, all these characteristics are largely heritable (passed on from generation to generation via genes) and share common genetic bases.

Stress, Personality, Psychopathology, and Smoking

Individuals with specific psychiatric problems and personality traits leading to frequent or intense personal distress are substantially more likely to smoke. Smoking rates are disproportionately high in individuals with psychiatric conditions, including major depressive disorder, various anxiety disorders, schizophrenia, antisocial personality disorder, attention deficit hyperactivity disorder (ADHD), and various substance abuse disorders, including alcoholism. The prevalence of smoking in individuals with a lifetime history of these conditions is two to three times higher than in unaffected individuals. The personality traits associated with the increased prevalence of smoking reflect dispositions that are similar in nature to psychiatric disorders. For example, the personality trait of neuroticism (the general tendency to experience negative affect and stress) has been found to be associated with higher prevalence of smoking. Smoking (and drug abuse more broadly) is also much more prevalent among individuals high in impulsiveness or sensation-seeking traits. In addition to finding relations between these traits and smoking among adults, longitudinal studies have shown that children and adolescents with these traits are more likely to smoke as adults (as well as to use other drugs). Taken together, these data suggest that smoking behavior is not randomly distributed in the adult population and also support the notion that nicotine plays some role in the psychological life of the smoker beyond simple addiction or withdrawal alleviation.

Identical Genes Related to Smoking, Psychopathology, and Personality Traits

Results from family, twin, and molecular genetic studies demonstrate that genetic factors play an important role in smoking behavior and stress responses. Genes account for approximately half of the variability in who will smoke and who will not. Further, many of the same genes that predispose individuals to smoke are also responsible, in part, for predisposing individuals to the stress-related personality traits and psychiatric disorders previously mentioned. For instance, the same genes that contribute to a vulnerability to neuroticism also appear to dispose individuals to clinical depression and to smoking. Similarly, the same genes that contribute to impulsivity and sensation seeking also contribute to a variety of compulsive behaviors, including drug abuse, antisocial behavior, and smoking.

The identification of some of the many genes that contribute to smoking and smoking-related traits has been one of the major accomplishments of recent years. Genetically influenced biological differences between people in (1) brain neurotransmitter receptors and (2) liver enzymes related to nicotine metabolism appear to play roles in determining smoking. Some of the most exciting insights in this area are related to the neurotransmitter dopamine. Dopamine is intimately associated with coping, stress, natural reward, and the pleasurable effects of abused drugs, including nicotine. A number of genes combine to determine a person's brain dopamine system functioning. Those individuals with low dopamineric system functioning levels are more likely than others to smoke, abuse alcohol and other drugs, and have impulsive and sensation-seeking personality traits. Thus, these dopamine genes appear to contribute to the association of smoking with these personality traits and substance-abuse patterns.

Smoking as a Coping Response

These personality traits and psychiatric conditions are associated with distressing cognitive and emotional states. To the degree smoking is effective at ameliorating these undesirable cognitive or affective states, coping by means of smoking will occur and will be experienced as rewarding by a smoker. It is not surprising, then, that those individuals who frequently experience cognitive and affective states that can be improved by smoking are more likely than others to find smoking to be a useful and reinforcing tool (and thus smoke more often).

Although smokers as a group report smoking to reduce negative affect; cope with stress; reduce weight or appetite; and enhance stimulation, cognitive performance, and pleasure, the relative importance of these smoking motivations vary across (and also within) smokers. Consistent with the coping model, those who are depression prone are more likely to say they smoke to reduce depressive moods and thoughts, whereas those with attentional problems say they smoke more often to enhance attention and, in turn, those who are prone to anxiety are more likely to say they smoke to alleviate anxiety. Similarly, individuals who are motivated to keep from gaining weight value the fact that smoking helps maintain a lower body weight. Thus, the motivations to smoke are to some extent consistent with personality traits of the smokers. This tendency to smoke for reasons related to personality traits is called trait-adaptive responding because smoking reflects an adaptive coping response related to the smoker's specific personality traits (see **Figure 1**).

Smoking/Nicotine as a Coping Response

Withdrawal alleviation As previously suggested, one theory proposes that smoking alleviates stress only to the extent that nicotine withdrawal is stressful to smokers. These withdrawal alleviation theories are supported by the simple fact that smokers find abstinence from smoking stressful and smoking alleviates this stress. A related theory suggests that smokers so come to associate withdrawal-induced stress with negative states that any negative state – whether during withdrawal or not – cues smoking behavior.

Although withdrawal alleviation models of smoking and stress are compelling, they cannot provide a complete picture of nicotine dependence. The withdrawal alleviation model suggests the stress of withdrawal is temporary; once withdrawal subsides the now-ex-smokers will return to their presmoking affective and cognitive states. Indeed, many studies have reported temporary increases in negative affect, stress, and difficulty concentrating following quitting that return to or improve beyond prequit levels in a matter of weeks. However, these studies have been limited by a number of factors that might preclude accurate characterization of withdrawal in smokers. First, because these studies do not take into account data of smokers who relapse (i.e., smokers for whom quitting is most difficult), the findings minimize the negative affect and distress the majority of

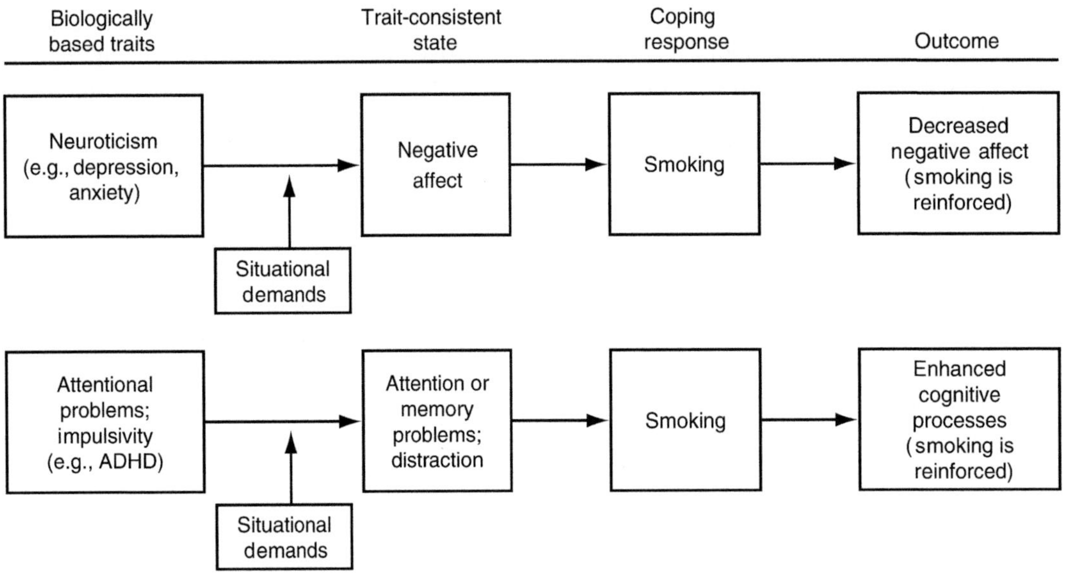

Figure 1 Biologically based traits increase the frequency and severity of trait-consistent states. To the extent that these states are improved by smoking/nicotine, smoking is reinforced.

smokers experience on quitting. Second, these studies have often not included a continuing-to-smoke control group, so other factors affecting mood and cognition, such as the passage of time, are also not accounted for.

When these two limitations are eliminated from research designs, a different picture of withdrawal emerges. Recent longitudinal studies that minimize relapse and include adequate control groups have observed transient increases in negative affect, stress, and difficulty concentrating that do not return to baseline levels, or the approximate levels of these symptoms in a continuing-to-smoke control group. These findings suggest that smokers may smoke, in part, to reduce underlying distressful cognitive and affective states that were present prior to becoming a smoker, which, on quitting smoking, are rerevealed. Thus, smokers may smoke in order to alleviate withdrawal symptoms to a degree, but also smoke in order to self-medicate underlying trait-based problems. It should be noted, however, that well-designed studies to date have accurately assessed the effects of quitting smoking on negative affect for only 45 days of abstinence. Thus, it is possible that after a longer period of time effects of quitting do resolve in most quitters.

Absolute inherent effects nicotine A growing body of research suggests that nicotine can, under specific situations, improve mood and cognitive performance, even in smokers who are only minimally deprived of nicotine or in nonsmokers. Laboratory studies show that smoking and other forms of nicotine delivery usually reduce negative moods and emotions in situations in which stressors are ambiguous and/or not dominant, such as situations in which an individual is anticipating experiencing stress. In contrast, when the context includes clear, immediate, and potent threat stimuli, negative moods are not impacted by smoking or nicotine.

Many experts and some experimental evidence suggest that nicotine can also indirectly promote positive affect and minimize negative affect in situations in which nicotine contributes to goal achievement. For example, when they need to concentrate for a long period of time to accomplish a goal, such as writing a paper, smokers say they smoke to sustain their concentration and thereby achieve their goal. Laboratory studies have also shown nicotine to facilitate cognitive functions, including vigilance and memory, in both habitual tobacco users and in individuals with no prior exposure to nicotine. In addition, other studies have shown that nicotine may improve affect and reduce stress by helping smokers focus on emotionally positive or neutral distractors. Research suggests that nicotine is especially effective at reducing stress when there is a substantial degree of choice as to whether or not to attend to stressful cues and when some of these nonstressful cues are emotionally positive.

A two-factor model of smoking A combined two-factor model proposes that smokers smoke in order to (1) prevent or alleviate withdrawal and (2) gain beneficial effects inherent in nicotine. Among heavy smokers, the acute effects of abstinence resolve across the first week or two of abstinence; thereafter, underlying psychological and pathological traits are rerevealed and greater stress, negative affect, and difficulty concentrating are experienced. Similarly, the attention and mood-enhancing effects of most habitually used stimulant drugs (caffeine, amphetamine, and cocaine) appear to reflect the combined influence of such inherent and withdrawal-alleviation mechanisms.

Habit, sensory aspects, and other factors Smokers may smoke for numerous reasons other than those already described. Many smokers find the sensory aspects of smoking pleasurable (e.g., the feel of smoke in lungs and the taste), and these sensory cues further reinforce smoking behavior. Further, many smokers, regardless of why they started smoking in the first place, may continue to smoke, largely out of habit. Finally, recent evidence suggests that nonnicotine chemicals in tobacco smoke may have anti-depressant qualities that may further ameliorate negative affect and reinforce smoking behavior.

Smoking Cessation, Stress, and Coping

Based on the empirical evidence showing that smoking cessation is frequently a stressful process resulting in more coping failures than successes, clinicians and researchers have spent much time and energy on minimizing smoking-cessation-related stress and maximizing coping.

Psychological and Behavioral Therapies for Smoking Cessation

Most of the widely used smoking cessation programs include several hours of skills training in cognitive and behavioral techniques designed to help the smoker cope not only with the cravings to smoke but also with negative mood states frequently associated with quitting and known to promote relapse to smoking. Such techniques include behavioral relaxation training and learning to think about stressful situations in a manner that is less likely to produce negative emotional states. Currently popular pharmacological treatments, such as nicotine gum, nicotine patches, and the antidepressant drug Zyban, also include a complex therapeutic package that includes behavioral relaxation and coping components, along with information about the cessation process and social support.

Antidepressant Medication Therapies for Smoking Cessation

Consistent with the view that smoking motivation and the effects of smoking cessation are mediated by brain mechanisms related to negative affect and depression, one antidepressant medication, Zyban, has been found to be beneficial in helping individuals maintain smoking abstinence. This U.S. Food and Drug Administration (FDA)-approved smoking-cessation drug is also marketed under a different brand name as an antidepressant medication.

The Psychobiology of Smoking, Coping, and Stress Diasthesis

During withdrawal from nicotine, smokers with depressive tendencies have been found to exhibit brain wave (via electroencephalogram, EEG) asymmetry profiles characteristic of depressed individuals. These abstinence-induced EEG asymmetries appear to last for at least a month after quitting. The EEG asymmetry seen in these individuals is a relatively greater EEG slowing of the left (compared to the right) frontal cortex subsequent to quitting. Left-hemisphere processing is associated with active coping, verbal behavior, and positive affect, whereas right-hemisphere processing is more associated with negative mood states and withdrawal. These and related findings suggest that nicotine may act as an antidepressant in part because in individuals prone to depression it tends to increase the activation more in the left than in the right frontal cortex. Overall, nicotine tends to increase brain activation as measured by EEG, whereas smoking abstinence tends to decrease EEG activity in both hemispheres, although to a greater extent in the left relative than in the right frontal cortex. This decrease in EEG activation corresponds to the sustained decrease in ability to concentrate also found to last for at least a month after quitting smoking.

The EEG-activating effects of smoking are thought to reflect the effects of nicotine on brain receptors for the neurotransmitter acetylcholine. Nicotine has the ability to stimulate cholinergic receptors throughout the body. The stimulation of these cholinergic receptors can result in a cascade of events, including increases in heart rate, blood pressure, blood cortisol concentrations and the activation of other neurotransmitter systems in the brain. Another important brain system influenced by nicotine uses dopamine as its neurotransmitter. Dopamine (DA) is associated with brain regions involved in attention, emotion, coping, and reward. DA is involved in coping in both positive and negative emotional states. Nicotine-induced increments in brain mesolimbic DA activity may increase the ability of the organism to avoid aversive stimuli and to obtain positive ones.

The effects of smoking on EEG, mood, and attention discussed so far have been found to be due primarily to the effects of nicotine; however, recent evidence suggests that an unidentified component of tobacco smoke (other than nicotine) inhibits monoamine oxidase (MAO) activity in the brain in the same manner as some antidepressant medications. Thus, it may be that some of smoking's antidepressant, mood-enhancing, and cognitive benefits come from the inhibition of MAO activity by something other than nicotine.

Summary

Environment, genetics, personality, and psychopathologic traits interact to determine smoker status and the type of smoker an individual becomes. Individuals genetically and otherwise predisposed to negative affect, sensation seeking, and/or suboptimal cognitive performance are more likely to be exposed to smoking environments, start smoking in order to seek negative affect relief or as an act of sensation seeking, and find smoking reinforcing. The widely held belief among smokers and nonsmokers that smoking reduces negative affect and enhances cognition leads predisposed individuals to experiment with smoking as a form of self-medication, to minimize negative affect, and to maximize cognitive functioning. The affect-modulating and cognitive-enhancing effects of nicotine are more reinforcing to those who need and value them the most – those in stressful circumstances and those with a vulnerability to cognitive and affective dysfunction. When individuals who are predisposed to smoking try to quit, they lose the beneficial effects of nicotine and are especially vulnerable to experiencing the cognitive or affective state to which they are predisposed. Thus, depression-prone individuals are more likely to become depressed, anxiety-prone individuals are more prone to anxiety, and attentionally disordered quitters are disposed to suffer more severe attention problems. The enhanced severity of cognitive and affective responses to quitting contributes to the failure of vulnerable individuals to maintain abstinence after efforts to quit smoking. Smoking in individuals who are vulnerable to smoking can thus be seen as an attempt to adapt to their situation by altering their cognitive and/or affective state.

However, affective and cognitive traits also alter the probability of smoking by more indirect mechanisms. Both affective and cognitive traits influence long-term goals by a number of indirect mechanisms. For example, risk-taking and other reward and sensation-seeking behaviors make certain individuals temperamentally insensitive to cues of potential punishment (e.g., health warnings about smoking) and promote cognitive, social, and behavioral sequences that reinforce smoking and other risk-taking behavior. The sensation-seeking life style, which includes smoking, drinking, and a focus on pleasure, may be so reinforcing to individuals with a strong genetic disposition that their cognitive motivational schemas include no plans to quit any risky behaviors. In contrast, negative-affect-prone individuals are likely to focus on the immediate relief of negative affect produced by smoking rather than on the long-term health consequences. Individuals who are more psychobiologically stable will see less benefit from smoking and be less inclined to take up or continue smoking because the perceived risks outweigh the perceived gains.

See Also the Following Articles

Alcohol, Alcoholism, and Stress: A Psychobiological Perspective; Comorbid Disorders and Stress; Drug Use and Abuse.

Further Reading

Comings, D. E., Ferry, L., Bradshaw-Robinson, S., et al. (1996). The dopamine D2 receptor (DRD2) gene: a genetic risk factor in smoking. *Pharmacogenetics* **6**, 73–79.

Gilbert, D. G. (1995). *Smoking: individual differences, psychopathology, and emotion.* Washington, DC: Taylor and Francis.

Gilbert, D. G. (1997). The situation x trait adaptive response (STAR) model of substance use and craving. *Human Psychopharmacology: Clinical and Experimental* **12**, S89–S102.

Gilbert, D. G., McClernon, F. J., Rabinovich, N. E., et al. (1998). Effects of smoking abstinence on mood and craving in men: influences of negative-affect-related personality traits, habitual nicotine intake, and repeated measurements. *Personality and Individual Differences* **25**, 399–423.

Gilbert, D. G., McClernon, F. J., Rabinovich, N. E., et al. (2002). Mood disturbance fails to resolve across 31 days of cigarette abstinence in women. *Journal of Consulting & Clinical Psychology* **70**, 142–152.

Gilbert, D. G., McClernon, F. J., Rabinovich, N. E., et al. (2004). Effects of quitting smoking on EEG activation and attention last for more than 31 days and are more severe with stress, dependence, DRD2 A1 allele, and depressive traits. *Nicotine & Tobacco Research* **6**, 249–267.

Kandel, D. B. and Davies, M. (1986). Adult sequelae of adolescent depressive symptoms. *Archives of General Psychiatry* **43**, 255–262.

Kassel, J. D. (1997). Smoking and attention: a review and reformulation of the stimulus-filter hypothesis. *Clinical Psychology Review* **17**, 451–478.
Kassel, J. D., Stroud, L. R. and Paronis, C. A. (2003). Smoking, stress, and negative affect: correlation, causation, and context across stages of smoking. *Psychological Bulletin* **129**, 270–304.
Kendler, K. S., Neale, M. C., MacLean, C. J., et al. (1993). Smoking and major depression: a causal analysis. *Archives of General Psychiatry* **50**, 36–43.
Levin, E. D., Conners, C. K., Sparrow, E., et al. (1996). Nicotine effects on adults with attention-deficit/hyperactivity disorder. *Psychopharmacology* **123**, 55–63.
Scarr, S. and McCartney, K. (1983). How people make their own environments: a theory of genotype x environment effects. *Child Development* **54**, 424–435.
Shiffman, S. A. (1986). Cluster analytic classification of smoking relapse episodes. *Addictive Behaviors* **11**, 295–307.

Drug Use and Abuse

J R Mantsch
Marquette University, Milwaukee, WI, USA

Glossary

Addiction A chronically relapsing neurobiological disease characterized by an inability to control drug use.

Craving An intense, consuming, and often uncontrollable desire to use a drug.

Neuroplasticity The ability of the brain to physically change in response to stimuli such as drugs.

Relapse The recurrence of drug use after a period of drug abstinence.

Withdrawal A broad range of adverse symptoms that emerge on the termination or reduction of drug use.

Stress and Drug Addiction

Drug addiction is a chronically relapsing condition that is characterized by an inability to self-regulate drug consumption. In an addicted individual, drug use is compulsive and occurs in spite of negative social, legal, financial, and medical consequences. Despite its prevalence and tremendous cost to society, little progress has been made in the development of effective addiction treatment strategies. One of the issues that makes addiction so difficult to treat is that not all addicts use drugs for exactly the same reasons. Thus, the factors that contribute to drug use by one individual may be quite different from those that underlie drug self-administration by another. In many individuals, drug use is a stress-driven behavior. This is especially problematic because the life of a drug addict is a particularly stressful one; even though many individuals initially turn to drugs in order to help them cope with stress, drug use by itself can generate and/or aggravate stress responses. The result of this circular relationship between stress and drug use appears to be a vicious cycle within which the onset of stress promotes drug use, which in turn generates more stress and therefore leads to further drug-seeking behavior. Breaking this self-perpetuating cycle by minimizing the influence of stress will probably provide a key to the successful treatment of many drug addicts.

People use drugs because of the effects that they have on the brain. Acutely, drugs produce their euphoric effects through the activation of the neural circuits that underlie natural reward. Such effects tend to offset the negative feelings typically associated with stress. With repeated drug exposure, changes in this neurocircuitry begin to emerge such that the brain of a drug addict is functionally different from that of a non-drug user or someone who only occasionally uses drugs. Significantly, when a drug is used repeatedly, the incentives and neurobiological events that drive drug use change such that the drug user enjoys the drug less but needs the drug more. These changes in brain function that emerge with repeated drug use are collectively referred to as neuroplasticity and appear to be long-lasting, if not permanent. The consequence of such long-lasting neuroplasticity is a diseaselike condition that is associated with a high risk for relapse in many individuals. For this reason, understanding how neuroplasticity that is pathogenic for addiction develops and is expressed is critical for the prevention and treatment of the condition. Similar to its role in the addiction cycle, the involvement of stress in addiction-related neuroplasticity is bidirectional. Stress promotes the onset of drug-induced neuroplasticity, the expression of which includes aggravated behavioral and hormonal stress responses.

Clinical Evidence

Clinical evidence for a role for stress in drug addiction is largely anecdotal and correlative. In general, stress is cited as a causative factor for drug use, and the inability to effectively cope with stress is predictive of drug relapse. In addition, there is a high incidence of stress-related comorbidity, including posttraumatic stress disorder (PTSD), panic attacks, and depression in drug-dependent populations. For example, it has been reported that up to 43% of cocaine-dependent individuals meet the *Diagnostic and Statistical Manual of Mental Disorders* (3rd edn. rev.; DSM III-R) criteria for lifetime PTSD. In one study, 95.5% of subjects with concurrent PTSD and cocaine dependence reported a functional relationship between cocaine use and their PTSD symptoms, with 86.4% indicating that their PTSD symptoms worsened with drug use.

More direct evidence that stress can lead to drug use is provided by clinical laboratory studies demonstrating that the personalized stress imagery scripts can increase subjective measures of craving for cocaine and alcohol in recovering addicts. In fact, these studies have shown that scripts describing stressful events can be just as effective at eliciting drug craving as scripts describing actual drug use. The ability to directly assess stress-induced craving in human addicts within a laboratory setting should provide a useful tool for testing the effectiveness of novel treatment approaches aimed at preventing stressor-induced drug use.

Animal Studies

The study of drug abuse has relied heavily on preclinical animal research. In particular, drug self-administration procedures in which rats are surgically implanted with intravenous catheters and required to perform a behavioral task, such as pressing a response lever, in order to receive drug infusions have been valuable for the preclinical study of drug abuse and addiction. The validity of such procedures arises from the observation that, with few exceptions, drugs that are abused by humans are also self-administered by rats. Variations of the self-administration procedure have been used to define a role for stress in different aspects of the addiction process. In particular, research has focused on the effects of stressors on the acquisition, escalation, and reinstatement of drug-seeking behavior. A brief summary of this research is provided next.

Acquisition

Not everyone who tries a drug for the first time will like it and will start using the drug on a regular basis. Individual differences in initial responsiveness to drugs exist and can be influenced by a number of variables. Some individuals are genetically predisposed toward drug abuse, whereas others are influenced by environmental factors such as stress. It is likely that for many, individual susceptibility to addiction arises from a complex interplay among genes, drug effects, and environment such that the genetic potential for addiction is realized only if the drug is used in the wrong environmental context.

Preclinically, factors that increase the likelihood that drug use will be initiated can be studied using acquisition self-administration models in which predisposition to engage in drug use is defined according to how readily drug-naïve subjects acquire the behavior of drug self-administration. Using such models, it has been reported that a variety of stressful stimuli ranging from very basic stressors (such as repeated tail pinch) to more complex stressors (such as social defeat) facilitate the acquisition of drug self-administration by rats. These effects of stress do not appear to be short-lived. In fact, it has been reported that when rats are exposed to a stressor during the first weeks of life (e.g., daily isolation) more rapid acquisition of drug self-administration can be observed months later during adulthood, suggesting that the onset of stress, especially at critical phases of life, may permanently increase individual susceptibility to drug addiction. Interestingly, it is not just stress but the ability to control stress that is important for its effects on acquisition. Rats exposed to electric foot-shock stress acquire cocaine self-administration at lower dose than nonshocked controls when they are unable to control shock delivery but not when the same amount of shock is delivered under response-contingent conditions. These findings parallel clinical reports that it is not the onset of stress *per se* that predicts drug use but rather the coping strategy that is used when an individual is confronted with a stressor. Understanding how stress serves as a determinant of the initiation of drug use will permit the identification of populations that are at risk for addiction and should aid efforts to prevent drug abuse.

Escalation

Just because someone uses a drug regularly does not mean that that person is addicted. It is the loss of control over drug use and its negative impact on other facets of a drug user's life that define addiction. This aspect of drug addiction has been studied using rodent drug self-administration models in which progressively escalating patterns of drug intake emerge when daily access to a drug is prolonged. The onset of escalating use patterns is thought to reflect the transition from controlled drug use to out-of-control drug addiction. For this reason, further characterization of the variables that promote escalating self-administration patterns in rodents should provide insight into factors that accelerate the onset of drug addiction. Recently, our laboratory has begun to examine the impact of chronic stress delivered across an extended period of ongoing cocaine self-administration. To date, our studies have shown that exposure to stress at the time of daily cocaine self-administration progressively escalates drug intake over a 14-day period, suggesting that, like prior exposure to cocaine, repeated stress can accelerate the onset of addiction. Significantly, these findings imply that in addition to acutely generating drug use, stress can aggravate addiction by promoting drug-induced neuroplasticity.

Reinstatement

In drug addicts, craving, or the intense desire to use a drug, typically precedes drug use. The onset of craving is often unpredictable and can suddenly occur even after months or years of drug abstinence, making it a formidable obstacle to the effective long-term management of drug addiction. Drug craving can be studied preclinically using reinstatement self-administration procedures in which the abilities of various stimuli to reinstate extinguished drug-seeking behavior are examined. With these procedures, drug self-administration is extinguished by replacing the drug with an inert substance. As a result, responding previously maintained by presentation of the drug declines. The restoration or reinstatement of extinguished behavior under various experimental stimuli is thought to reflect the onset of craving for that drug and therefore can be used to identify the risk factors for drug relapse. Using such procedures, it has been demonstrated that acute exposure to stressors can reinstate responding previously reinforced by a variety of abused drugs including cocaine, ethanol, heroin, and nicotine without increasing responding not previously associated with drug delivery. These findings parallel those from clinical studies showing that subjective stress imagery can increase measures of drug craving in recovering addicts and suggest that the inclusion of pharmacological and behavioral strategies aimed at reducing stress during drug abstinence is probably critical to the success of any addiction treatment program.

Effects of Drug Abuse on Stress Responses

In addition to acting as a causative factor for drug-seeking behavior, stress also emerges as a consequence of drug use. It is well known that for most drugs of abuse, intense stress and anxiety are prominent features of acute drug withdrawal. In animal studies, these withdrawal symptoms can be observed as exaggerated anxiety-like behaviors measured using a variety of behavioral tests following withdrawal from repeated drug exposure. Significantly, altered anxiety responses appear to persist long after other acute withdrawal symptoms dissipate. These augmented anxiety-like responses during late withdrawal probably translate into increased susceptibility to drug relapse during periods of stress. One way to examine the effects of prior drug use on relapse is to compare stressor-induced reinstatement during withdrawal in rats with different histories of drug exposure. When rats have a history of self-administering greater amounts of drug, they also display higher levels of reinstatement in response to stress, suggesting that the amount of prior drug use can alter responsiveness to stress in a way that contributes to further drug-seeking behavior. These findings are paralleled by the results of clinical studies showing that stress-induced cravings, anxiety, and physiological responses in abstinent cocaine users are augmented in individuals with a history of high-frequency cocaine use compared to individuals with a history of using the drug less frequently. Our own data indicate that the behavioral responses to stressors are not simply exaggerated as a consequence of drug self-administration but, rather, are qualitatively different such that rats with a history of cocaine self-administration appear to be more assertive when confronted with a stressful situation, possibly reflecting a maladaptive coping strategy during stress that may result from drug use.

Neurobiological Mechanisms

Like all factors that influence drug-seeking behavior, stressors exert their effects on drug use by altering the activity of the neurobiological systems within the brain that underlie motivated behavior. In particular, a critical role for a pathway in the brain consisting of nerve projections from the medial prefrontal cortex that release the amino acid neurotransmitter glutamate into the nucleus accumbens has been identified for drug-seeking behavior. This neural subcircuit is closely modulated by the neurotransmitter dopamine, released from nerves that originate in the ventral tegmental area (VTA) of the midbrain. Like other stimuli that acutely generate drug use, stress provokes drug-seeking behavior through the activation of this pathway. The mechanism through which this activation occurs during stress is not entirely clear, but it appears to require the stimulation of dopaminergic neurons in the VTA that project to the medial prefrontal cortex and almost certainly involves the neuropeptide corticotropin releasing hormone (CRH). Significantly, stress can intensify the responsiveness of this motivational pathway to subsequent stimulation by inducing a form of cellular neuroplasticity in dopaminergic cells in the VTA called long-term potentiation (LTP), thereby increasing vulnerability to the effects of abused drugs.

Corticotropin Releasing Hormone

In addition to its role as an initiator of the hormonal stress response through its actions in the pituitary gland, CRH exerts its effects within the brain, where it functions as a neuropeptide mediator of stress-related behavioral responses and anxiety. CRH administered directly into a number of brain regions, including the VTA, reinstates extinguished drug-seeking behavior, whereas CRH antagonists prevent stress-induced reinstatement. The exact mechanism through which CRH stimulates dopamine cells in the VTA is unclear, but it appears to require the association of CRH with its binding protein and the activation of a specific subtype of the CRH receptor, the CRH_2 receptor, which in turn facilitates cellular activation by the neurotransmitter glutamate. The likely role for CRH as a mediator of stress-induced drug-seeking behavior makes the peptide an obvious target for the development of pharmacotherapy aimed at promoting drug abstinence by preventing relapse during periods of stress. Although promising, clinical evaluation of the usefulness of drugs that interfere with the actions of CRH awaits the availability of selective nonpeptide CRH-receptor-blocking drugs that can readily penetrate the blood–brain barrier to reach sites of CRH action in the brain.

Glucocorticoids

Although the ability of acute stress to precipitate drug craving and use is problematic for addicts, it is chronic stress that can have an especially deleterious impact on the addiction process by producing or facilitating neuroplasticity that is pathogenic for addiction. Whereas the acute effects of stress on drug-seeking behavior appear to be mediated primarily through the actions of CRH in the brain, many of the effects of chronic stress on drug use appear to involve the release of glucocorticoid hormones from the adrenal gland. Glucocorticoids (such as cortisol in humans and corticosterone in rats) are critical mediators of the physiological and behavioral responses that enable an organism to adapt to and cope with stress. Such responses are beneficial for short-term adaptation to stressful stimuli, but, with constant activation, they can be detrimental to an organism, a consequence of chronic stress referred to as allostatic load. These allostatic effects appear to include adaptations in the motivational neurocircuitry of the brain that promote illicit drug use. Although glucocorticoids alone are capable of producing addiction-related neuroplasticity, it appears that in many cases these hormones work in concert with other stress-related molecules such as CRH to influence the addiction process. It is likely that many such interactions occur in the VTA, where stressor-induced neuroplasticity involving dopamine cells appears to be mediated by CRH and may require glucocorticoid receptor activation. Further research is needed to determine whether glucocorticoids and their receptors are viable targets for the pharmacotherapeutic management of drug addiction. A summary of one putative neurobiological

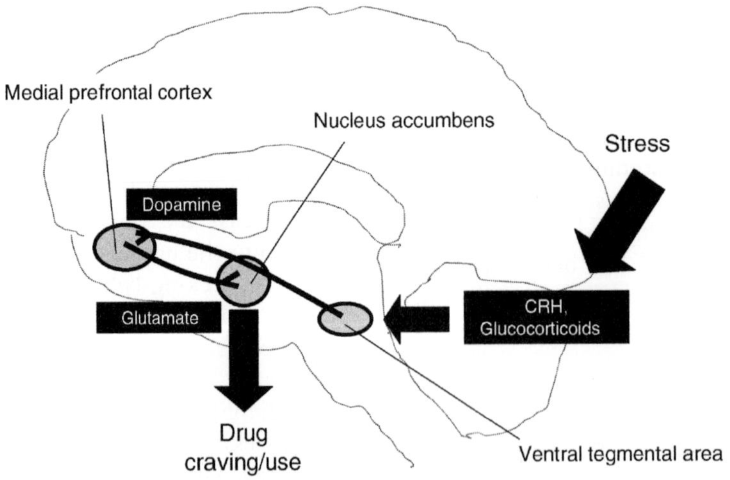

Figure 1 One putative neurobiological pathway through which stressful stimuli may influence drug-seeking behavior and addiction. The results of recent animal studies indicate that stressful stimuli increase brain corticotropin releasing hormone (CRH) levels, which, in concert with elevated glucocorticoids, exert effects on cells in the ventral tegmental area of the brain to increase dopaminergic neurotransmission in the medial prefrontal cortex and nucleus accumbens and facilitate the activity of neurocircuitry that underlies motivation and natural reward.

pathway through which stress influences drug-seeking behavior is provided in **Figure 1**.

Treatment Implications

The recognition that stress is a key contributor to drug abuse and addiction should highlight the need for the development and implementation of novel therapeutic strategies aimed at minimizing the contribution of stress to the addiction process, especially in subpopulations of addicts whose drug use is stress-driven. Identifying which addicts will benefit most from such approaches poses a challenge to drug-dependence treatment providers and will probably require the establishment of new assessment tools that permit the determination of the role of stress in drug use on an individual basis. Although available, cognitive and behavioral therapies aimed at helping recovering addicts manage their stress are underused and understudied. Further, many drugs that are traditionally used for the treatment of stress-related psychiatric conditions (e.g., antidepressants and benzodiazepines) are not commonly prescribed to treat addiction and, in many cases, are avoided even though they may be beneficial if used properly in the right individuals. The eventual development and approval of new drugs that block the actions of CRH in the brain will, it is hoped, provide important tools for the management of drug addiction. At the same time, basic preclinical research must continue to examine the neurobiological mechanisms through which stress influences drug addiction so that new targets (e.g., the orexins/hypocretins) can be discovered and more effective drugs can be developed.

See Also the Following Articles

Alcohol, Alcoholism, and Stress: A Psychobiological Perspective; Interactions Between Stress and Drugs of Abuse.

Further Reading

Back, S. E., Brady, K. T., Jaanimagi, U., et al. (2006). Cocaine dependence and PTSD: a pilot study of symptom interplay and treatment preferences. *Addictive Behaviors* **31**, 351–354.

Breese, G. R., Chu, K., Dayas, C. V., et al. (2005). Stress enhancement of craving during sobriety: a risk for relapse. *Alcoholism: Clinical and Experimental Research* **29**, 185–195.

Fox, H. C., Talih, M., Malison, R., et al. (2005). Frequency of recent cocaine and alcohol use affects drug craving and associated responses to stress and drug-related cues. *Psychoneuroendocrinology* **30**, 880–891.

Goeders, N. E. (2002). Stress and cocaine addiction. *Journal of Pharmacology and Experimental Therapeutics* **301**, 785–789.

Kalivas, P. W. and McFarland, K. (2003). Brain circuitry and the reinstatement of cocaine-seeking behavior. *Psychopharmacology* **168**, 44–56.

Koob, G. F., Ahmed, S. H., Boutrel, B. P., et al. (2004). Neurobiological mechanisms in the transition from drug use to drug dependence. *Neuroscience and Biobehavioral Reviews* **27**, 739–749.

Kreek, M. J., Nielsen, D. A., Butelman, E. R., et al. (2005). Genetic influences on impulsivity, risk taking, stress responsivity and vulnerability to drug abuse and addiction. *Nature Neuroscience* **8**, 1450–1457.

Marinelli, M. and Piazza, P. V. (2002). Interaction between glucocorticoid hormones, stress and psychostimulant drugs. *European Journal of Neuroscience* **16**, 387–394.

Saal, D., Dong, Y., Bonci, A., et al. (2003). Drugs of abuse and stress trigger a common synaptic adaptation in dopamine neurons. *Neuron* **37**, 577–582.

Sarnyai, Z., Shaham, Y. and Heinrichs, S. C. (2001). The role of corticotropin-releasing factor in drug addiction. *Pharmacological Reviews* **53**, 209–243.

Shalev, U., Grimm, J. W. and Shaham, Y. (2002). Neurobiology of relapse to heroin and cocaine seeking: a review. *Pharmacological Reviews* **54**, 1–42.

Sinha, R. (2001). How does stress increase risk of drug abuse and relapse? *Psychopharmacology* **158**, 343–359.

Vocci, F. J., Acri, J. and Elkashef, A. (2005). Medication development for addictive disorders: the state of the science. *American Journal of Psychiatry* **162**, 1432–1440.

Volkow, N. D. and Li, T. K. (2004). Drug addiction: the neurobiology of behaviour gone awry. *Nature Reviews Neuroscience* **5**, 963–970.

Wang, B., Shaham, Y., Zitzman, D., et al. (2005). Cocaine experience establishes control of midbrain glutamate and dopamine by corticotropin-releasing factor: a role in stress-induced relapse to drug seeking. *Journal of Neuroscience* **25**, 5389–5396.

Comorbid Disorders and Stress

S Sundram
Mental Health Research Institute of Victoria, Northern Psychiatry Research Centre, and University of Melbourne, Melbourne, Australia
Avril Pereira
Mental Health Research Institute of Victoria, Melbourne, Australia

Glossary

Comorbidity	The concurrence within the one individual of a substance use disorder and another psychiatric disorder.
Dopamine	A catecholamine neurotransmitter central to reward processes and psychiatric disorders.
Mesolimbic dopamine pathway	The trajectory within the brain of dopamine-releasing neurons from the ventral tegmental area to the nucleus accumbens, amygdala, hippocampus, and other related regions.
Nucleus accumbens	A brain region rich in dopamine neurons and believed to integrate reward responses and to be affected in substance use disorders.
Substance-use disorder (SUD)	The repeated uncontrolled use of a substance resulting in deleterious health and social outcomes; there are two forms, dependence and the less severe abuse.

Introduction

Comorbidity simply refers to the concurrent presence of two or more discrete disorders in the one individual. In psychiatry, it refers to at least one disorder being a recognizable *Diagnostic and Statistical Manual for Mental Disorders* (4th edn.; DSM-IV) or *International Classification of Diseases* (10th edn.; ICD-10) diagnosis and the second or subsequent disorders being either a physical medical illness or another psychiatric disorder. Commonly, however, the second disorder is substance-related, and it is in this context that comorbidity (also referred to as dual diagnosis) is discussed here.

Substance-related disorder refers to the consumption of a substance by an individual resulting in deleterious health, social, or psychological outcomes. This definition allows the exclusion of substance use within culturally determined or religious domains and the recognition that some substance use may not necessarily be harmful depending on the substance and volume of use. Nevertheless, this definition encompasses a broad and heterogeneous group of disorders that can be applied to any particular substance. These disorders can be classified into disorders induced by the substance and disorders of the regulation of substance use. The first category includes intoxication, withdrawal, and those disorders that mimic other psychiatric disorders: deliriums of intoxication and withdrawal; dementia; amnestic, psychotic, mood, anxiety, and sleep disorders; and sexual dysfunction. The second category incorporates dependence and abuse. Dependence, which is considered more severe than abuse, comprises three or more of the following: tolerance (needing an increased amount of the substance for the equivalent effect or a diminished effect with same amount), withdrawal (physiological response to the reduction of substance use), prolonged or excessive ingestion, unfulfilled desire to reduce use, excessive time spent on substance use to the detriment of other activities, and use in spite of deleterious health effects. Abuse emphasizes the persistent use of the substance in the face of work, social, or forensic problems when the criteria for dependence are not met.

Commonly used substances include alcohol, caffeine, nicotine, cannabis, amphetamines, opioids, cocaine, hallucinogens, phencyclidine and ketamine, inhalants, and benzodiazepines; most commonly the use of more than one substance (polysubstance use) is observed. The pattern of substance use generally follows social criteria so that legal substances, such as alcohol, nicotine, and caffeine are most widely used, followed by decriminalized substances, and then by the most readily available illicit substances. For example, alcohol-use disorders are relatively less common in religious and social groups that prohibit its use.

When we combine these lists of disorders and substances, a large number of permutations for substance-related disorders is possible. All substances must induce intoxication; however, not every substance causes every other disorder. This is dependent on its individual pharmacodynamic and pharmacokinetic properties and, thus, it is critical to emphasize the differences in the individual behavioral and neurobiological effects of each substance and their interaction with other psychiatric disorders. For example the sedating and myorelaxant properties of benzodiazepines contrast with the stimulating effects of amphetamine.

Given that comorbidity refers to coexisting but discrete disorders, the relationship between the disordered regulation of substance use and other psychiatric disorders and stress is of primary relevance here; SUD is used here to refer to disorders of substance-use regulation, namely dependence and abuse. This article outlines the observed relationships between SUD and other psychiatric disorders. It discusses the possible nature of these relationships with reference to the role of stress and details this in reference to major depression because of the well-documented effect of stress on relapses of both SUD and major depression.

Prevalence of Comorbidity

The lifetime prevalence of SUD in the general community has been estimated to be 16.7% (excluding nicotine and caffeine); the 12-month prevalence figures for any mental disorder is 26.2%. Thus, even if no relationship existed between the two clusters, comorbidity would be predicted to be 4% by chance alone. The reality is, however, that approximately 76% of men and 65% of women with SUD also have an additional psychiatric diagnosis, most commonly that of another SUD. Other, non-SUD psychiatric diagnoses also occur at rates greater than in the general community, and the reciprocal relationship is also true, suggesting that the two clusters of disorders are not independent. This high rate of comorbidity needs to be considered within the context of the various methods of ascertainment used (retrospective or prospective, structured interview, self-report, or caregiver report), the diagnostic systems used (DSM-III, DSM-III-R, DSM-IV, or ICD-10), and the sample populations (urban or rural; and psychiatric inpatient, outpatient, general community, drug treatment program, or correctional facility). This limits the extent to which studies may be compared across regions or over time. Given the diversity of substances and co-occurring disorders, the prevalence of comorbidity inevitably differs by diagnostic classification. Notwithstanding this, the incidence of comorbidity appears to have increased over the past 2 decades. In 1980 the United States National Center for Health Statistics reported that 12% of psychiatric inpatients treated that year had a SUD in addition to a non-substance-use psychiatric disorder. A decade later, the Epidemiological Catchment Area (ECA) study recorded that 48% of individuals with schizophrenia had a lifetime diagnosis of SUD. Subsequent estimates of the prevalence of such comorbidity range from 35 to 53% in community and inpatient settings, respectively. It is noteworthy that epidemiological surveys that estimate the lifetime and 12-month prevalence of psychiatric disorders in the general population such as the 1990–1992 National Comorbidity Survey (NCS) and the 2001–2003 NCS-2 and NCS-Replication have enabled the analysis of comorbidity rates unbiased by sample selections of affected individuals. These surveys, however, are also limited in that they underrepresent several population segments such as the homeless or those in institutions. The examination of the so-called low-prevalence psychotic disorders is also excluded. It is unsurprising, therefore, that prevalence estimates of comorbidity from community population surveys are generally lower than seen in clinical settings.

Substances

Unfortunately, unraveling comorbidity is complicated by polysubstance use, particularly of alcohol with other drugs. According to the NCS, 78% of alcohol-dependent men and 86% of women met the criteria for a lifetime diagnosis of another psychiatric disorder, including drug dependence. Furthermore, although demographic characteristics such as male gender, younger age, less education, history of incarceration, and symptoms of conduct disorder and antisocial personality disorder predict substance misuse, these are not consistently associated with the types of substances misused. For example, age is related to lifetime prevalence of cannabis and cocaine but not alcohol-use disorder. In addition, attempts to find demographic or clinical correlates related to the order of onset of substance use and psychiatric disorders have not detected consistent differences to demonstrate a causal relationship. A key point to note is that no psychiatric diagnosis is exclusively related to a specific type of SUD.

Alcohol

Consistent across several studies, alcohol is the most commonly abused substance (when nicotine and caffeine are not measured), followed by cannabis. Among individuals with psychotic illnesses, approximately 39% of men and 17% of women had a lifetime diagnosis of alcohol abuse or dependence compared with a 12-month prevalence in the general population of 9% and 4%, respectively (National Survey of Mental Health and Well-being). These data concur with the ECA study, which found that 47% of those with schizophrenia spectrum disorders met the criteria for at least one comorbid SUD (34% for alcohol, 28% for any drug use disorder). A high rate of alcohol comorbidity with affective illness is also described with adverse outcomes of mood destabilization and induction of depressive or manic episodes. In their 1990 review of studies on hospitalized alcoholics, Merikangas and Gelernter found that depressive symptomatology ranged from 16 to 59% and that this met a diagnosis of secondary major depression in 8–53% of cases. Although there is a consensus that a high comorbidity of alcohol abuse/dependence and depression occurs in clinical samples, there is far less agreement concerning the nature or direction (primary or secondary) of this relationship. This distinction is necessary in determining whether alcohol misuse and depression are different symptomatic expressions of a common dysfunctional neurobiological substrate or whether one condition induces the other. In contrast, alcohol abuse is also frequently comorbid with bipolar disorder and posttraumatic stress disorder, but in these cases it is usually temporally secondary.

Nicotine

In the case of nicotine, investigation of a subset of NCS participants found that psychiatric disorders predicted an increased risk for the first onset of daily smoking and subsequent nicotine dependence. Most notable are people with schizophrenia, who have smoking rates of between 70 and 90% (compared to approximately 25% for the general population), resulting in excess morbidity and mortality in this group. As well, nicotine dependence is twice as prevalent in patients with mood, anxiety, or personality disorders than in the general population. The reasons for this increased rate of use include self-medication to ameliorate the symptoms of the disorder or the side-effects of treatment.

Conversely, it has also been proposed that daily smoking is a causal factor in panic disorder and agoraphobia, conditions that for some individuals may be relieved by smoking cessation. Of interest also are data on twins centered on the familial aggregation of smoking and depression, indicating common or shared genes as a source of this association. Defining the interaction between genes and environment in such comorbidity is important in understanding why increased risk for substance use occurs.

Illicit Drugs

The risk relationship between illicit substance use and other psychiatric disorder appears to be reciprocal, with one predicting the increased likelihood of the other. Moreover, approximately one in five people report the use of more than one illicit drug. The substances most frequently misused include cannabis, amphetamines, opioids (heroin), cocaine, hallucinogens, ecstasy or MDMA (N-methyl-3,4-methylenedioxy-methamphetamine), and benzodiazepines (nonprescribed use). As may be anticipated, individuals with multiple dependencies experience the highest rates of psychiatric comorbidity. Most psychiatric illnesses including psychotic, mood, anxiety, or alcohol-use disorders are often comorbid with illicit SUDs. In such psychiatric cohorts, gender differences in drug use are commonly substance-type-specific. For example, men are twice more likely than women to meet the criteria for cannabis abuse or dependence; however, in cocaine and opioid abusers, the numbers are generally similar between the sexes. It is also prudent to highlight that differences in the availability of illicit drugs in the study location may explain the data gathered. Thus, whereas cocaine is the illicit drug most commonly used by incarcerated women in the United States, cannabis, opioids, and benzodiazepines were most frequently used in an Australian cohort.

Etiological Theories

Each class of abused drugs is chemically diverse and produces effects through actions at different specific cellular and molecular targets within the brain; nevertheless, the pathways underlying reward and dependence are thought to be similar. The common mode of action involves all drugs of abuse releasing dopamine, either directly or indirectly, within the shell of the nucleus accumbens. This dopamine is released from neurons that originate in the ventral tegmental area (VTA) and terminate in the nucleus accumbens, amygdala, the bed nucleus of the stria terminalis, and other regions and are termed the mesolimbic dopamine projection. This is thought to be the path for all natural rewards such as food and sex and also for other nondrug rewards such as gambling. However, repeated drug use that results in drug dependence is more complex than simple changes in extracellular dopamine or receptor sensitivity. Drug dependence comprises a number of aspects including the need for the drug, the motivation to use it, the reward or pleasurable aspect of the use, and the relief from withdrawal symptoms. The brain regions and neurochemical pathways underpinning these distinct behavioral processes differ and are not fully elucidated, although they are considered to be similar between drugs of abuse. How these pathways are involved with the manifestation of other psychiatric disorders and how the pathologies of both sets of disorders may interact and be modulated by stress are poorly understood. Hence, although there is convincing epidemiological evidence linking psychiatric disorder and SUDs and stress, direct biological evidence explaining this association is limited. Several competing theories have been proposed to explain this high co-occurrence.

Common Factor Models

Common factor models posit that comorbidity is the result of shared vulnerability to both disorders. Specific factors can independently increase the risk of developing both disorders and thus the increased comorbidity is explained. For example, common genetic predisposition may underlie both the index and the comorbid condition. Other possible common factors include social class of rearing, family disruption, cognitive functioning, and exposure to an environmental toxin (e.g., lead).

Genetics There is clear evidence that genetic factors play a role in both most major psychiatric disorders, including schizophrenia, bipolar disorder, and major depression, and in SUDs. The question is whether genetics contributes to comorbidity. Studies have shown that comorbid patients are more likely to have relatives with a SUD than patients without a dual diagnosis; however, this does not imply linked genetic factors. An alternative question is whether genetic vulnerability to one disorder increases the risk of exposure to the other disorder. Data addressing this point indicate that the genetic risk of schizophrenia is not associated with an increased risk of SUD in relatives, or vice versa. Such findings suggest that shared genetic factors do not explain the increased rates of comorbid substance use in schizophrenia. This conclusion is also supported by twin studies on the inheritability of schizophrenia and alcoholism, in which the rates of the disorders between monozygotic and dizygotic twins were compared and no correlation was found. A 2003 large multivariate modeling study using same-sex twins demonstrated that common genetic factors for SUDs loaded with adult antisocial behavior and conduct disorder but not with internalizing disorders such as major depression and anxiety disorders. These data contribute to dispelling notions of a common shared genetic vulnerability but not of disorder-specific interactions. Consequently, although there may be some genetic contribution to comorbidity, the problem remains of identifying which factors are inherited and how they interact with other personal traits and facets of the environment to elevate risk.

Secondary Substance Disorder Models

Several models postulate that psychiatric illness increases the vulnerability of a patient to developing a SUD. These models are broadly characterized into two types: the self-medication model and the supersensitivity model.

Self-Medication Model Self-medication denotes that individuals use specific substances to attenuate adverse states caused either by their psychiatric disorder or by its treatment. The underlying assumption is that substances are used in a selective manner based on their distinct pharmacological effects. Examples of symptom alleviation include the use of nicotine by people with schizophrenia to normalize deficits in sensory processing (attention) or the use of stimulant drugs (amphetamines and cocaine) by depressed patients to counter anergic symptoms (lack of energy and amotivation). An example of substance use mitigating the side-effects of psychotropic medications is nicotine relieving the extrapyramidal motor and dysphoric side-effects induced by antipsychotic medication; it is proposed that it releases dopamine to ameliorate the dopamine D2 receptor blockade induced by the medication. As intuitively appealing as the self-medication hypothesis is, the evidence is not supportive. First, much substance use, especially cigarette smoking, precedes the first symptoms of the psychiatric disorder, let alone the first treatment. Second, the factors most consistently associated with substance use in psychiatric patients, such as availability, cost, compliance with the peer group, facilitation of social interaction, intoxication, and relaxation, are the same as that observed in the general community. Similarly, patients seldom report self-medication as a reason for substance use. Finally, the choice of substance does not appear to be related to the psychiatric diagnosis or type or severity of symptoms.

The Supersensitivity Model This model contends that a combination of genetic and early environmental (pre- or postnatal) events interact with an environmental stressor to precipitate the onset or relapse of a psychiatric disorder in a vulnerable individual, where vulnerability is defined as a compromised biological sensitivity to stress. Therefore, whereas psychotropic medications can be protective or decrease vulnerability, substance abuse may increase it. This sensitivity may then make psychiatric patients more likely to experience negative consequences from using even small amounts of the substance. The assertion is that these negative outcomes of substance use, rather than the use itself, is what differentiates comorbid patients from the general population. Hence, given a similar volume of use, a greater proportion of people with psychiatric disorders will present with problematic use. Various observations provide support for this model, including the lesser amounts of substance used by comorbid patients, induction of clinical symptoms by low-dose drug (amphetamine) challenge tests, and negative effects such as relapse following the administration of small quantities of the substance. Similarly, a longitudinal examination of the course of drinking alcohol in a psychiatric cohort found that fewer than 5% were able to sustain symptom-free drinking over time without negative consequences, compared to approximately 50% within the general population.

Secondary Psychiatric Disorder Model

This model posits that the SUD induces the psychiatric disorder, based on observations of the psychotogenic effects of drugs such as stimulants (amphetamines and cocaine), hallucinogens (lysergic acid diethylamide), and cannabis and the depressive effects of alcohol. However, the complex interaction of neurobiological and psychosocial factors that underlie each disorder often makes the assignment of causality in this direction difficult.

Comorbidity between schizophrenia and cannabis use illustrates this point. Cannabis may induce a transient psychotic state characterized by hallucinations and agitation that may be difficult to differentiate from a primary psychotic disorder. Further, cannabis use commonly precedes the onset of schizophrenia. Trying to determine the issue of causality, however, is hard given that the available evidence is largely based on epidemiological studies. A 2002 meta-analysis concluded that cannabis use accounted for approximately 8% of the attributable risk for developing schizophrenia. This may account for the anecdotal clinical observations of cannabis causing schizophrenia and the conflicting prevalence data that frequently show no relation between the two disorders.

With respect to alcohol use and depression, the notion is that alcohol increases the risk and severity of depression, although no causal association has been established. This is complicated by the general observation that alcohol abuse and dependence develops after the onset of bipolar disorder, again emphasizing the need to carefully differentiate particular disorders and their comorbidity.

Bidirectional Models

Bidirectional models suggest interactional effects between psychiatric and SUDs that account for the high co-occurrence rates. For example, a SUD could trigger a psychiatric illness in a vulnerable individual, which is maintained by continued substance use due to cognitive factors, social conditioning, beliefs, and motivations. Despite evidence that substance misuse worsens the course of psychiatric illness, these postulates, although highly plausible, remain largely theoretical and untested.

Comorbidity and Stress

An extension of causal explanations for the co-occurrence of psychiatric and SUDs incorporates stress as central to the genesis and perpetuation of the comorbid state. It should be noted that the role of stress has already been well established independently in both SUDs and other psychiatric disorders. This is based on increasing evidence that these disorders are associated with maladaptive neurobiological changes in brain stress circuits that principally comprise the hypothalamic-pituitary-adrenal (HPA) axis, corticotropin releasing hormone (CRH), and noradrenergic systems. The primary stress mediators of this endocrine system include the glucocorticoids (adrenal steroids such as cortisol) and catecholamines (dopamine, norepinephrine, and epinephrine), which in the short term are vital for the adaptation and maintenance of homeostasis but which can act detrimentally with repeated long-term release. As previously mentioned, chronic drug use is linked with neuroadaptations in the brain reward pathways, predominantly involving mesolimbic dopamine projections. One possible mechanism of interaction could be that stress activation of the HPA axis causes the release of glucocorticoids that interact with mesolimbic dopamine release and stimulate neuronal pathways implicated in substance misuse. Neuroadaptations in stress and reward circuits may, accordingly, underlie the adverse states often associated with psychiatric disorders and SUDs. It is feasible therefore that common mechanisms influencing stress, motivation, and behavior may contribute to comorbidity.

Data indicate that stress plays a role in the development and relapse of comorbid disorders. For instance, high levels of exposure to adversity or stressful events have been causally related to the onset of depressive and anxiety disorders. Similarly, stressors may facilitate substance misuse by increasing the reinforcing efficacy of substances that ameliorate the anxiety and dysphoric symptoms induced by stress. Further support is obtained from animal studies in which stress can induce drug self-administration, increase the sensitivity to the reinforcing effects of drugs, and precipitate the reinstatement or relapse of substance use even after prolonged periods of withdrawal. Hence, from a theoretical perspective, stress has been proposed as a factor that links psychiatric disorders and SUDs. This model postulates that a chronic distress state due to repeated stress exposure underlies the severity of psychiatric symptoms and substance use. This adverse state is then associated with maladaptive responses such as drug use in order to maintain homeostasis. Maladaptive responses may, in turn, alter HPA or CRH circuits and various neurotransmitter systems to induce substance craving and poor behavioral or coping strategies, causing neuroadaptations in the brain stress and reward pathways. Increased drug use to levels characteristic of dependence leads to further changes in these circuits. Such alterations thereby promote the susceptibility to recurrent stress exposure in comorbid individuals. Supporting this paradigm is the notion that various genetic and environmental vulnerability factors (such as family history and social influences, individual differences in responsiveness to substances, specific personality traits, early life trauma, and poor cognitive functioning) aid development of distress states.

Major Depression, Substance Use Disorders, and Stress

A number of the issues discussed here may be usefully illustrated using the relationship among major depression (MD), SUDs, and stress. As previously noted, the high rate of MD in people with a primary SUD and vice versa underscores the increased risk of an individual with one disorder developing the other. Furthermore, there is considerable evidence relating stressors to the onset, perpetuation, and relapse to either MD or SUD. Hence, it may be that life stressors predispose to each disorder independently, that the stress in predisposing the individual to one disorder renders him or her vulnerable to the development of the other, or that underlying factors such as genes or early environment predispose the individual to experiencing stressors, MD, and SUDs. In parallel with understanding these interactions among MD, SUDs, and life stressors from a psychosocial epidemiological perspective, the involvement of CRH and the HPA axis in both MD and SUD suggests shared neural substrates.

Unraveling these associations is only just beginning; however, there is some clinical, biochemical, and neuroimaging evidence to this end. Clinically, MD and substance withdrawal share similarities, including dysphoria or lowered mood, irritability, anxiety, sleep and appetite changes, and impaired concentration. This is especially so for alcohol withdrawal, in which a depressive phase indistinguishable from MD is present initially in up to 80% of patients but commonly remits without antidepressant treatment.

In functional imaging studies using positron emission tomography or functional magnetic resonance imaging of MD reduced frontal metabolism, anterior cingulate hypoactivity and amygdala hyperactivity indicate altered frontolimbic functioning. Similarly, in people with SUDs, decreased frontal and anterior cingulate activity has been described, in particular in distressed cocaine-dependent subjects and methamphetamine abusers with mood and anxiety symptoms. This group of methamphetamine abusers also demonstrated amygdala hyperactivity, a finding noted in abstaining cocaine-dependent people with cravings induced by image cues. Although these data are not definitive, they indicate that MD and SUDs share common neural regions of dysregulation that are associated with negative affect and stress-related drug seeking.

In acute withdrawal from nicotine and cocaine, both the distress and depressive symptoms positively correlate with changes in CRH and HPA axis responses. Blunted ACTH and cortisol responses to CRH have also been described in people with SUDs, both with and without depressive symptoms. Consistent with this, individuals abstaining from nicotine, alcohol, or multiple substances demonstrated blunted cortisol responses to psychological stressors; D-fenfluramine induced a similar response in abstaining heroin users. These attenuated responses may indicate overactivity of the HPA axis and are commonly seen in MD. The role of this axis is supported by the observations in animal studies that the stress of repeated foot shocks precipitated a relapse to drug use that was prevented by CRH antagonists. In addition, the extrahypothalamic role of CRH in the bed nucleus of the stria terminalis and amygdala is important in mediating the effects of external stressors on relapses to drug use in animal models. Thus, overall increased CRH-related function has been implicated for substance withdrawal, at least for psychostimulants, opioids, ethanol, nicotine, and benzodiazepines. This same change is described in MD with increased CRH levels in the cerebrospinal fluid of depressed subjects and a decrease in CRH levels with antidepressant or electroconvulsive treatment. Hence, it may be that stress as reflected through the perturbation of CRH has a common effect on MD and substance withdrawal.

The most commonly noted neurochemical system changes in MD are the monoamines, especially serotonin and norepinephrine (NE), and CRH and the HPA axis. Some evidence supports a role for dopamine dysfunction; however, therapeutic strategies augmenting dopamine neurotransmission are of equivocal benefit. In contrast, for SUDs dopamine release in the nucleus accumbens is the central mechanism of reward and motivation for use and as previously noted CRH–HPA axis dysregulation appears during withdrawal. Therefore the neuroimaging findings of a shared frontolimbic circuit dysfunction in MD and SUDs probably involve other linking neural systems. Although speculative, one possibility is through CRH–HPA axis and NE, where either peripheral glucocorticoids cross the blood–brain barrier or NE from the locus coeruleus bind to its receptors in the nucleus accumbens and ventral tegmental area, enhancing DA release within the nucleus accumbens similar to drugs of abuse. Thus, a well-described finding in MD of altered CRH–HPA axis and NE activity can influence the central pathway involved in SUDs. This probably oversimplified schema suggests that a primary MD increases vulnerability to a subsequent SUD and that substance use may be compensatory in reestablishing homeostasis in a deficient reward–motivation pathway. Although it is problematic to extrapolate from clinical observations to neural mechanisms, this proposal is consistent with a much greater decrease in cocaine use in depressed cocaine users compared to nondepressed users when both were treated with antidepressants. Similar but more modest effects have been noted for both alcohol and nicotine users. Also, MD is known to sensitize smokers to stress, which increases the motivation for smoking. Moreover, for abstaining smokers with a psychiatric disorder, depression often accompanies nicotine withdrawal, with relief from these symptoms prompting a relapse. Smokers therefore anticipate that nicotine will provide partial relief from stress and depression, as it does from the symptoms of withdrawal. In support of this premise is the finding that stress and nicotine both induce synaptogenesis (synapse formation) in the VTA. Furthermore, increase in dopamine release caused by nicotine is suggested to improve anhedonia (loss of pleasure), often associated with depressive illness.

Conclusion

This article describes the high rate of comorbidity between SUDs and other psychiatric disorders, briefly outlines competing hypotheses to explain this observation, proposes how stress may contribute to this, and illustrates this with reference to major depression. However, despite the strong epidemiological evidence of a high rate of comorbidity between SUDs and other psychiatric disorders that is exacerbated by stress, the divergent pathologies of major psychiatric disorders and the limited understanding of the neuroadaptations involved in SUDs suggest that this interaction differs between the disorders. Moreover, although there is limited evidence to support the self-medication hypotheses, alternative explanatory hypotheses remain plausible. Thus, untangling the interaction of stress-related factors in the neurobiological findings in these disorders and their effects on the brain changes from substance dependence will be essential in determining the correct hypothesis of comorbidity. The result of this endeavor could have profound effects on the prevention and treatment of SUD and other psychiatric disorder comorbidity.

See Also the Following Articles

Alcohol, Alcoholism, and Stress: A Psychobiological Perspective; Schizophrenia.

Further Reading

Brady, K. T. and Sinha, R. (2005). Co-occurring mental and substance use disorders: the neurobiological effects of chronic stress. *American Journal of Psychiatry* **162**, 1483–1493.

Kessler, R. C., Chiu, W. T., Demler, O., et al. (2005). Prevalence, severity and comorbidity of 12-month DSM-IV disorders in the National Comorbidity Survey Replication. *Archives of General Psychiatry* **62**, 617–627.

Khantzian, E. J. (1985). The self-medication hypothesis of addictive disorders: Focus on heroin and cocaine dependence. *American Journal of Psychiatry* **142**, 1259–1264.

Lowinson, J. H., Ruiz, P., Millman, R. B. and Langrod, J. G. (eds.) (2004). *Substance abuse: a comprehensive textbook* (4th edn.). Philadelphia: Lippincott, Williams & Wilkins.

Mueser, K. T., Drake, R. E. and Wallach, M. A. (1998). Dual diagnosis: a review of etiological theories. *Addictive Behaviours* **23**, 717–734.

Nestler, E. J. (2005). Is there a common molecular pathway for addiction? *Nature Neuroscience* **8**, 1445–1449.

Swendsen, J. D. and Merikangas, K. R. (2000). The comorbidity of depression and substance use disorders. *Clinical Psychology Review* **20**, 173–189.

H. Autistic Spectrum Disorders

Neurodevelopmental Disorders in Children

N J Rinehart and B J Tonge
Monash University, Clayton, Victoria, Australia

Glossary

Pervasive developmental disorders (PDD) A group of serious neuro-developmental disorders affecting communication and social skills and behaviour.

Autism (autistic disorder) A PDD that involves delayed and deviant language development, impaired social skills and ritualistic and repetitive patterns of behaviour, usually associated with intellectual disability but a minority have normal IQ (high functioning).

Asperger's disorder A PDD characterised by normal intellectual ability and language development but the presence of impaired social skills and ritualistic and repetitive patterns of behaviour.

Autism spectrum disorder A term usually applied to represent autistic disorder, Asperger's disorder and atypical autism or PDD not otherwise specified (PDD-NOS) which share some common features of problems with communication and social skills and behaviour.

Attention-deficit/hyperactivity disorder (ADHD) A neuro-developmental disorder presenting with inattention, impulsiveness and motor hyperactivity excessive for the developmental age and usually associated with learning problems.

Autism and Asperger's Disorder

Autistic disorder (referred to as autism here) and Asperger's disorder are classified under the umbrella term pervasive developmental disorders (PDDs). PDD applies to children who share the core features of severe and pervasive impairment in social and communication skills, together with the presence of restricted and repetitive patterns of behavior and interest. Other disorders that are categorized as PDDs include Rett's disorder, childhood disintegrative disorder, and pervasive developmental disorder, not otherwise specified (PDD-NOS). These disorders have their onset within the first 3 years of life. This section focuses on the two main PDDs, autism and Asperger's disorder. The term autistic spectrum disorders (ASDs) is frequently used to a describe a group of individuals with either autism or Asperger's disorder and is used accordingly in this article.

Epidemiology

The prevalence of autism is around 10–12 per 10 000. There is no evidence that prevalence varies between countries or racial groups, and social class and level of parental education are not associated with autism. Autism is more common in boys than girls (4:1), and this gender distribution is even more marked in Asperger's disorder (10–13:1).

Clinical Features of Autism

Autism presents with delays and abnormalities in the development of language and social skills and the presence of rigid, repetitive, stereotyped play and behavior, often in association with intellectual disability (i.e., an IQ below 70) and a variety of neurological conditions such as epilepsy. A reliable diagnosis can be made from the age of 2 years. Parents usually first seek help because their child has language delay and a lack of nonverbal communication. About 50% of children with autism fail to develop functional speech and only slowly learn to compensate with gesture. Language development is often abnormal in the remainder, with echolalia, self-directed jargon, and the repetition of irrelevant phrases, for example, from a television show. The correct use of pronouns and the related development of a sense of self and others are delayed. Poor comprehension, problems expressing needs by words and gesture, and difficulty in social understanding are frequently the causes of stress, frustration, and disturbed behavior. Children who do develop functional language usually have difficulty in using language socially and in initiating or sustaining reciprocal conversations. In contrast to children with autism, young people with Asperger's disorder have no delay in the development of normal expressive and receptive language, including the use of communicative phrases by the age of 3. However, children with Asperger's disorder have problems in their social use of language, for example, being verbose and preoccupied with a favorite topic. Their speech may appear odd due to the use of an unusual accent or the presence of abnormalities in pitch and volume, leading, for example, to a flat and monotonous delivery.

The play, behavior, and daily life of children with autism is usually rigid and repetitive. Their ritualistic play lacks imagination and social imitation. The older children may develop preoccupations with themes such as train timetables or dinosaurs, and this will be the focus of their play, drawing, and conversation. Change or unexpected events can be a significant source of stress: for example, the change of a school timetable.

Approximately 80% of children with autism also have intellectual disability, and a range of other emotional and behavioral disturbances is common. Children with autism who have intellectual (thinking) abilities within the normal range are referred to as high functioning. In contrast, all children with Asperger's disorder have normal intellectual abilities.

High levels of inattentiveness and behavioral hyperactivity are common problems in children with autism and Asperger's disorder; for example, at least 13% of children with autism also meet criteria for ADHD (although a diagnosis of ADHD cannot be made concurrently with a diagnosis of ASD). The overlap of these disorders suggests that ASDs and ADHD share areas of brain dysfunction.

The Neuropsychology of ASDs

There are three main brain theories of autism: theory of mind, the executive dysfunction theory, and the theory of weak central coherence. A poor theory of mind refers to problems with understanding that other people have their own perspectives and thoughts; it is believed to be a reason why people with ASDs have difficulties understanding and relating to other people. The executive dysfunction theory accounts for the problems that people with ASDs experience with timing and planning and producing appropriate and relevant behavior (e.g., coping with changes in the school timetable, planning homework). This breakdown in the ability to effectively direct one's behavior is also thought to be related to the repetitive, stereotyped, and restricted behavioral patterns of ASDs. Weak central coherence refers to a problem with being unable to see the forest for the trees and is thought to be responsible for why people with ASDs tend to be obsessed with details and often miss the bigger picture.

Standardized tests have demonstrated that the neuropsychological profile of autism is characterized primarily by deficient cognitive flexibility and planning, but without problems in the ability to sustain and direct attention (problems attributed to the prefrontal regions of the brain). Research suggests that the kinds of problems that individuals with Asperger's disorder have in directing their behavior may be different from those observed in autism, for example, their problem may be more one of initiating behavior than moving effectively from one behavior to another, perhaps suggesting that different parts of the prefrontal brain are involved in each disorder. Neuromotor testing has found that the walking and upper body postural alignment of people with ASDs is similar to that observed in patients who have Parkinson's disease and patients with cerebellar ataxia, indicating the role of the basal ganglia and cerebellum in these disorders. Again, autism and Asperger's disorder may be associated with different kinds of motor problems, which would suggest the differential involvement of these brain regions.

Neuroimaging Studies in ASDs

Neuroimaging techniques that enable us to look at the structure and function of the brain (e.g., computed tomography [CT], magnetic resonance imaging [MRI], and functional magnetic resonance imaging [fMRI]) have been unsuccessful in revealing a part or function of the brain that is consistently abnormal in all children diagnosed with ASDs. Structural changes in the brains of individuals with autism include a slightly increased average brain volume, a reduction in neuronal integrity in prefrontal areas (an area important for executive functioning – see preceding), decreased gray matter volume in the limbic system (an area important for social understanding), reduced neuron numbers in the vermis of the cerebellum, and gross structural changes in the cerebellum (an area important for motor and cognitive functioning) and the parietal lobes (an area important for efficient attention). fMRI studies have shown decreased activation in the highly interconnected cortical and subcortical frontal structures, suggesting a disconnection between thinking and motor processors in the brain. In summary, the brain imaging research data showing multiple brain region involvement and inconsistencies between people with ASDs fits with the clinical definitions of these disorders as being psychiatrically and neurologically complex and heterogeneous.

Genetics

The cause of the majority of cases of ASD remains unknown, but they are almost certain to have a multifactorial and complex genetic basis. Autism is associated with defined environmental causes, such as rubella and cytomegalovirus, fetal infections, perinatal brain injury, toxins, and specific genetic abnormalities such as tuberous sclerosis and fragile X syndrome in less than 10% of cases. A higher incidence of prenatal stressors occurring between 21 and 32 weeks of gestation has been associated with the later development of autism. A suggested link between measles, mumps, and rubella vaccination and the use of thiomerosol in vaccines as a cause of the increased prevalence of autism has been discounted by several comprehensive studies.

Attention-Deficit/Hyperactivity Disorder (ADHD)

The symptoms of ADHD may vary in different settings, and diagnosis is often subdivided into the number of symptoms in each of the dimensions of inattention or hyperactivity/impulsiveness. Thus, a child may be diagnosed as ADHD predominately hyperactive type or predominantly inattentive type. Estimates of the prevalence of ADHD vary widely, ranging from 20 to 1–2% depending on the application of diagnostic criteria. The combined inattentive-hyperactive subtype is the most common presentation.

Epidemiology

The childhood prevalence of ADHD is approximately three times higher in males than in females. Symptoms usually reduce with maturation, but at least 30% of children with ADHD will continue to suffer from the disorder in adulthood.

Clinical Features of ADHD

The diagnosis of ADHD is based on a clinical judgment that there are sufficient symptoms of inattention and hyperactivity/impulsiveness, together with the decision that these symptoms cause significant impairment in daily functioning in at least two settings and are not consistent with the developmental level of the child. Therefore, diagnosis requires a careful and comprehensive history of the child's development and behavior from the parents and other informants such as the teacher, together with observation of the child's behavior.

Apart from showing high levels of distractibility and inattention, children with ADHD are disorganized and are usually unable to follow routine or complete tasks. They have difficulty monitoring their behavior and therefore often interrupt others, have difficulty following rules, and display inappropriate and impulsive behavior. Those who also suffer from hyperactivity are constantly restless and fidgety, have difficulty remaining seated, and behave as if they are driven by a motor. These behaviors are influenced by aspects of the environment, such as the degree of external stimulation and sensory complexity. Therefore, observers may report differences in behavior depending upon the context. For example, a teacher in a busy, noisy classroom setting is more likely to observe inattention than a teacher's aide who meets with the child for individual teaching in a quiet library environment. However, the symptoms and impairments are usually observed, at least to some extent, in all aspects of the child's daily life.

The Neuropsychology of ADHD

In common with ASDs, neurocognitive testing has revealed that ADHD involves deficiencies within the prefrontal regions of the brain described under the umbrella term of executive dysfunction. However, the type of prefrontal executive dysfunction differs between ASDs and ADHD. The classic ADHD profile is characterized by inhibitory deficits and problems with sustained attention, compared to planning and cognitive flexibility deficits in the cognitive profile of children with autism.

Neuroimaging Studies of ADHD

As is the case with ASDs, no consistent structural abnormalities have been recorded for individuals affected by ADHD. ADHD has been associated in some but not all studies with smaller whole brain volumes, right prefrontal anomalies, and structural anomalies in the basal ganglia, cerebellum, and corpus callosum. As is the case with ASDs, fMRI studies have shown decreased activation in the highly interconnected cortical and subcortical frontal structures, particularly in neural regions that subserve key attentional and inhibitory functions.

Genetics and Stressors

The inherited basis for ADHD has been estimated in around 80% of cases, with perinatal brain injury (e.g., caused by stress, alcohol, tobacco, and other substance abuse during pregnancy) responsible for the remainder. The cause in the inherited cases is likely to be a complex interaction of multiple genes, while in some individuals there will also be an interaction with perinatal brain injury or other environmental stressors such as fetal alcohol exposure or postnatal malnutrition. As is the case with ASDs, there has been a large number of candidate gene and linkage studies of ADHD. Genetic screening for ASDs and ADHD is not yet possible.

Stress Associated with Autism and ADHD

Neurodevelopmental disorders present a considerable stress and burden for the affected individual, parents, siblings, and caregivers in the community. The particular stressors change over time and therefore need to be considered in the context of a human life span approach.

Stress Issues from Birth to Preschool

The trajectory of the stress and devastation that accompany a diagnosis of a neurodevelopmental disorder begins for the parents when their child is between 1 and 3 years of age, when parents realize, either through their own observations or through those of others (e.g., extended family, maternal health nurse, general practitioner), that something is not quite right with their child's developmental progress, for example, behavioral deficits in the form of language or social delays, inattentiveness, or behavioral excesses in the form of increased motor activity and hypervigilance. This realization usually triggers a string of subsequent referrals for pediatric, audiological, psychological, and speech and language assessment. Incumbent in each of these referrals is set of neurobiological and developmental test protocols to rule out various diagnoses. For example, a pediatrician may request a series of metabolic (e.g., phenylketonuria) and genetic tests (e.g., fragile X). The psychologist may undertake behavioral and cognitive standardized assessments, while the speech pathologist may request standardized assessments of receptive (i.e., understanding) and expressive (communicative) language. Investigation and testing may occur over a period of 3–12 months, at which time the family will be referred to a specialist (e.g., child psychiatrist, clinical psychologist) or specialist clinic for final diagnostic confirmation. The time length and uncertainty about their child's diagnostic status that parents experience during the assessment process is often stressful.

The formal diagnosis of a neurodevelopmental condition will often trigger a significant grief reaction in parents, who may mourn the loss of their perfect child and be required to reconsider future plans they may have had for their child, e.g., attending particular schools. In the case of ASDs, or when the child has additional severe intellectual disability, there may be a sense of loss about not having grandchildren, as many people affected by these disorders do not go on to partner and have their own children. Furthermore, research has shown that mothers of children with autism are more likely to suffer from depression than mothers of children with other physical conditions (e.g., cystic fibrosis) and mental disabilities.

Parents are typically provided with information about the genetic component of neurodevelopmental disorders at the time of diagnosis. For example, in the case of ASDs, if an older sibling has autism, the risk that a subsequent sibling will have autism is 2–8%. This information is stressful for parents because it has implications for younger siblings and for future family planning.

After a formal assessment has taken place, parents will play an important advocacy role throughout the child's life, a role that requires a significant emotional and financial commitment to ensure that a high quality of life is maintained for their child at each developmental stage. During the preschool years, parental advocacy typically involves organizing appropriate early interventions (e.g., speech and language, occupational therapy, behavioral management). The process of dealing with often lengthy waiting lists to access public services, or self-funding private interventions places a considerable emotional and financial burden on families and may place stress on the larger family unit by increasing work hours for caregivers and reducing time and resources for other family members, in particular, unaffected siblings. Surveys of maternal stress levels have estimated that approximately two-thirds of mothers of children with ASDs experience clinically significant levels of stress when their child is between 2 and 7 years of age. Stress levels are particularly high when a child with ASD has high levels of maladaptive and disruptive behaviors.

Children with ADHD often have hostile interactions with other children (e.g., hitting and biting) during the preschool years. This places a considerable stress not only on parents, but also on the broader preschool community (e.g., parents of other children and teachers). Compared to fathers, mothers have reported that they find these behaviors to be significantly more stressful.

Receiving education about the disorder and skills training in managing problem behaviors, learning relaxation and stress management techniques, and increased social support (e.g., respite care and community support groups) have been found to be useful for improving parental mental health and reducing parental stress associated with having a child with a neurodevelopmental condition.

Stress Associated with the Primary School Years

Interventions put in place during preschool years will typically continue into the primary school years depending on the availability of community and privately funded resources. During the school years, parents often become concerned about their child's education and adverse school experiences such as being teased. They focus on advocating for appropriate educational modifications and placements to promote their child's ability to reach individual academic potential and to experience a safe and supportive school environment. This usually involves families again seeking out the services of psychologists and speech pathologists so that their child can have updated assessments of language and cognitive ability. This process is a burden for children and parents because it is time consuming and costly. In some cases, at the end of such assessment processes, children are deemed ineligible for education aide support or special consideration because of bureaucratic and funding reasons (e.g., the child's IQ is 72 points rather than 70 points). This issue sometimes requires higher levels of advocacy from involved health professionals to assist parents with appeal processes.

For children with autism who have good early intervention, focused on the parent (e.g., behavior management training, psychoeducation) as well as the child, disruptive behaviors are manageable, and the quality of life for the child and family is generally improved. For children who do not receive good early interventions, or when standard interventions are inadequate, perhaps due to additional neurobiological comorbidity and ongoing disruptive behaviors (e.g., stubbornness, self-injury, and aggression), there is an increased risk of failure in school and community activities, in some cases leading to more restrictive care. When psychological and behavioral interventions have not been successful in the management of disturbed emotions and behaviors, which may be underpinned by high levels of anxiety, treatment with neuroleptic medication (e.g., haloperidol, risperidone, imipramine, clomipramine, fluoxetine) that targets specific symptoms might prove helpful.

While the antisocial behavioral tendencies (e.g., biting and hitting) of children with ADHD may subside with good management during the preschool years, for older children poor management and associated comorbidity (e.g., conduct disorder and oppositional defiant disorder, learning disorders) increase the chances of school failure and peer rejection. Comorbidity with oppositional defiant disorder (e.g., clashing verbally with authorities) has been suggested at between 32 and 60%, while comorbidity with conduct disorder (e.g., engaging in theft) has been estimated at anywhere between 12 and 25%. Stimulant medications (e.g., methylphenidate and dexamphetamine) are effective treatments for the symptoms of ADHD. Side effects, which may include decreased appetite, insomnia, fatigue, irritability, and increase in pulse rate and blood pressure, may be a source of stress for the individual and for parents. Tricyclic antidepressants (imipramine) clonidine, or atomoxetine (an inhibitor of the presynaptic norepinephrine transporter) are alternative treatments for children who have intolerable side effects or are unresponsive to stimulant medication. Parents may be stressed by the uncertainty of potential long-term effects of placing their child on medication. Currently there is a lack of good long-term evidence for the effectiveness of stimulant medication on learning, but they may decrease the risk of later substance abuse.

Stress Associated with the Secondary School Years

In the normal scheme of development, the transition from a relatively protected and highly structured primary school setting to secondary school is often a time of stress for children and families; these concerns and issues are magnified when a child has a neurodevelopmental disorder. In contrast to primary school, secondary school is often larger and requires the young person to be independent, navigate the school timetable, and engage in homework. All of these activities require good executive functions, e.g., planning, preparation, and anticipation, skills classically affected by neurodevelopmental disorders.

Adolescence is a developmentally complex time defined by social and sexual development and identity formation. Because social understanding and adaptability are innately reduced in ASDs it is an especially complex time for these young people. The affected young person may be more stressed than their nonaffected peers as they go through puberty and deal with changes in physical body shape, development in their thinking and insight, and emerging sexuality. Stress is also elevated for those individuals who develop comorbid psychiatric conditions, particularly depression, during this time. Depression may manifest as mood disturbance and irritability, sleep and appetite disturbance, and thoughts of suicide that may be enacted. The increased vulnerability to depression during adolescence may be associated with self-awareness of the disability, pubertal brain development, and a family history of depression. Stress and anxiety have been associated with the onset of tic disorder, or Tourette syndrome, in young people with ASDs. There is also an increased risk of developing psychosis during adolescence or early adult life, particularly for young people with Asperger's disorder. Individuals with associated intellectual disability are at greater risk for developing epilepsy during the adolescent and early adult years.

In addition to ongoing issues that first emerge in the primary school years (e.g., associated learning difficulties estimated in up to 50% of children with ADHD) for young people affected by ADHD and their families, new hazards during secondary schooling revolve around ongoing and escalating child–parent conflicts, delinquent behavior, substance abuse (e.g., nicotine, alcohol, and illicit drug use), and an increased risk of being involved in car accidents, all of which may lead to school suspensions, community marginalization, and an increased risk of a breakdown of family relationships. It has been noted that increased marital discord when a child in the family has been diagnosed with ADHD may be influenced by the parents themselves having ADHD, given the associated genetic vulnerability. Young people who are treated with stimulant mediation for ADHD are less likely to use substances compared with adolescents with ADHD who are not receiving treatment.

In contrast to individuals with ADHD, individuals with ASDs often go to lengths not to use drugs and alcohol, an issue that may paradoxically cause stress and social conflict because the individual with ASD may feel driven to impose their rigid views about abstinence onto unsuspecting others, for example, taking a cigarette or alcoholic beverage out of the hand of a friend or restaurant patron.

Stresses during Adulthood

For people affected by ASDs, the adulthood stressors vary widely according the individual's intellectual ability, capacity for independent living, and provision of social, emotional, financial, and occupational support. It has been suggested that individuals with associated intellectual disability and epilepsy are at greater risk for deterioration during early adulthood, while there may be some improvement in functioning in normally intelligent young adults with ASDs. People with moderate to profound intellectual ability may be placed in special housing accommodation or residential care, depending on the family's emotional and financial ability to retain care within the family unit. This time of transition may be particularly stressful for the individual because it involves adaptation to a new environment and many changes in daily routine. Transition is stressful for family members involved in the decision-making process because they often feel a great sense of guilt and loss. Thus, the grieving process over the loss of the young person's potential, which begins for parents when they first come to terms with the diagnosis, is often revisited at this developmental point. Alternatively, the prospect of providing continuing care, without the hope of relief, is a source of anxiety for aging parents.

Even when young people with ASDs have relatively intact intellectual ability (e.g., ranging from mildly impaired to normally intelligent), they remain greatly impaired in their ability to process social information. Like the transition from primary school to secondary school, the transition to adulthood involves another leap of independence, involving a greater need for executive abilities (e.g., budgeting money, planning meals) and social adjustment. Indeed, the social rules may become even more perplexing for an adult with ASDs, as the immediate supports and supervision from parents, teachers, and school aides reduce or disappear as the young person is expected to live independently in the community. The transition to adulthood is perhaps more complex for individuals who have poorer adaptive and life skills, with a lack of early intervention and skills training and poor management of associated comorbid psychiatric conditions such as anxiety during the formative years.

Reduced social ability and obsessional characteristics associated with ASDs may put an individual at greater risk for being unwittingly involved in inappropriate or illegal behavior, for example, sexual offending or stalking, which may occur in the context of naive and inept attempts to make social contact. Similarly, there have been reports in the Australian and European media about individuals with ASDs stealing trams or trains to pursue an obsessional interest in the rail system. Interventions to manage these types of forensic issues may be punitive and inappropriate, particularly when the individual's diagnosis may not be known, leading to additional feelings of being rejected and further emotional and behavioral problems.

Adults with ADHD are usually less disruptive and hyperactive than children with ADHD, but usually remain somewhat impulsive, disorganized, inattentive, and restless or lack motivation. Young adults with comorbid conduct disorder and an inability to control their behavior are at increased risk for being in trouble with the law, ranging from accumulating multiple speeding fines to committing more significant crimes, such as robbery. The disinhibited, poorly focused, and overactive symptoms of those with ADHD may make it difficult to maintain employment and social and stable intimate relationships.

Conclusion

ASDs and ADHD are lifelong neurodevelopmental conditions, possibly involving overlapping brain regions, that are associated with numerous and accumulating individual stressors across the life span. Despite the many differences between ASDs and ADHD, there are many commonalities in the factors that may protect against or lessen the impact of these stressors. At the forefront of these is the availability of early interventions, parent support and guidance, and ongoing management at key developmental stages from health, education, and welfare services (e.g., general practitioners, psychologists, psychiatrists). These may prevent the accumulation of stressful events and related complications that significantly reduce the quality of life of the affected individual and family and are costly to society with an increased prospect of unemployment, family and relationship breakdown, legal issues, and psychiatric care.

See Also the Following Articles

Attention-Deficit/Hyperactivity Disorder, Stress and.

Further Reading

Barkley, R. A. (1998). *Attention deficit hyperactivity disorder: a handbook for diagnosis and treatment* (2nd edn.). New York: Guilford Press.

Bradshaw, J. L. (2001). *Developmental disorders of the frontostriatal system: neuropsychological, neuropsychiatric and evolutionary perspectives.* Hove, East Sussex, UK: Psychology Press Ltd.

Brereton, A. V. and Tonge, B. J. (2005). *Preschoolers with autism: an education and skills training program for parents.* London: Jessica Kingsley.

Cohen, D. J. and Volkmar, F. R. (eds.) (1997). *Handbook of autism and pervasive developmental disorders,* (2nd edn.). New York: Wiley & Sons.

Howlin, P. (2000). Outcome in adult life for more able individuals with autism or Asperger syndrome. *Autism* **4**(1), 63–83.

I. Behavioral disorders

Attention-Deficit/Hyperactivity Disorder, Stress and

L E Arnold
Ohio State University, Columbus, OH, USA
R L Lindsay
Arizona Child Study Center, Phoeniz, AZ, USA

This is a revised version of the article by L Eugene Arnold, Encyclopedia of Stress First Edition, volume 1, pp 262–267, © 2000, Elsevier Inc.

Glossary[1]

Amphetamine Generic name for a stimulant medicine approved by the Food and Drug Administration (FDA) for treatment of attention-deficit/hyperactivity disorder (ADHD). It has two main brands: Adderall and Dexedrine. It is available in immediate-release tablets and extended-release encapsulated beads of different durations (Adderall XR and Dexedrine Spansule).

Atomoxetine Generic name for a nonstimulant medicine approved by the FDA for treatment of ADHD. The brand name is Strattera. It is available only as an encapsulated powder.

Clonidine A blood pressure medicine often used in the treatment of ADHD, especially with co-occurring tics or sleep problems. The brand name is Catapres. It is not approved by the FDA for treatment of ADHD but is commonly used, often with one of the FDA-approved drugs. It has been replaced somewhat by guanfacine, a similar drug with longer duration and less sedation.

Combined type ADHD ADHD with both six or more symptoms of inattentiveness and six or more symptoms of hyperactivity and impulsivity.

Comorbid Pertaining to other disorders co-occurring with ADHD – i.e., in the same person at the same time

Conduct disorder (CD) A form of disruptive behavior disorder typified by a repetitive and persistent pattern of behavior in which the basic rights of others or major age-appropriate societal norms and rules are violated. Referred to by the juvenile justice system as delinquency.

Desipramine Antidepressant that has been shown effective for ADHD in controlled studies. The brand name is Norpramin. Used more in adults than children. Not FDA-approved for ADHD, but accepted by experts.

Disruptive behavior disorders (DBD) An array of psychiatric disorders marked by aggression, hostility, rule breaking, defiance of authority, and violation of social norms. The primary forms are oppositional defiant disorder (ODD) and conduct disorder (CD). Some authors include ADHD as a form of DBD.

Guanfacine A blood pressure medicine often used in ADHD, especially with tics. The brand name is Tenex. Although not approved by the FDA for this use, it is supported by a controlled study.

Hyperkinetic disorder An old term for ADHD in the United States that is still used in Europe. Hyperkinetic literally means overactive.

Impairment Interference with normal function or performance.

Methylphenidate Generic name for a stimulant medicine approved by the FDA for treatment of ADHD. It has several brands: Ritalin, Concerta, Metadate, and Methylin. It is available in immediate-release tablets and in several long-acting forms, including encapsulated beads of differing durations (Ritalin LA and Metadate CD) and an oral osmotic tablet (Concerta).

Operational criteria Steps that one can go through to see if experts would recognize a patient as having the disorder. If the patient meets all the operational criteria, one can be sure that clinicians anywhere who are familiar with the disorder would agree with the diagnosis.

Oppositional defiant disorder (ODD) A form of disruptive behavior disorder typified by a pattern of negativistic, hostile, and defiant behavior.

Pemoline Generic name for a stimulant medicine approved by the FDA for treatment of ADHD. The brand name is Cylert. It is not recommended as a first or second choice because of rare life-threatening liver damage.

Posttraumatic stress disorder (PTSD) A form of anxiety disorder in which a person who was exposed to a traumatic event persistently re-experiences the event, avoids things associated with the event, and has persistent arousal that was not present before the trauma.

Definition and Overview

Attention-deficit/hyperactivity disorder (ADHD) is a common disorder of cognition and behavior

[1] Adapted with permission from Arnold, L. E. (2004). *A Family Guide to Attention-Deficit/Hyperactivity Disorder.* Newtown, PA: Handbooks in Health Care. Copyright 2004, Handbooks in Health Care.

originating in childhood. According to the American Psychiatric Association's *Diagnostic and Statistical Manual of Mental Disorders,* 4th edition (DSM-IV), diagnosis requires, in addition to sufficient symptoms, that some of the symptoms must have caused impairment before age 7, some impairment is present in two or more settings, and there must be evidence of significant impairment in social, academic, or occupational functioning.

For the inattentive type, there must be six of the following nine symptoms:

1. Often failing to pay attention to details or making careless mistakes
2. Frequent difficulties sustaining attention
3. Often not seeming to listen
4. Often failing to follow instructions or failing to finish things
5. Frequent difficulty organizing
6. Often avoiding tasks that require sustained mental effort
7. Often losing necessary things for tasks
8. Frequent easy distraction
9. Frequent forgetfulness

For diagnosis of the hyperactive-impulsive type, six of the following nine symptoms are necessary:

1. Frequent fidgeting or squirming
2. Often leaving seat
3. Often running or climbing excessively
4. Frequent difficulty playing quietly
5. Often acting as if driven by a motor
6. Often talking excessively
7. Often blurting out answers before questions have been completed
8. Frequent difficulty awaiting turns
9. Often interrupting or intruding

For the combined type, the full-blown syndrome, there must be six symptoms from each cluster.

ADHD itself is not considered a stress disorder. However, it is related to stress in a number of ways. As with most disorders of health, both physical and mental, the symptoms can be aggravated by stress. Many of them can be mimicked by stress. Further, the symptoms of the disorder, especially if untreated, can cause stress both in the individual afflicted and in family members, especially parents, and in teachers, other caretakers, and peers. Later in life, residual symptoms of ADHD can stress spouses or significant others, employers, and co-workers. Finally, adults with residual ADHD can stress their children, whether or not the children also have ADHD. The following description assumes the untreated natural course of the full-blown disorder (combined type).

Aggravation, Complication, or Mimicking of ADHD Symptoms by Stress

Individuals with ADHD have a more tenuous functioning capacity than normal. They are more impulsive, less organized, less attentive to detail, less patient, more easily frustrated. They are also more likely to have additional problems, such as anxiety (about 30%), depression, or learning disorders (20–25%), which further compromise their functional abilities. They often have less adequate verbal memory or other perceptual, associative, or mnemonic ability. Some authorities believe that they are less easily rewarded by ordinary daily activities that normal people find sufficiently rewarding to maintain attention and interest, resulting in frequent boredom and lack of satisfaction. All this adds up to less coping ability. Consequently, the amount of stress needed to induce stress symptoms in these individuals is less than for other people. Since stress by itself can induce concentration and memory problems, it can add an extra increment of impairment to the attention and memory problems of ADHD. Similarly, stress-induced anxiety can add to the restlessness of ADHD, and impulse control often deteriorates further with stress.

Children who are suffering stress symptoms may appear to present with ADHD even if they do not have it. The hypervigilance, anxiety, restless sleep, and preoccupied inattention of posttraumatic stress disorder (PTSD) can mimic the distractibility, restlessness, and inattentiveness of ADHD. In a study of 117 children who appeared before a juvenile/family court secondary to experiencing significant child abuse and/or trauma, children with PTSD demonstrated concurrent ADHD, but not oppositional defiant disorder (ODD)/conduct disorder (CD). Indeed, children presenting with ADHD symptoms should be routinely assessed for traumatic experiences. There may be a bidirectional association between child maltreatment and ADHD/ODD, with head trauma from abuse aggravating or even causing ADHD, and ADHD symptoms inviting abuse.

The anxiety, misbehavior, withdrawal, depression, preoccupation, easy frustration, and impaired performance of an adjustment disorder can also mimic the inattentiveness, misbehavior, impaired performance, and restlessness of ADHD. The agitation, withdrawal, impaired concentration, and irritability of stress-induced depression can mimic the restlessness, inattentiveness, and impulsiveness of ADHD. Indeed, the final DSM-IV criterion for diagnosing ADHD is that the symptoms are not better explained by another mental disorder.

ADHD Symptoms as Stressors

Untreated symptoms of ADHD stress the persons who have the disorder, their family – parents, siblings, spouse, and children – teachers, employers, and peers.

ADHD as a Stressor of the Person Afflicted

Children or adults with ADHD, though of normal or even superior intelligence, find it difficult to achieve at a level commensurate with their ability. They have to try harder to achieve the same results as peers of the same intelligence. The impulsiveness of the disorder may repeatedly get either children or adults into trouble before they realize what has happened.

For example, a child with inattention may have to struggle for an hour or two to complete the same homework that a peer of normal attentional focus can complete in a half hour. Even then, he or she may forget to turn it in on time and thus not receive full credit for it. Similarly, inattention can interfere with sports performance, a source of the greatest interest and pride for many children, especially boys, who outnumber girls with the disorder two or three to one. Inattentively missing the catch of an easy pop fly, making impulsive mistakes, or failing to hear or carry out the coach's instruction, thus incurring the contempt of peers and coach, or being chosen 18th when sides are chosen, can all stress one's self-esteem. Even at home, children with ADHD may find their achievement and behavior compared unfavorably with those of siblings of equal potential. They may be acutely aware of parental (or teacher) disappointment in their performance or behavior and conclude that they are not loved, at least not as much as siblings or classmates. Needing more prompting by teachers (and parents) for daily function, they may feel picked on, nagged, and alienated from the usual sources of caregiver support. Thus, the developmental tasks of childhood, including acquisition of academic and social skills, basic skills of civilization, work habits, friendships, secure family relations, autonomous functioning, self-control, and self-confidence, are accomplished – if at all – at a more stressful price in the presence of ADHD.

In adolescence and young adulthood, the inattentiveness and impulsiveness of ADHD lead to poorer driving records than those of age mates (two to four times as many accidents). Parents are thus understandably reluctant to sign for a driving permit as early as the adolescent wishes, and are reluctant to allow use of the family car once a driver's license is obtained. Given the importance of a car for peer esteem and adolescent and young adult social life, this parental reluctance aggravates any family conflict, further cripples peer relations, and adds further increments of psychological stress. The impulsiveness and disorganization of the disorder also lead to a higher rate of teenage pregnancy in girls with ADHD and probably in girlfriends of boys with ADHD, not to mention greater exposure to sexually transmitted diseases. After all, precautions (including abstinence) require some reflection, organization, and impulse control. Thus, the interaction of ADHD with developmental issues of adolescence compound the ADHD-induced stresses from earlier childhood.

Adults with inattention become bored or frustrated with many jobs that others find tolerable or even interesting. They may wallow miserably in a lower-skilled job than their abilities deserve. Conversely, they may have an erratic work history, as their dissatisfaction and short attention span lead them to seek relief in job changes or even to impulsively quit without another job lined up. Employer dissatisfaction with poor attention to detail, restlessness, or failure to follow instructions may also lead to short tenures on many jobs. Thus, occupation, which should be one of the supports of self-esteem and satisfaction, may become an additional stressor economically and psychologically in the presence of ADHD. Similar patterns of frustration, boredom, restlessness, and difficulty sustaining commitment may dog social and intimate relationships of those with ADHD, who have lower rates of successful marriage. Failed love, separation, and divorce are well-documented stressors for anyone.

ADHD as a Stressor of Parents and Teachers

The constant activity, easy frustration, irritability, disorganization, tendency to lose things, and difficulty following instructions found in children with ADHD can stress any adult attempting to manage their behavior, structure their activities, or teach them. It is particularly frustrating to teachers when they recognize that the child has the intellectual ability but is not doing the work. Many teachers agonize over the wasted potential, or even blame themselves for the child's poor performance. An unsuccessful intelligent pupil is stressful to the teacher's self-image. Erroneous conclusions that the child is lazy or obstinate can poison the teacher–pupil relationship and stress both teacher and child. This stress can possibly spill over into the teacher–parent relationship and affect all three parties.

Parents are stressed by similar disappointments and child performance difficulties at home, which is less intense than at school, but more consistent and enduring (every day, every year). Neglected chores, disorganized messiness, impulsive accidents, poor judgment, hectic overactivity and intrusiveness, conflicts with siblings, undone homework, calls from school, poor report cards, and other stresses are not what most parents anticipate at their child's birth. Such disappointments make it hard for parents to love (or at least hard to like) the child, leading to feeling guilty for being a rejecting parent. Criticisms of the child's behavior and the parents' child-rearing practices by well-meaning friends and relatives may add to the parents' feeling of failure. The child's impulsive destructiveness and accident proneness, as well as chronic need for professional services, round out the picture of a high-maintenance child who stresses the parents economically, physically, and psychologically.

Research has confirmed the profound impact of the problems of the ADHD child on the parents. In a well-controlled study of parent–child interactions, the placebo condition showed the mothers of boys with ADHD to be very directive, commanding, and negative with the child, with little positive interaction; when a dose of stimulant medicine was given to alleviate the child's ADHD symptoms, the same mothers became much friendlier and more respectful of the child, allowed the child more autonomy, and gave many fewer negative messages to the child. This demonstrated that the negative parental attitude often seen toward ADHD children is not part of the parents' personality, but a response to the child's problems. ADHD tends to bring out the worst in those around the afflicted person.

The negativity often spreads into the marital relationship as the frustrated parents disagree about how to handle the child's problems. For example, the father may blame the mother because he can get the child to behave for short times (sometimes by heavy-handed means) and the mother cannot get the child to behave during the much longer intervals she is responsible for. The mother may feel that the father's disciplinary approach is abusive. Each may blame the other's genes. One parent may wish to medicate the child while the other objects to this. One parent may be enthusiastic about behavior modification but may find the system sabotaged by the other parent's failure to cooperate. In some cases one parent does not even recognize or admit there is a problem, while the other parent struggles with numerous complaints from school. One indicator of the marital stress engendered by a child with ADHD is the higher divorce rates reported for parents of such children. (This may be a partial cause as well as effect: divorce is stressful to children, and stress may nudge a subclinical case over the diagnostic threshold by aggravating otherwise mild symptoms.)

ADHD as a Stressor of Peers

Siblings, classmates, or teammates of children with ADHD are often unsung victims of the afflicted child's symptoms. The afflicted child's (proband's) needs for attention, supervision, and services tend to drain parent, teacher, and coach resources from siblings, classmates, and teammates. This relative neglect can sometimes be carried to the point of actual neglect, as all family efforts are focused on the impaired member. The whole family may have to forego outings that the proband cannot handle, or may cater to the proband, either out of pity or out of fear of impulsive tantrums. Older siblings' social life may be impacted by the need to monitor the proband, by embarrassment, or by the proband's intrusiveness. Younger siblings may be steamrollered by the proband's overactivity and inattentive thoughtlessness, or even be endangered by the proband's reckless impulsiveness.

Classmates or teammates may find their education, projects, activities, or games disrupted by the hyperactive child's impulsive intrusiveness, failure to wait a turn, failure to carry out an assigned part of the team's effort, need for excessive attention, failure to finish the activity, impulsive arguing, irritability, or other failure to be a good team player. It should be no surprise that children with ADHD typically fare poorly in peer sociometric ratings. Tragically, the hyperactive child's normal wish for friendships, implemented by clumsy, intrusive, impatient attempts to impose friendships, often only makes the situation worse. Thus, in the presence of ADHD, the normal need for peer relations stresses both the hyperactive child and available peers.

When ADHD persists into adulthood, the brunt of peer difficulties falls on the significant other, who may have to endure financial uncertainty as well as a disorganized lifestyle and interpersonal inconsistency and unpredictability. Again, the high rate of failed marriages and other relationships stresses both the direct victim of ADHD and the indirect peer victims. Employers and co-workers also suffer some stress from the ADHD worker's inconsistent performance, restlessness, disruptiveness, failure to listen to or follow instructions, and failure to carry out assigned parts of a project. In some cases the need for the unpleasant task of firing the ADHD worker adds to the employer's stress. Even when the ADHD employee quits voluntarily, there is the stress of finding and training a replacement.

ADHD as Stressor of the Hyperactive Adult's Children

An important but as yet largely unstudied area is the stress on children of having parents with ADHD. Theoretically, parenting characterized by inattentiveness, inconsistency, impatience, impulsiveness, and disorganization should be stressful for any child. Since ADHD is highly heritable, an adult with ADHD has a good chance of having a child with ADHD. Because ADHD children have a special need for parental support and structure, we might expect that they would be especially vulnerable to the inattentive, unstructured disorganization of an ADHD parent. Conversely, what parenting skills the ADHD parent has will be challenged by the additional stress of a child with ADHD, in a vicious cycle. Thus both parent and child would be stressed by their mutual handicap.

ADHD Treatment as Stressor

Despite considerable evidence as to the effectiveness of pharmacotherapy in ADHD, there are considerable misgivings about the increasingly widespread use of medications, which may contribute further to the stresses of living with ADHD or with a child with ADHD. Parents (and children) are bombarded by media messages stating that medications are harmful or unsafe and can lead to abuse (of the medication or of street drugs), and that ADHD is a myth created by intolerant teachers and parents in an effort to place a pharmacologic leash on the child who only requires more discipline.

Any medication strong enough to treat ADHD is also strong enough to harm. One of the stresses of having ADHD or a child with ADHD is the worry about the long-term effect of medications, which is aggravated by media sensationalism. Sudden death due to medications is a recurring concern. In the 1980s this was reported in several patients taking desipramine, a tricyclic antidepressant known to cause cardiac slowing or blocking and that had demonstrated benefit in ADHD. In the 1990s the combination of methylphenidate and clonidine (an antihypertensive) was reported to have contributed to the deaths of four children, all of whom had other complications such as preexisting cardiac disease (two cases), recent general anesthesia, or other medications. In 2005, Health Canada withdrew Adderall XR (an amphetamine stimulant) from the Canadian market, citing international safety information, including 14 reports of sudden deaths, heart-related deaths, and strokes in children and adults taking recommended doses of the medication. The Food and Drug Administration (FDA) in the United States reviewed the same data but had a very different interpretation and response than Health Canada. The FDA did not conclude that any immediate changes were needed in the approved use of this drug based upon its preliminary understanding of Health Canada's analyses of adverse event reports and the FDA's own knowledge and assessment of the reports received by the agency. However, because the stimulants are adrenergic agents, they can theoretically affect heart function, so a "black box" warning was added to the label as a safety precaution for the minority of patients who have a pre-existing cardiac abnormality. There is no evidence that the reported number of sudden deaths significantly exceeds those expected by chance, and Health Canada has reversed the ban, but the mere discussion is enough to worry many patients and parents.

Potential liver disease is another concern. By 1996, enough evidence had accumulated to confirm the risk of rare irreversible liver necrosis in association with pemoline, which was therefore demoted from a first-line drug to third-line. A recent report concerning a nonstimulant medication, atomoxetine, described liver enzyme elevations in two patients that resolved after the medication was discontinued. In a small, preliminary study, researchers found that after just 3 months, every one of a dozen children treated for ADHD with the drug methylphenidate experienced a threefold increase in levels of chromosome abnormalities – occurrences sometimes associated with increased risks of cancer and other adverse health effects. Even though no epidemiologic data have been found showing a higher rate of cancer in those who took methylphenidate (which has been on the market for 40 years), findings like this are still worrisome, adding to the natural stresses that the disorder brings.

Even nonmedical treatments can generate stress, especially if they are demanding or expensive, and thus stress family resources. For example, a systematic program of behavior modification requires considerable time and effort of the caregiver, who may feel that he or she has already given.

Conclusion

Untreated ADHD – and sometimes even treated ADHD – may be considered a stress generator, with a large ripple effect impacting practically all of society: the 35% of the population who have ADHD, their parents, siblings, teachers, classmates, teammates, mates, children, employers, co-workers, and even unknown other drivers. Thus, effective programs for preventing, curing, or controlling ADHD symptoms could ameliorate the fabric of stress throughout society.

See Also the Following Articles

Posttraumatic Stress Disorder in Children.

Further Reading

American Psychiatric Association (1994). *Diagnostic and Statistical Manual of Mental Disorders* (4th edn.). Washington, D.C.: American Psychiatric Press.

Famularo, R., Fenton, T., Kinscherff, R. and Augustyn, M. (1996). Psychiatric comorbidity in childhood post traumatic stress disorder. *Child Abuse and Neglect* 20(10), 953–961.

Ford, J. D., Racusin, R., Ellis, C. G., et al. (2000). Child maltreatment, other trauma exposure, and posttraumatic symptomatology among children with oppositional defiant and attention deficit hyperactivity disorders. *Child Maltreatment* 5(3), 205–217.

Weinstein, D., Staffelbach, D. and Biaggio, M. (2000). Attention-deficit hyperactivity disorder and posttraumatic stress disorder: differential diagnosis in childhood sexual abuse. *Clinical Psychology Review* 20(3), 359–378.

J. Eating disorders

Eating Disorders and Stress

D C Jimerson
Beth Israel Deaconess Medical Center and Harvard Medical School, Boston, MA, USA

This article is reproduced from Encyclopedia of Stress First Edition, volume 2, pp 4–8, © 2000, Elsevier Inc.

Glossary

Amenorrhea A symptom of anorexia nervosa in adolescent and adult women, characterized by the failure of menstrual cycles to occur during three or more consecutive expected cycle intervals.

Binge-eating episode consumption of an abnormally large amount of food in a discrete episode, during which eating feels out of control.

Hypothalamus A region in the lower part of the brain involved in the regulation of eating behavior, as well as the modulation of other metabolic and hormonal systems.

Neurotransmitter A naturally occurring neurochemical which participates in the selective transmission of signals in neuronal pathways modulating behavior and physiological functions.

Purging behaviors In patients with eating disorders, symptoms intended to control body weight by eliminating ingested foods and liquids; examples include self-induced vomiting and misuse of laxatives.

Restricting behavior In patients with eating disorders, a pattern of strict limitation of food intake in order to control body weight.

Serotonin A naturally occurring neurochemical which acts as a neurotransmitter in the central nervous system, including pathways modulating meal size and mood.

Clinical Overview of Eating Disorders

In recent years there has been increasing awareness of the prevalence of anorexia nervosa and bulimia nervosa, and the personal and social costs associated with these disorders. This awareness has been reflected in attention to these problems in the lay press and in professional publications. Clinical investigations have yielded new insights into the prevalence and symptom patterns of anorexia nervosa and bulimia nervosa. Although the etiology of these disorders is unknown, potential psychosocial and biological risk factors have been identified, and new treatment approaches have been developed. This article provides an overview of clinical characteristics of these disorders, and highlights several directions of recent research advances. Consultation with a medical and/or mental health professional is important for an individual seeking specific guidance regarding clinical evaluation and treatment.

Anorexia Nervosa

Clinical Characteristics

Anorexia nervosa is widely recognized as a syndrome of weight loss which is associated with fears of unwanted weight gain, and is not a consequence of other medical illness. Symptoms of anorexia nervosa were first described in the medical literature more than 100 years ago. Specific diagnostic features of the syndrome are outlined in the *Diagnostic and Statistical Manual of Mental Disorders, 4th edn.* (*DSM-IV*). The most prominent features of anorexia nervosa include weight loss below 85% of an individual's expected body weight, associated with an intense fear of excessive weight gain and abnormal perception of body-weight status. An additional characteristic of the disorder in adolescent and adult females is a period of amenorrhea, usually thought to be a consequence of low body weight. Approximately half of individuals with anorexia nervosa exhibit binge-eating or purging behaviors associated with efforts to maintain a low weight, while others engage predominantly in food restriction. Based on DSM-IV diagnostic categories, these individuals are grouped into binge eating-purging type and restricting type, respectively.

Anorexia nervosa is associated with a range of medical problems which are thought to be primarily related to malnutrition and weight loss. Among the more common problems are anemia, abnormalities in blood pressure and heart rhythm, and alterations in blood electrolyte levels. Activity in the hypothalamic-pituitary-adrenal axis is often increased, with malnutrition-related elevations in blood levels of the stress-related hormone, cortisol. Consistent with physiological adaptations to conserve energy, functional activity in the hypothalamic-pituitary-thyroid axis and the sympathetic nervous system are frequently decreased. Reduction in bone mineral density with increased risk of bone fractures is often a long-term consequence of severe malnutrition in anorexia nervosa.

Naturalistic follow-up studies indicate that at 5–10 years after initial assessment, about 40–60% of patients achieve stable weight recovery, while 10–20% of patients continue to have symptoms of the disorder. In general, it is difficult to predict an individual's long-term outcome based on initial symptomatology. The estimated mortality associated with anorexia nervosa is approximately 6% during the first 10 years after initial assessment, with variability in findings most likely reflecting the severity of initial symptomatology.

Epidemiology and Psychiatric Comorbidity

The average age of onset of anorexia nervosa is approximately 18 years, although a significant number of patients experience an early age of onset (i.e., at 8–14 years). Anorexia nervosa is approximately 10 times more prevalent in females than in males. Among young women, the group at highest risk for the disorder, the prevalence of anorexia nervosa has been estimated as approximately 0.5%. Although epidemiological data are limited, it is known that anorexia nervosa can occur in individuals of various ethnic backgrounds and socioeconomic classes.

Individuals with anorexia nervosa often have a history of additional psychiatric symptoms, particularly depression and anxiety disorders, including obsessive–compulsive disorder. It is of note that marked weight loss in healthy volunteers has been shown to result in depressive symptoms and preoccupation with food. Thus, for some anorexic patients, depressive symptoms may improve with nutritional stabilization and weight restoration.

Overview of Treatment Approaches

For patients with acute weight loss with life-threatening medical and psychiatric symptoms, hospitalization may be necessary. Following medical stabilization, inpatient treatment often includes a behaviorally oriented weight-restoration program with a gradual increase in caloric intake. Individual, group, and family psychotherapy (especially for younger patients) are commonly employed. For less severely ill patients, day hospital treatment or outpatient therapy is usually recommended. Available medication treatments appear to be of only limited benefit in achieving weight restoration, although they may be particularly helpful for symptoms of depression and anxiety. Following weight restoration, a significant number of individuals experience a relapse to low-weight episodes. Again, available medication treatments appear to have only limited benefit in preventing relapse.

Bulimia Nervosa

Clinical Characteristics

The hallmark symptom of bulimia nervosa is the binge-eating episode. In the *DSM-IV*, a binge-eating episode is characterized as consumption of an abnormally large amount of food in a discrete episode, during which eating feels out of control. Although binge eating had previously been recognized in patients with anorexia nervosa, during the 1970s clinicians noted a syndrome of binge eating that occurred in individuals in a normal weight range. Current diagnostic criteria for bulimia nervosa specify that binge-eating episodes, along with compensatory behaviors designed to avoid weight gain, occur on average at least twice a week over a period of at least 3 months. Additionally, body shape and weight play an excessively large role in influencing the individual's sense of self-worth. For some patients, compensatory behaviors include purging activities such as self-induced vomiting or laxative misuse, while for others, fasting or excessive exercise are the main weight control strategies.

Although nutritional abnormalities may result in medical symptoms in patients with bulimia nervosa, these are usually less marked than in anorexia nervosa. It has been recognized, however, that purging behaviors can contribute to significant alterations in blood levels of potassium and other electrolytes, potentially leading to serious heart arrhythmias. A range of other serious medical complications have also been reported. Abnormalities in neuroendocrine hormone levels are not infrequent in bulimia nervosa, being associated with such symptoms as abnormal menstrual cycle patterns in up to 50% of patients.

Follow-up studies ranging up to 10 years following initial assessment indicate that approximately 50–60% of patients with bulimia nervosa will have recovered from the disorder. Approximately one-third of individuals will have significant persisting symptoms, and 10–15% will still meet criteria for the disorder. It is not uncommon for individuals to have one or more relapses, particularly during the first 6 months following their initial recovery from symptoms.

Recently there have been a number of clinical studies of a syndrome provisionally identified as binge-eating disorder. Binge-eating disorder is similar to bulimia nervosa in that affected individuals have recurrent episodes of binge eating. In contrast to bulimia nervosa, individuals with binge-eating disorder do not engage in recurrent inappropriate compensatory behaviors designed to counteract the caloric intake associated with binge eating. Thus, binge-eating disorder is commonly associated with obesity. Further research is needed to clarify the role of psychosocial environment, stressful life situations, and biological characteristics as risk factors for binge-eating disorder.

Epidemiology and Psychiatric Comorbidity

Similar to anorexia nervosa, the average age of onset of bulimia nervosa is approximately 18 years, with a female to male ratio of approximately 10:1. Based on current diagnostic criteria, bulimia nervosa is estimated to occur in 1–3% of young women.

Approximately 50% of patients with bulimia nervosa have an episode of major depression, either concurrent with, or at a time separate from, the eating disorder. Other relatively common comorbid psychiatric symptoms in patients with bulimia nervosa include substance-use disorders and anxiety disorders.

Overview of Treatment Approaches

Patients with bulimia nervosa are most often treated in an outpatient setting, although life-threatening psychiatric symptoms (such as active suicidal ideation) or medical complications may lead to hospitalization. Clinical psychotherapy trials have focused primarily on structured short-term therapies (e.g., cognitive behavioral treatment or interpersonal treatment) lasting 4–5 months. These treatments generally achieve greater than a 50% decrease in binge frequency, with a substantial number of patients achieving abstinence from binge episodes. Additionally, placebo-controlled trials have shown that a range of antidepressant medications can significantly decrease frequency of bulimic episodes for many individuals. Current treatment research includes comparative trials of stepped-care approaches such as an initial trial of self-help guided by a health-care provider, and studies of sequential treatments for individuals who do not show evidence of improvement as psychotherapy proceeds.

Etiological Influences in Eating Disorders

Psychosocial and Biological Risk Factors

Although clinical investigations have identified important leads, specific etiological factors responsible for anorexia nervosa and bulimia nervosa remain unknown. Cultural factors leading to increased emphasis on slender appearance are generally thought to contribute to an increased prevalence of eating disorders. Stresses associated with school transitions and occupational demands have been suggested as possible contributors to the increased risk for the eating disorders among adolescents and young adults.

Clinical investigations have demonstrated increased ratings of perfectionistic character traits and depressive symptoms in anorexia nervosa. Research on risk factors suggests that perfectionism and low self-evaluation may be associated with the later development of anorexia nervosa.

The onset of bulimia nervosa is often preceded by extended periods of recurrent dieting occurring in the context of other psychosocial stressors. Other behavioral characteristics that have been identified in patients with bulimia nervosa include impulsivity and mood lability, and it is possible that these traits may contribute to the onset or perpetuation of symptoms in this disorder. Several psychological models of binge-eating behavior have been proposed. In one model, for example, an individual attempting to follow a reduced calorie diet may experience an abstinence violation effect following ingestion of modest amounts of snack foods, leading to a transient inclination to abandon dietary restraint altogether. Factors that may lead to dieting, such as parental or childhood obesity, have been identified as potential risk factors for the development of this disorder.

Psychobiological Models

Family studies have shown that there is an increased rate of eating disorders in first-degree relatives of individuals with anorexia nervosa and bulimia nervosa. Similarly, twin studies have shown a higher concordance for the eating disorders in monozygotic twins in comparison to dizygotic twins. These studies suggest that heritable biological characteristics contribute to the onset of the eating disorders, although the potential role of familial environmental factors must also be considered.

Biological factors are likely to contribute to one or more dimensions of symptomatology in eating disorders. Neurotransmitters, neuropeptides, and related neuromodulators have been shown to act in the central nervous system, particularly in the hypothalamus, to modulate hunger and satiety. Recent research has shown that peptides released from the gastrointestinal tract help to regulate eating behavior. For example, preclinical studies have shown that naturally occurring neurochemicals such as ghrelin can substantially increase food intake and body weight, while other neuropeptides such as cholecystokinin can decrease food intake. Thus, binge-eating episodes characteristic of bulimia nervosa may reflect the interaction of stressful psychosocial events with abnormalities in the release of meal-regulating peptides such as ghrelin and cholecystokinin. There has also been recent interest in the metabolic signaling protein, leptin, which is produced in adipose tissue and released into the circulation. Dieting and weight loss is associated with a decrease in leptin levels. It has been hypothesized that a marked reduction in blood leptin levels may play a role in menstrual cycle abnormalities commonly associated with anorexia nervosa.

The neurotransmitter serotonin has been the focus of considerable research in patients with anorexia nervosa and bulimia nervosa. Laboratory studies have shown that patients with eating disorders often experience abnormal patterns of hunger and satiety over the course of a meal. Serotonin plays an important role in postingestive satiety, and appears to be important in regulation of mood and anxiety-related symptoms. Preliminary findings suggest that impaired function in central nervous system serotonergic pathways may contribute to binge eating and mood instability in bulimia nervosa. Dieting behaviors may tax the adaptive capacities of serotonergic pathways. Therapeutic effects of antidepressant medications in bulimia nervosa are thought to be related to their capacity to restore more normal signaling patterns in serotonergic pathways.

Recent studies have also explored whether abnormalities in metabolic signals related to energy metabolism contribute to symptoms in the eating disorders. Several studies have suggested that patients with bulimia nervosa may have a lower rate of energy utilization (measured as resting metabolic rate) than healthy individuals. Thus, a biological predisposition toward greater than average weight gain could lead to preoccupation with body weight and food intake in bulimia nervosa.

Further Reading

Agras, W. S., Walsh, T., Fairburn, C. G., et al. (2000). A multicenter comparison of cognitive-behavioral therapy and interpersonal psychotherapy for bulimia nervosa. *Archives of General Psychiatry* **57**, 459–466.

American Psychiatric Association (2000). *Diagnostic and statistical manual of mental disorders, 4th edn., text revision.* Washington, D.C.: American Psychiatric Association.

American Psychiatric Association Workgroup on Eating Disorders (2006). Practice guideline for the treatment of patients with eating disorders. 3rd edn. *American Journal of Psychiatry* **163**, 1–54.

Eckert, E. D., Halmi, K. A., Marchi, P., et al. (1995). Ten-year follow-up of anorexia nervosa: clinical course and outcome. *Psychological Medicine* **25**, 143–156.

Fairburn, C. G., Cooper, Z., Doll, H. A., et al. (1999). Risk factors for anorexia nervosa: three integrated case-control comparisons. *Archives of General Psychiatry* **56**, 468–476.

Fairburn, C. G., Welch, S. L., Doll, H. A., et al. (1997). Risk factors for bulimia nervosa. A community-based case-control study. *Archives of General Psychiatry* **54**, 509–517.

Jimerson, D. C. and Wolfe, B. E. (2004). Neuropeptides in eating disorders. *CNS Spectrums* **9**, 516–522.

Jimerson, D. C., Wolfe, B. E. and Naab, S. (2006). Eating disorders. In: Coffey, C. E., Brumback, R. A., Rosenberg, D. R., et al. (eds.) *Pediatric neuropsychiatry*, pp. 307–320. Philadelphia: Lippincott, Williams & Wilkins.

Keel, P. K., Mitchell, J. E., Miller, K. B., et al. (1999). Long-term outcome of bulimia nervosa. *Archives of General Psychiatry* **56**, 63–69.

Kendler, K. S., MacLean, C., Neale, M., et al. (1991). The genetic epidemiology of bulimia nervosa. *American Journal of Psychiatry* **148**, 1627–1637.

Kishi, T. and Elmquist, J. K. (2005). Body weight is regulated by the brain: a link between feeding and emotion. *Molecular Psychiatry* **10**, 132–146.

Stoving, R. K., Hangaard, J., Hansen-Nord, M., et al. (1999). A review of endocrine changes in anorexia nervosa. *Journal of Psychiatric Research* **33**, 139–152.

Sunday, S. R. and Halmi, K. A. (1996). Micro- and macroanalyses of patterns within a meal in anorexia and bulimia nervosa. *Appetite* **26**, 21–36.

Zhu, A. J. and Walsh, B. T. (2002). Pharmacologic treatment of eating disorders. *Canadian Journal of Psychiatry* **47**, 227–234.

K. Endocrine – Psychopathy - Cushings

Cushing's Syndrome, Neuropsychiatric Aspects

M N Starkman
University of Michigan, Ann Arbor, MI, USA

This is a revised version of the article by M Starkman, Encyclopedia of Stress First Edition, volume 1, pp 621–625, © 2000, Elsevier Inc.

Glossary

Hippocampus	A brain structure that is part of the limbic system and key to learning and memory.
Libido	Desire for sexual activity.
Mental status evaluation	Standard bedside clinical tests used to examine mental functions.
Neuropsychological studies	Tests of various aspects of cognition, including verbal functions, visuospatial functions, learning, and memory.
Sleep electroencephalogram (EEG)	An electroencephalogram taken during sleep to measure brain electrical activity and study the structure of sleep.

Cushing's disease, the major type of spontaneous Cushing's syndrome, is the classic endocrine disease characterized by hypersecretion of cortisol. Intriguingly, emotional disturbances were already recognized as a feature of the disease in Harvey Cushing's original description in 1932. This association was then confirmed by retrospective chart reviews. More recently, studies of patients with spontaneous Cushing's syndrome examined prior to treatment have characterized the disturbance and shown that the majority manifest clinical features similar to those seen in patients with a primary psychiatric depressive disorder. Patients with Cushing's disease and syndrome exhibit a consistent constellation of symptoms, including abnormalities in mood (irritability and depression), vegetative functions (decreased libido and increased insomnia), and cognitive functions (decreased concentration, learning, and memory).

Neuropsychiatric Symptoms in Patients with Spontaneous Untreated Cushing's Syndrome

Mood and Affect

Irritability, a very frequent symptom seen in close to 90% of patients, is usually the earliest behavioral symptom to appear. It begins close to the onset of the earliest physical symptom (weight gain) and prior to the appearance of other physical manifestations of Cushing's syndrome. Patients describe themselves as feeling overly sensitive, unable to ignore minor irritations, and impatient with or pressured by others. In addition, overreactivity and easy development of anger occur. Patients feel that they are often on the verge of an emotional explosion and that the intensity of anger experienced is also increased.

Depressed mood is reported by 60–80% of patients. There is a range in the intensity of depressed mood. Some patients describe short spells of sadness; others experience feelings of hopelessness and giving up. Suicide attempts are infrequent but may occur. Hypersensitivity and oversentimentality lead to crying spells. For some, crying also occurs as the behavioral response to anger and frustration and feeling unable to respond effectively. Patients also experience spontaneous onset of depressed mood or crying in the absence of any proceeding upsetting thought or event.

The time course of the mood disturbances is noteworthy. Most patients report that their mood disturbances are intermittent rather than sustained. Sometimes they wake up depressed and remain depressed throughout the day or the next day as well. Alternatively, the onset of depressed mood and/or crying might occur during the day, often suddenly. The duration of each depressive episode is usually 1 to 2 days and is rarely longer than 3 days at a time. A frequent weekly total is 3 days per week. There is no regular cyclicity, however, so patients cannot predict when a depressive day will occur. Although there are intervals when they might not experience pleasure, these patients do not experience the unrelenting, unremitting inability to experience pleasure that is characteristic of patients with severe psychiatric depressive illness. There are intervals when patients retain the capacity for pleasure, finding enjoyment in hobbies and interpersonal relationships. At times, they may find it difficult to initiate such activities, although once others mobilize them, they are able to enjoy them. Some patients do experience decreased interest in their environment.

Social withdrawal is less common, but can occur. Sporadic withdrawal might occur because of the patient's need to remove him- or herself from a situation of overstimulation that elicits the fear of impending emotional dyscontrol. Guilt is infrequent; if present, it is not excessive, self-accusatory, or irrational, but is related to remorse about angry outbursts and inability to function well at work and in the family. Hopelessness is infrequent, but, if present, is attributed to the increasing physical and emotional disability that has puzzled the patient's physicians and been resistant to treatment interventions until the diagnosis of Cushing's syndrome is finally made.

A minority of patients experience episodes of elation-hyperactivity early in the course of the illness. These episodes of elation are described as a high. During these episodes, patients are more ambitious than usual and might attempt to do more than their ability and training make reasonable. Increased motor activity is present, with restlessness and rapidly performed activities. Patients report embarrassment that their speech is both loud and rapid. As the illness progresses and new physical signs of Cushing's syndrome begin to appear, this type of episode becomes rare or disappears entirely.

A percentage of patients report generalized anxiety. New-onset panic disorder has also been observed in patients with Cushing's syndrome. In addition, even patients who do not experience psychic anxiety describe episodic symptoms of autonomic activation such as shaking, palpitations, and sweating.

Biological Drives

Abnormalities in four areas of basic biological vegetative drives are present:

1. Fatigue. This is reported by 100% of patients.
2. Libido. A decrease in libido is very frequent and reported by close to 70% of patients. In fact, this is one of the earliest manifestations of Cushing's disease, beginning when the patient is experiencing the first onset of weight gain.
3. Appetite and eating behavior. More than 50% of patients have an alteration in their appetite; in 34% appetite is increased; in 20% it is decreased.
4. Sleep and dreams. Difficulty with sleep, particularly middle insomnia and late insomnia (early morning awakening), is found in more than 80% of patients. Difficulty with early insomnia (not falling asleep at bedtime) is not as frequent. One-third of patients report an alteration in the frequency or quality of their dreams, which are increased in their frequency and intensity and become bizarre and very vivid. Some patients report they have lost the ability to wake themselves out of a nightmare. Sleep EEG studies indicate that there are many similarities between Cushing's disease patients and patients with major depressive disorder. For example, both groups show significantly less total sleep time, lower sleep efficiency, and shortened rapid eye movement (REM) latency compared to normal subjects.

Cognition

Cognitive symptoms are a prominent part of the clinical picture. Most patients report difficulty with concentration, inattention, distractibility, and shortened attention span. Some patients report episodes of scattered thinking, while others note slow thinking. Thought blocking may occur in more severe instances. Patients may find themselves using incorrect words while speaking or misspelling simple words. Perceptual distortions are very rare.

Impairment of learning and memory is among the most frequent symptoms and is reported by 80% of patients. Patients report problems with registration of new information. They commonly repeat themselves in ongoing conversations. They easily forget items such as appointments made, names of people, and location of objects.

Most patients have no disorientation or overt clouding of consciousness, and their waking electroencephalographs (EEGs) are not characteristic of delirium. On mental status bedside clinical evaluation, difficulties with tests such as mental subtraction and recall of recent U.S. presidents are seen in close to 50% of the patients.

Detailed neuropsychological studies reveal that individuals vary in the severity of degree of cognitive dysfunction, with minimal or moderate to severe decrements in a variety of subtests seen in close to two-thirds of patients. Verbal functions and learning are particularly affected. Once learned, the percent retention of verbal material is not subnormal. The overall pattern of decrements in cognitive function suggests the involvement of both frontal lobe and hippocampus.

Specific Features of the Neuropsychiatric Symptoms

The psychiatric symptoms that develop in Cushing's syndrome are not simply a nonspecific response to severe physical illness. Irritability and decreased libido occur early, often before patients are aware that they have any physical problems other than weight gain. Later, when depressed mood appears, it is not simply the demoralization seen in the medically ill, but episodic sadness and crying, sometimes occurring in the absence of depressive thought content. The incidence of depressive disorders is greater than in comparison groups with other types of pituitary tumors or hyperthyroidism. Although they have difficulty with concentration and memory, patients with Cushing's syndrome are not delirious.

The overwhelming majority of patients with spontaneous Cushing's syndrome do not have very severe neuropsychiatric disturbances of a psychotic or confusional nature, as patients receiving corticosteroids for treatment of certain physical disorders sometimes may. This can be understood by considering that patients with spontaneous Cushing's syndrome differ from those receiving high-dose steroids in several respects. The level of circulating cortisol in the former is not as high as the equivalent amount of steroid administered to the latter. Patients with Cushing's syndrome also differ from those receiving exogenous steroids in that they are exposed to sustained elevated cortisol levels for months to years and are less subject to sudden acute shifts and rapid rates of change of steroid levels that occur during short-term treatment with high-dose corticosteroids.

Although similar in many respects to the major depressive disorders, the depression seen in Cushing's syndrome does have certain distinguishing clinical characteristics. Irritability is a prominent and consistent feature, as are symptoms of autonomic activation such as shaking, palpitations, and sweating. Depressed affect is often intermittent, with episodes lasting 1 to 3 days and recurring very frequently at irregular intervals. Patients usually feel their best, not their worst, in the morning. Psychomotor retardation, although present in many patients, is usually not so pronounced as to be clinically obvious and is usually apparent only in retrospect after improvement with treatment. The majority of these patients are not withdrawn, monosyllabic, unspontaneous, or hopeless. Their guilt, when present, is not irrational or self-accusatory and is primarily related to their realistic inability to function effectively. Significant cognitive impairment, including disorders of concentration, learning, and memory, is a very consistent and prominent clinical feature.

Improvement in Neuropsychiatric Symptoms after Treatment

Significant improvements in depression rating scores occur after treatment produces decreases in cortisol. In treated patients, improvements in depressed mood begin with a decrease in the frequency of days when the patient feels depressed. In addition, each episode lasts a shorter period of time, perhaps only a few hours instead of 1 to 2 days. The patients also describe a change in the quality of the depressive mood, so that they no longer experience it being as deep. They no longer feel depressed without some external precipitating reason. A mood change comes on gradually and abates gradually, rather than appearing suddenly as before. Crying becomes less frequent, is less easily elicited by environmental upsets, occurs only with some identifiable external precipitant, and is of shorter duration.

The time course of improvement in depressed mood compared to improvement in other neurovegetative symptoms is of interest. In patients with Cushing's disease who manifest depressed mood at initial evaluation and are subsequently studied during the first 12 months after treatment, improvement in symptoms other than depressed mood occur prior to improvement in depressed mood. Depressed mood is less likely than irritability and sleep, for example, to be among the first cluster of symptoms to improve. Interestingly, this lag is similar to that seen in psychiatric patients with depressive episodes treated with antidepressants, in whom improvements in sleep and psychomotor activity often occur prior to improvement in depressed mood.

Cognitive testing after treatment indicates improvement in many, but not all, affected functions. After cortisol levels decline to normal concentrations, verbal learning and verbal functions such as verbal fluency improve.

Antidepressant medication is more effective after treatment has normalized cortisol levels. When selective serotonin reuptake inhibitors are administered prior to treatment, patients report only partial effectiveness, so that only mood or only vegetative symptoms improve. After treatment, antidepressants can be helpful when depressed mood lingers or is exacerbated by the sharp and rapid decline in steroid levels.

The long-term impact of Cushing's disease on subjective well-being after cure has been studied by using validated health-related questionnaires that assess quality of life. While there is partial resolution of physical and psychosocial decrements after treatment, at long-term follow-up many report some decrease in quality of life.

Brain-Imaging Studies in Cushing's Syndrome

Brain-imaging technology has provided further information about the effects of cortisol on brain structure and function. The hippocampus is a brain structure key to learning and memory. During active Cushing's syndrome, greater elevations in cortisol are associated with smaller hippocampal formation volume. Reduced hippocampal formation volume is associated with lower scores for verbal learning and recall. After treatment reduces cortisol concentrations to normal, the hippocampal formation increases in volume more consistently and to a greater degree than other brain structures examined for comparison. Greater decreases from the initial pretreatment cortisol levels are associated with greater increases in hippocampal formation volume. Studies indicate that patients with Cushing's disease show a reduction in the metabolism of glucose in several brain regions. Studies using functional brain imaging in Cushing's syndrome indicate altered activation in the verbal learning (encoding) systems, including the hippocampus. In addition, accuracy of emotion processing is decreased, and altered activation patterns occur in the brain regions subserving it.

Mechanisms for the Behavioral Effects of Cortisol

The neuropsychiatric abnormalities seen in untreated Cushing's syndrome are related, at least in part, to the effect of elevated levels of cortisol. Cortisol has pleiotropic effects in the central nervous system. Possible mechanisms for the effect of cortisol on mood, cognition, and vegetative functions include those already shown to be actions of glucocorticoids in animals. These include a direct effect on receptors of central nervous system cells, the synthesis or function of neurotransmitters, effects on glucose metabolism and electrolytes, increasing sensitivity of the brain to other neuroactive substances such as excitatory amino acids, effects on nerve growth factors, and neurogenesis.

While this article has focused on a single adrenal steroid, cortisol, levels of other adrenal glucocorticoids as well as sex steroids produced by the adrenal, such as testosterone and dehydroepiandrosterone (DHEA), are also altered in patients with Cushing's syndrome. These substances likely modify the effect of cortisol on psychopathology, and their role remains to be elucidated.

Further Reading

Brunetti, A., Fulham, M. J., Aloj, L., et al. (1998). Decreased brain glucose utilization in patients with Cushing's disease. *Journal of Nuclear Medicine* **39**, 786–790.

Cohen, S. I. (1980). Cushing's syndrome: a psychiatric study of 29 patients. *British Journal of Psychiatry* **136**, 120–124.

Jeffcoate, W. J., Silverstone, J. T., Edwards, C. R. and Besser, G. M. (1979). Psychiatric manifestations of Cushing's syndrome: response to lowering of plasma cortisol. *Quarterly Journal of Medicine* **48**, 465–472.

Kelly, W. F., Checkley, S. A., Bender, D. A. and Mashiter, K. (1983). Cushing's syndrome and depression – a prospective study of 26 patients. *British Journal of Psychiatry* **142**, 16–19.

Lindsay, J. R., Nansel, T., Baid, S., Gumowski, J. and Nieman, L. (2006). Long-term impaired quality of life in Cushing's syndrome despite initial improvement after surgical remission. *Journal of Clinical Endocrinology and Metabolism* **91**, 447–453.

Loosen, P. T., Chambliss, B., DeBold, C. R., Shelton, R. and Orth, D. N. (1992). Psychiatric phenomenology in Cushing's Disease. *Pharmacopsychiatry* **25**, 192–198.

Mauri, M., Sinforiani, E., Bono, G., et al. (1993). Memory impairment in Cushing' s disease. *Acta Neurologica Scandinavica* **87**, 52–55.

Shipley, J. E., Schteingart, D. E., Tandon, R. and Starkman, M. N. (1992). Sleep architecture and sleep apnea in patients with Cushing's disease. *Sleep* **15**, 514–518.

Sonino, N., Fava, G. A., Belluardo, P., Girelli, M. E. and Boscaro, M. (1993). Course of depression in Cushing's syndrome: response to treatment and comparison with Grave's disease. *Hormone Research* **39**, 202–206.

Starkman, M. N. (1987). Commentary on M. Majewska: actions of steroids on neuron: role in personality, mood, stress and disease. *Integrative Psychiatry* **5**, 258–273.

Starkman, M. N. and Schteingart, D. E. (1981). Neuropsychiatric manifestations of patients with Cushing's syndrome: relationship to cortisol and adrenocorticotropic hormone levels. *Archives of Internal Medicine* **141**, 215–219.

Starkman, M. N., Schteingart, D. E. and Schork, M. A. (1981). Depressed mood and other psychiatric manifestations of Cushing's syndrome: relationship to hormone levels. *Psychosomatic Medicine* **43**, 3–18.

Starkman, M. N., Schteingart, D. E. and Schork, M. A. (1986). Cushing's syndrome after treatment: changes in cortisol and ACTH levels, and amelioration of the depressive syndrome. *Psychiatric Research* **17**, 177–188.

Starkman, M. N., Gebarski, S. S., Berent, S. and Schteingart, D. E. (1992). Hippocampal formation volume, memory dysfunction, and cortisol levels in patients with Cushing's syndrome. *Biological Psychiatry* **32**, 756–765.

Starkman, M. N., Giordani, B., Gebarski, S., Berent, S., Schork, M. A. and Schteingart, D. E. (1999). Decrease in cortisol reverses human hippocampal atrophy following treatment of Cushing's disease. *Biological Psychiatry* **46**, 1595–1602.

Starkman, M. N., Giordani, B., Berent, S., Schork, M. A. and Schteingart, D. E. (2001). Elevated cortisol levels in Cushing's disease are associated with cognitive decrements. *Psychosomatic Medicine* **63**, 985–993.

Starkman, M. N., Giordani, B., Gebarski, S. S. and Schteingart, D. E. (2003). Improvement in learning associated with increase in hippocampal formation volume. *Biological Psychiatry* **53**, 233–238.

Tucker, R. P., Weinstein, H. E., Schteingart, D. E. and Starkman, M. N. (1978). EEG changes and serum cortisol levels in Cushing's syndrome. *Clinical Electroencephalography* **9**, 32–37.

Whelan, T. B., Schteingart, D. E., Starkman, M. N. and Smith, A. (1980). Neuropsychological deficits in Cushing's syndrome. *Journal of Nervous Mental Diseases* **168**, 753–757.

L. Sleep disruption and psychiatric disorders

Sleep, Sleep Disorders, and Stress

A N Vgontzas, S Pejovic and M Karataraki
Penn State University College of Medicine, Hershey, PA, USA

This is a revised version of the article by A N Vgontzas, E O Bixler and A K Kales, Encyclopedia of Stress First Edition, volume 3, pp 449–457, © 2000, Elsevier Inc.

Glossary

Addison's disease	An endocrine disease that is associated with aldosterone and cortisol (hormones) by the adrenal glands.
Apnea	Cessation of breathing lasting at least 10 s.
Cataplexy	A brief and sudden loss of muscle control without loss of consciousness usually precipitated by strong emotions.
Continuous positive airway pressure (CPAP)	A small apparatus which through a soft plastic mask blows air gently through the nose into the throat to keep the airway open.
Cosinor analysis	Least square approximation of time series using a cosine function of known period.
Dihydroxy-phenylacetic acid (DOPAC)	A metabolite of dopamine.
Dihydroxy-phenylglycol (DHPG)	A metabolite of norepinephrine produced by the action of the enzyme monoamine oxidase (MAO) which can be measured in urine.
Hypersomnia	Disorder of excessive diurnal and nocturnal sleep.
Hypnagogic	Occurrence of an event while drifting into sleep.
Hypoxia	A pathological condition in which the body as a whole (generalized hypoxia) or region of the body (tissue hypoxia) is deprived of adequate oxygen supply.
Idiopathic	Of unknown causation.
Microneuro-graphy	A method to record the traffic of impulses in human nerves with percutaneously inserted needle electrodes.
Narcolepsy	Sleep disorder associated with excessive daytime sleepiness, involuntary daytime sleep episodes, disturbed nocturnal sleep, and cataplexy (sudden loss of muscle tone).
Parasomnia	Is any sleep disorder such as sleep-walking, teeth grinding, night terrors, rhythmic movement disorder, rapid eye movement (REM) behavior disorder, restless leg syndrome, and sleep talking, characterized by partial arousals during sleep or during transitions between wakefulness and sleep.
Polysomno-graphy	The continuous and simultaneous recording of physiological variables during sleep, e.g., electroencephalography, electro-oculography, electromyography, electrocardiography, respiratory flow, etc.
Pulsatile analysis	A global analysis of the mechanical function of the cardiovascular system, including the determinants of cardiac output.
Slow-wave sleep (SWS)	Sleep characterized by electroencephalogram waves of duration slower than 4 Hz and high amplitude.
Stage rapid eye movement (REM) sleep	The stage of sleep with highest brain activity characterized by enhanced brain metabolism and vivid dreaming.

Sleep appears to be an important element in maintaining equilibrium or homeostasis that is vital for the survival of living organisms. In this article, we review the association between sleep, sleep disorders, and stress, which has been defined as a state of disharmony, or threatened homeostasis.

Normal Sleep

Humans spend at least one-third of their lives asleep, yet there is little understanding of why we need sleep and what mechanisms underlie its capacities for physical and mental restoration. However, there has been a significant increase of empirical knowledge that is useful in the evaluation and management of most sleep complaints and their underlying disorder.

The interaction of circadian effects, i.e., usual time to go to sleep and amount of prior wakefulness (homeostatic response), determines the onset and amount of sleep. Natural sleep–wake rhythms cycle at about 25 h rather than coinciding with the solar 24-h schedule. As a result, many people depend on external cues to keep their diurnal cycle on time. The normal diurnal clock resists natural changes in its pattern by more than about 1 h per day, which explains the sleep difficulties that usually accompany adaptation to new time zones or switches in work shifts.

Individuals differ considerably in their natural sleep patterns. Most adults in nontropical areas are comfortable with 6.5–8.0 h daily, taken in a single period. Children and adolescents sleep more than adults, and young adults sleep more than older ones. Normal sleep consists of four to six behaviorally and electroencephalographically (EEG) defined cycles, including periods during which the brain is active (associated with rapid eye movements, called REM sleep), preceded by four progressively deeper, quieter sleep stages graded 1–4 on the basis of increasingly slow EEG patterns. Slow-wave sleep (SWS; also referred to as deep sleep; stages 3 and 4) gradually lessens with age and usually disappears in the elderly.

Sleep Disorders

Sleep disorders are common in the general population and are associated with significant medical, psychological, and social disturbances. Insomnia, the most common sleep disorder, most often reflects psychological disturbances. Excessive daytime sleepiness is the predominant complaint of most patients evaluated in sleep disorders clinics and often reflects organic dysfunction. Narcolepsy, idiopathic hypersomnia, and sleep apnea are the most common disorders associated with excessive daytime sleepiness. Narcolepsy and idiopathic hypersomnia are chronic brain disorders with an onset at a young age; sleep apnea occurs predominantly in middle-aged men and (to a lesser degree) women and is associated with obesity and cardiovascular complications. The parasomnias, including sleepwalking, night terrors, and nightmares, have benign implications in childhood but often reflect psychopathology or significant stress in adolescents and adults and organicity in the elderly.

Sleep, Sleep Disorders, and Physical and Emotional Stress

"Stress is life and life is stress" in Hans Selye's words. If it is a fact that there is no life without stress, it is also true that there is no life without sleep. Thus, it is not surprising that the association between sleep and physical and emotional stress has been long recognized. Hippocrates observed early on the relationship between mental and physical health and sleep and stated that sleeplessness is a sign of pain and suffering and may lead to mental illness while sleeping during the day (daytime sleepiness) is an indication of illness. Also, sleep has been an ancient remedy in the hands of physicians to combat emotional or physical stress, e.g., infection.

Acute or short-term sleep disturbance is usually associated with a variety of situational stresses (work-related, interpersonal, or financial difficulties) or with medical problems such as pain, cardiopulmonary or gastrointestinal disorders, or the febrile prodromes to influenza. Various drugs, including those that humans have been using for hundreds of years to decrease stress and dysphoria such as alcohol, nicotine, and caffeine, can affect adversely the quantity and quality of sleep. Stressful life events at the onset of sleep disorders are quite common, particularly in those disorders that appear to be of emotional origin, such as insomnia. It has been found that 75% of the chronic insomniacs had experienced some stressful life event at about the time insomnia began. Stressful life events are present, although to a lesser degree compared to insomniacs, in other sleep disorders, such as narcolepsy or sleep apnea, or adult sleepwalking, night terrors, and nightmares. The presence of stressful life events at the onset of organic disorders, such as narcolepsy or sleep apnea, is considered coincidental. However, it is interesting to note that, for example, it has been proposed that in narcolepsy it is the combination of genetic factors and stress, including emotional stress, which leads to the manifestation of the disorder. In this respect, a recent study showed that a majority of people with narcolepsy had a stressful life event at onset of their illness.

Psychological distress appears to be quite common among patients with sleep disorders. In some of these disorders, such as chronic insomnia or adult parasomnias, it appears to be primary or etiologic. In other sleep disorders, such as sleep apnea, narcolepsy, or idiopathic hypersomnia, it appears to be secondary or reactive to the chronic physical problems associated with the sleep disorder. Furthermore, it has been reported that in insomniacs, it is not only stress, but also how they handle stress that leads to chronic difficulties in initiating and maintaining sleep. In particular, insomniacs handle external stress and conflict by internalization of their emotions which results in a combination of emotional arousal and physiological activation. This mental and physiological hyperarousal leads to difficulty in initiating sleep, whether at the beginning of the sleep period or when returning to sleep following awakening. Fear of sleeplessness and performance anxiety further intensifies the emotional arousal. All of these factors through behavioral conditioning lead to a vicious circle that perpetuates insomnia.

Because of the high frequency of emotional distress associated with sleep disorders, stress management techniques are routinely recommended to all sleep-disorder patients. Specifically, in insomnia, besides recommending sleep hygiene measures, medication, or psychotherapy, a series of stress management measures are routinely recommended, such as: recognizing the association between stressful events and sleeplessness; ventilating conflict and anger to avoid internalization of emotions; addressing daily worries a few hours before bedtime; becoming tolerant of occasional sleeplessness; avoiding rumination over sleep difficulty; and relaxation techniques. Increasing empirical evidence suggests that cognitive behavioral therapy (CBT) for insomnia is the most effective nonpharmacological approach in the management of chronic insomnia. Besides using educational and behavioral techniques, CBT involves cognitive restructuring that aims at identifying and altering faulty beliefs and attitudes about sleep that in themselves are believed to perpetuate the vicious cycle of insomnia, fear of sleeplessness, emotional arousal, and further sleep disturbance. However, the CBT approach does not address long-term personality patterns such as internalization of psychological conflict and inhibition of emotions associated with insomnia. In the sleep disorders of organic origin, such as narcolepsy or sleep apnea, supportive therapy, including educating and advising patients and their families gently but honestly about the nature of the chronic disorder and that the symptoms are not under voluntary control, is of utmost importance. Furthermore, helping the patient to adjust his or her lifestyle to the changes imposed by the sleep disorder, i.e., sleep or cataplectic attacks in narcolepsy, or enhancing his/her compliance to the chronic use of cumbersome and often, anxiety-provoking therapies, such as continuous positive airway pressure (CPAP) in sleep apnea, is an important dimension of the overall management of the sleep-disorder patient.

Sleep disturbance is a very frequent symptom in most of the psychiatric disorders. Depression, anxiety disorders, and acute onset schizophrenia are frequently associated with sleep disturbance. Depression, in particular melancholia, is associated with early morning awakening, while sleep loss is the early sign of an acute onset schizophrenia or an early sign of relapse. In contrast, sleep disturbance or sleep loss can lead to mental illness. For example, it has been reported that chronic insomnia is associated with a higher incidence of major depression. Also, acute sleep loss can lead to a manic episode in a patient with bipolar disorder. Thus, it is not surprising that sleep therapy or hypnotherapy was very common in the practice of mental health professionals in the nineteenth and early twentieth centuries. Today, the improvement of the quality and quantity of sleep of a person under emotional distress is one of the therapeutic priorities of the practicing clinician.

Sleep and Stress System

In mammalian organisms, including humans, the stress system consists of components of the central nervous system (CNS), including: the corticotropin-releasing hormone (CRH) neurons of the hypothalamic paraventricular nucleus; and several, mostly norepinephric nuclei of the brain stem, and their peripheral limbs, the hypothalamic-pituitary-adrenal (HPA) axis and the peripheral autonomic system, whose main function is to maintain homeostasis, both in the resting and stress states.

Normal Sleep and Stress System

Although the association between stress and sleep has been noticed for hundreds of years, a more systematic and scientifically based approach in the relation between sleep and stress system has only existed since the 1980s. It was in 1983 that Dr. Weitzman and his colleagues reported that sleep, in particular SWS, appears to have an inhibiting influence on the HPA axis and cortisol secretion (**Figure 1**). Since then, several studies have replicated this finding. In a reverse mode, activation of the HPA axis and central administration of CRH can lead to arousal and sleeplessness. In normal sleepers, wakefulness and stage 1 sleep (light sleep) accompany cortisol increases, while SWS is associated with declining plasma cortisol levels. In addition, in healthy people, induced sleep disruption (continuous arousals) is associated with significant increases of plasma cortisol levels. Furthermore, mean plasma cortisol level was significantly higher in a group of subjects with a shorter total sleep time than another group with a longer total sleep time. Finally, it has been suggested that the effect of aging on the levels and diurnal variation of human adrenocorticotropic activity could be involved in the etiology of poor sleep in the elderly.

REM sleep, which is a state of CNS activation that resembles unconscious wakefulness (paradoxical sleep), appears to be associated with a higher activity of the HPA axis (**Figure 1**). An early study showed that urinary 17-hydroxy corticoids were increased during REM epochs in urological patients. One study in healthy, normal sleepers showed that the amount of REM sleep was positively correlated with 24-h urinary free-cortisol (UFC) excretion. These results are consistent with the co-existence of stress system activation, and REM sleep increases in patients with melancholic depression. In rats, chronic mild stress resulted in disruption of REM sleep, including a reduced latency to the onset of first REM period, providing support for the validity of the proposed association between stress and mechanisms underlying endogenous depression, including REM sleep alterations.

Although the effects of sleep on the sympathetic nervous system have been studied less frequently, it appears that in humans during sleep, catecholaminergic activity is decreased (**Figure 1**). In particular, catecholaminergic activity appears to be suppressed during SWS, while there is an activation of the sympathetic nervous system during REM sleep. It has

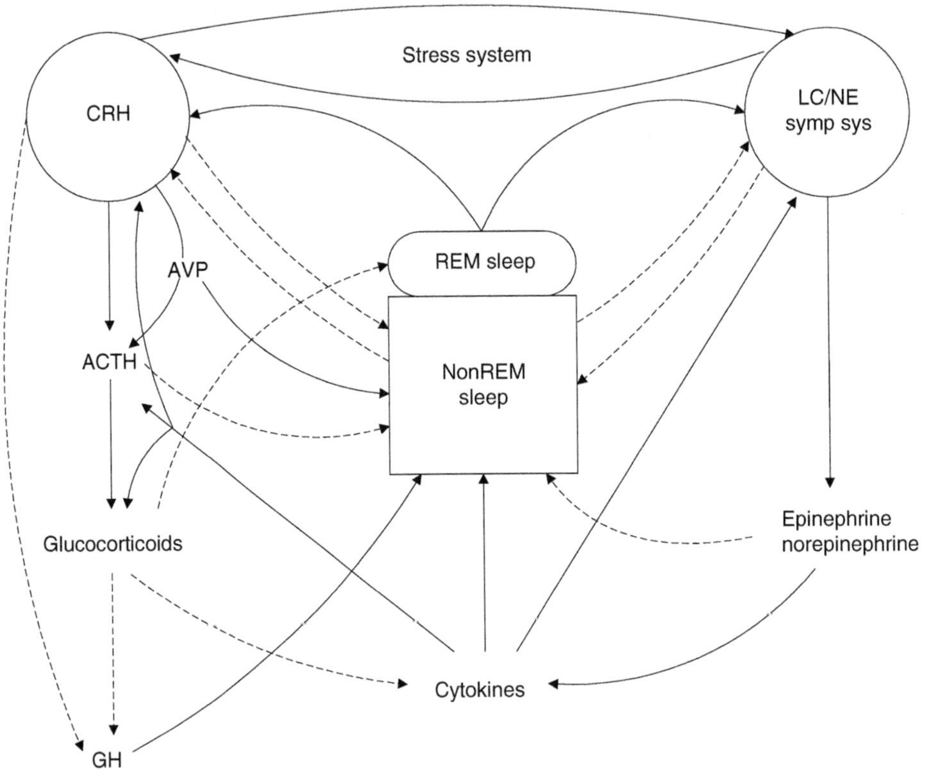

Figure 1 A simplified, heuristic model of the interactions between central and peripheral components of the stress system with sleep and REM sleep. CRH–ACTH cortisol and LC/NE systems are two main arousal systems that their activation leads to wakefulness. NonREM sleep is associated with an inhibitory effect on these two wakefulness promoting systems, whereas during REM there is an activation of both limbs of the stress system. ACTH, corticotropin; AVP, arginine vasopressin; CRH, corticotropin-releasing hormone; GH, growth hormone; LC/NE symp sys, locus ceruleus-norepinephrine/sympathetic system. A solid line denotes promotion/stimulation; a broken line denotes disturbance/inhibition.

been found that in healthy, normal sleepers, the amount of REM sleep correlated to 24-h excretion of urinary catecholamines while sympathetic-nerve activity measured using microneurography, was elevated during REM sleep. Interestingly, in rats, locus ceruleus (LC) neurons fire most frequently during waking, less during nonREM (NREM) sleep, and are silent during paradoxical sleep.

The stress system is closely linked with immune responses. In particular, three pro-inflammatory cytokines (tumor necrosis factor-α (TNF-α), interleukin (IL)-1, and IK-6) have a strong stimulating effect on HPA axis (**Figure 1**). Glucocorticoids, the endproducts of the HPA axis, inhibit the production of all three cytokines, while catecholamines, the other products of the stress system, stimulate IL-6 secretion. In animals, several studies have demonstrated the potential role of these cytokines, particularly IL-1 and TNF-α in sleep regulation. In humans, these cytokines appear to be increased at nighttime. A study in young, healthy, normal sleepers showed that the amount and quality (depth) of sleep correlated negatively with the overall daytime secretion of IL-6. These data suggest that a good night's sleep is associated with decreased secretion of IL-6, a good sense of wellbeing, and that good sleep is associated with decreased exposure of tissues to the pro-inflammatory and potentially detrimental actions of IL-6.

The role of corticotropin-releasing hormone in sleep–wake regulation CRH, which is produced and released from parvicellular neurons of the paraventricular nucleus, is the key regulator of the HPA axis. Release of CRH is followed by enhanced secretion of adrenocorticotropic hormone (ACTH) from the anterior pituitary and cortisol from the adrenal cortex. CRH exerts various influences on behavior, including wakefulness and sleep.

Several studies in animals have shown that intracerebroventricular administration (ICV) of CRH induces increased waking. Also, specific CRH receptor blockade reduces spontaneous awakening and rat strains deficient in the synthesis and secretion of hypothalamic CRH spend less time awake than do control counterparts. Finally, CRH concentration in the brains of rats exhibits circadian fluctuations and is highest when rats are most active. Several reports indicate that CRH is excitatory in the LC, hippocampus, cerebral cortex, and some portions of the hypothalamus. Spontaneous discharge rates in the LC are highest during arousal and lowest during sleep. Also, it has been reported that the brain β_1-adrenergic system is involved in the restraint stress-induced increase in arousal in rats.

In humans, the majority of studies suggest that the sleep of young individuals is rather resistant to the arousing effects of CRH. In contrast, middle-aged individuals responded to an equivalent dose of CRH with significantly more wakefulness and suppression of SWS compared to baseline. Based on these findings, we concluded that middle-aged men show increased vulnerability of sleep to stress hormones, possibly resulting in impairments in the quality of sleep during periods of stress. These findings suggest that changes in sleep physiology associated with middle-age play a significant role in the marked increase of prevalence of insomnia in middle-age. Also, peripheral administration of CRH is associated with REM suppression, which is stronger in the young than in the middle-aged. The administration of ACTH and its analogs in humans has been associated with general CNS activation consisting of a decreased sleep period time and sleep efficiency, and an increase of sleep latency. Continuous administration of ACTH produced a marked reduction in REM sleep.

Arginine vasopressin (AVP) is a peptide which acts as a co-factor of CRH in the activation of the HPA system. Several experiments in rats have suggested that the continuous administration of AVP causes sleep disturbance.

Steroid effects on sleep The administration of glucocorticoids has been reported to be associated with a robust suppression of REM sleep (**Figure 1**). Also, in some studies, it has been reported that the continuous or pulsatile nocturnal administration of cortisol paradoxically was associated with a modest increase of SWS in addition to the well-established decrease of REM sleep. The opposite effects of cortisol on SWS compared to CRH are believed to be mediated by a feedback inhibition of CRH from cortisol. In contrast, the glucocorticoid antagonist, mifepristone (RU-486), led to a significant worsening of sleep in normal controls. The administration of mineralocorticoids is not associated with significant changes of sleep structure.

A study in patients with Addison's disease recently demonstrated that an evening replacement dose of hydrocortisone was necessary for proper expression of REM sleep (*vide infra*) suggesting that glucocorticoids have some permissive action for this sleep parameter, possibly reflecting an inverse u-shaped dose–response curve.

Interestingly, in clinical practice, the use of glucocorticoids is associated with sleep disturbance. In fact, in a multicenter study in which steroids were used on a short-term basis, sleep disturbance was one of the most common side effects.

Aging, HPA axis, and sleep Old age is associated with marked sleep changes consisting of increased wakefulness, minimal amounts of SWS, declining amounts of REM sleep, and earlier retiring and rising times. Some studies have shown that older adults have elevated cortisol levels at the time of the circadian nadir and have higher basal cortisol levels than younger adults. It is difficult to discern whether the latter changes are associated with aging or increased medical morbidity common in this group. It has been suggested that the effect of aging on the levels and diurnal variation of human adrenocorticotropic activity could be involved in the etiology of poor sleep in the elderly. Higher evening cortisol concentrations are associated with lower amounts of REM sleep and increased wakefulness. More recently, it was shown that older women without estrogen replacement therapy (ERT), when subjected to mild stress, showed greater disturbances in sleep parameters than women receiving ERT, suggesting that female hormones protect women's sleep from external stressors.

Sleep Deprivation and Stress System

If sleep is important for our sense of wellbeing, then it is conceivable that sleep deprivation represents a stress to humans and should be associated with activation of the stress system. However, several studies that have assessed the effects of one night's sleep deprivation on the HPA axis have shown that cortisol secretion is either not or minimally affected by sleep following prolonged wakefulness. Two studies have reported somewhat antithetical results, with the one study showing that cortisol secretion is elevated the next evening following sleep deprivation, and the other study showing a significant decrease of plasma cortisol levels the next day and recovery night. The study that showed decrease of plasma cortisol levels following sleep loss indicated that this inhibition of the HPA axis activity was associated with an enhanced activity of the growth hormone axis. The finding that sleep deprivation leads to lower cortisol levels postdeprivation (primarily during the subsequent night of sleep) suggests that lowering the level of HPA activity, which is increased in depression, may be the mechanism through which sleep deprivation improves the mood of depressed individuals. Prolonged sleep deprivation that results in death is associated with increased plasma norepinephrine levels, and higher ACTH and corticosteroid levels at the later phase of sleep deprivation. It is postulated that these increases are due to the stress of dying rather than to sleep loss.

A recent study demonstrated that a week of partial sleep restriction did not affect significantly the 24-h cortisol secretion either in men or women. However, there was a significant effect in terms of the circadian secretory pattern of the hormone as indicated by the significant time effect, and the time and gender interaction effect. Specifically, the peak cortisol secretion in the morning was lower after sleep restriction than baseline and this difference was stronger in men than in women. In both genders, the peak of cortisol secretion was shifted by 2 h earlier than baseline (08.00 versus 06.00). Sleep restriction did not affect significantly the nadir value of cortisol secretion, neither the afternoon, nor evening presleep levels.

The inconsistency in cortisol secretion after total or partial sleep loss may be explained by methodological differences in these studies, i.e., nonstressful deprivation is not associated with increased cortisol secretion. Also, the higher evening cortisol levels reported in studies where sleep was curtailed at the beginning of the night may represent a change of the 24-h-secretory pattern, e.g., a shift of the nadir point later at night.

Although sleep deprivation appears to have beneficial effects on the mood of depressed individuals, in healthy individuals, sleep deprivation leads to next-day fatigue and somnolence, decreased concentration and attention, and increased vulnerability to accidents. These effects appear to be mediated partially by the increased levels of IL-6, which is related to the stress system. It has been shown that following sleep deprivation, there is an increase of IL-6 levels during the daytime and a decrease during the first night of sleep following sleep deprivation. The increased levels of IL-6 during the daytime can explain the somnolence and fatigue experienced by the individuals after one night's sleep loss, whereas the nighttime undersecretion of IL-6 might be responsible for the better quality (depth) of their sleep. The exact mechanisms of this elevation are not known. However, alterations of the stress system following sleep deprivation may be responsible for this elevation. For example, the decreased levels of cortisol postdeprivation and/or possible increase of catecholaminergic activity can lead to elevation of plasma IL-6 levels. It has been shown that sleep deprivation in humans appears to enhance norepinephrine and dopamine activity.

Sleep Disorders and Stress System

Although sleep disorders/disturbances with their various physical and mental effects on the individual should be expected to affect the stress system, information regarding the effects of sleep disorders/disturbances on this system is lacking.

Insomnia and stress system Insomnia, a symptom of various psychiatric or medical disorders, may also be the result of an environmental disturbance or a stressful situation. When insomnia is chronic and severe, it may itself become a stress that affects the patient's life so greatly that it is perceived by the patient as a distinct disorder itself. Either way, as a manifestation of stress or a stressor itself, insomnia is expected to be related to the stress system. There is a paucity of data regarding the activity of the stress system in insomniacs. Few studies have measured cortisol levels in poor sleepers or insomniacs, and those results are inconsistent. The majority of these studies reported no difference between controls and poor sleepers in 24-h cortisol or 17-hydroxy steroid excretion. In a study in 15 young adults with insomnia, it was demonstrated that 24-h UFC levels were positively correlated with total wake time (**Table 1**). In addition, 24-h urinary levels of catecholamines and their metabolites, dihydroxyphenyl glycol (DHPG), and 3,4-dihydroxy-phenylacetic acid (DOPAC) were positively correlated with percent stage 1 sleep and wake time after sleep onset. Norepinephrine tended to correlate positively with percent stage 1 sleep and wake time after sleep onset and negatively with percent SWS. It was concluded that in chronic insomnia, the activity of both limbs of the stress system, i.e., the HPA axis and the sympathetic system, relates positively to the degree of objective sleep disturbance.

Table 1 Sleep disorders and the stress system

Insomnia	Increased 24-h secretion of ACTH-cortisol, more intense in the evening; positive correlations between 24-h UFC and urinary catecholamines and polysomnographic indices of severity of the disorder
Sleep apnea	Increased excretion of urinary catecholamines; increased nighttime plasma catecholamines; increased daytime plasma IL-6 and TNF-α levels; mild hypercortisolemia compared to obese controls
Narcolepsy	Increased daytime plasma IL-6 and TNF-α levels
Idiopathic hypersomnia	Mild hypocortisolism; enhanced ACTH secretion to exogenous CRH; central CRH deficiency

ACTH, adrenocorticotropic hormone; CRH, corticotropin-releasing hormone; IL-6, interleukin-6; TNF-α, tumor-necrosis factor-α; UFC, urinary free-cortisol.

However, in this study also, the total amount of the 24-h UFC or catecholamines excretion was not different from normative values. The results on the positive correlation between urinary catecholamines and polysomnographic indices of sleep disturbance in chronic insomnia are consistent with previous studies that showed elevated urinary catecholamines in chronically stressed subjects who experience sleep disturbance or in healthy subjects whose sleep was affected by nocturnal aircraft noise.

In a recent controlled study in which objective sleep testing and frequent blood sampling was employed, 24-h ACTH and cortisol plasma concentrations were significantly higher in people with insomnia than matched healthy controls. Within the 24-h period, the greatest elevations were observed in the evening and first half of the night. Also, people with insomnia with a high degree of objective sleep disturbance (sleep time <70%) compared to those with a low degree of sleep disturbance secreted a higher amount of cortisol. Pulsatile analysis revealed a significantly higher number of peaks per 24 h in insomniacs than in controls ($p < 0.05$), while Cosinor analysis showed no differences in the circadian pattern of ACTH or cortisol secretion between people with insomnia and controls. Thus, insomnia is associated with an overall increase of ACTH and cortisol secretion, which, however, retains a normal circadian pattern. Also, this increase relates positively to the degree of objective sleep disturbance. These findings are consistent with a disorder of CNS hyperarousal rather than one of sleep loss, which is usually associated with no change or a decrease in cortisol secretion, or a circadian disturbance. Two recent studies found that cortisol was elevated in primary insomnia with objectively documented sleep disturbance during the evening and nighttime. However, another study found that people with insomnia without evidence of objective sleep disturbance did not report differences from controls. These findings suggest that objective sleep disturbance may be a useful index of the biological severity of the disorder.

Chronic activation or dysregulation of the stress system may play a significant role in the poor mental and physical health associated with chronic insomnia. Insomnia is associated with a higher risk of development of psychiatric disorders, such as major depression and anxiety disorders. Also, people with insomnia tend to have more health complaints than normal controls, both as children and adults, and they do appear to have poorer health in other respects. Psychosomatic-type illnesses, such as allergy, asthma, colitis, hypertension, migraine headaches, and ulcers, are reported by about twofold more people with insomnia than controls. Consistent with the above finding, a recent study that used a large general random sample of men and women (1754 people) reported that insomnia is independently associated with medical disorders such as hypertension. Also, nonspecific physical symptoms, such as headache, diarrhea, constipation, stomach discomfort, palpitations, shortness of breath, nonspecific pain, tiredness, and weakness, are also more common in people with insomnia. It can be hypothesized that these physical complaints, including those labeled as psychosomatic, reflect the chronic effects of an activation/dysregulation of the stress system in various body organs and functions. Furthermore, these data suggest that the therapeutic goal in insomnia should not be just to improve the quality or quantity of nighttime sleep. Rather, they suggest that the common practice of prescribing hypnotics only for patients with chronic insomnia at most is of limited efficacy. Sedative antidepressants alone or in combination with the newer antidepressants, e.g., selective serotonin reuptake inhibitors (SSRIs), appear to have a normalizing effect on measures, i.e., cortisol. Furthermore, the focus of psychotherapeutic and behavioral modalities, including sleep hygiene measures, should not be to just improve the emotional and physiological state of the people with insomnia pre- or during sleep, but rather to decrease the overall emotional and physiologic hyperarousal and its underlying factors, present throughout the 24 h sleep–wake period. Finally, objective measurements of sleep using simpler methods such as actigraphy may prove useful in predicting the severity of the disorders and, therefore, the urgency for medical intervention.

Disorders of excessive daytime sleepiness and stress system Obstructive sleep apnea, the most common sleep disorder associated with excessive daytime sleepiness and fatigue, is associated with nocturnal hypoxia and sleep fragmentation. The latter conditions should be expected to be associated with an activation of the stress system. Indeed, it has been shown that urinary catecholamines, as well as plasma catecholamines measured during the nighttime, are elevated in people with sleep apnea compared to controls (**Table 1**). Also, using microneurography, it has been shown that obstructive apneas are associated with a surge of sympathetic nerve activity. It has been proposed that sympathetic activation in sleep apnea is one of the mechanisms leading to the development of hypertension, a condition commonly associated with sleep apnea. With similar logic, it was expected that sleep apnea would be associated with an activation of the HPA axis also. However, the few studies that have assessed the plasma cortisol levels in people with sleep apnea have failed to show any differences from controls. Also, no differences were reported in the excretion of cortisol following the abrupt withdrawal of CPAP, a definitive treatment for sleep apnea. However, whether these results represent an adaptation of the HPA axis to a chronic physical stress or are a result of incomplete assessment of the HPA axis, remains open.

Narcolepsy and idiopathic hypersomnia are two primary sleep disorders of bipolar disorders currently treated with medication such as stimulants and modafinil. The association of the two other organic disorders of excessive daytime sleepiness, narcolepsy and idiopathic hypersomnia, with the stress system has not been assessed. Preliminary data from a study that assessed the responsiveness of plasma cortisol and ACTH to the exogenous administration of CRH in individuals with idiopathic hypersomnia indicated reduced 24-h UFC levels compared to controls while ACTH response to CRH tended to be significantly higher in the patients compared to controls (**Table 1**). These preliminary findings suggest a subtle hypocortisolism and inferred central CRH deficiency in patients with idiopathic hypersomnia. A central CRH deficiency in these patients is consistent with their clinical profile of increased daytime sleepiness and deep nocturnal sleep (generalized hypoarousal).

The stress related cytokines (TNF-α, IL-1, and IL-6) have been suggested as potential mediators of excessive daytime sleepiness (**Table 1**). In 1997, a report on the morning plasma levels of TNF-α, IL-1β, and IL-6 in patients with sleep apnea, narcolepsy and idiopathic hypersomnia showed that TNF-α was significantly elevated in people with sleep apnea and narcolepsy compared to that in normal controls. Plasma IL-1β concentrations were not different between the sleep disorder patients and controls, whereas IL-6 was markedly and significantly elevated in patients with sleep apnea compared to that in normal controls. The primary factor in the elevation of plasma TNF-α values was the degree of nocturnal sleep disturbance, whereas the primary determinant for IL-6 levels was body mass index. These findings suggest that TNF-α and IL-6 might play a significant role in mediating sleepiness and fatigue in disorders of excessive daytime sleepiness in humans. Also, it was hypothesized that IL-6 plays a role in mediating sleepiness in obese patients, even those without obstructive sleep apnea, who experience, as confirmed also in the sleep laboratory, a significant degree of daytime sleepiness and fatigue. In 1996, another study reported that the circadian rhythm of TNF-α was significantly altered in patients with sleep apnea and that the peak concentration that occurred during the night in normal control subjects was not present in patients. Rather, the patients exhibited increased TNF-α concentrations in the afternoon, the time period during which concentrations in normal control subjects were at a minimum. Furthermore, in this study, it was reported that the alteration in the cytokine profiles were not normalized by the CPAP therapy. Since then, several studies have confirmed that TNF-α and IL-6 are elevated in disorders of excessive daytime sleepiness, i.e., sleep apnea and narcolepsy independently of confounding variables such as obesity. Interestingly, a recent study reported that neutralizing TNF-α is associated with a significant decrease of sleepiness in patients with sleep apnea.

Conclusion

In conclusion, the collective findings on the association between sleep and stress system appear to suggest that sleep is a major antistress mechanism that is vital in the preservation of the physical and mental homeostasis of the human species. Also, sleep loss appears to be a physical and mental stress to humans, whereas sleep disorders/disturbances may lead to a significant dysregulation of the stress system. More knowledge on the association between sleep, sleep disorders, and stress system would lead to a better understanding of the mechanisms that underlie sleep's capacities for physical and mental restoration and to improve treatment of sleep disorders/disturbances.

Further Reading

Chrousos, G. P. (1995). The hypothalamic-pituitary-adrenal axis and immune-mediated inflammation. *New England Journal of Medicine* **332**, 1351–1362.

Chrousos, G. P. and Gold, P. W. (1992). The concepts of stress and stress system disorders. *JAMA* **267**, 1244–1252.

Edinger, J. D. and Means, M. K. (2005). Cognitive-behavioral therapy for primary insomnia. *Clinical Psychology Review* **25**, 539–558.

García-Borreguero, D., Wehr, T. A., Larrosa, O., et al. (2000). Glucocorticoid replacement is permissive for rapid eye movement sleep and sleep consolidation in patients with adrenal insufficiency. *Journal of Clinical Endocrinology and Metabolism* **85**, 4201–4206.

Kales, A. and Kales, J. (1984). *Evaluation and treatment of insomnia.* New York: Oxford University Press.

Krueger, J. M. and Obál, F. (1994). Sleep factors. In: Saunders, N. A. & Sullivan, C. E. (eds.) *Sleep and breathing*, pp. 79–112. New York: Dekker.

Opp, M. R. (1995). Corticotropin-releasing hormone involvement in stressor-induced alterations in sleep and in the regulation of waking. *Immunology* **5**, 127–143.

Rechtschaffen, A. and Kales, A. (1968). *A manual of standardized terminology, techniques, and scoring system for sleep stages of human subjects.* NIH Report No. 204. Bethesda, MD: National Institutes of Health.

Rechtschaffen, A., Bergmann, B. M., Everson, C. A., et al. (1989). Sleep deprivation in the rat: X. integration and discussion of the findings. *Sleep* **12**, 68–87.

Rodenbeck, A., Heuther, G., Ruther, E., et al. (2002). Interactions between evening and nocturnal cortisol secretion and sleep parameters in patients with severe chronic primary insomnia. *Neuroscience Letters* **324**, 154–163.

Rodenbeck, A., Cohrs, S., Jordan, W., et al. (2003). The sleep-improving effects of doxepin are paralleled by a normalized plasma cortisol secretion in primary insomnia. A placebo-controlled, double-blind, randomized, cross-over study followed by an open treatment over 3 weeks. *Psychopharmacology* **170**, 423–428.

Somers, V. K., Dyken, M. E., Mark, A. L., et al. (1993). Sympathetic-nerve activity during sleep in normal subjects. *New England Journal of Medicine* **328**, 303–307.

Steiger, A. and Holsboer, F. (1997). Neuropeptides and human sleep. *Sleep* **20**, 1038–1052.

Steiger, A., Antonijevic, I. A., Bohlhalter, S., et al. (1998). Effects of hormones on sleep. *Hormone Research* **49**, 125–130.

Van Cauter, E. (2005). Endocrine physiology. In: Kryger, M. H., Roth, T. & Dement, W. C. (eds.) *Principles and practices of sleep medicine* (4th ed., pp. 266–282). Philadelphia, PA: Elsevier Saunders.

VanCauter, E., Leproult, R. and Plat, L. (2000). Age-related changes in slow wave sleep and REM sleep and relationship with growth hormone and cortisol levels in healthy men. *JAMA* **284**, 861–868.

Vgontzas, A. N., Papanicolaou, D. A., Bixler, E. O., et al. (1997). Elevation of plasma cytokines in disorders of excessive daytime sleepiness: role of sleep disturbance and obesity. *Journal of Clinical Endocrinology and Metabolism* **82**, 1313–1316.

Vgontzas, A. N. and Kales, A. (1999). Sleep and its disorders. *Annual Review of Medicine* **50**, 387–400.

Vgontzas, A. N., Bixler, E. O., Lin, H.-M., et al. (2001). Chronic insomnia is associated with nyctohemeral activation of the hypothalamic-pituitary-adrenal axis: clinical implications. *Journal of Clinical Endocrinology and Metabolism* **86**, 3787–3794.

Vgontzas, A. N., Zoumakis, M., Bixler, E. O., et al. (2003). Impaired nighttime sleep in healthy old vs. young adults is associated with elevated plasma IL-6 and cortisol levels: physiologic and therapeutic implications. *Journal of Clinical Endocrinology and Metabolism* **88**, 2087–2095.

Vgontzas, A. N., Zoumakis, M., Bixler, E. O., et al. (2004). Adverse effects of modest sleep restriction on sleepiness, performance, and inflammatory cytokines. *Journal of Clinical Endocrinology and Metabolism* **89**, 2119–2126.

Night Shiftwork

T Åkerstedt and G Lindbeck
Karolinska institutet, Stockholm, Sweden

Introduction

Shiftwork may not be the typical stressor in the classic sense, but it affects the systems of stress and restitution in a very pronounced way and causes cardiovascular disease, gastroinstestinal disease, and insomnia, among other conditions. Here we review some of the connections. But before that we need to look at the phenomenon of shiftwork. This is an arrangement of work hours through which the daily duration of production/service extends to cover operation during 2–3 work days compressed into one 24-h period. Each day is called a shift. Normally, the first step of extension beyond a day shift is to introduce morning and evening shifts (6 a.m.–2 p.m. and 2 p.m.–10 p.m., respectively). When necessary, a night shift may also be used to cover the remaining 8 h. In Europe, workers often alternate among shifts, working the same shift two to four times in succession and then switching to a new shift. In transport, health care and the service sector, the shifts may be more variable in placement and duration, but the principle of alternating among different shifts remains. Even the permanent night worker alternates between a night shift and day life during his days off. Usually, the night shift is the most problematic, causing disturbed circadian rhythms, disturbed sleep, and excessive sleepiness and several diseases deriving from these disturbances.

The Mechanism

Shift work would not present a problem were it not for the biological clock that drives physiology and psychology through a 24-h cycle, with high and low periods of activity. The central oscillator is situated in the hypothalamus. It is a self-sustained oscillator and drives much of our physiology in an approximately 24-h cycle. It receives input from light and other stimuli that synchronize the pacemaker with the environmental light–dark cycle, called Zeitgebers, which entrain (influence) the biological clock to the light–dark changes of the normal environment. Essentially, light before the circadian trough (low) phase delays the biological clock (1–2 h) and light after the trough phase advances the clock.

The influence of the circadian cycle on sleep was demonstrated in monthlong isolation studies in which individuals could live according to their own preferred sleep–wake schedules. This led to the finding that some individuals developed a period of around 25 h, and that some individuals desynchronized, showing different period lengths for their sleep–wake rhythm and for their rhythm of metabolism (rectal temperature). However, the present estimate of the period length with control for light is 24.1 h. It was later shown that whenever the sleep–wake rhythm placed sleep around the acrophase (circadian maximum) of rectal temperature, sleep was shortened, and when sleep was placed around the circadian trough phase, sleep was promoted. Thus, the biological clock interfered with sleep and wakefulness.

Effects on Sleep

The dominant health problem reported by shiftworkers is disturbed sleep and wakefulness. At least three-quarters of the shift-working population is affected. When comparing individuals with a very negative attitude to shiftwork with those with a very positive one, the strongest discriminator seems to be the ability to obtain sufficient quality of sleep during the daytime. Electroencephalograph (EEG) studies of rotating shiftworkers and similar groups showed that day sleep is 1–4 h shorter than night sleep. The shortening is due to the fact that sleep is terminated after only 4–6 h without the individual being able to return to sleep. The sleep loss is primarily taken out of stage 2 sleep (basic sleep) and stage rapid-eye movement (REM) sleep (dream sleep). Stages 3 and 4 (deep sleep) do not seem to be affected. Furthermore, the time taken to fall asleep (sleep latency) is usually shorter. Night sleep before a morning shift is also reduced, but the termination is through artificial means and the awakening is usually difficult and unpleasant. Interestingly, day sleep does not seem to improve much across series of night shifts. It appears, however, that night workers sleep slightly better (longer) than rotating workers on the night shift.

As indicated previously, shiftwork sleep duration is approximately 5.5–6 h after the night shift, and several laboratory studies have found that this amount of sleep curtailment may affect sleepiness moderately. The 2003 study by Van Dongen and colleagues indicates that the critical point for the accumulation of fatigue is approximately 7 h of sleep per night. The circadian trough and extended wakefulness (often up to 20 h) are other powerful contributors.

Alertness

Night-oriented shiftworkers complain as much about fatigue and sleepiness as they do about disturbed sleep. The sleepiness is particularly severe on the night shift, appears hardly at all on the afternoon shift, and is intermediate on the morning shift. The maximum is reached toward the early morning (5 a.m.–7 a.m.). Frequently, incidents of falling asleep occur during the night shift. At least two-thirds of the respondents report that they have experienced involuntary sleep during night work. Ambulatory EEG recordings verify that incidents of actual sleep occur during night work in, for example, process operators. Other groups, such as train drivers or truck drivers, show clear signs of falling asleep while driving at night. This occurs toward the second half of the night and appears as repeated bursts of alpha and theta EEG activity, together with closed eyes and slow undulating eye movements. As a rule, the bursts are short (1–15 s) but frequent and seem to reflect let-downs in the effort to fend off sleep. Approximately one-quarter of the subjects recorded show the EEG/electrooculograph (EOG) patterns of fighting with sleep. This is clearly a larger proportion than is found in the subjective reports of episodes of falling asleep.

Performance

As may be expected, sleepiness on the night shift is reflected in performance. One of the classic studies in this area is by Bjerner and colleagues, who showed that errors in meter readings over a period of 20 years in a gas works had a pronounced peak on the night shift. There was also a secondary peak during the afternoon. Similar observations have been made for switchboard operators and other groups. Late-night shift performance capacity has been compared with performance following the ingestion of alcohol to a 0.08% blood alcohol level.

Accidents

If sleepiness is severe enough, interaction with the environment ceases, and if this coincides with a critical need for action, an accident may ensue. Most of the available accident data on night-shift sleepiness has been obtained from the area of transportation; the National Transportation Safety Board ranks fatigue as one of the major causes of heavy vehicle accidents.

Very little relevant data are available from conventional industrial operations, but fatal work accidents show a higher risk in shiftworkers and accidents in the automotive industry may exhibit night-shift effects. An interesting analysis has been put forward by the Association of Professional Sleep Societies Committee on Catastrophes, Sleep and Public Policy. Its consensus report notes that the nuclear plant meltdown at Chernobyl occurred at 1:35 a.m. and was due to human error (apparently related to work scheduling). Similarly, the Three Mile Island reactor accident occurred between 4 and 6 a.m. and was due not only to the stuck valve, which caused a loss of coolant water, but also, more important, to the workers' failure to recognize this event, which led to the near meltdown of the reactor. Similar incidents (although with the ultimate stage having been prevented) occurred in 1985 at the David Beese reactor in Ohio and at the Rancho Seco reactor in California. Finally, the committee also stated that the NASA Challenger space shuttle disaster stemmed from errors in judgment made in the early morning hours by people who had had insufficient sleep (because of partial night work) for days prior to the launch. Still, there is very limited support for the notion that shiftwork outside the area of transportation actually carries a higher over all accident risk.

As with sleep, the two main factors behind sleepiness and performance impairment are circadian cycle homeostatic factors. Alertness falls rapidly after awakening, but gradually levels out as wakefulness is extended. The circadian influence appears as a sine-shaped superimposition on this exponential fall in alertness. Akerstedt describes this as a three-process model of alertness regulation. Space does not permit a discussion of the derivation of these functions here.

Stress Indices

A number of studies have looked at the effect of shiftwork on endocrine and other stress-related parameters. The circadian pattern of cortisol, growth hormone, and melatonin is clearly affected by night work, but the adjustment to night work is only partial. We should also consider the increased cortisol levels and reduced insulin sensitivity following the reduction of sleep to 4 h. On the other hand, there do not seem to be any data on the long-term consequences of night work on stress indices, except perhaps for a suppression of testosterone in male nightworkers with a negative overall attitude to night shifts. Also, testosterone seems linearly related to sleep duration, as demonstrated in experimental studies of shifted sleep.

Gastrointestinal Effects

Gastrointestinal complaints are more common among night shiftworkers than among day workers. In a review of a number of reports covering 34 047 people with day or shiftwork, ulcers were found to occur in 0.3–0.7% of day workers, 5% of morning and afternoon shiftworkers, 2.5–15% of rotating shiftworkers with night shifts, and 10–30% of ex-shiftworkers. Several other studies have come to similar conclusions. Other gastrointestinal disorders, including gastritis, duodenitis, and dysfunctions of digestion are more common in shiftworkers than in day workers.

The pathophysiological mechanism underlying gastrointestinal diseases in shiftworkers is unclear, but one possible explanation is that intestinal enzymes and intestinal mobility are not synchronized with the sleep–wake pattern. Intestinal enzymes are secreted with circadian rhythmicity, and shiftworkers' intake of food is irregular compared with intestinal function. A high nightly intake of food may be related to increased lipid levels, and eating at the circadian low point may be associated with altered metabolic responses. In addition, reduced sleep affects lipid and glucose metabolism. Recently, an epidemiological study showed a large increase in ulcer risk in shiftworkers with complaints of sleep or excessive sleepiness.

Cardiovascular Effects

A number of studies have reported a higher incidence of cardiovascular disease, especially coronary heart disease, in shiftworkers than in those who work days. In a study of 504 paper-mill workers followed for 15 years a dose–response relationship was found between number of years of shiftwork and incidence of coronary heart disease in the exposure interval 1–20 years of shiftwork. A study of 79 000 female nurses in the United States gave similar results, as did studies of more than 1 million Danish men and of a cohort of Finnish workers. Again, disturbances of metabolic parameters such as lipids and glucose might contribute to this. The effects of shiftwork on metabolic changes do not seem as pronounced, however, as those of stress. Very few studies are available, but the prevalence of endocrine and metabolic diseases seems increased in shiftworkers, including increased insulin resistance.

Mortality

The mortality of shift- and day workers was studied by Taylor and Pocock, who studied 8603 male manual worker in England and Wales between 1956 and 1968. Day, shift-, and ex-shiftworkers were compared with national figures. The standardized mortality rate (SMR) can be calculated from observed and expected deaths reported in the paper. SMRs for deaths from all causes were 97, 101, and 119 for day, shift-, and ex-shiftworkers, respectively. Although the figures might indicate an increasing trend, the differences were not statistically significant. However, the reported SMR close to 100 is remarkable because the reference population was the general male population. Most mortality studies concerned with occupational cohorts reveal SMRs lower than 100, implying a healthy worker's effect. The same study showed a significantly increased incidence of neoplastic disease in shiftworkers (SMR 116).

Conclusion

Shiftwork (with night shifts) impairs sleep and alertness and increases the risk of cardiovascular and gastrointestinal disease. It also disturbs the circadian timing of the endocrine and other systems. Thus, it may serve as one form of stressor and may combine with traditional psychosocial stressors.

See Also the Following Articles

Sleep, Sleep Disorders, and Stress.

Further Reading

Åkerstedt, T. (2003). Shift work and disturbed sleep/wakefulness. *Occupational Medicine* 53, 89–94.

Bjerner, B., Holm, Å. and Swensson, Å. (1955). Diurnal variation of mental performance: a study of three-shift workers. *British Journal of Industrial Medicine* 12, 103–110.

Dijk, D.-J. and Czeisler, C. A. (1995). Contribution of the circadian pacemaker and the sleep homeostat to sleep propensity, sleep structure, electroencephalographic slow waves, and sleep spindle activity in humans. *Journal of Neuroscience* 15, 3526–3538.

Drake, C. L., Roehrs, T., Richardson, G., et al. (2004). Shift work sleep disorder: prevalence and consequences beyond that of symptomatic day workers. *Sleep* 27, 1453–1462.

Folkard, S. and Tucker, P. (2003). Shift work, safety and productivity. *Occupational and Environmental Medicine* 53, 95–101.

Harrington, J. M. (ed.) (1978). *Shift work and health: a critical review of the literature.* London: HMSO.

Hastings, M. H., Reddy, A. B. and Maywood, E. S. (2003). A clockwork web: circadian timing in brain and periphery, in health and disease. *Nature Reviews Neuroscience* 4, 649–661.

Knutsson, A. (2003). Health disorders of shift workers. *Occupational Medicine* 53, 103–108.

Mitler, M. M., Carskadon, M. A., Czeisler, C. A., et al. (1988). Catastrophes, sleep and public policy: consensus report. *Sleep* 11, 100–109.

Spiegel, K., Leproult, R. and Van Cauter, E. (1999). Impact of sleep debt on metabolic and endocrine function. *Lancet* 354, 1435–1439.

Taylor, P. J. and Pocock, S. J. (1972). Mortality of shift and day workers 1956–68. *British Journal of Industrial Medicine* 29, 201–207.

Tüchsen, F. (1993). Working hours and ischaemic heart disease in Danish men: a 4-year cohort study of hospitalization. *International Journal of Epidemiology* 22, 215–221.

Van Dongen, H. P., Maislin, G., Mullington, J. M., et al. (2003). The cumulative cost of additional wakefulness: dose-response effects on neurobehavioral functions and sleep physiology from chronic sleep restriction and total sleep deprivation. *Sleep* 26, 117–126.

Psychiatric Disorders Associated with Disturbed Sleep and Circadian Rhythms

E K Simon
Rosalind Franklin University of Medicine and Science, North Chicago, IL, USA

Introduction

Sleep disturbance is one of the most common complaints associated with the psychiatric syndromes described in the diagnostic and statistical manual of mental disorder-4th edition-text revision (DSM-IV-TR). The mood disorders, unipolar and bipolar together with anxiety disorders (generalized anxiety disorder (GAD) and posttraumatic stress disorder (PTSD)), have sleep disturbance in their criterion. Schizophrenia is also associated with poor sleep quality. Sleep and circadian disturbances influence the presentation and course of psychiatric illnesses, together with the quality of life, and in many cases help in predicting the outcome. Models developed from studies of sleep and circadian rhythms in psychiatric patients help us gain insight into the disease process itself. Proper diagnosis and treatment with emphasis on sleep and circadian rhythm lead to better understanding of the disorders, as well as an improved outcome.

Mood Disorders

Major Depressive Episode

The diagnostic criteria for major depressive episode (MDE) are shown in **Table 1**.

Sleep disturbance in MDE MDE is characterized by depressed mood, anhedonia, fatigue, psychomotor retardation or agitation, insomnia or hypersomnia, weight loss, guilt, sense of worthlessness, and suicidal ideations, plans, or acts (**Table 1**). Insomnia manifests as difficulty in falling asleep or staying asleep or waking up earlier than the usual schedule. Self-reports, questionnaires, and structured interviews from several studies reveal poor sleep quality and impaired daytime functioning in MDE. Hypersomnia is seen primarily in younger patients and in bipolar depressed patients.

According to the (DSM-IV-TR), 90% of inpatients and 40–60% of outpatients with MDE have polysomnography (PSG) abnormalities. They have delayed sleep onset, disturbed sleep continuity, and poor sleep efficiency (**Figure 1**). Slow-wave sleep (SWS and non-rapid eye movement (NREM) stages 3 and 4) is reduced particularly in the first half of the night. Rapid eye movement (REM) sleep shows decreased REM latency, increased REM density, and increased duration of REM sleep early in the night and increased duration of REM throughout the night.

Quantitative electroencephalography (EEG) shows decreased delta wave power and delta wave counts during sleep. The abnormalities in delta sleep are seen more in men than in women. PSG abnormalities are not prominent in adolescents and prepubertal children. In psychotic depression, the PSG findings are most marked and REM latency is very short. The REM sleep abnormalities are associated more with the first episode of depression, or seen earlier during the course of a depressive episode or in recurrence. The patients with significant life stressors preceding the onset of a depressive episode is less likely to have REM sleep abnormalities compared to patients without stressors. Reduced REM latency is associated with increased response to pharmacotherapy and electroconvulsive therapy (ECT) but not psychotherapy. Response to cognitive behavioral therapy (CBT) or interpersonal therapy (IPT) is significantly reduced in patients with reduced REM latency, increased REM density, and disturbed sleep continuity. Reduced REM latency and reduced SWS are trait markers of depression, as they persist after remission and are seen in twins and first-degree relatives of the patients.

Table 1 Diagnostic criteria for major depressive episode

A. Five (or more) of the following symptoms have been present during the same 2-week period and represent a change from previous functioning; at least one of the symptoms is either (1) depressed mood or (2) loss of interest or pleasure.

Note: Do not include symptoms that are clearly due to a general medical condition or mood-incongruent delusions or hallucinations.

1. Depressed mood most of the day, nearly every day, as indicated by either subjective report (e.g., feels sad or empty) or observation made by others (e.g., appears tearful). *Note:* In children and adolescents, can be irritable mood.
2. Markedly diminished interest or pleasure in all, or almost all, activities most of the day, nearly every day (as indicated by either subjective account or observation made by others).
3. Significant weight loss when not dieting or weight gain (e.g., a change of more than 5% of body weight in a month), or decrease or increase in appetite nearly every day. *Note:* In children, consider failure to make expected weight gains.
4. Insomnia or hypersomnia nearly every day.
5. Psychomotor agitation or retardation nearly every day (observable by others, not merely subjective feelings of restlessness or being slowed down).
6. Fatigue or loss of energy nearly every day.
7. Feelings of worthlessness or excessive or inappropriate guilt (which may be delusional) nearly every day (not merely self-reproach or guilt about being sick).
8. Diminished ability to think or concentrate, or indecisiveness, nearly every day (either by subjective account or as observed by others).
9. Recurrent thoughts of death (not just fear of dying), recurrent suicidal ideation without a specific plan, or a suicide attempt or a specific plan for committing suicide.

B. The symptoms do not meet criteria for a Mixed Episode.

C. The symptoms cause clinically significant distress or impairment in social,occupational, or other important areas of functioning.

D. The symptoms are not due to the direct physiological effects of a substance (e.g., a drug of abuse or a medication) or a general medical condition (e.g., hypothyroidism).

E. The symptoms are not better accounted for by bereavement (i.e., after the loss of a loved one), the symptoms persist for longer than 2 months or are characterized by marked functional impairment, morbid preoccupation with worthlessness, suicidal ideation, psychotic symptoms, or psychomotor retardation.

Source: American Psychiatric Association (2000) *Diagnostic and Statistical Manual of Mental Disorders*, 4th edn., Text Revision. Washington, DC: American Psychiatric Association.

Functional neuroimaging findings in MDE Functional neuroimaging studies of depressed patients during wakefulness show hypometabolism in the dorsolateral prefrontal cortex (DLPFC) and anterior cingulate regions and hypermetabolism in the amygdala, hippocampus, and the orbitofrontal cortex (ventral and medial) (**Figure 2**). The functional neuroimaging studies during sleep reveal differences between controls and patients during both NREM and REM sleep. An 18-fluorodeoxyglucose positron emission tomography ([^{18}F] FDG PET) study focusing on the first NREM sleep period in MDE showed a higher metabolic rate of glucose globally in comparison to controls. The glucose metabolic rate was high in the posterior cingulate, amygdala, hippocampus, occipital and temporal cortices, and the pons. Reduced glucose metabolism was found in the anterior cingulate, caudate, and medial thalamus compared to controls. Another [^{18}F] FDG PET study examining the transition from wakefulness to NREM sleep in MDE found that the metabolic rate remained relatively elevated in the frontoparietal regions and the thalamus (**Figure 2**). Examination of the relationship between regional cerebral glucose metabolism assessed by [^{18}F] FDG PET and beta EEG power, a marker of arousal, in patients with MDE and controls during NREM sleep showed that beta power is negatively correlated with subjective sleep quality. Both groups showed significant correlation between beta power and regional cerebral glucose metabolism in

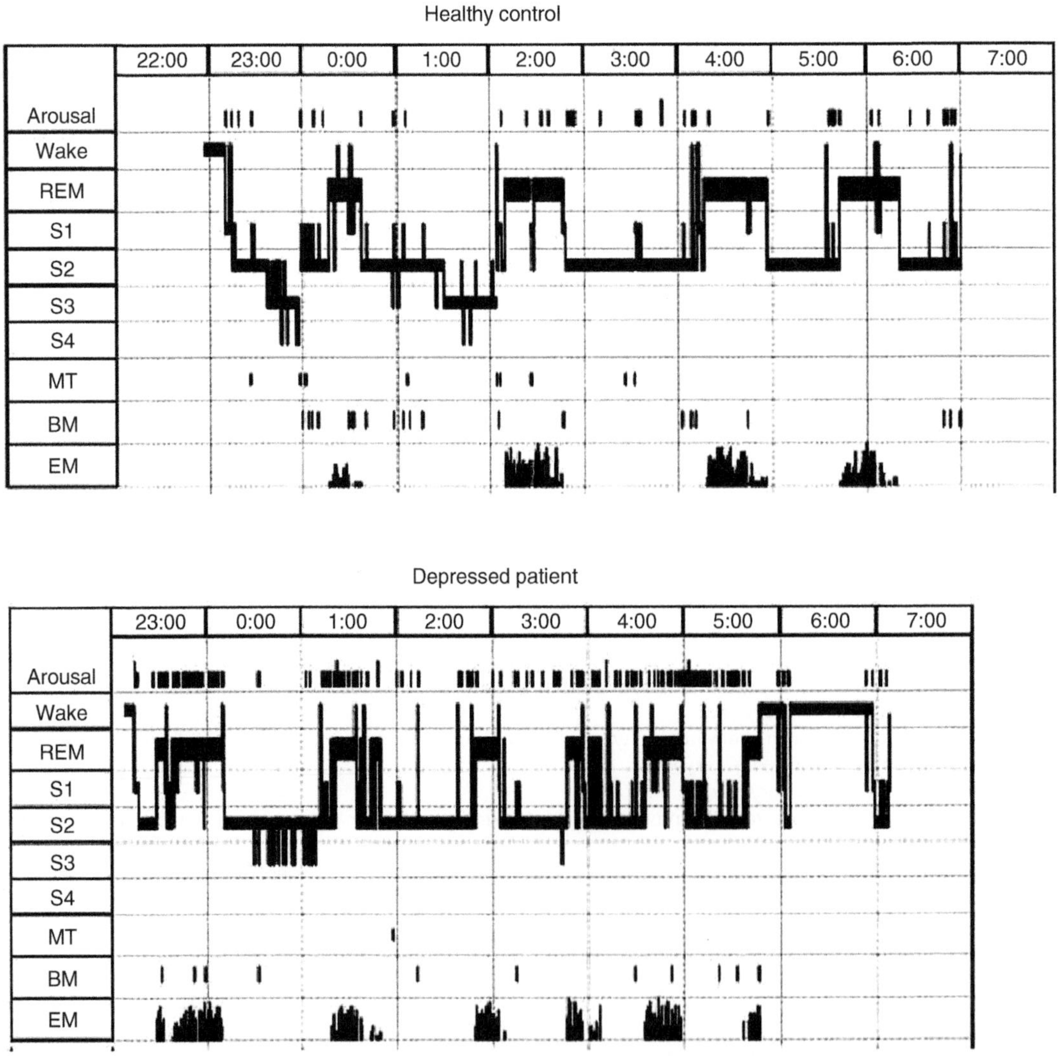

Figure 1 Sleep profile of a medication-free depressed female patient and a healthy female control. Compared with the healthy subject, the sleep profile of this patient shows many of the typical features of sleep in depression: impaired sleep continuity, disinhibition of REM sleep, and reduction of slow-wave sleep. W, wake; REM, rapid eye movement sleep; S1–4, sleep stages 1–4; MT, movement time; BM, body movement; EM, rapid eye movements. From Berger M, van Calker D, and Riemann D (2003) Sleep and manipulations of the sleep–wake rhythm in depression. *Acta Psychiatrica Scandinavica* 108(supplement 418): 84. Used with permission from Blackwell Munksgaard.

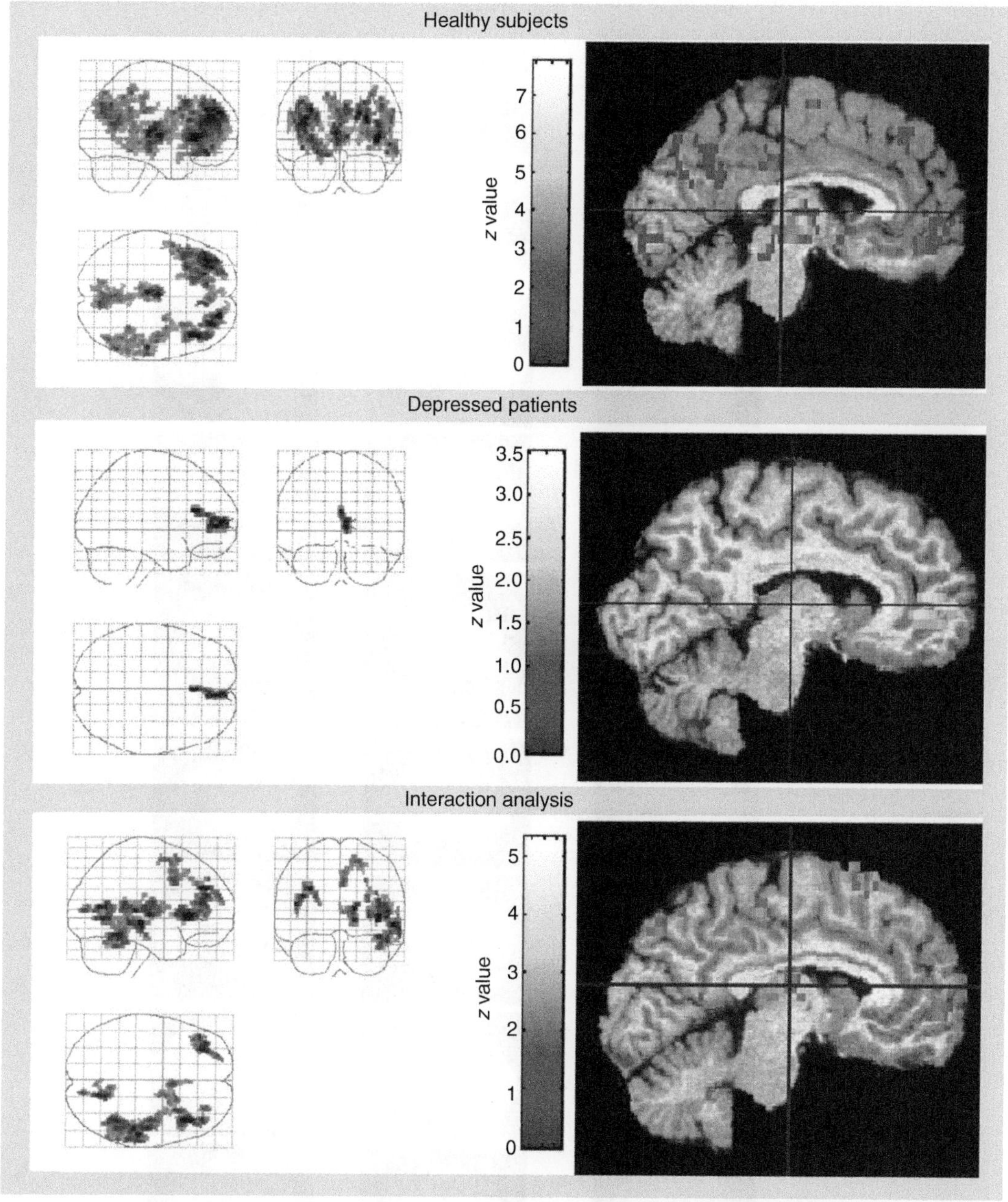

Figure 2 Areas of significant reduction in cerebral glucose metabolism from presleep wakefulness to NREM sleep in healthy subjects and depressed patients and between group differences in metabolic change. Region-of-interest analyses with small volume corrections show a reduction in regional cerebral glucose metabolism in the thalamus from presleep wakefulness to NREM sleep in both study groups. A bilateral metabolic decline in the thalamus was seen in the healthy subjects (left thalamus shown in figure; blue lines intersect at Talairach coordinates $x=-4$, $y=-22$, $z=8$), whereas the metabolic decline was limited to the right thalamus in depressed patients (blue lines intersect at Talairach coordinates $x=8$, $y=-16$, $z=8$). Areas where depressed patients exhibited less of a decline in regional cerebral glucose metabolism from presleep to NREM sleep relative to healthy subjects are presented in the bottom image: depressed patients showed less of a metabolic decline in the thalamus relative to healthy subjects (blue lines intersect at Talairach coordinates $x=-2$, $y=-14$, $z=4$). From Germain A, Nofzinger EA, Kupfer DJ, and Buysee DJ (2004) Neurobiology of non-REM sleep in depression: Further evidence for hypofrontality and thalamic dysregulation. *American Journal of Psychiatry* 161: 1859. Used with permission from American Psychiatric Publishing, Inc.

venteromedial PFC and right lateral inferior occipital cortex. The studies taken together suggest a dysfunction of arousal in the depressed patients.

Functional neuroimaging of REM sleep in the normal subjects show a pattern resembling wakefulness in the cortical metabolism (**Figure 3**). There is also increased metabolism in the limbic and paralimbic structure during REM sleep. This has been referred to as the anterior paralimbic REM activation axis. In patients with MDE, [^{18}F] FDG PET reveals an

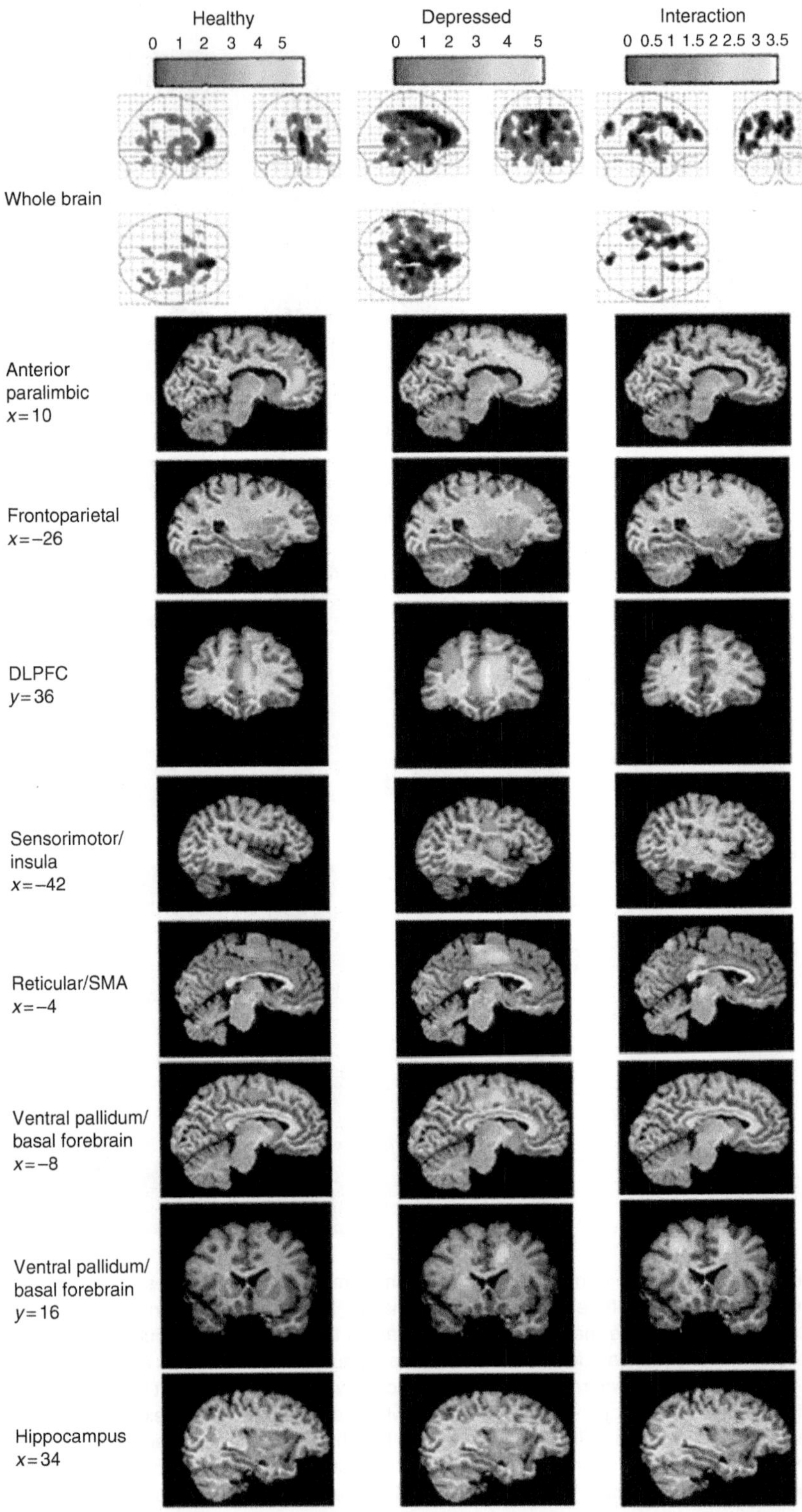

Figure 3 Waking to REM sleep activation, comparison between patients with MDE and healthy controls. Waking to REM sleep activations in healthy subjects (column 1), depressed subjects (column 2), and interactions showing regions where the depressed subjects' waking to REM activations are greater than those of healthy subjects (column 3). DLPFC indicates dorsolateral prefrontal cortex; SMA, supplementary motor area; and *x* and *y*, Talairach *x* and *y* coordinates, respectively. From Nofzinger EA, Buysee DJ, and Germain A, et al. (2004) Increased activation of anterior paralimbic and executive cortex from waking to rapid eye movement sleep in depression. *Archives of General Psychiatry* 61: 699. Used with permission from American Medical Association.

activation of the anterior paralimbic structures greater in area, spatially, compared to controls. They also show greater activation in bilateral DLPFC, left premotor, primary sensorimotor, and left parietal cortices, together with midbrain reticular formation. The increased paralimbic activation may be related to affective dysregulation and the increased activation of the DLPFC may be linked to cognitive dysfunction in depressed patients.

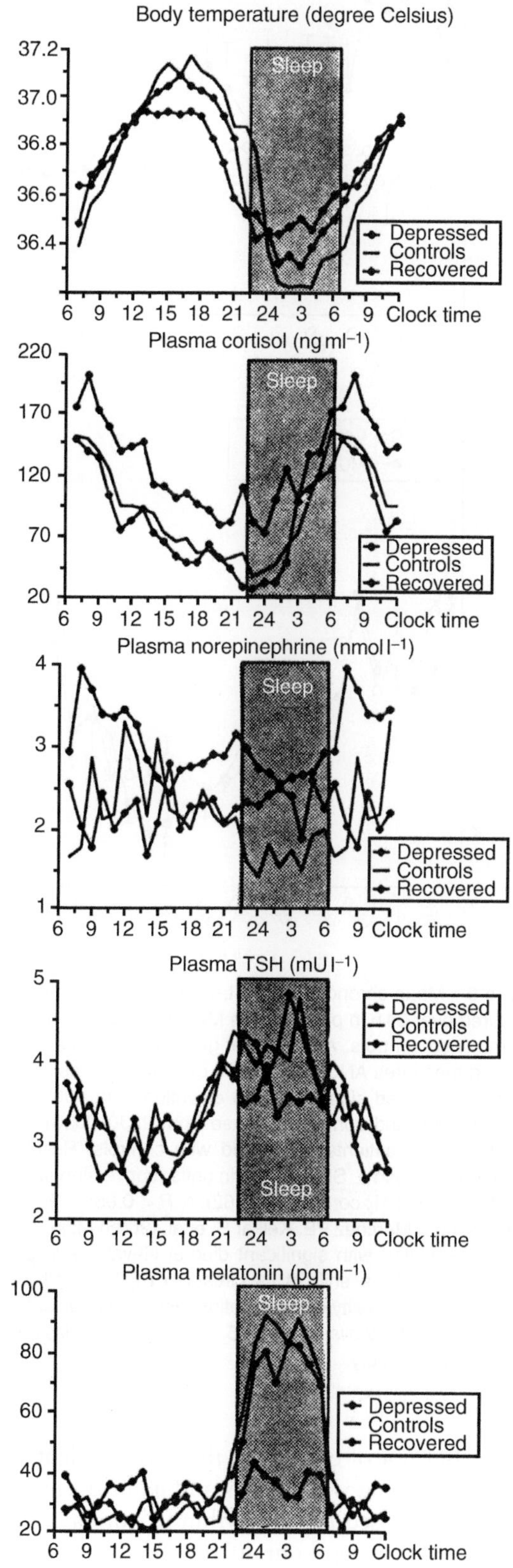

Figure 4 Comparison of circadian rhythms of temperature, cortisol, norepinephrine (NE), thyroid stimulating hormone (TSH), and melatonin between patients with endogenous depression, recovered patients, and healthy subjects. Circadian profiles approximating that of controls are noted in recovered patients. Adapted from Souetre E, Salvati E, Belugou J-L, et al. (1989) Circadian rhythms in depression and recovery: Evidence for blunted amplitude as the main chronobiological abnormality. *Psychiatry Research* 28: 266. Used with permission from Elsevier Scientific Publishers Ireland, Ltd.

Circadian rhythm disturbance in MDE *Methodological issues.* Most of the studies on circadian rhythm in MDE are of patients following a regular diurnal rhythm. Constant routine or other protocols used to avoid masking are seldom used. When employed, sleep deprivation, a necessary part of the procedure, can lead to remission or a switch into hypomania or mania, thus making interpretation difficult. The disorder itself can influence the circadian rhythm and lead to differences between controls and patients. The differences noted may be epiphenomena or they can actually precipitate or perpetuate the depression.

Standardized sleep–wake schedules that are used prior to protocols, such as constant routine, being therapeutic, alter the phenomenology of the illness. Even with these limitations, this strategy can eliminate the possibility that the observed differences are epiphenomena from the influence of the disordered sleep–wake cycle on the patient's circadian rhythms. Most studies recruit patients via ads or from tertiary centers, thereby reducing the generalizability of the findings. There is also the bias of self-selection. Use of a heterogeneous patient population has led to confounding of results in circadian studies (e.g., mixing bipolar and unipolar patients, inpatients and outpatients, melancholic and nonmelancholic patients). Homogenous patient samples, correctly matched for age and sex, with control groups, lead to better understanding of the disease and to valid, reproducible results.

Core body temperature rhythm in MDE. Early studies had reported a phase advance of core body temperature in MDE, but it was not consistently replicated by later studies. The most consistent finding was the reduced amplitude of the core body temperature (**Figure 4**). This was related to the reduced fall of temperature during sleep. The amplitude was lower among patients with reduced REM latency compared to patients with longer REM latency. The period and amplitude of core body temperature rhythm normalizes while in remission.

Melatonin in MDE. Melatonin exhibits blunted amplitude, as already noted, with temperature. Studies with highly specific assays did not validate the finding already discussed that resulted from older studies. Melatonin is also influenced by light, posture, and medications, factors not taken into account by older studies. Reduced concentration of melatonin in patients with MDE has been reported, but the studies have methodological flaws, such as small sample size, poor matching, and infrequent sampling. At reported temperature, the amplitude of melatonin normalizes with remission. Differing levels of nocturnal melatonin secretion have been observed during two different episodes of depression in the same patient. This finding should serve as a cautionary note while we attempt to interpret cross-sectional studies.

Hormonal rhythms in MDE. Among the rhythms studied, cortisol linked to the circadian rhythm has shown a decrease in amplitude and phase advance. Growth hormone secretion shows a reversal of its usual pattern, leading to more secretion in the day as opposed to the night. Thyroid-stimulating hormone also shows decreased amplitude. To sum up, decreased amplitude of various rhythms appears to be the most consistent observation in depression (**Figure 4**).

A recent study comparing patients with MDE with and without psychotic features suggests that each subtype is associated with distinct patterns of hypothalamic–pituitary–adrenal (HPA) axis activity. The patients with psychosis had significantly higher evening cortisol levels than healthy controls or nonpsychotic patients. This is consistent with earlier literature and is thought to be linked to reduced feedback inhibition of HPA axis in psychotic depression.

Diurnal variation in MDE. It has been known since antiquity that the symptoms of depression have a distinct diurnal pattern: worse in the morning and improving as the day progresses. This is especially true for the melancholics. Some studies suggest that the diurnal variation is also seen in other types of depression, other psychiatric disorders, and even in healthy subjects. It has been demonstrated that every pattern of diurnal variation can be observed in a population of depressed individuals on long-term follow-up (i.e., morning low, evening low, and indifferent type).

A recent study of patients with MDE compared with controls, matched for age, gender, body mass index (BMI), and menstrual cycle, found significant mean elevation of interleukin-6 (IL-6) in the patient group from 1000 to 1200 h and at 1500 h (**Figure 5**). They also found a 12 h shift in the circadian rhythm of IL-6 but not of cortisol in the MDE patients with the zenith during wake hours and nadir during sleep hours, as opposed to the rhythm in normal subjects (zenith during sleep hours (0100–0500 h) and nadir

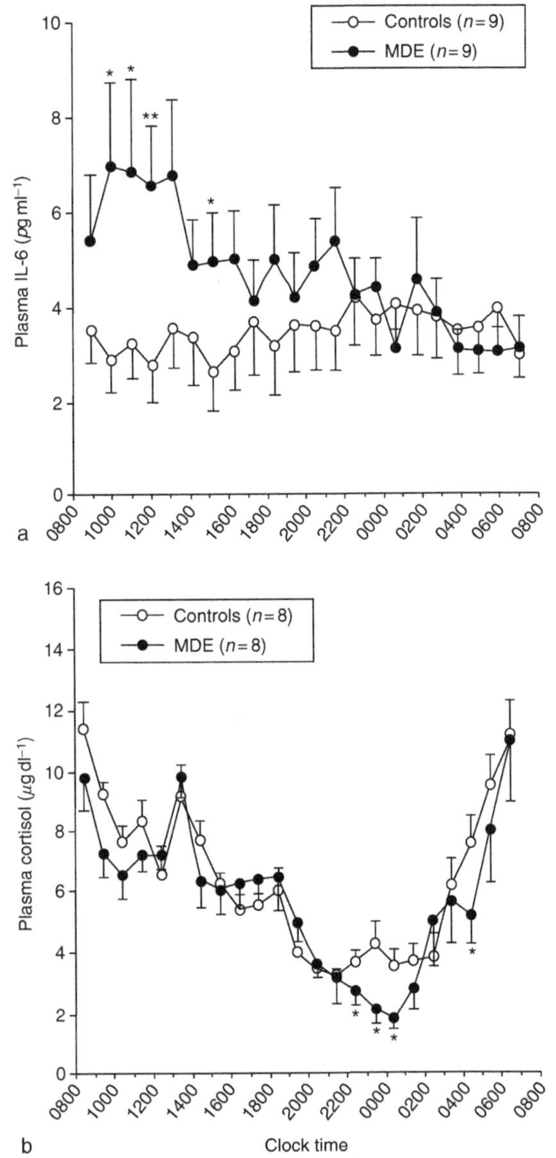

Figure 5 Mean chronograms of IL-6 (a) and cortisol levels (b) measured over 24 h in patients with MDE and age-, gender- and BMI-matched controls. A significant group-by-time interaction in repeated-measures ANOVA, followed by *post hoc t*-tests at each time point, showed significant IL-6 elevation from 1000–1200 h and at 1500 h, and cortisol decrease from 2230–0030 h and at 0430 h in MDE patients, compared with controls. Results are presented as mean ± SEM in metric units (conversion factors to SI units: IL-6, 0.131; cortisol, 27.5862). *, $P < 0.05$; **, $P < 0.01$. From Alesci S, Martinez PE, Kelkar S, et al. (2005) Major depression is associated with significant diurnal elevations in plasma interlukin-6 levels, a shift of its circadian rhythm, and loss of physiological complexity of its secretion. *Journal of Clinical Endocrinology and Metabolism* 90: 2525. Used with permission from the Endocrine Society.

during morning hours (0800–1000 h)). A striking finding of the study was the significant correlation found between fatigue and poor concentration with IL-6 levels in depressives, which could explain the diurnal variation of symptoms.

Social rhythms in MDE. The social *zietgeber* hypothesis posits that in patients who are vulnerable to affective disorder, changes in social *zeitgebers* can lead to disruption of circadian rhythms and eventually precipitate a mood episode, manic, or depressive (**Figure 6**). The event in question may be a *zeitstorer*, an active disrupter of social and familial life, such as the death of a spouse or the birth of a new baby. The *zeitstorer* leads to lack of regular activity or to uncoupling phenomena, where the regular activity fails to entrain the circadian rhythm and presentation of the disorder.

A recent study found that depressed and control groups were similar in levels of regular daily activity, done alone or with others. The regular pattern of daily activity was entraining the cortisol rhythm of healthy controls but not of the depressed patients, and the controls had a more normative decline in cortisol rhythm on the days they reported more activities involving others. In depressive patients the daily activity was not entraining the cortisol rhythm

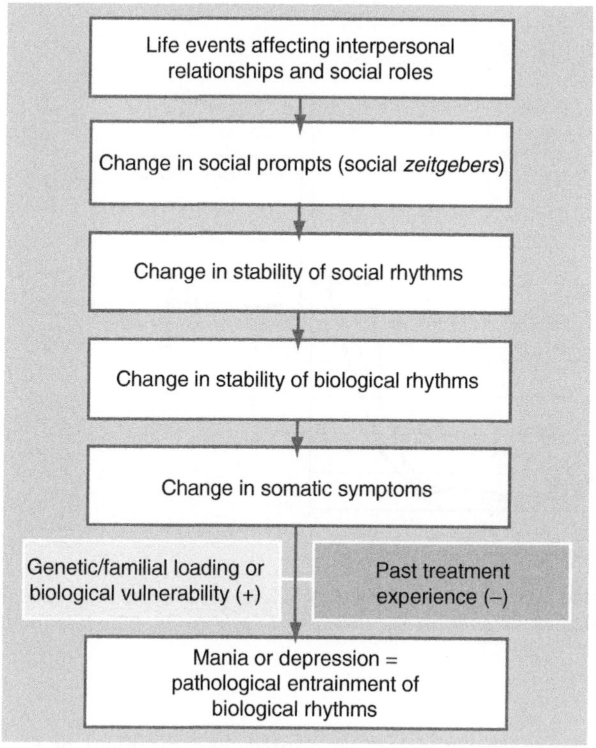

Figure 6 Social *zeitgeber* hypothesis. Adapted from Frank E (2005) *Treating Bipolar Disorder: A Clinician's Guide to Interpersonal and Social Rhythm Therapy.* Used with permission from Guilford Press.

and an uncoupling was observed. It should be noted that the patients were outpatients who had a score of 23 on Beck Depression Inventory without meeting the DSM criteria for MDE.

Psychotherapy helps re-entrain the disrupted rhythm of depressed patients by establishing regular routines and providing exposure to *zeitgebers*, both photic and otherwise. With cognitive behavior therapy, activity scheduling, in which the patient is asked to schedule and engage in preplanned activities, was found to be one of the critical components of the therapeutic action.

Seasonal Affective Disorder

In seasonal affective disorder (SAD), episodes of depression are temporally connected to a particular time of the year (e.g., depression in winter and remission in summer) (**Table 2**). Winter SAD shows prominent anergy, hypersomnia, overeating, weight gain, and carbohydrate craving. Less common is presentation of depression in the summer; summer SAD presents with insomnia, irritability, loss of appetite, and loss of weight. SAD can be a part of a unipolar or bipolar disease. It is more common in Bipolar II Disorder, in which the summer leads to hypomania. The prevalence of the disease increases with higher latitudes, young are at higher risk, and women comprise 60–90% of patients with SAD.

Self-report questionnaires and prospective sleep diaries show that the symptomatic SAD patients have significant increase in sleep duration and difficulty awakening in winter (**Figure 7**). Polysomnographic studies of SAD show reduced sleep efficiency, reduced NREM stage 3 and 4, and increased REM density, but less evidence of reduced REM sleep latency (SL). Actigraphic studies have found diminished levels of activity in both seasonal and nonseasonal depression.

A recent trial of bright light for those with SAD comparing patients who fulfilled the Rosenthal and DSM-IV-TR criteria for SAD with age and sex-matched healthy subjects found that the former had 33% lower total activity and 43% lower daylight activity in week 1 of the trial, as documented by actigraphy. The SAD patients also exhibited attenuation of the amplitude of sleep–wake cycle by 6%, a phase delay of almost 1 h, and lowered sleep efficiency. The bright light by week 4 led to increase in the total and daylight activity in the patients. The reduced amplitude of the circadian rhythm also increased and the delayed circadian rhythm advanced with improved sleep efficiency.

The above view is supported by another study that demonstrated that the prototypical SAD patient is phase delayed (71% in the study) whereas a subgroup may be phase advanced (29% in the study). The same

Table 2 Diagnostic criteria for seasonal pattern specifier

Specify if:

With Seasonal Pattern (can be applied to the pattern of Major Depressive Episodes in Bipolar I Disorder, Bipolar II Disorder, or Major Depressive Disorder, Recurrent)

A. There has been a regular temporal relationship between the onset of Major Depressive Episodes in Bipolar I or Bipolar II Disorder or Major Depressive Disorder, Recurrent, and a particular time of the year (e.g., regular appearance of the Major Depressive Episode in the fall or winter). *Note:* Do not include cases in which there is an obvious effect of seasonal-related psychosocial stressors (e.g., regularly being unemployed every winter).

B. Full remissions (or a change from depression to mania or hypomania) also occur at a characteristic time of the year (e.g., depression disappears in the spring).

C. In the last 2 years, two Major Depressive Episodes have occurred that demonstrate the temporal seasonal relationships defined in criteria A and B, and no nonseasonal Major Depressive Episodes have occurred during that same period.

D. Seasonal Major Depressive Episodes (as described above) substantially outnumber the nonseasonal Major Depressive Episodes that may have occurred over the individual's lifetime.

Source: American Psychiatric Association (2000) *Diagnostic and Statistical Manual of Mental Disorders*, 4th edn., Text Revision. Washington, DC: American Psychiatric Association.

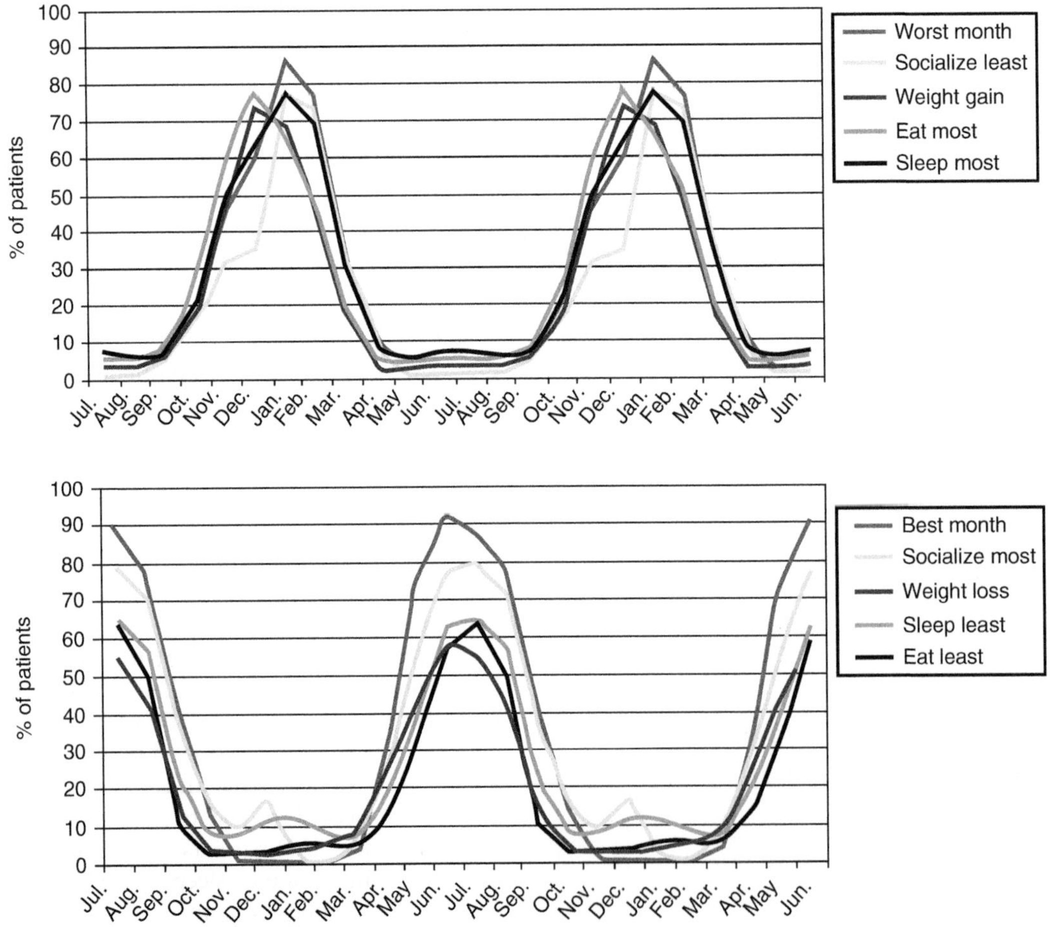

Figure 7 Seasonal change in symptoms of SAD ($n = 1042$). Adapted from Modell JG, Rosenthal NE, and Harriet AE et al. (2005) Seasonal affective disorder and its prevention by anticipatory treatment with bupropion XL. *Biological Psychiatry* 58: 663. Used with permission from Society of Biological Psychiatry.

study also found that the phase-delayed patient group responded to low-dose melatonin in the afternoon. The effect was pronounced as the phase angle difference (PAD) between dim light melatonin onset (DLMO) and midsleep approached the ideal of 6 h. The phase-advanced SADs showed a similar antidepressant response to low-dose melatonin when it was administered in the morning.

The treatment for SAD is bright light therapy, at an intensity of up to 10 000 lux, for a period of 30–60 min in the morning. Studies suggest that morning light is superior to evening light. The bright lights used currently are polychromatic. One recent study reports that blue light with short wave length (468 nm) from light-emitting diodes (LED) is comparable in efficacy to bright white light and is better than dim long-wavelength red light.

FDA approved bupropion extended release in 2006 for prevention of SAD. The pivotal studies were three randomized placebo controlled trials of patients ($n = 1042$) who had history of SAD, on average 13 prior episodes, who were treated with Bupropion XL 300 mg day^{-1}, in autumn prior to the onset of depression. At the end of 4–6 months, the treatment groups had 16% patients who had depression as opposed to the 28% in the placebo group. It should be noted that there was a significant placebo response, which was attributed to the close attention the placebo group received during the trial. Historically, the placebo response has been increasing in efficacy trials of depression.

Bipolar Disorder

Bipolar disorder is a severe disorder of mood manifested by recurrent episodes of mania and depression. The mania is characterized by persistently elevated, expansive, or irritable mood, with grandiosity, decreased need for sleep, pressure of speech, distractibility, flight of ideas, and increased involvement in goal-directed or high-risk activity (**Table 3**). Patients with bipolar disorder exhibit depression that resembles unipolar depression. Bipolar disorder is divided into slow cycling (fewer than four episodes a year) and rapid cycling (more than four episodes) forms. Rapid cycling bipolar disorder (RCBD) tends to be more common in women than in men. Bipolar disorder in which the switch happens multiple times a day has been called ultra rapid cycling.

Sleep disturbance in bipolar depression It has been suggested that bipolar depressed patients have hypersomnia, characterized by increased duration of sleep during the night and excessive daytime somnolence. Studies using measures such as the multiple sleep latency test (MSLT) found no signs of objective hypersomnia in bipolar depression as opposed to hypersomnia in obstructive sleep apnea (OSA) or narcolepsy.

PSG studies of sleep in bipolar depression have generally found results that are no different from those in unipolar depression (**Figure 8**). A recent review of PSG studies, seven in total, found no difference between unipolar and bipolar participants. The authors went on to reanalyze their own data of unipolar and bipolar patients, exactly matched for age, gender, and severity of depression, and found that bipolar depressed patients had more pronounced sleep abnormalities. They showed significant decrease in sleep efficiency, increase in number of wake periods, longer duration of early morning awakenings, and increased REM density, both in the first REM period and during the total duration of REM.

Sleep disturbances in mania There are few studies of sleep disturbance in manic patients compared to those

Table 3 Diagnostic criteria for manic episode

A. A distinct period of abnormally and persistently elevated, expansive, or irritable mood, lasting at least 1 week (or any duration if hospitalization is necessary).

B. During the period of mood disturbance, three (or more) of the following symptoms have persisted (four if the mood is only irritable) and have been present to a significant degree:

1. Inflated self-esteem or grandiosity
2. Decreased need for sleep (e.g., feels rested after only 3 h of sleep)
3. More talkative than usual or pressure to keep talking
4. Flight of ideas or a subjective experience that thoughts are racing
5. Distractibility (i.e., attention too easily drawn to unimportant or irrelevant external stimuli)
6. Increase in goal-directed activity (either socially, at work or school, or sexually) or psychomotor agitation
7. Excessive involvement in pleasurable activities that have a high potential for painful consequences (e.g., engaging in unrestrained buying sprees, sexual indiscretions, or foolish business investments)

C. The symptoms do not meet criteria for a Mixed Episode.

D. The mood disturbance is sufficiently severe to cause marked impairment in occupational functioning or in usual social activities or relationships with others, or to necessitate hospitalization to prevent harm to self or others, or there are psychotic features.

E. The symptoms are not due to the direct physiological effects of a substance (e.g., a drug of abuse, a medication, or other treatment) or a general medical condition (e.g., hyperthyroidism).

Note: Manic-like episodes that are clearly caused by somatic antidepressant treatment (e.g., medication, electroconvulsive therapy, and light therapy) should not count toward a diagnosis of Bipolar I Disorder.

Source: American Psychiatric Association (2000) *Diagnostic and Statistical Manual of Mental Disorders*, 4th edn., Text Revision. Washington DC: American Psychiatric Association.

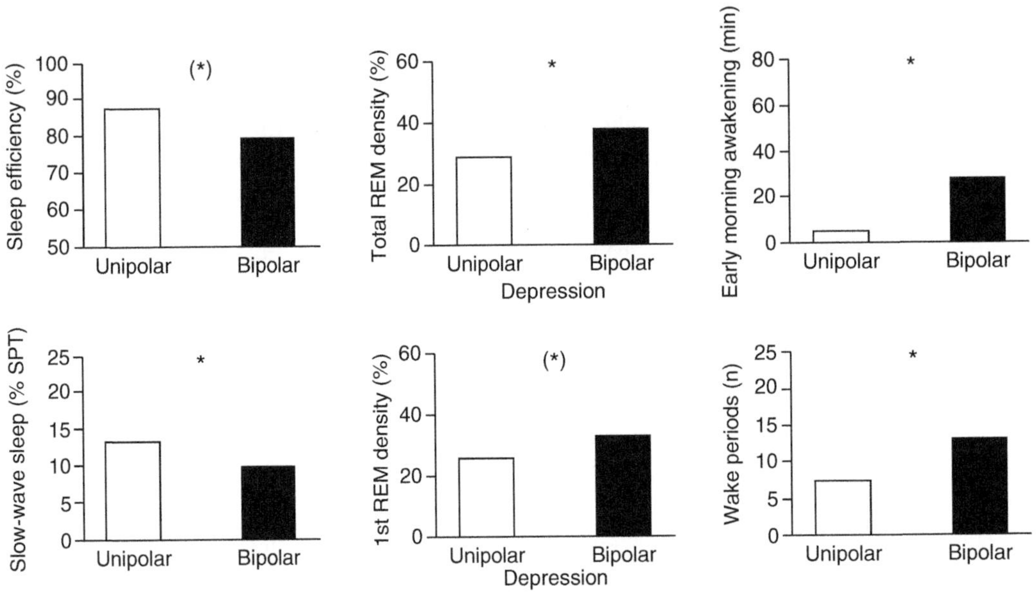

Figure 8 Polysomnographically recorded sleep variables in unipolar vs. bipolar depression ($n = 27$ patients per group). (*) $p < 0.10$, * $p < 0.05$. SPT; Sleep period time. From Riemann D, Voderholzer U, and Berger M (2002) Sleep and sleep–wake manipulations in bipolar depression. *Neuropsychobiology* 45(supplement 1): 9. Used with permission from Karger.

with depression because of the nature of the disorder, the difficulty in getting consent for a study, and the ethical issues involved in keeping patients unmedicated for the study period. Subjectively, manic patients report reduced need for sleep, with few hours of sleep at night and no deleterious effect on daytime functioning or energy. Some patients have total insomnia during the manic phase.

Studies using PSG in unmedicated patients have found more pronounced sleep continuity disturbances in mania compared to depressives. REM sleep findings were similar to depression, but the SWS was not found to be reduced.

Circadian rhythm disturbances in bipolar disorder Among the different types of bipolar disorder, rapid cycling bipolar disorder (RCBD) has been most associated with abnormality of the circadian rhythm. In patients with RCBD, the decrease in sleep duration heralds the onset of mania or the switch from depression into mania (**Figure 9**). Decreased sleep duration is more consistently associated with a shift to an earlier wake-up time. Diurnal variation, which is discussed prominently in depression literature, is also seen in RCBD. The patients with RCBD tend to switch up during the day from depression or euthymia into hypomania or mania, and switch down from mania or hypomania into depression or euthymia after overnight sleep. It is also observed in a handful of cases that DLMO is phase delayed early in the course of a depression episode in patients with RCBD. The phase advances slowly as the illness progresses, and the most advanced position is reached prior to a switch to hypomania or mania.

Social rhythm in bipolar disorder The social *zeitgeber* hypothesis mentioned earlier in the case of MDE holds good for bipolar disorder too (**Figure 6**). It has been noted that disruptive events (*zeitstorer's*) happen more frequently prior to manic or hypomanic episodes when compared with euthymic periods. In RCBD, significantly decreased social rhythm has been reported. Reduced social rhythm has been found in groups of adolescents who were at high risk of developing bipolar disorder in a sample of bipolar II patients compared to a control group. In a recent study conducted in Germany that examined social rhythm instabilities in adolescents and young adults at risk for affective disorders, participants from the bipolar risk group were found to have reduced social rhythm scores as measured by the Social Rhythm Metric when compared with a control group. The Social Rhythm Metric quantifies the stability of an individual's daily routine and lists activities that are identified as central to everyday life. The group with risk for unipolar depression defined by the high rigidity scores from the rigidity subscale of the Munich Personality Test did not show reduced social rhythm scores.

Schizophrenia

The diagnostic criteria for schizophrenia are shown in **Table 4**.

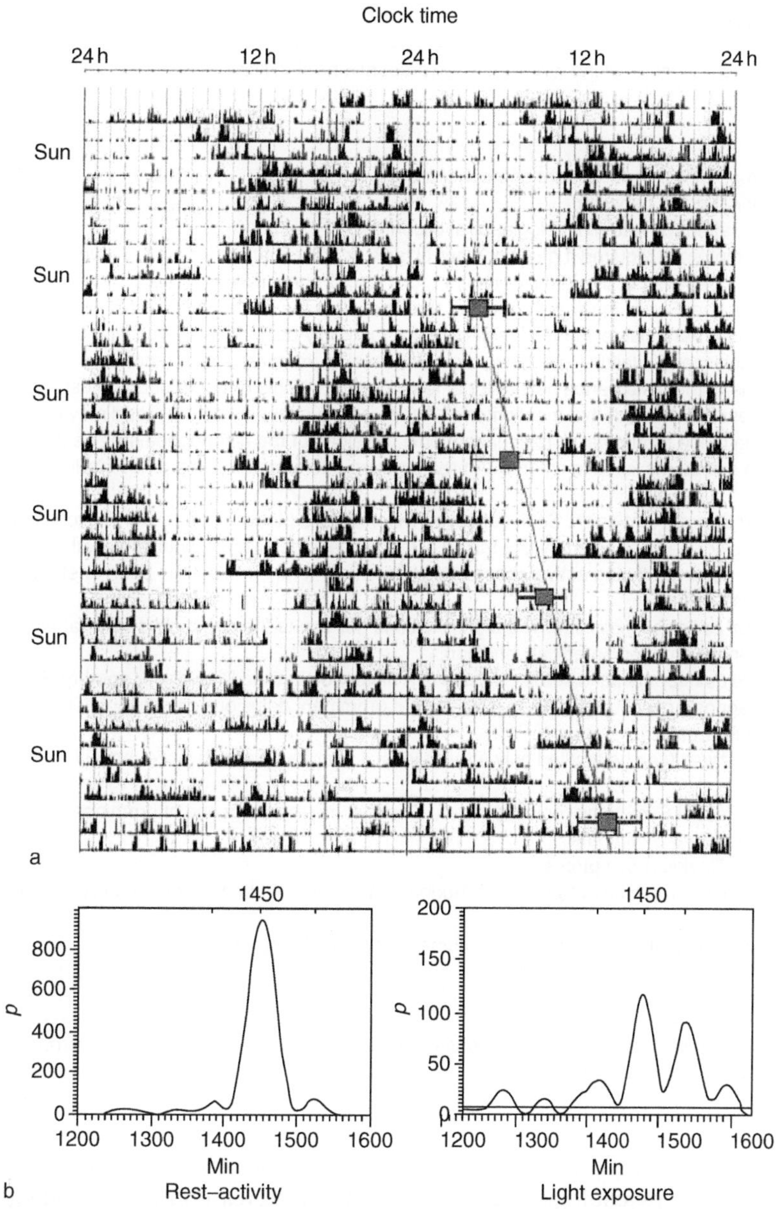

Figure 9 (a) Double-plotted actogram (consecutive days next and beneath each other) of a schizophrenic patient (27-year-old man), whose rest–activity patterns reveal extremely delayed rest and activity onsets, reversed day–night activities, and remarkably prolonged activity and rest phases. This person's weekly sleep onset times delayed from 00:00 to 06:40 h between week 1 and week 5, and his wake-up times delayed from 10:38 to 16:52 h. On average, he slept about 8:30 h (SD + 2:43 h) per 24 h, but sleep efficiency was low (75.9%, SD + 12.9%). Light–dark exposure (gray) also coincides with his rest–activity behavior, indicating an irregular light input to the clock. The phase of his melatonin peak (dark gray squares with 95% confidence interval) changes in synchrony with activity. Abscissa 1/4 days of measurements, Ordinate: clock time in hours. (b) Lomb-Scargle periodograms of the above data, detecting the dominant period at 1450 min (24.17 h) for both activity–rest and light–dark cycles. *p*, power; — indicates missing data. Medication: olanzapine, sodium valproate. From Wulff K, Joyce E, Middleton B, Dijk D-J, and Foster RJ (2006) The suitability of actigraphy, diary data, and urinary melatonin profiles for quantitative assessment of sleep disturbances in schizophrenia: A case report. *Chronobiology International* 23: 489. Used with permission from Taylor & Francis.

Sleep Disturbance in Schizophrenia

Schizophrenia is a chronic psychotic disorder characterized by delusions, hallucinations, disorganized speech, grossly disorganized behavior, and negative symptoms such as affective flattening, alogia, and avolition.

The sleep of the schizophrenic is characterized by increased latency and increased wake time after sleep onset. The latter may be a sign of impending relapse of the psychosis. In a study of 145 patients with schizophrenia, patients who reported poor subjective

Table 4 Diagnostic criteria for schizophrenia

A. *Characteristic symptoms:* Two (or more) of the following, each present for a significant portion of time during a 1-month period (or less if successfully treated):
  1. Delusions
  2. Hallucinations
  3. Disorganized speech (e.g., frequent derailment or incoherence)
  4. Grossly disorganized or catatonic behavior
  5. Negative symptoms, i.e., affective flattening, alogia, or avolition

Note: Only one criterion A symptom is required if delusions are bizarre or hallucinations consist of a voice keeping up a running commentary on the person's behavior or thoughts, or two or more voices conversing with each other.

B. *Social/occupational dysfunction:* For a significant portion of the time since the onset of the disturbance, one or more major areas of functioning such as work, interpersonal relations, or self-care are markedly below the level achieved prior to the onset (or when the onset is in childhood or adolescence, failure to achieve expected level of interpersonal, academic, or occupational achievement).

C. *Duration:* Continuous signs of the disturbance persist for at least 6 months. This 6-month period must include at least 1 month of symptoms (or less if successfully treated) that meet criterion A (i.e., active-phase symptoms) and may include periods of prodromal or residual symptoms. During these prodromal or residual periods, the signs of the disturbance may be manifested by only negative symptoms or two or more symptoms listed in criterion A present in an attenuated form (e.g., odd beliefs, unusual perceptual experiences).

D. *Schizoaffective and mood disorder exclusion:* Schizoaffective Disorder and Mood Disorder with Psychotic Features have been ruled out because either (1) no major depressive, manic, or mixed episodes have occurred concurrently with the active-phase symptoms; or (2) if mood episodes have occurred during active-phase symptoms, their total duration has been brief relative to the duration of the active and residual periods.

E. *Substance/general medical condition exclusion:* The disturbance is not due to the direct physiological effects of a substance (e.g., a drug abuse or a medication) or a general medical condition.

F. *Relationship to a pervasive developmental disorder:* If there is a history of Autistic Disorder or another Pervasive Developmental Disorder, the additional diagnosis of schizophrenia is made only if prominent delusions or hallucinations are also present for at least a month (or less if successfully treated).

Classification of longitudinal course (can be applied only after at least 1 year has elapsed since the initial onset of active-phase symptoms):

Episodic with Interepisode Residual Symptoms (episodes are defined by the reemergence of prominent psychotic symptoms); also specify if with Prominent Negative Symptoms

Episodic with No Interepisode Residual Symptoms

Continuous (prominent psychotic symptoms are present throughout the period of observation); also specify if with Prominent Negative Symptoms

Single Episode in Partial Remission; also specify if with Prominent Negative Symptoms

Single episode in Full Remission

Other or Unspecified Pattern

Source: American Psychiatric Association (2000) *Diagnostic and Statistical Manual of Mental Disorders*, 4th edn., Text Revision. Washington, DC: American Psychiatric Association.

sleep quality had lower perceived quality of life, more depressive symptoms, more psychological distress, and adverse events to medications. Some schizophrenics complain of total or near total insomnia although PSGs document objective sleep. The subjective perception of insomnia may be incorporated by schizophoenic patients into their delusional belief system.

Patients with schizophrenia show a decrease in continuity of sleep, SWS, REM sleep, and reduced REM latency. A recent review of never-medicated or previously medicated schizophrenics found that the majority of the studies reported reduced SWS and REM latency together with unchanged duration of REM sleep. The never-medicated group had increased latency to stage 2, wake time after sleep onset (WASO), and total number of awakenings and reduced total sleep time (TST) and sleep efficiency (SE), with pronounced decrease in REM latency but unchanged REM duration. Similar findings were found for patients in first episode or acute exacerbations. Two studies did not find a decrease in SWS. Findings for chronic schizophrenics were also similar, except for a significant increase in the latency to stage 2 sleep. To sum up, sleep in patients with schizophrenia, irrespective of exposure to psychotropics or clinical course, shows initial and middle insomnia and reduced SWS.

Reduced SWS is consistently seen in studies using quantitative methods of EEG analysis but not always in studies using visual. SWS decrease is associated with the negative symptoms and has been consistently replicated in many studies. It is stable over the course of the disease (1 year follow-up) and predicts poor outcome at years 1 and 2. It also is associated with impaired attention in schizophrenia. The findings regarding REM sleep are harder to interpret, as studies have variously reported an increase, decrease, and no change in the total REM sleep. Only previously treated patients show an increase in total REM, which may be due to the effects of withdrawal from medication or related to the state of the disease (acute exacerbation). Two studies have noted an association between increased REM sleep and suicidality in schizophrenia. The negative symptoms have also been inversely associated with the REM SL.

Methodological Issues

Most studies follow a small number of schizophrenic patients who are heterogeneous regarding the course and subtype of the illness. The control groups include patients with neurological disorders or other medical disorders. The use of differing criteria for diagnosis and lack of clarity regarding the process of diagnosis makes it difficult to compare results across studies. Some studies have not used the latest scoring criteria for sleep, thus putting the validity of findings at risk. The age and gender of the patients also influence the results (increased incidence of OSA or periodic limb movement disorder (PLMD) with age or insomnia in women). Many studies fail to rule out the primary sleep disorder, thereby leading to abnormal findings falsely attributed to schizophrenia. Patients exposed to psychotropics, especially on a chronic basis, have changes in sleep continuity, NREM, and REM sleep that can act as confounding factors. Another factor noted is the first-night effect that reduces the REM and SWS sleep, particularly stage 4, leading to a lack of difference between patient and control group. This is obvious when the values of the control group are compared with similar controls.

Circadian Rhythm Disturbance in Schizophrenia

The studies in this area are few, follow a small number of patients, and have methodological issues as already described in the section on PSG. Studies of schizophrenia have not used techniques such as temporal isolation or constant routine. Body temperature and hormonal rhythms generally show a pattern similar to that of the normal subjects, as opposed to the findings in MDE. The cortisol levels in one study showed higher levels in early sleep but a normal overall pattern. Growth hormone secretion shows inconsistent results across studies, with both normal and decreased values reported.

A recent case report of a 27-year-old man with schizophrenia (monitored by wrist actigraphy, light detection, diary records, and urinary 6-sulfatoxymelatonin (aMT6s) measurements) showed phase shifts, highly delayed sleep-onset and offset, and irregular rest activity phases (**Figure 9**). The period of the rest activity rhythm, melatonin rhythm, and light–dark (L-D) cycle were longer than 24 h. In another study, the second-generation antipsychotic (SGA), clozapine, led to highly ordered rest–activity cycles, when compared to first-generation antipsychotics (FGA) (e.g., haloperidol; **Figure 10**). This was the first study that reported the differential effect of FGA and SGA on the circadian rhythm.

Anxiety Disorders

The anxiety disorders that are described in the DSM-IV-TR are panic disorder, phobias (specific and social), obsessive compulsive disorder (OCD), PTSD, and GAD. Among these disturbed sleep is mentioned as a criterion for PTSD and GAD. Epidemiological studies have noted the links between insomnia and anxiety disorders. The treatments, pharmacologic and psychotherapeutic, used for anxiety disorders are also useful for insomnia, thus implying a common basis for these disorders.

Sleep and Circadian Rhythm Disturbance in Panic Disorder

Panic disorder is characterized by recurrent panic attacks and anticipatory anxiety, together with avoidance (**Tables 5** and **6**). It may present with or without agoraphobia. Sleep is of poor quality, interrupted, or restless as reported in surveys of patients with panic disorder when compared to controls. Among patients with panic disorder, 68% have difficulty falling asleep and 77% have restless sleep. Nocturnal panic attacks are reported by patients (33–71%) that resemble the daytime attacks. Patients report waking up “like a jolt” and experience a full-blown attack. Patients with nocturnal panic have early age of onset, comorbid depression, severe symptomatology, and increased suicidal ideation. It has been noted in case reports that panic disorder is associated with sleep-related breathing disorder.

PSGs show decreased sleep efficiency and total sleep duration. However, studies that excluded patients with comorbid depression did not show these changes. Normal amounts of REM and SWS are seen. The REM latency is reported either as normal or reduced. Increased movement time is also seen with panic disorder. The panic attacks appear while transitioning from stage 2 to SWS in the first half of night. Nocturnal panic attacks can be induced by infusing caffeine during SWS. Two groups have reported cardiopulmonary instability in patients with panic disorder, one by infusing lactate during sleep and the other by demonstrating greater variability in the heart rate during NREM sleep.

There have been few studies regarding panic disorder and circadian rhythm. Circadian rhythms of cortisol

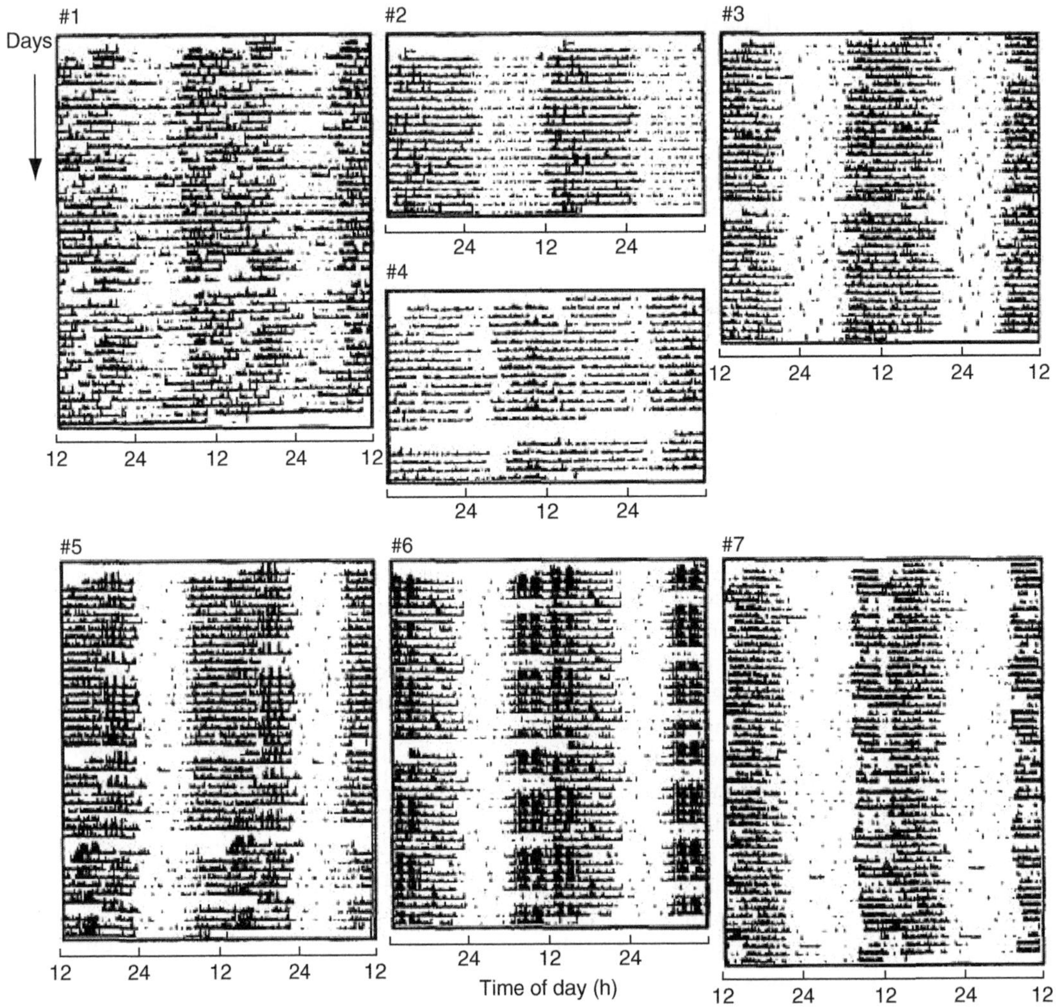

Figure 10 Actograms of seven schizophrenia patients on monotherapy for at least a year. All patients were hospitalized except patient 3 (day patient) and patient 4 (ambulatory). Patients 1–4 were treated with classical neuroleptics (haloperidol or flupentixol); patients 5–7 were treated with clozapine. Motor activity is registered in black (1-min bins) and graphed as a double 24 h plot over 48 h (first line, days 1 and 2, second line, days 2 and 3, etc.). Occasional missing data are left blank. From Wirz-Justice A, Haug H-J, and Cajochen C (2001) Disturbed circadian rest–activity cycles in schizophrenia patients: An effect of drugs? *Schizophrenia Bulletin* 27: 499. Used with permission from Oxford University Press.

and adrenocosticotropin (ACTH) may be abnormal in panic disorder. Elevated nocturnal cortisol secretion has been reported, as well as increased ultradian secretory episodes. The CRF has variable phase and changes in mean level has been noted.

Sleep and Circadian Rhythm Disturbance in Social and Specific Phobia

Social and specific phobia are both characterized by fear and avoidance (**Tables 7** and **8**). Subjective reports show poor sleep quality, daytime impairment, and increased SL, but these findings were not reported by one study that used PSG. In another study, sleep architecture was no different between patients having MDE with or without phobias. The TST, SL, and SE were similar between patients and controls. The measure of REM SL, density, duration, and distribution was also normal in phobias.

Sleep and Circadian Rhythm Disturbance in Generalized Anxiety Disorder

GAD is characterized by excessive worry (**Table 9**). Patients have sleep disturbance as one of the criterion in the DSM-IV-TR, namely initial or middle insomnia with restless or unsatisfying sleep. The latter occurs in 60–70% of patients. Patients may report a variety of sleep complaints clinically. PSG studies show sleep initiation and maintenance difficulties. NREM stage

Table 5 Diagnostic criteria for panic attack

Note: A Panic Attack is not a codable disorder. Code the specific diagnosis in which the panic attack occurs (e.g., **300.21** Panic Disorder with Agoraphobia).

A discrete period of intense fear or discomfort, in which four (or more) of the following symptoms developed abruptly and reached a peak within 10 min.

1. Palpitations, pounding heart, or accelerated heart rate
2. Sweating
3. Trembling or shaking
4. Sensations of shortness of breath or smothering
5. Feeling of choking
6. Chest pain or discomfort
7. Nausea or abdominal distress
8. Feeling dizzy, unsteady, lightheaded, or faint
9. Derealization (feelings of unreality) or depersonalization (being detached from oneself)
10. Fear of losing control or going crazy
11. Fear of dying
12. Paresthesias (numbness or tingling sensations)
13. Chills or hot flushes

Source: American Psychiatric Association (2000) *Diagnostic and Statistical Manual of Mental Disorders*, 4th edn., Text Revision. Washington, DC: American Psychiatric Association.

Table 6 Diagnostic criteria for panic disorder

Diagnostic criteria for panic disorder without agoraphobia

A. Both (1) and (2):
   1. Recurrent unexpected Panic Attacks.
   2. At least one of the attacks has been followed by 1 month (or more) of one (or more) of the following:
      a. Persistent concern about having additional attacks
      b. Worry about the implications of the attack or its consequences (e.g., losing control, having a heart attack, 'going crazy')
      c. A significant change in behavior related to the attacks

B. Absence of Agoraphobia.

C. The Panic Attacks are not due to the direct physiological effects of a substance (e.g., a drug or abuse a medication) or a general medical condition (e.g., hyperthyroidism).

D. The Panic Attacks are not better accounted for by another mental disorder, such as Social Phobia (e.g., occurring on exposure to feared social situations), Specific Phobia (e.g., on exposure to a specific phobic situation), Obsessive–Compulsive Disorder (e.g., on exposure to dirt in someone with an obsession about contamination), Posttraumatic Stress Disorder (e.g., in response to stimuli associated with a severe stressor), or Separation Anxiety Disorder (e.g., in response to being away from home or close relatives).

Diagnostic criteria for panic disorder with agoraphobia

A. Both (1) and (2):
   1. Recurrent unexpected Panic Attacks.
   2. At least one of the attacks has been followed by 1 month (or more) of one (or more) of the following:
      a. Persistent concern about having additional attacks
      b. Worry about the implications of the attack or its consequences (e.g., losing control, having a heart attack, and 'going crazy')
      c. A significant change in behavior related to the attacks

B. The presence of Agoraphobia.

C. The Panic Attacks are not due to the direct physiological effects of a substance (e.g., a drug abuse or a medication) or a general medical condition (e.g., hyperthyroidism).

D. The Panic Attacks are not better accounted for by another mental disorder, such as Social Phobia (e.g., occurring on exposure to feared social situations), Specific Phobia (e.g., on exposure to a specific phobic situation), Obsessive–Compulsive Disorder (e.g., on exposure to dirt in someone with an obsession about contamination), Posttraumatic Stress Disorder (e.g., in response to stimuli associated with a severe stressor), or Separation Anxiety Disorder (e.g., in response to being away from home or close relatives).

Source: American Psychiatric Association (2000) *Diagnostic and Statistical Manual of Mental Disorders*, 4th edn., Text Revision. Washington, DC: American Psychiatric Association.

2 is increased while SWS is decreased in GAD. GAD patients do not show the decreased REM latency seen in MDE. This may help differentiate one from the other. Patients with GAD have lower levels of activity as documented by SRM (social rhythm metric) in one study.

Sleep and Circadian Rhythm Disturbance in Posttraumatic Stress Disorder

PTSD is characterized by persistent reexperiencing of the trauma, with avoidance and hyperarousal (**Table 10**). Nightmares and initial and middle

Table 7 Diagnostic criteria for specific phobia (formerly known as simple phobia)

A. Marked and persistent fear that is excessive or unreasonable, cued by the presence or anticipation of a specific object or situation (e.g., flying, heights, animals, receiving an injection, seeing blood).
B. Exposure to the phobic stimulus almost invariably provokes an immediate anxiety response, which may take the form of a situationally bound or situationally predisposed Panic Attack.
Note: In children, the anxiety may be expressed by crying, tantrums, freezing, or clinging.
C. The person recognizes that the fear is excessive or unreasonable.
Note: In children, this feature may be absent.
D. The phobic situation(s) is avoided or else is endured with intense anxiety or distress.
E. The avoidance, anxious anticipation, or distress in the feared situation(s) interferes significantly with the person's normal routine, occupational (or academic) functioning, or social activities or relationships, or there is marked distress about having the phobia.
F. In individuals under age 18 years, the duration is at least 6 months.
G. The anxiety, Panic Attacks, or phobic avoidance associated with the specific object or situation, are not better accounted for by another mental disorder, such as Obsessive–Compulsive Disorder (e.g., fear of dirt in someone with an obsession about contamination), Posttraumatic Stress Disorder (e.g., avoidance of stimuli associated with a severe stressor), Separation Anxiety Disorder (e.g., avoidance of school), Social Phobia (e.g., avoidance of social situations because of fear of embarrassment), Panic Disorder With Agoraphobia, or Agoraphobia without History of Panic Disorder.

Specify type:
Animal Type
Natural Environment Type (e.g., heights, storms, and water)
Blood-Injection-Injury Type
Situational Type (e.g., airplanes, elevators, and enclosed places)
Other Type (e.g., fear of choking, vomiting, or contracting an illness; in children, fear of loud sounds or costumed characters)

Source: American Psychiatric Association (2000) *Diagnostic and Statistical Manual of Mental Disorders*, 4th edn., Text Revision. Washington, DC: American Psychiatric Association.

Table 8 Diagnostic criteria for social phobia (social anxiety disorder)

A. A marked and persistent fear of one or more social or performance situations in which the person is exposed to unfamiliar people or to possible scrutiny by others. The individual fears that he or she will act in a way (or show anxiety symptoms) that will be humiliating or embarrassing. *Note*: In children, there must be evidence of the capacity for age-appropriate social relationships with familiar people and the anxiety must occur in peer settings, not just in interactions with adults.
B. Exposure to the feared social situation almost invariably provokes anxiety, which may take the form of a situationally bound or situationally predisposed Panic Attack. *Note*: In children, the anxiety may be expressed by crying, tantrums, freezing, or shrinking from social situations with unfamiliar people.
C. The person recognizes that the fear is excessive or unreasonable. *Note*: In children, this feature may be absent.
D. The feared social or performance situations are avoided or else are endured with intense anxiety or distress.
E. The avoidance, anxious anticipation, or distress in the feared social or performance situation(s) interferes significantly with the person's normal routine, occupational (academic) functioning, or social activities or relationships, or there is marked distress about having the phobia.
F. In individuals under age 18 years, the duration is at least 6 months.
G. The fear or avoidance is not due to the direct physiological effects of a substance (e.g., a drug abuse or a medication) or a general medical condition and is not better accounted for by another mental disorder (e.g., Panic Disorder with or without Agoraphobia, Separation Anxiety Disorder, Body Dysmorphic Disorder, a Pervasive Developmental Disorder, or Schizoid Personality Disorder).
H. If a general medical condition or another mental disorder is present, the fear in criterion A is unrelated to it, e.g., the fear is not of Stuttering, trembling in Parkinson's disease, or exhibiting abnormal eating behavior in Anorexia Nervosa or Bulimia Nervosa.

Specify if:
Generalized: if the fears include most social situations (also consider the additional diagnosis of Avoidant Personality Disorder)

Source: American Psychiatric Association (2000) *Diagnostic and Statistical Manual of Mental Disorders*, 4th edn., Text Revision. Washington, DC: American Psychiatric Association.

insomnia are reported subjectively. Nightmares are found in 59–68% of patients. There are anxious arousals that occur in relation to both REM and NREM sleep. The arousals lead to excessive motor activity and awakenings. PSG documents decreased sleep efficiency and decreased TST with increased movement time. REM sleep in PTSD is reported as resembling depression in some studies. Reduced or prolonged latency is shown, depending on the studies reviewed, and reduced duration of REM sleep. Comorbid MDE, SRBD (sleep-related breathing disorder), or SUD (substance use disorders) may confound results. Although nightmares are reported in both REM and NREM sleep, the majority of studies support an association with REM sleep. Increased REM density has been described in combat veterans with chronic PTSD.

Table 9 Diagnostic criteria for generalized anxiety disorder (includes overanxious disorder of childhood)

A. Excessive anxiety and worry (apprehensive expectation), occurring more days than not for at least 6 months, about a number of events or activities (such as work or school performance).
B. The person finds it difficult to control the worry.
C. The anxiety and worry are associated with three (or more) of the following six symptoms (with at least some symptoms present for more days than not for the past 6 months). *Note:* Only one item is required in children.
   1. Restlessness or feeling keyed up or on edge
   2. Being easily fatigued
   3. Difficulty concentrating or mind going blank
   4. Irritability
   5. Muscle tension
   6. Sleep disturbance (difficulty falling or staying asleep, or restless unsatisfying sleep)
D. The focus of the anxiety and worry is not confined to features of an Axis I disorder, e.g., the anxiety or worry is not about having a Panic Attack (as in Panic Disorder), being embarrassed in public (as in Social Phobia), being contaminated (as in Obsessive–Compulsive Disorder), being away from home or close relatives (as in Separation Anxiety Disorder), gaining weight (as in Anorexia Nervosa), having multiple physical complaints (as in Somatization Disorder), or having a serious illness (as in Hypochondriasis), and the anxiety and worry do not occur exclusively during Posttraumatic Stress Disorder.
E. The anxiety, worry, or physical symptoms cause clinically significant distress or impairment in social, occupational, or other important areas of functioning.
F. The disturbance is not due to the direct physiological effects of a substance (e.g., a drug abuse or a medication) or a general medical condition (e.g., hyperthyroidism) and does not occur exclusively during a Mood Disorder, a Psychotic Disorder, or a Pervasive Developmental Disorder.

Source: American Psychiatric Association (2000): *Diagnostic and Statistical Manual of Mental Disorders,* 4th edn., Text Revision. Washington DC: American Psychiatric Association.

Table 10 Diagnostic criteria for posttraumatic stress disorder

A. The person has been exposed to a traumatic event in which both of the following were present:
   1. The person experienced, witnessed, or was confronted with an event or events that involved actual or threatened death or serious injury, or a threat to the physical integrity of self or others
   2. The person's response involved intense fear, helplessness, or horror. *Note:* In children, this may be expressed instead by disorganized or agitated behavior.
B. The traumatic event is persistently reexperienced in one (or more) of the following ways:
   1. Recurrent and intrusive distressing recollections of the event, including images, thoughts, or perceptions. *Note:* In young children, repetitive play may occur in which themes or aspects of the trauma are expressed.
   2. Recurrent distressing dreams of the event. *Note:* In children, there may be frightening dreams without recognizable content.
   3. Acting or feeling as though the traumatic event were recurring (includes a sense of reliving the experience, illusions, hallucinations, and dissociative flashback episodes, including those that occur on awakening or when intoxicated). *Note:* In young children, trauma-specific reenactment may occur.
   4. Intense psychological distress at exposure to internal or external cues that symbolize or resemble an aspect of the traumatic event
   5. Physiological reactivity on exposure to internal or external cues that symbolize or resemble an aspect of the traumatic event
C. Persistent avoidance of stimuli associated with the trauma and numbing of general responsiveness (not present before the trauma), as indicated by three (or more) of the following:
   1. Efforts to avoid thoughts, feelings, or conversations associated with the trauma
   2. Efforts to avoid activities, places, or people that arouse recollections of the trauma
   3. Inability to recall an important aspect of the trauma
   4. Markedly diminished interest or participation in significant activities
   5. Feeling of detachment or estrangement from others
   6. Restricted range of affect (e.g., unable to have loving feelings)
   7. Sense of a foreshortened future (e.g., does not expect to have a career, marriage, children, or a normal life span)
D. Persistent symptoms of increased arousal (not present before the trauma), as indicated by two (or more) of the following:
   1. Difficulty falling or staying asleep
   2. Irritability or outbursts of anger
   3. Difficulty concentrating
   4. Hypervigilance
   5. Exaggerated startle response
E. Duration of the disturbance (symptoms in criteria B, C, and D) is more than 1 month.
F. The disturbance causes clinically significant distress or impairment in social, occupational, or other important areas of functioning.

Specify if:
Acute: duration of symptoms is less than 3 months
Chronic: duration of symptoms is 3 months or more
Specify if:
With Delayed Onset: onset of symptoms is at least 6 months after the stressor

Source: American Psychiatric Association (2000): *Diagnostic and Statistical Manual of Mental Disorders,* 4th edn., Text Revision. Washington DC: American Psychiatric Association.

Patients with PTSD have increased excretion of 24 h catecholamines. The ratio of nocturnal to diurnal urinary catecholamines is increased relative to controls. The hypersecretion of cortisol during the night is not seen in the PTSD, as opposed to patients with depression.

Conclusion

There is strong evidence that disturbances of sleep are central to many psychiatric disorders. The strongest evidence is with mood disorders, both unipolar and bipolar. The REM and SWS abnormalities noted are biologic markers, both state and trait. They are also strong predictors of response to treatment and outcome in MDE. SAD is increasingly being recognized, and the new treatment modalities that are being developed will go a long way in treating and preventing it. Treatments of bipolar disorder, which take into account the circadian component, would bolster the current therapies. Studies of sleep in schizophrenia help us understand the disease and improve the quality of life in patients by managing sleep and circadian rhythms optimally. Anxiety disorders present hand in hand with sleep disturbance, and findings regarding sleep help us delineate anxiety from depression and devise better management strategies.

Further Reading

Alesci, S., Martinez, P. E., Kelkar, S., et al. (2005). Major depression is associated with significant diurnal elevations in plasma interlukin-6 levels, a shift of its circadian rhythm, and loss of physiological complexity of its secretion. *Journal of Clinical Endocrinology and Metabolism* **90**, 2522–2530.

Benca, R. M. (2005). Mood disorders. In: Kryger, M. H., Roth, T. & Dement, W. C. (eds.) *Principles and Practice of Sleep Medicine* (4th edn., pp. 1311–1327). Elsevier Saunders: Philadelphia.

Boivin, D. B. (2000). Influence of sleep–wake and circadian rhythm disturbances in psychiatric disorders. *Journal of Psychiatry and Neuroscience* **25**, 446–458.

Buysse, D. J., Nofzinger, E. A., Keshavan, M. S., Reynolds, III C. F. and Kupfer, D. J. (1999). Psychiatric disorders associated with disturbed sleep and circadian rhythms. In: Turek, F. W. & Zee, P. C. (eds.) *Regulation of Sleep and Circadian Rhythms*, pp. 597–641. New York: Marcel Dekker.

Halaris, A. (1987). *Chronobiology and Psychiatric Disorders*. New York: Elsevier.

Leibenluft, E. and Frank, E. (2001). Circadian rhythm in affective disorders. *Handbook of Behavioral Neurobiology* **12**, 625–644.

Lewy, A. J., Lefler, B. J., Emens, S. J. and Bauer, V. K. (2006). The circadian basis of winter depression. *Proceedings of the National Academy of Sciences of the United States of America* **103**, 7414–7419.

Mellman, T. A. (2003). Sleep aspects of anxiety disorders. In: Nutt, D. J. & Ballenjer, J. C. (eds.) *Anxiety Disorders*, pp. 125–133. Cambridge, Mass: Blackwell Publishing.

Meyer, T. D. and Maire, S. (2006). Is there evidence for social rhythm instability in people at risk of affective disorders? *Psychiatry Research* **141**, 103–114.

Monti, J. M. and Monti, D. (2005). Sleep disturbance in schizophrenia. *International Review of Psychiatry* **17**, 247–243.

Nofzinger, E. A. (2005). Functional neuroimaging of sleep. *Seminars in Neurology* **25**, 9–18.

Nofzinger, E. A. and Keshavan, M. A. (2002). Sleep disturbances associated with neuropsychiatric disease. In: Davis, K. L., Charney, D., Coyle, J. T. & Nemeroff, C. (eds.) *Neuropsychopharmacology: The Fifth Generation of Progress*, pp. 1945–1959. Philadelphia: Lippincott Williams & Wilkins.

Stetler, C., Dickerson, S. S. and Miller, G. E. (2004). Uncoupling of social zeitgebers and diurnal cortisol secretion in clinical depression. *Psychoneuroendocrinology* **29**, 1250–1259.

Wehr, T. A. and Goodwin, F. K. (1983). Circadian rhythms in psychiatry. *Psychobiology and Psychopathology*, (vol. 2. Pacific Grove, CA: Boxwood Press.

Wirz-Justice, A. (1994). Biological rhythms in mood disorders. In: Bloom, F. E. & Kupfer, D. J. (eds.) *Psychopharmacology: The Fourth Generation of Progress*, pp. 999–1017. New York: Raven Press.

Relevant Websites

http://www.aasmnet.org – American Academy of Sleep Medicine.

http://www.acnp.org/default.aspx?Page=Home – American College of Neuropsychopharmacology.

http://www.psychiatryonline.com – American Psychiatric Publishing, Inc.

http://www.northwestern.edu – Center for Sleep and Circadian Biology at Northwestern University.

http://www.hhmi.org – Howard Hughes Medical Institute.

http://www.sleepmedtext.com – *Principles and Practice of Sleep Medicine* (the authoritative text on sleep medicine).

http://www.npi.ucla.edu – Siegel Lab at the University of California Los Angeles.

http://www.wpic.pitt.edu – Sleep Neuroimaging Research Program, University of Pittsburgh Medical Center, Western Psychiatric Institute and Clinic, Pittsburgh.

http://www.sltbr.org – Society for Light Treatment and Biological Rhythms.

http://med.stanford.edu – Stanford University Center for Excellence for the Diagnosis and Treatment of Sleep Disorders.

M. Dementia – Alzheimer's Disease

Neurodegenerative Disorders

M F Mendez and A M McMurtray
West Los Angeles Veteran's Affairs Medical Center and University of California, Los Angeles, CA, USA

Glossary

Alzheimer's disease	A progressive neurodegenerative dementia affecting memory and other cognitive functions.
Hippocampus	Area of the brain concerned with encoding and storage of new declarative memory.
Neuron	Single cell functional unit of the nervous system.
Parkinson's disease	Progressive neurodegenerative disorder affecting movement, balance, and postural stability.
Substantia nigra	Area of the brain principally affected in Parkinson's disease containing a high concentration of dopaminergic neurons.

Overview of Neurodegenerative Disorders

Neurodegenerative disorders are characterized by a gradual loss of neurons, often leading to death. The term encompasses a broad range of clinical diseases, including progressive dementing conditions, of which the most common are Alzheimer's disease (AD), movement disorders, exemplified by Parkinson's disease (PD), and a range of other neurological disorders. Neurodegenerative disorders have in common a gradual loss of neurons and synaptic connections, usually occurring in later life. Specific diseases are distinguished by the presence of characteristic symptoms that depend on the location at which neuronal loss is occurring in the brain. Typically, the degree of neuronal loss correlates directly with the appearance and progression of the clinical symptoms. In AD, neuronal loss occurs early in the hippocampus, a brain region concerned with declarative episodic memory. In PD, the characteristic clinical triad of tremor, bradykinesia, and postural instability only become evident after 70–80% of dopaminergic neurons in the substantia nigra are lost.

The gradually progressive nature of these disorders, often combined with a long preclinical course before the development of symptoms, allows ample time and opportunity for environmental factors such as stress to contribute to disease development and progression. These features, however, make detection of environmental factors with disease-modifying effects by traditional epidemiological methods difficult. Prospective studies attempting to identify associations between stress beginning early in life and a clinical syndrome many years later in middle or even late life are hindered by the long length of time between exposure and disease onset, while retrospective studies are hampered by trying to quantitate environmental stress and account for the large fluctuations that occur over the course of a lifetime. Additionally, definitive diagnosis of most neurodegenerative disorders requires inspection of brain pathology after death, further complicating study of patients during life. Consequently, most knowledge concerning the relationship of stress to neurodegenerative disorders originates either from studies of animal models or from changes in stress-related hormones in those with neurodegenerative disorders compared to those without.

Despite the limitations, the scientific literature substantially supports an association of psychological and physiological stress with the risk of neurodegenerative disease. This article describes the clinical and neuropathological findings of AD and PD, as illustrative of the most common neurodegenerative disorders. It describes the effects of stress on animal models of neurodegenerative disorders and evidence for alterations in stress hormones in the setting of neurodegenerative disease.

Neurodegenerative Dementias: Alzheimer's Disease

AD is the most common neurodegenerative disorder and a major health-care problem that will continue to increase in importance as the U.S. population ages. Currently, more than 4 million Americans have a diagnosis of AD, resulting in enormous economic and social costs for their care, with a total in the United States alone approaching $100 billion per year.

AD occurs primarily but not exclusively in the elderly, with onset in most patients occurring after age 65. More rarely, onset may occur as early as the fourth decade of life, particularly in those with a familial form of the disease. Overall, prevalence for AD among the elderly (age 65 or greater) is about 6%, doubling approximately every 5 years after age 60, affecting between 26 and 45% of those age 85 or older. The annual incidence of new cases of AD per 100 000 people in the United States also rises with advancing age, one reason why investigators predict that AD will affect an increasingly large number of persons in the coming years, as the average age of the U.S. population increases. Some have predicted that in the United States the number of people with this disease may reach 14 million by the year 2050.

In the absence of a definitive clinical test or biomarker, the clinical diagnosis of AD depends on clinical criteria. The diagnosis of clinically probable AD by National Institute of Neurologic and Communicative Disorders and Stroke and the AD and Related Disorders Association Work Group (NINCDS-ADRDA) criteria requires impairment in at least two cognitive domains, progressive deterioration, absence of delirium, onset between 40 and 90 years of age, and lack of evidence for other dementing diseases after a standard work-up. Besides memory, other cognitive domains that may be affected include language, visuospatial perception or constructions, calculations, praxis, and executive functions. Patients meeting these criteria typically display progressive impairment in activities of daily living such as driving, buying groceries, preparing meals, doing laundry, and basic functions such as walking safely and maintaining personal hygiene. The diagnosis of clinically probable AD using NINCDS-ADRDA criteria reportedly results in correct identification at autopsy in 85 in 95% of cases. Like other neurodegenerative disorders, gradual deterioration until death is typical, with a mean survival after symptom onset of 10.3 years.

The definitive diagnosis of AD requires clinicopathological correlation. One hallmark of the disorder is the presence of intracellular neurofibrillary tangles (NFTs) containing the microtubule associated tau protein in an abnormal phosphorylated state. Another hallmark of AD is the presence of extracellular senile or neuritic plaques greater than expected for the patient's age. The central core of these plaques is composed of β-amyloid peptides such as Aβ42. Around this amyloid core are degenerating dendrites and axons, some of which contain paired helical filaments like those found in NFTs. In addition to NFTs and neuritic plaques, the neuropathology of AD, like all neurodegenerative disorders, includes a progressive loss of neurons and their synaptic connections.

Both familial and environmental risk factors exist for development of AD. First, the development of AD at an early age (younger than age 65) often occurs as a result of autosomally dominantly inherited mutations in genes such as presenilin 1 and 2 and the amyloid precursor protein. Second, presence of an apolipoprotein E genotype with at least one ε4 allele results in an earlier age of onset of the disorder. Apolipoproteins are cholesterol-bearing proteins that mediate neuronal protection and repair and may participate in Aβ42 deposition. Third, women appear to be at slightly greater risk for AD, even when accounting for their greater longevity over men. Fourth, in addition to age, risk for AD increases with traumatic head injury, small head size, and low education, presumably on the basis of decreased neuronal reserve. Finally, later age of symptom onset, prominent psychiatric symptoms, and comorbidity such as cerebrovascular disease, heart failure, a history of heavy alcohol use, excessive weight loss, and institutionalization all may have a negative impact on clinical progression and eventually survival. In contrast, environmental and familial risk factors such as ethnic background and marital status are not proven to affect survival or rate of disease progression.

More recent evidence implicates psychological stress as an additional risk factor for the development of AD. Several studies show that patients with a high susceptibility to distress are more prone to AD in later life. When patients are followed to autopsy, those with a high susceptibility to distress as indicated by the personality trait of neuroticism are twice as likely as those without this susceptibility to have the NFTs and neuritic plaques of AD. Those with high distress proneness have a greater than 10-fold increase in episodic memory decline compared to those with low distress proneness. Other studies indicate that everyday hassles and challenging life events may exacerbate age-related declines on episodic memory tests. These findings implicate accelerated damage to the hippocampi as the mediator of the effects of stress on memory.

Much data indicate that the hippocampal region is involved in the response to stress. Animal and human studies indicate memory deficits associated with hippocampal damage after chronic stressful experiences. Corticosteroid receptors are abundant in the hippocampus, and high, stress-induced concentrations of glucocorticoids become toxic to the hippocampal neurons. Studies have reported high concentrations of cortisol in association with hippocampal atrophy in patients with dementia, as well as in posttraumatic stress disorder and major depression.

Many studies suggest abnormal function of the hypothalamic-pituitary-adrenal (HPA) axis in patients with AD. There are reports of increased serum cortisol levels and reduced feedback inhibition of cortisol secretion in patients with AD. Corticosteroid hypersecretion may downregulate the hippocampal corticosteroid receptors, which in turn dampens the feedback inhibition of the HPA, leading to further hypersecretion and eventual hippocampal neuronal loss. Other studies have focused on abnormal neuroendocrine responses to challenge with a chemical agent. Several studies report that AD patients demonstrate elevated cortisol levels relative to nondemented controls after challenge by a dexamethasone suppression test. In these studies, cortisol levels after administration of dexamethasone correlated directly with dementia severity. Another study compared cortisol and prolactin responses to administration of naltrexone, an opiate antagonist, in AD patients and normal elderly controls. In this study, normal control patients demonstrated a significantly greater increase in cortisol levels after a single dose of naltrexone compared to the AD patients, with no difference in prolactin response between the groups. Finally, cortisol levels have been shown to directly correlate with severity of cognitive decline and degree of hippocampal atrophy in AD patients.

One further mechanism for stress-induced injury in AD is vascular. The neuropathology of AD and the cerebrovascular changes may be synergistic. Higher stress-induced systolic and diastolic blood pressure (BP) reactivity, including variability in BP on 24-h ambulatory monitoring, has been associated with decreased performance in verbal memory and executive tests. The relation of BP reactivity to decreased cognitive function may be mediated by silent cerebrovascular changes from cerebral hypoperfusion. Repeated episodes of stress-induced BP reactivity can result in white matter changes or other silent cerebrovascular lesions on neuroimaging. Finally, life may also produce a hypercoagulable state that could contribute to cerebrovascular disease.

Neurodegenerative Movement Disorders: Parkinson's Disease

PD is an extrapyramidal movement disorder of unknown etiology, with onset between the ages of 50 and 65 years, and is more common in males than females with a ratio of 3:2. PD is fairly common, with a prevalence of approximately 100 to 180 per 100 000 population. Disease course is shorter on average than AD, with an 8-year mean duration of illness. Patients with PD have a two- to fivefold increased mortality compared to nondemented people in the same community. Risk of mortality directly relates to symptom severity, with death typically occurring due to aspiration pneumonia, urinary tract infection, or unrelated conditions of the elderly.

Clinically, PD has five primary characteristics: resting tremors, rigidity, bradykinesia, postural instability, and responsiveness to treatment with dopaminergic agents. In any particular patient some components may be evident and others not, and components are commonly asymmetric at onset. Of the primary clinical characteristics, presence of tremor is most suggestive of PD as opposed to other parkinsonian disorders. The tremor is classically present at rest, occurring at approximately four to eight cycles per second, and may develop in one upper extremity before spreading to involve all four limbs, face, and tongue. Bradykinesia contributes to the expressionless or masked face, sialorrhea, and micrographia. The gait is festinating, with abnormal righting reflexes and a slightly flexed posture. Eye movements may have subtle abnormalities in voluntary gaze, pursuit, and convergence. Many patients develop autonomic symptoms including postural hypotension, impotence, atony of the large bowel with constipation, and esophageal spasm.

Characteristic pathological changes of idiopathic PD typically occur in the pars compacta of the substantia nigra. Classically, there is marked depigmentation and neuronal loss, with presence of Lewy bodies in this region. As a consequence of these changes, dopaminergic neurons in the substantia nigra pars compacta are lost, affecting projections to the corpus striatum. Less pronounced changes are evident in a variety of other brain stem and diencephalic nuclei, including the locus ceruleus, dorsal vagal nucleus, and sympathetic ganglia. Although depletion of dopamine is the classic neurotransmitter deficit in PD, levels of norepinephrine, glutamate decarboxylase, GABA, methionine-enkephalin cholestokinin, and serotonin are also decreased in the substantia nigra of PD patients. No evidence supporting or suggesting a link between stress and neurotransmitter levels has been reported in PD.

Lewy bodies are characteristic of PD. Certain sites show a predilection for development of Lewy bodies, including the entorhinal region, the CA2 sector of the hippocampal formation, limbic nuclei of the thalamus, anterior cingulate, agranular insular cortex, amygdale, ventromedial divisions both of the basal and accessory basal nuclei, and central nucleus. Lewy bodies are composed of aggregates of α-synuclein, suggesting a possible central role for this protein in the pathogenesis of PD. Further evidence in the form of dopaminergic loss and inclusion body formation in α-synuclein mice reinforces a causal role for α-synuclein in this disorder. The proposed pathological mechanism starts with a reduction in the solubility of α-synuclein, resulting in the formation of filaments, which then aggregate into the cytoplasmic inclusions called Lewy bodies that contribute to the dysfunction or death of the glial cells and neurons in which they form in PD patients. However, no evidence for a relationship between degree of pathological changes or presence of Lewy bodies and stress has been reported in PD.

Environmental risk factors for PD include age, family history, and rural living possibly related to pesticide exposure. A genetic component to risk for development of PD is suggested by some studies reporting an increased prevalence rate of PD in relatives of PD patients compared to the general population. This has not been confirmed in twin studies, which failed to demonstrate increased concordance among identical twin pairs. Exposure to environmental toxins may be a rare cause of PD, such as from exposures to pesticides or herbicides and well water consumption. In contrast to AD, most studies do not find that APOE e4 is a risk factor for PD or PD dementia; however, PD patients show a trend toward slightly higher APOE e4 allele frequencies (12.5 to 17%) compared to normals (10 to 12.5%). One study showed that the APOE e4 allele frequency was significantly higher for PD dementia compared to PD and may affect an earlier age of onset for PD. Additionally, while female gender is associated with an increase risk of developing AD, male gender is associated with increased risk of PD.

Stress is probably an additional risk factor for PD. When compared to levels in unaffected spouses and siblings, cortisol levels in untreated patients with idiopathic PD are elevated. Other neuroendocrine abnormalities such as elevated levels of prolactin and decreased levels of growth hormone and adrenocorticotropic hormone have been demonstrated in patients with PD compared to normal controls. The clinical understanding of HPA axis dysfunction in PD, however, is often complicated by medical treatment, since selegiline, a medication used in treating patients with PD, may lower cortisol levels. Investigators have studied neuroendocrine abnormalities in a dog model of PD, using 1-methyl-4-phenyl-1,2,3,6-tetrahydropyridine (MPTP)-treated animals. After MPTP treatment, which damages neurons in the substantia nigra, plasma ACTH and cortisol are elevated in the treated dogs compared to untreated controls. In these animals, elevated cortisol levels result in excessive stimulation of neuronal glucocorticoid receptors, contributing to excitotoxic cell death. Excitatory stimulation of postsynaptic glutamate (NMDA) receptors in nigrostriatal neurons increases intracellular concentrations of calcium, possibly leading to disruption of the cell cytoskeleton or activation of caspase pathways leading to programmed cell death. Increased oxidative stress at the cellular level is also important in the pathogenesis of PD. Oxidative stress, through the depletion of glutathione and other free radical detoxificant enzymes, impaired mitochondrial complex I activity, or enhanced iron-mediated free radical production may contribute directly to neuronal loss in PD.

Conclusions

In summary, stress and its physiological effects may play a role in the progressive loss of neurons that occurs in neurodegenerative disorders. Increased cortisol levels due to both acute and chronic stress have demonstrated associations with hippocampal degeneration and memory impairment. This may be particularly relevant in the study of neuronal loss in AD, a disorder in which hippocampal degeneration occurs early in the disease course. Stress-induced alterations in BP and consequent vascular injury may further predispose to AD. In PD, elevated cortisol levels result from abnormalities of the function of the HPA axis, possibly contributing to loss of dopaminergic neurons in the substantia nigra by a variety of mechanisms, including excitotoxic cell death, increased intracellular calcium levels, and increased oxidative stress. Much more research is vitally needed in order to more clearly characterize and understand the contributions of stress to AD, PD, and the many other neurodegenerative disorders.

See Also the Following Articles

Alzheimer's Disease.

Further Reading

Belanoff, J. K., Gross, K., Yager, A., et al. (2001). Corticosteroids and cognition. *Journal of Psychiatric Research* 35, 127–145.

Bremner, J. D. (1999). Does stress damage the brain? *Biological Psychiatry* **45**, 797–805.

Deshmukh, V. D. and Deshmukh, S. V. (1990). Stress-adaptation failure hypothesis of Alzheimer's disease. *Medical Hypotheses* 32, 293–295.

Fratiglioni, L., Paillard-Borg, S. and Winblad, B. (2004). An active and socially integrated lifestyle ion late life might protect against dementia. *Lancet Neurology* **3**, 343–353.

Kirschbaum, C., Wolf, O. T., May, M., et al. (1996). Stress- and treatment-induced elevations of cortisol levels associated with impaired declarative memory in healthy adults. *Life Science* 58, 1475–1483.

McEwen, B. S. (2002). Sex, stress and the hippocampus: allostasis, allostatic load and the aging process. *Neurobiology of Aging* 23, 921–939.

Meyer, J. S., Rauch, G., Rauch, R. A., et al. (2000). Risk factors for cerebral hypoperfusion, mild cognitive impairment, and dementia. *Neurobiology of Aging* **21**, 161–169.

Nasman, B., Olsson, T., Viitanen, M., et al. (1995). A subtle disturbance in the feedback regulation of the hypothalamic-pituitary-adrenal axis in the early phase of Alzheimer's disease. *Psychoneuroendocrinology* **20**, 211–220.

Sapolsky, R. M. (1999). Glucocorticoids, stress, and their adverse neurological effects: relevance to aging. *Experimental Gerontology* **34**, 721–732.

Sapolsky, R. M., Romero, L. M. and Munck, A. U. (2000). How do glucocorticoids influence stress responses?

Integrating permissive, suppressive, stimulatory, and preparative actions. *Endocrinology Review* **21**, 55–89.
VonDras, D. D., Powless, M. R., Olson, A. D., et al. (2005). Differential effects of everyday stress on the episodic memory test performances of young, mid-life, and older adults. *Aging and Mental Health* **9**, 60–70.
Waldstein, S. R. and Katzel, L. I. (2005). Stress-induced blood pressure reactivity and cognitive function. *Neurology* **64**, 1746–1749.
Waldstein, S. R., Siegel, E. L., Lefkowitz, D., et al. (2004). Stress-induced blood pressure reactivity and silent cerebrovascular disease. *Stroke* **35**, 1294–1298.
Wilson, R. S., Evans, D. A., Bienias, J. L., et al. (2003). Proneness to psychological distress is associated with risk of Alzheimer's disease. *Neurology* **61**, 1479–1485.
Wilson, R. S., Barnes, L. L., Bennett, D. A., et al. (2005). Proneness to psychological distress and risk of Alzheimer disease in a biracial community. *Neurology* **64**, 380–382.

Alzheimer's Disease

A E Roth
Nathan S. Kline Institute for Psychiatric Research, Orangeburg, NY, USA
W M Greenberg and N Pomara
Nathan S. Kline Institute for Psychiatric Research, Orangeburg, NY, and New York University School of Medicine, New York, NY, USA

Glossary

Amyloid precursor protein (APP) A protein that is normally cut into smaller lengths by enzymes, resulting in the peptides amyloid beta (A-β)-40 and A-β-42. A-β-42 may circulate in small clumps (oligomers) and is believed to be neurotoxic and to be involved in the causation of Alzheimer's disease. The A-β peptides may be found later in Alzheimer's disease in larger clumps deposited in the brain, known as amyloid plaques.

Corticosteroid hormones Hormones produced by the adrenal gland as part of the stress response (principally cortisol in humans and corticosterone in rodents).

Declarative memory Memories of facts and words (semantic memory) and personal events (episodic memory) that can be consciously recalled, as opposed to nondeclarative, implicitly learned procedural skills.

Delirium A disturbance in consciousness, manifested by difficulties in focusing, sustaining, or shifting attention, with cognitive deficits. A delirium usually develops over a brief period of time and tends to fluctuate over the course of a day. It is directly caused by an active medical condition, such as an infection with a high fever, electrolyte disturbance, or liver or kidney failure.

Dementia A syndrome of significant memory impairment compared with previous functioning, occurring with other cognitive deficits and not existing only during a period of delirium.

Hypothalamic-pituitary-adrenal (HPA) axis The system that orchestrates the body's response to stress using hormones, with negative feedback mechanisms to allow the organism to return to baseline activation.

The Clinical Picture of Alzheimer's Disease

Dementia is a syndrome defined as the development of significant memory deficits together with other cognitive impairments, not occurring exclusively during a delirium. Of those diagnosed with dementia, between 50–60% have dementia of the Alzheimer's type, also called Alzheimer's disease (AD), a disorder characterized by symptoms with gradual onset but a relentlessly progressive course. Early symptoms most prominently involve difficulties remembering recent events and forming new memories, and these are often accompanied by visuospatial and language problems. As the disease progresses, individuals slowly lose the ability to perform the activities of daily living, such as managing finances and driving a car. Eventually, attention, verbal ability, problem solving, reasoning, and all forms of memory become seriously impaired. Personality changes associated with the progression of AD may include increased apathy, anger, dependency, aggressiveness, and occasionally inappropriate sexual behavior; paranoid thinking is also not uncommon. In the latter stages of this disorder, individuals may be mute, completely confused, and bedridden. At this time, available treatments usually offer, at most, a temporary slowing of the symptomatic deterioration.

Early-onset AD is defined as a case in which the onset of dementia occurs at or prior to age 65; when symptoms first appear later in life it is referred to as late-onset AD. Somewhat complicating diagnostic specificity, AD may often co-exist with dementia or cognitive impairment due to another cause, most frequently vascular dementia (i.e., related to small or large strokes). Although making a probable diagnosis of AD is often not very difficult, it is a diagnosis that is only confirmed on autopsy. The prevalence of AD increases with age, from less than 1% of those age 65 to conservatively 13% of those age 85 and 23% of those age 90. As more individuals live to older ages, putting them at higher risk for this serious disorder, the economic burden of providing nursing home and other medical care to afflicted individuals, coupled with the tragic toll it takes on lives of the sufferers, their families, and other caretakers, constitutes a problem of ever-increasing magnitude.

Risk Factors for Alzheimer's Disease

Early-onset AD is infrequent, making up approximately 10% of AD cases seen in clinical practice. Most cases of early-onset AD are familial; they have been linked to specific identifiable mutations and have an autosomal-dominant pattern of inheritance with nearly full penetrance. Mutations in the Alzheimer precursor protein (APP) gene on chromosome 21, the Presenilin-1 gene on chromosome 14, and the Presenilin-2 gene on chromosome 1 have been identified, and they account for approximately 50% of all cases of early-onset familial AD. Also, most individuals who have trisomy-21 (Down syndrome), and therefore three APP genes instead of two, develop AD at relatively early ages, supporting the theory that the overexpression of the APP protein may be involved in causing AD.

In contrast, only a small number of late-onset AD cases are familial and no deterministic genetic mutations have yet been identified for late-onset sporadic AD, which accounts for more than 90% of AD cases. Clearly, genetic factors are not the sole cause of late-onset sporadic AD because the concordance rate for AD in monozygotic twins ranges from 31 to 59%. Instead, it appears that a number of genetic and environmental factors may increase the risk for this disorder. To date, the only genetic factor that has been associated with increased risk for late-onset AD is a form of the apolipoprotein E gene known as the APOE ϵ4 allele, which has a prevalence of approximately 25% in the general Caucasian population. Having one ϵ4 allele increases the risk of developing late-onset AD, and having two alleles (homozygosity) further increases the risk. In nondemented individuals, the APOE ϵ4 allele has been associated with poorer performance on delayed recall tasks and greater hippocampal atrophy compared with controls. The environmental risk factors for late-onset AD are diverse and incompletely characterized. Significant head trauma (i.e., with a loss of consciousness for an extended period) is a predisposing risk factor; higher education is an example of a protective factor. Women appear to be at a slightly higher risk of developing AD.

The Pathophysiology of Alzheimer's Disease

The characteristic features associated with AD include brain atrophy, amyloid plaques, and neurofibrillary tangles, and these abnormalities generally affect the medial temporal lobes the earliest and most intensely. Currently, there is compelling evidence that all types of AD, irrespective of age of onset, result from the neurotoxic effects of increased brain levels of soluble oligomeric forms of A-β peptides, derived from the amyloid precursor protein (APP), and from its aggregated forms (amyloid) as present in senile plaques and in the walls of small cerebral vessels. In cases of early-onset familial AD caused by genetic mutations, the increase in A-β is secondary to the increased production of the peptides A-β-40 and, especially, A-β-42 through the increased activity of β and γ secretases, two cleavage enzymes for APP. In contrast, in sporadic late-onset AD, it has been generally thought that decreased clearance of A-β is the proximate cause. In support of this hypothesis, brain regions associated with increased amyloid deposits in sporadic AD show lower levels of VPS26 and VPS35, two retromer proteins involved in the intracellular compartmental trafficking of the A-β peptides. Interestingly, there is recent evidence that the APOE ϵ4 allele may also increase A-β peptide production, raising the possibility that increased A-β production contributes to the development of sporadic AD in elderly individuals with this allele. There is evidence that increased A-β peptide levels facilitate the abnormal phosphorylation of the τ protein, which in turn leads to its forming intracellular neurofibrillary tangles. This supports the general belief that the neurofibrillary tangles are a secondary phenomenon; however, memory deficits correlate more with the presence of neurofibrillary tangles than with plaques. The earliest pathological alterations of AD are usually seen in the entorhinal cortex and nearby CA1 subfield of the hippocampus, both structures in the medial temporal lobe critical for the formation of new memories, thereby explaining the prominent memory symptoms that are typically present as an initial symptom of AD.

AD is eventually accompanied by the pronounced degeneration of cholinergic neurons in the nucleus basalis with associated reduced levels of acetylcholine, and this loss seems to contribute significantly to memory dysfunction. The degeneration of dopaminergic neurons in the noradrenergic nucleus locus ceruleus, the serotonergic dorsal raphe nucleus, and the dopaminergic substantia nigra and the significant reductions in somatostatin-like immunoreactivity and corticotropin releasing hormone (CRH) immunoreactivity in the neocortical brain regions have also been demonstrated in AD and might contribute to the noncognitive symptoms associated with this disease.

Paradoxically, there is evidence, albeit indirect, that AD may be accompanied by overactivity of neuronal synapses using the neurotransmitter glutamate, possibly secondary to the loss of the high-affinity glutamate transporters that has been reported in AD. The overactivation of glutamate *N*-methyl-D-aspartate (NMDA) receptors produces excitotoxic effects, especially in areas such as the hippocampus and entorhinal cortex, in which the density of these receptors is high. These brain regions have been implicated in learning and memory and show profound abnormalities, including atrophy even in the earliest stages of AD, supporting a possible role for disturbances in glutamatergic neurotransmission in the cognitive and degenerative alterations associated with this disorder. There is also some empirical support for oxidative stress and inflammation having etiological roles in the pathogenesis of AD.

The Hypothalamic-Pituitary-Adrenal Axis in Normal Brain Functioning

The HPA manages the body's response to stress and is necessary for normal survival. When this system is activated, the paraventricular nucleus in the hypothalamus releases CRH; this both activates the sympathetic nervous system and stimulates cells in the anterior pituitary to secrete adrenocorticotropic hormone (ACTH), which stimulates cells in the adrenal cortex to synthesize and release corticosteroid hormones into the bloodstream. This complex orchestrated response acutely inhibits anabolic activity (growth-promoting functions), increases the opposite catabolic activities, and initiates the fight-or-flight reaction. This fight-or-flight reaction includes increases in heart rate and blood pressure, inhibition of the immune system, and experiential and behavioral activation. The corticosteroid secretion by the adrenal glands (principally cortisol in humans and corticosterone in rodents) provides negative feedback at the levels of both the hypothalamus and pituitary. Another important influence keeping this system in homeostatic balance is modulation provided by the hippocampus in the medial temporal lobe, a structure also critically responsible for acquiring and consolidating new declarative memories (semantic memories of facts and words and episodic memories of personal events, as opposed to nondeclarative, implicitly learned procedural skills).

Two types of corticosteroid receptors exist on the surface of neurons: type I or mineralocorticoid receptors (MRs), which have a higher affinity for corticosteroids, and type II or glucocorticoid receptors (GRs), which have a lower affinity. Under normal, nonstressful conditions, with low levels of circulating corticosteroids, mostly the higher-affinity MRs are stimulated, with GRs remaining mainly unaffected.

Stress and the Hypothalamic-Pituitary-Adrenal Axis

In the hippocampus, when the MRs are predominantly activated, the formation of new declarative memories is supported by the mechanism of long-term potentiation. Under low levels of acute stress, there may even be some improvement in this function. However, when stress levels and the associated increases in circulating corticosteroid levels cause more activation of the GRs, there is interference with forming new memories. This pattern of low levels of stress improving performance and higher levels of stress disrupting performance has sometimes been descriptively referred to as an inverted-U relationship. Slight elevations in stress hormones are also associated with enhanced attention and motivation, both important for performing well on memory and higher-order cognitive tasks but impairing the recall of previous memories. These latter actions appear to be mediated by both β-adrenergic and cholinergic receptors in the basolateral complex of the amygdala.

Stress and the Hypothalamic-Pituitary-Adrenal Axis in Animal Studies

Prolonged HPA overactivity is also associated with cognitive decline and hippocampal atrophy in rats. Rodents exposed to stress paradigms or administered large doses of corticosterone have been reported to have atrophy of the hippocampal neurons and increased sensitivity to toxins, but this could not be replicated in pigtailed macaque monkeys exposed to high doses of cortisone for 12 months. Species differences may be important because these primates proportionately have far fewer hippocampal GRs than rodents.

Stress and Hypothalamic-Pituitary-Adrenal Axis in Normal Aging

The hippocampus plays a major role in learning and memory performance, in particular in declarative (conscious and voluntary) memory. It is susceptible to damage from intense prolonged stress. Cortisol production increases during stress, and long-term exposure to high levels of cortisol causes atrophy and impaired neurogenesis in the hippocampus. There is also evidence of hippocampal atrophy as a function of aging, and HPA overactivity is associated with cognitive decline and hippocampal atrophy in normal elderly.

There are a variety of measures of HPA activity: simple plasma cortisol and salivary cortisol measures have been used, but there is much variation in these over the course of a day. Urinary cortisol may be a more reliable measure of cortisol secretion over time, and some studies have determined that cerebrospinal fluid (CSF) cortisol more accurately reflects cortisol levels in the central nervous system. Another widely used measure of HPA activity is the dexamethasone (DST) test (DST is a synthetic glucocorticoid). DST is typically administered to individuals in the evening, and plasma cortisol levels are measured the following day in the morning or afternoon. Ordinarily, DST suppresses the HPA axis, and plasma cortisol levels will be low the day after DST administration. Failure to suppress the HPA axis (nonsuppression) is evidence of a loss of normal feedback control and homeostasis.

There is some evidence suggesting gender differences in the role of cortisol overproduction in cognitive and memory dysfunction in normal elderly individuals. One study has found that increases in urinary cortisol excretion are significantly associated with declines in memory performance over 2.5 years in healthy elderly women but not in men. Furthermore, women who showed a decrease in urinary cortisol excretion showed significant improvement in memory performance over time. These findings highlight the possibility that damage to the structure and functioning of the brain from hypercortisolemia might be reversible, at least for healthy elderly women, although it is believed that prolonged and repeated exposure to glucocorticoids increases the risk of irreversible damage.

Indeed, longitudinal examinations of cortisol levels and declarative memory performance reveal that elderly individuals with high and increasing cortisol levels over periods ranging from 1 to 3 years show significantly greater impairments in declarative memory performance and significantly greater hippocampal atrophy than do individuals who show decreases or low and smaller increases in cortisol levels over time. The amount of hippocampal atrophy in elderly individuals with high and increasing levels of cortisol was found to be equivalent to that of older adults exhibiting mild cognitive impairment (MCI). Although cortisol levels, on average, increase with aging, there is much interindividual variability in cortisol production in the elderly, with some individuals actually showing decreases in cortisol levels over time.

Stress and Alzheimer's Disease

Because older age, hypercortisolemia, and hippocampal atrophy are all associated with AD, the role of stress in AD pathology and memory dysfunction has logically attracted some attention. According to the glucocorticoid cascade hypothesis, hippocampal degeneration in AD might result in increased cortisol secretion, due to the loss of normal negative hippocampal feedback to the HPA axis. In turn, the overactive HPA system evident in AD could lead to additional neuronal degeneration, thereby inducing progressive cognitive impairment – potentially a vicious circle.

Memory deficits have also been found in the presence of other disorders that are associated with persistent HPA activation and high cortisol levels, such as Cushing's disease and major depressive disorder. One investigator found that, compared to matched controls, women with histories of recurrent major depression had smaller hippocampal volumes, the size of which were correlated with their lifetime duration of depression, and did more poorly on tests of verbal memory.

Most studies of individuals with AD have found them to have elevated post-DST cortisol levels compared to healthy controls. Increased HPA activity, as evidenced by elevated basal cortisol levels, elevated glucocorticoid activity, increased CSF cortisol levels, and hippocampal atrophy, have also been usually found to be positively associated with the degree of cognitive impairment in elderly individuals with AD. A relevant variable also appears to be the presence of agitation, found to be more frequent in DST nonsuppressors. In one small study that followed AD patients for up to 3 years, increased basal plasma cortisol levels were found to linearly correlate with decline in cognitive functioning.

A recent study demonstrated a relationship between APOE genotype and CSF cortisol levels in individuals with AD. Specifically, in analyses controlling for age, it was found that individuals with AD who had the APOE $\epsilon4$ genotype had significantly higher cortisol levels than did individuals without the $\epsilon4$ allele. Similar analyses performed with nondemented elderly individuals revealed only a trend for individuals with the $\epsilon4$ allele to have higher CSF cortisol levels. These findings suggest that the APOE $\epsilon4$ genotype might contribute to HPA axis dysfunction. However, CSF cortisol levels were not significantly correlated with measures of global cognitive status, although it is possible that CSF cortisol levels might be associated with more subtle changes in cognitive functioning.

Psychological Stress and the Hypothalamic-Pituitary-Adrenal Axis in Alzheimer's Disease

The evidence of a direct role of stress in AD onset remains limited and inconclusive. As previously noted, there are many studies reporting a significant association between acute and chronic stress with memory impairment, yet few studies have considered the role of elevated stress levels in the development of AD. In a longitudinal analysis of subjects' proneness to psychological distress and AD onset, investigators found that in analyses that accounted for depressive symptoms, for each 1-point increase on the distress-proneness scale there was a corresponding 6% greater risk of AD onset. Proneness to psychological distress was measured with a well-established index of neuroticism. Furthermore, greater proneness to psychological distress was associated with poorer levels of, and a greater decline in, global cognitive functioning. Additional analyses revealed an association between greater psychological distress and greater decline in episodic memory functioning. Specifically, decline was 16% greater for each 1-point increase on the distress proneness scale in episodic memory functioning. However, proneness to psychological distress was not associated with pathological AD as examined postmortem.

In a similar analysis examining distress-proneness and AD onset in a community sample of Caucasian and African American (49.8%) elderly individuals, it was found that individuals who scored in the ninetieth percentile or higher on a neuroticism index were 2.4 times more likely to develop AD over the course of 3–6 years. Additional analyses accounting for depressive symptoms or excluding individuals with depression at baseline did not alter the results. Although the researchers did not have postmortem data for AD pathology, the APOE genotype (a potential risk factor for AD) was available; and the researchers found no significant association between APOE genotype and distress-proneness in the full sample. Interestingly, the magnitude of the association between distress-proneness and AD onset was significantly different in Caucasian versus African American individuals. In the Caucasian sample, with each 1-point increase on the distress-proneness scale the odds of developing AD increased 12%. In contrast, the odds of developing AD in the African American sample increased only 2% for every 1-point increase on the distress-prone scale. These findings highlight the possibility of sociocultural differences in the association between stress and AD onset.

Other studies examining psychosocial stressors and AD onset have reported similar findings. For example, in a longitudinal analysis of psychosocial stressors and AD onset, when accounting for demographic factors, including education, individuals who reported psychosocial stressors as far back as childhood were found to have significantly higher rates of AD onset relative to individuals with fewer or no psychosocial stressors. Specifically, the incidence rate of AD over 9 years in individuals reporting no psychosocial stressors was 1.7%, and this rose to 5% in individuals reporting one or two and to 8.3% for individuals reporting three or more psychosocial stressors. The psychosocial stressors or risk factors that were considered included events from childhood (i.e., death of a parent and poverty), adulthood (i.e., death of a spouse, arduous manual labor, and serious illness in a child), and old age (i.e., deterioration in financial status and physical illness). Psychosocial stressors that were significantly associated with AD onset included the death of a parent during childhood, arduous manual labor, physical illness in a spouse during old age, and serious illness in a child (offspring). Possibly relevant to this finding is an earlier study reporting that, when accounting for education and alcohol consumption, men who had occupations involving manual labor were 5.3 times more likely to be diagnosed with late-onset AD than were men in nonarduous occupations. The finding that psychosocial stressors earlier in the life span might contribute to dysfunction in later life is also congruent with research using animal models in which earlier experiences altered noradrenergic and serotonergic functions in adulthood and the rate of aging.

A Possible Treatment Approach

An interesting avenue in exploring the role of stress hormones in AD is the potential therapeutic utility of corticosteroid receptor antagonists such as mifepristone (RU-486). In a pilot study in which participants were randomized to placebo or treatment with RU-486 for 6 weeks, participants taking RU-486 improved on measures of memory, whereas participants in the placebo condition declined. Other studies have also revealed that short-term use of RU-486 improves memory performance in bipolar patients but not for individuals with schizophrenia. Indeed, using a corticosteroid receptor antagonist to try to delay the onset or slow the progression of cognitive impairment and AD deserves further consideration.

Conclusion

Studies examining HPA dysfunction, cortisol levels, and indices of psychological distress have found significant associations with memory impairment, memory decline, AD, or AD onset. Although it appears that psychological distress, independent of depression, may play a role in AD onset, research on the biological mechanisms linking stress to AD onset remains inconclusive. HPA overactivity and high or increasing levels of cortisol seem to be associated with cognitive dysfunction and brain changes associated with AD, but it is unclear whether these impairments precede AD onset or are a function of the illness. Longitudinal research examining the biological mechanisms of stress and AD onset would be fruitful for further understanding the link between psychological stress and AD.

Further Reading

Davis, K. L., Davis, B. M., Greenwald, B. S., et al. (1986). Cortisol and Alzheimer's disease. I: Basal studies. *American Journal of Psychiatry* **143**, 442–446.

Fratiglioni, L., Ahlbom, A., Viitanen, M., et al. (1993). Risk factors for late-onset Alzheimer's disease: a population-based, case-control study. *Annals of Neurology* **33**, 258–266.

Li, S., Mallory, M., Alford, M., et al. (1997). Glutamate transporter alterations in Alzheimer's disease are possibly associated with abnormal APP expression. *Journal of Neuropathology and Experimental Neurology* **56**(8), 901–911.

Lupien, S. J., DeLeon, M., DeSanti, S., et al. (1998). Longitudinal increase in cortisol during human aging predicts hippocampal atrophy and memory deficits. *Nature Neuroscience* **1**, 69–73.

Lupien, S. J., Nair, N. P. V., Brière, S., et al. (1999). Increased cortisol levels and impaired cognitive cognition in human aging: implication for depression and dementia in later life. *Reviews in Neuroscience* **10**, 117–139.

Nemeroff, C. B., Kizer, J. S., Reynolds, G. P., et al. (1989). Neuropeptides in Alzheimer's disease: a post-mortem study. *Regulatory Peptides* **25**(1), 123–130.

Peskind, E. R., Wilkinson, C. W., Petrie, E. C., et al. (2001). Increased CSF cortisol in AD is a function of APOE genotype. *Neurology* **56**, 1094–1098.

Pomara, N., Singh, R., Deptula, D., et al. (1992). Glutamate and other CSF amino acids in Alzheimer's disease. *American Journal of Psychiatry* **149**(2), 251–254.

Pomara, N., Doraiswamy, P. M., Tun, H., et al. (2002). Mifepristone (RU 486) for Alzheimer's disease. *Neurology* **58**(1), 1436–1437.

Pomara, N., Greenberg, W. M., Branford, M. D., et al. (2003). Therapeutic implications of HPA axis abnormalities in Alzheimer's disease: review and update. *Psychopharmacology Bulletin* **37**(2), 120–134.

Sapolsky, R. M., Krey, L. and McEwen, B. S. (1986). The neuroendocrinology of stress and aging: the glucocorticoid cascade hypothesis. *Endocrine Reviews* **7**, 284–301.

Seeman, T. E., McEwen, B. S., Singer, B. H., et al. (1997). Increase in urinary cortisol excretion and memory declines: MacArthur studies of successful aging. *Journal of Clinical Endocrinology and Metabolism* **82**(8), 2458–2465.

Sheline, Y. I., Sanghyavi, M., Mintun, M. A., et al. (1999). Depression duration but not age predicts hippocampal volume loss in medically healthy women with recurrent major depression. *Journal of Neuroscience* **19**, 5034–5043.

Small, S. A., Kent, K., Pierce, A., et al. (2005). Model-guided microarray implicates the retromer complex in Alzheimer's disease. *Annals of Neurology* **58**, 909–919.

Wilson, R. S., Barnes, L. L., Bennett, D. A., et al. (2005). Proneness to psychological distress and risk of Alzheimer's disease in a biracial community. *Neurology* **64**, 380–382.

Diabetes Type 2 and Stress: Impact on Memory and the Hippocampus

A Convit
Department of Psychiatry, New York University School of Medicine, Millhauser Laboratories, New York, and Nathan Kline Institute, Orangeburg, NY, USA
M Rueger
New York University School of Medicine, New York, NY, USA
O T Wolf
University of Bielefeld, Bielefeld, Germany

Introduction

The aim of this article is to present our understanding of how the abnormalities in peripheral glucose control and elevations in cortisol levels associated with type 2 diabetes mellitus (T2DM) may give rise to medial temporal lobe (MTL) pathology and dysfunction. The article falls into four main sections: Memory and aging, effects of glucocorticoid functioning on the brain, impact of diabetes on the brain, and, finally, an integrative model that attempts to explain how the specific MTL dysfunction may come about. First, we give a brief introduction on normal and pathological changes in the aging brain before we explain how hypothalamic–pituitary–adrenal (HPA) axis functioning, that is, cortisol secretion and control, can affect brain and cognition. Next, we summarize evidence that insulin resistance and type 2 diabetes can contribute to a reduced integrity of the MTL memory system. In this context we highlight the multiple interactions between the glucoregulatory system and the neuroendocrine stress system. The last section presents an explanatory model of how we conceptualize the above-mentioned processes give rise to the MTL impairments, and provides a framework for the generation of specific hypotheses for future research in this area.

Memory in Aging: Normal Changes, Mild Cognitive Impairment, and Dementia

Cross-sectional studies of human aging have consistently reported that, relative to younger individuals, normal elderly show performance reductions in memory, attention, visual–spatial function, abstraction, and problem solving. Longitudinal studies provide a refinement by demonstrating that over time the most salient declines are in tests sensitive to frontal lobe function, namely working memory (requiring the short-term storage and manipulation of information prior to responding), psychomotor efficiency, word knowledge, attention, learning, and problem solving. Although the majority of this literature suggests that most cognitive deficits are related to frontal dysfunction, some research suggests that MTL, which includes structures such as the hippocampus, amygdala, and entorhinal cortex, may also be involved. In normal aging cognitive deficits do not generally result in impairments in everyday functioning.

Memory impairments have been recognized for many years as the most reliable early clinical symptom in dementia of the Alzheimer's type, and both the pathology – namely the distribution of neurofibrillary tangles (one of the two types of brain pathology that are necessary for a brain diagnosis of Alzheimer's disease (AD)) – and the *in vivo* imaging literature indicate that the earliest lesions are in the MTL. In addition, among elderly individuals who demonstrate subtle impairments in functioning and who may be considered at higher risk for significant cognitive decline and AD, those who have so-called mild cognitive impairment (MCI), demonstrate predominantly MTL pathology in the earliest stages of cognitive deterioration. With that being said, most middle age and elderly individuals who present with memory and other cognitive impairments, but with no impairments in overall functioning, will not go on to develop dementia.

Links between Diabetes and Dementia

There is evidence from longitudinal population-based studies that the risk of dementia is higher among individuals with diabetes than among those without it. The risk seems to be higher for individuals with the Apo E ε 4 genotype or receiving insulin treatment. The Apo E gene, which has a polymorphic distribution in the population, codes for a protein that is important in lipid transport and metabolism. Individuals with one or two copies of the Apo E ε 4 allele have a higher risk for cardiovascular disease. However, findings have been inconsistent as to whether this increased risk is specific for AD, multi-infarct dementia (MID), or dementia in general. Although the associations between diabetes and dementia are intriguing, none of these studies has directly assessed the impact of T2DM-related factors. For example, the impacts of hypertension and cardiovascular disease, conditions associated with T2DM, cognitive decline, and dementia, have not been evaluated. Although diabetes is often associated with vascular pathology ranging from micro-vessel disease to hypertension and stroke, studies to date have not provided sufficiently detailed data on those diabetes-associated factors to better ascertain how they may mediate or modulate the risk for dementia associated with diabetes.

The magnitude of the risk for AD related to diabetes is only modest and smaller than that of some nonspecific risk factors, such as low education or history of head trauma. It is possible that the impact of diabetes, analogous to that of low education and head trauma, is to reduce the brain reserve of affected individuals, and thus the associations observed between diabetes and AD may also be nonspecific. This position is supported by the extant pathology literature. Out of the autopsy series available, most fail to find increased Alzheimer's pathology in those individuals with diabetes (with some studies actually finding reduced AD pathology among diabetics), and only one series found a nonsignificant increase among Apo E ε 4 diabetics. However, based on indirect evidence some investigators have speculated that diabetes may be 'mechanistically' linked to AD. This hypothesis is based on observations that insulin acutely enhances memory in healthy older subjects, but is less able to do so in AD patients. In addition, insulin might increase levels of inflammatory cytokines and amyloid beta in the brain. Future research will test these hypotheses.

The Impact of Cortisol on Cognition and the Brain

Stress is conceptualized as a perceived challenge to the organism's balance or homeostasis, and the resulting processes intended to return the organism to equilibrium are termed 'allostasis.' The most prominent of these processes is the activation of the HPA axis. This activation results in the release of glucocorticoids (GCs) and the activation of the sympathetic nervous system (SNS), leading to the release of catecholamines (epinephrine and norepinephrine). In the presence of an acute stress these responses protect and allow the organism to adapt to its changed internal or external environment. However, when the stress becomes chronic or the organism responds inappropriately (e.g., poor habituation or a failure of negative feedback), multiple systems, including the brain, are negatively impacted. This state has been called 'allostatic load.'

GCs, depending on their timing, can have positive or negative acute effects on memory. For example, stress (or an acute increase in GCs) during learning, or immediately thereafter, leads to enhanced memory consolidation. In contrast, an equivalent rise in GCs shortly before delayed retrieval causes impaired retrieval. Animal and human studies suggest that both the positive and negative GC effects are mediated by interactions between amygdala and hippocampus, two limbic structures central in emotional processing and memory formation.

Chronic stress leads to negative consequences in both animals and humans. In animals, chronic stress causes structural alterations of neurons (dendritic atrophy or dendritic remodeling) in hippocampus and prefrontal regions. In addition, stress negatively impacts neurogenesis and alters cholinergic, serotonergic, and dopaminergic systems. These changes are associated with impaired memory performance, although the mediating mechanisms remain unclear. For example, both rats and tree shrews subjected to repeated stress develop impairments in hippocampal-based memory tasks. In contrast, amygdala-mediated tasks, such as fear conditioning, are enhanced. Age affects the organism's response to stress. Although there is large individual variability, aged individuals have increased GC levels as well as impairments in HPA axis negative feedback, both of which have been associated with cognitive impairments. For example, rodents with age-associated increases in HPA activity had impairments in memory performance, whereas those with normal levels did not. Moreover, pharmacological or behavioral interventions that stabilized HPA activity throughout life offered protection from those age-associated memory problems.

In the human, conditions leading to substantially elevated cortisol levels are characterized by impairments in memory, attention, and mood. For example, the hypercortisolemia present in Cushing's disease is associated with reductions in memory performance and hippocampal atrophy, deficits that are at least partly reversible upon successful reduction of the supraphysiological cortisol levels. Elevations in basal GC levels within the normal range have also been associated with cognitive dysfunction; older individuals with higher cortisol levels show poorer memory and faster cognitive decline. However, the causal order of these associations remains unsettled. The behavioral impairments may be secondary to cortisol-induced hippocampal atrophy. However, given the importance of the hippocampus on cortisol feedback inhibition, the cortisol elevations may be the result rather than the cause of hippocampal atrophy. Nevertheless, some recent studies offer indirect support for primacy of cortisol elevations leading to hippocampal damage. For example, self-reported stress proneness is associated with an increased risk for dementia, a disease that involves hippocampus and other MTL structures in its initial stages. Further indirect support is offered by the finding that individuals with genetically determined increases in tissue GC bioavailability have a higher risk for AD.

HPA axis dysregulation, in addition to possible direct effects on the hippocampus, may affect memory through its impact on other related systems also known to affect memory. For example, GCs can impair insulin sensitivity or lead to enhanced visceral fat deposition and altered food intake, which in turn can lead to problems with glucose control, conditions known to be associated with reductions in memory performance. Interestingly, the adverse consequences of stress on the hippocampus occur faster in diabetic animals, suggesting an increased vulnerability of the diabetic brain. The interactions between the HPA axis and the glucoregulatory system will be illustrated in the following section.

Interactions between Cortisol, Insulin Function, and Type 2 Diabetes

Research conducted during the past decade has demonstrated that the HPA axis and the glucoregulatory system interact at multiple levels. Examples can be found for interactions at the behavioral and system level as well as on particular aspects of neuronal or transporter functioning.

Cortisol secretion and peripheral glucose regulation are closely linked. For example, we know that physiologically increased cortisol acutely inhibits insulin release, and that pharmacological doses of GCs cause reductions in glucose disposal (insulin resistance). In addition, in animal models GCs reduce the amount of insulin transported across the blood–brain barrier (BBB), and in large doses inhibit neuronal and glial glucose uptake in the hippocampus but not in other brain regions (e.g., hypothalamus, cerebellum, or cortex). Similar effects have been noted in the human; we have shown that acute cortisol administration leads to a specific *in vivo* hippocampal reduction in glucose utilization as seen with positron emission tomography. It is noteworthy that the hippocampus is the brain area with greatest co-localization of cortisol and insulin receptors. It is possible that the GC-mediated reductions in memory performance are due to their impact on hippocampal energy status.

Chronic stress in animals leads to effects at a behavioral level. Investigators have documented that chronic stress, through a facilitating effect on the HPA axis, leads to changes in eating habits. These animals seek more 'comfort' food and the GC elevations promote visceral fat deposition. In the human, chronic stress, with the associated hyperactivity of the SNS and HPA systems, can lead to the metabolic syndrome, which is characterized by central obesity, impairments in glucose regulation, hypertension, and abnormal lipid profiles.

Problems with peripheral glucose control may potentiate the deleterious effects that cortisol exerts on the brain. For example, when diabetic rats are stressed, they develop extensive hippocampal damage in one-third the time it takes nondiabetic animals to develop equivalent stress-mediated damage. It has also been shown that diabetic rats have chronic elevations of basal GCs and have greater and more prolonged responses to stress. We also know that reduced hippocampal integrity may lead to impaired cortisol feedback inhibition, and thus to elevated cortisol secretion. Adding support to the notion that the stress and the glucoregulatory systems interact in their influence of cognition during aging are observations from the MacArthur Study on Successful Aging. These investigators reported that summary measures of allostatic load, consisting of a combination of stress hormone measures and metabolic syndrome measures, were a superior predictor of cognitive and functional decline in older individuals.

Although it is difficult to ascertain cause and effect, it may be that abnormal glucose tolerance causes hippocampal dysfunction, which then affects cortisol feedback control, which in turn may result in elevated cortisol levels, thus contributing to a vicious cycle of further hippocampal damage.

Impact of Diabetes on the Brain

Neurons neither synthesize nor store glucose and are hence dependent on external sources to meet their energy demands. For a long time it was thought that the brain sat in a privileged position and that its glucose supply was independent of what was happening in the periphery. Only in recent years has this view changed, and it has become apparent that glucose transport into the brain is affected by the peripheral environment and that insulin, insulin receptors, and insulin-sensitive glucose transporters (GLUTs) are all present in brain, although their function remains unclear.

Under normal physiological circumstances the metabolism of glucose borne by the blood accounts for 99% of the brain energy needs. Although glia and astrocytes contain glycogen, the contributions of this glycogen to the overall energy demands of the brain are not known. (Note: It is our opinion that understanding the role of glycogen in brain will be an area of great interest in the near future. This opinion is based on the fact that upon restoration of euglycemia after an episode of hypoglycemia, glycogen deposition in brain goes up markedly, perhaps protecting the brain from subsequent hypoglycemic episodes. In addition, experimental animals subjected to weekly episodes of significant hypoglycemia perform better than sham animals on memory tests during euglycemia, and this improved memory performance is preserved in these animals in old age. Whether these memory-enhancing and protective effects are due to hypoglycemia-based improved transport of glucose across the BBB or to increased deposition of brain glycogen, or both, has yet to be established.)

Despite the fact that the brain depends on peripheral glucose, up until 10 years or so ago, it was commonly believed that the brain was able to obtain all the metabolic substrate it needed, irrespective of what was happening in the periphery. Although the transport of glucose across the BBB remains poorly understood, we now know that the peripheral environment can exert significant influences on BBB transport. For example, the BBB glucose transporter can be up- or downregulated, dependent on the sustained peripheral glucose levels. Additional potential links between systemic and brain glucose control and metabolism are offered by the presence of insulin and insulin-sensitive glucose transporters (GLUT4) in the brain. In peripheral tissues insulin regulates glucose homeostasis through effects on GLUT4, the glucose transporter highly expressed in fat and muscle. GLUT4 is also expressed in brain, including the hippocampus. However, it is not known if insulin affects glucose uptake into the hippocampus. Moreover, it remains to be seen how brain GLUT4 behaves in a state of peripheral insulin resistance. Regardless, it is clear is that glucose uptake and utilization in the brain are complex and that their regulation is yet to be understood.

Because impaired insulin function (or absence of sufficient insulin) and the resulting hyperglycemia are at the core of diabetes, it is likely that these fluctuations will have an impact on the brain and its functioning. There is mounting evidence that diabetes, whether it is type 1 or type 2, has a negative impact on both cognition and brain. However, the resultant adverse effects may vary by the type of diabetes. A straightforward assessment of the differential impact of type 1 and type 2 diabetes on cognition and brain is complicated by the fact that most studies only contrast one type of diabetic patient against controls and do not control for comorbid conditions or possible mediating factors such as hypertension, vascular disease, and depression, which are often associated with diabetes.

Adults with type 1 diabetes mellitus (T1DM), when contrasted to nondiabetic controls, show reduced performance on several cognitive domains, including psychomotor efficiency, intelligence, visual and sustained attention, and speed of information processing. The majority of studies of adults with T1DM demonstrate that the presence of macrovascular disease, but not glycemic control or the number of hypoglycemic episodes, contributed to the lower cognitive performance described. Cognitive deficits are also observed in children and adolescents with T1DM, but there's no consensus in the literature as to whether age of onset or disease duration affects the severity of those cognitive deficits. Furthermore, it remains unclear whether the cognitive impairments worsen with age. In addition, the nature of the impact on cognitive functioning of episodes of either hypoglycemia or hyperglycemia remains unclear. Different studies have evaluated study participants of various ages and have used different test batteries, which do not permit a straightforward comparison across studies.

In contrast to the findings in T1DM, studies of T2DM show mostly impairments in verbal memory and processing speed, whereas other cognitive domains, such as visuospatial function and attention, remain preserved. There is also evidence that in T2DM, glycemic control might influence the cognitive deficits; improvements in glucose control by either pharmacological or behavioral interventions have been associated with attenuation of the cognitive deficits. Additionally, cognitive deficits seem to be augmented by factors associated with T2DM, such as hypertension, depression, and vascular disease. Some studies suggest that severe memory impairments are only seen in older T2DM populations and that the cognitive deficits seen in T2DM represent an acceleration of normal brain aging.

There are only a few *in-vivo* imaging studies in diabetes, and existent studies have not contrasted T1DM and T2DM. The overall findings are that type 1 diabetes leads to general brain atrophy, whereas T2DM seems to preferentially involve MTL structures, and that these findings may be independent of vascular complications. In our own work we have demonstrated that among relatively young individuals with well-controlled T2DM, only reductions in memory, performance, and hippocampal volume separate them from age-, gender-, and education-matched normal controls. In addition, we have described very similar cognitive and imaging findings among normal middle-aged and elderly nondiabetic individuals with impairments in glucose tolerance. Few studies evaluate the brain in T1DM, and there is only one study of adults with T1DM that looked at both cognition and brain with magnetic resonance imaging (MRI). One small pilot study in adults with longstanding T1DM observed reductions in psychomotor speed and selective attention which was accompanied by global cerebral atrophy (increase in cerebrospinal fluid and decrease in total brain volume). However, no evidence for hippocampal volume reductions and memory impairments were detected.

In recent years, paralleling the obesity epidemic, the prevalence of T2DM within the population has risen even among children and adolescents. To date there are no reports in the literature evaluating cognition and brain status among children with T2DM. Preliminary pilot data from our group shows widespread cognitive impairments among obese adolescents with T2DM when contrasted with age-, gender-, and education-matched obese controls.

The precise mechanisms by which diabetes and impaired glucose regulation affect memory are not clear, but the risk factors that are often associated with insulin resistance and that are part of the metabolic syndrome, namely hypertension and dyslipidemia, might play a role. In the next section we outline a model of how diabetes directly affects brain structures that are central for memory process, that is, the hippocampus.

Possible Mechanisms for the Cognitive Impairments Seen in T2DM

Glucose is transported across the BBB by GLUT1, a glucose transporter highly expressed in the vascular endothelial cells of the BBB. Although the regulation of glucose transport into the brain is not well understood, GLUT1 has very high affinity for glucose and is saturated at normal blood glucose levels. Previous work in animal models has established that long-term elevations in peripheral glucose result in decreased transport of glucose across the BBB, whereas the opposite is true for chronic hypoglycemia, in which there is an increase in transport across the BBB. In both these circumstances it is believed that the amount of GLUT1 expressed at the BBB is responsible for the changes in glucose transport.

During brain activation, there are measurable shifts in the local concentrations of available glucose.

For example, visual stimulation reduces visual cortex glucose concentrations as seen with MRI-based spectroscopy. Brain glucose levels can be measured directly with microdialysis probes in free-moving rats. Using these techniques there is evidence that glucose is compartmentalized in brain, and that different brain areas control their glucose levels locally. For example, glucose drops are restricted to the hippocampus when the animal is performing a memory test, and are present despite constant peripheral glucose levels.

The BBB glucose transporter, GLUT1, is saturated at normal physiological glucose concentrations. Therefore, to acutely increase net glucose flux across the BBB, the number of GLUT1 proteins exposed to the blood must be increased. Dilatation of the capillary bed will expose more endothelial cells, with their corresponding GLUT1, to the blood, and thus increase the acute transport of glucose into the brain. However, the mechanisms responsible for regulating the rapid changes in local blood flow that are associated with brain activation are not yet well characterized. What is currently well described is that both individuals with T2DM and individuals with insulin resistance short of diabetes show impairments in endothelial-dependent vasodilatation. Consequently, given that cognitive testing leads to activation (and drops in the interstitial glucose levels in the areas activated), this endothelial dysfunction may lead to a 'functional hypoglycemia' and contribute, at least in part, to the cognitive deficits associated with diabetes and insulin resistance.

It is not known whether elevated cortisol levels affect glucose transport at the BBB (**Figure 1**). However, we know from animal studies that glucocorticoid exposure inhibits glucose transport into hippocampal neurons and glia. We also know that individuals with T2DM (and insulin resistance) have abnormalities in the HPA axis, particularly in feedback control. Consequently, we propose that, analogous to the reduced ability to locally increase glucose flux across the BBB with activation due to the reduced vascular reactivity in T2DM and insulin resistance, among individuals with elevated cortisol levels, there may also be a 'functional hypoglycemia,' this time at the neuronal level, also contributing to the cognitive deficits.

We propose that although this aggregate 'functional hypoglycemia' may be widespread in the brain, its damaging consequences may be at first more apparent in the hippocampus because of its high vulnerability to damage from hypoglycemia or other noxious influences. This hypothesized chronic low-grade 'functional hypoglycemia' may, in the long run, lead to hippocampal damage and volume loss.

It is also possible that chronic hyperglycemia is toxic to the microvascular endothelial cells, thus impairing transport of glucose across the BBB. Also, chronic hyperglycemia may be toxic to hippocampal cells directly by the increased production of damaging oxidative species resulting from increased metabolism based on increased intracellular glucose. However, this model, proposed by Brownlee to explain the tissue damage resulting from diabetes, does not offer an explanation for the damage associated with milder forms of insulin resistance, when glucose levels are still normal and there is only an elevation in fasting insulin levels. Future research will need to approach the problem more comprehensively, by evaluating multiple systems in the same individuals so as to better determine the relative contribution of each in the phenomenology expressed.

Summary

Americans are living longer, which has contributed to the rising rate of age-associated diseases such as type 2 diabetes and dementia. This, coupled with the

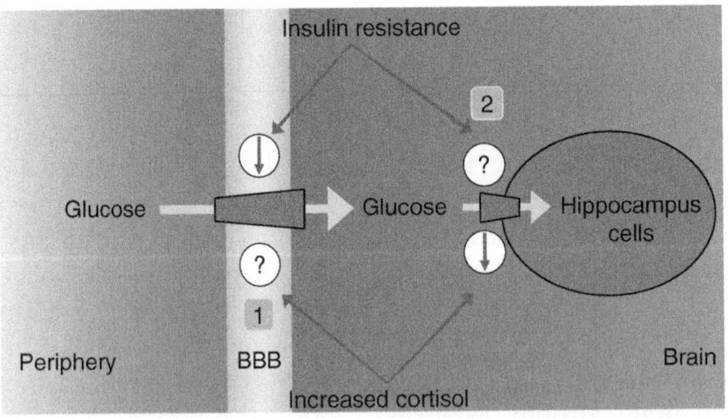

Figure 1 Representation of the blood and the brain compartments separated by the BBB. The green trapezoids represent the GLUTs. Reduced glucose transport across the BBB (step 1) and/or into the cells in the hippocampus (step 2), particularly during activation, may result in functional hypoglycemia and impaired memory performance. The sections of the bidirectional arrows pointing to the down red arrows represent known negative influences on glucose transport, and those pointing to the question marks represent a proposed negative influence that remains to be shown.

epidemic of obesity in industrialized nations, which will further add to an increasing number of T2DM cases within the overall population, makes improving our understanding of how type 2 diabetes affects the aging brain indispensable. In this article, we have reviewed the existing literature on brain aging, diabetes, and the stress regulatory system. There is increasing evidence that dysregulation of the stress and glucoregulatory systems interacts at multiple levels to exert a negative impact on human health in general, and on the aging brain in particular. Although a consensus has not yet gelled within the literature on the exact brain areas affected by the dysregulation of those systems, it is now clear that the MTL is likely the major brain region affected. Within the MTL, the hippocampus, a structure crucially involved in recent memory, appears to be particularly sensitive to these neuroendocrine abnormalities. Since MTL atrophy is also of relevance for MCI and AD, this might explain some of the recently reported associations between dementia and type 2 diabetes. An enhanced understanding of the underlying pathological processes will allow the development of behavioral and pharmacological approaches targeted to protect the integrity of the hippocampus in older individuals. But there is much work to be done and additional progress in this research area is clearly warranted.

Further Reading

Awad, N., Gagnon, M. and Messier, C. (2004). The relationship between impaired glucose tolerance, type 2 diabetes, and cognitive function. *Journal of Clinical and Experimental Neuropsychology* **26**, 1044–1080.

Biessels, GJ., Staekenborg, S., Brunner, E., Brayne, C. and Scheltens, P. (2006). Risk of dementia in diabetes mellitus: A systematic review. *The Lancet Neurology* **5**(1), 64–74.

Brownlee, M. (2001). Biochemistry and molecular cell biology of diabetic complications. *Nature* **414**, 813–820.

Burke, SN. and Barnes, CA. (2006). Neural plasticity in the ageing brain. *Nature Reviews* **7**, 30–40.

Cervos-Navarro, J. and Kater, SB. (1991). Selective vulnerability in brain hypoxia. *Critical Reviews in Neurobiology* **6**, 149–182.

Convit, A. (2005). Links between cognitive impairment in insulin resistance: An explanatory model. *Neurobiology of Aging* **26S**, S31–S35.

Convit, A., Wolf, OT., Tarshish, C. and de Leon, M. (2003). Reduced glucose tolerance is associated with poor memory performance and hippocampal atrophy among normal elderly. *Proceedings of the National Academy of Sciences of the United States of America* **100**(4), 2019–2022.

Dallman, MF., Pecoraro, N., Akana, SF., et al. (2003). Chronic stress and obesity: A new view of "comfort food." *Proceedings of the National Academy of Sciences of the United States of America* **100**, 11696–11701.

Den Heijer, T., Vermeer, SE., van Dijk, EJ., et al. (2003). Type 2 diabetes and atrophy of medial temporal lobe structures on brain MRI. *Diabetologia* **46**, 1604–1610.

Desrocher, M. and Rovet, J. (2004). Neurocognitive correlates of type 1 diabetes mellitus in childhood. *Child Neuropsychology* **10**, 36–52.

Gold, SM., Dziobek, I., Sweat, V., et al. (2007). Specific hippocampal damage and memory impairments as possible early brain complications of type 2 diabetes. *Diabetologica* **50**(**4**), 711–719.

Lobnig, BM., Kromeke, O., Optenhostert-Porst, C. and Wolf, OT. (2005). Hippocampal volume and cognitive performance in long-standing type 1 diabetic patients without macrovascular complications. *Diabetic Medicine* **23**, 32–39.

McEwen, BS. (2002). Sex, stress and the hippocampus: Allostasis, allostatic load and the aging process. *Neurobiology of Aging* **23**, 921–939.

McEwen, BS., Magarinos, AM. and Reagan, LP. (2002). Studies of hormone action in the hippocampal formation: Possible relevance to depression and diabetes. *Journal of Psychosomatic Research* **53**, 883–890.

McNay, EC., McCarty, RC. and Gold, PE. (2001). Fluctuations in brain glucose concentration during behavioral testing: Dissociations between brain areas and between brain and blood. *Neurobiology of Learning and Memory* **75**(3), 325–337.

Pardridge, WM., Triguero, D. and Farrell, CR. (1990). Downregulation of blood-brain barrier glucose transporter in experimental diabetes. *Diabetes* **39**, 1040–1044.

Roozendaal, B., Okuda, S., de Quervain, DJ. and McGaugh, JL. (2006). Glucocorticoids interact with emotion-induced noradrenergic activation in influencing different memory functions. *Neuroscience* **138**, 901–910.

Rosmond, R. (2005). Role of stress in the pathogenesis of the metabolic syndrome. *Psychoneuroendocrinology* **30**, 1–10.

Tooke, JE. and Goh, KL. (1998). Endotheliopathy precedes type 2 diabetes. *Diabetes Care* **21**(12), 2047–2049.

Vivian, EM. (2006). Type 2 diabetes in children and adolescents: The next epidemic? *Current Medical Research and Opinion* **22**(2), 297–306.

Wolf, OT. (2003). HPA axis and memory. *Best Practice and Research: Clinical Endocrinology and Metabolism* **17**, 287–299.

Chaperone Proteins and Chaperonopathies

A J L Macario and E Conway de Macario
New York State Department of Health and The University of Albany (SUNY), Albany, NY, USA

Glossary

Chaperone machine — A functional chaperoning complex formed by the chaperone Hsp70(DnaK), the co-chaperones Hsp40(DnaJ), and a nucleotide-exchange factor, for example, GrpE in prokaryotes and BAG-1 (BCL2-associated pathanogen, where BCL2 stands for B cell lymphoma 2) and HspBP1 (Hsp70-binding protein 1) in eukaryotes.

Chaperonin — A molecular chaperone belonging to the 60-kDa family.

Chaperonin system type (group) I — A chaperoning complex formed by the 60-kDa chaperonin and a 10-kDa co-chaperonin (e.g., GroEL and GroES, respectively, in bacteria) that is present in bacteria, in the bacterial-related eukaryotic-cell organelles, and in some archaea.

Chaperonin system type (group) II — A chaperoning complex formed by subunits of the 60-kDa family in archaea (i.e., the thermosome subunits) and by related proteins of various sizes in the eukaryotic cell cytosol.

Molecular chaperone — A molecule that assists polypeptides in the process of folding to achieve a final functional conformation or to regain such conformation after reversible denaturation. The prototype is the stress protein called Hsp70(DnaK).

Phylogenetic domain — The highest order of classification of all living cells (domain, kingdom, phylum, class, order, family, genus, species) that represents the major evolutionary lines of descent, or phylogenetic lineages. Three domains have been identified: Bacteria (or eubacteria), Archaea (archaebacteria), and Eucarya (eukarya, eukaryotes); the former two are prokaryotes.

Stress (heat shock) proteins — The products of the stress (heat shock) genes. Many of these are molecular chaperones, for example, the components of the chaperone machine.

Stress (heat shock) response — The series of intracellular events caused by cell stressors. One of the most prominent of these events is the induction of the stress (heat shock) genes, resulting in the production of stress (heat shock) proteins.

Proteins

A protein molecule is a chain whose links are amino acids. The number, type, and order of amino acids in the chain are specified by the gene that encodes the protein, and they determine the primary structure. To reach a functional status, a protein must acquire higher levels of complexity. It must fold onto itself to achieve secondary and tertiary levels of structure. In addition, some proteins must associate with others to form a quaternary structure before they can become fully functional.

The functional conformation of a protein, once acquired, may be partially or completely lost in a process called protein denaturation. This can happen when a cell is stressed. There are a number of cell stressors of a physical or chemical nature that cause protein denaturation. Although the information necessary to achieve a final functional conformation is contained in the primary structure, many proteins need assistance to fold properly or to refold after reversible denaturation. This assistance is provided by molecular chaperones.

Definition

Chaperone proteins, or molecular chaperones, are proteins that assist others to fold properly during or after synthesis, to refold after partial denaturation, and to translocate to the cellular locales at which they reside and function. Chaperones are also involved in the regulation of their own genes and in the presentation of proteins destined for degradation by proteases. Some chaperones are themselves proteases.

Many chaperones are stress (heat shock) proteins, in that they increase in quantity on cell stress (also termed heat shock, although heat is not the only stressor known) so as to counteract the protein-denaturing effects of stressors (e.g., heat, alcohol, ischemia-hypoxia, heavy metals, and hypersalinity). For this reason, stress proteins and molecular chaperones are usually treated together, as a single large group of heterogeneous components, termed Hsp (for heat shock protein). Thus, there are many cell stressors that cause stress or heat shock and many stress or heat shock proteins, but not all of the latter are molecular chaperones. Likewise, not every molecular chaperone is a stress protein.

As may be inferred from their multiplicity of function, molecular chaperones are promiscuous; they interact with a variety of molecules. They are also ubiquitous; they occur in all cells, tissues, and organs, with very few known exceptions. Furthermore, molecular chaperones are present in the various compartments of the eukaryotic cell, nucleus, cytosol, and organelles such as mitochondria and choloroplasts; they are also present in the prokaryotic cell cytoplasm and periplasm.

Classification

Stress proteins, including the chaperones, are grouped into families on the basis of similarities in molecular masses (**Tables 1** and **2**). The genes encoding most of these proteins are stress-inducible, but they are also expressed constitutively (i.e., in the absence of stress) at lower levels.

The best studied are the Hsp70 and Hsp60 families, but considerable progress has also been made in the investigation of proteins belonging to other families, for example, Hsp40 and Hsp90, the high-molecular-weight proteases, and the small heat shock proteins (sHsp).

Biology

Chaperones and stress proteins can be viewed from an evolutionary-phylogenetic standpoint, while keeping in mind that the separation between prokaryotes and eukaryotes is not absolute, inasmuch as the eukaryotic cell contains components of prokaryotic ancestry. For instance, the mitochondrion is the remnant of an ancient alpha-proteobacterium that entered into a symbiotic association with a primitive eukaryotic cell. Similarly, the chloroplast descends from a primitive symbiotic cyanobacterium. Even the eukaryotic nucleus contains, in its DNA, genes that were derived from bacteria. In this regard, genes encoding chaperones of the Hsp60 and Hsp70 families are of particular interest. These chaperones are present in the mitochondria, chloroplasts, endoplasmic reticulum (ER), and other organelles (see **Table 2**), but their genes reside in the nucleus. These genes are transcribed in the nucleus, but the chaperones are synthesized in the cytosol and are finally translocated to the destination organelle. In fact, it has been the comparative analyses of Hsp70 and Hsp60 amino acid sequences that have convincingly shown the origin of the genes that encode these proteins and have provided strong support for the idea that the eukaryotic cell is an assemblage of diverse parts, several of which are prokaryotic in origin.

Phylogenetic Domains

Since the late 1970s, the idea that all living cells can be sorted into three main lines of evolutionary descent, or phylogenetic domains, has gained acceptance, although many points remain controversial and the boundaries between domains at the beginning of evolution are less well-defined than was initially believed. Nevertheless, it is helpful to think of stress proteins and chaperones within the context of the three domains, Bacteria (eubacteria), Archaea (archaebacteria), and Eucarya (eukaryotes) – the former two being prokaryotes. Why is this helpful? Because archaea (i.e., the members of the domain Archaea) are indeed different from bacteria and eucarya or

Table 1 Stress (heat shock) proteins and chaperones in prokaryotes

Family		*Examples*	
Name(s)	*Mass (kDa)*	*Bacteria*	*Archaea*
Heavy; high molecular weight; Hsp100	100 or higher	Clp	No[a]
Hsp90	81–99	HtpG	No
Hsp70; DnaK; chaperones	65–80	DnaK; Hsc66	Hsp70(DnaK)[b] (only some species)
Hsp60	55–64		L
Chaperonins group I		GroEL	GroEL (only some species)
Chaperonins group II		No	TF55; thermosome subunits (up to five)
Hsp40; DnaJ	35–54	DnaJ	Hsp40(DnaJ) (only some species)
Other	≤34		
small Hsp; sHsp		sHsp: Hsc20; Hsp15; alpha-crystallin family; other	sHsp: Hsp16.5; α-crystallin family; other
miscellanea		Hsp33; GroES; GrpE; PPIase; PDIase; IbpA/B; SecB; other	GroES (only some species); GrpE (only some species); PPIase; PDIase; prefoldin, 1 or 2 subunits; Sso7d

[a] No indicates not yet found, or not yet investigated in many species.
[b] Archaeal species with Hsp70(DnaK) also have Hsp40(DnaJ) and GrpE; no species has yet been found having only one or two of these three chaperones.

Table 2 Stress (heat shock) proteins and chaperones in eukaryotes[a]

Family		*Examples*			
Name(s)	*Mass (kDa)*	*Cytosol*	*Mitochondrion*	*Endoplasmic reticulum*[b]	*Chloroplast*
Heavy; high molecular weight; Hsp100	≥100	Hsp101 (Hsp102); Hsp104; Hsp105 alpha and beta; Hsp110	ClpXP/Hsp100	Hsp170 (Grp170)	
Hsp90	81–99	Hsp90(Hsp82; Hsp83; Hsp90 alpha and beta); Grp94	No	Hsp90 (GRP94; Grp94; endoplasmin; gp96))	Hsp93 (atHsp93-III; atHsp93-V)
Hsp70; chaperones	65–80	Hsp70(Hsp72); Hsc70 (Hsp73); SSA1-4; SSB1-2	mhsp70; SSC1; mt-Hsp70 (Grp75); Hsp78;Ssq1; Ecm10	BiP(Grp78); Erp72; SSi1p; Kar2p; Lhs1p	Hsp70(DnaK) Hsp70B; Hsc70-2
Hsp60	55–64				
chaperonins group I		No	Cpn60 (mtGroEL; mtHsp60)	No	Cpn60 (Rubisco binding protein)
chaperonins group II		CCT (TRiC; TCP1 complex): up to 9 subunits	No	RBP	No
Hsp40; DnaJ	35–54	Hsp40; Hdj1(MAS5); Hdj2 (DjA1; HSDJ); DjA4; Sis1p; Ydj1p	Hsp40; Mdj1p; Mdj2p; DjA3	Hsp40; Hsp47; Sec63p; Erdj3; Scj1p; JEM1p	Hsp40(DnaJ); ANJ1; TLP40; CDJ2
Other	≤34				
small Hsp; sHsp		alpha-crystallin family; Hsp10; Hsp20(Hsp26); Hsp22; Hsp27	Hsp10(Cpn10; mtGroES)	Cpn20	
miscellanea		PPlase; PDIase; prefoldin (Gim)(up to 6 subunits);	GrpE(mtGrpE;Yge1; Mye1p); PPlase; Atp12p; Hep1	Cpn20; PPlase; PDIase	GrpE; Hsp18; Hsp25; Hsp26; Cpn10; Cpn20; atAcd

[a]Chaperones build multimolecular assemblies to exercise their functions. These assemblies are formed by identical or different chaperone molecules (subunits) and by cofactors. In addition, theses chaperone complexes interact with other chaperone complexes (networking) and with the protein-degradation machinery (e.g., the ubiquitin–proteasome system) to integrate the protein quality-control system of the cell. Synonyms are given in parentheses. No indicates not yet found, or not yet investigated in many species.
[b]In addition to the chaperones listed in the endoplasmic reticulum column, this organelle also has Grp58(Erp57) and lectins (calreticulin and calnexin, approximately 45 and 60 kDa, respectively) that assist, together with associated factors, the folding and oligomerization of many glycoproteins.

eukaryotes (i.e., the members of the domains Bacteria and Eucarya, respectively) in terms of the Hsp70 and Hsp60 chaperones. For example, bacteria possess the Hsp70 (also named DnaK), Hsp40 (also named DnaJ), and GrpE stress proteins that constitute the molecular chaperone machine (KJE) and the Hsp60–Hsp10 molecules that constitute the GroEL/S or chaperonin group I system. In contrast, many archaea do not have the chaperone KJE or GroEL/S, and eukaryotes have GroEL/S homologs only inside their organelles. It is noteworthy that many archaea do not have KJE because this machine is present in all bacteria and eukaryotes without any known exception. Also remarkable is the presence of GroEL/S in some archaea because until recently it was thought that this chaperoning complex was exclusive to the bacteria and bacteria-related organelles.

The structures and functions of the molecular chaperone machine and of the chaperonin system type I are relatively well characterized in the bacterium *Escherichia coli*. There is also considerable information on the eukaryotic Hsp70 complex and on the chaperonin system type II. Intriguingly, some archaea either do not have an identifiable chaperone machine or have one of bacterial type with the Hsp70(DnaK), Hsp40(DnaJ), and GrpE components, but they all have a type II chaperonin system. The fact that archaea have a eukaryotic type of chaperonin system is remarkable because archaea, like bacteria, are prokaryotes.

Also interestingly, eukaryotes have the bacterial type of Hsp60 chaperonin system in their organelles, bearing witness to the bacterial origins of the latter. Thus, one of the most exciting fields of biology at present is the analysis of chaperonins and chaperones in organisms representing the three phylogenetic domains and domain branches to understand the evolution of these molecules and also to elucidate the relationships among species, and between organelles and their prokaryotic ancestors.

Another point of great interest, from both the evolutionary and the physiological standpoints, is that a number of archaeal species do not have Hsp70 (DnaK) or the other components of the chaperone machine, Hsp40(DnaJ) and GrpE. This peculiarity is remarkable because it represents the only exception known to the rule that every organism has an Hsp70 system (in fact, Hsp70 is considered one of the most highly conserved proteins in nature). The absence of the gene triad that encodes the components of the chaperone machine is noteworthy also because it raises the issue of how these organisms can achieve protein biogenesis and survive stress without the molecular chaperone machine.

Physiology

Prokaryotes, with few exceptions, have only a single *hsp70(dnaK)* gene, which is active under normal physiological conditions and is activated further by stressors. In the latter case, an increase in Hsp70 (DnaK) over the basal or constitutive levels is observed; it may be due to increased transcription and/or translation, and/or decreased mRNA and/or Hsp70(DnaK) degradation. In contrast, eukaryotes have more than one *hsp70(dnaK)* gene. Essentially, one gene is active physiologically and responds to physiological signals (it is said to be constitutively induced), whereas the other gene is induced by stressors. The former gene is designated cognate *hsp70*, abbreviated *hsc70*, and the protein is termed Hsc70. In fact, eukaryotic cells may have more than one representative of the two types of the *hsp70* gene, and both types may respond to physiological stimuli, such as stimuli derived from cell-cycle and cell-differentiation events. Therefore, *hsp70(dnaK)* is also interesting from the point of view of cell physiology during development and histogenesis and is an important player in pathology and disease.

Pathology and Medicine

Molecular chaperone genes and proteins, as well as chaperonins and other stress genes and proteins, are being studied at the present time to determine their roles in the maintenance of health and in the development of disease. It is conceivable that the failure of the chaperoning processes due to a defective chaperone (chaperonopathy) will lead to the accumulation of misfolded proteins that do not function or to misplaced proteins that do not reach their destination in the cell to function properly. In both instances, the accumulation of nonfunctional proteins will encumber the cell and disturb its normal physiology. This is why protein degradation is also an important cellular process, part of which depends on molecular chaperones.

Chaperonopathies may be caused by genetic defects (e.g., chaperone–gene mutation) or by posttranslational modifications of the chaperone molecule, such as those observed in the elderly as a manifestation of the aging process, which is characterized by a progressive accumulation of biochemical damage in many proteins.

Molecular chaperones may be exploited as tools for preventing protein denaturation or for restoring partially denatured proteins (e.g., during surgery) when ischaemia-hypoxia (a strong cell stressor) is unavoidable. The use of chaperones for prevention and treatment of pathological conditions is emerging as a new medical field: chaperonotherapy.

Mechanism

The mechanism of action of chaperones at the molecular level has not been fully elucidated for any organism or any particular family of chaperones, but there is considerable information on the Hsp70(DnaK) and Hsp60 (chaperonin) systems in *E. coli*. How do chaperones interact to help a polypeptide to acquire its final three-dimensional (native) configuration, based on its primary structure? It is known that chaperones neither provide steric information nor form part of the final product. The Hsp70(DnaK) system in the cytosol is believed to bind nascent polypeptides so as to prevent their aggregation, either among one another or with other polypeptides in the immediate vicinity. In this manner, the Hsp70(DnaK) machine maintains the newly made polypeptide in a folding-competent status. In contrast, the Hsp60 (chaperonin) system GroEL/S acts posttranslationally and assists in the folding of polypeptides ranging in size from 25 to 55 kDa. Hence, without chaperones, most polypeptides would aggregate and the few that would proceed in the right direction toward achieving a physiologically active conformation would do so very slowly and inefficiently. Within this context, it is easy to realize that chaperones and chaperonins, and other stress proteins such as the sHsp, play a critical role in cell survival during stress, when the tendency toward protein denaturation and aggregation is strong.

The binding of polypeptides to, and their release from, Hsp70(DnaK) is ATP-dependent and involves the other members of the Hsp70(DnaK) machine, Hsp40(DnaJ), and a nucleotide-exchange factor (e.g., GrpE in prokaryotes). Hsp40 binds the polypeptide in need of assistance and presents it to Hsp70–ATP complex. As this complex binds the Hsp40-tagged polypeptide, Hsp40 catalyzes ATP hydrolysis, which increases the strength of the binding between Hsp70–ATP and the polypeptide. GrpE then comes into action and catalyzes the exchange of ATP for ADP on Hsp70. When Hsp70 is once again complexed with ATP, its affinity for the polypeptide diminishes and the latter is released, either because it has folded correctly or because it has to be processed further by the Hsp60 system GroEL/S.

The GroEL/S complex in *E. coli* is a cylindrical barrel. GroEL (the Hsp60 component) forms two heptameric rings with a central cavity. GroES (the Hsp10 subunit) forms a single heptameric ring and serves as a lid for the two-ring GroEL barrel. The polypeptide-folding mechanism is believed to be as follows. The unfolded polypeptide reaches the entrance to the GroEL barrel either unassisted or ushered by the chaperone machine, enters into the cavity, and binds to hydrophobic patches in the wall of the barrel. The GroES ring, together with ATP, then binds to the GroEL cylinder, thereby closing it. Thus, a hydrophilic folding chamber (also called cage) is created, and the polypeptide is in an environment in which it becomes soluble and can fold correctly. ATP binding to the other GroEL ring releases GroES, opening the barrel, and this allows the folded polypeptide to escape into the cytosol. The cycle is repeated if the folding process was incomplete.

The details just described have been inferred from experiments *in vitro* with *E. coli*. It is not known to what extent the *in vitro* findings reproduce the *in vivo* mechanisms. Also, the mechanism of Hsp70–Hsp60 chaperoning in locales other than the cytosol, for example, in the mitochondria, differs from the mechanism described earlier. Similarly, the mechanisms of action of the other families of chaperones are also different in many details.

We may conclude, from studies pertaining to the *E. coli* cytoplasm, that, whereas the Hsp70(DnaK) chaperone machine intervenes early in protein synthesis (during translation) to prevent aggregation of the majority of the nascent polypeptides, the Hsp60 chaperonin system acts later. The GroEL/S complex intervenes posttranslationally and only to assist that fraction of the new polypeptides that reach it either unassisted or ushered by the chaperone machine. The rest of the newly made polypeptides in *E. coli* do not use the GroEL/S chaperonin system, and they probably fold in the cytosol assisted only by the chaperone machine.

To Fold, Refold, or Degrade

The protein content and quality of a cell vary according to the cell's needs imposed by physiological (e.g., cell cycle or differentiation stage) and environmental changes (e.g., nutrient limitation, pH drop, or temperature or osmolarity upshift). The diverse array of proteins and the quantities of each of these must be adjusted precisely to the requirements of every moment of the cell's life. This delicate balance is achieved by various complementary, coordinated mechanisms that effectively either increase or decrease the concentration of any given protein in its native functional conformation in any given cell locale. Also, when proteins are damaged by stressors, they must be restored to normality (native as opposed to denatured or unfolded, or misfolded, status) or they must be eliminated if the damage is too severe and beyond repair.

Stress proteins, particularly those that are molecular chaperones, play a key role not only in protein biogenesis and in restoring partially damaged proteins to a functional pool, but they are also involved in eliminating molecules that cannot be recovered. For the latter purpose, stress proteins act in conjunction with proteases or they use their own proteolytic power (many stress proteins are proteases, and some are both chaperones and proteases). Because of this dual role – assistance in the generation and recovery of polypeptides, as well as in their destruction – stress proteins are essential tools by which the cell maintains its protein balance.

Proteins for degradation are either normal or abnormal. Many normal proteins have a short life span; they are naturally unstable, as required by their transient tasks inside the cell. Examples are transcription regulatory factors, termed activators, that need to be eliminated to downregulate the expression of certain genes. The same is true for some repressors, which have to be removed when the gene that they regulate must be upregulated or induced. Many abnormal (denatured) proteins are generated by stress, as noted earlier. In addition, abnormal proteins may appear in the cell in the absence of stress, as a result of genetic mutations or of transcriptional, translational, and/or processing errors.

Whatever the case, unfit or unnecessary proteins must be either eliminated or restored to a functional status; for each one, the cell must make the decision as to whether to try to fold, or refold, or to degrade. In the last alternative, the cell will not only be freed from potentially detrimental molecules or molecular debris, but it will at the same time acquire building blocks to synthesize new molecules. Proteins destined for degradation must be recognized by proteases; for this purpose, they have tags that are seen by the proteolytic enzymes. Some molecular chaperones provide the tag and present the protein for degradation to the protease.

In conclusion, molecular chaperones not only assist in the generation of protein molecules, but they also contribute to the elimination of proteins when they are potentially dangerous or no longer necessary (dispensable) to the cell.

See Also the Following Articles

Chaperonopathies.

Further Reading

Deuerling, E. and Bukau, B. (2004). Chaperone-assisted folding of newly synthesized proteins in the cytosol. *Critical Reviews in Biochemistry and Molecular Biology* **39**, 261–277.

Ferrari, D. M. and Soeling, H-D. (1999). The protein disulphide-isomerase family: unraveling a string of folds. *Biochemical Journal* **339**, 1–10.

Hartl, F. U. and Martin, J. (1995). Molecular chaperones in cellular protein folding. *Current Opinion in Structural Biology* **5**, 92–102.

Jackson-Constan, D., Akita, A. and Keegstra, K. (2001). Molecular chaperones involved in chloroplast protein import. *Biochimica et Biophysica Acta: Molecular Cell Research* **1541**, 102–103.

Kovacheva, S., Bedard, J., Patel, R., et al. (2005). *In vivo* studies on the roles of Tic110, Tic40, and Hsp93 during chloroplast protein import. *The Plant Journal* **41**, 412–428.

Lee, A. S. (2001). The glucose-regulated proteins: stress induction and clinical applications. *Trends in Biochemical Sciences* **26**, 504–510.

Macario, A. J. L. and Conway de Macario, E. (2001). The molecular chaperone system and other anti-stress mechanisms in Archaea. *Frontiers in Bioscience* **6**, d262–283 [online].

Macario, A. J. L. and Conway de Macario, E. (2004). The pathology of anti-stress mechanisms: a new frontier. *Stress* **7**, 243–249.

Macario, A. J. L., Malz, M. and Conway de Macario, E. (2004). Evolution of assisted protein folding: the distribution of the main chaperoning systems within the phylogenetic domain Archaea. *Frontiers in Bioscience* **9**, 1318–1332 [online].

Martin, J. (2004). Chaperonin function – effects of crowding and confinement. *Journal of Molecular Recognition* **17**, 465–472.

Martin, J., Gruber, M. and Lupas, A. N. (2004). Coiled coils meet the chaperone world. *Trends in Biochemical Sciences* **29**, 455–458.

Maruyama, T., Suzuki, R. and Furutani, M. (2004). Archaeal peptidyl prolyl *cis*-transisomerases (PPIases): update 2004. *Frontiers in Bioscience* **9**, 1680–1700. [online].

Morano, K. A., Liu, P. C. C. and Thiele, D. J. (1998). Protein chaperones and the heat shock response in *Saccharomyces cerevisiae. Current Opinion in Microbiology* **1**, 197–203.

Riggs, D. L., Cox, M. B., Cheung-Flynn, J., et al. (2004). Functional specificity of co-chaperone interactions with Hsp90 client proteins. *Critical Review in Biochemistry and Molecular Biology* **39**, 279–295.

Scharf, K-D., Siddique, M. and Vierling, E. (2001). The expanding family of *Arabidopsis thaliana* small heat stress proteins and a new family of proteins containing alpha-crystallin domains (Acd proteins). *Cell Stress & Chaperones* **6**, 225–237.

Schlicher, T. and Soll, J. (1997). Chloroplastic isoforms of DnaJ and GrpE in pea. *Plant Molecular Biology* **33**, 181–185.

Spiess, C., Meyer, A. S., Reissmann, S., et al. (2004). Mechanism of the eukaryotic chaperonin: Protein folding in the chamber of secrets. *Trends in Cell Biology* **14**, 598–604.

Townsend, P. A., Stephanou, A., Packham, G. and Latchman, D. S. (2005). BAG-1: A multifunctional prosurvival molecule. *International Journal of Biochemistry and Cell Biology* **37**, 251–259.

Wimmer, B., Lottspeich, F., van der Klei, I., et al. (1997). The glyoxysomal and plastid molecular chaperones (70-kDa heat shock protein) of watermelon cotyledons are encoded by a single gene. *Proceedings of the National Academy of Sciences USA* **94**, 13624–13629.

Zhao, Q., Wang, J., Levichkin, I. V., et al. (2002). A mitochondrial specific stress response in mammalian cells. *EMBO Journal* **21**, 4411–4419.

Chaperonopathies

A J L Macario and E Conway de Macario
New York State Department of Health and The University of Albany (SUNY), Albany, NY, USA

Glossary

Acquired chaperonopathy	A chaperonopathy that is due to a structural defect in a molecular chaperone acquired during the life of the individual and that is not passed on to the offspring, i.e., is not hereditary.
Chaperone complex	A team of two or more chaperones, cochaperones, and cofactors assembled to carry out the chaperoning process.
Chaperone networking	The interaction of a chaperone complex with another, distinct chaperone complex, or with a protein-degrading complex.
Chaperonopathy	A pathological condition in which a molecular chaperone is abnormal.
Client polypeptide or substrate	A polypeptide recognized by a chaperone or chaperone complex as needing assistance for folding or refolding, or as destined for degradation.
Dysregulatory chaperonopathy	Increase or decrease in the levels of a molecular chaperone caused by up- or downregulation, respectively, of its parent gene.
Genetic chaperonopathy	A chaperonopathy characterized by a structural defect in a molecular chaperone due to a genetic (hereditary) cause, such as a gene mutation.
Genetic polymorphism	The occurrence, in a population of organisms of the same species, of more than one allele or genetic marker at the same locus. A polymorphism is distinguished by the fact that the least frequent allele or marker occurs more often than if it were due only to mutation.
Primary chaperonopathy	A condition in which the molecular chaperone pathology is not the consequence of another pathological disorder.
Proteinopathy	A pathological condition characterized by the occurrence of an abnormal protein molecule, usually with a tendency to misfold, aggregate, and precipitate.
Secondary chaperonopathy	A condition in which a molecular chaperone pathology is associated with another disorder and is the consequence of it, rather than its cause.

Definitions and Classifications

A chaperonopathy can be defined as a pathological entity characterized by a defect in a chaperone or cochaperone. In structural chaperonopathies, the structure of the chaperone molecule is altered because its parent gene is mutated, or because of another mechanism acting beyond the DNA, namely, during or after gene transcription. An example of the latter post-DNA mechanisms resulting in a structural defect in the chaperone molecule is an aberrant posttranslational modification.

Other chaperonopathies do not involve a structural modification of the chaperone molecule itself, but rather are characterized by quantitative (increase or decrease) and spatial (distribution in cells and tissues) changes. Levels of chaperones may be elevated or decreased in cells in certain diseases compared with levels in the same cells from healthy individuals. Likewise, the distribution pattern of a chaperone inside a cell (e.g., within the cytosol, or within organelles), or in various cell types and tissues, may differ from that typical of healthy counterparts.

Quantitative alterations may be caused by up- or downregulation of the chaperone gene or by other posttranscriptional mechanisms such as increased (or decreased) stability of mRNA and/or protein or translation rate.

In the case of chaperones whose parent genes are stress inducible, i.e., genes that respond to stressors and are active in the stress response, quantitative changes may be due to up- or downregulation of stress gene regulators such as the HSF (heat shock factor) genes in eukaryotes. If a chaperone gene is up- or downregulated by its own regulatory mechanisms, the resulting pathologic entity will be a dysregulatory chaperonopathy.

From another standpoint, chaperonopathies may be characterized as primary or secondary. The former are due to defects inherent in the chaperone molecule, defects that have an impact on cells and tissues, and thus becomes a central part of pathogenesis. Examples of primary chaperonopathies are those due to inherited defects in the chaperone-encoding genes.

Secondary chaperonopathies are the consequence of a disease rather than the reverse; the defective chaperone is not a primary factor in pathogenesis, but it may contribute to it. Among these are chaperonopathies associated with the process of aging and chaperonopathies caused by stressors that damage the chaperone molecule. Likewise, some quantitative chaperonopathies may be classified as secondary.

Another cause of chaperone failure may reside not in the chaperone itself, but in the client polypeptide. At least two causes have been recognized. (1) The substrate is genetically defective and lacks the segment of sequence that would be recognized by

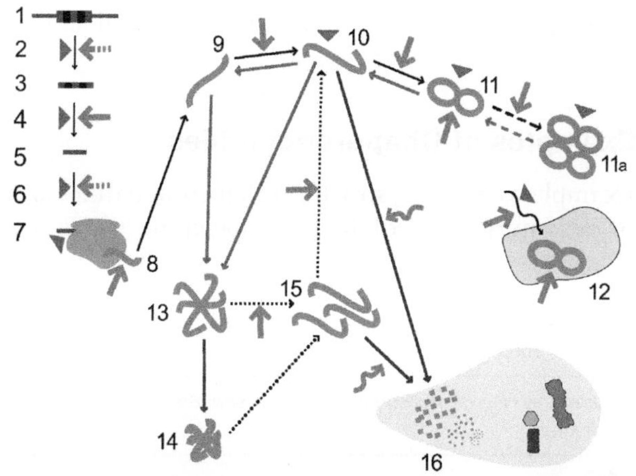

Figure 1 Schematic (not to scale) of the life of a protein, from parent gene to fully folded molecule to degradation, in a eukaryotic cell. Crucial steps that require chaperone assistance, and sites of stress impact whose adverse effects might enhance senescence and/or disease development, are noted. 1, Protein-coding gene (brown rectangle) with two introns (black). 2, Transcription. 3, Primary transcript (pre-mRNA), still with the two introns. 4, Pre-mRNA processing, including intron removal and exon splicing. 5, Mature mRNA (brown rectangle). 6, mRNA transport from nucleus to cytosol via nuclear pore complex. 7, mRNA translation on the ribosome (light blue). 8, Nascent polypeptide (orange, thick wavy line) emerging from the ribosome, when folding begins, assisted by ribosome-associate chaperones. 9, Newly made polypeptide released by the ribosome on its way to posttranslational folding. 10, The same polypeptide farther along the folding pathway. 11, New protein, correctly folded into its tertiary structure (native, functional conformation); some proteins achieve a functional status by forming oligomers (quaternary structure), 11a. 12, Some proteins are translocated into organelles (e.g., mitochondrion; yellow) through the organellar membranes. 13, Aggregate, formed by unfolded or misfolded polypeptides. 14, Precipitate of aggregated polypeptides (protein deposit or inclusion body). 15, Unfolded or partially folded polypeptides freed from the aggregates by the action of aggregate-dissolving mechanisms involving chaperones. 16, Protein degradation products, depicted inside a shaded area that symbolizes a dynamic graveyard, in which degradation proceeds from oligopeptides of decreasing lengths down to individual amino acids, which will ultimately be recycled as building blocks for new proteins, in step 8. Some of the known proteolytic machineries found in prokaryotic and eukaryotic cells are depicted: the proteasome-ubiquitin system (magenta), tricorn protease (light green), and other proteases (dark blue). Also, the proteasome (immunoproteasome) generates short antigenic peptides by cleaving large protein antigens for use by antigen-presenting cells. Black solid arrows: physiological route from gene to functional protein. Black wavy arrow: translocation pathway from cytosol into an organelle, for example a mitochondrion. Green solid arrows: critical steps that require chaperone assistance. Green broken arrows: critical steps for which chaperone assistance is probably needed but not yet fully documented. Red arrowheads: molecule (or structure, function, pathway) adversely affected by stress. Red arrows: route from unfolded, partially folded, or misfolded proteins toward aggregation; this route is followed by abnormal proteins even in the absence of stress, and by normal and abnormal proteins that have been denatured by stress. Blue solid arrow: route from protein aggregation toward precipitation of aggregates (inclusion body formation). Violet arrows: routes to protein degradation followed by normal proteins in physiological cellular processes (e.g., in gene regulation, via activator or repressor degradation) and by abnormal proteins that cannot be folded or rescued (refolded) by chaperones (there should also be a similar arrow from 9 to 16, which was omitted for the sake of clarity). Green wavy arrows: participation of chaperones in protein degradation pathways. Black dotted arrows: recovery route from aggregate to free polypeptides to refolding; possibly this route is very actively utilized in proteinopathies, as the chaperoning systems attempt to rid the organism of pathologic aggregates, and to avoid protein deposition. A similar course of events may occur during senescence, with the caveat that the required chaperoning systems probably become less and less efficient with age. Black discontinuous (squares alternating with solid circles) arrow from 14 to 15: possible but improbable recovery route from protein deposit toward the release of free, re-foldable polypeptides. Note that the need for chaperone assistance and the stress-sensitive sites are widespread. Modified from Macario, A. J. L. and Conway de Macario, E. (2002). Sick chaperones and ageing: a perspective. *Ageing Research Reviews* **1**, 295–311, with permission.

the chaperone machine to proceed with folding; consequently, the client polypeptide remains unfolded and malfunctional. (2) The substrate does interact with the chaperone, but because the substrate has certain biochemical-biophysical characteristics, this interaction inhibits rather than initiates the chaperoning process that leads to folding.

Similarly, chaperonopathies may be classified as genetic or acquired. The former are due to a genetic defect, e.g., mutation in the chaperone-encoding gene itself or in the gene encoding a chaperone gene regulator (e.g., the HSF gene). Polymorphisms in these genes may also account for some chaperonopathies.

A genetic chaperonopathy can be described at any of several levels: (1) a locus, gene, or exon that is altered, causing the absence of a chaperone molecule, or its structural abnormality, leading to malfunction; (2) a gene product, from primary transcript to protein (pre-mRNA, or mRNA, or protein, **Figure 1**) can be structurally and functionally abnormal; (3) a chaperone complex or chaperone network that is structurally and functionally deficient due to a defect in one of the components, e.g., a chaperone or cochaperone molecule; (4) a cell, tissue, or organ abnormality that is the consequence of the chaperone deficiency; and (5) developmental and clinical manifestations, i.e., the phenotype.

Acquired chaperonopathies are those that are not heritable; they feature defects, quantitative or structural, in the chaperone molecule due to posttranscriptional aberrations. Acquired chaperonopathies can be described at various levels, as for the genetic chaperonopathies, except that in the acquired conditions the DNA (locus, gene, exon) does not carry hereditary defects.

The chaperones discussed in this article are proteins; hence, the chaperonopathies can be considered a subset of the proteinopathies. In these conditions, a protein is structurally and functionally altered, and it usually has a tendency to misfold, aggregate, and precipitate. Abnormal chaperones can also follow this fate.

Molecular Pathology

Structural defects, genetic or acquired, in a chaperone molecule may affect one or more of the chaperone's functional domains and may have an impact on one or more of its functions.

A chaperone molecule must be able to recognize the client polypeptide in need of assistance for folding or refolding, and it must also be able to interact with the other members of the chaperone complex (the actual chaperoning machine). Furthermore, a chaperone must be able to interact with other chaperoning machines and with protein-degrading machines (to build the chaperone networks involved in protein quality control). Interaction with protein-degrading machines is necessary when the client polypeptide cannot be folded properly and has to be eliminated. Chaperone complex formation and networking involve distinct segments (molecular domains) of the chaperone molecule. If one of these segments is altered because of a mutation or a posttranslation modification, the particular interaction in which the affected segment is involved will not occur, will be ineffective, or will proceed at a slower than normal rate. This perturbation will affect the functioning of the entire molecule, and also the structure and function of the whole chaperone complex and network of which the affected molecule is part. As the chaperone complex is affected, so will all of those cellular processes that require the complex; pathology will ensue.

Impact of Defective Chaperones

Figure 1 shows the life history of a typical protein molecule, from the production of the message (transcription of its parent gene) encoding the amino acid sequence to its final functional form. The figure also shows the points of impact of cell stressors along the way from transcription to the final native conformation, including migration and translocation to the cell locale in which the mature protein molecule resides and functions, and the consequences of misfolding, aggregation, and deficient structure, which lead to degradation.

Deficient chaperones can cause pathological disorders of various severities in any cell, tissue, or organism, whether animal or plant. They can also affect prokaryotic cells, rendering them vulnerable to environmental changes and other agents.

Examples of Chaperonopathies

Examples of genetic, structural chaperonopathies and of polymorphisms of human chaperone genes are

Table 1 Genetic chaperonopathies and human chaperone gene polymorphisms[a]

Chaperone Hsp gene/protein affected	*Disease/syndrome*
sHsp	
Hsp27	Williams
	Charcot-Marie-Tooth
	Distal hereditary motor neuropathy
Alpha crystallins	Childhood cataracts
Alpha-B-crystallin	Desmin-related myopathy
Hsp22	Distal motor neuropathy
Chaperone cofactors for microtubule biogenesis	
Cofactor C (RP2)	X-linked retinitis pigmentosa
Cofactor E	Sanjad-Sakati and Kenny-Caffey
	Progressive motor neuronopathy
Chaperonin of group I, Hsp60	
Mitochondrial Hsp60 (Cpn60)	Hereditary spastic paraplegia
Chaperonin of group II, CCT subunits	
Alpha subunit	McKusick-Kaufman and Bardet-Biedl
Delta subunit	Hereditary sensory neuropathy
Peptidyl-prolyl *cis-trans* isomerase (FKBP)	Leber congenital amaurosis
Genetic polymorphism	*Abnormality/disease*
hsp70-1 promoter region, allele (A)-110	Does not favor longevity in women
hsp70-Hom, T247C, threonine instead of methionine at position 493	Does not favor longevity
hsp70-1, promoter region, allele (C)-110	Associates with Parkinson's disease in Taiwanese

[a]For explanations and references, see Macario, A. J. L., Grippo, T. M. and Conway de Macario, E. (2005). Genetic disorders involving molecular-chaperone genes: a perspective. *Genetics in Medicine* **7**, 3–12; and Macario, A. J. L. and Conway de Macario, E. (2005). Sick chaperones, cellular stress, and disease. *New England Journal of Medicine* **353**, 1489–1501.

Abbreviations: CCT, chaperonin containing TCP-1 (see footnote to **Table 3**); FKBP, FK506-binding protein (FK506 is a compound that affects the immune system so that immune responses are suppressed).

Table 2 Examples of chaperonopathies associated with aging[a]

Hsp/chaperone/HSF	*Experimental-clinical observation*	*Conclusion*
Alpha-A-crystallin	Low levels and PTM and truncation in aged retina	Senescence-associated quantitative and qualitative changes
Alpha crystallins	Decreased solubility and PTM in the eye lens	Senescence-associated qualitative changes
Hsp70 and Hsc70	Aged cultured hepatocytes, melanocytes, and skin fibroblasts, and fibroblasts from old humans: low response to heat shock	Senescence-associated quantitative and functional changes
Hsc70	Low levels in retinas from aged humans and monkeys	Same as above
Hsp27, Hsp70, Hsc70,	High basal levels in aged, cultured, RMHS-treated fibroblasts from humans	Quantitative and functional changes due to aging and chronic stress
Hsp90	Decreased with RMHS and aging in human skin fibroblasts	Same as above
Hsp90	Low levels and chaperone capacity in the cytosol of aged hepatocytes	Functional changes associated with aging
HSF-1	Low levels in aged fibroblasts in culture and from the elderly	Senescence-associated quantitative and functional changes

[a]For source of data, explanations, and references, see Macario, A. J. L. and Conway de Macario, E. (2005). Sick chaperones, cellular stress, and disease. *New England Journal of Medicine* **353,** 1489–1501.
Abbreviations: PTM, posttranslational modification; RMHS, repeated mild heat shock; HSF, heat shock factor (a regulator of transcription of heat shock genes in eukaryotes).

Table 3 Examples of disease-associated chaperonopathies[a]

Hsp/chaperone	*Experimental-clinical observation*	*Disease*
Alpha-B-crystallin	High in IBM muscle fibers	IBM
Alpha-B-crystallin	High in glial inclusions	Tauopathies (CBD, PSP, FTDP-17)
Hsp25	Decreased in motoneurons	ALS (mouse model)
Alpha-B-crystallin, Hdj1, Hdj2, Hsp70, alpha and beta SGT proteins	Low in brain	Huntington's
Hsp72	High in plaques and tangles, and in brain cortex	Alzheimer's
Grp78	High in neurons that are otherwise normal	Alzheimer's
Hsp60, Hsp70RY, Hsc70, alpha-B-crystallin, Grp75, Grp94	Altered distribution pattern in several regions of the brain	Alzheimer's

[a]For source of data, explanations, and references, see Macario, A. J. L. and Conway de Macario, E. (2005). Sick chaperones, cellular stress, and disease. *New England Journal of Medicine* **353,** 1489–1501.
Abbreviations: IBM, inclusion body myositis; CBD, corticobasal degeneration; PSP, progressive supranuclear palsy; FTDP-17, frontotemporal dementia with parkinsonism linked to chromosome 17; ALS, amyotrophic lateral sclerosis; SGT, small glutamine-rich tetratricopeptide repeat containing (protein).

listed in **Table 1**. Chaperonopathies associated with senescence and with disease are listed in **Tables 2** and **3**, respectively.

See Also the Following Articles

Chaperone Proteins and Chaperonopathies.

Further Reading

Bloemendal, H., de Jong, W., Jaenicke, R., et al. (2004). Aging and vision: structure, stability and function of lens crystallins. *Progress in Biophysics and Molecular Biology* **86**, 407–485.

Chapple, J. P., Grayson, C., Hardcastle, A. J., et al. (2001). Unfolding retinal dystrophies: a role for molecular chaperones? *Trends in Molecular Medicine* 7, 414–421.

Cloos, P. A. C. and Christgau, S. (2004). Post-translational modifications of proteins: Implications for aging, antigen recognition, and autoimmunity. *Biogerontology* 5, 139–158.

Csermely, P. (2001). Chaperone overload is a possible contributor to 'civilization disease.' *Trends in Genetics* 17, 701–704.

Jackson, P. K. (2004). Post-translational control and ubiquination. In: Epstein, C. J., Erickson, R. P. & Wynshaw-Boris, A. (eds.) *Inborn errors of development*, pp. 804–814. Oxford, UK: Oxford University Press.

Macario, A. J. L. and Conway de Macario, E. (2001). Molecular chaperones and age-related degenerative disorders. *Advances in Cell Ageing Gerontology* 7, 131–162.

Macario, A. J. L. and Conway de Macario, E. (2002). Sick chaperones and ageing: a perspective. *Ageing Research Reviews* 1, 295–311.

Macario, A. J. L. and Conway de Macario, E. (2004). The pathology of cellular anti-stress mechanisms: a new frontier. *Stress* 7, 243–249.

Macario, A. J. L. and Conway de Macario, E. (2005). Sick chaperones, cellular stress, and disease. *New England Journal of Medicine* **353**, 1489–1501.

Macario, A. J. L., Grippo, T. M. and Conway de Macario, E. (2005). Genetic disorders involving molecular-chaperone genes: a perspective. *Genetics in Medicine* 7, 3–12.

Nardai, G., Csermely, P. and Soti, C. (2002). Chaperone function and chaperone overload in the aged: a preliminary analysis. *Experimental Gerontology* **37**, 1257–1262.

Slavotinek, A. M. and Biesecker, L. G. (2001). Unfolding the role of chaperones and chaperonins in human disease. *Trends in Genetics* **17**, 528–535.

Soti, C. and Csermely, P. (2003). Aging and molecular chaperones. *Experimental Gerontology* **38**, 1037–1040.

Verbeke, P., Fonager, J., Clark, B. F. C. and Rattan, S. I. S. (2001). Heat shock response and aging: mechanisms and applications. *Cell Biology International* **25**, 845–857.

N. Suicide

Adolescent Suicide

M Berk, R Suddath and M Devich-Navarro
University of California, Los Angeles, CA, USA

Glossary

Serotonin (or 5-hydroxytryptamine; 5-HT) An indole amine that is a key chemical neurotransmitter in the nervous system. Disordered serotonin transmission is implicated in depression, suicide, schizophrenia, anxiety and other mental disorders.

Serotonin receptors Receptors are docking sites for bioactive molecules such as serotonin. There are more than 15 serotonin receptor subtypes all located in the cell membrane. With the exception of the 5-HT_3 receptor, a ligand gated ion channel, all other 5-HT receptors are G protein coupled seven transmembrane (or *heptahelical*) receptors that activate an intracellular second messenger cascade. The different subtypes subserve different functions and are targets for different drugs. Thus, for example, the 5-HT2A receptor is the docking target for the hallucinogen, Lysergic acid diethylamide (LSD).

Serotonin transporter The serotonin transporter (SERT) is a 12-transmembrane protein that mediates serotonin uptake (back into the neuron) and thus reduces extracellular serotonin levels in the brain and especially at synapses. SERT is a major target for therapeutic intervention, and the selective serotonin reuptake inhibitors (SSRIs) are the most frequently prescribed antidepressants worldwide. Increased synaptic serotonin concentrations generated by SSRIs are thought to alleviate depression.

Adolescent suicide is a serious public health problem. According to the most recent statistics, suicide is the third leading cause of death among 10- to 24-year-olds in the United States, accounting for 11.7% of all deaths in this age group. Nonfatal suicide attempts are also a significant concern in their own right. In 2002, approximately 124 409 visits to U.S. emergency departments were made after attempted suicide or other self-harm incidents among people ages 10–24 years old. According to data obtained as part of the Youth Risk Behavior Survey, a national survey administered to high school-age youth in 2003, approximately 17% reported having seriously considered attempting suicide, 16.5% reported having made a plan for suicide, 8.5% reported having attempted suicide, and 2.9% reported having made a suicide attempt that required treatment by medical professionals. Suicide attempts can lead to injury, place youth at increased risk for death by suicide and future suicide attempts, place burden on the health-care system, and are associated with a range of adverse outcomes including substance abuse, high-risk sexual acts, school drop-out, poor academic performance, and delinquency.

Risk Factors for Suicide in Adolescents

Prior suicide attempts are the biggest risk factor for a subsequent suicide attempt or completed suicide. Psychopathology is a risk factor for suicide attempts. Approximately 90% of suicide victims have a psychiatric illness at the time of their death. Significant increases in the risk of suicidal behavior are associated not only with depression but also with psychosis, substance abuse, disorders that involve impaired impulse control, and a variety of other psychiatric disorders.

Epidemiological studies of adolescent suicide have demonstrated an increased risk of suicidal behavior with age and significant gender effects that depend entirely on the distinction between completed suicide and suicide attempts. Suicide is relatively uncommon before age 12, and incidence rates rise in the late teens and early twenties. Suicidal ideation and suicide attempts are more common among females than males. In contrast, completed suicide is three to five times more common among males than females. The higher rate of completed suicide in males has been attributed to a variety of factors, including the use of more lethal methods (such as firearms) and higher rates of aggression and substance abuse. The most common way that females attempt suicide is to overdose. In some countries where more lethal drugs are accessible or where emergency medical care is less effective, the rate of completed suicide in females exceeds that of males. Race has been demonstrated as a risk factor for completed suicide. Completed suicide is more common in Whites than African Americans in the United States. The highest rates are among Native Americans and the lowest are among Asian/Pacific Islanders. Similar rates have been described for suicide attempts and recent data suggest that some groups, such as Hispanic females, may be exhibiting more frequent suicide attempts over recent years.

When evaluating an adolescent's risk for suicide, late adolescent age, male gender, and Native American race suggest a higher risk. The presence of significant psychiatric illness, substance abuse/intoxication, and particularly past suicide attempts also increase an individual's risk. In addition, the presence of significant family conflict, dysfunction with peers, or hopelessness increases the risk of suicide.

Neuroscientific Findings in Adolescent Suicide

Several psychiatric disorders now have a significant and growing body of evidence supporting genetic susceptibility to the disorder and underlying neurological or neurochemical abnormalities. Distinct findings in suicidal patients independent of a specific psychiatric diagnosis have been described. For example, structural brain abnormalities identified as white matter hyperintensities on magnetic resonance imaging (MRI) have been associated with suicide attempts in depressed adolescents. Several studies have described abnormalities present in the serotonin neurotransmitter systems in both suicide attempters and completers. Specifically, decreased serotonin transporter binding and increased serotonin receptor density have been reported in a number of studies and may represent a possible mechanism for a heritable risk for suicidal behavior.

Treatments and Possible Effects of Antidepressants

The U.S. Food and Drug Administration has issued warnings of a possible increase in suicidal behavior in individuals being treated with antidepressant medications. These warnings originated as a result of analyses of published and unpublished data on the use of antidepressants in adolescents that indicated approximately a 2% increase in the rate of suicidal behaviors (but not completed suicides) in treated versus placebo groups. These warnings contrast with other findings, including a clear decrease in the overall suicide rate beginning with the widespread use of antidepressants, the absence of antidepressant medication in the majority of the postmortem analyses of completed suicides, and the demonstrated efficacy of antidepressants in adolescent depression. Current practice guidelines include enhanced monitoring for suicidal behaviors during the initial weeks of antidepressant therapy.

Research into psychotherapeutic treatments targeting suicidal behavior in adolescents has demonstrated benefits for family- and community-based interventions and for cognitive-behavioral interventions that target preventing repeat suicidal behavior by improving adolescents' problem-solving skills, decreasing hopelessness and negative cognitions, and improving their ability to regulate negative emotions. Common factors in treatment approaches to suicidal adolescents involve identifying and treating risk factors such as underlying depression, substance abuse, and family stressors. Acutely suicidal patients are treated first for any injuries they have sustained and next with inpatient hospitalization or some equivalent level of supervision to assure their safety. When patients are no longer in danger, medication and psychotherapy can be provided on an outpatient basis, with the goal of preventing a future suicide attempt.

See Also the Following Articles

Depression and Manic–Depressive Illness; Suicide, Biology of; Suicide, Psychology of; Suicide, Sociology of.

Further Reading

Centers for Disease Control (2004). Methods of suicide among persons aged 10–19 years – United States, 1992–2001. *Morbidity and Mortality Weekly Report* 53, 473–474.

Centers for Disease Control (2004). School-associated suicides – United States, 1994–1999. *Morbidity and Mortality Weekly Report* 53, 476–477.

Centers for Disease Control (2004). Suicide attempts and physical fighting among high school students – United States, 2001. *Morbidity and Mortality Weekly Report* 53, 474–475.

Gould, M. S., Greenberg, T., Velting, D. M., et al. (2003). Youth suicide risk and preventive interventions: a review of the past 10 years. *Journal of the American Academy of Child and Adolescent Psychiatry* **42**(4), 386–405.

Mann, J. J., Brent, D. A. and Arango, V. (2001). The neurobiology and genetics of suicide and attempted suicide: a focus on the serotonergic system. *Neuropsychopharmacology* **24**, 467–477.

Mann, J. J., Emslie, G., Baldessarini, R., et al. (2006). ACNP task force report on SSRIs and suicidal behavior in youth. *Neuropsychopharmacology* **31**, 473–492.

Suicide, Biology of

M A Oquendo
Columbia University and New York State Psychiatric Institute, New York, NY, USA
L Giner
Fundacion Jimenez Diaz and Universidad Autonoma de Madrid. Madrid. Spain
J J Mann
Columbia University and New York State Psychiatric Institute, New York, NY, USA

This is a revised version of the article by M A Oquendo and J J Mann, Encyclopedia of Stress First Edition, volume 3, pp 538–543, © 2000, Elsevier Inc.

Glossary

5-Hydroxy-indoleacetic acid (5-HIAA) A metabolite of serotonin.

Cerebrospinal fluid 5-hydroxyindoleacetic acid (CSF 5-HIAA) The concentration of 5-HIAA found in the cerebrospinal fluid. The concentration of 5-HIAA in the cerebrospinal fluid is considered a reflection of serotonergic function in the central nervous system.

Major depression A temporary or chronic mental disorder characterized by the occurrence of five of the following symptoms during a 2-week period or longer: feelings of sadness, inability to enjoy things, sleep disturbance, appetite disturbance, psychomotor changes, fatigue, difficulty concentrating, and suicidal ideas.

Model for understanding suicidal behavior An explanation of how suicide risk factors contribute to suicidal behavior by creating a predisposition to suicidal behavior (lowering the threshold for suicidal acts) or by acting as triggers or stressors precipitating suicidal acts.

Psychosis A temporary or chronic mental condition characterized by an inability to distinguish between reality and nonreality.

Serotonin A neurotransmitter with multiple effects throughout the brain and with a role in a variety of psychiatric disorders and symptoms, including depression, anxiety, aggression, and suicidal behavior.

Stress A force that disrupts the equilibrium or normal functioning of an individual's mental or physical state. Different types of stressors may precipitate suicidal behavior.

Suicide Self-inflicted death committed by an individual with the intention to end his or her life.

This article describes how stressors interact with a low threshold for acting on suicidal ideas. The types of stress that may lead to suicidal behavior are discussed, and factors influencing the threshold for suicidal behavior are described. Stressors that contribute to suicidal behavior include negative events, social conflict, acute psychiatric conditions, acute intoxication, and contagion. Risk factors that lower the threshold for suicidal behavior include family history of suicidal behavior, low serotonergic functioning, comorbid psychiatric conditions, dysfunction of the stress-reactivity hormonal system, marital isolation, early parental loss, and a history of sexual or physical abuse. Factors that raise the threshold for suicidal behavior include religious affiliation, moral constraints, concerns about social disapproval, and feelings of responsibility toward family. An understanding of the risk factors for suicidal behavior and stressors is crucial in developing methods for the prevention of suicide attempts and completion. Because it is a combination of these psychiatric, biological, and environmental risk factors that ultimately leads to an individual's suicide, interventions that address both the role of stressors and raise the threshold for acting on suicidal impulses are critical to prevention.

Introduction

Suicide is a self-inflicted death by an individual with the intention of ending his or her life. As the eleventh leading cause of death in the United States, it accounts for approximately 30 000 deaths a year in the United States and almost 1 million deaths worldwide. In the United States, suicide is the third leading cause of death in people ages 15–24 years and the second leading cause of death in those ages 24–35 years. The World Health Organization has noted a 60% increase in suicide deaths in the past 45 years. Although the actual number of suicide attempts is more difficult to quantify, it is estimated to be 10–20 times that of completed suicides.

Psychiatric, biological, and environmental factors contribute to suicidal behavior and ultimately to suicide completion. Among environmental contributors, stress has long been recognized as having a role in the timing of suicide. However, stress may also be mediated by psychiatric or biological factors. In addition, stress alone, although important, is not a sufficient condition for suicidal behavior. Suicidal behavior also requires a vulnerability for acting on such impulses. Thus, risk factors for suicide can be understood using a model that integrates the role of stress and the threshold for acting on the resulting suicidal impulse.

A Model for Understanding Suicidal Behavior

We have described a model in which suicidal behavior is the outcome of the interaction between an individual's threshold for suicidal acts and stressors that serve as triggers for suicidal behavior. In this model, which is illustrated in **Figure 1**, the threshold is trait-related and refers to the propensity for suicidal behavior. In contrast, stressors, which may be considered state-related, are triggers that determine the timing and contribute to the probability of suicidal acts. Consequently, risk factors that contribute to suicidal behavior may be categorized according to whether they affect the threshold or act as stressors.

Stressors: Triggers for Suicidal Behavior

Stressors may be environmental, behavioral, biological, or a combination of these, as listed in **Table 1**.

Environmental Stressors

Environmental triggers can be categorized as negative events or as contagion. Negative events may include financial difficulties, interpersonal loss (death of a family member or a loved one), loss of property, conflict with parents, or other interpersonal conflict. Contagion refers to the effects of suicides in the community on an individual's decision to commit suicide. These triggers may contribute to the timing of the suicidal act.

Negative events, specifically the loss or lack of a significant relationship, have been suggested to play a key role in the deaths of (1) suicide victims without mental health care, (2) suicide victims with alcohol abuse, (3) suicide victims with personality disorders, and (4) suicide victims with mood disorders. In addition, suicide is associated with financial troubles, homelessness, and job problems. The number of adverse life events appears to play a role as well. However, stressors or negative events related to suicide may vary depending on the culture studied. Most studies published in English have been conducted in Western cultures. Similarities regarding the precipitants of suicide in Eastern and Western cultures exist, such as the number of adverse life events; the presence of severe, acute stress at the time of death; high chronic stress in the year before death; and poor quality of life in the month before death. Yet differences in terms of the type of events that may precipitate suicide have been reported. In China, for example, loss of face, described as an unexpected insult to one's reputation, is a stressor associated with suicide not generally observed in Western cultures. As such, it appears that in different cultures the sensitivity to particular environmental stressors differs.

It is possible that negative events lead to suicide at least in part by disrupting the person's social support network; this network often plays a major role in suicide prevention by providing supervision and emotional support. For example, loss of a loved one is a negative event that leads to an immediate decrease in social support, and this can trigger suicidal behavior. Similarly, social support may be acutely lowered when there is conflict with family and can thereby trigger suicidal acts. Consistent with this idea, the social networks that attempters have seem to be weaker than those of nonattempters, as measured by

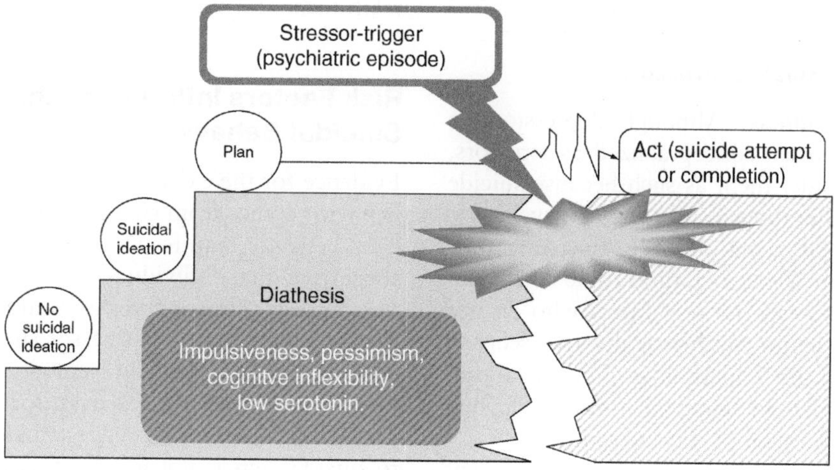

Figure 1 The diathesis–stress model for understanding suicidal behavior.

marital status, living alone, interactions with family members, frequency of recent moves, and the number of close friends.

Another important environmental trigger is contagion, also known as the Werther effect, which was named by Philips in 1974 after Goethe's *The Sorrows of Young Werther.* The Werther effect has been documented as a meaningful contributor to suicidal behavior in both adolescent populations and older populations. Recent outbreaks of suicide in adolescent and elderly populations have raised concerns about media coverage of suicides and the potential for precipitating more suicidal acts within communities. Presumably, individuals with a lower threshold for acting on suicidal thoughts are more likely to act on them after learning of a suicide or an assisted suicide on television or in the newspaper. Moreover, the judicial environment may affect the risk for suicidal behavior in contagion situations by changing public attitudes about the acceptability of suicide. Although there is limited data available, it is possible that the extensive media coverage of physician-assisted suicide and its legalization in one state of the United States, as well as in some European countries, has increased the rate of suicide across diagnoses, including major depression, and specifically in those who are chronically ill and depressed. In fact, physician-assisted suicides and euthanasia contribute to significant underreporting of suicides (as much as 20%) in countries such as the Netherlands, where these procedures are often not reported.

Thus, environmental factors or stressors that play a role in suicidal behavior include the disruption of social support networks, negative events, and interpersonal conflict as well as the altering of perceptions about the acceptability of suicide. These stressors are not causal, however, because the majority of individuals exposed to them do not commit suicide. Nonetheless, they may contribute to the timing and occurrence of suicidal acts in vulnerable people.

Biological and Psychiatric Stressors

Acute psychiatric illness Although depression or psychosis are not often conceptualized as stressors, it is useful to consider them as such because suicide rarely occurs in the absence of a major psychiatric disorder. The rate of mental illness in suicide victims varies from 90% in Western cultures to 60% in Eastern ones. However, even those subjects who do not meet criteria for a major psychiatric disorder seem to have some form of psychopathology. The most common mental disorders in suicide victims are depression and substance abuse, particularly alcoholism.

However, psychiatric illness alone is not sufficient to trigger suicidal behavior. Between 2 and 15% of subjects who suffer from unipolar depression ultimately commit suicide. Schizophrenia also carries a high risk of 10–15%. In bipolar disorder, the risk for suicide is generally considered to be approximately 19%; however, whereas some propose that it is nearly 50%, others question whether even 19% is an overestimate. Nonetheless, despite the high rate of suicide associated with these psychiatric conditions, most patients with these conditions do not commit suicide or even attempt suicide. Thus, the presence of a single stressor such as a psychiatric condition appears to be a necessary, but not sufficient, cause for suicidal behavior.

Acute intoxication Substance and alcohol abuse greatly increase the risk of suicide, an effect that is especially pronounced in youth suicide. Acute substance intoxication can be considered a trigger associated with suicidal behavior. In fact, a recent review of acute alcohol use and suicidal behavior noted that 37% of completed suicides and 40% of attempted suicides involved acute alcohol use. Moreover, acute alcohol use was more prevalent among those who used violent methods of suicide such as self-immolation or gunshot.

To the extent that some individuals respond to environmental stress by using substances, acute intoxication may mediate suicidal responses to stress. The consequences of acute intoxication appear to be biological and behavioral in nature. The biological consequences of acute intoxication with alcohol include, for example, an acute increase of serotonin release, although the long-term consequence is lower serotonin function. In addition, the disinhibiting behavioral effects of intoxication may also play an important role in its association with suicidal behavior. Individuals may be more likely to act on a suicidal impulse when acutely intoxicated than when sober. Thus, acute alcohol intoxication has a complex relationship to suicidal acts.

Risk Factors Influencing the Threshold for Suicidal Behavior

Evidence for the existence of a threshold for suicidal behavior comes from two general findings. First, suicidal behavior manifests early in the course of illness, suggesting that individuals with a vulnerability for this behavior (lower threshold) are likely to express it early in the face of a stressor such as a depressive episode. Second, suicidal behavior runs in families independently of familial risk for mood disorders. Together, these factors suggest that the vulnerability to suicidal acts is not merely related to the presence of a mood disorder or to demoralization secondary

Table 1 A model for understanding suicidal behavior

	Stressors precipitating suicidal behavior	*Factors affecting the threshold for acting on suicidal ideation*
Environmental	Negative events (social, financial, or family crisis) Contagion	Marital isolation Lack of religious affiliation Low self-esteem Fewer perceived responsibilities toward family Fewer perceived reasons for living
Behavioral	Judicial environment Acute substance intoxication	Alcohol or substance abuse
Biological	Major psychiatric episode Acute substance intoxication	Genetic and familial factors Low serotonergic activity (aggression) Stress response (childhood history of physical and sexual abuse) Comorbidity (alcohol or substance abuse, cluster B personality disorder, posttraumatic stress disorder)

to prolonged illness. Rather, suicidal behavior relates to a threshold, predisposition, or diathesis toward acting on suicidal urges. This threshold for suicidal behavior is influenced by risk factors that may be categorized as familial/genetic, biological, or environmental, as listed in **Table 1**.

Familial/Genetic Influences on the Threshold for Suicidal Behavior

Evidence for the presence of genetic risk factors include the presence of a family history of suicide. Although this risk factor could be thought of as facilitating suicidal behavior due to identification or contagion, it includes a genetic component as well. Adoption studies have found that, independent of the transmission of a major psychiatric disorder, adoptees who commit suicide have a sixfold higher rate of suicide among their biological relatives than do matched adoptees who do not complete suicide (None of the adopting relatives committed suicide.) Moreover, there appears to be greater concordance for suicide in monozygotic than in dizygotic twins. Other evidence for the genetic component of suicide is that the familial transmission of suicide risk to offspring appears to be independent of the transmission of psychiatric conditions. A study of Old Order Amish families has shown that family loading for mood disorders alone is not predictive of completed suicide. Rather, individuals with both a mood disorder and a family history of suicide have an increased risk for suicide.

Most genetics studies of suicidal behavior have focused on seven genes: the serotonin transporter (SERT), tryptophan hydroxylase (TPH) 1 and 2, three serotonin receptors (5-HTR1A, 5-HTR2A, and 5-HTR1B), and the monoamine oxidase promoter (MAOA), all of which are key proteins in the maintenance of serotonin function. Although there are no clear findings, the following are most promising:

1. The SERT promoter gene has two polymorphisms or variants, a short and a long form. The short form has been associated with suicidal behavior in different subpopulations, such as violent attempters and female suicide attempters. In a recent meta-analysis, suicidal behavior was reported to be more common in those with the short variant of the SERT promoter gene (OR = 1.17, CI 1.04–1.32; $p = 0.009$). Moreover, the short form has been reported to have an interaction with current life events, making those with this variant vulnerable to suicidal behavior when exposed to stress.
2. The 5-HTR1A gene encodes the 5-HT_{1A} receptor, which in depressed suicide victims has been found to have altered binding in the ventral prefrontal cortex, the region of the brain involved in decision making and restraint, among other functions.
3. The 5-HTR1B gene, which encodes the $5HT_{1B}$ receptor, appears to be related to impulsivity and aggressive behavior. This gene has two identified variants, both associated with 20% fewer receptors in the postmortem brain, although these variants were found at the same frequency in suicide and control subjects.
4. A low expressing version of the MAO gene has been reported to interact with exposure to childhood abuse, resulting in aggression in adult males and indicating that the effect of this gene is only manifested if there are negative environmental conditions or, in other words, is dependent on a gene–environment interaction.

Thus, genetic and familial contributions to the diathesis for suicidal behavior require further inquiry but hold promise in the elucidation of suicide risk in individuals who carry the relevant variants of these genes.

Neurobiological Influences on the Threshold for Suicidal Behavior

The relationship of abnormal monoamine function to suicide risk has been studied for over 30 years. CSF 5HIAA is a metabolite of serotonin and its concentration in the cerebrospinal fluid (CSF) is considered a reflection of serotonergic function in the central nervous system (CNS). Patients with major depression who have made suicide attempts have lower levels of 5-HIAA in their CSF compared to depressed patients who do not have a history of suicide attempts. The reduction in CSF 5-HIAA appears to be more pronounced in depressed patients making planned, highly lethal attempts that more closely resemble failed suicide. Furthermore, CSF 5-HIAA correlates with characteristics of the most lethal attempt in the patient's lifetime, even when the suicide attempt is not temporally close to CSF measurements. In addition, CSF 5-HIAA seems to predict the risk of future suicide. These findings, together with those from animal studies in which the heritability and stability of CSF 5-HIAA on test–retest has been demonstrated, suggest that serotonergic dysfunction is trait-related and thus can reasonably be considered a factor that lowers the threshold for acting on suicidal thoughts.

Other measures of serotonergic function also indicate decreased serotonergic function in the CNS of suicide attempters. Fenfluramine has been widely used as a serotonin-releasing agent. Its effects on serotonin include reuptake inhibition, release from presynaptic storage granules, and possibly direct stimulation of postsynaptic receptors. We have reported that a fenfluramine challenge test elicited a lower serotonin-mediated prolactin response in patients with a major depressive episode who had a lifetime history of high-lethality suicide attempts compared with depressed patients who had a lifetime history of only low-lethality attempts. Moreover, using positron emission tomography and radioactively tagged glucose, we have reported that high-lethality suicide attempters exhibit low metabolism in the prefrontal cortex, the brain area associated with decision making and restraint. They also show impaired serotonergic responsivity. Both of these abnormalities are proportional to the lethality of their suicide attempt and are related to suicide intent and impulsivity and thus may influence lethality via these parameters. In addition, the postmortem examination of brains from suicide victims found reduced binding to the serotonin transporter sites, which was especially pronounced in the ventral and dorsal prefrontal cortex. The increased binding or number of postsynaptic 5-HT_{1A} and 5-HT_{2A} receptors in prefrontal cortex, postulated to reflect an accommodation to low serotonin, has been reported in most studies as well. Studies of brain stem, from which CNS serotonin neurons emanate, have found reduced concentrations of serotonin or 5-HIAA in suicide victims. Together, these findings suggest that serotonin dysfunction in the CNS is associated with severe and lethal suicidal behavior.

Lower serotonergic functioning may have other effects on suicidal behavior as well and may mediate the association between suicide and behaviors such as aggression and alcoholism. Among depressed individuals, those who have made suicide attempts tend to be more aggressive. Several studies show that in humans and in nonhuman primates, aggression is linked to low serotonin function. Similarly, the biological underpinnings of the predisposition to abusing alcohol, including a low serotonin function and lower CSF 5-HIAA in alcoholics during abstinence compared to immediately after the discontinuation of drinking, have been shown. Thus, individuals predisposed to alcoholism or aggression may have biological parameters, such as low central serotonergic functioning, that are also associated with suicidal behavior.

In summary, serotonergic dysfunction may influence the threshold for both attempted and completed suicide. Moreover, serotonergic function may be a mechanism whereby genetic factors influence the suicide threshold. Clearly, the relationship among genetic endowment, suicide, and serotonin functioning needs further study.

Stress Response and Suicidal Behavior

Childhood physical and sexual abuse has been associated with suicidal behavior. Those who experience corporal punishment in adolescence are reported to be at increased risk of depressive symptoms, suicidal ideation, and alcohol abuse. Suicidal ideation increases markedly with the frequency of adolescent corporal punishment for both males and females. In fact, adolescent suicide attempters are three to six times more likely than controls to have had contact with the social services department. They also commonly had notations in their chart about child abuse. In a college sample, 16% of men and 24% of women reported sexual abuse as children. Such a history predicted depression, chronic self-destructiveness, suicidal ideation and attempts, self-mutilation, and substance abuse. The younger the person was at time of first abuse, the higher the number of suicide attempts reported. Similarly, in a sample of depressed individuals, suicide attempters were more likely to have experienced sexual abuse themselves as children, and their offspring were also at increased risk for being sexually abused and for being suicide attempters, than were depressed individuals who were not suicide attempters. These findings support the link between childhood abuse and subsequent suicidal behavior.

Childhood physical and sexual abuse has been linked to abnormalities in the stress response as mediated by the hypothalamic-pituitary-adrenal (HPA) axis. The HPA axis, with its intricate two-way interaction with the serotonergic system, has been proposed to play a key role in the correlation between early stress exposure and later impulsivity, aggression, and suicidal behavior. Indeed, suicidal behavior seems to be related to hyperactivity of the HPA axis. Among depressed individuals, those with a hyperactive HPA axis, as demonstrated by an inability to suppress cortisol in the face of external steroid administration (dexamethasone suppression test), have been reported to have a ninefold elevation in risk for suicide. Moreover, suicide victims have larger adrenal glands, which produce stress hormones and low prefrontal cortex corticotropin releasing hormone binding, consistent with a hyperactive HPA axis.

Influence of the Presence of Multiple Psychiatric Diagnoses on the Threshold

Comorbid conditions that increase the risk for attempted suicide include alcohol abuse, substance abuse, posttraumatic stress disorder, and cluster B personality disorders. In depressed inpatients, these conditions are more common among suicide attempters.

Studies have suggested that when alcoholism and depression are comorbid, suicide attempt risk is greatly increased, even when the presence of an antisocial personality disorder or other personality disorders are controlled for. Furthermore, depressed alcoholics usually report more suicidal ideation than nonalcoholic depressed patients, even when the severity of other depressive symptoms is similar. Apart from the biological pathways previously noted, other mechanisms may mediate the relationship between alcohol and suicide. For example, alcoholism may lead to unemployment, financial problems, and interpersonal problems. Psychologically, it may increase loneliness and aggression and it may inhibit coping mechanisms, all of which may lower the threshold for suicidal behavior.

Suicide attempts are also reported to be more common in depressed patients with comorbid borderline personality disorder (BPD) than in depressed patients without BPD. Moreover, subjects with major depression and comorbid borderline personality disorder are more likely to make multiple suicide attempts, and the attempts are no less medically damaging than those made by patients with major depression alone. Thus, the potential lethality of suicide attempts in patients with comorbid disorders and/or BPD should not be underestimated.

Posttraumatic stress disorder (PTSD) is frequently comorbid with depression, and when they co-occur the risk for suicidal behavior is enhanced. The relationship between PTSD and suicidal behavior appears to be mediated by the presence of cluster B personality disorder (CBPD), with both PTSD and CBPD arising as a result of earlier traumatic experiences. The assessment and treatment of comorbid conditions such as PTSD and CBPD in the context of depression may contribute to the reduction of suicide risk in this vulnerable population.

Environmental and Psychological Influences on the Threshold for Suicidal Behavior

There are environmental and psychological effects on the threshold for suicidal behavior. Environmental conditions that lower social support, such as marital isolation or living alone, are associated with suicide risk. Indeed, married women have a lower rate of completed suicide than women who are not married. In the same vein, an association between committing suicide in the context of a major affective disorder and not living with a child under the age of 18 has been reported.

However, there are clinical variables that increase the threshold for suicide attempts. These include religious or moral constraints, concerns about social disapproval, and coping and survival skills. In particular, religious affiliation seems to be associated with less suicidal behavior in depressed inpatients, and this protective effect may be mediated through moral objections to suicide and feelings of responsibility toward family. In fact, for a woman, the likelihood of completed suicide decreases as the number of children she has increases.

A variable not easily classified as influencing either threshold or trigger is low self-esteem. Although low self-esteem can be an enduring trait, it is also a symptom of depression that can be exacerbated during depressive episodes. In patients with recurrent major depressive disorder without comorbid personality disorders, those who reported feeling like a failure were significantly more likely to have made a suicide attempt than those not reporting such feelings. In agreement with this finding, we have found that a factor of the Beck Depression Inventory that captures self-blame is associated with a history of suicidal behavior. Thus, low self-esteem may decrease the threshold for acting on suicidal thoughts in general, and its effect may be magnified during acute episodes of depression.

In summary, environmental factors related to social support and psychological attitudes, such as self-esteem or moral constraints against suicidal behavior, are important contributors to the threshold for suicide.

Summary

Risk factors can facilitate suicide by either acting as stressors or lowering the threshold for suicide. These stressors may be environmental, biological, or psychiatric in nature. Environmental stressors include negative events and contagion. Psychiatric stressors often have biological underpinnings, and acute psychiatric illness is a prominent stressor that is present in 60–90% of suicides. Acute intoxication also increases the risk of suicidal behavior by causing changes in serotonergic function and by disinhibiting the individual, making it more likely that he or she will act on suicidal impulses. These stressors act as triggers and precipitate suicidal acts.

However, whether psychiatric, environmental, or biological, stressors do not act alone in influencing suicidal behavior. Other risk factors influence suicidal behavior as well by lowering an individual's threshold for acting on suicidal ideation. Risk factors that lower the threshold for suicide can also be distinguished by three major categories: biological, psychiatric, and environmental.

Many studies of familial transmission of suicidal behavior have suggested that there is a genetic component to suicidal behavior. The strongest findings are related to the serotonin transporter gene (SERT), although there are promising results for other serotonin-related genes. Neurochemical risk factors such as lower CSF 5-HIAA levels and hyperactivity of the HPA axis are also associated with suicidal behavior and appear to be biochemical traits. These biological factors may potentially become useful predictors of suicidal behavior.

Psychiatric comorbidity may also lower the threshold for suicidal behavior. Studies suggest that in depressed patients, the presence of alcohol abuse, substance abuse, PTSD, or CBPD can increase the propensity to act on suicidal thoughts. Environmental influences that lower the threshold for suicidal behavior include marital isolation, early childhood parental loss, and a childhood history of physical or sexual abuse. An individual's threshold for suicide is also lowered by feelings of low self-esteem. Several factors appear to raise the threshold for suicidal behavior. These protective factors include religious affiliation, moral constraints, concerns about social disapproval, coping and survival skills, and family responsibility. These attitudes may act as an incentive not to commit suicide.

This article describes a comprehensive model for categorizing risk factors for suicidal behavior into those that act as stressors and those that lower the threshold for acting on suicidal ideas. This model may guide research into methods of prevention and treatment of suicidal behavior and, ultimately, save lives.

Acknowledgments

This work was supported by PHS Grant MH46745 and MH59710. We thank Ms. Ansley Roche and Sadia Chaudhury for their assistance in the preparation of this manuscript.

Further Reading

Anguelova, M., Benkelfat, C. and Turecki, G. (2003). A systematic review of association studies investigating genes coding for serotonin receptors and the serotonin transporter. II: Suicidal behavior. *Molecular Psychiatry* **8**, 646–653.

Caspi, A., Sugden, K., Moffitt, T. E., et al. (2003). Influence of life stress on depression: moderation by a polymorphism in the 5-HTT gene. *Science* **301**, 386–389.

Cherpitel, C. J., Borges, G. L. and Wilcox, H. C. (2004). Acute alcohol use and suicidal behavior: a review of the literature. *Alcoholism, Clinical and Experimental Research* **28**, 18S–28S.

Egeland, J. A. and Sussex, J. N. (1985). Suicide and family loading for affective disorders. *Journal of the American Medical Association* **254**, 915–918.

Grunebaum, M. F., Keilp, J., Li, S., et al. (2005). Symptom components of standard depression scales and past suicidal behavior. *Journal of Affective Disorders* **87**(1): 73–82.

Linehan, M. M. and Shearin, E. N. (1998). Lethal stress: a social–behavioral model of suicidal behavior. In: Fisher, S. & Reason, J. (eds.) *Handbook of life stress, cognition and health*, pp. 265–285. New York: John Wiley & Sons.

Malone, K. M., Haas, G. L., Sweeney, J. A., et al. (1995). Major depression and the risk of attempted suicide. *Journal of Affective Disorders* **34**, 173–185.

Mann, J. J. (2003). Neurobiology of suicidal behaviour. *Nature Reviews: Neuroscience* **4**, 819–828.

Mann, J. J., Malone, K. M., Psych, M. R., et al. (1996). Attempted suicide characteristics and cerebrospinal fluid amine metabolites in depressed inpatients. *Neuropsychopharmacology* **15**, 576–586.

Mann, J. J., Oquendo, M., Underwood, M. D., et al. (1999). The neurobiology of suicide risk: a review for the clinician. *Journal of Clinical Psychiatry* **60**(supplement 2), 7–11.

Mittendorfer-Rutz, E., Rasmussen, F. and Wasserman, D. (2004). Restricted fetal growth and adverse maternal psychosocial and socioeconomic conditions as risk factors for suicidal behaviour of offspring: a cohort study. *Lancet* **364**, 1135–1140.

Oquendo, M. A., Friend, J. M., Halberstam, B., et al. (2003). Association of comorbid posttraumatic stress disorder and major depression with greater risk for suicidal behavior. *American Journal of Psychiatry* **160**, 580–582.

Oquendo, M. A., Malone, K. M. and Mann, J. J. (1997). Suicide: risk factors and prevention in refractory major depression. *Depression and Anxiety* **5**, 202–211.

Oquendo, M. A., Placidi, G. P., Malone, K. M., et al. (2003). Positron emission tomography of regional brain metabolic responses to a serotonergic challenge and lethality of suicide attempts in major depression. *Archives of General Psychiatry* **60**, 14–22.

Phillips, M. R., Yang, G., Zhang, Y., et al. (2002). Risk factors for suicide in China: a national case-control psychological autopsy study. *Lancet* **360**, 1728–1736.

Relevant Websites

Centers for Disease Control. http://www.cdc.gov.
World Health Organization. http://www.who.int.

Suicide, Psychology of

D Lester
Richard Stockton College of New Jersey, Pomona, NJ, USA
R L Walker
University of South Carolina, Columbia, SC, USA

This is a revised version of the article by D Lester, Encyclopedia of Stress First Edition, volume 3, pp 544–548, © 2000, Elsevier Inc.

Glossary

Assisted suicide	Suicidal acts in which the individual is assisted. This may take the form of a prescription being written for a lethal dose of a medication or of someone else administering the lethal dose/injection.
Attempted suicide	A suicide act that the individual survives. At the lower end of medical lethality, attempted suicide may be difficult to distinguish from self-mutilation. In Europe, the trend has been to call suicidal acts that are not life-threatening parasuicide or deliberate self-harm.
Completed suicide	A suicidal act that results in the death of the individual. It is sometimes called fatal suicide.

The study of suicide is complicated by difficulties in determining intentionality, or whether the suicidal person has engaged in intentional self-harm. Recently, suicide nomenclature has evolved such that clinicians, researchers, and others can now use a common language to understand the suicide-related behavior. Beyond assisted suicide, attempted suicide, and completed suicide, suicidal ideation, defined as any self-reported thoughts of engaging in suicide-related behavior, is also commonly used. In addition, parasuicide is used rather than attempted suicide to describe self-destructive behavior in the absence of clear intent of suicide. The term suicidality should be avoided because it refers to a broad range of suicide-related behaviors.

The 2001 National Strategy for Suicide Prevention noted that 650 000 people receive emergency care for suicide attempts and 30 000 die by suicide each year in the United States. Given the loss of life and impact on families and communities, suicide has been declared a serious public health problem. The goals of the National Strategy are to (1) promote awareness of suicide as a public health problem; (2) develop broad-based support for suicide prevention; (3) develop and implement strategies to reduce the stigma associated with mental illness, substance abuse, and suicide; (4) develop and implement community-based suicide prevention programs; (5) promote efforts to reduce access to lethal methods of self-harm; (6) implement effective training to assess at-risk individuals and provide effective intervention; (7) develop clinical and professional practices; (8) increase access to mental health services; (9) improve the reporting and media portrayal of suicide-related behavior; (10) promote research on suicide and suicide prevention; and (11) improve and expand surveillance systems. The overarching objective is a comprehensive and integrated approach to reducing the loss associated with suicide and related behaviors. Many other nations have also developed national strategies for reducing the incidence of suicide.

The 2002 Institute of Medicine (IOM) report for the United States is an excellent and comprehensive resource for understanding suicide's history; impact;

manifestations across gender, ethnic, age, and other demographic groups; and protective factors or suicide buffers. For example, although African Americans were previously thought to be protected from suicide, studies show that in the 1980s and 1990s Black men ages 25–34 years demonstrated suicide rates comparable to that of White men in the same age group. The most recent data and trends are cited in the IOM report, including the cost to society due to medical expenses for emergency intervention and treatment, lost productivity, and reduced wages. The value of lost productivity alone was estimated to be $11.8 billion in 1998.

Suicide can be studied at the societal or at the individual level. Sociological research has focused primarily on the societal rate of completed suicide, a rate that is relatively stable over time. At the individual level, in contrast, both completed and attempted suicides have been studied and both behaviors are difficult to predict. Suicide is rare, with the completed suicide rate, for example, seldom rising above 40 per 100 000 per year in any nation. The rarity of suicidal behavior means that prediction instruments (typically based on personal data and psychiatric and psychological measures) will have a high rate of false positives (people predicted to be suicides who, in fact, will not kill themselves). Differences between the predictability of suicide at societal and individual levels has an analogy in radioactive decay, in which the half-life of a mass of, say, uranium is easily determined and constant, whereas predicting which particular uranium atom will decay next is impossible.

Suicide fits well with the diathesis–stress model of psychiatric disorder, in which only those individuals with a predisposition (diathesis) to develop a disorder do so when faced with particular stressors. It should be noted, however, that both factors can influence one another – a diathesis can make it more likely that a person will encounter stressors and a stressor can strengthen a diathesis. For example, a stress such as the loss of a loved one can be more stressful for a person who has few friends than for someone without that diathesis. Likewise, a tendency to have few friends may be increased by the experience of interpersonal losses.

Diathesis

Many predisposing factors for suicide have been identified by research.

1. Neurophysiological dysfunction, especially problems in serotonergic pathways, may underlie the psychiatric disorders for which the risk of suicide is high.
2. The majority of suicides are found to have been suffering from a psychiatric disorder. In particular, suicide is common in those suffering from affective disorders such as a major depressive disorder or a bipolar affective disorder (manic–depression), substance abuse (both drug and alcohol abuse), and schizophrenia.
3. Childhood experiences such as the loss of a parent (or other primary caregiver) through death, especially if the death is from suicide, or divorce and physical or sexual abuse are commonly found in the personal histories of suicides. Lester studied 30 suicides famous enough to have a biography written about them (such as Ernest Hemingway) and found that exactly half had experienced the loss of a parent or other loved one. Fourteen of the 15 suicides who had experienced such a loss had experienced this loss between the ages of 6 and 16. However, it is not clear whether such experiences increase the risk of suicide directly or whether they increase the risk of psychiatric disorders, which in turn increases the risk of suicide. For example, a history of physical and sexual abuse is associated with a wide spectrum of later psychiatric disorders, including depression, anxiety, eating disorders, and substance abuse, in addition to suicidal behavior.
4. The mood of potential suicides is characterized by depression. Suicidal individuals obtain high scores on self-report measures of depression, and the level of depression of those attempting suicide increases with the seriousness of their suicidal intent. Depression includes many components: physical symptoms (such as sleep and appetite problems), mood symptoms (such as depression and guilt), and cognitive symptoms (such as hopelessness). Suicidal individuals tend to be hopeless, believing that things will not improve and will probably worsen in the future. Aaron Beck has found that self-report measures of hopelessness are stronger predictors of suicidal intent than self-report measures of depression. Edwin Shneidman has called the psychological pain experienced by potential suicides psychache.
5. Suicidal individuals appear to think differently from nonsuicidal individuals. Research has found that suicidal individuals have a reduced ability to generate alternatives other than death for the problems they are facing; they tend to think in dichotomous categories, polarizing their evaluations into extremes, such as good versus bad or right versus wrong; and they tend to think rigidly.
6. In addition, the risk of suicide is strongly associated with simple demographic characteristics. Suicide rates in the United States are higher in

men than in women, in the elderly than in the young, in Whites than in African Americans, and in the divorced and widowed than in the single and married. These demographic correlates of suicide risk vary from country to country, however.

In 2005, Joiner developed a comprehensive interpersonal-psychological theory of attempted and completed suicide and hypothesized that suicidal people must (1) be capable of lethal self-injury, (2) perceive that they are a burden to loved ones, and (3) believe that they are not connected to a valued group or relationship. These three necessary precursors answer the question of why people do or do not die by suicide. For example, few people die by suicide, relatively speaking, and interpersonal-psychological theory suggests that the acquired ability to inflict self-harm requires courage, fearlessness, and habituation to self-harm. Joiner asserted that individuals must also see themselves as ineffective and burdensome to loved ones. In contrast, a sense of belonging to a valued group acts as a suicide buffer. In sum, the confluence of three factors must be in place. However, those who engage in repeated attempts at suicide are at high risk for suicide.

Joiner's theory explains several research findings. For example, the relatively low rate of suicide despite the high lifetime prevalence of lifetime suicide thoughts is explained by the absence of two or more factors (such as the incapability of self-injury and a sense of connectedness). Thus, not everyone who considers suicide or feels hopeless will attempt suicide. Note that those who die by suicide use more lethal means and therefore demonstrate a stronger propensity to self-harm. Although women are less likely to die by suicide than men, those women who die are as likely as men to use very lethal methods (e.g., a gun and hanging). The role of neurophysiological factors in suicide is related to the impact of neurotransmitters on negative emotionality, which may, in turn, incite feelings of burdensomeness and contributes to a lesser feeling of belongingness.

Stress as a Precipitant of Suicide

Suicides are found to have experienced higher levels of stressful events in the past year than nonsuicidal individuals. Not only is the level of stressful events higher, but typically there is a further increase in this already high level in the weeks immediately prior to the suicide. These conclusions are based on retrospective studies of the lives of completed suicides in the hours, days, weeks, and months prior to their death – a procedure called a psychological autopsy. In a psychological autopsy, mental health professionals, usually guided by an interview schedule, seek out and interview friends, colleagues, and relatives of the suicide and inquire into the suicide's recent behaviors and psychological state.

Commentators have suggested that men become suicidal more as a reaction to performance failure, whereas women become suicidal more as a reaction to romantic conflict. However, research has indicated few differences between the stressors encountered by female and male suicides. Large differences in precipitating stressors by age have been observed. Stressors experienced by adolescent and young adult suicides tend more often to involve negative interpersonal events, such as friction and break-ups with loved ones and problems involving work, finances, and the criminal justice system. In contrast, stressors of elderly suicides tend more often to involve medical problems and intrapsychic states such as depression. These differences by age are found both in psychological autopsy studies and in content analyses of suicide notes.

Similar differences have been observed in attempted suicides and those thinking about the possibility of killing themselves, who also are found to have experienced more recent stressful events than nonsuicidal psychiatric patients or general medical patients. Two studies from the 1990s illustrate the role of stress. Paul Dean and colleagues found that suicidal ideation in college students was positively associated with self-ratings of negative life events in the past year and, in addition, depression, hopelessness, and perfectionism, and was negatively associated with scores on a reasons-for-living scale. John Reich and colleagues found that suicidal ideation in a sample of elderly adults (mean age 70 years) was associated with worsening health in the prior 6 months and, in addition, self-reported feelings of helplessness, fatalism, confused thinking, and low self-esteem.

The Adequacy of Stressors

Older adults who commit suicide are typically seen as having experienced more adequate stressors than younger adults and adolescents who kill themselves. Elderly suicides are frequently suffering from medical problems, often severe, and have experienced a succession of losses (of loved ones and friends, of employment and work, and of physical abilities). Thus, the precipitants of their suicides appear to involve severe stress. Most of the examples of rational suicide involve such cases, and indeed assisted-suicide laws passed in the United States and other nations are usually restricted to those who are terminally ill. In contrast, the precipitants of suicide in adolescents and young adults are sometimes seen as inadequate causes of suicide.

Such suicides are, therefore, viewed as impulsive and not rational and are less predictable.

The Situation

The situation in which potential suicides find themselves may also play a role in precipitating their suicides. The easy availability of lethal methods for suicide may play a role. Research on the effects of restricting easy access to methods for suicide (such as detoxifying domestic gas, placing emission controls on cars, and restricting the number of pills prescribed for psychiatric disorders) has shown that this can be an important tactic for preventing suicide.

The publicity given to suicides, especially suicides by celebrities, has been shown to lead to an increase in the suicide rate in the following few days, especially among those of the same age and sex as the celebrity. Suicide among peers can have a contagion effect, precipitating suicidal behavior in those with those characteristics that predispose the individual to suicide. Suicides occurring in schools have aroused particular concern, and there are now guidelines for staff in responding to the suicide of a student.

Survivors

The experience of having a loved one complete suicide can be extremely traumatic for those left behind. In addition to the normal grieving process, there is additional stress from feelings of guilt and responsibility (could something have been done to help the suicide and prevent their death?), anger (over their suicide), and stigma from others who may view the survivors with suspicion or simply not know how to respond.

In addition, some suicides kill themselves in such a way that their loved ones discover the body. The discovery of the body of a loved one drowned, hanging from a hook, with cut wrists, or, even worse, grossly disfigured by a bullet is extremely traumatic. It creates a final picture of the loved one that is difficult to exorcize.

Survivors have become very active in their communities and in professional organizations devoted to suicide prevention. They have formed self-help groups, sometimes with the involvement of clinicians, to meet and assist one another in dealing with the complicated grief that accompanies the suicide of a loved one. Books have been written for survivors and the membership of the American Association of Suicidology has a large contingent of survivors.

Assisted Suicide

The reluctance of people to kill themselves with violent methods and the desire of suicidal individuals to have others assist them in their suicides have led to widespread debate about assisted suicide. Derek Humphry published the book *Final Exit*, which details the medications and dosages for suicide – a do-it-yourself book that became a best seller in the United States. Similar books in other nations (such as France) have been banned.

In physician-assisted suicide, typically the goal is to have physicians provide a sufficient amount of a lethal medication for the client to complete suicide. In most regions that have legalized this process (e.g., in Oregon and the Netherlands), this process is restricted to those who are terminally ill, and there is a detailed procedure for those applying for physician-assisted suicide that must be followed.

However, on occasion, physicians and relatives have assisted the suicidal individual in the actual killing, for example, by administering the lethal injections or by shooting the person. This is illegal in almost all nations and jurisdictions, and those assisting in the actual killing can be, and indeed sometimes are, charged with murder. Nevertheless, such incidents have occurred and continue to occur. The line between assisting someone to commit suicide and murdering someone is, therefore, blurred in these cases, and society is vigorously debating these issues at the present time.

Preventing Suicide

The prevention of suicide uses several strategies. Many communities now have suicide prevention centers that maintain telephone counseling services staffed primarily by well-trained lay people who can provide crisis counseling for those who are suicidal. The American Association of Suicidology has a directory of such centers in the United States and also inspects and certifies the centers if asked to do so. Befrienders International, Life Line, and the International Federation of Telephone Emergency Services are three international organizations that have established and coordinated crisis counseling and suicide prevention services in other nations.

Educational programs have been established to inform students in school about suicide, especially about recognizing signs of suicidal intent in their peers, and to provide them with resources to which they can refer their suicidal peers. Educational programs have also occasionally been established for general practitioners and family physicians so that they can diagnose depression in their patients more accurately and prescribe antidepressants more effectively.

Clinicians have been developing counseling techniques especially designed for suicidal clients to supplement the general systems of psychotherapy (such as transactional analysis and reality therapy) that guide therapists. These new techniques have been primarily in the field of cognitive therapy and are based on the results of research on the cognitive processes of suicidal individuals discussed earlier.

The 2002 report from the IOM examined prevention and medical and psychosocial intervention, but also looked at barriers to research, treatment, and effective prevention. For example, suicide is more likely to occur within 1 month after discharge from psychiatric institutions than at other times. The report noted that a significant gap in clinical trials is the absence of high-risk patients. Because effective treatments (psychopharmacological and psychosocial) involve long-term maintenance in which the individual is required to have contact with a health-care professional, adequate health-care insurance coverage is essential. School-based programs that target high-risk school-age children are essential for suicide prevention among youth and seem to result in increased social support, self-efficacy, and self-esteem among youth at risk for suicide, but research on these intervention programs is complicated by poor control groups and limited long-term follow up.

See Also the Following Articles

Depression and Manic–Depressive Illness; Suicide, Biology of; Suicide, Sociology of.

Further Reading

Clark, R. V. and Lester, D. (1989). *Suicide: closing the exits.* New York: Springer-Verlag.

Dean, P. J., Range, L. M. and Goggin, W. C. (1996). The escape theory of suicide in college students. *Suicide and Life-Threatening Behavior* **26**, 181–186.

Freeman, A. and Reinecke, M. A. (1993). *Cognitive therapy of suicidal behavior.* New York: Springer.

Henry, A. F. and Short, J. F. (1954). *Suicide and homicide.* New York: Free Press.

Humphry, D. (1991). *Final exit.* Eugene, OR: The Hemlock Society.

Institute of Medicine of the National Academies. (2002). *Reducing suicide: a national imperative.* Goldsmith, S. K., Pellmar, T. & Bunney, W. E. (eds.). Washington, DC: The National Academies Press.

Joiner, T. (2005). *Why people die by suicide.* Cambridge, MA: Harvard University Press.

Leenaars, A. A. and Wenckstern, S. (eds.) (1991). *Suicide prevention in schools.* New York: Hemisphere.

Lester, D. (1997). *Making sense of suicide.* Philadelphia: Charles Press.

Lukas, C. and Seiden, H. M. (1987). *Silent grief.* New York: Scribners.

O'Carroll, P. W., Berman, A. L., Maris, R. W., et al. (1996). Beyond the Tower of Babel: a nomenclature for suicidology. *Suicide and Life-Threatening Behavior* **26**, 237–252.

Reich, J. W., Newson, J. T. and Zaura, A. J. (1996). Health downturns and predictors of suicidal ideation. *Suicide and Life-Threatening Behavior* **26**, 282–291.

Shneidman, E. S. (1996). *The suicidal mind.* New York: Oxford University Press.

U.S. Department of Health and Human Services (2001). *National strategy for suicide prevention: goals and objectives for action.* Rockville, MD: Public Health Service.

Suicide, Sociology of

D Lester
Richard Stockton College of New Jersey, Pomona, NJ, USA
R M Fernquist
Central Missouri State University, Warrensburg, MO, USA

This is a revised version of the article by D Lester, Encyclopedia of Stress First Edition, volume 3, pp 549–552, © 2000, Elsevier Inc.

Glossary

Attempted suicide — A suicide act that the individual survives. Attempted suicide is at the lower end of medical lethality and may be difficult to distinguish from self-mutilation. In Europe, the trend has been to call suicidal acts that are not life-threatening parasuicide or deliberate self-harm.

Completed suicide — A suicidal act that results in the death of the individual. It is sometimes called fatal suicide.

Sociological research into suicide has focused primarily on the rate of completed suicide in regions (nations or regions within nations), a rate that is relatively stable over time. Ecological studies examine suicide rates of a set of regions at one point in time, usually to see which social characteristics of the regions predict the suicide rates. Time-series studies examine suicide rates of one region each year for a period of time, usually to see which social characteristics predict the yearly suicide rate. Time-series cross-sectional studies examine suicide rates of a number of different countries simultaneously for a period of time. Here multivariate ecological studies of suicide are reviewed. Three major theories of suicide are presented: Emile Durkheim's, Andrew Henry and James Short's, and Raoul Naroll's. The role of culture conflict in increasing the rate of suicide is illustrated. Finally, the possibility of sociological studies of nonfatal suicide is discussed.

Durkheim's Theory

The first major theory of the social suicide rate was proposed in 1897 by Emile Durkheim. Durkheim argued that two broad social characteristics are responsible for determining the social suicide rate: social integration and social regulation. Social integration is the extent to which the members of the society are bound together in social networks. Very high levels of social integration lead to high rates of altruistic suicide, whereas very low levels lead to high rates of egoistic suicide. Social regulation is the extent to which the desires and behavior of the members of the society are restricted by social norms and customs. Very high levels of social regulation lead to high rates of fatalistic suicide, whereas very low levels lead to high rates of anomic suicide.

There has been a great deal of research purporting to test this theory, for example, exploring the association between divorce rates and suicide. Divorce is presumed to weaken the extent of social integration and reflect weak social regulation, and therefore higher divorce rates should be positively associated with higher suicide rates. Both ecological studies and time-series studies have confirmed this predicted positive association between divorce rates and suicide rates.

However, research rarely examines the roles of both social integration and social regulation separately, partly because it is difficult to operationalize the two social characteristics independently of one another. The few studies that have attempted to do so have found that measures of social integration are stronger correlates of suicide rates than measures of social regulation.

Furthermore, no research has attempted to classify suicides in the societies under study into Durkheim's four types. Durkheim proposed, for example, that low levels of social integration result in high levels of egoistic suicide. Therefore, a proper test of Durkheim's theory requires the dependent variable to be the rate of egoistic suicide. The rate of egoistic suicide is not identical to the total social suicide rate, which is, instead, the combined rate of all four of Durkheim's types of suicides.

Henry and Short's Theory

Henry and Short proposed a theory based on both psychoanalytic theory and the frustration–aggression hypothesis. They assumed that the primary target of aggression for a frustrated individual is another person. What inhibits this other-oriented aggression and results in the aggression being directed inward onto the self?

Henry and Short proposed that the primary factor was the strength of external restraints on behavior. When behavior is required to conform rigidly to the demands and expectations of others, the role of others in the responsibility for the self's frustration and misery is strong. As a consequence, other-oriented aggression is legitimized. When external restraints are weak, the self must bear the responsibility for the frustration and misery. Thus, other-oriented aggression is not legitimized, and self-directed aggression becomes more likely.

These proposals lead to interesting predictions, many of which have been confirmed. The oppressed in a society have clear external sources to blame for their misery – their oppressors. Therefore, other-oriented aggression is legitimized for them, and they will tend to have higher rates of assault and, in the extreme, homicide. In contrast, the oppressors in the society have fewer external sources to blame for their misery because, as the dominant group, they have tremendous opportunities for advancement and gratification. Therefore, the oppressors in the society will tend to have higher rates of depression and, in the extreme, suicide. These predicted differences in the suicide and homicide rates are found for African Americans and Whites in the United States.

Henry and Short's theory can also explain the positive association between the quality of life and suicide rates. When the quality of life in a nation is high, there are few external sources to blame for one's misery, and so suicide will tend to be more common. This association has been confirmed in ecological studies both of nations and of U.S. states.

Naroll's Theory

Raoul Naroll, an anthropologist, proposed a theory of social suicide rates that has relevance to stress. Naroll proposed that suicide was more likely in those who were socially disoriented, that is, in those who lack or lose basic social ties (such as those who are single or divorced). Because not all socially disoriented people commit suicide, there must be a psychological factor that makes suicide a more likely choice when a person is socially disoriented, and Naroll suggested that it was the person's reaction to thwarting disorientation contexts. Such contexts involve a weakening of the person's social ties as a result of the actions of other people or him- or herself (but not as a result of impersonal, natural, or cultural events). Being divorced by a spouse or murdering one's spouse are examples of such contexts, but storm damage to property or losing a spouse to cancer are not. In thwarting disorientation contexts, some people commit protest suicide, which Naroll defined as voluntary suicide committed in such a way as to come to public notice (and, therefore, excludes unconsciously motivated suicides and culturally motivated suicides such as suttee).

Durkheim's theory of suicide refers more to steady-state characteristics of the society as major explanatory variables, whereas Naroll's theory suggests the role of sudden, acute changes in a society – societal stressors. Furthermore, Narroll's theory is phrased in a way that makes it more usefully applied to individuals as well as to societies as a whole.

Culture Conflict

Cultures often come into conflict, a source of stress that may increase the suicide rate. For example, the conflict between traditional Native American culture and the dominant Anglo-American culture has often been viewed as playing a major role in precipitating Native American suicide. Philip May reviewed three hypotheses that might have relevance here. In the social disorganization hypothesis, the dominance of the Anglo-American culture is viewed as forcing Native American culture to change and as eroding traditional cultural systems and values. This changes the level of social regulation and social integration, important causal factors for suicide in Durkheim's theory of suicide.

A second hypothesis focuses on cultural conflict. The pressure from the educational system and mass media on Native Americans, especially on youth, to acculturate, a pressure that is opposed by their elders, leads to great stress for the youth. A third hypothesis focuses on the breakdown of the family in Native American tribes. Parents are often unemployed, substance abusers, and in trouble with the law, and divorce and desertion of the family by one or both parents are common. The suicide rates of three groups of Native Americans in New Mexico, the Apache, Pueblo, and Navajo (whose suicide rates were 43.3, 27.8, and 12.0 per 100 000 per year, respectively), were in line with their levels of acculturation as rated by May (high, moderate, and low, respectively).

Measuring Regional Stress

Linsky and co-workers measured the stress level of each of the U.S. states in three areas. For economic stress, they used business failures, unemployment claims, strikes, bankruptcies, and mortgage foreclosures. For family stress, they used divorces, abortions, illegitimate births, and fetal and infant deaths. For community stress, they used disasters, new housing starts, new welfare recipients, high school dropouts, and interstate migration. They found that states with higher levels of stress also had higher suicide rates. Interestingly, however, the ratings of the stress level of each state based on responses from a national survey, which asked residents about their perceived level of stress, were not associated with the state suicide rates.

Multivariate Studies of Regional Suicide Rates

The accuracy of official national and regional rates of suicide has been questioned by Jack Douglas and others, who have argued that these rates are biased by the values of the local coroners and medical examiners and of the resident populations. However, despite the fact that regions do have different standards for classifying a death as suicide, Peter Sainsbury and Brian Barraclough showed that the suicide rates of immigrants to one country from different nations are in almost the same rank order as the suicide rates of nations of origin.

The suicide rates of 71 nations reporting to the World Health Organization are shown in **Table 1** for males and females. An inspection of the table reveals two basic findings: (1) in all countries, males have higher suicide rates than females, which suggests that differential gender socialization (e.g., males are socialized to be more aggressive and to keep their feelings inside) significantly impacts suicide rates; and (2) suicide rates vary significantly among the 71 countries, which suggests that cultures differ in the degree to which suicide is viewed as an acceptable behavior. Cutright and Fernquist term this phenomenon the culture of suicide.

Simpson and Conklin identified two clusters of variables that were associated with national suicide rates: (1) a cluster that had the highest loading from the percentage of Muslims in the population and (2) a cluster that seemed to assess economic development. Suicide rates were lower in nations with less economic development and where Islam was a more important religion. Two other clusters (Christianity and the Eastern bloc) were not associated with suicide rates.

Table 1 Suicide rates around the world[a]

Country	*Year reported*	*Males*	*Females*	*Country*	*Year reported*	*Males*	*Females*
Lithuania	2002	80.7	13.1	Norway	2001	18.4	6.0
Russian Federation[b]	2002	69.3	11.9	Canada	2000	18.4	5.2
Belarus	2001	60.3	9.3	Chile	2001	18.2	3.0
Kazakhstan	2002	50.2	8.8	United States	2000	17.1	4.0
Latvia	2002	48.4	11.8	Hong Kong	2000	16.1	10.1
Estonia	2002	47.7	9.8	Northern Ireland	2002	15.9	3.5
Ukraine	2002	46.7	8.4	Puerto Rico	2000	15.2	1.4
Hungary	2002	45.5	12.2	Turkmenistan	1998	13.8	3.5
Slovenia	2002	44.4	10.5	Thailand	2000	13.5	3.7
Japan	2002	35.2	12.8	Argentina	2001	13.4	3.5
Finland	2002	32.3	10.2	Netherlands	2003	12.7	5.9
Belgium	1997	31.2	11.4	Spain	2001	12.2	3.7
Austria	2002	30.5	8.7	Uzbekistan	2000	11.8	3.8
Croatia	2002	30.2	10.0	El Salvador	1999	11.6	5.4
Uruguay	2000	29.0	5.5	Costa Rica	2002	11.6	2.0
France	2000	27.9	9.5	Singapore	2001	11.5	6.9
Moldova, Republic of[c]	2002	27.9	5.2	Italy	2001	11.1	3.3
Switzerland	2000	27.8	10.8	England and Wales	2002	9.8	2.8
Poland	2002	26.6	5.0	Israel	1999	9.8	2.3
Bulgaria	2002	25.6	8.3	Venezuela	2000	8.8	1.5
Korea, Republic of	2002	24.7	11.2	Panama	2000	8.4	1.3
Czech Republic	2002	24.5	6.1	Columbia	1999	8.1	2.4
Romania	2002	23.9	4.7	Bahrain	2000	7.2	0.3
Slovakia	2000	22.6	4.9	Brazil	2000	6.4	1.6
Trinidad & Tobago	1998	22.2	4.7	Mexico	2001	6.3	1.3
Cuba	2001	21.4	8.0	Ecuador	2000	6.0	2.6
Denmark	1999	21.4	7.4	Albania	2001	5.5	2.3
Ireland	2001	21.4	4.1	Greece	2001	5.3	0.9
Germany	2001	20.4	7.0	Armenia	2002	4.0	0.7
Australia	2001	20.1	5.3	Paraguay	2000	3.9	1.7
New Zealand	2000	19.8	4.2	Georgia	2001	3.4	1.1
Scotland	2002	19.7	5.9	Guatemala	1999	3.4	0.8
Kyrgyzstan	2002	19.1	4.0	Philippines	1998	1.8	0.6
Sweden	2001	18.9	8.1	Azerbaijan	2002	1.8	0.5
Portugal	2002	18.9	4.9	Egypt	2000	0.1	0.0
Mauritius	2000	18.8	5.2				

[a]Rate per 100 000 population from latest year reported, ranked according to male suicide rates.
[b]Excluding Chechnya.
[c]Excluding Transdinestria.
Source: World Health Organization Statistical Information Systems website.

In similar study of the social correlates of national suicide rates, Lester identified 13 orthogonal (independent) factors for social variables, only one of which was associated with suicide rates, a factor that seemed to measure economic development (with high loadings from such social variables as low population growth and high gross domestic product per capita). Thus, these two studies agreed in finding that economic development is associated with higher suicide rates. Cutright and Fernquist reported that classical Durkheimian variables measuring social integration (i.e., divorce, fertility, and religiosity), as well as female labor-force participation, were strong predictors of cross-national suicide rates for both males and females of different age groups.

For the United States, a similarly designed study conducted by Lester identified a cluster of variables that seemed to measure social disintegration (high divorce and interstate migration rates, low church attendance, and high per capita alcohol consumption), and this was the strongest correlate of the suicide rates of the states.

Nonfatal Suicide Behavior

Almost all sociological research and theories have hitherto been proposed for fatal (completed) suicide. Nonfatal suicidal behavior has been relatively ignored. It is important that better epidemiological studies of attempted suicide and suicidal ideation be conducted so that sociologists can develop theories of these behaviors. The World Health Organization has sponsored a comparative epidemiological study of attempted suicide in 15 sites. Unfortunately, the sites are limited to cities in European nations and do not encompass these nations as a whole. However, the study is innovative and may lay the groundwork for more comprehensive epidemiological studies in the future. Linsky and colleagues have obtained estimates of the incidence in the previous year of suicidal ideation in U.S. states and sought social correlates of this. Thus, such research is possible, and it is to be hoped that more studies are planned along these lines.

See Also the Following Articles

Affective Disorders; Suicide, Biology of; Suicide, Psychology of.

Further Reading

Cutright, P. and Fernquist, R. M. (2000). Effects of societal integration, period, region, and culture of suicide on male age-specific suicide rates: 20 developed countries, 1955–1989. *Social Science Research* **29**, 148–172.

Cutright, P. and Fernquist, R. M. (2000). Societal integration, culture, and period: their impact on female age-specific suicide rates in 20 developed countries, 1955–1989. *Sociological Focus* 33, 299–319.

Cutright, P. and Fernquist, R. M. (2003). The gender gap in suicide rates: an analysis of twenty developed countries, 1955–1994. *Archives of Suicide Research* 7, 323–339.

Douglas, J. D. (1967). *The social meanings of suicide.* Princeton, NJ: Princeton University Press.

Durkheim, E. (1897). *Le suicide.* Paris: Felix Alcan. [English edition: (1951). *Suicide.* New York: Free Press.]

Henry, A. F. and Short, J. F. (1954). *Suicide and homicide.* New York: Free Press.

Lester, D. (1988). *Why women kill themselves.* Springfield, IL: Charles Thomas.

Lester, D. (1989). *Suicide from a sociological perspective.* Springfield, IL: Charles Thomas.

Lester, D. (1994). *Patterns of suicide and homicide in America.* Commack, NY: Nova Science.

Lester, D. (1994). *Patterns of suicide and homicide in the world.* Commack, NY: Nova Science.

Lester, D. (1995). Thwarting disorientation and suicide. *Cross-Cultural Research* **29**, 14–26.

Linehan, M. (1973). Suicide and attempted suicide. *Perceptual and Motor Skills* **37**, 31–34.

Linsky, A. S., Bachman, R. and Straus, M. A. (1995). *Stress, culture, and aggression.* New Haven, CT: Yale University Press.

Sainsbury, P. and Barraclough, B. M. (1968). Differences between suicide rates. *Nature* **220**, 1252.

Simpson, M. E. and Conklin, G. H. (1989). Socioeconomic development, suicide and religion. *Social Forces* **67**, 945–964.

Van Winkle, N. W. and May, P. A. (1986). Native American suicide in New Mexico, 1959–1979. *Human Organization* **45**, 296–309.

Relevant Website

World Health Organization Statistical Information Systems website. http://www3.who.int/whosis/menu.cfm.

IV. NEUROPSYCHOLOGICAL

Disease, Stress Induced

H S Willenberg and S R Bornstein
University Hospital, Duesseldorf, Duesseldorf, Germany

This is a revised version of the article by H S Willenberg, S R Bornstein and G P Chrousos, Encyclopedia of Stress First Edition, volume 1, pp 709–713, © 2000, Elsevier Inc.

Glossary

Adrenocorticotropic hormone (ACTH)	Is known under its scientific term "corticotropin". Regulates adrenal steroidogenesis, specifically glucocorticoid synthesis and cortisol release.
Adaptive response	Complex set of an organism's reactions to reestablish homeostasis.
Apoptosis	Cell death initiated by several mechanism in a regulated process. It is also termed "programmed cell death." Cells with this fate undergo a sequence of changes typical for this process.
Arginine-vasopressin (AVP)	Peptide hormone, which stimulates pituitary ACTH release
Corticotropin-releasing hormone (CRH)	Also termed "corticotropin-releasing factor" (CRF) or "corticoliberin." Main regulator of ACTH.
Homeostasis	State of dynamic equilibrium.
LC/NE system	Locus ceruleus / norepinephrine system.
Proopiomelanocortin (POMC)	Polypetide secreted by pituitary cells which is the basis for several hormones of the pituitary that are yielded by alternative processing, including corticotropin, melanocyte-stimulating hormones (MSH), and endorphins.
Sympathetic-adrenomedullary system (SA system)	Part of the autonomic neural system.
Stress	State of threatened homeostasis.
Stressor	Forces that threaten to destroy the state of homeostasis.

The continuation of life depends on the ability of an organism to maintain a state of dynamic equilibrium or homeostasis. Homeostasis is constantly disturbed by entropic forces, the stressors; the state of threatened homeostasis is called stress. A complex set of behavioral and physical reactions, the adaptive response, is employed by the organism to reestablish balanced physiological conditions. At the beginning of the twentieth century, Walter Cannon and Hans Selye developed these modern concepts of stress and discussed the relation between stress and disease. In antiquity, Hippocrates regarded health as the harmonious balance of the four key elements of life – water, fire, air, and earth – and defined states of imbalance among these elements as disease. He also described the adaptive response as the "healing power of nature." (Chrousos et al.)

The actual term stress was originally adopted from physics by Hans Selye. In physics, it describes the resistance of a body to applied pressure, following Hook's law of elasticity. An acting force may distort a body elastically in a linear fashion or, if applied excessively in quality, quantity, or time, may produce nonlinear deformations. Similarly, stress may be a transient and time-limited state, well balanced by the adaptive responses of the organism, whereas excessive and prolonged stress may alter the physiological and behavioral defense mechanisms, rendering them inefficient or deleterious.

Anatomy and Physiology of the Stress System

Structures that include components of a network of neural and endocrine responses that are activated adaptively during stress have been collectively called the stress system. On the cellular level, molecules such as the highly conserved heat shock proteins (hsp) are primitive key elements of the cellular stress response. They comprise several families of proteins that are found across species and are classified depending on their molecular size (kilodaltons) into hsp16–30, hsp60, hsp70, and hsp90. They have been shown to regulate cell and tissue homeostasis and to be protective when this is threatened by stressors.

The central components of the stress system are located in the hypothalamus and the brain stem, the phylogenetically oldest parts of the brain. These centers receive information inputs of internal and external origins and compute the appropriate responses, which are effected by two main pathways: the endocrine hypothalamic-pituitary-adrenal (HPA) axis and the neural systemic sympathetic-adrenomedullary (SA) and parasympathetic systems. Their central regulators and peripheral end products, corticoropin releasing hormone (CRH), glucocorticoids, and catecholamines, are key hormones in the reestablishment and maintenance of cardiovascular, metabolic, immune, and behavioral homeostasis.

The Hypothalamic-Pituitary-Adrenal Axis and Stress

CRH, the principal central regulator of the HPA axis, is mainly produced by parvocellular neurons of the hypothalamus in the paragigantocellular and parabranchial nuclei of the medulla and in the central nucleus of the amygdala. Its action on the pituitary gland is supported by arginine vasopressin (AVP), also secreted by parvocellular neurons of the paraventricular hypothalamic nuclei (PVN). CRH induces the production and secretion of adrenocorticotropic hormone (ACTH) from the pituitary, a hormone whose main target is the cortex of the adrenal gland. The intracerebroventricular administration of CRH causes the activation of the stress system and behavioral patterns similar to those observed during stress.

The adrenal gland, as the end organ of the HPA axis, is subject to functional changes of the stress system. It responds quite rapidly to sustained stimulation with hypertrophy and hyperplasia, which can be monitored on the macroscopic, microscopic, ultrastructural, and molecular levels. Whereas in acute stress high blood concentrations of glucocorticoids and ACTH can be found, in chronic stress high levels of glucocorticoids and relatively low levels of ACTH are frequently observed. This dissociation between the central activation of the HPA axis and adrenal cortex function represents an adaptation of the stress system whereby medullary input and hypertrophy-hyperplasia of the zona fasciculata of the adrenal cortex sustain elevated glucocorticoid secretion in the presence of low normal ACTH concentrations. In addition, although ACTH is a potent secretagogue for adrenal steroids, this peptide does not seem to mediate the hyperplasia of the adrenal cortex during stress. Other pituitary factors are under discussion, especially N-terminal fragments of proopiomelanocortin (POMC).

Glucocorticoids exert their pleiotropic effects through ubiquitously distributed intracellular receptors in almost all tissues of the body. In addition, they participate in their own regulation of secretion through a classic negative feedback mechanism by binding to high-affinity mineralocorticoid and low-affinity glucocorticoid receptors in the frontal cortex, amygdala, hippocampus, hypothalamus, and pituitary. Exposure to pathologically elevated levels of glucocorticoids causes neurons to slow down their metabolism, although these neurons may undergo death by apoptosis. Therefore, this loop of HPA axis regulation serves to terminate or suppress an excessive response of the stress system.

The Systemic Sympathetic-Adrenomedullary and Parasympathetic Systems

This axis originates from mostly norepinephrine cell groups of the locus ceruleus, medulla, and pons (LC/NE). Efferent projections of these neurons terminate throughout the brain and spinal cord as well as in the peripheral ganglia of the autonomic nervous system. Through a complex neural network, a wide spectrum of physiological functions can be controlled. These include cardiovascular tone, respiration, skeletal muscle and adipose tissue metabolic activity, and gastrointestinal function. The adrenal medulla is an effector organ of this system, supplying the systemic circulation with epinephrine and norepinephrine. These catecholamines also potentiate ACTH-stimulated cortisol production by the adrenocortical cells.

Coordination and Communication of Hypothalamic-Pituitary-Adrenal Axis and LC/NE System

The organization and implementation of a qualitatively and quantitatively appropriate stress response depends on the fine-tuning of both the regulatory centers of the stress system and the response of target organs. Indeed, a complex network of neurons, neuronal and hormonal factors, and other cell mediators is at interplay at each level of interactions. The secretion of CRH and central catecholamines is controlled by the neurons of the frontal cortex, mesocortical/mesolimbic system, and the amygdala–hippocampus complex. Neuronal pathways that produce γ-aminobutyric acid (GABA), substance P, and β-endorphin inhibit CRH-producing neurons. CRH is not only responsible for the activation of the HPA axis but also for the stimulation of LC/NE neurons in the brain stem.

The adrenal gland unites the HPA and SA axes under a common capsule. A great degree of intermingling of cortical and medullary cells increases the area of contact between these systems. In addition to the stimulation through ACTH, ACTH-independent mechanisms seem to be involved in the adaptation to chronic stress. The stimulation of chromaffin cells leads to the potentiation of glucocorticoid secretion, whereas glucocorticoids enhance catecholamine production by medullary cells.

Interplay of the Stress System with Major Endocrine, Immune, and Other Systems

The activation of the stress system helps the organism to overcome the influence of stressors and, therefore, postpones all functions that may interfere with the chance of the individual to survive. The stress system stimulates the mesocorticolimbic system, influencing motivation and reward phenomena. The stress system also stimulates the amygdala and hippocampus. The former generates fear and anxiety, whereas the latter participates in the negative feedback control of the HPA axis; both recall implicit emotion-laden memories. Neurons of the arcuate nucleus of the hypothalamus produce POMC-derived peptides. Two of these, α-melanocyte-stimulating hormone (-MSH) and β-endorphin inhibit the activity of the stress system. Projections to the brain stem and spinal cord elevate the gain threshold, producing so-called stress-induced analgesia.

The activation of the stress system leads to the inhibition of a number of endocrine axes. These include the gonadal, growth, and thyroid axes. The direct inhibition of central neural circuits is supported by the peripheral suppressive actions of glucocorticoids.

Other profound consequences of stress system activation are observed in the immune system. However, the adrenal cells express toll-like receptors, making the adrenal cortex sensitive to registering the activations of the innate immune system. Further important participants in the immunological homeostasis are cytokine signals from cells of the immune tissue. All three major inflammatory cytokines – tumor necrosis factor α, interleukin 1, and interleukin 6 – produced at sites of inflammation in a cascade-like fashion, exert stimulatory effects on the HPA axis. Their actions are directed to all three levels of the HPA axis. The most potent mediator among them is interleukin 6; it causes elevation of CRH, AVP, ACTH, and the glucocorticoids. Indirect actions of the inflammatory cytokines on the HPA axis are also attained through the stimulation of the noradrenergic centers in the brain stem. In chronic hypoactivation of the HPA axis, increased serum levels of interleukin 6 can be observed.

The stress system uses additional mechanisms to affect immune homeostasis. In addition to the suppressive effect of glucocorticoids on the production of tumor necrosis factor α, interleukin 1, and interleukin 6, the glucocorticoids also inhibit the target tissue responses to cytokines through the suppression of nuclear transcription factor-κB and activator protein 1 (AP-1). Glucocorticoids also cause a switch from type 1 T-helper cytokine profile to type 2 T-helper cytokine profile by inhibiting interleukin 12 and by stimulating interleukin 10. In this way, a shift from a cellular to a humoral immune response is promoted. In addition, the glucocorticoids initiate apoptosis in the eosinophils and in some lymphocytes.

Stress and Disease

Stress plays an important role in individual and species survival, but it also participates in the development and aging of every individual. The quality, intensity, and duration of stress are important in determining the positive or negative effects on the organism.

There are two main conditions of the stress system that lead to pathology: an excessive and prolonged or a defective adaptive response to a stressor. In both cases, the dose–response relation between the potency of a stressor and the adaptive response of the organism is shifted to the left or right, respectively. Excessive or defective reactions to stressors that are associated with pathological or physiological states are summarized in **Table 1**. More than half of the variance determining the stress response is due to inherited factors, whereas the remaining half is due to early-life constitutional factors and concurrent environmental input.

Table 1 Pathological conditions associated with altered activity of the HPA axis

Increased HPA activity	*Decreased HPA activity*	*Disrupted HPA activity*
Severe chronic disease	Atypical depression	Cushing's syndrome
Melancholic depression	Seasonal depression	Glucocorticoid deficiency
Anorexia nervosa	Chronic fatigue syndrome	Glucocorticoid resistance
Obsessive-compulsive disorder	Hypothyroidism	
Panic disorder	Adrenal suppression	
Chronic excessive exercise	Obesity (hyposerotinergic forms)	
Malnutrition	Nicotine withdrawal	
Diabetes mellitus	Vulnerability to inflammatory disease (Lewis rat)	
Hyperthyroidism	Rheumatoid arthritis	
Central obesity	Premenstrual tension syndrome	
Childhood sexual abuse	Postpartum mood and inflammatory disorders	
Pregnancy	Vulnerabilty to alcoholism	

In the syndrome of major melancholic depression, a disproportionate activation of the generalized stress response is chronically manifested. Central activation with consequent elevation of CRH is followed by a blunted ACTH response of the pituitary to exogenous CRH, probably due to the downregulation of CRH receptors and/or increased glucocorticoid feedback. At autopsy, these patients have an increased number of CRH and AVP neurons in the parvoventricular nucleus of the hypothalamus and hippocampal atrophy. In addition, imaging and morphometric studies have shown that the pituitary and adrenals are enlarged. The sequelae of hypercortisolism include pseudo-Cushing's syndrome manifestation, osteoporosis, and opportunistic infections. Similar observations were made in patients with chronic active alcoholism, with anorexia nervosa, who were sexually abused in their youth, and with obsessive-compulsive disorders.

Another example of hyperactivation of the stress system is critical illness. When entering a chronic state, interleukin 6 and possibly other cytokines synergize with ACTH to maintain increased stimulation of the adrenal cortex. In this condition, a dissociation between ACTH and cortisol levels occurs. As in melancholic depression, these patients escape full HPA axis suppression following dexamethasone.

In the autoimmune-inflammatory syndrome of rheumatoid arthritis, a hypoactive HPA axis has been reported. It appears that a defective glucocorticoid response to inflammation is an important factor in the pathogenesis of this disease.

Disease and Stress

There are pathological conditions of the stress system leading to disease and, *vice versa*, diseases that alter the activity of the stress system in a pathological fashion.

Stress System Disorders

The adaptive response to stress has three components. First, stress has to be sensed. Sensory neural and hormonal pathways have developed to connect the outside world and the rest of the body to the central nervous system. Hypersensitivity or hyposensitivity to stressors may cause disproportionate responses, resulting in pathology. Therefore, disorders characterized by altered perception of signals to the stress system cause inefficient responses to natural challenges, with the consequent development of secondary diseases.

The second component covers the calculation and integration of the information input, and the third component covers the response. Disorders of the central nervous system that influence these responses interfere with the stress system and develop pathology related to this interference.

The activation of the stress system is necessary to overcome homeostasis-threatening events, but excessive and prolonged activation may be self-destructive. Transient hypercortisolemia is necessary during surgery, sepsis, and other severe conditions, but hypercortisolemia also leads to hyperglycemia, hyperlipidemia-increased catabolism, and immune suppression – all states that, if chronically present, have major adverse effects on the body.

Diseases That Directly Influence the Stress System

Diseases generally disturb homeostasis and should be regarded as stressors. Conversely, every stressful influence that alters homeostasis of the organism in a long-term fashion could be regarded as a process that may cause disease.

Cushing's syndrome or Addison's disease leads to the disintegration of the stress system, which then fails to mount an adaptive response. In addition, severe sepsis leads directly to the activation of the stress system. Patients with these conditions develop multisystem disorders that result from excessive or defective cortisol effects on systems, whose proper function depends on optimal glucocorticoid activity.

Further Reading

Bornstein, S. R. and Chrousos, G. P. (1999). Adrenocorticotropin (ACTH)- and non-ACTH-mediated regulation of the adrenal cortex – neural and immune inputs. *Journal of Clinical Endocrinology and Metabolism* **84** (5), 1729–1736.

Bornstein, S. R. and Ehrhart-Bornstein, M. (1999). Interactions of the stress system in the adrenal: basic and clinical aspects. In: Bolis, C. L. & Licinio, J. (eds.) *Stress and adaptation: from Selye's concept to application of modern formulations*, pp. 89–108. Geneva: World Health Organization.

Chrousos, G. P. (1998). Stressors, stress, and neuroendocrine integration of the adaptive response: the 1997 Hans Selye memorial lecture. *Annals of the New York Academy of Sciences* **851**, 311–335.

Chrousos, G. P., Loriaux, D. L. and Gold, P. W. (1988). The concept of stress and its historical development. *Mechanisms of physical and emotional stress. Advances in Experimental Medical Biology* **245**, 3–7.

Somatic Disorders

F Creed
University of Manchester, Manchester, UK

This is a revised version of the article by F Creed, Encyclopedia of Stress First Edition, volume 3, pp 483–485, © 2000, Elsevier Inc.

Glossary

Anxiety disorder	A disorder of mood characterized by tension and worry, often accompanied by physical symptoms of tension, including palpitations, butterflies in the stomach, and breathing difficulties.
Chronic social difficulties	Ongoing environmental stressors such as unemployment, serious financial or health difficulties, and ongoing serious difficulties in close relationship.
Depressive disorder	A disorder of mood accompanied by sleep, appetite disturbance, lack of energy and concentration, and possibly ideas of suicide.
Life event	A discrete change in the person's immediate environment, such as a bereavement or a marital separation.
Medically unexplained symptoms	Symptoms of pain or function (e.g., bowel or breathing disturbances) that cannot be explained on the basis of underlying organic disease.
Organic disease	A physical disease understood on the basis of recognized tissue damage.
Psychosomatic medicine	The study of biological, psychological, and social aspects of all diseases.

Psychosomatic Disorders

Psychosomatic disorders were previously thought to be a separate group of disorders in which stress and psychological distress led to disease. Examples were peptic ulcer, arthritis, and dermatitis. It is now recognized that all diseases may have social, psychological, and behavioral aspects as well as physical organic features. The World Health Organization defines psychosomatic medicine as "the study of biological, psychological and social variables in health and disease."

This is best illustrated by the example of heart disease. Heart disease is caused by many factors. These include inherent biological factors, including age, sex, and genetic enhancement, that increase the chances of a heart attack; physiological factors, such as raised blood pressure, smoking, alcohol consumption, and increased blood cholesterol level; and psychological and social factors, which include depression, anxiety, and certain forms of stress, which are associated with an increased chance of developing a heart attack or increased chance of dying thereafter. Stress may lead to anxiety or depressive disorders, which can lead to a fast heart rate and increased chance of irregular heart beats, which may be fatal soon after a heart attack. Lack of social support – in the form a close person with whom all difficulties or problems can be shared – also contributes to increased chance of further heart attacks.

Thus, the modern view of psychosomatic mechanisms includes a role for stress, depression, and lack of social support alongside biological factors in the causation or outcome of disease. The relative importance of environmental stress varies in different conditions.

Stress and the Onset of Organic Disorders

Stress is much less important than the other biological or physical causative factors in the development of a heart attack. There is no clear link between stressful life events (e.g., marital separation and loss of job) and having a heart attack. There is a link with more chronic stress – 40% of heart attack patients have experienced a chronic social difficulty concerning work, money, or housing compared to 17% of healthy controls. The greatest difference seems to be in the excessive hours worked and lack of proper holidays. This seems to be something that individuals bring on themselves by working excessively hard (i.e., the type A personality).

In other diseases, different patterns have been reported. In peptic ulcer, for example, life events are important, especially those that engender goal frustration. These events involve working hard toward a particular goal for many years and then being thwarted by a change of circumstances at the last moment. Such an event occurred in over half (54%) of people with peptic ulcer, compared to only 9% of healthy comparison groups.

Another stress is that of a major earthquake. There was an increase in the number of people with stomach ulcer after the Hanshin-Awaji earthquake; for most people, the ulcer developed in conjunction with an infectious agent in the stomach, *Helicobacter pylori*, but among those physically injured following the earthquake stomach ulcers developed independently of this infectious agent. Thus, there is a clear relationship with stress, which must be considered alongside other risk factors for peptic ulcer – *H. pylori* infection, drugs taken for arthritis smoking, and an inherited predisposition.

There is a discernible increase in environmental stress prior to the onset of stroke, but the effect is weak – the biological factors listed as risk factors for heart disease are much more important. In one study, 24% of stroke patients and 12% of controls had experienced a severe life event in the year prior to the stroke. This is a much smaller difference than that found in peptic ulcer.

It is easy to assess life events prior to the onset prior of a heart attack or a stroke because these conditions develop at a clear point in time. In multiple sclerosis, however, the onset is much less clearly defined. It does appear that the experience of a severe life event during the 6 months prior to the onset of multiple sclerosis is very considerable – 62% of multiple sclerosis patients had experienced such an event, compared to only 15% of a control group. If this result is confirmed, it suggests that the experience of stress probably interacts with the immune system, which may have been sensitized by exposure to an infection during childhood or early adulthood.

Stress and the Immune System

One of the most likely ways that stress leads to the onset of organic disease is by the modification of the immune system. This has been shown in very well-controlled studies of susceptibility to infection with the cold virus. An impressive feature is the dose–response relationship between an index of psychological stress and chance of infection; that is, the more stress experienced, the greater likelihood that a cold will develop after experimental exposure to the virus. The psychological stress in these studies comprised a combination of stressful life events (environmental stress) and the degree of distress (symptoms of anxiety and depression).

In order to exclude the interference with biological variables, these studies controlled for a number of variables that might explain the stress–infection association: smoking, alcohol, exercise, diet, quality of sleep, number of white cells in the blood, and total immunoglobular levels. The researchers also excluded the effect of personality variables of low self-esteem, personal control, and degree of extroversion and introversion. When this is done, there is a clear link between the stress levels of the caregivers of people with Alzheimer's disease and immune response, measured by the antibody response to influenza vaccination.

Medically Unexplained Symptoms

By contrast to the pattern observed in organic disease, there seems to be a very clear increase in stress just before the onset of certain disorders in which no organic disease can be found to explain the symptom. Typical disorders are irritable bowel syndrome, chronic fatigue syndrome, and fibroymalgia. The symptoms may be severe (e.g., pain) and may lead to an operation, such as an appendectomy although the appendix appears to be quite normal The pain may also lead to many investigations that fail to reveal any recognized organic disease to explain it. Approximately two-thirds of such patients have experienced recent environmental stress, compared to less than one-quarter of people with organic disease or healthy control subjects. This pattern of recent stress is similar to the stress that occurs prior to depressive disorders.

Anxiety and Depressive Disorders

The most common reaction to environmental stress is depression or anxiety, which, if severe and/or prolonged, amounts to anxiety or depressive disorder. Bereavement is a typical environmental stress that may be followed by the onset of depression; it may also be associated with the increased onset of serious physical illness. The mortality of widowers has been shown to increase 40% during the 6 months following the loss of their wives.

This means that the combination of a physical (organic) disorder and concurrent anxiety or depressive disorder is common; approximately one in five people with a serious and/or disabling physical illness have concurrent anxiety or depression. Depressed people with physical illness experience more severe pain, view their illness more seriously, and feel that the chance of recovery is lower. This view of the illness can lead to a delay in the return to normal activities, such as return to work or resuming a normal sexual relationship after a heart attack.

A woman with rheumatoid arthritis, for example, whose husband also has a disabling illness can be described as being under stress, partly because of her own illness and partly because of her husband's illness. These two stresses may lead to depression, in which case the pain worsens and the illness appears to be worse. Her going to a rheumatology clinic may lead to a change in the treatment for her rheumatoid arthritis, but only if the depression is recognized and treated will the patient's health begin to return. For this reason, modern medicine is increasingly keen to identify anxiety and depressive disorders in patients with chronic diseases, as well as the accompanying environmental stress.

Further Reading

Creed, F. H. (1993). Stress and psychosomatic disorders. In: Goldberger, L. & Breznitz, S. (eds.) *Handbook of stress: theoretical and clinical aspects*, pp. 496–510. New York: Macmillan.

Cohen, S., Tyrrel, D. A. J. and Smith, S. P. (1991). Psychological stress and susceptibility to the common cold. *New England Journal of Medicine* **325**, 606–612.
Dickens, C. M., McGowan, L., Percival, C., et al. (2004). Lack of a close confidant, but not depression, predicts further cardiac events after myocardial infarction. *Heart* **90**(5), 518–522.
Frasure-Smith, N., Lesperance, F. and Talajic, M. (1993). Depression following myocardial infarction: impact on 6-month survival. *Journal of the American Medical Association* **270**, 1819–1825.
Hemingway, H. and Marmot, M. (1993). Evidence based cardiology: psychosocial factors in the aetiology and prognosis of coronary heart disease. Systematic review of prospective cohort studies. *British Medical Journal* **318**, 1460–1467.
Matsushima, Y., Aoyama, N., Fukuda, H., et al. (1999). Gastric ulcer formation after the Hanshin-Awaji earthquake: a case study of Helicobacter pylori infection and stress-induced gastric ulcers. *Helicobacter* **4**, 94–99.
Vedhara, K., Cox, N. K., Wilcock, G. K., et al. (1999). Chronic stress in elderly carers of dementia patients and antibody response to influenza vaccination. *Lancet* **353**, 627–631.
World Health Organisation (1964) *Psychosomatic Disorders. Thirteenth Report of the WHO Expert Committee on Mental Health.* Geneva: World Health Organisation.

Arthritis - Psychological

J W Younger and A J Zautra
Arizona State University, Tempe, AZ, USA

Glossary

Adrenocorticotropic hormone (ACTH)	A hormone secreted by the pituitary that stimulates the adrenal gland to produce cortisol.
Arthritis	An inflammatory condition, primarily involving joints and surrounding tissue, that causes pain and may restrict mobility.
Catecholamines	Chemicals that serve as stress neurotransmitters in the nervous system and that are also secreted as hormones by the adrenal gland.
Cortisol (hydrocortisone)	A primary glucocorticoid that mobilizes energy for stress responses and serves as a potent anti-inflammatory and immunosuppressant.
Epinephrine (adrenaline)	One of the catecholamines responsible for the sympathetic (fight-or-flight) response.
Flare	Sharp but transient increases of inflammation and pain in some types of arthritis.
Hypothalamic-pituitary-adrenal (HPA) axis	A major neuroendocrine system involved in stress responses and responsible for production of catecholamines and cortisol.
Pannus	An abnormal growth of synovial tissue that is associated with joint destruction.
Proinflammatory cytokines	Intercellular immune messengers that increase inflammatory responses.
Synovium	A fluid-filled membrane that surrounds joints and provides joint protection, lubrication, and nutrition.

Definition

Arthritis is a term that covers over 100 inflammatory and degenerative joint conditions. The most common forms include osteoarthritis, rheumatoid arthritis, gout, ankylosing spondylitis, juvenile arthritis, psoriatic arthritis, and systemic lupus erythematosus. Despite having different etiologies, including infection, autoimmune pathology, and physical trauma, these conditions are tied together by common characteristics of chronic pain and impairment in daily functioning. Stress–arthritis research has focused mainly on the two most common forms: rheumatoid arthritis (RA) and osteoarthritis (OA).

Stress and Rheumatoid Arthritis

RA affects approximately 3 million people in the United States and is three times more likely to occur in women than men. This autoimmune disorder is characterized by the inflammation of the synovium surrounding joints. The disease is typically symmetric, affecting the same joints on both sides of the body.

Symptoms include swollen and/or tender joints as well as fatigue, low-grade fever, and general malaise. Many individuals with RA also experience episodic flares, in which symptoms are intensified. RA progresses from initial synovial inflammation to abnormal growth of the synovial tissue (pannus), which overgrows the joint area and breaks down surrounding bone and cartilage through the release of enzymes. RA can be severely disabling because of chronic pain and restricted joint flexibility.

Does Stress Exacerbate Rheumatoid Arthritis Symptoms?

Some evidence supports the view that stress may contribute to the onset of RA, but methodological challenges of retrospection diminish confidence in a number of these findings. A much stronger case has been made, however, for stress as being an aggravating factor in RA disease course. Minor stressors and daily hassles have, in particular, been linked to both self-reported pain and objective markers of inflammation. Both work stress and interpersonal stress predict increases of disease severity, and depression may further elevate stress-related inflammatory processes. Major acute stressors such as the sudden death of a spouse, on the other hand, may actually diminish the inflammatory response during the period of stress adaptation.

Biological support for stress–RA relations have focused mainly on proinflammatory cytokines, intercellular messengers responsible for triggering inflammatory immune responses. Many cytokines, including interleukin (IL)-1, IL-6, and tumor necrosis factor alpha (TNF-α) are stimulated by infection, physical trauma, and psychological stress. These stress-activated cytokines are also implicated in RA pathophysiology to the extent that many pharmaceutical treatments are designed to suppress either the general immune system or specific cytokines. Biological response modifiers, the newest class of RA drugs, bind to proinflammatory cytokines and prevent their interaction with cell-surface receptors, thus inhibiting inflammatory immune responses.

In healthy individuals, the anti-inflammatory hormone cortisol (hydrocortisone) acts as an immunomodulator, suppressing both the production and activity of proinflammatory cytokines. Cortisol production may be induced through a stress response or triggered by increased levels of IL-6, serving as a modulating feedback loop. When endogenous cortisol levels are low, proinflammatory cytokine levels and disease activity are high. Daily circadian dips of cortisol in the early morning and late evening are associated with higher joint pain. Also, as cortisol levels diminish through late adulthood and old age, RA joint pain worsens. The recognition of hydrocortisone's anti-inflammatory properties led the wide use of externally administered glucocorticoids for managing RA symptoms.

Given that some stress hormones such as cortisol reduce proinflammatory cytokine activity, it may appear contradictory that stress increases pain in RA patients. It is important to note, however, that both pro- and anti-inflammatory agents are released during the stress response. Some stress hormones, such as prolactin, are proinflammatory.

The central pathophysiology of RA, then, may lie in the relative underactivity of anti-inflammatory agents compared with pro-inflammatory agents. This hypothesis is supported by observed dysregulations in the HPA axis. In RA, the HPA axis is probably underactive, leading to insufficient production of cortisol. Specifically, decreased cortisol secretion has been linked to diminished adrenal responsiveness to ACTH stimulation. RA patients may also exhibit abnormal responses to stress-induced catecholamines. In particular, it has been observed that externally administered epinephrine decreases cortisol in RA patients but not in healthy controls. If internal, stress-induced production of epinephrine similarly suppresses cortisol in RA patients, a proinflammatory state may be created, leading to the clinical observations of joint swelling and tenderness.

In addition to direct effects on peripheral sites of pain, stress may influence central processes involved in the affective responses to pain. Under periods of high stress and distress, RA symptoms and pain may be more salient. Conversely, positive emotion may buffer RA patients from the negative affective responses to pain, lowering stress reactivity and thus indirectly diminishing inflammatory processes.

Cognitive and Affective Factors in Rheumatoid Arthritis Stress–Pain Cycles

Given the exacerbating role of stress on RA symptoms, it is important to note that the disease itself may be a significant source of stress for afflicted individuals. In addition to pain, RA patients can suffer extensive physical limitations, which may lead to depressive symptoms and increased dependence on others. Activity limitations due to motion restriction and pain can affect every part of a person's life, impairing his or her ability to work, limiting recreational/social activities, and straining familial relationships. These physical and psychosocial stressors may further exacerbate pain and affect the disease course, potentially leading to a cycle of ever-increasing pain and stress. Not everyone is adversely affected by the disease, however, and many cognitive factors have been found to partially determine the impact of

RA on a person's life. Premorbid depression, beliefs about the consequences of arthritis, and coping style all predict a more severe disease course. Resilient personality features and a strong social support network may sustain quality of life and forestall disability even among those with active disease. Positive emotion has also been associated with a reduction in proinflammatory cytokine activity and pain, suggesting that greater attention to emotion regulation may foster resilience.

The discovery of modulating cognitive factors has led to many psychological interventions for RA. Cognitive-behavioral interventions for arthritis management increase self-efficacy, reduce maladaptive coping styles, and decrease helplessness. By changing personal mastery, these therapies reduce negative interpretations of the disease and prevent an accumulation of stress that could further advance disease severity.

Stress and Osteoarthritis

OA is the most common form of arthritis, affecting nearly 30 million individuals in the United States. Symptoms of OA include joint pain, stiffness, and loss of mobility. Affected joints may include the knees, hips, lower back, neck, fingers, and the base of the thumb and big toe. Pain and stiffness is usually the most severe following long periods of inactivity, such as on waking in the morning. The disease is characterized by abnormalities in the cartilage, beginning first with a loss of elasticity. This initial stage is followed by the damage to surrounding bone, including the formation of growths and cysts. These malformations interfere with joint movement and cause pain. In later stages, the synovium may become inflamed, leading to immune involvement and further cartilage damage and pain.

Although the pathophysiological profile of OA is very different from RA, many OA patients also suffer from considerable pain and physical limitation. OA sufferers complain of many daily stressors: pain, disability, and dependence on others. Fluctuations of OA pain are, like RA, influenced by daily stress. Unlike RA, there is little evidence that stress affects the disease processes.

Cognition and emotion regulation may serve as modulators between physical limitation/pain and consequent distress, however, and a number of factors can increase life satisfaction in those with OA. Greater self-efficacy and strong perceived social support both predict increased life satisfaction. Effective interventions often target these factors. Behavioral and cognitive-behavioral approaches may also help increase activities such as exercise that ease joint pain, increase mobility, and provide psychophysiological stress-buffering effects. Newer emotion-regulation interventions such as mindfulness meditation also show promise as a means of reducing the distress associated with pain episodes. These interventions may enhance psychological well-being, even for those with substantial disease.

A Special Case: Arthritis in Children

Individuals with juvenile arthritis (JA) suffer from complaints very similar to adult RA and OA. As with adult arthritis, there are associations between significant life stress and the development of JA, although a conclusive link cannot yet be drawn. Further, the same cognitive/coping factors seem to play important roles in determining the disease impact on life satisfaction.

Despite similarities, JA may be distinguished from adult arthritis by the added impact of the disease on social and psychological development. Children with JA most often complain of the disease hampering their performance in class, limiting their extracurricular activities, and limiting their activities with peers. Stress resulting from diminished social activities during critical development periods may have an impact on long-term psychological adjustment. Disease severity, however, is not always associated with psychological adjustment, suggesting that some variables play moderating roles. In particular, the child's attitude toward illness (positive or negative) can moderate the relationship between stress and adjustment, buffering the development of depression and strengthening the capacity for resilience. Major tasks for both parents and therapists, then, may be to teach alternative ways to interpret the disease, increase self-efficacy, and further the development of emotional maturity. These strategies for disease management should be maintained even when the child needs support for the physical tasks in everyday life.

See Also the Following Articles

Pain.

Further Reading

Astin, J. A., Beckner, M., Wright, K., et al. (2002). Psychological interventions in rheumatoid arthritis: a meta-analysis of randomized control trials. *Arthritis Care and Research* **47**, 291–302.

Crofford, L. J. (2002). The hypothalamic-pituitary-adrenal axis in the pathogenesis of rheumatic diseases. *Endocrinology and Metabolism Clinics of North America* **31**, 1–13.

Cutolo, M. and Masi, A. T. (2005). Circadian rhythms and arthritis. *Rheumatic Diseases Clinics of North America* **31**, 115–129.
Cutolo, M., Sulli, A., Pizzorni, C., et al. (2003). Hypothalamic-pituitary-adrenocortical and gonadal functions in rheumatoid arthritis. *Annals of the New York Academy of Sciences* **992**, 107–117.
Herrmann, M., Scholmerich, J. and Straub, R. H. (2000). Stress and rheumatic diseases. *Rheumatic Diseases Clinics of North America* **26**, 1–27.
LeBovidge, J. S., Lavigne, J. V., Miller, M. L., et al. (2005). Adjustment to chronic arthritis of childhood: the roles of illness-related stress and attitude toward illness. *Journal of Pediatric Psychology* **30**, 273–285.
McEwen, B. S., Biron, C. A., Brunson, et al. (1997). The role of adrenocorticoids as modulators of immune function in health and disease: neural, endocrine and immune interactions. *Brain Research and Brain Research Review* **23**, 79–133.
Raison, C. L. and Miller, A. H. (2003). When not enough is too much: the role of insufficient glucocorticoid signaling in the pathophysiology of stress-related disorders. *American Journal of Psychiatry* **160**, 1554–1565.
Sharpe, L., Sensky, T. and Allard, S. (2001). The course of depression in recent onset rheumatoid arthritis: the predictive role of disability, illness perceptions, pain and coping. *Journal of Psychosomatic Research* **51**, 713–719.
Straub, R. H., Dhabhar, F. S., Bijlsma, J. W., et al. (2005). How psychological stress via hormones and nerve fibers may exacerbate rheumatoid arthritis. *Arthritis & Rheumatism* **52**, 16–26.
Straub, R. H., Kittner, J. M., Hiejnen, C., et al. (2002). Infusion of epinephrine decrease serum levels of cortisol and 17-hydroxyprogesterone in patients with rheumatoid arthritis. *Journal of Rheumatology* **29**, 1659–1664.
Wilder, R. L. (2002). Neuroimmunoendocrinology of the rheumatic diseases: past, present, and future. *Annals of the New York Academy of Sciences* **966**, 13–19.
Zautra, A. J. (2003). *Emotions, stress, and health.* New York: Oxford University Press.
Zautra, A. J., Smith, B. W. and Yocum, D. (2002). Psychosocial influences on arthritis-related disease activity. In: Sivik, T., Byne, D., Lipsitt, D. R., Christodoulou, G. N. & Dienstfrey, H. (eds.) *Psycho-neuro-endocrino-immunology (PNEI):. a common language for the whole human body*, pp. 201–207. Amsterdam: Elsevier.
Zautra, A. J., Yocum, D. C., Villanueva, I., et al. (2004). Immune activation and depression in women with rheumatoid arthritis. *Journal of Rheumatology* **31**, 457–463.

Diet and Stress, Psychiatric

V March and M H Fernstrom
University of Pittsburgh Medical Center, Pittsburgh, PA, USA

Glossary

Behavioral modification — A specific set of counseling techniques using specific tools to change an individual's behavior by altering habitual thoughts and activities in specific situations.

Body mass index (BMI) — The formula of weight (in kilograms)/height (in meters) squared that is used to quantitate medical overweight and obesity. Healthy BMI = 18.5–24.9; Overweight = 25–29.9; Class I Obesity = 30–34.9; Class II Obesity = 35–39.9; Class III Obesity = 40 and above.

Central adiposity — Body fat concentrated in the abdomen; even in the absence of overweight or obesity, this may alone increase cardiovascular risk.

Lifestyle changes — The stepwise substitutions of unhealthful behaviors with more healthful ones, with the goal of improving health, including weight management.

Readiness — An index of individual willingness and motivation to make lifestyle changes leading to better health.

Stress — A biological condition altering brain and metabolic functions as the body responds to a noxious or life-threatening stimulus.

Stress eating — Overeating with a perceived lack of control in response to behavioral stressors; also called emotional eating.

Introduction

Over the past 3 decades, the surging numbers of overweight and obese individuals worldwide have prompted the use of the term obesity epidemic to describe this phenomenon. Not only adult but also young children and adolescents are affected, putting these populations at risk for obesity-related comorbidities, including sleep apnea, hypertension, and type II diabetes. Many hypotheses have been proposed to explain the increasing rate of obesity, including both biological and environmental factors. Although larger portions, readily available food, and lack of activity all contribute to weight gain, the perception of a stressful environment is often raised by patients, both adults and children, as a major reason for overeating and weight gain. The term stress eating, also called emotional eating, has been used to describe eating behavior in which an individual responds to a mentally stressful situation with uncontrolled eating of high-calorie foods, even in the absence of hunger.

Stress can be loosely defined as a physical or emotional response by which the organism attempts to protect itself. A stressor, whether environmental (exogenous) or biological (endogenous), can cause certain physiological changes to occur. These changes, both biochemical and hormonal, permit an organism to adapt in survival mode. The adrenal hormones epinephrine, norepinephrine, and cortisol modulate the metabolic stress response in animals. During this fight-or-flight reaction, these hormones modify blood flow by increasing circulation to the heart, lungs, and skeletal muscle to facilitate escape while decreasing circulation to nonessential areas, including the splanchnic vasculature supplying the gastrointestinal tract. This classic stress response is not compatible with eating.

However, excessive cortisol secretion alone seems to stimulate appetite in certain individuals and has been shown to be a factor in visceral and abdominal fat distribution in humans. This is illustrated in the extreme in (1) Cushing's syndrome and Cushing's disease, disorders that both involve an overproduction of cortisol by the adrenal glands, and (2) people receiving high-dose corticosteroid therapy. Because of this pattern of appetite increase and fat deposition, some investigators have postulated that stress in animals (including humans) causes high cortisol levels, which, in turn, lead to stress-eating responses. Data supporting this hypothesis have been inconsistent, which is not surprising given the complexity of hypothalamic and gut signaling of hunger and fullness control, as well as the newly discovered role of adipocytes in appetite regulation.

In this article, we summarize the most recent research on stress eating in animal models and in humans. We also discuss environmental and psychosocial factors contributing to overeating and weight gain. Our clinical experience serves as a resource to identify practical strategies for the clinical management of stress eating in overweight and obese patients.

Biological Basis of Stress Eating

Current medical literature is replete with articles on both the psychological and physiological responses to stress. The animal literature typically exposes animals to noxious stimuli (including isolation, tail pinch, electric shock, cold water immersion) and examines food consumption. The results of these studies have been diverse. Following the stressors, both eating response and the weight of subjects have been variable, either increasing or decreasing compared to controls. A recent series of studies in rats using restraint as a stressor measured caloric intake, caloric efficiency, body weight, intra-abdominal fat, and hormonal levels including adrenocorticotropic hormone (ACTH), insulin, and leptin. The results indicated that, although weight tended to vary after stress, the deposit of abdominal fat and the consumption of comfort foods (lard and sucrose-sweetened beverages) in proportion to chow increased. The authors suggested that the ingestion of comfort foods appeared to decrease stress hormone responses. They further speculated that the same type of response might occur in humans.

Human studies have typically addressed the interaction of stress and overeating by examining the hypothalamic-pituitary-adrenal axis. In controlled laboratory studies, stress is induced with either physiological or environmental manipulations, and hormonal measurements and/or eating behavior are measured. A blunting of the usual adrenal cortisol response to the pituitary-stimulating hormone ACTH is often reported. Other studies have indicated that laboratory stressors produced increases in serum cortisol response that could be positively correlated with the increased consumption of sweet and high-fat foods.

The discordant conclusions of both the animal and human studies have prompted more questions than answers. Nonetheless, there is general acknowledgment that stress-eating behavior exists and that it may pose a significant barrier to the treatment of obesity. If we are to treat obesity effectively, practical recommendations for treatment of stress eating are needed even before a complete understanding of the neurological and metabolic basis for this phenomenon is reached.

Practical Treatment of Stress Eating

A key element of stress eating is the consumption of food in the absence of physical hunger, often to the point of being uncomfortably full. Frequently, stress eating results in a sensation of uncomfortable fullness followed by feelings of guilt, self-hatred, and self-disgust.

The pattern of stress-related overeating is heterogeneous both among and within individuals and may include constant grazing, binge-eating, and nighttime eating. During an episode of stress eating, significant quantities of comfort foods are consumed, uniformly described as palatable and most often sugar–fat or salty–fat combinations. Left untreated, regular stress eating may contribute to the obesity.

Following an incident of stress eating, an individual may attempt to compensate by consciously curtailing food intake. This restrained eating, in turn, may trigger more stress eating. Stress eating may be continuous over variable stretches of time or brief, depending on the intensity and duration of the stressor. Many environmental factors that increase anxiety may contribute to stress eating in both children and adults. These include frightening world events, financial worries, and occupational or domestic demands. Habitual exercise, which could help offset stress-eating through both regular calorie expenditure and stress reduction, is often avoided because of time constraints, concerns for personal safety, reductions in gym classes for youths, and increasing dependence for entertainment on more passive activities, such as television, computer and video games.

Despite the increased incidence of obesity, there remains the societal pressure to be thin. The quest for thinness at any cost abounds, but the ideal body type promoted in the media is not realistic for most people. A vicious cycle may occur when the failure of attempts at quick weight loss lowers an individual's self-esteem and increases frustration, inciting further episodes of stress eating. In order to break this cycle, active intervention is required. What is effective intervention? The health-care community must help refocus our society's expectations by helping the individual set realistic goals for achieving a healthy weight. People tend to do well when very small yet incremental behavioral changes are adopted initially. The goal of better health, not a specific weight, should be emphasized; as little as a 5% reduction in weight can improve health significantly. Motivational interviewing, a form of nonthreatening history-taking, enables the practitioner to identify unhealthful eating behaviors in a patient while simultaneously permitting a collaborative interaction in which the patient determines the course of action and the clinician serves as a facilitator. To best assist a patient, the health-care provider should become familiar with some basic behavioral modification techniques.

Overview of Lifestyle Change

Stress eating may be considered one of several types of nonhunger eating, that is, eating that is unrelated to physiological hunger. Rarely do stress-eaters complain of hunger symptoms (e.g., sweating, headache, poor concentration, irritability, lightheadedness, racing pulse, and hypotension) prior to food consumption. In fact, most of these individuals acknowledge no feelings of hunger when feeling the urge to stress eat. Although there is no consensus about treatment, the National Weight Control Registry has been tracking a cohort of 3000 individuals who have lost at least 30 pounds and kept it off for at least 1 year. Started in 1994, the Registry has identified five behaviors contributing to long-term weight loss: (1) maintaining high levels of physical activity; (2) following a low-fat, low-calorie high-carbohydrate diet; (3) monitoring food intake and weight; (4) possessing coping skills enabling the continuation of weight-loss strategies despite stressful situations or cravings; and (5) eating breakfast. Although it is not known whether these recommendations will help for stress eating by itself, it is reasonable to use these tools to manage weight over the long term.

Overcoming Therapeutic Barriers

Many health-care professionals, even when provided with materials, do not discuss weight control with their patients. The reasons for this are unclear, but there are probably at least two: (1) The discussion of lifestyle change is time-consuming and cannot easily be accommodated by the typical 10- to 20-min patient visit and (2) clinicians may hesitate to broach the subject of weight because many of them are overweight or obese themselves, they are afraid they might insult the patient, and they may feel incompetent to discuss weight management because the medical education curricula today generally do not incorporate courses related to weight control. Nonetheless, it is quite possible to include brief patient education sessions about weight management into a primary-care office visit, especially in the context of a longitudinal clinician–patient relationship. For a clinician who cannot or will not spend time on this topic during the office visit, important weight management concepts can be assimilated into patient handouts that can be distributed without discussion or left in the examination and waiting rooms for patients to peruse at their leisure. In addition, the use of a physician-extender can be considered to help guide the weight-loss process.

Use of the Prescription Pad

The clinician's role as medical expert and prescriber of treatment can be a powerful catalyst of change. Patients are likely to take a written prescription more seriously than other modes of medical advice, including verbal instruction and guidance. The use of the prescription pad for dietary and exercise recommendations can be a very useful tool because it lends further credibility to lifestyle change as an actual treatment recommendation. (When necessary, more traditional prescriptions for laboratory testing, weight-loss medications, and/or a surgical consultation can be added.) Moreover, the patient is more likely to remember what has been written down, particularly if there are multiple instructions.

Basic Recommendations for the Primary-Care Clinician

Recommendations, such "eat less; exercise more," although logical, are unhelpful because they are both condescending and too general. The majority of obese individuals are well aware that in order to lose weight, they must eat less and exercise more; however, they do not know how to accomplish this. Therefore, the clinician's suggestions should be specific and individualized.

A clinician can first teach a patient to become more cognizant of the physical signs of hunger and satiety by making the following suggestions.

1. Use a three-point hunger scale to rate feelings of hunger (1 = hungry; 2 = content; 3 = stuffed).
2. Determine when the desire to eat coincides with higher stress levels, with signs of physical hunger, or both.
3. Attempt to delay eating during high levels of stress, particularly if no physical hunger is sensed.
4. Eat slowly – it takes 20 min for the stomach to signal fullness to the brain.
5. After a 100- to 200-Cal snack, find a distraction to help postpone further eating for at least 1 h (encourage noneating, stress-reducing activities).
6. Repeat the phrase, "I can always have more later"; this can reassure an individual who becomes anxious if food is unavailable.
7. Avoid liquid calories; this is a crucial piece of advice because patients often ignore beverages in their calculations of daily calories consumed.

A sense of deprivation often occurs when people eliminate favorite foods from their daily diet. Historically, such foods have been judgmentally referred to as illegal, off-limits, not allowed, and even bad. The avoidance of these foods, in and of itself, can cause mental stress while the forbidden nature of these foods may increase their desirability and thus provide a powerful trigger for stress eating. The uncontrolled eating of allowed foods is a common way to overcompensate for not being permitted to eat the desired food, but this most often results in an overconsumption of total daily calories because the mental hunger has not been fulfilled. Instead, stress-eaters should be given permission to eat their favorite foods in the context of a healthful diet. If no foods are excluded from stress-eaters' diets, compensatory overeating is more likely to be better managed. A caloric allowance for favorite foods should be considered in a day's food intake equation.

Nearly all patients are well aware that insufficient physical activity presents a significant barrier to weight control. Regular physical activity, because it can relieve stress, helps to reduce the need to stress eat. Activity also modestly increases the expenditure of calories, making long-term weight loss success more likely. After medical clearance, the exercise prescription for all sedentary individuals should emphasize a gradual increase in duration and intensity of activity. For sedentary individuals reluctant or unable to exercise, increasing the activities of daily living can provide an alternate route for augmenting calorie expenditure. Activity goal-setting can be accomplished with the use of a pedometer, a small digital instrument which, when clipped to an individual's waistband, records the number of steps taken per day. By demonstrating that simple changes can make a significant difference in overall activity level, a pedometer can also be a motivational tool. The daily step number may be increased with such modifications as parking farther away from work or the store, choosing a more distant bus stop, taking the stairs instead of the elevator, using the manual channel-changer instead of the remote, pacing while talking on the phone, and walking for 5 min during a lunch break.

Other Behavioral Techniques

Many weight management programs, whether commercial or medical center-based, apply the principles of cognitive-behavioral therapy directed at lifestyle change. In the case of lifestyle change related to weight control, these principles can help people strike a more healthful balance in their behaviors relating to both eating and activity. These include self-monitoring, bartering, cognitive restructuring, preplanning, positive self-talking, imaging, and asserting.

- Self-monitoring, one of the most important tools for the stress-eater, has been proven to lead to sustained success. The technique involves recording periodic (i.e., daily or weekly) weights, daily activity, and food intake. Despite the proven efficacy and relative ease of this method, many individuals seem to have difficulty sustaining the effort involved in logging.

• Bartering in behavioral modification terms means making choices. Substitutions, trade-offs, and banking calories are different types of bartering.

• Cognitive restructuring is a technique that allows replacing eating and rumination about food with another behavior. As a cognitive-restructuring exercise, the patient may generate a list of stress-reducing activities. Such activities might include taking a bubble bath, talking to a friend, watching a movie, reading, getting a massage, participating in community or other volunteer work, becoming occupied with a hobby, taking a class, cleaning out drawers, shopping, or rekindling intimacy with a partner.

• Preplanning is a method of preparing for events in which stress eating is likely to occur. Through this process, many patients have been able to retrieve a sense of control over their eating.

• Positive self-talk is another effective way to interrupt the stress-eating pattern. Negative thoughts seem to exacerbate stress eating and should be discouraged; the switch to a more affirmative cognitive process often takes practice. One exercise incorporates patients' transcribing negative thoughts in one column and positive replacement statements in an adjacent column. A variation on this method is for patients to speak aloud or write down all their accomplishments, recent or past, or to congratulate themselves on accomplishments related to weight loss, for example, to say "I am a size smaller than I was 2 months ago" or "I rode the stationary bike for half an hour three times this week." Repeating these sorts of sentences may not only change the patients' thought processes but also help relieve stress, both of which will subsequently promote behavior change.

• Imaging is mental rehearsal. By envisioning an upcoming stressful scenario, individuals may also imagine an appropriate response to the stressor that can later be put into action. Another strategy is to recommend imagining a relaxing situation (e.g., lying on a beach or getting a massage) during a stressful event, a process that, through mitigating the feelings that induce stress eating, may minimize the odds of an actual stress-eating response.

• Asserting is an invaluable tool for the stress-eater. Because individuals stress eat in order to avoid confrontation, teaching strategies to gradually increase self-assertiveness are important. The phrase "I need" is central to learning self-assertiveness. For example, people can be given the homework of becoming assertive in a relatively nonthreatening situation, such as informing a demanding young child, "I need to go take a shower now, and I need privacy while I am doing this."

Understanding and Addressing Failure in a Stress-Eater

The breaking of any unhealthful habit (or addiction) carries with it the risks of lapse, relapse, and collapse. In fact, when the habit is ingrained, lapses are almost inevitable and should be considered a normal part of the habit-changing process.

A lapse is an isolated episode of recurrence of the old habit or behavior. Lapses often occur when people have not planned for an unusual occasion, but they can happen even with the most detailed calculation. A relapse is several episodes in succession of the old pattern of behavior. Vacation commonly provokes a relapse, which, for some, is difficult to reverse. Collapse, a complete abandonment of healthful behaviors, is less likely if the stress-eater, after a single lapse, is able to get right back on the track of a palatable and manageable weight-loss plan. In the event of a lapse or relapse, the stress-eater should be encouraged to bring all behavioral methods to bear, return for weight management visits in order to get the necessary reinforcement, and garner support from friends and family.

Other Therapies: Pharmacotherapy and Surgery

Weight-loss medication should be considered a tool to make the lifestyle effort easier. It is not a replacement for lifestyle, nor should it be viewed as a cure for obesity. Some prescription medications can be used in stress-eaters who exhibit great difficulty with behavior change related to eating and activity. Medications such as sibutramine and buproprion (in depressed obese patients) exert more subtle effects on hunger and satiety and can therefore be employed as teaching devices. However, even with the medications, the signals can be ignored and an individual can eat through the effects of the medications. Therefore, the importance of a complete explanation by the practitioner about the use of these or other weight-loss medications cannot be overemphasized. Sibutramine is approved for long-term use in weight loss, and although active weight loss seems to last for approximately 6–9 months for responders, the weight maintenance effects of the drug may continue for at least 2 years. Bupropion, which is FDA-approved as an antidepressant and as a smoking-cessation adjunct – and not FDA-approved for weight loss – has sometimes been used for weight management in depressed patients. Sibutramine, used either intermittently or continuously, can help promote both weight loss and maintenance. Another medication, orlistat, a pancreatic lipase inhibitor, also has behavioral effects, but not by acting directly on the brain; this medication works by inhibiting the absorption of dietary fat from the intestine. When orlistat is taken as directed and a high-fat meal is consumed, bloating, diarrhea, flatulence, and leakage of foul-smelling stools will occur as a consequence of the decreased dietary fat absorption. The medication allows weight loss in part due to a reduction in the absorption of calories but primarily via its role as a negative reinforcer because the consumption of high-fat comfort foods results in unpleasant side effects. Because this medication has no effect on carbohydrate or protein absorption, total calorie intake may not be reduced.

Bariatric surgery, including both the roux-en-y gastric bypass and laparoscopic gastric banding, is initially considered by many patients to be the cure for obesity. When a severely obese individual (BMI 40 or greater) has been unable to maintain weight loss even with sustained effort, weight loss surgery should be considered. For these patients, either restriction (gastric banding) or a combination of restriction and malabsorption (gastric bypass) can be the missing tool in the weight management toolbox. Obesity surgery allows the motivated patient to sustain a lifestyle effort that results in long-term weight-loss success. The lifestyle after surgery is quite demanding, and patients need to be taught that even after surgery it is possible to regain weight with poor eating habits – including grazing throughout the day and consuming high-calorie liquids. The stress-eater must be taught new behavioral modification techniques to manage stress without food, with these concepts being reinforced after surgery for at least 2–3 years.

Conclusion

Stress can produce both biochemical and behavioral responses in certain individuals, often resulting in stress eating and subsequent weight gain. Stress eating may be an important contributor to the current obesity epidemic. Although the understanding of stress eating is rudimentary at this time, certain behavioral techniques seem to be effective treatments, at least for some patients; many of these therapies are outlined in this article. These strategies can be easily initiated by a wide range of health-care providers during routine outpatient office visits and need not be time-consuming. Although all patients will not respond, many patients will benefit from a brief review of treatment options.

Changing eating behavior is difficult, but it is possible when a stress-eater is motivated to change and is willing to put in the effort. Assistance from health-care providers may facilitate lifestyle changes sufficient for many patients to achieve long-term weight-loss success. A basic understanding of simple behavioral modification will allow a more effective treatment of obesity in the primary-care setting. In certain individuals who are refractory to such methods alone, referral to a comprehensive weight management program may be necessary, particularly for the coordination of the more complex modalities of cognitive-behavioral methods, diet and exercise education, and the judicious use of medications and surgery.

Further Reading

Dallman, M. F., Pecoraro, N., Akana, S. F., et al. (2003). Chronic stress and obesity: a new view of "comfort food." *Proceedings of the National Academy of Sciences USA* **100**, 11696–11701.

Epel, E., Lapidus, R., McEwen, B., et al. (2001). Stress may add bite to appetite in women: a laboratory study of stress-induced cortisol and eating behavior. *Psychoneuroendocrinology* **26**, 37–49.

Habib, K. E., Gold, P. W. and Chrousos, G. P. (2001). Neuroendocrinology of stress. *Endocrinology & Metabolism Clinics of North America* **30**, vii–viii, 695–728.

Jessop, D. S., Dallman, M. F., Fleming, D., et al. (2001). Resistance to glucocorticoid feedback in obesity. *Journal of Clinical Endocrinology and Metabolism* **86**, 4109–4114.

Klem, M. L., Wing, R. R., McGuire, M. T., et al. (1997). A descriptive study of individuals successful at long-term maintenance of substantial weight loss. *American Journal of Clinical Nutrition* **66**, 239–246.

Kouvonen, A., Kivimaki, M., Cox, S. J., et al. (2005). Relationship between work stress and body mass index among 45,810 female and male employees. *Psychosomatic Medicine* **67**, 577–583.

Lichtman, S. W., Pisarska, K., Berman, E. R., et al. (1992). Discrepancy between self-reported and actual caloric intake and exercise in obese subjects. *New England Journal of Medicine* **327**, 1893–1898.

Lowe, M. R. and Levine, A. S. (2005). Eating motives and the controversy over dieting: eating less than needed versus less than wanted. *Obesity Research* **13**, 797–806.

Pecoraro, N., Reyes, F., Gomez, F., et al. (2004). Chronic stress promotes palatable feeding, which reduces signs of stress: feedforward and feedback effects of chronic stress. *Endocrinology* **145**, 3754–3762.

Stafford, R. S., Farhat, J. H., Misra, B., et al. (2000). National patterns of physician activities related to obesity management. *Archives of Family Medicine* **9**, 631–638.

Yin, Z., Davis, C. L., Moore, J. B., et al. (2005). Physical activity buffers the effects of chronic stress on adiposity in youth. *Annals of Behavioral Medicine* **29**, 29–36.

Diet and Stress, Non-Psychiatric

J Wardle
University College London, London, UK
E L Gibson
Roehampton University, London, UK

This is a revised version of the article by J Wardle, Encyclopedia of Stress First Edition, volume 1, pp 694–698, © 2000, Elsevier Inc.

Glossary

Dieting	Deliberate modification of food intake in order to lose weight.
Disinhibition	Acute loss of cognitive control over food intake.
Emotional eating	Eating in response to emotional cues.
Hyperphagia	Eating more than usual.
Hypophagia	Eating less than usual.
Restrained eating	The chronic tendency to try to exert control over food intake. It was first measured with the Restraint Scale, which in addition to items reflecting attempts to diet, included loss of control over eating and weight fluctuation. More recent measures of restraint have placed greater emphasis on the dieting component, conceptualizing the episodes of loss of control as forms of disinhibition of restraint, rather than part of the core concept.

Introduction

There is a widespread belief that stress influences eating behavior, but considerable uncertainty about the direction of the effect, i.e., whether stress increases or decreases food intake. An analysis of the physiology of stress would lead us to expect decreased eating, because stress slows gastric emptying and increases energy substrate levels, which should reduce appetite. Stress also promotes behaviors designed to cope with or escape from the source of stress, and under these circumstances, eating might be accorded a lower priority. In contrast, the literature on human reactions to stress suggests that it can be associated with increased food intake or a shift toward a higher fat diet.

Our knowledge of stress and eating comes from diverse areas of research, including clinical studies on the etiology of obesity and eating disorders, laboratory studies on dieting and the regulation of food intake, surveys of stress and health-related behaviors, and animal work on stress responses. The diversity of this literature means that there is great variation in the sources and intensity of the stressors that have been examined, the circumstances in which food is consumed, the quality of dietary information that can be gathered, and the populations that have been studied. On this basis, it may not be surprising to find that the links between stress and eating appear to be complex.

Animal Research into Stress and Eating Behavior

Animal research appears to offer the ideal opportunity to examine the general, physiologically mediated effect of stress on food intake. Animals can be exposed to stress or a control condition; stressors can vary in quality, intensity, or duration; the animal's deprivation state can be manipulated; and the type of food supplied can be varied. However, to date, this research has produced an extraordinarily inconsistent set of results. Much of the early work used rats as the experimental subjects and tail pinch as the stressor and typically found that food intake was increased by this procedure. However, tail pinch is now thought to represent an atypical stressor, if it is even stressful at all, and increased eating may be part of a general increase in oral behaviors, rather than a specific behavioral response. Other stressors have included electric shock, noise, immobilization, isolation, housing changes, cold water swims, and defeat in fights, with varied effects on food intake from study to study, ranging from substantial increases in food intake in some studies to substantial decreases in other studies. Attempts to relate the direction of the effect on eating to the characteristics of the stressor have so far been unsuccessful, partly because many of the stressors have been used in only a handful of studies, whereas electric shock, which has been used often, shows inexplicable variation. To date, the only possible consistencies are that chronic stressors appear to be more likely to have a hyperphagic effect and social stressors may be more hyperphagic than physical stressors.

Recent animal research has provided some more fruitful results by considering individual differences in susceptibility to stress. For example, rats that are resistant to dietary-induced obesity seem to be hyperresponsive to stress, at both the neurohormonal and behavioral level, compared to those rats that become obese when allowed to overeat. Intriguingly, it has recently been shown that it is the ability to choose from separate sources of energy-dense palatable foods that confers stress resilience, rather than an increase in energy-dense food intake per se.

Human Research into Stress and Food Intake

Human research on stress and food intake has come from several research traditions. Naturalistic studies usually investigate community samples and attempt to gather information on food intake at high- and low-stress periods of life. The focus in these studies, as in most of the animal research, has been on the general effect of stress on eating over the short or medium term. Laboratory studies usually administer a stressful procedure in parallel with an eating task, then covertly assess food intake. The emphasis therefore is on the acute effects of stress. Most of the laboratory studies have taken an individual differences perspective, examining stress-related eating in relation either to weight or dietary restraint.

Naturalistic Studies

There is a variety of naturally occurring, but predictable, stressful circumstances that can provide an experimental context in which to study stress-related variations in diet. School or university examinations have been used as the stressor in several studies, and periods of high work stress in others. Food intake is recorded either in a diary record kept by the study participants or with a 24-h recall procedure. The food records are then analyzed to obtain estimates of intake of energy and nutrients. Biological measures such as weight or blood lipids have been included in some studies to provide another indicator of dietary change.

Among the published studies there is one element of consistency, namely, none of them has found lower food intake, on average, during the higher stress time. Likewise, there is little evidence for lower weight or lower serum cholesterol under stress. Otherwise, the results have been divided. In some of the studies, both overall energy intake and intake of fat are higher at the high-stress time. In other studies, there is enormous individual variability, but no average difference in energy intake between low- and high-stress periods. In a recent study, mood and eating were sampled at random intervals in students awaiting an exam in a few days. They reported more negative moods, together with an increase in reported eating for distraction, relative to an exam-free control group. However, no differences were found for food intake or choice. In another study, which unlike many naturalistic studies was not confounded by the passage of time, high workload in department store workers was associated with higher fat, sugar, and total energy intake, but only in people who habitually restrained their food intake.

In a recent survey of a large number of U.S. teenagers, depressive symptoms were associated with perceived barriers to healthy eating, meal skipping, and more disordered eating, although the only significant change in diet appeared to be increased consumption of soft drinks in more depressed school children. In a Finnish population-based study of adults, stress-driven eaters ate more energy-dense high-fat foods and had higher body mass indices. Other studies have suggested a link between stressful life events and higher body weight. However, this does not necessarily imply increased eating, since reduced physical activity may also be an important contributor. For example, parents of a child recently diagnosed with cancer gained more weight over 3 months compared to parents with a healthy child. However, since they also reported both less physical activity and lower energy intake, it is likely that most of the weight gain was attributable to a stress-induced reduction in activity.

The balance of evidence so far has to be that stress in everyday life rarely appears to have a hypophagic effect, and it may, in some people and some circumstances, have a hyperphagic effect.

One explanation for the variability in results is the poor validity and reliability of measures of food intake. Keeping a food diary is an onerous task, so compliance is poor, and even among those who return a diary there are likely to be errors: people forget foods, are not able to assess quantities accurately, and often complete the diary well after the eating event. Diary keeping is also reactive, i.e., it is likely to influence the behavior being monitored, because of either the increased attention or the wish to present a good record to the experimenter. Unscheduled 24-h recalls avoid the problem of reactivity, but are still susceptible to forgetting and misreporting, as well as providing a much more restricted snapshot of food intake. Methodological problems also arise from translating typical information on food intake (e.g., "I had a medium-sized cheese sandwich, but I am not sure if the bread was spread with butter or margarine, or what type of cheese it was") into any meaningful value for energy and nutrient intake. Even expert dietitians are reduced to estimating and guessing a good deal of the time. The poor data quality means that any results must be evaluated cautiously, and results from small samples could easily give a misleading impression.

A second explanation for variability in the results is the different kinds of stressor. The animal literature suggests that physical stressors might be more likely to elicit hypophagia, and social stressors, hyperphagia. In human experiences, the stress of surgery for a hernia, which was used in one study, is qualitatively and quantitatively different from the stress of an examination or a period of long working hours used in others, and this difference could well have an effect on food intake. Some stressors could occur together with changes in circumstances that enforce a change in eating behavior even if there is no direct effect of the stress on appetite. However, at present there are too few human studies to make any systematic analyses of the differential effects of different types of stressor.

The third explanation is that individuals might vary in their response to stress, and the admixture of response types could differ from study to study. Few naturalistic studies have taken an individual difference perspective, but those that do indicate that there are important individual differences that need to be considered in examining the effects of stress. In one study, middle-aged men and women kept daily stress diaries over several weeks and at the same time recorded whether, on that day, they had eaten more, the same, or less than usual. The pattern of results showed that most individuals were consistent in their reactions to stress, with some consistently eating more on higher stress days, and others consistently eating less. Over the sample as a whole, the hypophagic response predominated. Similarly, in surveys that ask respondents about how stress affects their eating, the majority report some effect of stress, with approximately equal proportions saying that they eat more and eat less while under stress.

Laboratory Studies

Most laboratory studies have been based on the idea that the biologically natural response to stress is hypophagia, but that individuals who are either overweight or highly restrained eaters are unresponsive to their internal signals. Participants are therefore characterized according to these features and hypothesized to respond differently to stress.

Laboratory studies have used a range of stressors, including unpleasant films, false heart rate feedback, and threat of public speaking. In the typical design, participants are exposed either to the stressor or to a control procedure, and food intake is assessed covertly, often disguised as a taste test in which participants are asked to taste and rate some flavors of a palatable food such as ice cream. The amount that is eaten is recorded accurately by preweighing then reweighing the food containers.

Obesity and stress-induced eating The clinical interest in stress-related eating stemmed from the psychosomatic theory of obesity, which suggested that for the obese, eating met emotional rather than nutritional needs, and that the tendency toward emotional eating explained why they had become obese in the first place. Eating was hypothesized to provide reassurance, and hence stress was predicted to trigger higher-than-usual food intake, so-called emotional eating. There is no doubt that many obese people report that they eat more under stress, but these clinical reports need to be examined in controlled studies, both to establish their validity and to see whether stress-related eating is specific to obesity.

In practice, laboratory studies on stress-related eating in the obese have produced mixed results, with some finding higher intake under stress in the obese and others not. There has also been variability in naturalistic studies, but on balance, there is probably enough evidence to conclude that obesity is an indicator of a higher risk of stress-induced hyperphagia, or at least a lower likelihood of stress hypophagia.

The other side of the psychosomatic theory was that eating would have an anxiolytic effect, and this has received less support. Clinically, many obese people admit that any solace they derive from eating is transient and rapidly followed by shame and regret at not having showed more self-control. In laboratory studies there has been no evidence that eating successfully reduces emotional arousal. These observations have largely discredited the basic idea of the psychosomatic theory, the idea that obesity represents a disorder of emotional reactions. However, there is still interest in the idea that the obese have a reduced sensitivity to internal satiety cues, and the fact that they do not show stress hypophagia may be a consequence of this lack of internal responsiveness.

Stress, restraint, and emotional eating In 1972, a radical alternative to the psychosomatic theory of obesity was proposed, namely, that any abnormalities of eating observed in the obese were not pre-existing tendencies, but a consequence of the steps that they were taking to reduce their weight. At first the emphasis was on the effects of maintaining a body size below the hypothesized set-point. This was superseded by Restraint Theory, which proposed that one of the important determinants of food intake regulation was the tendency toward restrained eating – the combination of concern about eating and weight fluctuation. Most obese people and a significant proportion of normal-weight adults, particularly women, are constantly trying to restrict their food intake in order to reduce their weight. The habit of trying to restrict food intake could have the effect of changing people's relationship with food, such that the usual cues to hunger and fullness become less effective in regulating their eating behavior. Restrained eaters were found to limit their food intake at times when external or emotional pressures were low, but at other times, they would abandon restraint and eat to capacity, so-called disinhibition.

One of the early observations on restrained eating was that, among individuals who experienced anxiety in response to a stressor, food intake was increased among the restrained eaters and decreased among unrestrained eaters. This general pattern, involving an interaction between stress and restraint in predicting food intake, has proved extremely robust. Across many different studies, with a wide range of stressors, restrained eaters almost always eat more in the stressed than in the unstressed condition. In contrast, unrestrained eaters show more variation, sometimes eating the same amount and sometimes eating less while under stress. The results of these laboratory studies have been strikingly consistent in an area in which most of the work is notable for its inconsistency.

There is now a growing interest in examining the role of restraint in predicting individual differences in responses to stress in real-life studies, and so far the results are consistent with the laboratory studies in showing that restrained eaters are more likely to report stress-induced hyperphagia, whereas unrestrained eaters are more likely to report hypophagia. These findings are supported by results from quantitative studies using psychometric measures of restraint and emotional eating, which found that higher restraint was associated with higher levels of emotional eating.

Recently there has been a resurgence of interest in the role of negative affect and emotional eating as predictors of problematic eating and poor control of weight. One reason for this has been the realization that earlier psychometric measures to some extent conflated restrained and emotional eating. Dietary restraint was measured in most studies by the Restraint Scale, which includes the tendency for eating to be disinhibited by emotional states. In one laboratory study, when separate scales were used to measure restraint and emotional eating (Dutch Eating Behaviour Questionnaire), the latter was the better predictor of stress-induced eating. That study tested the effects of public-speaking stress on intake of a variety of foods from sweet, salty, and bland taste categories, and in addition, high- and low-fat examples within those sensory groups. Analyzing effects by taste category may be important because stress and mood have been shown to affect taste perception. The food was presented as a buffet-style meal during preparation of the speech task. Stress did not alter overall intake; however, stressed emotional eaters ate more sweet, high-fat foods (chocolate and cake), and a more energy-dense meal, than either unstressed emotional eaters or nonemotional eaters in either condition. This supports the survey findings that sweet, fatty foods such as chocolate may be preferentially sought during stress or negative affect, at least in a subgroup of susceptible individuals (see next section).

Emotional eating may underlie previous reports that dietary restraint or female gender predicts stress-induced eating. Moreover, emotional eaters may be more susceptible to effects of stress: women who ate more from a selection of snack foods after a stressful task also showed the greatest release of the stress-sensitive hormone, cortisol, and more stress-induced negative affect. These high reactors also showed a preference for sweet foods. So it seems that emotional eaters may be more likely to experience mood disturbance when challenged.

Emotional and disinhibited eating and dietary restraint could interact: the latter seems to contribute to stress-induced eating of sweet, fatty foods by women classified as disinhibited eaters. Recently, it was shown that highly restrained/low emotional eaters ate more chocolate after both ego-threatening and cognitively demanding tasks, whereas low restraint/high emotional eaters ate more chocolate only after the ego threat.

Emotional responses to food may also be sensitive to expectations. In a laboratory study, women were asked to rate various emotions immediately after eating small amounts (5 g) of nine different foods, three being low in energy, three medium, and three high in energy (in counterbalanced order). Intensity of negative moods (sad, ashamed, anxious, sleepy) increased with increasing energy density of the foods, and more so for overweight than for normal-weight women. Moreover, medium- and high-energy foods were rated less healthy and more dangerous than low-energy foods. These effects were independent of rated pleasantness of the foods. It is probable that these effects were psychological rather than physiological in nature, given the small amounts of food eaten and the immediacy of the ratings. The negative effects of the high-energy foods presumably reflect concerns about their impact on health and weight gain. Interestingly, though, stronger increases in negative mood were seen for women reporting greater tendencies to eat in response to emotional state.

These results are similar to the finding that self-identified chocolate addicts felt guiltier after eating chocolate than a control group. The chocolate addicts also reported worse mood before eating the chocolate. By contrast, in another study in healthy men, experimental induction of sadness decreased appetite, whereas when the men were cheerful, the chocolate tasted more pleasant and stimulating and more of it was eaten. This gender difference is likely to be confounded by dispositional and attitudinal differences.

Stress and Food Choice

Human studies on stress and meal patterns/food choice Studies of stress and eating usually focus on the amount of food consumed, but stress might also affect food choices or meal patterns. In the naturalistic studies that showed increased energy intake, there was also an increase in the proportion of energy from fat. This could reflect an increased preference for fatty foods, or alternatively a different meal pattern. In most Western countries the proportion of fat in meal-type foods tends to be lower than in snack-type foods. If stress induced a shift from meals to snacks, this would be reflected in a higher fat intake and might also increase the total energy intake, since higher fat foods have a higher energy density.

In most naturalistic studies, it is not possible to distinguish meal pattern changes from food choice changes, because the data are presented in terms of daily intake of nutrients, without any information either on foods eaten or timing of consumption. Most laboratory studies have also failed to address the food choice issue, because they present only a single type of food. However, there is some evidence that sweet, high-fat foods are the ones most likely to show an increase (see previous section), whereas fruit and vegetables appear to be avoided during stress. In a study of health behaviors in 11- to 13-year-old schoolchildren in London, greater perceived stress was associated with more fatty food intake, less fruit and vegetable intake, more snacking, and a reduced likelihood of daily breakfast consumption.

A survey of possible changes in food choice during stress among 212 students revealed an interesting pattern of effects of stress, which was partly independent of whether participants were grouped as reporting eating more, the same, or less overall when stressed. That is, sweets and chocolate were reported to be eaten more under stress by all groups, even those eating less overall; conversely, intakes of fruit and vegetables, and meat and fish, were reported as less or unchanged under stress in all groups. The changes for the staple food, bread, matched the overall group self-perceptions of changes in eating due to stress. These data imply that mechanisms governing effects of stress on food choice may be somewhat separate from those influencing overall appetite under stress and that foods such as sweets and chocolate may be particularly selected in stressful circumstances.

Chocolate: A unique mood-enhancing food? Chocolate does seem to have a special place in the relationship between food choice and mood: it is a widely liked food, and people often report choosing to eat chocolate during stress. Indeed, experimenters frequently choose chocolate or chocolate-containing foods as the test foods in studies looking at stress-induced eating, reflecting a cultural awareness of its value as a mood enhancer. There are popular notions, perpetuated both in the lay and scientific media, that chocolate contains psychoactive chemicals, such as phenylethylamine and cannabinoids, that are responsible for its effect on mood. However, for reasons of quantity and availability to the brain, these compounds are not likely to alter mood when obtained from chocolate. Nevertheless, it has recently been shown that the methylxanthines in chocolate, caffeine, and theobromine can indeed improve mood (hedonic and energetic dimensions) as well as mental function. Perhaps the effects of these compounds underlie a curious recent report showing that mothers who said they ate chocolate every day during pregnancy subsequently rated their babies' temperaments more positively when aged 4–9 months. These mothers did not appear to have distinctive personality traits that might otherwise explain the rating difference.

Chocolate has other characteristics that could be mood enhancing. It is high in fat and sugar and so would be likely to activate opioidergic hedonic and dopaminergic reward pathways (see next section). It is also low in protein (3–6% of energy), so if eaten in sufficient amounts on an empty stomach might conceivably enhance mood via increased synthesis of the brain neurotransmitter serotonin, as outlined in a later section. Finally, chocolate could also acquire secondary reinforcing or mood-enhancing properties by association with its use as a treat or gift and convivial social interaction. However, it should be remembered that in those who may consider chocolate to be a dangerous temptation that threatens their weight control, eating it can have negative consequences for mood.

Mechanisms Relating Stress to Eating

Neurohormonal Pathways

Eating food activates brain pathways involved in reward, and so might be expected to have a positive effect on mood. Furthermore, some of the ingested nutrients could alter the function of neurohormonal systems involved in coping with stress. We now consider the main pathways that appear to underlie such effects.

Opioids Endogenous opioid neuropeptides are released during stress and are known to be important for adaptive effects such as tolerance of pain. They are also involved in motivational and reward processes in eating behavior, such as stimulation of appetite by palatable foods. This would tend to suggest that there would be a link between opioid action, stress, and food choice. Perhaps the best evidence for opioid involvement in an interaction between stress and eating is the finding that, in animals and human infants, ingestion of sweet and fatty foods, including milk and even a nonnutritive sweetener, alleviates crying and other behavioral signs of distress. This stress-reducing effect of sweet taste has been shown to depend on opioid transmitter systems.

In human neonates, sucking on a pacifier (dummy) or brief exposure to breast milk is also very effective in reducing signs of pain or spontaneous crying. Interestingly, as babies grow older, sweet taste becomes less effective at calming than pacifier sucking, which might reflect a maturational separation of taste and emotion or a difference in opportunities to learn the instrumental emotional value of the two experiences.

The extent to which adults (whether rat or human) retain an analgesic effect of sweet taste remains controversial. Using the cold pressor test (holding the hand in very cold water), pain threshold latency was extended by concurrent sweet taste in 8- to 11-year-old children. In adults, pain tolerance, but not threshold, was increased by prior tasting of a sucrose solution. However, perceived palatability (liking) may be important, since in one study it was found that only highly liked foods (chocolate chip cookies), and not bland or disliked foods, were able to increase pain tolerance in female students when eaten beforehand. It is tempting but speculative to conclude that adults may select sweet, fatty, palatable foods for opioid-mediated relief of stress.

Dopamine The neurotransmitter dopamine is thought to be the major chemical messenger for reward in the brain. The availability of dopamine receptors (D_2) in part of the brain reward pathway, the striatum, has been shown to be inversely correlated to body mass index. This finding has led to the suggestion of a neurochemical trait that elicits overeating of palatable foods so as to enhance dopamine release – a neural predisposition for comfort eating. In support of this, energy-dense snack foods appear to reinforce greater effort to obtain them in obese than in non-obese women. Young children of obese parents also show greater enjoyment of food as well as higher preference for high-fat energy-dense foods than offspring of non-obese parents. It may also be relevant that binge eating and other eating disorders are associated with greater risk of substance abuse, as well as susceptibility to negative affect, possibly linked by the fact that dopamine also mediates stress sensitivity, depression, and reinforcement of drug-taking habits.

Serotonin The neurotransmitter serotonin has been implicated in mood disorders, anxiety, and stress coping, as well as in eating behavior. Synthesis of serotonin (or 5-hydroxytryptamine [5-HT]) depends on dietary availability of the precursor essential amino acid, tryptophan (TRP), due to a lack of saturation of the rate-limiting enzyme, tryptophan hydroxylase, which converts TRP to the intermediate compound 5-hydroxytryptophan.

An important complication is that TRP competes with several other amino acids, the large, neutral, primarily branched chain amino acids (LNAA), for the same transport system from blood to brain. If the protein content of a meal is sufficiently low, such as 5% or less total energy as protein, then relatively few amino acids will be absorbed from the food in the gut. At the same time, insulin will stimulate tissue uptake of competing amino acids from the circulation, and the plasma ratio of TRP to those amino acids (TRP/LNAA) will rise, favoring more TRP entry to the brain. Conversely, a high-protein meal, which would be less insulinogenic, results in absorption of large amounts of competing amino acids into the blood, especially the branched-chain amino acids, leucine, isoleucine, and valine. On the other hand, TRP is scarce in most protein sources and is readily metabolized on passage through the liver; thus, the plasma ratio of TRP to competing amino acids falls after a protein-rich meal.

The possibility that a carbohydrate-rich, low-protein meal could raise 5-HT function gave rise to the proposal that some depressed people may self-medicate by eating high proportions of carbohydrate. It was suggested that this would lead to increased 5-HT release in a manner reminiscent of antidepressant drugs, which enhance aspects of 5-HT function by inhibiting removal of 5-HT from the synaptic cleft between nerve cells. For the most part, early behavioral and pharmacological evidence for such a phenomenon was not very convincing.

Nevertheless, recent research provides some further support for beneficial effects of carbohydrate-rich, protein-poor meals on mood and emotion in some people. When participants were divided into high or low stress-prone groups, as defined by a questionnaire measure of neuroticism, carbohydrate-rich, protein-poor meals (which raised plasma TRP/LNAA ratios) prior to a stressful task were found to block task-induced depressive feelings and release of the glucocorticoid stress hormone cortisol, but only in the high stress-prone group. This finding was replicated using high- vs. low-TRP-containing proteins (α-lactalbumin and casein, respectively). It was argued that because stress increases 5-HT activity, the poor stress coping of this sensitive group might indicate a deficit in 5-HT synthesis that is improved by this dietary intervention.

Neuroendocrine systems A critical neurohormonal system mediating the effects of stress on energy flux and appetite is the hypothalamic-pituitary-adrenocortical (HPA) axis. Neural stimulation of selected nuclei in the hypothalamus of the brain leads to corticotropin-releasing hormone (CRH) acting on the pituitary gland to release adrenocorticotropic hormone (ACTH), which in turn stimulates release of the steroid glucocorticoid hormone cortisol from the adrenal glands. In animals, CRH is known to mediate the suppression of food intake by severe stressors. On the other hand, exogenous glucocorticoids stimulate appetite by acting on the hypothalamus to inhibit CRH release.

The involvement of the HPA axis in the influence of stress on eating behavior seems likely for several reasons, including (1) glucocorticoid hormones substantially affect energy substrate mobilization and metabolism, increasing lipolysis, proteolysis, and gluconeogenesis while protecting hepatic glycogen stores; (2) the circadian rhythm of HPA axis responsivity is dependent on patterns of food ingestion; (3) normal meals containing at least 10% protein as energy activate the HPA axis and release cortisol in humans; and (4) acute food deprivation suppresses the HPA axis response to stress.

Furthermore, most animal models of obesity, genetic or otherwise, depend on an intact HPA axis, and disruption of its function may underlie at least some human obesity, in particular increased visceral adiposity, especially among obese patients suffering from anxiety and depression. The eating disorders bulimia and anorexia nervosa are also associated with hypercortisolemia and disrupted HPA axis activity even in the absence of undernutrition. An inability to cope with stress, coupled with chronic activation of appetite-suppressing CRH, is one psychobiological model proposed for anorexia nervosa.

Another hormone that may be involved in integrating HPA axis activity and food intake is the adipocyte hormone leptin. Leptin is synthesized in adipose tissue, and plasma levels correlate strongly with fat mass in humans, with consistently higher levels in women than in men independent of body composition. In genetic rodent models, obesity has been shown to be associated with the absence of either leptin (ob/ob mice) or its receptor (db/db mice; fa/fa rats). Glucocorticoids administered to humans cause gradual and sustained increases in plasma leptin, and leptin in turn seems to inhibit the activity of the HPA axis. Indeed, normal release of leptin and activity of the HPA axis are inversely related. Leptin may contribute to the regulation of energy balance in part by inhibiting activity of neuropeptide Y, which is known to stimulate feeding via an action in the hypothalamus. However, acute physiological changes in neither glucocorticoids nor short-term food intake seem directly to alter circulating leptin levels. Instead, leptin may be important for longer term regulation of food intake. Moreover, chronic stress may disrupt the balance between leptin and the HPA axis, leading to abnormal eating. The precise nature of the change in eating under chronic stress – under- or overeating – may depend on individual predispositions (see next section).

In stressed people, raised levels of cortisol contribute to abdominal obesity, which in turn promotes insulin resistance. However, insulin resistance may increase the likelihood that high-carbohydrate, low-protein foods would raise brain TRP and 5-HT levels because of increased levels of plasma free fatty acids, which, by competing for binding to albumin, could result in more unbound TRP in plasma. This might underlie recent findings that insulin-resistant people are less prone to suicide and depression, both of which are believed to be increased by low 5-HT function. However, animal studies suggest that this could also depend on normalization of HPA axis function and release of cortisol by feedback from increased abdominal adiposity and intake of high-carbohydrate, energy-dense foods, with a possible resultant improvement in mood. Similarly, in humans, patients with seasonal affective disorder (a form of depression) show increased insulin resistance in the winter, together with a greater predilection for sugar-rich foods, both of which might help alleviate their mood symptoms. Unfortunately, despite this possible protective effect, insulin resistance is a substantial risk to health by promotion of cardiovascular disease.

Biobehavioral Pathways

Theoretical considerations and empirical results indicate that the mechanisms linking stress to changes in food intake are far from straightforward. **Figure 1** illustrates the three principal pathways that have been implicated in the work in this area. In the center is the simple biological pathway whereby the physiological effects of stress inhibit the physiological features of hunger (or perhaps mimic the effects of satiety) and hence modify appetite and food intake. Animal research has generally been used to test this pathway since it is assumed that animals' food intake is more directly controlled by the basic drives of hunger and satiety. From present evidence it would seem that some stressors probably induce hypophagia and others hyperphagia, implicating a more complex pathway from stress to food intake even in animals. Humans have the advantage as research subjects that they can tell us about their subjective experience, yet few studies have incorporated measures of hunger or satiety to address this issue. At present, therefore, there is little direct evidence for

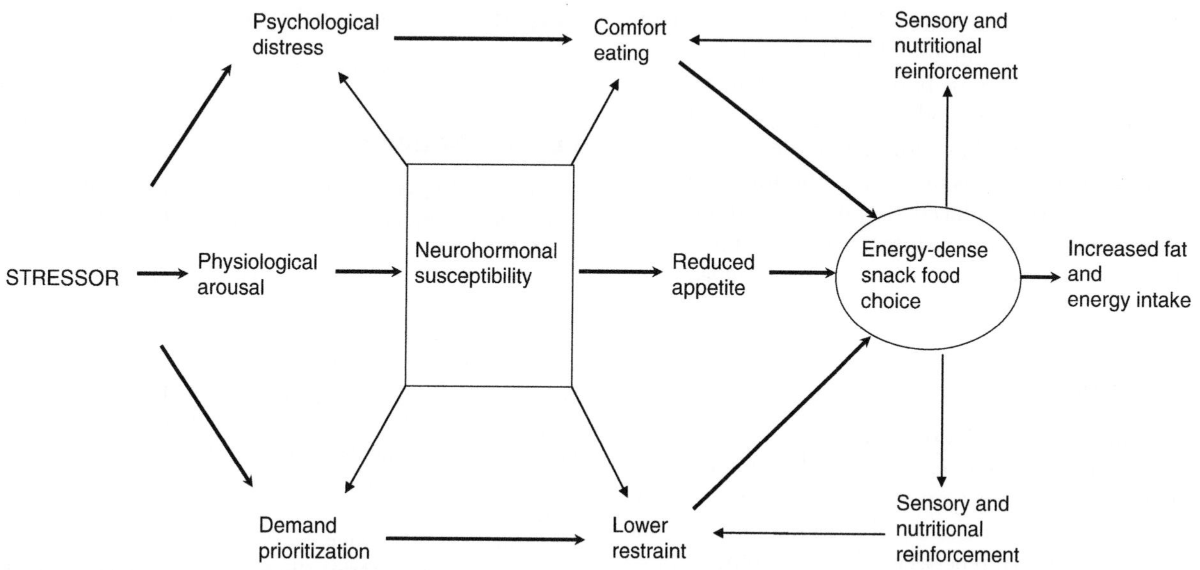

Figure 1 Biobehavioral pathways linking stress and diet.

the hypothesized physiological depression of hunger. The best evidence available from human studies comes from the studies of food intake among normal-weight, nonrestrained eaters. In the laboratory, unrestrained eaters either are unaffected by stress or eat slightly less, which is somewhat supportive of a reduction in appetite, at least in some situations, and for some foods.

A second pathway (shown at the bottom of **Figure 1**) results from consideration of the broader effects that stressors have across a range of aspects of life. In real life, stress motivates people to deploy resources toward dealing with the source of stress (so-called problem-focused coping). This may mean that longer term goals like dieting or healthy eating are temporarily set aside, with consequent effects on food choices. Food intake should increase most in those who were normally restrictive, so women, healthy eaters, and dieters should show the strongest hyperphagic response to stress. This idea is given some support from the higher food intake in stressed restrained eaters, the higher fat and energy intake under stress among women in some of the naturalistic studies, and the observation that energy intakes increase most among those who normally have a low energy intake.

The third pathway, shown at the top of **Figure 1**, relates to the fact that stress also comes with an emotional coloring, so coping efforts are deployed to deal not only with the source of stress, but also with the emotional state (emotion-focused coping). For some people, especially those who are usually self-denying with food, food may have a significant reward value and may be used to provide emotional comfort. Women in particular often describe food in terms of treats and rewards, and the potential comfort to be derived from sweet foods is deeply enshrined in contemporary culture. Clearly this idea has echoes of the discredited psychosomatic theory of obesity, but it should be remembered that it was rejected not because of the absence of emotional eating, but because eating did not appear to be a successful anxiolytic. Other emotional coping strategies are equally unsuccessful in the longer term (e.g., alcohol, smoking), but that does not prevent the smokers, drinkers, and stress eaters from feeling that their habits serve a comforting role. In the field of eating disorders, excessive eating has been hypothesized to provide escape from self-awareness, which is especially valued in response to ego-threatening stressors, so the idea that eating has a role, functional or dysfunctional, as an emotional coping strategy may have been rejected prematurely. If emotional eating is part of a stress-coping repertoire, it should be more common in restrained eaters, for whom food has a higher emotional value, and that of course is observed in all of the laboratory studies.

Figure 1 also depicts a likely final outcome of stress on diet, as discussed in the previous sections. That is, for multiple reasons, including sensory pleasure, modulation of neurotransmitter control of mood, and stress coping, susceptible stressed people may end up choosing energy-dense, sweet, fatty foods that will lead to a less healthy diet and possibly weight gain.

Finally, in real life, stresses are not usually single, transient, and novel, as they are in the laboratory. They are prolonged or repeated, they wax and wane, and they can become a familiar part of the landscape. This means that stress reactions are likely to be modified over time. Adaptational processes should be triggered to protect body fat stores; if stress induces hypophagia in the short term, then in the longer term, the loss of body fat should upregulate appetite and restore food intake to normal levels. Few human studies have looked at the effect of repeated stress exposures on eating, but animal studies show that stress-induced hypophagia diminishes with repeated stress exposures. The inclusion of this dynamic perspective adds yet another dimension to an already complex process.

Summary

In summary, the relationship between stress and eating is a complex one, moderated in humans not only by the type of person, the type of stress, and the types of foods that are available, but also by the dynamic relationship between the internal milieu and behavior over time. There is increasing evidence to support the view that some people are particularly susceptible to eating more sweet, fatty, energy-dense foods during stress. Possible explanations can be found at both the psychological and physiological level, but in either case it is probable that such a change in eating behavior helps the individual to cope with stress. Unfortunately, this change in diet may also result in weight gain, particularly abdominal obesity, and increased risk of cardiovascular disease.

This fascinating area is likely to challenge clinicians and researchers for some time to come, but it also provides one of the richest areas for demonstrating the importance of integrating biology and psychology to understand human behavior.

See Also the Following Articles

Diet and Stress, Psychiatric.

Further Reading

Cartwright, M., Wardle, J., Steggles, N., et al. (2003). Stress and dietary practices in adolescents. *Health Psychology* **22**, 362–369.

Dallman, M. F., Pecoraro, N., Akana, S. F., et al. (2003). Chronic stress and obesity: a new view of "comfort food". *Proceedings of the National Academy of Sciences USA* **100**, 11696–11701.

Greeno, C. G. and Wing, R. R. (1994). Stress-induced eating. *Psychological Bulletin* **115**, 444–464.

Heatherton, T. F. and Baumeister, R. F. (1991). Binge-eating as escape from self-awareness. *Psychological Bulletin* **110**, 86–108.

Herman, C. P. and Polivy, J. (1984). A boundary model for the regulation of eating. In: Stunkard, A. J. & Stellar, E. (eds.) *Eating and its disorders*, pp. 141–156. New York: Raven Press.

Markus, R., Panhuysen, G., Tuiten, A. and Koppeschaar, H. (2000). Effects of food on cortisol and mood in vulnerable subjects under controllable and uncontrollable stress. *Physiology and Behavior* **70**, 333–342.

Robbins, T. W. and Fray, P. J. (1980). Stress-induced eating: fact, fiction or misunderstanding. *Appetite* **1**, 103–133.

Rogers, P. J. (1995). Food, mood and appetite. *Nutrition Research Reviews* **8**, 243–269.

Slochower, J. A. (1983). *Excessive eating: The role of emotions and environment.* New York: Human Sciences Press.

Stone, A. R. and Brownell, K. D. (1994). The stress-eating paradox: multiple daily measurements in adult males and females. *Psychology and Health* **9**, 425–436.

Depersonalization: Systematic Assessment

M Steinberg
Northampton, MA, USA

Glossary

Amnesia — A specific and significant block of past time that cannot be accounted for by memory.

Depersonalization — Detachment from one's self, e.g., a sense of looking at one's self as if one were an outsider.

Derealization — A feeling that one's surroundings are strange or unreal. Often involves previously familiar people.

Dissociation — Disruption in the usually integrated functions of conscious memory, identity, or perception of the environment. The disturbance may be sudden or gradual, transient or chronic.

Identity alteration — Objective behavior indicating the assumption of different identities, much more distinct than different roles.

Identity confusion — Subjective feelings of uncertainty, puzzlement, or conflict about one's identity.

Depersonalization is characterized by a sense of detachment from the self. The symptom itself may manifest in a variety of axis I or axis II psychiatric disorders. The *Diagnostic and Statistical Manual of Mental Disorders,* 4th edition (DSM-IV) prefers to define depersonalization not in functional or nosologic terms, but phenomenologically, as in an alteration in the perception or experience of the self. The sense of detachment itself may be experienced in various ways. Commonly it appears as out-of-body experiences giving a sense of division into a participating and an observing self, resulting in the sense of going through life as though one were a machine or robot. In some cases, there exists a feeling that one's limbs are changing in size or are separated from the body.

It is important to distinguish between recurrent severe depersonalization that is characteristic of the dissociative disorders, including depersonalization disorder, and mild or moderate episodic depersonalization sometimes observed in patients with other nondissociative axis I or II disorders, and the isolated episode experienced by persons in the healthy population (normal controls).

Definition and Characteristics

Although depersonalization was first described in 1872, it was not named until 1898, when Dugas contrasted the feeling of loss of the ego with a real loss. In 1954, Ackner remedied the lack of clear-defined boundaries of the symptom by describing the four salient features: (1) feeling of unreality or strangeness regarding the self, (2) retention of insight and lack of delusional elaboration, (3) affective disturbance resulting in loss of all affective response except discomfort over the depersonalization, and (4) an unpleasant quality that varies in intensity inversely with the patient's familiarity with the symptom. Steinberg defined depersonalization as one of five core symptoms of dissociation (see above), the other four consisting of amnesia, derealization, identity confusion, and identity alteration. Each of the five dissociative disorders has characteristic symptom profiles of these core dissociative symptoms. For this reason, it is essential that the symptom of depersonalization is evaluated within the context of the other dissociative symptoms and not as an isolated symptom.

Episodes of depersonalization accompany or even may precipitate panic attacks and/or agoraphobia; they may also be associated with dysphoria. Chronic depersonalization frequently results in the patient's acceptance of the symptoms, in a manner of resignation. Patients experience difficulty putting their experience into words, but often compare their feelings to such states as being high on drugs, seeing themselves from the outside, or floating in space and watching themselves. Other descriptions of depersonalization include feelings of being unreal, or in severe cases, include the feeling of being numb or dead, or the lack of all feeling, which may be attributed to and/or misdiagnosed as depression.

Depersonalization has been reported to be the third most common complaint among psychiatric patients, after depression and anxiety. Incidence of actual depersonalization has been difficult to determine because of (1) the relative strangeness of the symptoms, (2) the difficulty patients experience in communicating them, and (3) the lack, until recently, of diagnostic tools for the systematic assessment of depersonalization. Detection is further complicated by the fact that depersonalization is not accompanied by altered external or social behavior, but by an altered state of perception on the part of the patient.

Etiology

Various biological and psychodynamic theories have been advanced for the etiology of depersonalization: (1) physiological or anatomical disturbance, with feelings of depersonalization produced by temporal lobe function and various metabolic and toxic states, (2) the result of a preformed functional response of the brain to overwhelming traumata, (3) a defense against painful and conflictual affects such as guilt, phobic anxiety, anger, rage, paranoia, primitive fusion fantasies, and exhibitionism, (4) a split between the observing and the participating self, allowing the patient to become a detached observer of the self, and (5) the result of a child's being raised in an environment that systematically fails to know some part of the child, who then experiences that part as tentative and as a result is unable to accurately assess the self.

Depersonalization has been reported to be a normal reaction to life-threatening events, such as accidents, serious illnesses, near-death experiences, anaphylactic reactions, and complications of surgery. Depersonalization is frequent among victims of sexual abuse, political imprisonment, torture, and cult indoctrination. Symptoms of depersonalization are often associated with hypnosis, hypnogogic and hypnopompic states, sleep deprivation, sensory deprivation, hyperventilation, and drug or alcohol abuse.

The development of specialized tests for the assessment of dissociation has led to an increase in investigations furthering our understanding of depersonalization. Depersonalization, as a brief, isolated symptom, is nonspecific and not necessarily pathognomonic of any clinical disorder. Research indicates that it is the persistence and nature of depersonalization that differentiates depersonalization in normal subjects versus persons with dissociative and nondissociative disorders. **Table 1** is useful for distinguishing between normal and pathological depersonalization. **Table 2** summarizes the spectrum of depersonalization.

The differential diagnosis tree of depersonalization (**Figure 1**) illustrates procedures for distinguishing between depersonalization disorder and other disorders that may resemble it. The differential diagnosis of patients experiencing recurrent or persistent depersonalization should include the dissociative disorders, various other psychiatric disorders, and possible medical disorders/organic etiology, most commonly acute head trauma, seizure disorders, and migraines.

Assessment with the SCID-D-R

The Structured Clinical Interview for DSM-IV Dissociative Disorders – Revised (SCID-D-R) is a diagnostic tool for the comprehensive assessment of dissociative symptoms and disorders, including the systematic identification of depersonalization. Developed in 1985 and extensively field tested, it is the only diagnostic instrument enabling a clinician to detect and assess the presence and severity of five core dissociative symptoms and the dissociative disorders (dissociative amnesia, dissociative fugue, depersonalization disorder, dissociative identity disorder, and dissociate disorder not otherwise identified) as defined by DSM-IV criteria. The SCID-D-R is a semistructured diagnostic interview with good-to-excellent inter-rater and test–retest reliability and discriminant validity. Guidelines for the administration, scoring, and interpretation of the SCID-D-R are reviewed in the *Interviewer's Guide to the SCID-D-R*. Severity rating definitions were developed to allow clinicians to rate the severity of symptoms in a systematic manner and are included in the guide.

Table 1 Distinguishing between normal and pathological depersonalization

Common mild depersonalization	*Transient depersonalization*	*Pathological depersonalization*
Context		
Occurs as an isolated symptom	Occurs as an isolated symptom	Occurs within a constellation of other dissociative or nondissociative symptoms or with ongoing interactive dialogue
Frequency		
One or few episodes	One or few episodes that are transient	Persistent or recurrent depersonalization
Duration		
Depersonalization episode is brief; lasts seconds to minutes	Depersonalization of limited duration (minutes to weeks)	Chronic and habitual depersonalization lasting up to months or years
Precipitating factors		
• Extreme fatigue • Sensory deprivation • Hypnagogic and hypnopompic states • Drug or alcohol intoxication • Sleep deprivation • Medical illness / toxic states • Severe psychosocial stress	• Life-threatening danger. This is a syndrome noted to occur in 33% of individuals immediately following exposure to life-threatening danger, such as near-death experiences and auto accidents (Noyes et al., 1977) • Single, severe psychological trauma	• Not associated with precipitating factors in column 1. • May be precipitated by a traumatic memory. • May be precipitated by a stressful event, but occurs even when there is no identifiable stress. • Occurs in the absence of a single immediate severe psychosocial trauma.

Reprinted with permission from Steinberg M: Handbook for the Assessment of Dissociation: A Clinical Guide. Washington, DC, American Psychiatric Press, Inc., 1995.

Table 2 The spectrum of depersonalization on the SCID-D-R

DID and DDNOS	*Non-dissociative and personality disorders*	*No psychiatric disorder*
Depersonalization questions elicit descriptions of identity confusion and alteration	No spontaneous elaboration	No spontaneous elaboration
Includes interactive dialogues between individual and depersonalized self	No interactive dialogues	No interactive dialogues
Recurrent–persistent	None–few episodes	None–few episodes

Note: DID = Dissociative Identity Disorder, DDNOS = Dissociative Disorder, Not Otherwise Specified.
Reprinted with permission from: Steinberg M: Interviewer's Guide to The Structured Clinical Interview for DSM-IV Dissociative Disorders – Revised. Washington, D.C. American Psychiatric Press, Second Edition, 1994.

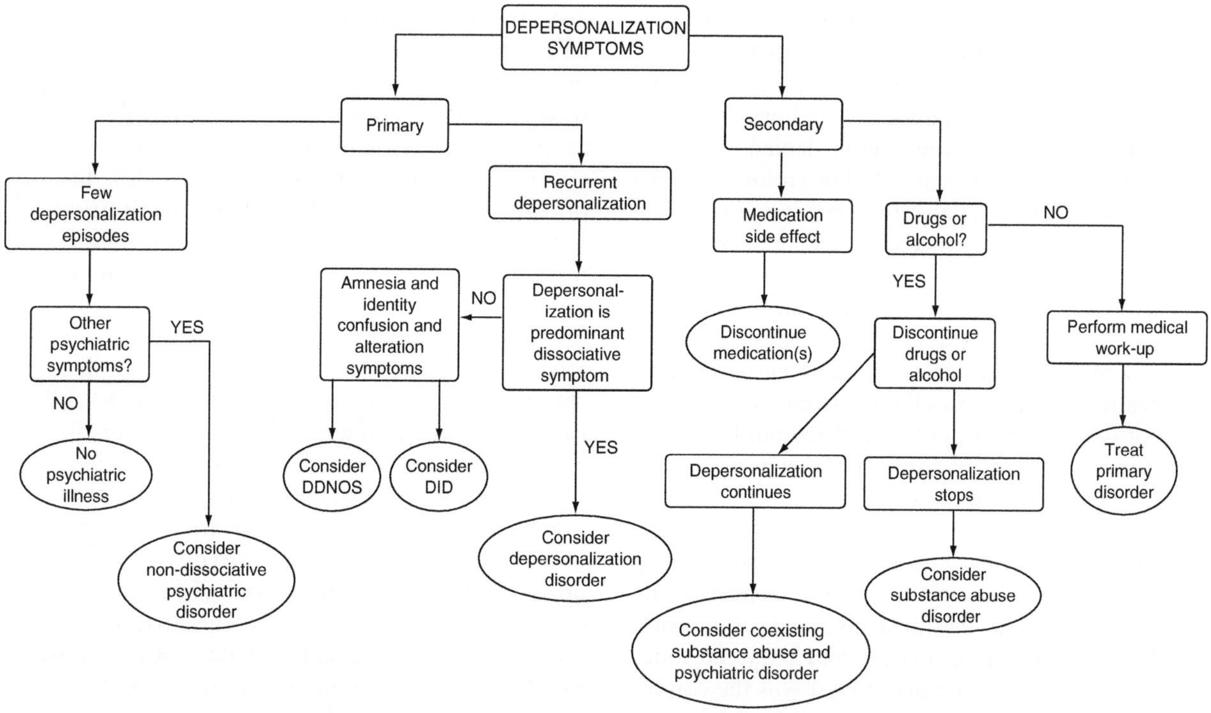

Figure 1 Differential diagnosis decision tree of depersonalization. Reprinted with permission from Steinberg, M (1994). *Interviewer's Guide to the Structured Clinical Interview for DSM-IV Dissociative Disorders – Revised.* Washington, DC: American Psychiatric Press.

The SCID-D-R can be used for symptom documentation and for psychological and forensic reports. Early detection of dissociative disorders, including depersonalization disorder, can be realized from the use of this specialized instrument, the format of which includes open-ended questions designed to elicit spontaneous descriptions of endorsed dissociative symptoms. The SCID-D-R has been demonstrated to be a valuable tool in differential diagnosis with patients of different ages (it can be used in adolescents as well as adults), backgrounds, previous psychiatric histories, and presenting complaints. It also plays a useful role in treatment planning, patient follow-up, and symptom monitoring.

Correct diagnosis is vital to proper treatment of the disorder. If the depersonalization is secondary to an underlying primary disorder, the symptom may be alleviated by treatment of the underlying illness. In instances in which patients experience only occasional episodes of depersonalization in the context of other nondissociative symptoms, the clinician may consider a diagnosis of nondissociative psychiatric disorder. The presence of depersonalization disorder itself will be characterized by recurrent depersonalization.

Case Study

The process of differential diagnosis of depersonalization may best be illustrated by presenting a case study. The study demonstrates the utility of the SCID-D-R in diagnostic assessment, patient education, and treatment planning. For space reasons, conventional formatting and content have been abbreviated.

Sample SCID-D-R Psychological Evaluation

Demographic information and chief complaint: Susan Walker is a 31-year-old administrative assistant at a community college who presented with the complaint of feeling detached from herself since adolescence.

Past psychiatric history: Although the patient had no history of hospitalization for psychiatric disturbance, she began treatment for an episode of depression that interfered with her employment and social relationships. Although admitting to past casual use of marijuana, she had never been in treatment for substance abuse disorder.

Family history: Susan had a younger sibling; both children grew up in an intact but emotionally unsupportive family. Patient reported that both parents suffered mood swings and unpredictable temper outbursts.

Mental status exam: Susan answered questions with relevant replies; although she seemed slightly depressed, her affect appeared full range. She denied hallucinations, both auditory and visual, and evidenced no psychotic thinking. She denied acute suicidal or homicidal ideas.

SCID-D-R evaluation: The SCID-D-R was administered to systematically evaluate the patient's dissociative symptoms and was scored according to prescribed guidelines. Significant findings from the SCID-D-R interview follow. Susan denied experiencing severe episodes of amnesia, but endorsed a persistent sense of depersonalization, resulting in distress and interference with occupational and personal functioning. This feeling of depersonalization had been chronic and occurred all the time rather than episodically. Although the feeling varied in intensity with her overall stress level, the experience of depersonalization was always characterized by a general sense of detachment from life, rather than by disturbances in body image or a split between participating and observing parts of the self. Only a single isolated out-of-body experience had occurred. Susan experienced feelings of derealization that varied in intensity with the depersonalization, but she reported the depersonalization as the most distressing symptom. She described recurrent anxiety and panic episodes triggered by the depersonalization; it was the combination of depersonalization and panic attacks that led to the depression that brought her into therapy. Susan reported that the depersonalization has eroded her sense of control over her occupational functioning and other significant areas of her life, but she did not attribute feelings of loss of control to identity confusion or alteration. She denied having internal dialogues, feelings of possession, or acquiring unexplained possessions or skills. Her descriptions of internal struggle were focused on her feelings of unreality, not on conflicts between different aspects of her personality or different personalities within herself.

Assessment: Susan's symptoms are consistent with a primary diagnosis of a dissociative disorder based on DSM-IV criteria and ICD-10 criteria. Specifically, in the absence of substance abuse disorder or other organic etiology, her severe chronic feelings of unreality toward herself and the accompanying dysfunction (in the absence of other dissociative symptoms such as identity confusion and alteration) are consistent with a diagnosis of depersonalization disorder.

Recommendations: Although detailed discussion of treatment for depersonalization disorder is beyond the scope of this article, it would be standard practice to conduct a follow-up interview to review the findings of the SCID-D-R evaluation, to educate the patient regarding her symptoms, and to begin the process of individual psychotherapy.

Conclusions

Recent advances in the development of reliable diagnostic tools allow for early detection and accurate differential diagnosis of depersonalization. Research based on the SCID-D-R indicates that depersonalization occurs in individuals without psychiatric illness who experience none to few brief episodes, as well as in individuals with dissociative disorders who experience recurrent to ongoing episodes. In addition to the frequency of the depersonalization, the nature, severity, and context also distinguish cases of dissociative disorder from other nondissociative disorders. Further research is necessary in the form of controlled double-blind studies comparing the efficacy of pharmacotherapeutic agents as well as psychotherapeutic techniques. As the SCID-D-R allows for the assessment of the severity of depersonalization based on operationalized criteria, pharmacotherapy trials can now be systematically performed and can evaluate baseline and postmedication severity levels of depersonalization. Given the frequency of misdiagnosis in patients suffering from depersonalization and other dissociative symptoms, earlier detection of dissociative disorders using the SCID-D-R can allow for rapid implementation of effective treatment.

Further Reading

Ackner, B. (1954). Depersonalization I.: aetiology and phenomenology. *Journal of Mental Science* **100**, 838–853.

American Psychiatric Association. (1994). *Diagnostic and Statistical Manual of Mental Disorders* (4th edn.). (DSM-IV). Washington, D.C.: American Psychiatric Association.

Baker, D., Hunter, E., Lawrence, E., et al. (2003). Depersonalization disorder: clinical features of 204 cases. *British Journal of Psychiatry* **182**, 428–433.

Bowman, E. S. and Markand, O. (1996). Psychodynamics and psychiatric diagnoses of pseudoseizure subjects. *American Journal of Psychiatry* **153**(1), 57–63.

Dugas, L. (1898). Un cas de depersonalization (A case of depersonalization). *Revue Philosophique* **45**, 500–507.

Lambert, M., Sierra, M. and Phillips, M. D. (2002). The spectrum of organic depersonalization: a review plus four new cases. *Journal of Neuropsychiatry and Clinical Neuroscience* **14**(2), 141–154.

Noyes, R., Jr. and Kletti, R. (1977). Depersonalization in response to life-threatening danger. *Comprehensive Psychiatry* **18**, 375–384.

Simeon, D., Gross, S., Guralnik, O., Stein, D. J., Schmeidler, J. and Hollander, E. (1997). Feeling unreal: 30 cases of DSM-III-R depersonalization disorder. *American Journal of Psychiatry* **154**, 1107–1113.

Steinberg, M. (1994). *The structured clinical interview for DSM-IV dissociative disorders – revised (SCID-D)* (2nd edn.). Washington, D.C.: American Psychiatric Press.

Steinberg, M. (1994). *The interviewers' guide to the structured clinical interview for DSM-IV dissociative disorders – revised* (2nd edn.). Washington, D.C.: American Psychiatric Press.

Steinberg, M. (1995). *Handbook for the assessment of dissociation: a clinical guide.* Washington, D.C.: American Psychiatric Press.

Steinberg, M. (1995). Advances in the clinical assessment of dissociation: the SCID-D-R. *The Bulletin of the Menninger Clinic* **59**, 221–231.

Steinberg, M. and Hall, P. (1997). The SCID-D diagnostic interview and treatment planning in dissociative disorders. *Bulletin of the Menninger Clinic* **61**(1), 108–120.

Steinberg, M. and Schnall, M. (2001). *The stranger in the mirror: dissociation—the hidden epidemic.* HarperCollins: New York.

Steinberg, M., Rounsaville, B., Buchanan, J., Raakfeldt, J. and Cicchetti, D. (1994). Distinguishing between multiple personality and schizophrenia using the Structured Clinical Interview for DSM-IV Dissociative Disorders. *Journal of Nervous and Mental Disorders* **Sept. 1994**, 495–502.

Learning and Memory, Effects of Stress on

M Lindau
Uppsala University, Uppsala, Sweden
O Almkvist
Karolinska Institutet and University of Stockholm, Stockholm, Sweden
A H Mohammed
Karolinska Institutet, Stockholm, and Växjö University, Växjö, Sweden

This is a revised version of the article by M Lindau, O Almkvist, and A H Mohammed, Encyclopedia of Stress First Edition, volume 2, pp 603–609, © 2000, Elsevier Inc.

Glossary

Stressor — Stimuli that puts an extra demand on the organism.

Stress hormones — Hormones of the adrenal glands that serve to maintain bodily homeostatis in response to challenging external and emotional environment. These hormones are the glucocorticoids and epinephrine.

Corticosterone — A steroid hormone in many species including rodents produced by the adrenal cortex and involved in response to stress and immune reaction.

Cortisol — A steroid hormone in humans produced by adrenal cortex, involved in response to stress and has direct influence on the nervous system.

Hippocampus — A region of the cerebral cortex lying in the basal medial part of the temporal lobe thought to be important for learning and memory.

Amygdala — A group of nuclei involved in the medial anterior part of the temporal lobe regulating emotion and certain types of learning.

Emotion — Mental state of arousal.

Memory — Encoding of information, storage and recall.

Learning — A relatively permanent change in cognition as a consequence of the acquisition of new information and experience, directly influencing behaviour.

Introduction

Conceptually, the term stress describes a load on the organism. A stressful situation puts extra demands upon the system for cognitive or physical productivity. A stressor, which might be external or internal, can be anything that puts extra demands upon the system, such as a specific problem, issue, challenge, or personal conflict. A stress reaction is the individual's response to a given stressor on the physiological, cognitive, and/or emotional plane. Strain occurs when the organism is overloaded, exposed to prolonged stress, or placed in situations that the system can not cope with. The psychological consequence of strain is fatigue or exhaustion. Traumatic, salient memories that the individual would like to forget but can not may result in a neurotic fixation on the memories of the trauma, i.e., posttraumatic stress disorder (PTSD).

Physiologically, stress might be defined as a state of physiological and emotional arousal of the organism. It leads to the activation of the autonomic nervous system and the hypothalamic-pituitary-adrenal axis. The main signaling hormones of these systems are (nor)adrenaline, corticotropin-releasing hormone, and cortisol (corticosterone in most rodents).

It is generally accepted that stress affects learning and memory processes and that stress might improve as well as impair the acquirement of information. How is this possible? One answer to this question is that there are at least three types of stressors, physical, cognitive, and emotional, which affect different regions of the brain. Another answer lies in the progress that has been made in the knowledge of the effects of stress on the different stages of learning and memory processing.

Although the mnemonic system in animals is considerably more restricted than that in humans, much complementary knowledge about the effects of stress on learning and memory in humans has been gained through animal studies. The following section gives an account of some of the basic research about this topic in animals.

Effects of Stress on Learning and Memory in Animals

Animals learn about the relationship or association between two events. In classical conditioning, the animal learns to associate a stimulus such as a tone (conditioned stimulus) with food (unconditioned stimulus). In operant or instrumental conditioning, the animal learns to associate a response, for instance, pressing a lever (instrumental response), with food reward (reinforcement). It has been suggested by some researchers (e.g., Anthony Dickinson) that associative learning mechanisms have been shaped by evolution to enable animals to detect and store information about real causal relationships in their environment.

Stress Hormones and Learning

The impact of stress hormones in modulating associative learning and cognitive function in animals has been a subject of continued investigation. The studies that have documented the relationship of levels of the stress hormones with cognitive function, such as attention, perception, and memory, have been done mostly in rodents, in which investigators have examined the influence of stress hormones on acquisition, consolidation, and retrieval of information. Glucocorticoids are the stress hormones secreted by the adrenal glands in animals. In primates and dogs, the naturally occurring glucocorticoid is cortisol, whereas in rodents and birds it is corticosterone.

Fluctuations in corticosterone levels can be said to reflect emotional states related to stress. In experimental animals, changes in hormonal levels can be achieved by pharmacological means or environmental manipulations and their effects assessed. Several studies have shown that stress and glucocorticoids influence cognitive function.

The administration of low levels of corticosterone improves performance in learning tasks in animals. However, whereas short-term exposure to low levels of corticosterone can enhance cognitive function, it is known that short-term exposure to higher levels as well as long-term effects of high levels of corticosterone (e.g., through sustained exposure to restraint stress) have deleterious effects on learning, memory, and cognitive function. The biphasic effects of corticosterone on memory formation have been demonstrated in behavioral studies performed in chicks and rats.

Young chicks have a tendency to peck spontaneously at small salient objects in the environment. This natural behavior of chicks has been exploited to study learning. Chicks will peck spontaneously at bright beads, and if the bead is dipped in a distasteful substance, the chicks will peck once at the bead and show a strong disgust response. Subsequently, they will avoid pecking a similar but dry bead and learn this avoidance behavior. The strong emotional fear component involved in this passive avoidance response in chicks prompted Sandi and Rose to explore the role of stress hormones in learning in the chick. In tests of passive avoidance learning in the chick, they found that an inverted U-shaped curve emerged, in which low levels (0.1 μg) and higher levels (2 μg) of corticosterone were without effect, whereas an intermediate dose (1 μg) improved learning. Similarly, in rodents, an inverted U shape is seen between the dose of administration of corticosterone and performance in learning tasks. It has thus been seen that low doses of corticosterone can improve learning, whereas continuous exposure to glucocorticoids results in neuronal death in the hippocampus and in impaired learning ability. Aged rats that are impaired in cognitive function have elevated levels of corticosterone and increased hippocampal neuronal loss when they are compared with aged rats that are not impaired in cognitive function.

The effects of corticosterone on cognitive function are mediated through binding of the stress hormones to specific receptors in the brain. These receptors, known as glucocorticoid receptors, have been found to be abundant in the hippocampus, a brain region that is critically involved in modulating learning and memory. Another region in the brain that participates in cognitive function is the amygdala, which also has moderate amounts of receptors for corticosterone. The actions of corticosterone in the hippocampus and amygdala can be induced by the administration of selective drugs that interact with the glucocorticoid receptors. Drugs include those that enhance the effects of corticosterone (glucocorticoid agonists) or those that block or attenuate the effect of corticosterone (glucocorticoid antagonists). These drugs have provided powerful tools in dissecting the role of stress hormones in the hippocampus and amygdala in modulating cognitive functions in rodents. Pharmacological or environmental manipulation of the glucocorticoid receptors influences cognitive function in rats.

Hippocampus and Learning in Animals

Considerable evidence shows that the hippocampus mediates spatial learning in rodents. Spatial learning in rodents can be examined by the use of a water maze, known as the Morris maze. The procedure involves placing an experimental animal in a large pool of water of about 1.5 m in diameter. The animal has to use spatial cues in the experimental room to locate an invisible escape platform that is hidden 2 cm below the surface of the opaque water. After a few days of testing, the animals learn to locate the platform within seconds. It has been demonstrated that rats perform poorly in this test if hippocampal function is impaired. Thus, aged rats with pathological changes in the hippocampus show impaired spatial learning in the water maze compared to aged rats that do not show pathological hippocampal changes. Aged rats that had been exposed to repeated restraint stress have a reduction in glucocorticoid receptors in the hippocampus. This results in, among other things, an impaired spatial learning ability. In contrast, animals that have higher levels of glucocorticoid receptors in the hippocampus show an increased ability for spatial learning. Administration of a glucocorticoid receptor antagonist in the brain appears to impair information processing during spatial learning.

To sum up, spatial memory in animals is dependent on hippocampal function. Through their action in the hippocampus, stress hormones facilitate spatial information processing so that low levels of corticosterone improve learning, whereas higher levels impair performance.

Amygdala and Learning in Animals

Many studies have concentrated on the effects that stress hormones have on the hippocampus and its relationship to learning. Work by James McGaugh and colleagues has begun to explore the role of stress hormone receptors in the amygdala on learning. The amygdala is a region of the brain that plays a crucial role in acquisition and expression of fear responses. This brain region is thought to influence memory storage processes in other brain regions, such as the hippocampus and cortex. An interaction of stress hormones and amygdala nuclei appears to be important in modulating memory consolidation for emotional events. Binding of glucocorticoid receptors in the basolateral nucleus is known to affect memory storage. It was found that administration of the glucocorticoid receptor agonist in this area immediately after training enhanced retention of a passive avoidance response. Many studies have examined the effects of glucocorticoids on the acquisition of newly acquired information. In a test of memory retrieval of long-term spatial learning memory, it was found that stress caused impaired performance, and this impairment could be related to circulating levels of corticosterone. These findings point to a critical involvement of the amygdala in regulating stress hormone effects on learning and memory.

To conclude, the amygdala is a region of the brain known to be importantly involved in emotions. Stress hormones can affect the memory storage of emotional events by their actions on the amygdala. The impact of stress on the hippocampus and amygdala is highlighted by emerging evidence from animal studies that revealed that stress causes changes in hippocampal plasticity and can thus modify the information storage mechanism in the hippocampus and that the amygdala is involved in the emergence of stress-associated changes in the hippocampus.

Summary

Stress hormones have biphasic effects on learning and memory in animals. Low levels of stress hormones improve performance, whereas higher levels have a deleterious effect on learning. Two brain regions important in regulating learning and memory are the hippocampus and amygdala, which contain receptors for stress hormones. The effects of stress hormones on learning are mediated by these receptors in the hippocampus and amygdala. Research in rodents has revealed that emotional arousal regulates learning through the action of stress hormones, which activate receptors in the hippocampus and amygdala to affect memory formation.

Memory, Learning, and Their Anatomical Bases in Humans

Conceptualization of Learning and Memory

The contemporary conceptual frameworks of learning and memory emanate from experimental psychology. According to this model, human memory is not a unitary system, but is composed of a series of interdependent brain systems characterized by different features in terms of time for the registration of new information (immediate/extended in time), type of information (implicit/declarative or explicit), accessibility (immediate/search), amount of information stored (limited/unlimited), spontaneous duration of information in memory (limited/unlimited), and awareness of information (yes/no). These distinct memory systems appear to be subserved by separate neural networks, as shown by brain behavior studies and prior studies demonstrating specific effects on memory due to lesions in the brain.

One major division of memory is that between implicit or nondeclarative memory and declarative (explicit) memory. Nondeclarative memory includes procedural memory, classical conditioning, the perceptual representation system, and priming. In line with phylogenesis and ontogenesis, one early type is procedural memory, which is expressed as skilled behavior or motor procedures, which appear to be subserved by regions in the basal ganglia. One division of procedural memory is classical conditioning, which is the same as a stimulus–response connection. The hippocampus and certain parts of the cerebral cortex have been identified as important areas for this memory system. Another type of implicit memory is the perceptual representation system, which is concerned primarily with the acquisition and use of perceptual objects of the world. The predominantly responsible brain areas are the primary association cortices. Another branch of implicit memory is priming, which refers to an unconscious ability to process a stimulus due to prior exposure. Declarative memory can be described as the conscious recollection of facts and events (Krystal et al., 1995). To this memory system belongs short-term memory or working memory, semantic memory, and verbal as well as visuospatial episodic memory. Short-term or working memory processes and stores temporarily a very limited amount of information. Semantic memory covers acquisition and use of factual knowledge about the world and is mapped by association areas in the brain. Information unique in time, location, and person is involved in storage and recall of information from episodic memory, for which the medial temporal lobes are one crucial point of the subserving neural networks. Another important aspect of memory is learning. Some authors equate long-term storage with learning, for example, calling it the process by which information that may be needed again is stored for recall on demand (Peterson, 1967). A broader definition is that learning is the same as the modification of behavior according to earlier experiences.

The Anatomy of Human Memory

The hippocampus thus plays an important role in several of the subdivisions of the two main memory systems. In the hippocampus, stimuli from the external world are classified and stored, momentarily in short-term memory and for longer periods of time in long-term memory, and the spatial and temporal dimensions of the experiences are recorded. It is doubtful, however, that the hippocampus is responsible for the more permanent consolidation of memories. Adjacent to the hippocampal system is the amygdala, which plays an important role in the processing of emotional information in the brain. The amygdala consists of several distinct nuclei, whose functional properties vary. The basolateral amygdaloid complex appears to be the nucleus that is involved most crucially in memory performance. However, it is not critical for the consolidation of a memory trace per se. Instead, it has been suggested that the amygdala assigns emotional meaning to incoming free-floating feelings, integrates this emotionally meaningful information with associated emotional memories, and, through projections to the hypothalamus, hippocampus, and basal forebrain, directs emotional behavior. The amygdala also contributes to the enhancement of a memory trace that is related to emotional responses such as stress.

The frontotemporal area is the center for the executive function, short-term memory, and personality. This area of the brain has an elaborate network of connections to most other regions of the brain and a high concentration of stress hormone receptors, which has been found to assure the role of the frontal lobes in stress, learning and memory.

Vulnerability of Human Memory

The current conceptualization of human memory posits that the order of memory acquisition during ontogenesis, as described earlier, is reversed when the brain is exposed to various adverse influences such as aging, toxins, inflammatory agents, and stress. The meaning of this is that more sophisticated memory systems, such as declarative memory, are hit at an early stage, whereas more basic and ontogenetically earlier systems, such as procedural memory, are afflicted later on. Of course, the reversed order of degradation does not hold when there is a highly localized attack on the brain, as is the case for brain trauma. However, it is well known that episodic memory is highly sensitive for aging as well as for disease processes such as Alzheimer's disease. The next section describes changes that take place in relation to memory performance when humans are exposed to stress.

Encoding in Stressful Situations

Encoding is closely connected with attention and vigilance, which both influence the encoding of information into declarative as well as nondeclarative memory. Attention, like vigilance, is highly sensitive to stress. To be able to encode an all-embracing picture of an event, it is necessary that attention be unrestricted. During a stressful situation the attentional span tends to be narrowed to the most salient stimuli in the situation, whereas more peripheral stimuli are neglected. It has also been suggested that the hippocampus seems to shut down under severe stress, which may contribute to an incomplete encoding of the stressful situation. It has been demonstrated experimentally that people who have been exposed to pictures of a bloody car accident tend to remember central trauma-related items better than more peripheral details. This laboratory finding is related to a real-world phenomenon called weapon focusing. Witnesses to crimes committed with visible weapons have sharper memories of the weapon than of other aspects of the situation, including the face of the perpetrator, for which the memories are more diffuse. The explanation for this is that the gun is the carrier of the most emotionally salient information and therefore captures the attention at the expense of other aspects. This phenomenon has been found to be particularly pronounced in people reacting with anxiety at the sight of weapons.

Short-term memory, which demands that information be held in consciousness momentarily, has been found to be extra sensitive to stress because the situation demands a focus on stress-relevant stimuli and therefore attention tends to be biased. On the contrary, overlearned abilities, such as procedural memory, for which the memory traces are well consolidated, are found to be more stress resistant than recently acquired memories, which are destroyed more easily. In a laboratory test of declarative memory, spatial thinking, and procedural memory tested with a word stem priming task, high levels of cortisol impaired declarative memory and spatial thinking, whereas procedural memory was spared.

One reason why overlearned skills are more difficult to erase is that repetition contributes to a better memory. Thus, it appears that more recently registered material in long-term storage and short-term memory is more sensitive to stress.

Effects of Anticipated Stress on Memory

It is not always being in the stressful situation that causes emotional arousal; the anticipation of the incoming stressor may have the same effect. In an experiment by Lupien and colleagues, a group of 14 healthy elderly persons was given a nonstressful task and a stressful task. The nonstressful condition consisted of a computer task. The stressful condition consisted of a videotaped public-speaking task, for which the discourse was said to be evaluated by experts. Before and after each condition subjects were given a declarative memory task and a nondeclarative word completion task. Results showed that in the responders (individuals who react to stress with an increase in cortisol levels), high levels of cortisol were secreted long before the stressful condition, which was not the case in the nonresponders (no change in cortisol level due to stress). This signifies that the anticipation of the incoming stressor played a more important role in the secretion of cortisol than the actual stressor. The responders also performed worse on the declarative memory task than the nonresponders, indicating that even the anticipation of stress has a detrimental effect on declarative memory. Nondeclarative memory was spared. The stress did not affect the nondeclarative memory significantly, either in the whole group or in the subgroups.

One concluding remark about the effects of stress on learning and memory is that stress seems to influence the modulation of memories through its effects on attention and vigilance during the encoding of information. This may be true both for being in a stressful situation and for anticipating of a fear-provoking event. Knowledge about the biological and psychological mechanisms behind the effects of stress on attention and memory storage may help individuals gain control over these processes in order to perhaps make use of the positive effects of stress on memory and learning and avoid the negative.

Possible Mechanisms of the Relation between Stress and Memory

It is possible to differentiate among physiological, cognitive, and emotional stress, which sometimes may partly overlap. These types of stress might be analyzed from two angles: context and time, and whether the stress is good or bad for learning and memory. Two types of learning that are enhanced by stress are classical fear and eyeblink conditioning, as well as processes related to learning about threatening stimuli. In the standard paradigm of eyeblink conditioning, the Pavlovian eyeblink conditioning, a human is exposed to an air puff to the eye, which evokes an involuntary eyeblink reflex as an unconditioned response (UR). When the air puff is directly preceded by a sound as the conditioned stimulus (CS), the human learns the association between the tone and the air puff and blinks in response to the tone, thus anticipating the air puff. The blink is the conditioned response (CR) and is an example of associative learning. Here we are dealing with a physiological stressful event that generates, not disturbs, new associative learning. Physical stressors are generally said to activate lower brain regions involved in, e.g., pain responses, whereas psychological stressors engage the limbic structures.

Concerning the effects of stress on cognition, particularly learning and memory, one of the greatest challenges for neuropsychological research today is to determine the effects of stress on the different stages of the memory process. It is suggested that stress has differential effects on distinct phases of the learning and memory processes. Consolidation of information is found to be enhanced by stress if the stress occurs concomitantly in time and in the same context as the thing to be remembered. The recall of information is impaired, however, if the system is exposed to stress shortly before the retrieval of information. One illustrative example of these conjunctions is given by Joëls et al. People passing a stressful examination may have difficulties in recalling the earlier learned, required information (impaired retrieval), but at the same time the traumatic experience of not remembering is burned deeply into their memories (enhanced consolidation). Retrieval difficulties have been interpreted as a negative consequence of the release of corticosteroid hormones. Inversely, the release of corticosteroid hormones facilitate new learning, which tends to compete with or overwrite the earlier acquired information. The competition between the access to earlier information and current challenges has been conceived as a kind of fruitful adaptation, since knowledge about new threats (i.e., risk of failure on the examination) may enhance the chances of future survival, in this context a better preparation for the next examination.

These findings are congruent with results showing that exposition for a psychological stressor preserves or enhances the memory for the emotional aspect of an event, while it simultaneously disrupts the memory for non-emotional or neutral aspects of the same event. This pattern may be explained by the fact that emotional and non-emotional memories are modulated by different structures of the brain. Encoding and retrieval of emotional memories are associated with the amygdala, whereas the encoding and retrieval of non-emotional memories are associated with the hippocampal formation. This pattern might also explain the gaps in memory and general memory impairment seen in patients suffering from traumatic memories.

Summary

Stress refers to an extra load on the organism. Neuroendocrinologically, stress reactions are characterized by the release of the stress hormones corticosterone in animals and cortisol in humans. Normally, increasing demands lead to increasing performance. However, this relationship holds up to a certain optimal level; thereafter, increasing demands lead to decreasing performance. This appears to be true for animal as well as human behavior in the domain of learning and memory. The mnemonic process in animals is characterized by associations between a few or several elements. Memory and learning in humans are more complex and may be analyzed in two main systems: declarative and nondeclarative memory. In animals as well as in humans, the same cerebral structures have been identified as crucial in the mnemonic process: the hippocampus and the amygdala. The hippocampus is critical for learning and memory, whereas the amygdala is responsible for the transmission of emotional information during the mnemonic process. Stress hormone receptors in the hippocampus and amygdala make these cerebral structures responsive to stress. The frontal lobes are also involved in the memory process, through the region's accumulation of stress hormone receptors and rich connections to other parts of the brain. It is possible to differentiate among physiological, cognitive, and emotional stress, which might be analyzed from a time and context perspective and with respect to whether they are gold or bad for memory. Generally, declarative memory is more sensitive to stress than nondeclarative memory. Stress has different effects on the declarative memory depending on which phase in the memory process that it occurs.

Further Reading

de Quervain, D. J., Roozendaal, B. and McGaugh, J. L. (1998). Stress and glucocorticoids impair retrieval of long-term spatial memory. *Nature* **394**, 787–790.

Joëls, M., et al. (2006). Learning under stress: how does it work? *Trends in Cognitive Science* **10**, 153–158.

Kim, J. J., Song, E. U. and Kosten, T. A. (2006). Stress effects in the hippocampus: synaptic plasticity and memory. *Stress* **9**, 1–11.

Krystal, J. H., et al. (1995). Toward a cognitive neuroscience of dissociation and altered memory functions in posttraumatic stress disorder. In: Friedman, M. J., Charney, D. S. & Deutch, A. Y. (eds.) *Neurobiological and clinical consequences of stress*, p. 249. Philadelphia, PA: Lippincott-Raven.

Lazarus, R. S. and Folkman, S. (1986). Cognitive theories of stress and the issue of circularity. In: Appley, M. H. & Trumbull, R. (eds.) *Dynamics of stress*, p. 63. New York: Plenum.

McEwen, B. S. and Sapolsky, R. M. (1995). Stress and cognitive function. *Current Opinion in Neurobiology* **5**, 205–216.

Payne, J. D., et al. (2006). The impact of stress on neutral and emotional aspects of episodic memory. *Memory* **14**, 1–16.

Peterson, L. R. (1967). Short-term memory. In: McGaugh, J. L., Weinberger, N. M. & Whalen, R. E. (eds.) *Psychobiology: readings from Scientific American*, pp. 141. San Francisco, CA: Freeman.
Pryce, C., Mohammed, A. H. and Feldon, J. (eds.) (2002). Environmental manipulations in rodents and primates: insights into pharmacology, biochemistry and behaviour. *Pharmacological and Biochemical Behavior* **73**, Special Issue.
Sandi, C. and Rose, S. P. (1994). Corticosterone enhances long-term retention in one-day-old chicks trained in a weak passive avoidance learning paradigm. *Brain Research* **647**, 106–112.
Shalev, A. Y. (1996). Stress versus traumatic stress. In: van der Kolh, B. A., McFarlane, A. C. & Weisaeth, L. (eds.) *Traumatic stress*, pp. 93. New York: Guildford Press.
Shors, T. J. (2006). Stressful experience and learning across the lifespan. *Annual Review of Psychology* **57**, 55–85.
Yerkes, R. M. and Dodson, J. D. (1908). The relation of strength of stimulus to rapidity of habit-formation. *Journal of Computational and Neurological Psychology* **18**, 459–482.

Pain

H J Strausbaugh and J D Levine
University of California, San Francisco, CA, USA

This article is reproduced from Encyclopedia of Stress First Edition, edition, volume 3, pp 115–118, © 2000, Elsevier Inc.

Glossary

Analgesia	A decreased perception of pain.
Hyperalgesia	An increased perception of pain.
Nociception	A perception of pain.
Opioid	Any of three families of endogenous peptides (i.e., as endorphin, enkephalin, and dynorphin) that induce analgesia by binding to μ, δ, or κ opioid receptors.

Introduction

Definition and Measurement of Pain

Pain has been defined as an aversive sensation originating from a noxious stimulus in a defined area of the body. Such intense, potentially tissue-injurious stimuli activate nociceptive sensory neurons (nociceptors), which transmit signals via the spinal cord to the brain that are perceived by the organism as pain. The central nociceptive processing areas include the thalamus, hypothalamus, mesencephalic tegmental area, mesolimbic areas, parabrachial nuclei, amygdala, bulbopontine reticular formation, and the somatosensory cortex. Pain has two components: a sensory or discriminate component and an affective or emotional component. Because pain involves both of these components, simply recording from peripheral nociceptors does not provide a sufficient measurement of pain because the affective component of pain is not assessed in this manner. To circumvent this problem, behavioral measures of pain are used. If animals display characteristic behaviors after application of a noxious stimulus, including withdrawal of the area to which the stimulus is applied, licking of the affected area, vocalization, or escape behavior, it is inferred that the animal is experiencing pain. A commonly used behavioral test for the measurement of pain in animals and the test upon which much of the current information on stress effects on pain is based is the tail flick test. In this test, an animal is lightly restrained and its tail is exposed to a heat source intense enough to produce pain in humans. The time it takes for the animal to remove its tail from the heat source is recorded as tail flick latency; the more painful the stimulus, the shorter the latency. An additional tool used to identify pain is the administration of opioid analgesics such as morphine. Morphine activates an endogenous pain control circuit to block the transmission of nociceptive signals. Therefore, if a noxious stimulus-induced behavior is blocked by morphine, it is considered to be painful.

Definition and Measurement of Stress

Stress is generally defined as any stimulus to which the organism is not adapted. Like pain, stress involves a perceptual component and is therefore difficult to assess in laboratory animals. To circumvent this problem, hormonal measurements are commonly used. Stressful stimuli activate three neuroendocrine circuits: the hypothalamic-pituitary-adrenocortical (HPA) axis, the sympathoadrenal axis, and the sympathetic neural axis. Although different stressors may activate these axes to varying degrees, all axes are activated by most stressful stimuli. Therefore, the hormonal measurement of activation of one of these axes, generally the HPA axis, is used as an operational definition of stress. Both adrenocorticotropic hormone (ACTH) and corticosterone are secreted rapidly into the blood upon activation of the HPA axis. Stimuli that evoke increases beyond normal circadian levels in either of these hormones are considered stressful.

How do these broad, somewhat overlapping concepts, pain and stress, relate to each other? One of the first written observations of the relationship between pain and stress comes from observations made by field doctors in Europe during World War II. These doctors observed that up to 70% of soldiers presenting with severe battle wounds would not report significant levels of pain. This apparent insensitivity to pain was short-lived; 24 h later, all soldiers reported significant levels of pain. Reports such as these suggested that the perception of pain could be modified cognitively. Because stress seemed to be a common factor in all of these reports, the question arose as to whether stress could affect pain perception. In 1976, a decreased perception of pain after exposure to a stressor was shown in laboratory experiments for the first time and was termed stress-induced analgesia. Although less well studied, it has also been shown that stress can enhance pain perception in some circumstances. This phenomenon has been termed stress hyperalgesia and is generally referred to as stress-induced hyperalgesia.

Stress-Induced Analgesia

Stress-induced analgesia refers to the well-established phenomenon that exposing humans or animals to a wide variety of stressors induces the suppression of pain perception. Although electric foot shock and cold water swim have been the most well-studied eliciting stressors, others include rotation, immobilization, and food deprivation. The decrease in pain sensitivity in these studies is usually measured as an increase in tail flick latency to noxious thermal stimuli. However, other pain sensitivity tests such as paw withdrawal, paw licking, and escape behavior in response to exposure to electrified grids or hot plates are also used.

Although the mechanisms of stress-induced analgesia are not completely understood, two subtypes of stress-induced analgesia – endogenous opioid dependent (opioid mediated) and opioid independent (nonopioid mediated) – can be distinguished. Opioid-mediated stress-induced analgesia is defined as stress-induced analgesia that either is blocked by the opiate receptor antagonist naloxone or is cross-tolerant to opioid agonists such as morphine. Cross-tolerance is determined by treating an animal for several days with morphine until the drug no longer produces analgesia. A stressful stimulus is then applied, and if the analgesia is blocked, then it is considered cross-tolerant to morphine. The nonopioid-mediated type of stress-induced analgesia is unaffected by these treatments. Characteristics of the stressor, including the temporal pattern of administration and severity, seem to predict whether opioid or nonopioid analgesia will be induced. In general, stressors that are intermittent and less severe produce opioid-mediated analgesia, whereas stressors that are continuous and of greater severity produce nonopioid-mediated analgesia. Both forms can be classically conditioned.

The distinct nature of opioid- and nonopioid-mediated subtypes of stress-induced analgesia is supported by the fact that they are not cross-tolerant. In fact, a collateral inhibition model has been proposed by Bodnar and colleagues in which activation of one form of stress-induced analgesia would actively inhibit the other form. These investigators have shown that, if administered closely in time, nonopioid-mediated analgesia inhibits opioid-mediated analgesia. This is in contrast to the well-established phenomenon that distinct elicitors of opioid-mediated stress-induced analgesia synergize to produce greater analgesia. Bodnar and colleagues propose that collateral inhibition allows the animal to use its most adaptive system in response to potentially widely varying stressful situations presented by the environment.

The mechanism of opioid-mediated stress-induced analgesia is thought to involve both central and peripheral sources of opioids as well as both central and peripheral sites of action. Stress activates endogenous opioidergic neural circuits in the midbrain, which then transmit signals through the dorsolateral funiculus to inhibit pain transmission circuits in the dorsal horn of the spinal cord. Stress also induces the release of opioids from peripheral sources, including the pituitary gland and the adrenal medulla, and, during inflammation, from leukocytes. These opioids may act by binding to receptors on terminals of nociceptive peripheral sensory nerves and inhibiting noxious stimulation-induced activation or sensitization of these neurons. It is important to note that while these opioidergic pathways are a key element in mediating this type of analgesia, other neurotransmitters (e.g., serotonin, norepinephrine, acetylcholine), neuropeptides (e.g., cholecystokinin), and hormones (e.g., corticosterone) may also participate in this pathway.

Although it is clear that distinct pathways mediate opioid and nonopioid forms of stress-induced analgesia, there is some evidence that there may also be some pathways in common. Similar to opioid-mediated forms of stress-induced analgesia, both midbrain structures and the dorsolateral funiculus of the spinal cord are involved in mediating nonopioid stress-induced forms of analgesia. Additionally, mouse strains have been developed that express high or low levels of stress-induced analgesia. This phenotype is present whether the animals are exposed to stressors that characteristically induce opioid- or nonopioid-mediated analgesia. However, in the absence of specific gene products, this is not strong evidence for an overlap in the mechanism but does offer a promising avenue for future studies. In contrast to opioid-mediated stress-induced analgesia, vasopressin, thyrotropin-releasing hormone, and histaminergic systems are involved in mediating nonopioid-mediated stress-induced an algesia. Some forms of nonopioid-mediated stress-induced analgesia (e.g., continuous cold water swim) are mediated by the HPA axis and, in particular, by the adrenocortical system, whereas other forms (e.g., continuous foot shock of short duration) are not. Additionally, dopaminergic and cholinergic systems may play a role in mediating continuous cold water swim analgesia. Clearly, further research is required to elucidate the pathways that mediate nonopioid-mediated stress-induced analgesia.

Stress-Induced Hyperalgesia

Stress-induced hyperalgesia is defined as an increased sensitivity to noxious stimuli or a decrease in analgesia after exposure to stress. In the laboratory, an increased sensitivity to noxious stimuli is usually indicated by a decreased tail flick latency to noxious heat stimulation. Stress-induced hyperalgesia has been observed in animals after exposure to a variety of stressors, including ether, mechanical oscillation, vibration, a novel environment, and repeated exposure to cold temperatures. Stress-induced hyperalgesia has been much less well studied than stress-induced analgesia, and consequently the mechanisms of stress-induced hyperalgesia are still poorly understood. However, a general concept is emerging that an induction of stress-induced hyperalgesia is due to changes in the central, possibly perceptual, processing of nociceptive information by the organism and not due to changes in the processing of noxious stimuli at the level of the peripheral nociceptive pathways as may contribute to stress-induced analgesia. This emerging concept is based on several lines of evidence. First, electrophysiological recordings from nociceptive sensory neurons in the peripheral nerves indicate no change in sensitivity to the noxious stimulus before and after stress-induced hyperalgesia is elicited. Second, stress-induced hyperalgesia can be classically conditioned such that even when a noxious stimulus is not applied, a neutral stimulus that had been paired previously with the noxious stimulus can elicit hyperalgesia. Third, emotional characteristics of the rat can determine whether stress-induced hyperalgesia is induced. Although it is difficult to assess the emotional state of a rat, studies have shown that rats displaying behaviors thought to indicate anxiety (e.g., vocalization, agitation) during exposure to stress and the noxious stimulus display stress-induced hyperalgesia, whereas rats not displaying these behaviors and exposed to identical stimuli do not show stress-induced hyperalgesia. This concept is supported by the fact that administering antianxiety drugs (e.g., clonidine, diazepam) to these rats blocks stress-induced hyperalgesia, whereas administering anxiety-producing drugs (e.g., yohimbine) enhances and prolongs stress-induced hyperalgesia. Finally, clinical studies indicate that anxious patients display an increased sensitivity to pain. Of course, in these studies it is difficult to assess whether patients are more sensitive to pain because they are anxious or whether they are anxious because they are perceiving more pain. Further investigation will be required to elucidate the factors that elicit and the mechanisms that produce stress-induced hyperalgesia. Additionally, it has been shown that stress may inhibit the analgesic effects of drugs as well as enhance pain perception; however, the relationship between these two effects is currently unknown. Further investigation will be required to distinguish these two phenomena.

Further Reading

Amit, Z. and Galina, Z. H. (1986). Stress-induced analgesia: adaptive pain suppression. *Physiological Reviews* **66**, 1091–1120.

Bardiani, A. and Pavone, F. (1991). Reduction of oxotremorine-induced analgesia after chronic but not acute restraint stress. *Psychopharmacology (Berlin)* **104**, 57–61.

Bodnar, R. J. (1990). Effects of opioid peptides on peripheral stimulation and "stress"-induced analgesia in animals. *Critical Reviews in Neurobiology* **6**, 39–49.

Foa, E. B., Zinbarg, R. and Rothbaum, B. O. (1992). Uncontrollability and unpredictability in post-traumatic stress disorder: an initial model. *Psychological Bulletin* **112**, 218–238.

Gamaro, G. D., Xavier, M. H., Denardin, J. D., et al. (1998). The effects of acute and repeated restraint stress on the nociceptive response in rats. *Physiology and Behavior* **63**, 693–697.

Gue, M., Del Rio-Lacheze, C., Eutamene, H., Theodorou, V., Fioramonti, J. and Bueno, L. (1997). Stress-induced visceral hypersensitivity to rectal distension in rats: role of CRF and mast cells. *Neurogastroenterology and Motility* 9, 271–279.

Kelly, D. D. (ed.) (1986). *Stress-induced analgesia.* Annals of the New York Academy of Sciences (Vol. 467). New York: New York Academy of Sciences.

King, T. E., Crown, E. D., Sieve, A. N., Joynes, R. L., Grau, J. W. and Meagher, M. W. (1999). Shock-induced hyperalgesia: evidence forebrain systems play an essential role. *Behavioural Brain Research* **100**, 33–42.

Madden, J., Akil, H., Patrick, R. L. and Barchas, J. D. (1977). Stress-induced parallel changes in central opioid levels and pain responsiveness in the rat. *Nature* **265**, 358–360.

Mogil, J. S., Sternberg, W. F., Marek, P., Sadowski, B., Belknap, J. K. and Liebeskind, J. C. (1996). The genetics of pain and pain inhibition. *Proceedings of the National Academy of Sciences USA* **93**, 3048–3055.

Murison, R. and Overmier, J. B. (1993). Parallelism among stress effects on ulcer, immunosuppression and analgesia: commonality of mechanisms? *Journal of Physiology (Paris)* **87**, 253–259.

Nijenhuis, E. R., Vanderlinden, J. and Spinhoven, P. (1998). Animal defensive reactions as a model for trauma-induced dissociative reactions. *Journal of Trauma and Stress* **11**, 243–260.

Simone, D. A. (1992). Neural mechanisms of hyperalgesia. *Current Opinion in Neurobiology* **2**, 479–483.

Vidal, C. and Jacob, J. J. (1982). Stress hyperalgesia in rats: an experimental animal model of anxiogenic hyperalgesia in human. *Life Sciences* **31**, 1241–1244.

Watkins, L. R. and Mayer, D. J. (1982). Organization of endogenous opiate and nonopiate pain control systems. *Science* **216**, 1185–1192.

Migraine

N M Ramadan
Rosalind Franklin University of Medicine and Science, North Chicago, IL, USA

This is a revised version of the article by N M Ramadan, Encyclopedia of Stress First Edition, volume 2, pp 757–770, © 2000, Elsevier Inc.

Glossary

Cephalad — Toward the head.

Channelopathy — A condition resulting from many scenarios (membrane ion channels that open when they should not, channels that do not open very well or at all, channels that stay open too long, misplaced channels, and a lack of channels or too many channels) that potentially can be deleterious.

Comorbidity — The association between migraine and another condition that is unlikely to be random or causal.

Cortical spreading depression — A local neuronal phenomenon that is elicited by chemical, physical, or electrical stimuli; characterized by a short burst of neuronal electrical activity and followed by a short-lived (minutes) marching wave of slow neuronal suppression.

Incidence — The proportion of new cases of an illness in a defined population over a set time period.

Migraine — A primary headache disorder manifesting as episodic, usually unilateral severe head pain with nausea, vomiting, and light and noise sensitivity.

Neurogenic inflammation — A sterile inflammatory response that is caused by an injurious stimulus of peripheral neurons and that leads to the release of substances (e.g., neuropeptides) that alter vascular permeability.

Phonophobia — An unpleasant feeling when exposed to noise.

Photophobia — An unpleasant feeling when exposed to light.

Prevalence — The proportion of a given population with a disease over a defined period of time. Lifetime prevalence of migraine is the proportion of individuals in the general population who have ever had migraine during their life. Prevalence is the average disease incidence multiplied by its duration.

Trepanation — An old surgical procedure in which a hole is drilled or scraped into the skull, leaving the membrane around the brain intact.

Introduction

Migraine is a painful and disabling headache disorder that has plagued humanity for thousands of years. Julius Caesar, England's Queen Mary, Thomas Jefferson, Claude Monet, Vincent van Gogh, Georges Seurat (visual disturbances of migraine aura, the Seurat effect), Alexander Graham Bell, Friedrich Nietzsche, Peter Tchaikovsky, and Sigmund Freud all suffered from migraine. Over the centuries, migraine has been transformed from a disease that is caused by evil spirits to a vascular and then a neurovascular disorder with well-defined epidemiology, pathology, pathophysiology, pharmacology, therapeutics, and genetics. Several thousand years BC, trepanation was a common practice used to relieve migraine by releasing demons from the head. Egyptians bound a clay crocodile, holding grain in its mouth, to the head of headache patients, using a strip of linen that bore the Gods' names. Galen considered migraine a visceral pain disorder when he said, "How constantly do we see the head attacked with pain when yellow bile is contained in the stomach: as also the pain forthwith ceasing when the bile has been vomited." (Koehn, 1826) Tenth century Arabian physicians used garlic and hot iron on temple incisions (two-site venesection) to relieve head pain.

More recently, Sir Thomas Willis believed that migraine was caused by vasodilatation, arguing that headache symptoms were related to slowly ascending spasms beginning at the peripheral ends of the nerves. Similarly, Erasmus Darwin (Charles Darwin's grandfather) believed in vasodilation-induced migraine and proposed to treat it with centrifugation in order to force the blood from the head to the feet. Edward Liveing commented in "On Megrim, Sick-headache, and Some Allied Disorders" that the migraine, similar to epilepsy, is a malady of the nervous system caused by nerve-storm, which may be the first account of cortical spreading depression (CSD) as an initiator of migraine. Sir William Gowers proposed dividing the treatment of headache into prophylactic and episodic. He advocated continuous treatment with drugs to render attacks less frequent and treatment of the attacks themselves. In the late 1800s, the potent neurotoxin ergot, which comes from a fungus that grows on rye, was used to treat unilateral headache. Later in the early 1900s, the active chemical ergotamine was discovered and became the preferred treatment for migraine.

The modern understanding of migraine started with the work of Harold Wolff, a migraine sufferer himself, who performed elegant clinical experiments that supported the vascular theory of headache. Wolff and Ray published in 1940 a detailed map of pain-sensitive structures in the brain, which provided the basis for the link between arterial pathology and referred head pain. Contemporaneously, Leao discovered CSD in animals, which later was equated with human visual aura. Today, this phenomenon can be imaged and measured, and it is forming the backbone for the development of several classes of potential antimigraine drugs. To this end, it is important to mention seminal research from Boston (Cutrer and Sanchez del Rio), Detroit (Welch and Cao), Los Angeles (Woods), and elsewhere, which provided us with a window for analyzing and quantifying CSD in humans.

In the 1960s and beyond, Sicuteri, Lance, and Anthony stressed the role of serotonin in migraine. Their work was later amplified by Saxena, Humphrey, Martin, and others, who discovered the triptans. Also, the Copenhagen group led by Olesen drew attention to a mismatch between cerebral blood flow (CBF) changes and symptoms of migraine, which challenged the vasoconstriction–vasodilation theory. The same group evaluated the role of nitric oxide (NO) in inducing headache, and now NO synthase (NOS) inhibition is becoming a prime target in averting migraine.

The understanding of migraine mechanisms and therapeutics evolved over the last 2 decades with experiments that Moskowitz and fellow researchers conducted. The activation of the trigeminal system in animals was shown to induce plasma protein extravasation and neurogenic inflammation, and many antimigraine therapies blocked this response. Similarly, the initial work of Edvinsson and Goadsby was amplified in the last 10–15 years, culminating in advancing calcitonin gene-related peptide (CGRP) antagonists for migraine. Also, important work from Detroit, Michigan, and Bologna, Italy, supported the theory that the brain-energy metabolism in migraine sufferers is defective and that magnesium deficiency may contribute to the disease. These observations opened the field to testing magnesium, co-enzyme Q10 (CoQ10), and riboflavin (B2) for migraine prevention. Apropos, John Graham modernized the preventive treatment of migraine with the introduction of methysergide, Oscar Reinmuth's group drew attention to the role of propranolol in migraine, and recent studies from Welch and colleagues and Ferrari and coworkers suggested that migraine may be a progressive disorder that may warrant early and aggressive preventive therapy. Finally, the potential role of peripheral and central sensitization in migraine, which Burstein and colleagues are unfolding, is opening new windows into migraine therapeutic strategies.

Migraine is not an orphan in the era of genomic discoveries. French and Dutch researchers led the effort demonstrating that some forms of migraine result from defective calcium trafficking across its channels and provided a new avenue for exploring migraine mechanisms and therapies. A knockin model of abnormal mutations now provides a model of familial hemiplegic migraine and susceptibility to CSD. Also, the discovery of mutations in the Na-K adenosine triphosphatase (ATPase) gene is steering us to new pathophysiological and pharmacological directions. Indeed, excessive synaptic glutamate (Glu) is a by-product of these mutations, which predisposes the migraine brain to hyperexcitability, sensitization, and/or neuronal cell death.

Epidemiology

Prevalence estimates of headaches vary significantly among studies. For example, the prevalence of headache disorders in Europe and the United States ranges from 13% (1-year prevalence in people with serious headaches) to 93% (lifetime prevalence in the United Kingdom, based on a telephone interview). Several factors contribute to the observed variability, including the time periods used for estimating prevalence (e.g., 1-year vs. lifetime), targeted age range and other sociodemographic factors, methods of ascertaining headache diagnoses, and cooccurrence of different headache types. Regardless of the study methods, the majority of population-based studies of headache disorders in adults indicate a female preponderance, which is not unexpected because most chronic pain disorders with a remitting and relapsing course (e.g., fibromyalgia and irritable bowel syndrome) are more prevalent in women.

Rasmussen et al. conducted a large 1991 epidemiological study (1000 people, 25–64 years old) on the prevalence of headache disorders in Copenhagen County, Denmark. Tension-type headache was the most common, followed by fasting headache, migraine, and headache attributed to nose or sinus disease (**Table 1**).

Table 1 Lifetime prevalence of headache disorders in Denmark[a]

Type	*Prevalence (%)*
Primary headache disorders	
Tension-type headache	78.0
Migraine	16.0
Secondary headache disorders	
Fasting	19.0
Nose and sinus disease	15.0
Head trauma	4.0
Nonvascular intracranial disease (e.g., brain tumor)	0.5

[a]From Rasmussen, B. K., Jensen, R., Schroll, M., et al. (1991), Epidemiology of headache in a general population – a prevalence study, *Journal of Clinical Epidemiology* **44**, 1147–1157.

Epidemiology of Migraine

Few longitudinal studies have investigated the incidence of migraine. A 12-year follow-up of a Dutch general population sample ($n = 549$) determined that the incidence of migraine was 8.1 per 1000 person-years (male : female = 1 : 6). Data from a 2005 prevalence study in people 12–29 years old revealed slightly higher numbers – the incidence of migraine with aura was 14.1 per 1000 person-years and that of migraine without aura was 18.9 per 1000 person-years.

The incidence of migraine is two to three times higher in females than in males, and the peak age of onset is 5–9 years in males and 12–13 years in females for migraine with aura. For migraine without aura, the figures are 10–11 years for males and 14–17 years for females. The incidence of migraine may be increasing, particularly in women 10–49 years old.

In contrast to the paucity of studies of migraine incidence, several reports from various countries across the globe addressed migraine prevalence and established that it is a common disorder with particular predilection to Whites and women. Prior to 1988, population estimates of migraine prevalence varied from 3 to 35%. The application of the International Headache Society (IHS) 2004 diagnostic criteria led to more robust and consistent data on migraine epidemiology and allowed a better assessment of demographic influences such as race, socioeconomic status, gender, and geographical location. Indeed, several studies have now provided gender-dependent estimates of the 1-year prevalence of migraine: approximately 3–22% in women and 1–16% in men. The prevalence of migraine is highest in North America and lowest in Africa (**Figure 1**).

Population studies have confirmed that migraine is more prevalent in females than in males older

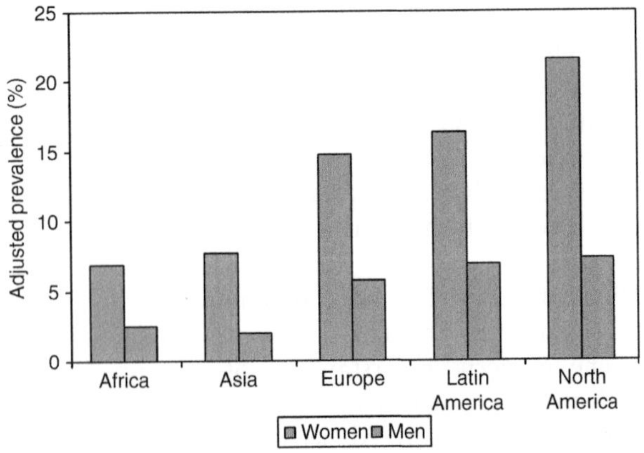

Figure 1 Prevalence of migraine across continents. From Lipton, R. B. and Bigal, M. E. (2005), Migraine: epidemiology, impact and risk factor for progression, *Headache* **45**(supplement 1), S3–S13.

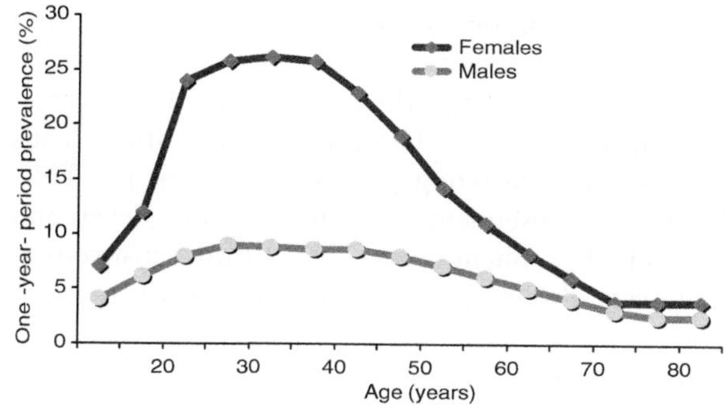

Figure 2 Prevalence of migraine by age. From Stewart, W. F., Lipton, R. B., Celentano, D. D., et al. (1992), Prevalence of migraine headache in the United States: relation to age, income, race, and other sociodemographic factors, *Journal of the American Medical Association* **267**, 64–69.

than 12 years (female : male = 2–3 : 1), regardless of race or geographical location. Migraine in children is almost as prevalent in boys as it is in girls.

The prevalence of migraine follows an inverted-U curve with advancing age (**Figure 2**). This phenomenon is significantly more pronounced in females. The peak prevalence of migraine is in the fourth and fifth decades; it declines substantially thereafter.

Migraine varies with race. Whites are more commonly affected (prevalence = 20.4% in women and 8.6% in males) than African Americans (16.2% in women and 7.2% in men) or Asian Americans (9.2% in women and 4.2% in men). Contrary to a widely held belief, migraine is more common in low-socioeconomic groups and in less-educated individuals. The use of care data indicate, however, that people in higher social strata and better-educated migraine sufferers are more likely to seek medical advice.

Neural Basis of Head Pain

Triggers of head pain in different headache disorders may vary, but the substrates for pain generation, stimulus conduction through the peripheral and central nociceptive pathways, recognition and perception of the experience, and memory and reaction to pain are largely similar whether the type of headache is primary (e.g., migraine) or secondary (e.g., trauma). A discussion of trigger mechanisms is beyond the scope of this article, but a brief overview of the final common pathways in pain are described next.

Neuroanatomy

The pathways of head pain can be anatomically dissected into four distinct locales (**Figure 3**):

1. Sensing organs such as the skin and blood vessels.
2. Sensory-discriminative regions, which include the trigeminal nucleus caudalis (TNC), thalamus, and the primary (S1) and secondary (S2) sensory cortices.
3. Emotion, memory, and behavioral response networks. These include the insula and hippocampus, which encode the memory and recognition of pain; cingulate, which modulates the affective and motivational aspects of pain; and precentral cortex, cerebellum, and cingulated, which are involved in the reaction to the painful experience.
4. Modulatory, predominantly inhibitory regions such as the hypothalamus, basal forebrain, and various brain-stem structures.

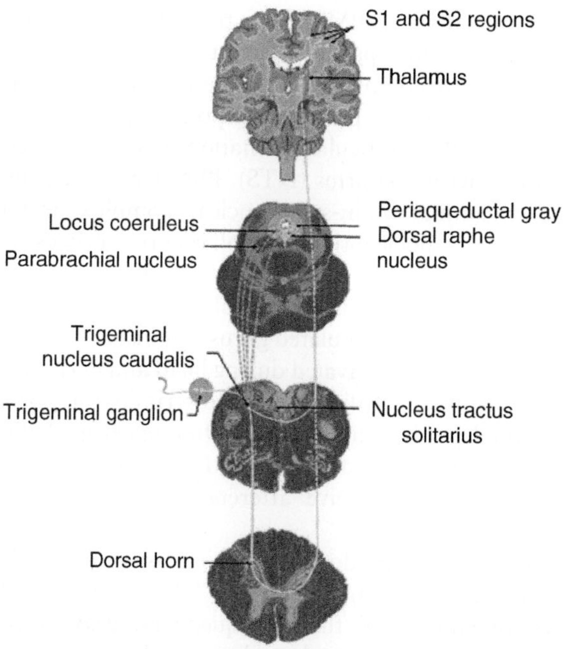

Figure 3 Nociceptive and modulatory pathways. Pathways in yellow represent afferent projections subserving pain; pathways in orange represent descending, mainly inhibitory projections.

Head pain is generated when pain-sensitive intracranial structures are stimulated. These include vascular structures such as the circle of Willis and proximal middle cerebral arteries, neuronal structures including the trigeminal and glossopharyngeal nerves, and the cranial meninges, particularly the perivascular components of the dura. Pain signals are transmitted from these nociceptive structures cephalad, mostly via Aδ and C fibers that contain neurotransmitters such as Glu, CGRP, substance P (SP), and neurokinin A (NKA). Middle meningeal artery nociceptive fibers travel through the first division of the trigeminal nerve (V1) to the ipsilateral trigeminal ganglion (TG), whereas fibers from the middle cranial fossa dura run in V3 to the ipsilateral TG. First-order neuron fibers in TG then project centrally onto secondary sensory neurons in the TNC, which in turn send their projections to the contralateral nucleus ventralis posteromedialis (VPM) of the thalamus. Projections of the nociceptive pathway from the trigeminal brain-stem nuclear complex include the trigeminal lemniscus, hypothalamic projections, pontine parabrachial nucleus (PBN), reticular formation, and the nucleus of the tractus solitarius (NTS). PBN feeds back into the trigeminal brain-stem nuclear complex and is involved in nociceptive control. Central processing of incoming pain signals beyond the thalamus include cortical areas such as the cingulate, insular, S1, and S2, as well as the cingulated gyrus and insula. Cortical neurons that are activated during head and peripheral pain include localizing and discriminating pain neuronal pools, which receive afferents from VPM, and those involved in the effective components of pain, which receive afferents from the medial thalamus.

Descending, predominantly inhibitory neuronal fibers project from the frontal lobe cortex to the hypothalamus and the periaqueductal gray (PAG) and from there descend to the rostral ventromedial medullary nuclear complex (RVM, the raphe magnus and adjacent reticular formation), which ultimately projects to the medullary and spinal dorsal horns.

Neurochemistry

The PAG–RVM system contains serotonin (5-HT) excitatory neurons that activate inhibitory interneurons of the substantia gelatinosa and lamina II of the spinal trigeminal nucleus. Electrical stimulation of either PAG or RVM or the exogenous injection of opioids, which activate the 5-HT system, results in inhibitory activity in the nociceptive neurons in the dorsal horn. Independently of PAG–RVM, a diffuse noxious inhibitory control (DNIC) system (not shown in **Figure 3**) directly reduces the firing of wide-dynamic range (WDR) neurons of the medullary dorsal horn cells following noxious stimulation from parts of the body that are remote from their receptor field.

The neurochemicals that are involved in pain derive from the vascular endothelium of nociceptive structures, which contains both vasoconstrictive (e.g., thromboxane, superoxide ions, and endothelin) and vasodilator substances (e.g., NO and prostacyclin), and from the adventitia–media junction of intracranial vessels, which are rich in neuropeptide-positive terminals (e.g., CGRP and SP).

Neurophysiology

Nociceptive activation induces peripheral sensitization, which is predominantly mediated by enhanced Na channels opening. This process perpetuates discharges along the nociceptive terminals and into TG with an ongoing cycle of enhanced Na-channel opening, excitatory neurotransmitter release, and further neuronal activation. With time, peripheral sensitization, perhaps through excessive *N*-methyl-D-aspartate (NMDA) Glu receptor activation, leads to a central sensitizing process initially at the TNC level and subsequently at the thalamic level and beyond. The phenomenon of central sensitization manifests physiologically as spontaneous activity in otherwise quiescent neurons, reduced threshold to activation, and expansion of the neuronal receptor field following distal stimulation.

Peripheral and central sensitization could continue unless various protective neuromodulatory mechanisms become operant. Modulation is mediated peripherally through the presynaptic inhibition of neurotransmitter release or centrally through several possible mechanisms, including the inhibition of afferent input. At the peripheral level, serotonergic presynaptic receptors of the 5-HT_{1D} and 5-HT_{1F} types and some metabotropic Glu receptors participate in suppressing neurotransmitter release. Centrally, TNC neurons are inhibited by local inhibitory interneurons (e.g., GABAergic), by activation of presynaptic inhibitory receptors (5-HT_{1D}, 5-HT_{1F}, 5-HT_{1B}, and metabotropic), or by descending inhibitory fibers (e.g., noradrenergic, adenosinergic, glutamatergic, serotonergic, and GABAergic). The descending modulatory system itself is under the control of various hypothalamic-pituitary outputs, such as estrogen levels, and melatonin cycles, which have direct relevance to the roles of sleep and menstrual cycles in migraine and other painful disorders.

Genetics

The genetics of most headache disorders remain elusive. On the other hand, some major advances in the genetics of migraine have been published in the last decade or so.

There is mounting evidence that a subform of migraine (familial hemiplegic migraine, FHM) is due to a membrane ion channelopathy or ionopathy (**Table 2**). A net gain of function of the calcium channel leads to an excessive intracellular calcium influx into the presynaptic glutamatergic terminal, Glu release, and persistent postsynaptic activation that predisposes to cortical spreading depression (CSD). Indeed, a knockin mouse model of a CACNA1A mutation that predisposes animals to CSD and transient hemiplegia has been developed. Alternatively, a defective Na pump reduces the efficiency of Glu transporters in clearing Glu, resulting in excessive Glu at the synaptic cleft and subsequently in continued postsynaptic excitation. Interestingly, a heterozygous mutation on the gene encoding for the Glu

Table 2 Some genetic defects in familial hemiplegic migraine that might predispose to hyperexcitable neurons[a]

Chromosome	*Gene mutations locale*	*Potential biological or physiological consequence*
19p13	CaCNA1A ($Ca_v2.1$)	↑ Ca^{2+} into presynaptic neuron, causing neurotransmitter release (e.g., glutamate)
1q23	$\tilde{\alpha}_2$ subunit of Na^+/K^+ ATPase	Defective clearing of glutamate from synaptic cleft
2q24	Neuronal Na channel	Enhanced EPSP
5p13	EAAT1 glutamate transporter	Defective clearing of glutamate from synaptic cleft

[a]CaCNA1A, α_1 subunit of calcium channel gene; ATPase, adenosine triphosphatase; Na, sodium; EPSP, excitatory postsynaptic synapse; EAAT1, excitatory amino acid transporter type 1.

transporter excitatory amino acid transporter type 1 (EAAT1) was discovered in 2004 in a patient with seizures, migraine, and alternating hemiplegia. Last, hyperexcitability can be caused by a neuronal Na-channel mutation, reported in 2005.

Genetic defects in FHM might not be extrapolated to the more common forms of migraine with and without aura, especially with the absence of consistent evidence of genetic mutations or functional polymorphism at the known FHM sites, but nearby loci are implicated. Furthermore, a 2005 genomewide scan of people with common forms of migraine confirmed genetic susceptibility at sites previously reported with FHM. In addition, new susceptibility loci were reported (3q and 18p11), which deserve further exploration.

Migraine Mechanisms

The mechanisms of migraine pain and its associated neurological, gastrointestinal, and autonomic manifestations are multiple and complex. Attacks could manifest as an isolated symptom (e.g., migraine aura without headache) or a sign and symptom complex (e.g., migraine with aura), which could take on a range of phenotypic expressions (e.g., emotional lability as part of a premonitory symptom complex followed by pain or a full-blown multiphasic attack manifesting as depressive symptoms, followed by a visual aura followed by pain with nausea and photophobia and phonophobia, and terminating with social-withdrawal feelings and tiredness). Therefore, deciphering migraine mechanisms requires a comprehensive understanding of the isolated manifestations and explanations for the event sequences.

Migraine is a neurobiological disorder of altered neuronal excitability and defective adaptive mechanisms to stressors of the system. The susceptibility to migraine is an interplay between genetic factors and environmental elements (e.g., stress and weather change). The migraine cascade can be conceptualized as a sequence of events occurring in a series, starting with the activation of hypothalamic pathways that trigger the premonitory symptoms and followed by cortical neuronal activation and CSD. Neuronal activation releases various substances such as hydrogen ions and NO, which in turn activate nociceptive terminals that, on the one hand, cause the release of substances such as CGRP and, on the other hand, transmit neuronal impulses into the medulla to the thalamus and up to the cortex for perception and reaction to the headache. CGRP, SP, and NKA participate in neurogenic vasodilation and inflammation, leading to peripheral sensitization and an abnormal response to previously innocuous stimuli (e.g., blood-vessel pulsations becoming painful). Often, peripheral sensitization can culminate in central sensitization with the activation of ancillary trigeminal nociceptive (e.g., allodynia in the distribution of the first division of the trigeminal nerve) and paratrigeminal pathways (e.g., photophobia and phonophobia).

The female preponderance of migraine sufferers provides some insight into the mechanisms of headache and pain. A discussion of the role of sex hormones and migraine mechanisms is quite complex and beyond the scope of this article, but a few highlights are noteworthy. Women detect trigeminal pain at a lower threshold than men, and their tolerance for the painful stimulus may be lower. Some researchers observed that these gender differences may be related to higher sensory-receptor density on the peripheral nerve terminals in women. Furthermore, estrogen receptors (ERs) are distributed on various neuronal pools that participate in migraine pain trafficking (e.g., TNC, hypothalamus, amygdala, PBN, and PAG). Lastly, ERs modulate neuropeptides in the trigeminal system that are involved in migraine (e.g., CGRP, SP, and NKA).

Migraine is comorbid with psychiatric conditions such as generalized anxiety disorders and depression (**Table 3**), and migraine attacks often are triggered by stress and lack of sleep. It has been suggested that bidirectional signal transmission through the trigeminovascular system accounts for both the migraine symptoms and the induction of these symptoms by triggers such as stress. Also, migraine shares similar mechanisms with chronic pain when comorbid psychiatric conditions such as depression could result from functional alterations in the reward–aversion pathways.

Migraine patients have some personality traits such as neuroticism, which could lead to altered coping mechanisms. Indeed, one study suggested that a migraine sufferer's coping mechanisms include amplified physical symptoms, social litigation, and preoccupation with stress. Also, migraine patients are less calm, more irritable, do not relax as well as a nonmigraine healthy controls, and often respond to physical symptoms, including pain, with internal tension.

Table 3 Comorbidity of migraine and systemic and psychiatric disorders

System	*Condition*
Gastrointestinal	Irritable bowel syndrome
Neurological	Epilepsy
	Multiple sclerosis
Psychiatric	Affective disorders
	Anxiety disorders
	Neuroticism
	Sleep disorders
	Substance abuse
	Suicide
Pulmonary	Asthma
Vascular and cardiovascular	Hypertension
	Hypotension
	Ischemic stroke
	Myocardial infarction
Others	Allergies
	Raynaud's phenomenon

Classification of Headache Disorders

The development of a headache disorder classification that is intuitive, psychometrically robust, and easy-to-use enables a better understanding of conditions associated with headache, improves patients' management, and provides a standardized approach to headache research. Headache disorders can be classified broadly as primary (e.g., migraine), and secondary (e.g., posttraumatic). Indeed, the *International Classification for Headache Disorders* (2nd edn.; ICHD-II) recognizes this dichotomy (**Table 4**). Primary headaches are classified largely on the basis of symptoms, whereas secondary headaches are grouped etiologically. Both acute and chronic forms of primary and secondary headache disorders are recognized (e.g., chronic migraine and chronic posttraumatic headache).

Clinical Presentations and Differential Diagnosis of Migraine

Migraine is characterized by episodes of head pain that is aggravated by movement, with associated nausea, photophobia, and phonophobia. Head pain

Table 4 Second International Classification for Headache Disorders (ICHD-II)[a]

Category	*Type*
Primary headache disorders (categories 1–4)	Migraine, tension-type headache, cluster headache and other trigeminal cephalgias, other primary headache (e.g., primary stabbing headache, primary cough headache)
Secondary headache disorders (categories 5–12)	Posttraumatic headache; headache attributed to cranial or cervical vascular disorders; headache attributed to nonvascular intracranial disorder; headache associated with substances or their withdrawal; headache attributed to infection; headache attributed to disorder of homeostasis; headache or facial pain associated with disorder of cranium, neck, eyes, ears, nose sinuses, teeth, mouth, or other facial or cranial structures; headache attributed to psychiatric disorder
Cranial neuralgias and central causes of facial pain (category 13)	Trigeminal neuralgia; glossopharyngeal neuralgia; nervus intermedius neuralgia; superior laryngeal neuralgia; nasociliary neuralgia; supraorbital neuralgia; occipital neuralgia; neck-tongue syndrome; external compression headache; cold stimulus headache; constant pain caused by compression, irritation or distortion of cranial nerves or upper cervical roots by structural lesions; optic neuritis; ocular diabetic neuropathy; head and facial pain attributed to herpes zoster; Tolosa-Hunt syndrome; ophthalmoplegic migraine; anesthesia dolorosa; central poststroke pain; facial pain attributed to multiple sclerosis; persistent idiopathic facial pain; burning mouth syndrome
Other headache, cranial neuralgia, central or primary facial pain	Headache unspecified

[a]From the Headache Classification Subcommittee, International Headache Society (2004), *Special issue on the international classification of headache disorders (2nd edn.), Cephalalgia* **24**(supplement 1).

in migraine is unilateral in approximately 60% of patients and throbbing in many but not all. Up to one-third of migraine patients experience transient neurological symptoms (i.e., aura) that herald or accompany the pain. Most migraine attacks last approximately 1 day (4–72 h in adults; they are of shorter duration in children), and their frequency is quite variable. The frequency of migraine is approximately once per month in population-based studies and three times per month in clinic-based cohorts. In the general population, 2–3% suffer chronic migraine, which is defined as attacks that recur more than 15 times per month. Last, the majority of migraine sufferers are disabled with their attacks.

A careful history and appropriate physical and neurological examination establish most causes of headache disorders. For example, the presence of associated symptoms (e.g., nausea and photophobia) helps to differentiate migraine from tension headache. Important elements of the history that help in establishing the diagnosis include (1) age of onset; (2) duration; (3) time to peak severity; (4) severity and headache-related disability; (5) frequency; (6) location; (7) preceding and accompanying symptoms, if any; (8) precipitating and aggravating factors; (9) circadian or diurnal patterns; and (10) relieving factors. It is also crucial to obtain a full headache medication history, including over-the-counter remedies.

The clinical presentations of migraine with and without aura are often characteristic (**Table 5**). On the other hand, the clinical presentations of secondary headache types mimicking migraine with aura are not unique (**Table 6**), with a few exceptions (e.g., benign or idiopathic intracranial hypotension). Also, the symptom complex of migraine and that of other primary headaches and secondary headaches overlap (**Table 7**). An algorithm that helps in the differentiation between primary and secondary headache disorders uses red flags (called SSNOOPs, an acronym based on the first letter of items in the

Table 5 Diagnostic criteria for migraine[a]

Migraine without aura	A. At least five attacks fulfilling B–D B. Headache attacks lasting 4–72 h (untreated or unsuccessfully treated) C. Headache has at least two of the following characteristics: unilateral location, pulsating quality, moderate or severe pain intensity, aggravation by or causing avoidance of routine physical activity (e.g., walking or climbing stairs) D. During headache at least one of the following: nausea and/or vomiting, photophobia and phonophobia E. Not attributed to another disorder
Migraine with typical aura	A. At least two attacks fulfilling B–C B. Aura consisting of at least one of the following, but no motor weakness: fully reversible visual symptoms including positive features (e.g., flickering lights, spots, or lines) and/or negative features (i.e., loss if vision), fully reversible sensory symptoms including positive features (e.g., pins and needles) and/or negative features (i.e., numbness), fully reversible dysphasic speech disturbance C. At least two of the following: headache [1.21] fulfilling criteria B–D for migraine without aura; begins during the aura or follows aura within 60 min; headache [1.22] that does not fulfill criteria B–D for migraine without aura; begins during the aura or follows aura within 60 min; headache [1.23] does not occur during aura nor follows aura within 60 min D. Not attributed to another disorder

[a]From the Headache Classification Subcommittee, International Headache Society (2004), *Special issue on the international classification of headache disorders (2nd edn.), Cephalalgia* **24**(supplement 1).

Table 6 Differential diagnosis of headache with transient neurological symptoms mimicking migraine with aura[a]

Cerebrovascular disease	Dissection, ischemic stroke and transient ischemic attacks, hemorrhagic stroke, AVM, primary CNS vasculitis, cerebrovenous sinus/dural thrombosis, postpartum angiopathy
Drug-induced	Nitric oxide-releasing compounds (e.g., nitroglycerin, sildenafil), illicit drugs
Endocrine/metabolic disorders	Hypoglycemia
Inherited/genetic disorders	CADASIL, MELAS, OTC deficiency
Nonvascular intracranial disorders	Focal encephalitis and aseptic meningitis, primary or metastatic brain tumors, idiopathic intracranial hypertension, HANDL (PLP), systemic vasculitis (e.g., SLE and aPL syndrome), HIV
Traumatic disease	Posttraumatic headache, postwhiplash injury
Others	Ictal headaches, whiplash injury, cervicogenic headache, chiari malformation type I, glaucoma

[a]aPL, antiphospholipid; AVM, arteriovenous malformation; CADASIL, cerebral autosomal dominant arteriopathy with subcortical infarcts and leukoencephalopathy; CNS, central nervous system; HANDL, headache, neurologic deficits, and cerebrospinal fluid lymphocytosis; HIV, human immunodeficiency virus; MELAS, mitochondrial encephalopathy with lactic acidosis and strokelike episodes; OTC, ornithine transcarbamylase; PLP, pseudomigraine with lymphocytic pleocytosis; SLE, systemic lupus erythematosus.

Table 7 Overlap in symptoms of migraine pain and secondary headaches

Symptom	*Some examples of headache conditions*
Unilateral headache	Trauma, cluster headache, trigeminal autonomic cephalgia, migraine, cerebrovascular disease, idiopathic jabbing headache, sinusitis, eye/jaw disease, cervical spine disease, giant cell arteritis
Throbbing pain	Migraine, cerebrovascular disease, hypertensive headaches
Exacerbation with movement	Migraine, headache attributed to conditions that increase intracranial pressure, posttraumatic headache, Chiari malformation type I, benign cough headaches
Photophobia	Migraine, cluster headache, meningitis, posttraumatic headache, subarachnoid hemorrhage
Nausea, vomiting	Headache attributed to conditions that increase intracranial pressure, meningitis, intracranial hemorrhage, trauma

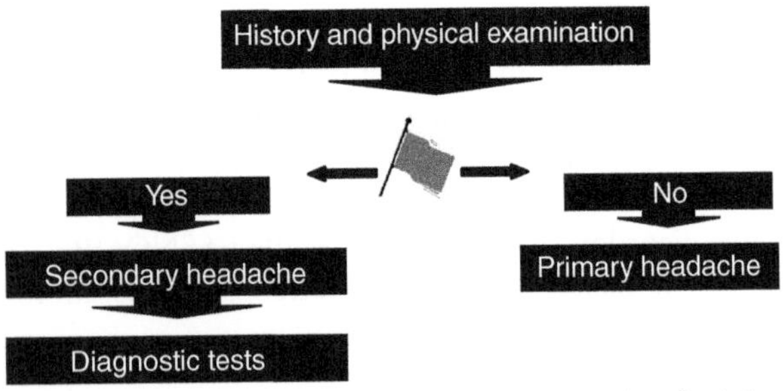

Figure 4 Approach to the diagnosis of headache. Red flag represents any of the SSNOOPs. Adapted from the Neurology Ambassador Program with permission.

following list) as the major branching point (**Figure 4**). SSNOOPs are:

- Systemic symptoms (fever or weight loss)
- Secondary risk factors: underlying disease (HIV or systemic cancer)
- Neurological symptoms or abnormal signs (confusion, impaired alertness or consciousness, neck stiffness, clumsiness, or weakness)
- Onset: sudden, abrupt, or split-second (first or worst)
- Older: new onset and progressive headache, especially in middle age (>50 years old)
- Previous headache history or headache progression: pattern change, first headache or different (change in attack frequency, severity, or new clinical features).

A variation of SSNOOP is SSNOOPP, which considers pain with local tenderness (e.g., jaw or temporal artery) as an additional red flag.

General medical and surgical histories, social and family histories, medications intake, and review of systems may provide clues to the diagnosis. For example, transient visual obscuration and intracranial noises may point to idiopathic intracranial hypertension. An antecedent motor vehicle accident within 6–12 months of the headache onset may indicate posttraumatic headache or whiplash headache. General and neurological examinations are an integral component of the assessment of patients with headaches. Papilledema, carotid bruits, neck limitation of motion, second trigeminal nerve branch or occipital triggers, tender temporal artery, and focal or lateralizing signs can all provide important clues to the diagnosis.

Once the characteristic symptoms of a migraine headache are identified and red flags are not elicited, imaging studies are likely to reveal a significant intracranial abnormality in only approximately 0.2% of patients. A magnetic resonance imaging (MRI) study is the preferred test when imaging is indicated.

Management

General Principles

General management strategies for migraine follow the TEEM© principles, which are:

- Trust and establish a strong rapport with the patient.
- Educate the patient about the disease/condition, treatment plan, and compliance. A major reason for failed therapy in headache disorders is noncompliance and/or unmatched or unrealistic expectations (e.g., expecting a cure for migraine).
- Empower the patient.
- Measure.

It is crucial to establish an accurate diagnosis based on a detailed history and physical examination and aided in special circumstances by neuroinvestigative techniques such as an MRI. It is also very important to systematically assess and follow up on the disease severity and disease-related disability by encouraging patients to maintain headache diaries in order to identify headache patterns, triggers, associated symptoms, response to intervention, and so on. The elicitation during the history of migraine comorbid conditions (**Table 3**) provides either opportunities to simplify treatment regimens (e.g., valproate for migraine and bipolar disease) or limitations on the use of certain medications (e.g., propranolol for migraine sufferers with asthma).

Pharmacotherapy of Migraine

Migraine pharmacotherapy can be divided into (1) the treatment of acute pain, (2) the treatment of associated symptoms, (3) traditional preventive agents, and (4) preemptive approaches when attacks have predictable triggers (e.g., menstruation). Preventive therapy for migraine is indicated for patients with (1) frequent or disabling attacks, (2) a prolonged aura, or (3) a poor response or intolerance to acute therapy.

Current acute therapy (**Table 8**) for migraine includes simple analgesics (e.g., acetaminophen) and compound analgesics (e.g., combined acetaminophen, aspirin, and caffeine; acetaminophen with codeine), nonsteroidal anti-inflammatory drugs (NSAIDs, e.g., ibuprofen), migraine-specific therapies such as ergots (ergotamine and dihydroergotamine, DHE) and triptans (serotonin type-1B and 1D, 5-$HT_{1B/D}$, agonist), and adjuvant therapies such as metoclopramide for gastrointestinal disturbances. Over-the-counter nonspecific therapies are well suited for low-severity migraine, but patients with more disabling attacks are better served by using migraine-specific agents. When at-home therapy fails, parenterally administered drugs such as DHE, which is often combined with other drugs such as prochloperazine or metoclopramide, may be needed. The choice of acute or preventive therapy should be guided by evidence, when available.

Preventive therapy is ideally aimed at reducing attack frequency, severity, duration, and overall impact and at achieving synergy with abortive therapy to improve its effectiveness. Pharmacological prevention includes β-adrenergic blockers, anticonvulsant or antiepileptic drugs, antidepressants, calcium channel blockers, and NSAIDs. Evidence supports the use of group 1 drugs (**Table 9**) as the first-choice therapies in migraine prevention.

Nonpharmacological complementary and alternative (integrative) migraine therapy includes trigger-avoidance and physical and behavioral interventions. A systematic review in 2000 led to the conclusion that relaxation training, biofeedback, and cognitive-behavioral therapy are proven treatments for migraine, but the evidence for physical treatments such as cervical manipulation and transcutaneous electrical nerve stimulation (TENS) is not as strong. Largely uncontrolled clinical trials support a role for acupuncture in migraine prevention, but two recent randomized trials failed to demonstrate that acupuncture is more effective than sham intervention.

Summary

Significant advances in the acute and prophylactic management of migraine headaches have emerged in recent years, providing relief for millions of migraine sufferers. Given that approximately 6% of men and

Table 8 Acute migraine pharmacotherapy[a]

Drug class/mechanism	*Drug/compound*	*Daily dose range (mg)*
Analgesics, simple	Acetaminophen	1000
Analgesics, compound	Acetaminophen + ASA + caffeine	600 + 400 + 200
	Acetaminophen + codeine	(250–500) + 30
	Isometheptane + dichloralphenazone + acetaminophen	(65–130) + (100–200) + (325–650)
Ergots	Nasal dihydroergotamine	2–4
	Ergotamine	1–6
Nonsteroidal anti-inflammatory drugs	Aspirin (ASA)	650–1000
	Diclofenac	50–100
	Flurbiprofen	100
	Ibuprofen	400–1200
	Ketoprofen	75–150
	Mefenamic acid	500
	Naproxen	750–825
	Rofecoxib	25–50
	Tolfenamic acid[b]	200
Triptans	Almotriptan	6.25–12.5
	Eletriptan	40–80
	Frovatriptan	2.5–5.0
	Naratriptan	1.0–2.5
	Rizatriptan	5–10
	Sumatriptan	25–100
	Zolmitriptan	2.5–5.0

[a]Oral and nasal therapies with at least one randomized controlled trial demonstrating efficacy of the active compound versus either placebo or another comparator. Reprinted from Ramadan, N. M. and Buchanan, T. M. (2006), New and future migraine therapy, *Pharmacology & Therapeutics* **112**(1), 199–212, with permission from Elsevier.
[b]Not available in the United States.

Table 9 Migraine preventive therapy[a]

	Group				
	1	2	3	4	5
Efficacy	+++	+ to ++	+++	+++	–
Evidence	Good	Limited	Consensus	Good	Good
Adverse events	Mild to severe	Mild to moderate	Mild to concerning	Concerning	
Examples	Amitriptyline, valproate, propranolol, topiramate, timolol	Verapamil, vitamin B_2, candesartan	Nortriptyline, phenelzine	Methysergide	Nifedipine

[a]+ indicates efficacy established (+++ is highest); – indicates that there is no evidence for efficacy as migraine prophylaxis. Adapted from Buchanan, T. M. and Ramadan, N. M. (2006), Prophylactic pharmacotherapy for migraine headaches. Data from the American Academy of Neurology. Used with permission.

17% of women experience migraines, many untreated patients may benefit from proper diagnosis and treatment. Various treatment regimens for the prevention of migraines have proved effective, but long-term prognosis remains less well delineated.

Acknowledgment

The authors wish to thank Ms. Joyce Lenz for her editorial assistance in preparing this manuscript.

See Also the Following Article

Pain.

Further Reading

Aizenman, E. and Sanguinetti, M. C. (2002). Channels gone bad: reflections from a Tapas bar. *Neuron* **34**, 679–683.

Borsook, D., Becerra, L., Carlezon, W. A., Jr., et al. (2006). Reward-aversion circuitry in analgesia and pain: implications for psychiatric disorders. *European Journal of Pain* **11**, 7–20.

Buchanan, T. M. and Ramadan, N. M. (2006). Prophylactic pharmacotherapy for migraine headaches. *Seminars in Neurology* **26**(2), 188–198.

Burstein, R. (2001). Deconstructing migraine headache into peripheral and central sensitization. *Pain* **89**, 107–110.

Burstein, R. and Jakubowski, M. (2005). Unitary hypothesis for multiple triggers of the pain and strain of migraine. *Journal of Comparative Neurology* **493**, 9–14.

Buzzi, M. G. and Moskowitz, M. A. (2005). The pathophysiology of migraine: year 2005. *Journal of Headache Pain* **6**, 105–111.

Dichgans, M., Freilinger, T., Eckstein, G., et al. (2005). Mutation in the neuronal voltage-gated sodium channel SCN1A in familial hemiplegic migraine. *Lancet* **366**, 371–377.

Goadsby, P. (1997). Pathophysiology of migraine: a disease of the brain. In: Goadsby, P. J. & Silberstein, S. D. (eds.) *Headache*, pp. 5–24. Boston: Butterworth-Heinemann.

Headache Classification Subcommittee, International Headache Society (2004). *Special issue on the International Classification of Headache Disorders* (2nd edn.) *Cephalalgia* (supplement 1).

Hu, X. H., Markson, L. E., Lipton, R. B., et al. (1999). Burden of migraine in the United States: disability and economic costs. *Archives of Internal Medicine* **159**, 813–818.

Jen, J. C., Wan, J., Palos, T. P., et al. (2005). Mutation in the glutamate transporter EAAT1 causes episodic ataxia, hemiplegia, and seizures. *Neurology* **65**, 529–534.

Koehn, C. G. (ed.) (1826). *Claudii Galeni opera omnia. vol. xii. De loci affectis.* Leipzig: In officina Car. Cnoblochii.

Lea, R. A., Nyholt, D. R., Curtain, R. P., et al. (2005). A genome-wide scan provides evidence for loci influencing a severe heritable form of common migraine. *Neurogenetics* **6**, 67–72.

Lipton, R. B. and Bigal, M. E. (2005). Migraine: epidemiology, impact and risk factor for progression. *Headache* **45**(supplement 1), S3–S13.

Lyngberg, A. C., Rasmussen, B. K., Jorgensen, T., et al. (2005). Incidence of primary headache: a Danish epidemiologic follow-up study. *American Journal of Epidemiology* **161**, 1066–1073.

Martin, V. T. and Behbehani, M. M. (2001). Toward a rational understanding of migraine trigger factors. *Medical Clinics of North America* **85**, 911–941.

Quality Standards Subcommittee, American Academy of Neurology (1994). The utility of neuroimaging in the evaluation of headache patients with normal neurologic examinations. *Neurology* **44**, 1353–1354.

Ramadan, N. M. and Buchanan, T. M. (2006). New and future migraine therapy. *Pharmacology & Therapeutics* **112**(1), 199–212.

Rasmussen, B. K., Jensen, R., Schroll, M., et al. (1991). Epidemiology of headache in a general population – a prevalence study. *Journal of Clinical Epidemiology* **44**, 1147–1157.

Stewart, W. F., Lipton, R. B., Celentano, D. D., et al. (1992). Prevalence of migraine headache in the United States: relation to age, income, race, and other sociodemographic factors. *Journal of the American Medical Association* **267**, 64–69.

Stovner, L. J. and Scher, A. I. (2006). Epidemiology of headache. In: Olesen, J., Goadsby, P. J., Ramadan, N. M., Tfelt-Hansen, P. & Welch, K. M. A. (eds.) *The headaches* (3rd edn., pp. 17–25). Philadelphia: Lippincott Williams & Wilkins.

van den Maagdenberg, A. M., Pietrobon, D., Pizzorusso, T., et al. (2004). A Cacna1a knockin migraine mouse model with increased susceptibility to cortical spreading depression. *Neuron* **41**, 701–710.

Relevant Websites

Campbell, J. K., Penzien, D. B. and Wall, E. W. (2000). Evidence based guidelines for migraine headache: behavioral and physical treatments. http://www.aan.com.

Frishberg, B. M., Rosenberg, J. H., Matchar, D. B., et al. (2000). Evidence-based guidelines in the primary care setting: neuroimaging in patients with non-acute headache. http://www.aan.com.

Asthma

A A Kaptein
Leiden University Medical Center, Leiden, The Netherlands

This is a revised version of the article by A A Kaptein, Encyclopedia of Stress First Edition, volume 1, pp 255–257, © 2000, Elsevier Inc.

Glossary

Asthma	Chronic inflammation of the airways, with reversible airway obstruction.
Psychoanalysis	School of thought in psychiatry that emphasizes the role of the unconscious in the etiology and course of psychological and somatic diseases.
Psychology	Study of the behavior of humans.
Self-management	An individual's ability to manage the symptoms, treatment, physical and psychological consequences, and lifestyle changes that are inherent in living with a chronic condition.

Asthma is a respiratory disease, defined as "... a chronic inflammatory disorder of the airways ... the chronic inflammation causes an associated increase in airway hyperresponsiveness that leads to recurrent episodes of wheezing, breathlessness, chest tightness, and coughing. These episodes are usually associated with widespread but variable airflow obstruction that is often reversible either spontaneously or with treatment." (Clark, 2002). The hallmark of asthma is its reversibility: stimuli, such as stress, elicit episodes of shortness of breath that disappear, either spontaneously or following the administration of medication. Asthma is a highly prevalent disorder: some 10% of the population in industrialized societies is diagnosed with asthma. It now seems that the increase in asthma prevalence has reached its plateau.

Various stimuli lead to asthma attacks in susceptible persons. Stress is one of these stimuli. But there are also others, such as tobacco smoke, cat dander, aspirin, cold air, and exertion. It is the genetic and immunological factors that determine susceptibility to asthma in an individual. Asthma attacks translate into symptoms that lead to limitations in daily functioning, psychological morbidity, and negative social consequences.

Stress has been and still is conceptualized as potentially (1) contributing to the causes of asthma, (2) contributing to the inception of an asthma attack, (3) contributing to the clinical course of asthma, and (4) representing a target for therapeutic interventions in order to reduce the impact of asthma on the daily life of the affected patient. These four topics are discussed below.

Stress as a Cause of Asthma

Asthma is currently viewed as a multicausal disorder; the medical and scientific communities still do not have a perfect understanding of potential causal factors and their interrelations. Patients with asthma report that stress is one of the major eliciting factors of asthma attacks, and that stress worsens the severity of their asthma attacks. Historically, these clinical observations have often informed past studies on whether stress is a causal factor in the etiology of asthma.

This research took place within a psychoanalytic and psychosomatic paradigm, en vogue in the first decades of the twentieth century. In this paradigm it was assumed that asthma was merely the somatic expression of an underlying source of stress: a psychological conflict within the patient or between the patient and a significant other. Asthma was conceived of as a symptom that symbolically expressed an anxiety neurosis: asthma nervosum could be traced back to the overhearing of the affected child of sexual activities between adults. In psychosomatic views on asthma, specific personality characteristics in combination with a specific interpersonal conflict or stress (centering on dependence vs. autonomy) were seen as the ultimate and main causes of asthma.

Empirical support for these views is not available, and therapeutic strategies following from these views (i.e., psychoanalytic therapy) failed to lead to improvements, with regard to either the disappearance of asthma altogether or reductions in the impact of asthma on the sufferer. However, some of the psychodynamic notions on asthma still seem to have survived. In a recent study on views of general practitioners (GPs) on asthma in various European countries, a GP remarked that "... as children these people very often have overprotective mothers (...) and when they've become adults they often live in circumstances where they do not want to share the air with other people." (Wahlström et al., 2001).

Research on the relation between stress or emotional arousal and changes in pulmonary function continues, but it remains unclear whether stress-induced airway obstruction really exists, let alone whether stress causes asthma. It seems safe to conclude that there is no evidence for the view that stress is an etiological factor in asthma.

Stress Brings on Asthma Attacks

Various stimuli and situations may elicit an attack of asthma in asthma patients. It is difficult for patients themselves, and for their partners and their physicians, to pinpoint exactly the stimulus or stimuli that caused or elicited a particular asthma attack. This, of course, complicates preventive or therapeutic measures. Quite frequently, patients attribute their asthma attacks to stress.

Experimental studies on stress and asthma assign short-term stressful tasks to be performed by healthy controls and people with asthma, in order to examine their effects on various physiological processes, e.g., pulmonary function. In children with asthma, performing the stressful task of talking into a tape recorder for a 5-min period about a stressful or embarrassing incident led to increases in airway resistance of up to 20%, which is a clinically meaningful change. Observational studies in children and adults with asthma demonstrate that severely negative life events often increase the risk of the occurrence of asthma attacks over the coming few weeks.

Laboratory studies in a small sample of adult patients with asthma show that there is a close connection between the processes of inflammation in asthma and emotional factors, as measured with functional magnetic resonance imaging (fMRI). A recent study demonstrated that neural circuitry underlying stress and emotion can regulate inflammation, and peripheral inflammatory mediators can influence mood and cognition.

Stress Affects the Course of Asthma

As in almost any (chronic) illness, there are great variations in clinical outcome of asthma. Some patients are hardly affected by their asthma; in other patients, asthma appears to completely dominate their lives. A consistent research finding on these observations is that measures of objective severity of asthma are hardly associated with differences in outcome or course of asthma. The stress coping paradigm allows for the explanation of at least some of those differences.

Researchers in Denver, Colorado have developed the psycho-maintenance hypothesis, which pertains to psychological factors maintaining the course and consequences of a (chronic) physical disorder. The researchers examined relationships in hospitalized patients with asthma among objective indicators of asthma severity, psychological characteristics, and outcome measures. Length of hospitalization, frequency of rehospitalization, and severity of medication at discharge turned out not to be determined by objective asthma severity indicators, but by stress-related characteristics. Anxiety (panic-fear) as a personality characteristic, and as a transient state related to dyspnea perception, in combination with various attitudes toward asthma (e.g., optimism, stigma), however, did predict those outcome measures. These findings have been replicated in other settings and other countries.

In addition to stress and attitudes toward asthma, psychiatric morbidity is associated with outcome. Achieving a good control of one's asthma and adequate functional status often appears to be negatively influenced by higher levels of depression, panic disorder, and social phobia. This relation again is hardly mediated by objective severity of asthma.

Symptom perception in asthma is also related to stress. Patients with higher levels of stress (negative affectivity) associate a wide range of nonspecific symptoms with their asthma, thereby altering the perception of the severity of asthma, which in turn influences their use of medication. These findings have great relevance for the topic discussed in the next paragraph: self-management skills for patients with asthma.

Stress Reduction Improves Asthma Outcomes

Teaching patients how to manage stress associated with asthma has a quite long history. Patients themselves indicate that when they become short of breath, they attempt to relax, which leads to subjective reductions in dyspnea. Behavioral scientists and medical professionals have examined the effects of relaxation training in patients with asthma to a great extent. However, the clinical wisdom of asthma patients has not been supported by empirical research. Relaxation therapies, biofeedback, and breathing retraining do not result in objective improvements in pulmonary function; neither do they affect clinical outcomes such as use of health-care services or medication.

Stress management training, however, appears to produce positive effects. Cognitive-behavioral stress management training leads to clinically meaningful and statistically significant improvements in children and adults with asthma. Cochrane Reviews reveal that medical care that encompasses teaching patients to perceive respiratory symptoms accurately, to respond to impending asthma attacks appropriately, and to cope well with the stress associated with dyspnea episodes and with asthma in daily social circumstances is associated with less disruption of daily activities, a better quality of life, and less use of health-care services.

Recently, two new areas of research pertaining to self-management of asthma have received much attention. The first is studying and examining the effects of expressive writing in adult patients with asthma. Patients have been encouraged to write about the most stressful event of their lives in the experimental condition, and about emotionally neutral topics in the control condition. Clinically meaningful improvements in pulmonary function were observed in the experimental condition. The second new area is research on illness representations, which pertains to studying the cognition of asthma patients of their respiratory condition and its treatment in relation to various outcome measures. Patients' own ideas, objectively correct or not, turned out to be predictors of the clinical course of asthma. Future research will make clear to what extent these two new topics will be integrated into stress management programs for patients with asthma. Another challenge is to ensure that effective components of self-management training programs will be incorporated into guidelines for health-care providers and applied for the patient's benefit.

See Also the Following Articles

Somatic Disorders.

Further Reading

Chrousos, G. P. (2000). Stress, chronic inflammation, and emotional and physical well-being: concurrent effects and chronic sequelae. *Journal of Allergy and Clinical Immunology* **106**, S275–S291.

Clark, J. H. (chair) (2002). *Global strategy for asthma management and prevention.* Bethesda, MD., NIH, National Heart, Lung, and Blood Institute.

Gibson, P. G., Coughlan, J., Wilson, A. J., et al. (2000). Self-management education and regular practitioner review for adults with asthma (Cochrane review). *The Cochrane Library* 4. Oxford: Update Software.

Kaptein, A. A. and Creer, T. L. (eds.) (2002). *Respiratory disorders and behavioral medicine.* London, UK: Martin Dunitz Publishers.

Kaptein, A. A., Scharloo, M., Helder, D. I., et al. (2003). Respresentations of chronic illnesses. In: Cameron, L. D. & Leventhal, H. (eds.) *The self-regulation of health and illness behavior,* pp. 97–118. New York and London: Routledge.

Kinsman, R. A., Dirks, J. F. and Jones, N. F. (1982). Psychomaintenance of chronic physical illness. In: Millon, T., Green, C. & Meagher, R. (eds.) *Handbook of clinical health psychology,* pp. 435–466. New York: Plenum Press.

Lavoie, K. L., Cartier, A., Labrecque, M., et al. (2005). Are psychiatric disorders associated with worse asthma control and quality of life in asthma patients? *Respiratory Medicine* **99**, 1249–1257.

Main, J., Moss-Morris, R., Booth, R., Kaptein, A. A. and Kolbe, J. (2003). The use of reliever medication in asthma: the role of negative mood and symptom reports. *Journal of Asthma* **40**, 357–365.

McQuaid, E. L., Fritz, G. K., Nassau, J. H., et al. (2000). Stress and airway resistance in children with asthma. *Journal of Psychosomatic Research* **49**, 239–245.

Rietveld, S., Everaerd, W. and Creer, T. L. (2000). Stress-induced asthma: a review of research and potential mechanisms. *Clinical and Experimental Allergy* **30**, 1058–1066.

Ritz, T. and Roth, W. T. (2003). Behavioral interventions in asthma. Breathing retraining. *Behavior Modification* **27**, 710–730.

Rosenkranz, M. A., Busse, W. W., Johnstone, T., et al. (2005). Neural circuitry underlying the interaction between emotion and asthma symptom exacerbation. *Proceedings of the National Academy of Sciences USA* **102**, 13319–13324.

Sandberg, S., Paton, J. Y., Ahola, S., et al. (2000). The role of acute and chronic stress in asthma attacks in children. *Lancet* **356**, 982–987.

Smyth, J. M., Stone, A. A., Hurewitz, A. and Kaell, A. (1999). Effects of writing about stressful experiences

on symptom reduction in patients with asthma or rheumatoid arthritis. *Journal of the American Medical Association* **281**, 1304–1309.
Wahlström, R., Lagerløv, P., Stålsby Lundborg, C., et al. (2001). Variations in general practitioners' views of asthma management in four European countries. *Social Science and Medicine* 53, 507–518.
Wolf, F. M., Guevera, J. P., Grum, C. M., Clark, N. M. and Cates, C. J. (2003). Educational interventions for asthma in children (Cochrane review). *The Cochrane Library* 2. Oxford: Update Software.
Wright, R. J., Rodriguez, M. and Cohen, S. (1998). Review of psychosocial stress and asthma: an integrated biopsychosocial approach. *Thorax* 53, 1066–1074.

Cancer

D Spiegel
Stanford University, Stanford, CA, USA

This is a revised version of the article by D Spiegel, Encyclopedia of Stress First Edition, volume 1, pp 368–375, © 2000, Elsevier Inc.

Glossary

Allostatic load	The physiological burden undertaken by the body to maintain allostasis, or internal stability, through environmental change evoked by a series of stressors.
Glucocorticoid	A class of stress hormones that mobilize glucose into the blood.
Hypothalamic-pituitary-adrenal (HPA) axis	One of the major stress response systems in the body; designed to maintain adequate glucose in the blood to help the brain and muscles respond to stressors.
Psychoneuroimmune connections	The relationship among the mind, brain, and components of the immune system.
Psychosocial factors	Psychological and social factors that affect cancer patients or may be a component of supportive care.

Mind–Body Interactions and Cancer

Cancer research has productively focused on the pathophysiology of the disease, emphasizing aspects of tumor biology as predictors of disease outcome at the expense of studying the role of the body's psychophysiological reactions to tumor invasion. These reactions are mediated by brain–body mechanisms, including the endocrine, neuroimmune, and autonomic nervous systems. Although a large portion of the variance in any disease outcome is accounted for by the specific local pathophysiology of that disease, some variability must also be explained by host-resistance factors, which include the manner of response to the stress of the illness.

That the stress of cancer is felt psychologically is indicated by the fact that as many as 80% of breast cancer patients report significant distress during initial treatment. Estimates of the prevalence of psychiatric disorders among newly diagnosed cancer patients has ranged from 30 to 44%, and 20–45% of patients exhibit emotional morbidity 1–2 years later. Even though the majority of women diagnosed with breast cancer do not meet the criteria for a psychiatric diagnosis, the vast majority experience the diagnosis of cancer as a major stressor, and 10% have severe maladjustment problems as long as 6 years later. Thus, breast cancer is a disease that causes considerable psychological stress.

Stress and Cancer Incidence and Progression

There is mixed evidence regarding whether social stress, such as divorce, loss of a job, or bereavement, is associated with a greater likelihood of incidence or relapse of cancer. Three recent meta-analyses have reached rather different conclusions. The first, which relied heavily on the European literature, concluded that stress has no effect on cancer incidence. It also reported that bereavement had no effect among 11 studies (odds ratio, OR, 1.06; 95% confidence interval, CI, 0.95–1.18, not significant) but that other stressors had a twofold effect (OR 2.63; 95% CI 2.34–2.96). However, the researchers based their final null conclusion on six studies they deemed to be of higher quality because of the use of population controls, blinding of interviewers to disease status, and other methodological issues. In these six studies, stress had no effect on cancer incidence. Although this meta-analysis clearly raised important questions about the stress–cancer link, it did so only after dismissing the findings of the majority of studies in the field. The second meta-analysis found that both stressful life events, in general, and those that involve loss and separation, in particular, are associated with breast cancer incidence. The authors of the third meta-analysis reported a modest yet statistically significant association between exposure to stress and the incidence of breast cancer, although they suggested that this association may be an artifact of publication bias.

It may well be that the factors that influence cancer progression are quite different from those affecting incidence. Although this may seem counterintuitive because the tumor burden is much greater as disease advances (by the time of death, a typical cancer patient may have approximately 1 kg of tumors in his or her body), the setting of disease progression is one in which physiological resources are stretched to their limit due to the higher tumor burden and cumulative effects of disease-related distress and disability. Even minor variations in somatic response to stress may have an effect on disease course at this point.

A large prospective study in Finland involving 10 808 subjects found that major life stressors such as divorces or death of a loved one in the preceding 5 years predicted a significantly elevated risk of subsequent breast cancer. However, another study found that reports of subjectively evaluated stress actually predicted lower subsequent breast cancer incidence. One way to interpret this apparent inconsistency in the literature involves the difference between experiencing and reporting stress. Given that the literature associates the repression of distress with a possibly elevated cancer risk, the studies of reported stress classify repressers with those subject who report no stress and therefore as being potentially at a higher cancer risk than if they actually had experienced objective stressors. Clearly more research is needed in this intriguing area.

Coping Style and Cancer Incidence and Progression

Coping-style variables that have been associated with higher cancer incidence include anger suppression and restrained aggression and introversion. Variables associated with slower progression include fighting spirit, expressed distress, assertive uncooperativeness, and assertiveness (being non-type C). Being emotionally reserved has been found to increase substantially the risk of mortality (odds ratio of 3.9) among lung cancer patients as well. Although the solidity of the evidence for these relationships varies, it is of interest that the styles putatively associated with cancer incidence and more rapid progression are similar emotional suppression and nonassertiveness.

Antoni and Goodkin found that a passive coping style is related to the promotion of cervical neoplasia. In another study, they also found that breast cancer patients were more likely to employ a repressive coping style than noncancer patients. Measures of this construct (repression/sensitization as a defensive style) have been reported as accounting for as much as 44% of the variance in the progression of breast cancer. Although stress may weaken the body's capacity to resist the progression of cancer, coping well with stress may counteract this effect. Work on psychological stress suggests that lack of control is a key factor in the magnitude of the physiological stress responses. People who feel helpless in response to stress may exhibit more exaggerated physiological evidence of stress, whereas those with greater self-efficacy in coping may dampen the effects of stress. In breast cancer patients, the belief that they could control the course of disease was significantly associated with good adjustment. Indeed, several studies have shown that it is not so much the intensity of the stressor as its perceived controllability that determines its effects. Changes in coping styles have been associated with changes in immune function, even over periods of less than a month. For example, in a study of the effects of emotional disclosure, subjects who discontinued their avoidance and engaged more fully in discussions of a stressful or traumatic topic exhibited decreases in antibody titers to the Epstein–Barr virus, indicating more successful surveillance of the latent virus by lymphocytes.

Expression, rather than suppression, of emotion has been postulated to reduce stress by discharging physiological arousal. Stress-related immune fluctuations due to the threat or onset of illness have also been shown to be reduced in those with an increased ability to cope with changes in their life through assertive communication. Active coping through openly expressing concerns and emotions is one factor that may influence the endocrine and immune alterations that may be related to disease progression.

Social Support as a Stress Buffer

Psychosocial treatments appear to buffer the effects of stress on endocrine function. For example, one intervention study found that biofeedback and cognitive therapy were associated with reduced cortisol levels in newly diagnosed breast cancer patients. Social support provided by the intervention may ameliorate the effect of stress on endocrine function. Indeed, providing social support during stress can profoundly alter the endocrine consequences of the stressor. Levine modeled this effect in squirrel monkeys. Although the animals produced large elevations in plasma cortisol concentrations when they were stressed when alone, stress-induced elevations were reduced by 50% when animals had one friend present and they disappeared when five friends were present. Thus, interventions that provide social support have the potential to ameliorate endocrine stress responses.

Thus, the social environment can have a buffering effect on stress. Being socially embedded is associated with less autonomic arousal than social isolation. Indeed, social connection has profound consequences for health. Being well integrated socially reduces all-cause age-adjusted mortality by a factor of two, approximately as much as having low versus high serum cholesterol levels or being a nonsmoker. Furthermore, people's positions in the social hierarchy (including relatively higher status even within the same social class) have health consequences. People are statistically more likely to die after than before their birthdays and important holiday, which are usually important times for social bonding and companionship.

Thus, the presence of adverse emotional events such as traumatic stressors seems to have negative potential health consequences, whereas good social relations seem to be associated with positive health outcomes.

There is evidence from 5 of 11 published randomized trials that psychosocial support is associated with longer survival for patients with breast cancer, malignant melanoma, and lymphoma. One component of the effective interventions is dealing directly with emotional distress associated with fears regarding disease progression.

There is evidence that resilience to stress, including disease-related distress, is associated with emotional style. Indeed, finding meaning in the midst of experiencing a distressing situation has been linked with a positive psychological state. Better adaptation does not involve being persistently upbeat or rigidly maintaining a positive attitude but, rather, dealing directly with negative affect as well. Positive and negative emotions are not merely opposite sides of a single dimension. The suppression of negative emotion tends to reduce the experience of all emotion, positive and negative. There is evidence that breast cancer patients who express more negative emotion (including anger and uncooperativeness) or realistic optimism (fighting spirit) may live longer.

Physiological Mechanisms of Stress and Support-Related Effects on Cancer Progression

Identifying the physiological mechanisms by which emotional expression and social support may influence survival time for patients with cancer is an intriguing problem. Possibilities range from body maintenance activities such as diet, sleep, and exercise to interactions with physicians and better adherence to medical treatment regiments to stress and support-mediated effects on endocrine and immune function. These systems, which are part of routine somatic control and maintenance functions in the body, are influenced by psychological and social variables and are also involved in host resistance to tumor progression.

There is a long history of research linking stress to increased cancer risk. In a series of classic experiments, crowded living conditions accelerated the rate of tumor growth and mortality in rats. In an authoritative 1998 review of the human stress literature, McEwen documented the adverse health effects of cumulative stressors and the body's failure to adapt the stress response to them. The activation of the HPA axis is an adaptive response to acute stress, but over time, in response to cumulative stress, the system's signal-to-noise ratio can be degraded so that it is partially on all the time; this leads to adverse physiological consequences, including abnormalities in glucose metabolism, hippocampal damage accumulation of abdominal fat, and depression. Depression has been associated with more rapid cancer progression in 19 of 24 recent studies, although it has little relationship to cancer incidence. Abnormalities of HPA axis function, including glucocorticoid receptor hypersensitivity, have also been found to be associated with posttraumatic stress disorder. Thus, adverse events ranging from traumatic stressors to cumulative minor ones and responses to them, including depression, are associated with HPA axis dysregulation. Persistently elevated or relatively invariant levels of cortisol may, in turn, stimulate tumor proliferation. Possible mechanisms include the differential gluconeogenesis response of normal and tumor tissue to glucocorticoid signals to secrete glucose into the blood, the activation of hormone receptors in tumors, and immunosuppression. Indeed, glucocorticoids are potently immunosuppressive, so the effects of acute and chronic stress and hypercortisolemia may include functional immunosuppression as well, as has been shown extensively in animals. There is a growing body of evidence of stress-induced immunosuppression in humans as well. This, in turn, could influence the rate of cancer progression.

Stress Reactivity and Disease Progression

Allostatic load has been defined as the price that the body has to pay for maintaining allostasis (stability through environmental change). Recently, it has been suggested that increased allostatic load, which may occur through the cumulative build-up of stress over a lifespan, may significantly hinder the functioning of different physiological systems. Cancer itself constitutes a series of stressors: the threat to life and health, the disruption of social activities, and the rigors and side effects of treatment. A given individual's psychological and physiological response pattern to stress in general is likely to be exacerbated by the diagnosis and treatment of cancer, thereby intensifying mind–body interactions mediated by the stress response system.

Reactivity to stressors involves not only the initial response but also the system's ability to reset itself after stress. Older organisms seem to reset themselves after a stressor less readily, leaving stress response systems more tonically upregulated for longer periods of time after cessation of the stressor. Cancer particularly affects older people, and chronic disease-related stressors are likely to further decrease the flexibility of stress response mechanisms. Sapolsky and colleagues found that stressed older animals not only had persistently elevated cortisol levels after the stress was over but also had much more rapid growth of implanted tumors. This finding was confirmed in a Ben-Eliyahu and coworkers, who also identified the suppressive effects of stress hormones on natural killer (NK) cells as one potential mediator of the effect. The magnitude of stress-induced elevation of corticosteriods may not be as important in cancer outcomes as the duration or persistence of the elevation.

Circadian Rhythm Disruption, Stress, and Cancer

Recurrence or metastasis of cancer can be considered a severe chronic stressor. Both short-term and long-term alterations in psychological state (e.g., major depression) are known to be correlated with endocrine changes. Stress is associated with increased sympathetic nervous system (SNS) and HPA axis activity. Catecholamines and cortisol (released during SNS and HPA axis activity) are elevated in cancer patients as well as in bereaved and depressed subjects. Abnormalities in the circadian rhythm of cortisol have been observed in subjects undergoing psychological stress (e.g., depression, unemployment, and posttraumatic stress disorder) and some types of physical stress (e.g., shift work and excessive workloads). Studies in humans by Sephton and coworkers and in animals by Filipski and coworkers have shown that abnormal diurnal patterns of cortisol (which is typically four to five times higher in the morning on waking than in the evening in humans) predict earlier cancer mortality. Furthermore, women who engage in nighttime shift work are at higher risk for developing breast cancer. Thus, the disruption of circadian patterns of sleep and related hormones, including cortisol and melatonin, are associated with an elevated risk of cancer incidence and progression.

Psychoendocrinology and Cancer

There are considerable data indicating that the HPA axis constitutes a likely connection between psychosocial factors and disease progression. Stress is processed through central nervous system (CNS) neurotransmitter systems such as norepinephrine, dopamine, and endorphins, which regulate hypothalamic releasing factors such as corticotropin releasing hormone (CRH), pituitary hormones such as prolactin and adrenocorticotropic hormone (ACTH), and, through these, adrenocortical steroids and medullary hormones. Cortisol is the classic stress hormone; it is elevated in response to stress for prolonged periods and is immunosuppressive.

The role of endogenous corticosteroids in breast cancer progression is worthy of further exploration because (1) steroid hormone levels are responsive to psychosocial stressors through the HPA axis via CRH, ACTH, and the response of the adrenal in producing them and (2) because breast cancer is a hormone-sensitive tumor, as evidence by the effectiveness of steroid receptor blockers such as tamoxifen in delaying progression. Although the specific receptors blocked involve estrogen and progesterone, cross-reactivity with androgenic steroids and the dedifferentiated state of tumor tissue make corticosteroids of potential interest.

High levels of stress hormones such as cortisol may be associated with worse disease prognosis because breast cancers are often hormone-sensitive. In a study of patients operated on for breast and stomach carcinoma, the failure of morning cortisol levels to decrease within 2 weeks after admission was associated with shorter survival times. Direct evidence for effects of the HPA axis in the development of breast cancer comes from a study in which high serum levels of dehydroepiandrosterone (DHEA), a correlate of HPA axis activity, predicted the subsequent development of breast cancer 9 years later in normal postmenopausal women who had donated blood for a serum bank. Thus, correlational evidence suggests that physiological stress responses associated with poor adjustment to cancer may, indeed, speed disease progression.

Mechanisms have been proposed whereby the neuroendocrine correlates of stress may promote neoplastic growth. Stress hormones may suppress immune resistance to tumors or act via differential effects on gluconeogenesis in healthy versus tumor cells. Tumor cells may become resistant to the catabolic action of cortisol, which inhibits the uptake of glucose in numerous cell types. In such cases, energy is preferentially shunted to the tumor and away from normal cells by cortisol. Several studies found an association between the stress-related elevation of glucocorticoids and more rapid tumor growth in animals. Another hypothesis suggests that hormones of the HPA axis may actually promote the expression of breast cancer oncogenes. In addition, because stress-related increases in SNS and HPA axis activity are known to have generally suppressive effects on immune function, it is certainly plausible that immune functions important in resistance to breast tumor growth are thereby suppressed. The elevation of glucocorticoids is associated with clinically significant immunosuppression, and the enhanced secretion of norepinephrine during stress has also been associated with suppression of lymphocyte function.

Other hormones that are elevated by stress, such as prolactin, growth hormone, and thyroid hormones, may also influence the course of disease. Prolactin is of special interest because of its role as both a tumor promoter and a stress hormone. There is evidence that a majority of breast carcinomas have prolactin receptors and that the presence of prolactin stimulates the growth of such tumors in tissue culture at physiological levels, perhaps by stimulating the development of estrogen receptors. Prolactin has been found to stimulate prostate carcinoma growth as well. Indeed strong positive correlations between prolactin and both estrogen and progesterone receptor levels in breast tumors have been noted. The surgical stress of radical mastectomy results in transiently elevated serum prolactin levels, perhaps through the removal of target tissue and a disruption in feedback mechanisms. Prolactin levels rise in response to other stressful stimuli as well. Because other pituitary hormones such as ACTH clearly reflect stress, it is possible that prolactin secreted in response to stress can thereby promote tumor growth. Thus, there is evidence for facilitative effects on tumor growth by stress hormones via several different mechanisms. Acute medical illness is associated with the increased secretion of ACTH and cortisol, and surgical stress is associated with lower DHEA/cortisol ratios (i.e., a combination of relatively low DHEA and relatively high cortisol levels) and higher prolactin levels.

Psychoneuroimmunology and Cancer

Many of these hormones are immunosuppressive when elevated. In spousal bereavement, cortisol levels are elevated, whereas NK cytotoxicity is decreased. Furthermore, there is no reason why disease-related stresses, including social isolation, death anxiety, pain, and sleep disturbance, should not affect immune function at the clinically observable level, for example in defenses against the progression of viral infection. Yet little is known about these mechanisms or their effects on clinical infection. Cohen showed that vulnerability to systemic infection by rhinovirus is significantly mediated by stress and that people with larger social networks are less susceptible to viral infection. This model might well apply as well to vulnerability to cancer progression.

There is a growing body of research that provides evidence of associations between psychological factors and immune function. The work of the Glasers has shown that subjects experiencing such stressors as being a caregiver for an Alzheimer's patient, undergoing divorce or bereavement, or being in a poor relationship have been shown to have greater distress and lower helper/suppressor cell counts and ratios, lower total T-lymphocyte numbers, lower NK cell activity, and poorer response to Epstein–Barr virus.

Further evidence comes from work showing that immune organs such as the spleen are heavily innervated and that there are receptors for a variety of neurotransmitters on the cell membranes of lymphocytes. Stress hormones are known to influence cell adhesion molecules on lymphocytes, providing a possible mechanism by which stress may alter lymphocyte trafficking and therefore immune function. There is good evidence for this hypothesis in work by Dhabhar, who demonstrated that stress and the circadian corticosterone rhythm induce significant changes in leukocyte distribution in animals. Moreover, he showed that acute stress significantly enhances a cutaneous delayed-type hypersensitivity (DTH) response (an *in vivo* measure of cell-mediated immunity). In contrast, chronic stress significantly suppresses DTH responses, and stress-induced trafficking of leukocytes to the skin may mediate these changes of immune function. Most interestingly, he was able to mimic the effects of acute and chronic stress on DTH responses by the administration of corticosterone at doses similar to physiological levels following either acute or chronic stress, suggesting that glucocorticoids may be an important mediator of DTH responses during stress.

Thus, there is growing evidence for links among psychological stress, glucocorticoid responses, and immunosuppression. In rats, for example, stress significantly decreased NK cytotoxicity, increased levels of cortisol and ACTH, and increased the metastatic spread of mammary tumor to lung tissue. In stage I and II breast cancer patients, higher perceived social support and active seeking of social support were related to increased NK cell activity, and lower NK cell activity has been shown to predict disease recurrence. Thus, psychological factors have been associated with changes in immune measures, and these changes are markers of cancer progression.

Psychosocial Interventions and Immune Function

Psychosocial treatments designed to improve coping and assist in stress reduction have been associated with improvements in both immune function and physical health in cancer patients. Supportive relationships seem to modulate stress-induced immunosuppression, for example, among medical students undergoing examination stress. Even the disclosure of traumas in journals has been associated with better immune function. Stress-related immunosuppression may be mitigated by active coping styles or social support. After a 6-week psychiatric intervention for newly diagnosed malignant melanoma patients conducted by Fawzy, α-interferon-augmented cytotoxic activity of NK cells was elevated in the intervention subjects 6 months later and a survival benefit was observed, although there was no direct relationship between changes in NK cell activity and survival time. NK cells are known to kill tumor cells of many different types when tested either *in vitro* or in animal studies and may be particularly prone to stress-induced suppression.

Immune Function and Disease Progression

It is not always clear whether changes in serum immune or endocrine measures are a cause of or result from changes in disease status. Indeed, the immune surveillance theory of cancer development and progression has been questioned. Cancer is not, after all, an immunodeficiency disease, and immunosuppressed patients such as those with acquired immunodeficiency syndrome (AIDS) are at higher risk only for rare cancers such as Kaposi's sarcoma. However, research in animals as well as humans suggests that immunosuppression may be a factor in the rate of disease progression, and *in vitro* measures of immune function that are salient to disease progression are affected positively by social support and adversely by stress.

There is evidence from nonclinical populations that social integration buffers against the stress-induced suppression of NK cell activity. It thus makes sense that the addition of intensive social support in groups for women undergoing substantial medical and other stressors might have a similar buffering effect. Thus, although definitive clinical links have not been made, there is evidence that NK call activity is associated with the rate of breast cancer progression. This immune parameter, which is affected by stress and social support, also varies with disease progression, making it a reasonable candidate for investigations into the mediators of the effects of group support on the rate of breast cancer progression.

Stress and Autonomic Responses

Cacioppo and colleagues examined the effects of psychological stress on autonomic responses including heart rate reactivity and cardiac vagal reactivity (as indexed by respiratory sinus arrhythmia reactivity). They found that individuals who demonstrated greater autonomic responses to brief laboratory stress also showed higher stress-related increases in ACTH and cortisol. Thus, autonomic tone may be a good index of the reactivity of the HPA axis to acute stress, and autonomic measures are less invasive than the repeated blood sampling that is required to measure short-term changes in HPA axis activity. The results of psychoneuroimmunological studies have shown that heart rate reactivity after a stressor was also related to changes in NK cell activity, suggesting that the measurement of stress-induced changes in autonomic tone may be of value in defining the possible mechanisms underlying psychosocial effects on immune function. Failures to mount a corticosteroid response to stress may place an undue burden on other stress response mechanisms, such as the autonomic nervous system. The loss of vagal tone is often seen in poor stress responders, leading to cardiovascular burden and possibly to immune effects as well. Autonomic tone has not only been associated with stress, but also with emotion regulation. Indeed, the baseline levels of cardiac vagal tone and vagal tone reactivity have been associated with behavioral measures of reactivity and the expression of emotion; thus, cardiac vagal tone can also serve as an index of emotion, and parasympathetic influences on heart rate may be influenced by emotional expression, for example as a means of coping with stressors.

Conclusion

The literature reviewed here provides evidence that people's manner of responding to disease-related stress may affect the rate of disease progression as well as their psychological adjustment. The stress response system is most effective when it is on when needed and off when it is not. Variance in the rate of cancer progression may be accounted for by more or less adaptive stress response systems. This effect of stress and stress response on cancer progression may be mediated by the endocrine, immune, or autonomic nervous systems or by some combination of the three. There is evidence that stress is a uniform part of the experience of cancer and its treatment, that various coping styles affect stress-mediated physiological effects, and that these in turn my affect the somatic response to cancer progression. Furthermore, various psychosocial interventions have proven effective in enhancing coping with this stress, and some have demonstrated an effect on disease progression. This evidence suggests that assistance with stress management can contribute to effective cancer treatment.

Further Reading

Fawzy, F. I., Canada, A. L. and Fawzy, N. W. (2003). Malignant melanoma: effects of a brief, structured psychiatric intervention on survival and recurrence at 10-year follow-up. *Archives of General Psychiatry* **60**(1), 100–103.

Lillberg, K., Verkasalo, P. K., Kaprio, J., et al. (2003). Stressful life events and risk of breast cancer in 10,808 women: a cohort study. *American Journal of Epidemiology* **157**(5), 415–423.

McEwen, B. S. (1998). Protective and damaging effects of stress mediators. *New England Journal of Medicine* **338**(3), 171–179.

Sapolsky, R. M. (1996). Why stress is bad for your brain. *Science* **273**(5276), 749–750.

Sephton, S. E., Sapolsky, R. M., Kraemer, H. C. and Spiegel, D. (2000). Diurnal cortisol rhythm as a predictor of breast cancer survival. *Journal of the National Cancer Institute* **92**, 994–1000.

Sephton, S. and Spiegel, D. (2003). Circadian disruption in cancer: a neuroendocrine-immune pathway from stress to disease? *Brain, Behavior & Immunity* **17**(5), 321–328.

Spiegel, D. and Classen, C. (2000). *Group therapy for cancer patients: a research-based handbook of psychosocial care.* New York: Basic Books.

Cardiovascular Disease, Stress and

G P Chrousos and G Kaltsas
University of Athens, Athens, Greece

Glossary

Catecholamines — Norepinephrine (norepinephrine), epinephrine (adrenaline), and dopamine are the mediators through which the autonomic nervous system responds to stressors and controls a wide variety of system functions, such as arousal, arterial blood pressure, glucose levels, etc.

Circadian rhythm — Many functions of living creatures are subject to periodic or cyclic changes mainly influenced by the nervous system. These changes are instrinsic to the organism independent of the environment and are driven by a biologic "clock". When they have a period of approximately 24 hours these rhythms are called circadian (around a day).

Cytokines — Substances secreted from a number of different immune, including activated macrophages and lymphocytes, and nonimmune cells. According to their subtype they may exert a pro- or anti-inflammatory effect and activate the stress response.

Cushing's syndrome — The presence of symptoms and signs associated with prolonged exposure to inappropriately elevated levels of free plasma glucocorticoids.

Glucocorticoids — The final endocrine effectors of the hypothalamic-pituitary-adrenal (HPA) axis. They are steroid pleiotropic hormones that exert their effects through ubiquitously distributed intracellular receptors. Glucocorticoids are crucial for the maintenance of resting and stress-related homeostasis, regulating and assuring the integrity of cardiovascular, metabolic, behavioral and immune homeostasis.

Metabolic syndrome — A clustering of factors closely associated with the development of atherosclerotic cardiovascular disease. The most recent definition includes central obesity, hypertriglyceridemia, low high-density lipoprotein (HDL) cholesterol levels, hypertension, and increased fasting glucose levels or diabetes mellitus type 2.

Stress State of threatened or perceived threatened homeostasis. Stress can be of either physical, social and/or psychological origin. During stress, a coordinated adaptive response of the organism is activated that is crucial in achieving and maintaining homeostasis. If this response is excessive and prolonged or defective and inadequate, the organism is in dyshomeostasis, or allostasis (allo = different) or cacostasis (caco = bad). The main components of the adaptive response are the corticotropin-releasing hormone (CRH) and the locus-caeruleus-norepinephrine (LC-NE)/arousal and autonomic nervous systems and their peripheral effectors, HPA axis and the systemic and adrenomedullary limbs of the autonomic system.

Sympathetic nervous system The SNS along with the parasympathetic system consist the autonomic nervous system. The SNS is under direct control from the CNS, allowing rapid onset of actions of short duration either exhitatoty or inhibitory) as a result of the abbreviated half-lifes of catecholamines.

Prevalence of Atherosclerosis – Cardiovascular Disease

Atherosclerotic lesions (atheroma) consist of asymmetric focal thickening of the innermost layer of the artery, the intima. Pathologic changes caused by atherosclerosis in the cardiovascular system, such as coronary heart disease, aneurisms of the aorta and brain, or peripheral limb ischemia, currently represent the most profound threat to the quality and expectancy of life in developed countries. It has been estimated that cardiovascular diseases (CVD) cause 38% of all deaths in North America and are the most common cause of death in European men under 65 years of age and the second most common cause in women. Ischemia of the myocardial and cerebral circulation – leading to myocardial infarction and stroke, respectively, develops when the atheromatous process prevents blood flow through the involved arteries either as a result of plaque rupture or endothelial erosion. Common risk factors for developing atherosclerosis are hyperlipidemia, hypertension, and disorders of carbohydrate homeostasis, such as glucose intolerance and diabetes mellitus type 2 (DM2). The spectrum of these traditional risk factors has lately been incorporated under the entity of the metabolic syndrome, which also includes visceral obesity, insulin resistance, and/or blood hypercoagulation. Patients with the metabolic syndrome are at increased risk for developing atherosclerosis and, therefore, constitute a group for early intervention. Over the past two decades, there has been a striking increase in the number of people with the metabolic syndrome; this increase is associated with the global epidemic of obesity and DM2. There is an urgent need for strategies to prevent the emerging global epidemic of metabolic syndrome along with the elevated risk not only of DM2 but also of CVD.

Established and Evolving Risk Factors of Atherosclerosis

When traditional risk factors are taken into consideration, not all cases of CVD can be attributed to their presence. Studies, such as the Framingham Heart Study, have shown that approximately 50% of coronary heart disease cases can be explained by the three major cardiovascular risk factors – elevated serum cholesterol, hypertension, and smoking. In addition, although rigorous treatment of hypercholesterolemia and hypertension was expected to substantially decrease CVD, these diseases still remain the main cause of death globally and are expected to increase further owing to a rapidly increasing prevalence of obesity in developing countries and Eastern Europe and the continuing rise in the incidence of obesity and diabetes in the western world. To explain these observations, additional pathogenetic mechanisms have been thought to contribute, among which is the effect that chronic stress may exert in the development of the metabolic syndrome and the concurrent presence of systemic smoldering inflammation.

Common effector pathways appear to mediate the pathogenesis of metabolic syndrome, atherosclerosis and CVD. These include activation of the hypothalamic-pituitary-adrenal (HPA) axis, the systemic/adrenomedullary sympathetic nervous systems (LC-NE-SNS) and the inflammatory/immune response. These systems, either alone or in combination, can initiate and/or promote mechanisms related to the development of atherosclerosis, such as mobilization of low-density lipoprotein (LDL), which is manufactured and secreted into the circulation by the liver, as a carrier of cholesterol to peripheral tissues. Macrophages, a major component of the immune system, contribute to the vascular accumulation of cholesterol by absorbing the oxidized forms of LDL and adhering to inflamed endothelium to ultimately form stenosis-causing plaques. Macrophages and the cytokines they produce can also be activated by the stress system, whereas cytokines are also a major link between obesity and endothelial dysfunction. Furthermore, alterations of cortisol secretion, effect, and dynamics have been thought to be related either directly and/or indirectly, through inhibition of systems that exert a protective effect, in the development of atherosclerotic lesions.

Alterations of the Function of the Stress System Leading to the Development of Atherosclerosis and Cardiovascular Disease

The Stress System

During stress, adaptive behavioral and peripheral responses are activated that optimize the ability of the organism to adjust homeostasis. Stress is associated with increased activity of the HPA axis and the LC-NE-SNS, which result in systemic elevations of their endocrine end-effectors, the glucocorticoids (cortisol) and the catecholamines (CAs). These compounds, together with other products of the stress system, such as for instance the cytokine interleukin (IL)-6, influence a variety of adaptive responses. The activation of the HPA axis is regulated by glucocorticoid negative-feedback control through glucocorticoid receptors (GR) in the central nervous system (CNS). Normally, there is a diurnal secretory pattern of cortisol with elevations in the early morning and decreases in the afternoon and evening hours. This basal activity is modified by stressful stimuli, which can be either physical (extreme environmental alteration, trauma, and toxins) and/or events that are perceived as unpleasant, demanding, scary, or threatening. The latter can include recalls of previously experienced or unpleasant or pleasant events which either positively or negatively influence the regulation of the HPA axis. Thus, stress leads to increased integrated cortisol and CA secretion, which can be of short or long duration depending on the severity and duration of the stressor. Following repeated exposure to stressors there is great interindividual variation in the extent of cortisol response habituation. Although studies have been conflicting with some showing activation and others attenuation of the HPA axis function in chronic stress, in both situations abnormalities of cortisol secretory dynamics are evident defining a chronic hyperactivation or hypoactivation of the stress system.

Overt or Subtle Hypercortisolism and Cardiovascular Disease

Excessive and sustained cortisol secretion or chronic administration of pharmacological doses of glucocorticoids (endogenous or exogenous Cushing's syndrome (CS), respectively) have been associated with the entire spectrum of the metabolic syndrome, including visceral obesity, insulin resistance/carbohydrate intolerance/DM2, dyslipidemia, dyscoagulation, and hypertension, along with their morbid sequelas of atherosclerosis and CVD. The causal association between chronic psychosocial stress, hypercortisolism, and metabolic syndrome-related manifestations has been shown experimentally only in cynomolgus monkeys. Major melancholic depression, a state of chronic and sustained hyperactivation of the stress system is also associated with hypercortisolism and such patients have a markedly decreased life expectancy due to increased mortality from CVD (2–3 risk of gender- and age-matched controls). Thus, sustained hypercortisolism, as encountered in CS and melancholic depression, is associated with increased prevalence of atherosclerosis, hypertension, and all the clinical and biochemical features of the metabolic syndrome and an overall increased in mortality from CVD.

The conspicuous similarities between CS and the metabolic syndrome and the development of atherosclerosis in both conditions suggest that hypercortisolism may be involved in the pathogenesis of the latter. There is some evidence that hypercortisolism may be directly related to the pathogenesis of the metabolic syndrome, as in such patients, alterations of the secretory pattern and turnover of glucocorticoids has been noted. Such patients may also have depressive (a severe form of chronic psychological stress) symptomatology and be at increased risk for developing a severe form of metabolic syndrome, depending on genetic, developmental and/or environmental factors. Indeed, some patients with depressive symptomatology and/or chronic active alcoholism associated with visceral obesity and insulin resistance and accompanied by increased cortisol secretion may occasionally be difficult to differentiate from those with frank endogenous CS. The term pseudo-Cushing syndrome has been employed to describe such patients. As depression is highly prevalent, affecting up to 10–15% of the population, a considerable number of patients with pseudo-Cushing are among us.

Increases in body mass index (BMI), blood pressure, and dyslipidemia in nonCushingoid middle-aged men have been correlated with the degree of stress perception and cortisol secretion. It is probable that similar parallel alterations of the other peripheral component of the stress system, the SNS, are also present.

CAs are important modulators of corticotropin-releasing hormone (CRH) and adrenocorticotropic hormone (ACTH) secretion, particularly during acute and chronic stress and their effects are mediated by both the $\alpha 1$ and $\alpha 2$ subtypes of adrenoceptors. Activation of the $\alpha 2$ subtype may represent a negative-feedback mechanism that prevents excessive glucocorticoid responses to internal and external stressors. Indeed, following α2 inhibition, the ACTH response after combined stimulation with CRH and antidiuretic hormone (AVP) was significantly higher in obese (visceral obesity) compared to normal weight individuals. This finding suggests that obese individuals with abdominal fat distribution may escape the physiologic α2-adrenoceptor control of their stress system, thus favoring inappropriate HPA axis and SNS excitation (**Table 1**).

Analyzing further the dynamics of cortisol secretion, it is evident that a nonstressed HPA axis is characterized by an increased variance of circadian cortisol secretion and an appropriate suppression of the morning cortisol levels in response to low-dose dexamethasone administration. In contrast, a chronically stressed HPA axis is characterized by a decreased diurnal variance, mostly due to evening elevation, mild morning decreases of cortisol levels, and inadequate suppression of morning cortisol by overnight dexamethasone. These findings suggest the presence of chronic hypersecretion of CRH in chronically stressed individuals and a reset of their HPA axis leading to an increase of total time-integrated cortisol secretion. In the presence of a properly functioning glucocorticoid negative-feedback system, these alterations of cortisol secretion are minimized resulting in amelioration of the manifestations of chronic hypercortisolism (**Tables 1** and **2**).

Table 1 Somatic consequences of chronic stress system activation/target tissue effects with respect to the development of CVD

HPA axis – cortisol	*Locus caeruleus/ norepinephrine CAs, IL-6*
CNS effects	
Potentiation of amygdala/fear – mesocorticolimbic dopaminergic system dysfunction (↑)	↑CAs
Leptin actions ↓	
GH/IGF-1 ↓	
LH/Testosterone – estadiol ↓	
TSH/thyroxine ↓	↓IL-6
Hypertension	
Vasoconstriction (↑) (CAs, angiotensin II, arginine-vasopressin/endothelin)	↑CAs
Vasodilatation (↓) (kallikrein, prostacyclin, NO-synthase, inflammatory cytokines)	
Salt retention ↑, Renin substrate↑	↑Renin, CAs
Visceral fat syndrome (↑)	
Insulin resistance (↑)	
Gluconeogenesis (↑), peripheral glucose disposal (↓), insulin concentration (↑), carbohydrate intolerance (↑),LDL-cholesterol and small dense LDL, FFA, TG (↑), coagulation process (↑),	↑CAs, ↑IL-6

↑, stimulation, ↓, inhibition; CA, catecholamine; CNS, central nervous system, FFA, free fatty acid; HPA axis, hypothalamo-pituitary-adrenal axis; GH, growth hormone; IGF, insulin growth factor; IL, interleukin; LDL, low-density lipoprotein; LH, luteinizing hormone; NO, nitric oxide; TG, triglyceride; TSH, thyroid-stimulating hormone. Adapted from *International Journal of Obesity* **24**, The role of stress and the hypothalamic pituitary adrenal axis in the pathogenesis of the metabolic syndrome: neuroendocrine and target tissue related causes. 2000, S50–S55, with permission.

Table 2 Abnormalities of the hypothalamic-pituitary-adrenal (HPA) axis associated with the metabolic syndrome and cardiovascular disease

Function	*Type of alteration of the HPA axis*
Cortisol metabolic clearance rate	↑
Cortisol production in peripheral tissues (adipose) – ↑ 11β-HSD1 activity	↑
Daily urinary free cortisol excretion	↑
Number of secretory pulses of ACTH	↑
Amplitude of secretory pulses of ACTH	↓
ACTH and cortisol response to ACTH	↑
ACTH and cortisol response to CRH and AVP	↑
ACTH and cortisol response to acute stress	↑
Cortisol response to meals	↑
HPA sensitivity to increased noradrenergic tone	↑
Cortisol suppression by dexamethasone	↓

↑, increased; ↓, decreased; ACTH, adrenocorticotropic hormone; AVP, antidiuretic hormone; CRH, corticotropin-releasing hormone; HPA, hypothalamic-pituitary adrenal; 11β-HSD1, 11β-hydroxysteroid dehydrogenase type 1. Adapted from *International Journal of Obesity* **24**, Activity of the hypothalamo-pituitary-adrenal axis in different obesity phenotypes. 2000, S47–S49, with permission.

The ability of the glucocorticoid negative-feedback system to limit the production of cortisol during stress can be impaired by early life stress and by exposure of the organism to chronic physical/emotional stress. The sensitivity of target tissues to glucocorticoids, of course, also plays a major role in both influencing the negative-feedback system and the actions of glucocorticoids on their other target tissues. Studies examining the presence of polymorphisms of the glucocorticoid receptor gene described the presence of a correlation between particular polymorphisms and the development of hypertension and/or visceral obesity, whereas others demonstrated that increased dermal tissue glucocorticoid sensitivity was associated with an increased blood pressure, insulin resistance, and hyperglycemia. Interestingly, the same subjects also exhibited an enhanced secretion of cortisol and impaired conversion of cortisol to inactive metabolites implying a direct or an indirect effect of stress on tissue active hormone availability.

Recent studies have shown alterations of 11β-hydroxysteroid dehydrogenase (11β-HSD) type 2, which converts cortisol to inactive cortisone, particularly in the kidney. However, the metabolic clearance rate of cortisol is mostly influenced by its regeneration from inactive cortisone in the liver, fat, and skeletal muscle by 11β-oxoreductase type 1. Consistent with animal studies, 11β-HSD2 appears to be a constitutive rather than a hormonally regulated enzyme, in contrast to 11β-HSD1 which is downregulated by insulin and estrogens and appears to be dysregulated in obesity. The activity of 11β-HSD1 in the omental fat of obese people is significantly higher than in lean individuals and the activity of the enzyme is further increased by exposure to cortisol and insulin. The inappropriate constant exposure of fat, particularly visceral fat, to cortisol may be important in determining its differentiation and mass increase leading to visceral obesity and the manifestations of the metabolic syndrome. In addition, it may modify the secretion of other adipose tissue hormones, such as leptin, IL-6, and/or adiponectin, and thus modify the output of adipose cells and influence the information they convey to satiety centers regarding fuel homeostasis.

High circulating cortisol levels or sustained alteration of the normal diurnal pattern of cortisol secretion also suppress the growth, thyroid and reproductive axes and lead to elevation of Ca^{2+}-stimulated cytokine production (and particularly IL-6) contributing further to the exacerbation of the metabolic syndrome by inducing lipolysis and utilization of protein for glyconeogenesis. Activation of the stress system is associated with suppression of growth hormone secretion and resistance of somatomedin C and other growth factor effects on their target organs. The reproductive axis is also inhibited at several levels by various components of the HPA axis. Either directly or via β-endorphin, CRH suppresses luteinizing hormone releasing hormone (LHRH) neurons, and thus gonadotropin secretion from the pituitary gland, whereas glucocorticoids exert inhibitory effects at the levels of LHRH neurons, pituitary gonadotrophs and the gonads and render target tissues of sex steroids resistant to these hormones. These effects and similar ones observed in the thyroid axis, counteract the beneficial effects these hormones may exert in body distribution and fuel homeostasis contributing further to the development of visceral obesity and the metabolic syndrome by antagonizing fat-tissue catabolism and inhibiting muscle and bone anabolism.

Although alterations of the LC-NE-SNS have not been studied in such detail as those of the HPA axis, it is quite likely that SNS hyperactivity, either as a result of a generalized activation of the stress system or as a compensatory mechanism in cases of a faltering HPA axis activity, also participates in the pathogenesis of cardiovascular disorders. A consequence of elevated SNS activity may be through elevated free fatty acid levels which can induce insulin resistance in muscle and amplify the metabolic perturbations of patients with pathological regulation of their HPA axis (**Table 1**).

Systemic Inflammation and Cardiovascular Disease

Over the last decade, there is mounting evidence that inflammation plays a major role in the development of CVD. Several studies have documented that elevated concentrations of IL-6 or the downstream acute phase reactant C-reactive protein (CRP) predict the development of CVD over many years, suggesting that inflammation makes a contribution to the earlier stages of the disease. Elevated IL-6 levels can predict total and cardiovascular mortality over a 5-year follow-up, the association being independent of prevalent vascular disease, smoking, and traditional risk factors. The predictive value of IL-6 is in fact stronger than that of CRP. This cytokine is not produced only as a result of inflammation but as a component of noninflammatory stress, while a large proportion of total circulating levels of IL-6 may originate from the adipose tissue. IL-6 participates in the development of CVD through different mechanisms, including induction of endothelial dysfunction, hepatic fibrinogen release, and adhesion molecule expression by endothelial cells and circulating leukocytes. Il-6 also decreases insulin sensitivity of peripheral tissues and increases circulating nonesterified fatty acids, inducing a metabolic syndrome phenotype. Psychological stress can elevate IL-6 levels through Ca^{2+} hypersecretion, possibly from liver Kupfer cells or from the adipose tissue itself. Il-6 is also a potent stimulator of the HPA axis leading to cortisol hypersecretion and the development of the metabolic syndrome through this path as well. It is possible that genetic variations of the IL-6 and other related genes involved in its signaling system modulate the body's response to stress and obesity.

Obesity as a Chronic Inflammatory State

Obesity is the most common and costly nutritional problem in the United States, affecting approximately 33% of the adult population while its incidence among children and adolescents is also rising. Obesity, particularly the visceral type, is the most important potentially preventable factor that substantially increases the risk for developing DM2, CVD, and certain types of cancers. Adipose tissue secretes large amounts of tumor necrosis factor (TNF)-α and IL-6 in a neurally, hormonally, and metabolically regulated fashion. The plasma levels of these cytokines are proportional to the BMI and are further elevated in patients with visceral obesity. The secretion of inflammatory cytokines has a circadian pattern, with elevations in the evening and in the early morning hours. This pattern is maintained in obese subjects, albeit at a higher level, is affected by the quality and quantity of sleep, and correlates with manifestations of the sickness syndrome. Thus, in obesity, hypercytokinemia is frequently associated with sleepiness and fatigue, as well with an activated acute-phase reaction. Obesity, especially the visceral type, can be considered as a chronic inflammatory state, with many of the behavioral, immune, metabolic and cardiovascular manifestations and sequelas of such a state.

Psychosocial Stress and Cardiovascular Disease

There has been considerable information relating alterations in the activity of the stress system and conventional risk factors in developing CVD, the major cause of morbidity and mortality in western societies. A consistent and continuous gradient between socioeconomic status (SES) and the prevalence of CVD has been found, with people from lower SES having more disease. In some studies the ratio of death rates from the lowest to the highest professional grade may be as high as 3 to 1. Although an inverse relation between SES and cigarette smoking has been noted, this is not obvious when total cholesterol and/or blood pressure are considered; however, an inverse relation between SES and BMI and visceral obesity was noted as well. Not surprisingly, physical inactivity was clearly linked to obesity and lower SES and this combination may contribute further to the SES-disease gradient. In favor of these observations is the finding of the Gothenberg Primary Prevention Study, which demonstrated an odds ratio of CVD morbidity of 2.2, which changed to only 1.9 after adjusting for established risk factors (including blood pressure, smoking, cholesterol, BMI, and exercise habit). The inability of traditional risk factors to explain more than 25% of the SES–CVD gradient suggests that additional factors related to the working conditions might contribute.

The ability to monitor surrogate markers of CVD and also to visualize atherosclerotic plaques directly has helped to evaluate the biologic pathways through which SES may exert its effects. An analysis of psychological factors and blood pressure reactivity (measured as the anticipatory increase in blood pressure before an exercise test) exhibited a clear relation to progression of atherosclerosis. Chronic psychosocial stress directly through the stress system and its hormones and/or indirectly through changes in health-related behaviors may be the main culprit connecting poverty and CVD.

Further Reading

Banks, J., Marmot, M., Oldfield, Z., et al. (2006). Disease and disadvantage in the United States and in England. *JAMA* **295**, 2037–2045.

Bjontrop, P. and Rosmond, R. (2000). The metabolic syndrome – a neuroendocrine disorder? *British Journal of Nutrition* **83**, S49–S57.

Charmandari, E., Tsigos, C. and Chrousos, G. (2005). Endocrinology of the stress response. *Annual Reviews of Physiology* **67**, 259–284.

Chrousos, G. P. (1998). Stressors, stress and neuroendocrine integration of the adaptive response: 1997 Hans Selye Memorial Lecture. *Annals of the New York Academy of Sciences* **851**, 311–335.

Chrousos, G. P. (2000). The role of stress and the hypothalamic pituitary adrenal axis in the pathogenesis of the metabolic syndrome: neuroendocrine and target tissue related causes. *International Journal of Obesity* **24**, S50–S55.

Chrousos, G. P. and Gold, P. W. (1992). The concepts of stress and stress system disorders. *JAMA* **267**, 1244–1252.

Eckel, R. H., Grundy, S. M. and Zimmet, P. Z. (2005). The metabolic syndrome. *Lancet* **365**, 1415–1428.

Fang, J., Madhavan, S. and Alderman, M. H. (1996). The association between birth-place and mortality from cardiovascular causes among black and white residents of New York City. *New England Journal of Medicine* **335**, 1545–1551.

Habib, K. E., Gold, P. W. and Chrousos, G. P. (2001). Neuroendocrinology of stress. *Endocrinology Metabolics Clinics North America* **30**, 695–727.
Hanson, G. K. (2005). Inflammation, atherosclerosis and coronary artery disease. *New England Journal of Medicine* **352**, 1685–1695.
Lynch, J. W., Kaplan, G. A., Cohen, R. D., et al. (1996). Do cardiovascular risk factors explain the relation between socioeconomic status, risk of all-cause mortality, cardiovascular mortality, and acute myocardial infarction? *American Journal of Epidemiology* **144**, 934–942.
McEwen, B. S. (1998). Protective and damaging effects of stress mediators. *New England Journal of Medicine* **338**, 171–179.
Pasquali, R. and Vicennati, V. (2000). Activity of the hypothalamo-pituitary-adrenal axis in different obesity phenotypes. *International Journal of Obesity* **24**, S47–S49.
Rosenbaum, M., Leibel, R. and Hirsch, J. (1997). Obesity. *New England Journal of Medicine* **396**, 396–407.
Rosmond, R., Lapidus, L. and Bjontrop, P. (1996). The influence of occupational and social factors on obesity and body fat distribution in middle-aged men. *International Journal of Obesity Related Metabolic Disorders* **20**, 599–607.
Yudkin, J. S., Kumari, M., Humphries, S., et al. (2000). Inflammation, obesity, stress and coronary heart disease: is interleukin-6 the link? *Atherosclerosis* **148**, 209–214.

Psychosomatic Heart Disease: Role of Sympathetic and Sympathoadrenal Processes

G W Lambert
Baker Heart Research Institute, Melbourne, Victoria, Australia
T Dawood
Baker Heart Research Institute and Monash University, Alfred Hospital, Melbourne, Victoria, Australia

Glossary

Neurogenic essential hypertension Elevated blood pressure initiated and sustained by a characteristic elevation in sympathetic nervous activity.

Major depressive disorder A common and severe mental illness characterized by feelings of hopelessness, helplessness, and worthlessness; often accompanied by suicidal thoughts.

Panic disorder A distressing and disabling condition with patients experiencing recurrent episodes of unexpected intense anxiety of sudden onset.

> I was walking along the road with two of my friends. Then the sun set. Then the sky became a bloody red and I felt a tinge of melancholy, a sucking pain beneath my heart. I stopped, leaned against the railing, dead tired. Over the blue-black fiord and city hung blood and tongues of fire. My friends walked on and I stood again trembling with fright. And I felt as if a loud unending scream were piercing nature. – Edvard Munch

Mechanisms Underlying Coronary Heart Disease and Myocardial Infarction and Possible Relationship to Stress and Behavior

Over recent years, substantial advances have been made in delineating the causes of coronary heart disease. At a community level, the importance of high blood pressure, tobacco smoking, and abnormal blood lipids as causal factors is well established. Recent epidemiological studies also point to an association between psychosocial stressors and increased risk of development of acute myocardial infarction. Mechanistically, the relevant issues linking psychosocial stress and acute cardiac events are whether stress, in one of its numerous forms, can (1) lead to the development of hypertension, (2) cause or aggravate atherosclerosis, and/or (3) trigger a cardiac event in the presence of existing atherosclerosis.

Relation of Stress to the Development of Hypertension

The importance of hypertension in the development of left ventricular hypertrophy, myocardial infarction, heart failure, and sudden death is well established. Indeed, over 90% of patients with heart failure in the Framingham study had a history of hypertension. The longitudinal studies of Timio and colleagues, examining hypertension development and cardiovascular morbidity and mortality in cloistered nuns, provide persuasive evidence linking the stress of daily life to the development of high blood pressure. Essential hypertension is commonly neurogenic, initiated and sustained by the sympathetic nervous system. While activation of the sympathetic nervous system outflows to the kidneys, heart, and skeletal muscle in hypertensive patients has been well documented, a second neural mechanism, reduced reuptake of the sympathetic neurotransmitter, norepinephrine, is also operative. Reuptake of norepinephrine into sympathetic nerves after its release terminates the neural signal. A fault in transmitter inactivation augments the effects of sympathetic nerve traffic. For the sympathetic nerves of the heart, approximately 95% of released norepinephrine is recaptured, so that the heart is more sensitive than all other organs to impediments in transmitter reuptake. Other cardinal signs of stress common to patients with neurogenic essential hypertension include activation of brain noradrenergic pathways and epinephrine release from the heart.

Relation of Stress to the Development of Atherosclerosis

There exist numerous population studies indicating that psychological disturbances, particularly anxiety and chronic stress, can contribute to atherosclerosis development. In the workplace, insufficient self-regulation of workload, deadlines, and planning and direction of the work have been linked to risk of developing atherosclerosis. Low socioeconomic status or employment level is associated with increased plasma fibrinogen and von Willebrand factor concentrations. Endothelial function is considerably impaired following acute experimental stress.

Relation of Stress to the Triggering of a Cardiac Event

Cardiac sympathetic nerves are preferentially activated by mental stress It is important to realize that sympathetic nervous activity at rest and in response to stress is regionalized. For instance, with even relatively mild experimental mental stress, such as that induced in the laboratory by performing difficult mental arithmetic, the sympathetic nerves of the heart are markedly and preferentially activated, whereas activation of muscle vasoconstrictor sympathetic fibers predominates during the cold pressor test. Mental stress in patients with existing coronary artery disease has been demonstrated to cause anginal chest pain and inadequate blood supply to the heart. The effect of mental stress on cardiac sympathetic nervous activation is greater in the elderly. The importance of cardiac sympathetic activation in these contexts is highlighted by the demonstration, in experimental animals with narrowing of the coronary arteries, that direct electrical stimulation of the cardiac sympathetics is capable of causing electrical instability of the myocardium, triggering disturbances of heart rhythm and cardiac arrest.

General relation between activity of the sympathetic nerves of the heart and sudden death In a range of clinical contexts, stimulation of the cardiac sympathetic outflow has been demonstrated to contribute to myocardial infarction, ventricular arrhythmias, and sudden death. Activation of the sympathetic outflow to the heart is common in patients unexpectedly developing ventricular tachycardia and ventricular fibrillation. Furthermore, myocardial stunning due to sudden emotional stress is associated with exaggerated sympathetic stimulation. Similarly, in patients with heart failure, there is a high level of stimulation of the cardiac sympathetic nerves, which is a proven determinant of sudden death. β-adrenergic blockers have been recently shown to increase survival in heart failure patients.

Direct relation between mental stress and sudden death in certain circumstances In a rare inherited heart condition, long QT interval syndrome, there is electrical instability of the heart muscle. Mental stress is one proven immediate cause of cardiac arrest in sufferers. Some research linking mental stress to sudden death is disputed because of disagreement over what constitutes a stress, and whether stress can be accurately measured. Recent research showing that rates of sudden, nontraumatic death in people with underlying coronary disease were markedly increased during catastrophic events is free of this criticism, as no finessing is needed in the psychological measurement of stress.

Sympathoadrenal Function in Panic Disorder

Debilitating episodes of recurring, often inexplicable anxiety afflict as many as 12% of the population. These attacks typically are unpleasant and may be accompanied by physical symptoms such as sweating, palpitations, tremor, and a sensation of suffocation. Given the prominent signs of sympathetic activation that occur during a panic attack, panic disorder patients find themselves at the nexus between cardiovascular and psychiatric medicine. It has until recently been felt that although panic disorder is distressing and disabling, it does not constitute a risk to life.

Sufferers often fear that they have heart disease because of the nature of their symptoms, but have been reassured that this is not the case. Epidemiological studies, however, indicate that there is an increased risk of myocardial infarction and sudden death in patients with anxiety disorders. This increased risk extends even to premenopausal women, who in general have low coronary risk.

Somatic Sensitization as a Panicogenic Factor

Patients with panic disorder often exhibit hypervigilance to somatic sensations such as an irregular heartbeat or lightheadedness. Given the convergence of neural networks involved in processing viscerosensory and contextual information and their links with brain regions pivotal in the fear network, it is possible that somatic sensation may be capable of triggering panic attacks. Such a concept is not without precedent. It has been known for some time that the presence of abnormalities of heart rhythm, supraventricular tachycardia in particular, can pre-date and in fact cause panic disorder. More recently, a very high rate of development of panic disorder was observed in patients with implanted cardiac defibrillators. Indeed, factors at play here seem to include the presence of cardiac symptoms and the enhanced vigilance that accompanies them.

Sympathetic and Adrenomedullary Function in Panic Disorder

Resting whole body, cardiac, and muscle vasoconstrictor sympathetic activity is normal in patients with panic disorder. While adrenal medullary secretion of epinephrine, measured by isotope dilution, is typically normal in these patients, there occurs a demonstrable release of epinephrine from the heart. It is probable that during the surges of epinephrine secretion that accompany panic attacks the cardiac sympathetic neuronal vesicles become loaded with epinephrine that is continuously co-released with norepinephrine in the interim periods between attacks. *In situ* synthesis of epinephrine, through activation within the heart of phenylethanolamine-n-methyltransferase (PNMT), perhaps induced by repeated cortisol responses during panic attacks, may also occur. In experimental models of stress, PNMT activation in the heart and other extra-adrenal organs has been demonstrated.

Norepinephrine Reuptake in Panic Disorder

As mentioned previously, reuptake of norepinephrine into sympathetic nerves after its release terminates the sympathetic neural signal. A phenotypic defect in norepinephrine transporter function has been described in patients with panic disorder. Such an abnormality in neuronal norepinephrine reuptake could sensitize the heart to sympathetic activation. The mechanism underpinning the defect in norepinephrine transporter function, and whether treatment modifies the activity of the norepinephrine transporter, remains unknown.

Sympathetic and Adrenomedullary Function during a Panic Attack

During panic attacks triggered cardiac arrhythmias, recurrent emergency room attendances with anginal chest pain and ECG changes of ischemia, coronary artery spasm in attacks occurring during coronary angiography, and myocardial infarction associated with coronary spasm and thrombosis have been documented. The recurrent episodes of unexpected intense anxiety that characterize a panic attack are accompanied by a pronounced activation of the sympathetic nervous system and adrenomedullary secretion of epinephrine. A concomitant elevation in blood pressure and heart rate also occurs. The characteristic chest pain that occurs during an attack is additionally accompanied by the release of neuropeptide Y into the coronary sinus. Neuropeptide Y is a potent vasoconstrictor with the capacity to cause coronary artery spasm.

Sympathoadrenal Function in Major Depressive Disorder

Central Nervous System Neuronal Activity

The etiology of major depressive disorder (MDD) has been linked, variously, to brain monoaminergic neuronal dysfunction, alterations in monoamine receptor sensitivity, and stress-induced activation of the hypothalamic-pituitary-adrenal axis. The lack of demonstrated relationships between different clinical presentations and biochemical abnormalities has hampered the development of sensitive biochemical markers for MDD. A major difficulty in commonly used peripheral indices of a neurotransmitter (or neurotrophic factor) as an indicator of brain dysfunction is that these compounds are also produced outside the brain. For this reason, venous blood is directly sampled from the brain to study central nervous system (CNS) neurotransmitter turnover, using central venous catheters placed high in an internal jugular vein. Under these circumstances, arteriovenous differences in neurotransmitter concentrations can be extrapolated to estimates of brain production. The observation of global (i.e., noradrenergic, dopaminergic and serotonergic) reduction in both subcortical monoamine turnover and cerebral glucose utilization in patients with MDD is consistent with a reduction in CNS neurotrophic support in patients with MDD.

Depression as a Risk Factor for the Development of Cardiac Disease

There is strong evidence that patients with MDD are at increased risk of developing coronary heart disease. This elevated risk is independent of classical risk factors such as smoking, obesity, hypercholesterolemia, diabetes, and hypertension. The association is present in males and females, across different age groups and in subjects living in different countries. The risk of coronary heart disease is increased 1.5- to 2-fold in those with minor/subsyndromic depression and 3- to 4.5-fold in subjects with major depression. To put this into perspective, the strength of the association between coronary heart disease and MDD is similar to that with smoking and hypercholesterolemia. Also conclusively demonstrated is the adverse effect of depression in patients with heart failure and in patients following myocardial infarction, which materially increases mortality.

Sympathoadrenal Activity in MDD

While the mechanism of increased cardiac risk attributable to MDD is at present uncertain, activation of the sympathetic nervous system may be of prime importance. Chronic stress has been linked with MDD. Examination of indices of sympathetic nervous function in MDD has yielded conflicting results. Some studies indicate a tendency for both the urinary excretion and cerebrospinal fluid level of norepinephrine and its metabolites to be diminished, whereas other reports document elevated plasma levels of norepinephrine and increased rates of norepinephrine spillover to plasma in patients with MDD. It is likely that sympathoadrenal activation is present only in a subset of patients with MDD. Indeed, Gold and colleagues recently demonstrated elevated norepinephrine levels in both the CSF and plasma of patients with melancholic depression.

In addition to possible effects on blood pressure and myocardial stability, sympathetically mediated neural vasoconstriction may exert metabolic effects in skeletal muscle, impairing glucose delivery to muscle and causing insulin resistance and hyperinsulinemia, and in the liver, retarding postprandial clearing of lipids and contributing to hyperlipidemia. A trophic effect of sympathetic activation on cardiovascular growth, contributing to the development of left ventricular hypertrophy, may also occur. Left ventricular hypertrophy is an independent risk factor for cardiovascular morbidity and mortality.

Further knowledge of the mechanisms responsible for generating cardiac risk may pave the way for novel and perhaps relatively simple therapeutic strategies (e.g., low-dose aspirin, β-blockers) to be administered to those with MDD in order to modify cardiac risk. Indeed, defining therapeutic interventions that reduce cardiac risk will be an important step forward in alleviating the burden of depressive illness on the community.

See Also the Following Articles

Hypertension.

Further Reading

Bunker, S. J., Colquhoun, D. M., Esler, M. D., et al. (2003). "Stress" and coronary heart disease: psychosocial risk factors. *Medical Journal of Australia* **178**, 272–276.

Esler, M., Jennings, G., Lambert, G., et al. (1990). Overflow of catecholamine neurotransmitters to the circulation: source, fate, and functions. *Physiological Reviews* **70**, 963–985.

Gold, P. W., Wong, M. L., Goldstein, D. S., et al. (2005). Cardiac implications of increased arterial entry and reversible 24-h central and peripheral norepinephrine levels in melancholia. *Proceedings of the National Academy of Sciences USA* **102**, 8303–8308.

Lambert, G., Johansson, M., Agren, H., et al. (2000). Reduced brain norepinephrine and dopamine release in treatment-refractory depressive illness: evidence in support of the catecholamine hypothesis of mood disorders. *Archives of General Psychiatry* **57**, 787–793.

Leor, J., Poole, W. K. and Kloner, R. A. (1996). Sudden cardiac death triggered by an earthquake. *New England Journal of Medicine* **334**, 413–419.

Matsuo, T., Suzuki, S., Kodama, K., et al. (1998). Hemostatic activation and cardiac events after the 1995 Hanshin-Awaji earthquake. *International Journal of Hematology* **67**, 123–129.

Musselman, D. L., Evans, D. L. and Nemeroff, C. B. (1998). The relationship of depression to cardiovascular disease: epidemiology, biology, and treatment. *Archives of General Psychiatry* **55**, 580–592.

Rosengren, A., Hawken, S., Ounpuu, S., et al. (2004). Association of psychosocial risk factors with risk of acute myocardial infarction in 11119 cases and 13648 controls from 52 countries (the INTERHEART study): case-control study. *Lancet* **364**, 953–962.

Schlaich, M. P., Lambert, E., Kaye, D. M., et al. (2004). Sympathetic augmentation in hypertension: role of nerve firing, norepinephrine reuptake, and angiotensin neuromodulation. *Hypertension* **43**, 169–175.

Spieker, L. E., Hurlimann, D., Ruschitzka, F., et al. (2002). Mental stress induces prolonged endothelial dysfunction via endothelin-A receptors. *Circulation* **105**, 2817–2820.

Timio, M., Saronio, P., Venanzi, S., et al. (1999). Blood pressure in nuns in a secluded order: a 30-year follow-up. *Mineral and Electrolyte Metabolism* 25, 73–79.
Wilkinson, D. J., Thompson, J. M., Lambert, G. W., et al. (1998). Sympathetic activity in patients with panic disorder at rest, under laboratory mental stress, and during panic attacks. *Archives of General Psychiatry* 55, 511–520.

Relevant Website

www.beyondblue.org.au *beyondblue* is a national, independent, not-for-profit organisation working to address issues associated with depression, anxiety and related substance misuse disorders in Australia.

Hypertension

A Steptoe
University College London, London, UK

This is a revised version of the article by A Steptoe, Encyclopedia of Stress First Edition, volume 2, pp 425–430, © 2000, Elsevier Inc.

Glossary

White-coat hypertension	Blood pressure that is elevated when measured in the clinic by a physician or nurse but normal when measured in other situations.
Hypertension	Sustained elevated blood pressure.
Left ventricular hypertrophy	The enlargement of the left ventricle of the heart, one of the adverse effects of hypertension.
Normotension	Blood pressure below the criteria for hypertension.

Prevalence

Hypertension is the condition of sustained elevated arterial blood pressure. The criteria for defining hypertension are somewhat arbitrary because the distribution of blood pressure level in the population is continuous. The current definition of hypertension is a systolic blood pressure $\geq$ 140 mmHg and diastolic pressure $\geq$ 90 mmHg. Most authorities regard a blood pressure in the range 130–139/85–89 mmHg as high-normal, although the Joint National Committee on Prevention, Detection, Evaluation, and Treatment of High Blood Pressure has defined levels of 120–139/80–89 mmHg as prehypertensive. Risk of coronary heart disease and stroke is directly related to blood pressure level, so hypertension defines those individuals who are at an especially elevated risk.

The prevalence of hypertension in the United States is approximately 29% in men and 30.5% in women. Recent figures from the United Kingdom indicate that approximately 37% of men and 34% of women are hypertensive. However, blood pressure tends to rise with age, so these overall figures disguise the substantial increase in hypertension in middle age. Thus, in the United States, the prevalence rises from 8.1% in men and 2.7% in women ages 20–34 years to 44.9% and 53.9% in those ages 55–64 years. There are also striking ethnic variations, with high rates in African Americans and in African Caribbean people in the United Kingdom.

Between one-third and one-half of hypertensives are not diagnosed and are unaware of their condition. Because hypertension is not consistently associated with symptoms, it is frequently identified only during routine screening, so it may continue for many years before detection. The number of diagnosed hypertensives who are not treated is substantial, whereas as many as 50% of patients who are prescribed antihypertensive medication do not have their blood pressure controlled adequately. The problem of hypertension is therefore considerable.

Etiological Factors

The etiology of hypertension is complicated. In a minority of cases, high blood pressure is associated with a specific pathological abnormality such as pheochromocytoma or a renovascular disorder. However, in most cases there is no single identifiable cause, and the condition is regarded as multifactorial. This condition was once known as essential hypertension because an elevated pressure was considered necessary to drive blood through partially blocked arteries. Now, cases without a single cause are sometimes called primary hypertensives to distinguish them from individuals whose hypertension is secondary to another disease. Hypertension typically develops over many years, with blood pressure gradually increasing until it reaches threatening levels. The most consistent predictors of future hypertension are a positive family history, a blood pressure in childhood or early adult life that is above average, and elevated body weight. High salt and alcohol intake also contribute.

The primary reason for considering stress to be an etiologic factor relates to the influence of the autonomic nervous system and neuroendocrine factors in hypertension. There is clear evidence of increased sympathetic nervous system activity in hypertension, as documented through raised levels of plasma norepinephrine. Microneurographic studies have shown elevated sympathetic nervous traffic to muscle. Hypothalamic activation may be responsible for these sympathetic responses, which in turn lead to inhibition of baroreceptor reflex sensitivity, peripheral vasoconstriction, and alterations of renal blood flow. Reduced parasympathetic activity may also be associated with the etiology of hypertension, together with the impairment of opioid-mediated counterregulatory processes. Abnormalities of adrenocortical function have been described in some cases of hypertension, and pro-inflammatory processes may contribute as well.

The hypothesis underlying much research on this topic is that the stress-induced activation of sympathetic and other pathways occurs repeatedly over months and years in susceptible individuals, leading to hemodynamic adjustments that increase hypertension risk. Evidence relevant to this hypothesis derives from several sources, including animal and human experimental studies and investigations of the impact of adverse life experiences, chronic stressors, and psychological characteristics.

Experimental Evidence

Animal Studies

Evidence that permanently elevated blood pressure can be produced with behavioral stress in animals is controversial. Although it is clear that acute hypertensive episodes can be induced, the development of sustained hypertension is more elusive. Aversive conditions such as restraint stress, unpredictable shock, and approach–avoidance conflict produce chronic hypertension in some studies but not others. Effects vary across species and are more prominent in the presence of risk factors such as a genetic predisposition and heightened salt sensitivity. Some of the most compelling evidence comes from studies carried out by Henry and coworkers on the effects of social conflict in CBA mice. Male mice raised in isolation were placed in complex colonies that encouraged conflict. There were immediate blood pressure increases that reverted to control levels after their removal from the colony. However, irreversible hypertension developed with prolonged exposure to conflict, accompanied by alterations in catecholamine synthesis and myocardial fibrosis and degeneration. Species differences are apparent in primates as well, although hypertension can be induced by prolonged shock avoidance in rhesus monkeys.

Cardiovascular Reactivity to Acute Behavioral Stress in Humans

Blood pressure increases acutely in response to a variety of behavioral stressors in humans, ranging from problem-solving tasks and emotionally laden interviews to painful stimuli such as the cold pressor test. The increase in blood pressure is typically accompanied by tachycardia, inotropic stimulation of the heart, vasodilatation in skeletal muscle and adipose tissue, and reduced blood flow to the kidneys, skin, and viscera.

The issue of whether these responses are involved in hypertension has been the subject of much research, stimulated in the 1950s by Jan Brod. Compared with normotensives, hypertensives typically show enhanced blood pressure responses to acute behavioral stress, accompanied by greater renal vasoconstriction and increased norepinephrine turnover. However, it is possible that this exaggerated cardiovascular responsivity is the result of the complex physiological adjustments that occur in hypertension and is not primary. Attention has therefore shifted to people with normal blood pressure who are at increased risk, for example, because of genetic factors. Results have again been variable, but a meta-analysis of this literature suggests that a proportion of people with a positive family history of hypertension are more reactive to tasks involving active behavioral responses (e.g., difficult problem solving) than are those without family histories. Young people with positive family histories may also have elevated blood pressure during their everyday lives, as assessed using automated ambulatory monitoring techniques.

Longitudinal studies have also been reported, testing the hypothesis that high reactivity to behavioral stress predicts future rises in blood pressure over 5–10 years. Most trials have found evidence in favor of this hypothesis. Impaired poststress recovery in blood pressure has also been shown to predict future increases. But such effects are not always observed, probably for two reasons. First, the investigation of acute responses to behavioral stress is complex and requires the careful standardization of procedures.

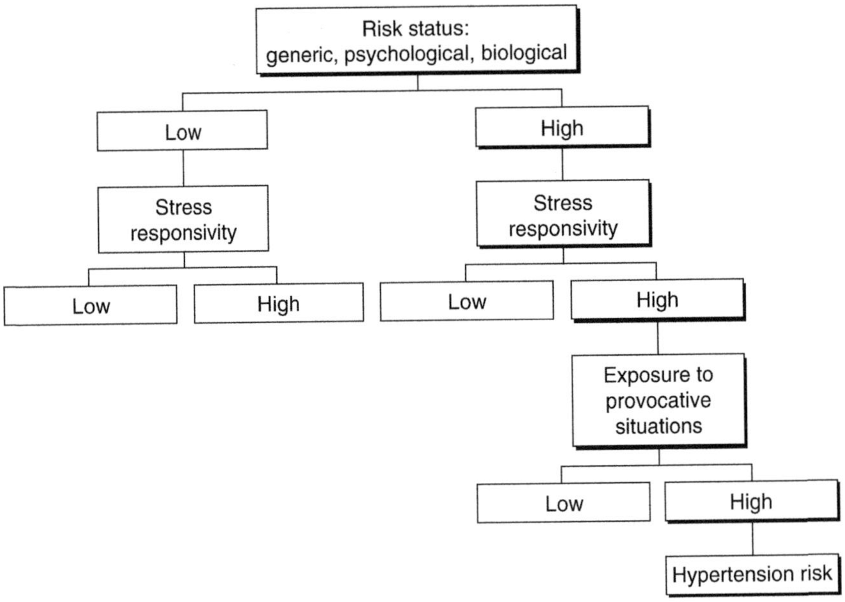

Figure 1 Schematic outline of the way in which acute cardiovascular and neuroendocrine stress responsivity might contribute to hypertension risk. Highlighted boxes indicate the highest risk group. The combination of high risk status, high stress responsiveness, and prolonged exposure to situations that provoke appropriate physiological responses is necessary.

Different types of stimuli elicit different patterns of physiological response. For instance, some tasks such as mental arithmetic elicit blood pressure responses that are primarily sustained through increased myocardial contractility and cardiac output, whereas others predominantly elicit increases in peripheral vascular resistance. These response profiles may not all be equally relevant to hypertension. Second, the nature of the hypothesized relationship between stress responsivity and hypertension should be considered. **Figure 1** outlines the presumed sequence of events. Heightened cardiovascular responses to acute stress *per se* will not increase the risk of hypertension. Such responses are relevant only if they are representative of the individual's experience during daily life. Stress-related factors are most likely to contribute to hypertension if reactive individuals are exposed over months or years to environments that elicit damaging patterns of intense response. This interaction has only been evaluated in a few studies to date. It should also be kept in mind that stress is only one of many factors contributing to hypertension and does not affect all those at risk in the same fashion.

Psychological Characteristics

The many comparisons that have been made between hypertensive patients and controls in terms of personality typically suffer from two limitations. First, the diagnostic label of hypertension may cause psychological distress and lead to changes on psychological tests. Second, because much hypertension is not diagnosed, any differences observed may be restricted to those who seek medical attention. Population-based studies involving measurements of blood pressure and psychological factors are therefore required.

Some population studies have shown prospective associations between tension or anxiety and future hypertension, but effects are small and inconsistent. A more persuasive body of evidence has linked hypertension with the ways that people cope with angry and hostile feelings. This notion was stimulated in the mid-1970s by research on hypertension and urban stress in Detroit. It was found that hypertension was more prevalent and that blood pressure was generally higher among black men living in high-stress areas (defined by population density, crime rate, and family instability) who also inhibited anger expression. Subsequent research has supported the link between anger inhibition and high blood pressure in a number of populations. However, it has also been found that the expression of anger is related to blood pressure, so perhaps the appropriateness of anger display and hostility management is more critical.

Hypertension is associated with mild deficits of cognitive function, as assessed by measures of memory, attention, and abstract reasoning. These effects vary with age, education, and whether blood pressure is being treated. The extent to which these impairments affect the performance of daily activities is not known. They may be the result of central nervous system neurophysiological sequelae of high blood pressure.

Lifestyle and Adverse Life Experience

What types of real-life stressful experience are likely to be associated with hypertension? If the inferences from laboratory studies are correct, they are experiences that are repeated or sustained over years and elicit active efforts to cope and maintain control. Acute traumatic events would not be expected to stimulate appropriate long-term cardiovascular and neuroendocrine responses, and indeed there is little evidence that acute life events are associated with the development of hypertension. In contrast, some forms of chronic stress are associated with sustained increases in blood pressure. Experiences such as caring for demented relatives, marital conflict, and the experience of racism in ethnic minorities have been related to increased blood pressure. Interesting results have emerged from studies of migrants from traditional, isolated, rural cultures to modernized, developing and developed societies. For example, increases in blood pressure have been recorded among young adults from the Luo tribe in western Kenya who migrated to Nairobi. The blood pressure rise was associated with a higher salt intake and greater body weight, but stress-related increases in the sympathetic nervous stimulation may also have been involved. Similarly, studies of migrants from the isolated Pacific Tokelau islands to New Zealand have shown that blood pressure increases are greater among those who establish extensive contact with non-Tokelauans compared with individuals who maintain traditional ethnic affiliations.

Blood pressure has been shown in several studies to be associated inversely with the size of social networks and the extent of social support. A striking illustration of the protective effects of a tranquil lifestyle and supportive environment is illustrated in **Figure 2**. This shows results from a long-term study of Italian nuns in a secluded order compared with nonsmoking, age-matched women living in local communities. It can be seen that the typical age-related increases in blood pressure were attenuated among the nuns, which was coupled with a significantly lower incidence of fatal and nonfatal cardiac events.

Work and Hypertension

Some types of work might be expected to have the characteristics that would lead to acute stress-induced increases in blood pressure and sympathetic activation, thereby heightening the risk of hypertension. An important early study by Cobb and Rose of air traffic controllers demonstrated an increased incidence and earlier onset of hypertension among men working in this highly demanding occupation compared with controls. Subsequently, an automated ambulatory recording apparatus has been used to measure blood pressure repeatedly as people go about their everyday lives. Blood pressure is typically higher at work than at home, and it is elevated in people who work in

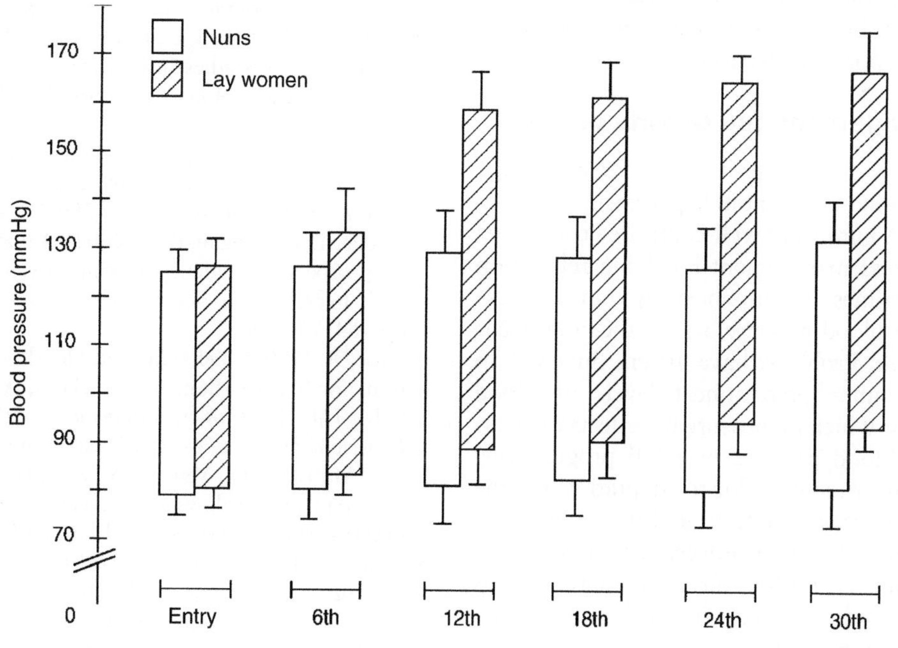

Figure 2 Results from a 30-year longitudinal study of 144 nuns from a secluded Catholic order and 138 age-matched nonsmoking women from the local community. The absence of age-related increases in blood pressure in the nuns is clear. Reproduced with permission from Timio et al. (1997). Blood pressure trend and cardiovascular events in nuns in a secluded order: a 30-year follow-up study. *Blood Pressure* **6**, 81–87. © Scandinavian University Press.

high-demand, low-control jobs. For instance, in the Work Site Blood Pressure Study in New York City, job strain (high demand, low control) was an independent predictor of hypertension after controlling for age, body mass index, type A behavior, 24-h sodium excretion, physical activity at work, education, smoking, and alcohol consumption. Longitudinally, individuals exposed to more years of high job strain had higher blood pressure. This is consistent with the evidence that lack of control over challenging situations is associated with heightened physiological activation.

White-Coat Hypertension

White-coat hypertension is the phenomenon of transiently raised blood pressure during measurement in the clinic by a physician or nurse compared with blood pressure as recorded at home or using an ambulatory recording apparatus. The definition of white-coat hypertension is somewhat arbitrary, but one study found that 20% of patients referred with a diagnosis of hypertension, whose diastolic pressure remained in the range of 90–104 mmHg on several occasions in the clinic, were normotensive during ambulatory monitoring. The phenomenon is clearly stress-related, in that it is dependent on physiological responses to the threatening clinical situation. People who exhibit white-coat effects do not have unusual psychological profiles, but do show heightened blood pressure responses to stressful behavioral tasks. There is also limited evidence that white-coat hypertension is associated with the secondary effects of hypertension such as left ventricular hypertrophy. However, the boundaries and the significance of the problem remain poorly understood.

Stress Management and Quality of Life

Despite research over the past quarter of a century, the use of stress management in hypertension remains controversial. A number of well-controlled trials have shown that stress management involving relaxation training (sometimes accompanied by biofeedback) can reduce the blood pressure and medication needs of hypertensives. Problems have arisen, however, in establishing genuine pretreatment levels of blood pressure against which to measure the effects of stress management. Blood pressure may fall progressively with repeated measurement due to adaptation and the habituation of white-coat effects, and these phenomena may be confused with the effects of stress management. The evidence for specific techniques such as transcendental meditation reducing the blood pressure of hypertensives is inconclusive.

The pharmacological treatment of hypertension is a complex and continuously developing field. Older treatments, such as β-adrenergic blockade and diuretics, have been joined by calcium antagonists and angiotensin-converting enzyme inhibitors. Some hypertensive medications have side effects that lead to impairments in the health-related quality of life. Stress management may play a role in particular types of cases. One is the individual whose blood pressure is only mildly elevated (e.g., 170/100 mmHg), who might be able to reduce blood pressure without recourse to lifetime medication. The second is the established hypertensive who is already medicated but who wishes to try alternative methods to reduce drug intake or because their blood pressure is poorly controlled. Other behavior changes also benefit hypertensives, including weight loss, increased physical exercise, and restriction of salt and alcohol intake. Stress management should therefore be applied in the context of these other aspects of behavior modification.

Further Reading

Chobanian, A. V., Bakris, G. L., Black, H. R., et al. (2003). The seventh report of the Joint National Committee on Prevention, Detection, Evaluation, and Treatment of High Blood Pressure: the JNC 7 report. *Journal of the American Medical Association* **289**, 2560–2572.

Eisenberg, D. M., Delbanco, T. L., Berkey, C. S., et al. (1993). Cognitive behavioral techniques for hypertension: are they effective? *Annals of Internal Medicine* **118**, 964–972.

Henry, J. P. and Stephens, P. M. (1977). *Stress, health, and the social environment.* New York: Springer-Verlag.

Muldoon, M. F., Terrell, D. F., Bunker, C. H., et al. (1993). Family history studies in hypertension research: review of the literature. *American Journal of Hypertension* **6**, 76–88.

Pickering, T. G., James, G. D., Boddie, C., et al. (1988). How common is white coat hypertension? *Journal of the American Medical Association* **259**, 225–228.

Rutledge, T. and Hogan, B. E. (2002). A quantitative review of prospective evidence linking psychological factors with hypertension development. *Psychosomatic Medicine* **64**, 758–766.

Steptoe, A. (1997). Behavior and blood pressure: implications for hypertension. In: Zanchetti, A. & Mancia, G. (eds.) *Handbook of hypertension – pathophysiology of hypertension*, pp. 674–708. Amsterdam: Elsevier Science.

Timio, M., Lippi, G., Venanzi, S., et al. (1997). Blood pressure trend and cardiovascular events in nuns in a secluded order: a 30-year follow-up study. *Blood Pressure* **6**, 81–87.

Waldstein, S. R. and Elias, M. F. (2001). *Neuropsychology of cardiovascular disease.* Mahwah, NJ: Lawrence Erlbaum.

Williams, D. R., Neighbors, H. W. and Jackson, J. S. (2003). Racial/ethnic discrimination and health: findings from community studies. *American Journal of Public Health* **93**, 200–208.

C-Reactive Protein

W J Kop and A A Weinstein
Uniformed Services University of the Health Sciences, Bethesda, MD, USA

Glossary

Acute coronary syndrome — A general term indicating a group of clinical symptoms compatible with acute myocardial ischemia, including myocardial infarction and unstable angina pectoris.

Acute-phase response — Complex series of biological reactions in response to infection, physical trauma, malignancy, or other physical challenges, involving blood clotting and inflammatory parameters. The acute-phase response can be initiated short-term (within min) and may last several days.

Antibody — Protein produced by the immune system that recognizes and helps fight infections and other foreign substances in the body.

Atherosclerotic plaque — Atherosclerosis is the hardening (loss of elasticity) and narrowing of medium or large arteries. The plaque is also called an atheroma, which involves the abnormal inflammation-dependent accumulation of white blood cells, lipids, and other cells within the arterial walls.

C-reactive protein (CRP) — A marker of inflammation and the acute-phase response that can be measured in blood samples.

Cytokine — A wide range of small proteins released by cells that have specific effects on cell interactions and cell function. Cytokines include the interleukins (ILs; e.g., IL-6), lymphokines, and cell signal molecules (e.g., tumor necrosis factor and interferons). Cytokines may stimulate (pro-inflammatory) or inhibit (anti-inflammatory, e.g., IL-4) the inflammation response. Cytokines that are bound to antibodies have a stronger effect on the immune system than unbound cytokines.

Lymphocyte — One of the white blood cell types involved in the immune response. The two major types of lymphocytes are T cells and B cells.

Monocyte — One of the white blood cell types that ingests microorganisms, other cells, or foreign substances. When a monocyte enters tissue, it develops into a macrophage (which surrounds, kills, and removes microorganisms).

Myocardial ischemia — Insufficient blood flow to part of the heart muscle, reflecting an imbalance between blood supply and cardiac demand.

Pathogen — An organism that causes disease in another organism, such as viruses and bacteria.

Phagocytosis — The process of ingesting and destroying microorganisms or other foreign substances by phagocytes. Phagocytes are cells that can ingest and destroy these foreign substances.

Vital exhaustion — A state characterized by unusual fatigue and loss of energy, increased irritability, and feelings of demoralization. Often precedes cardiac events. In the original conceptualization of the exhaustion construct, the term vital was included to reflect the far-reaching consequences of this condition on daily life function (similar to vital depression). We will refer to this construct as "exhaustion" in the remainder of this chapter.

C-Reactive Protein: Function and Measurement

C-reactive protein (CRP) is a member of the pentraxin protein family (molecular weight 120 kD) and a well-established inflammation marker. In the early 1930s, Tillett and Francis discovered CRP in the serum of patients with acute inflammation as a protein that reacted with the C polysaccharide of pneumococcus. Subsequent research has indicated that elevated CRP is a characteristic indicator of the acute-phase response in inflammatory disorders. The acute-phase response involves a shift in the plasma proteins released by the liver (including a decrease in albumin and an increase in CRP). The three acute-phase reactants that have been most extensively investigated are CRP, fibrinogen, and serum amyloid A (SAA), and these acute-phase proteins are well-documented inflammatory markers and mediators of atherosclerosis.

CRP is released from hepatocytes and its release is primarily stimulated by the cytokine interleukin (IL)-6. CRP mimics the function of an antibody, and is capable of complement activation. More specifically, CRP interacts with phagocytic cells at an injury site, binding to the phosphorylcholine of cell-wall polysaccharides from a wide range of bacteria and fungi. When CRP binds to a bacterium, the pathogen will become vulnerable for phagocytosis, and the immunological complement cascade will be activated. Unlike antibodies, CRP and other acute-phase reactants have no structural diversity and are not specifically released or targeted. In addition to the usual hepatic storage and release, CRP can also be stored in the hepatic endoplasmic reticulum, and this storage diminishes during inflammation thus leading to more efficient CRP secretion. CRP may also be released from other sources, including atherosclerotic plaques, vascular tissue, lymphocytes, and monocytes. CRP is a primary marker of the acute-phase reaction because of its rapid (24–28 h) and marked response to a wide variety of inflammatory conditions. Thus, CRP is part of the innate (nonadaptive) host response to infection and other pathogens.

CRP can be measured by a variety of methods including radioimmunoassay, immunonephelometry, immunoturbidimetry, immunoluminometry, and enzyme-linked immunosorbant assay (ELISA). Methods that enable precise measurements at low CRP concentrations have been defined as high sensitivity (hs) CRP assays. High sensitivity CRP is necessary to enable assessments in apparently healthy individuals using a lower limit of approximately 0.3 mg l^{-1}, with an assay imprecision of less than 10% at a CRP concentration of less than 1.0 mg l^{-1}. Based on the biological variability of CRP, the proposed allowable analytical error has been proposed to lie between 15% and 32%. Additional standardization is still necessary for some of the available assays, but a few well-established commercial hsCRP assays are available. CRP has a long half-life (approximately 19 h), and levels are relatively stable over time, with a 5-year correlation of approximately 0.4.

Diseases with a clinically significant inflammatory component are commonly associated with CRP levels exceeding 10 mg l^{-1}. However, the elevated CRP-related risk for cardiovascular disease is documented to occur at levels between 3.0 mg l^{-1} and 10.0 mg l^{-1}. Such low-grade elevations occur in approximately one-third of the adult population, primarily in the following settings: (1) diseases with tissue dysfunction or minor damage that are not primarily inflammatory (e.g., hypertension and atrial fibrillation); (2) conditions related to metabolic or hypothalamic pituitary dysregulation (e.g., obesity, insulin resistance, sleep apnea, exhaustion, and depression); and (3) adverse health behaviors (cigarette smoking, low physical activity, and high-fat diet).

Twin studies suggest a substantial genetic component (monozygotic concordance for CRP = 0.40). Multiple genetic polymorphisms for elevated CRP levels have been documented, but none are associated with an altered CRP amino acid sequence. A wide range of relatively minor environmental challenges (e.g., secondary smoke inhalation, pollutants, and estrogen-containing substances) and inflammatory stimuli related to minor injuries (e.g., dental problems and minor respiratory infection) are known to elicit low-grade CRP responses. Depending on the nature of the research question and study sample, these background factors need to be taken into account by statistical methods or research design.

Relationship between C-Reactive Protein and Cardiovascular Disease

Epidemiological studies have demonstrated that CRP and other acute-phase reactants predict incident and recurrent cardiovascular events. Based on population studies, clinical cut-off points for CRP have been set as: low (<1 mg l^{-1}), moderate (1–3 mg l^{-1}), and high (>3 mg l^{-1}). CRP levels of more than 10 mg l^{-1} should lead to referral for noncardiac diagnosis because of the high likelihood of an active inflammatory disorder. Three processes are important to consider in the relationship between CRP and cardiovascular disease: (1) the role of inflammation in the onset and gradual progression of atherosclerosis; (2) immune system involvement in acute atherosclerotic plaque rupture; and (3) secondary increases in inflammatory parameters following transient myocardial ischemia and/or myocardial infarction, or damage to the vasculature.

CRP may reflect early stages of atherosclerosis characterized by cell adhesion and engulfment of lipids and T cells. CRP may promote these gradual immune system-related processes. Elevated CRP levels have long-term predictive value for adverse cardiovascular outcomes, although some evidence suggests that the predictive value is most pronounced in the first 2 years of follow-up. The predictive value of CRP is statistically independent of other inflammatory predictors of cardiovascular disease (IL-6 and tumor necrosis factor (TNF)-α), and standard cardiovascular risk factors such as cholesterol.

In advanced coronary atherosclerosis, CRP may also promote transient increases in the risk of plaque rupture by promoting plaque instability and activation. Plaque rupture is associated with activation of the blood clotting process, which is linked to inflammatory parameters. The resulting sudden obstruction of coronary blood flow may lead to sustained myocardial ischemia and infarction.

In addition to promoting gradual atherosclerosis and plaque instability, elevated CRP levels may also reflect secondary inflammatory responses in patients with cardiovascular disease. Myocardial tissue damage or transient ischemia, infection, and mechanical cell injury are all known to activate numerous biological pathways, including the cytokine and coagulation systems. CRP levels tend to peak at 48–54 h postmyocardial infarction, and the increase is proportional to the magnitude of myocardial damage as documented by troponin levels.

Recent meta-analyses have confirmed the significant association between CRP and adverse cardiovascular risk, although the magnitude of risk is lower (odds ratio 1.58, 95% confidence interval 1.48 to 1.68) than originally reported. In addition, recent Mendelian randomization studies indicate that although genetic polymorphisms give rise to elevated CRP levels, these genetic factors are not associated with increased cardiovascular risk. These findings suggest that CRP may be a marker of the underlying atherosclerotic process and/or a measure that partly reflects other risk indicators. Additional studies are needed to further establish the epidemiological and experimental evidence for the role of CRP and other inflammatory markers in adverse cardiovascular disease progression. At present, CRP is not used to directly guide clinical practice in cardiovascular medicine.

Stress-Related Psychosocial Cardiovascular Risk Factors and C-Reactive Protein

Because of the well-documented predictive value of CRP for adverse cardiovascular health outcomes, we will primarily focus on stress-related psychological factors that are known to be associated with atherosclerotic disease progression. Chronic and acute psychological factors are associated with increased risk of coronary artery disease and its clinical manifestations as acute coronary syndromes, including myocardial infarction. These psychological constructs are characterized by increased levels of perceived stress and/or exposure to potentially stressful environmental challenges. The pathophysiological mechanisms accounting for the relationship between psychological factors and coronary disease progression are likely to involve inflammatory processes. This section selectively reviews the interplay between psychological factors and CRP. A detailed review on the psychoneuroimmunological processes in cardiovascular disease has been presented by Kop and Cohen (2007: 921–943).

Prior investigations have shown that psychological risk factors for coronary disease can be classified into three broad categories, based on their duration and temporal proximity to coronary syndromes: (1) chronic factors, such as negative personality traits (e.g., hostility) and low socioeconomic status (SES); (2) episodic factors with a duration of several months up to 2 years, among which are depression and exhaustion; and (3) acute factors, including mental stress and outbursts of anger. Accumulating evidence indicates that the stage of coronary disease is a major determinant of the inflammatory mechanisms involved in coronary disease progression and acute coronary syndromes.

Chronic Psychosocial Risk Factors and C-Reactive Protein

The chronic psychological factors discussed here are low SES and hostility, because of their well-documented relationship with coronary disease and the emerging evidence that these measures are also related to CRP. Both factors are associated with elevated levels of distress as a result of the purported increased exposure to challenging environmental circumstances and reduced resources to cope with such challenges.

SES can be defined based on a combination of education, income, job status, as well as other dimensions. Low SES is associated with elevated levels of CRP. For example, Owen et al. (2003: 286–295) documented elevated CRP levels among lower versus higher SES participants (1.18 ± 0.75 versus 0.75 ± 0.8 mg l^{-1}, $p = 0.002$) independent of sex, age, body mass, waist-to-hip ratio, smoking status, alcohol consumption, and season of the year. This finding has been replicated in larger epidemiological studies. The main potentially confounding factor in the association between SES and CRP is overweight. Nonetheless, most studies support a relationship between SES and CRP, even when statistically adjusting for body mass and other potentially confounding factors. However, because low SES is associated with a wide range of health behaviors, environmental exposures to pollutants and infectious agents, and psychological contextual factors, further studies are needed to clarify the role of SES in inflammatory factors such as CRP.

Hostility is a psychological trait characterized by a mixture of anger and disgust, and is associated with emotions such as resentment, indignation, and contempt. Hostility is predictive of long-term cardiovascular events, and this personality trait has been described as the toxic component of the type A behavior pattern. Research suggests modest (r values between 0.2 and 0.4) correlations between hostility and CRP levels. Measures of aggressive behavior are stronger predictors of CRP than general hostile attitudes. The mechanisms by which trait hostility, and particularly aggression, result in elevated inflammatory factors may involve stress-activated neurohormonal and autonomic nervous system pathways. Noradrenergic stimulation may increase gene expression for various inflammatory cytokines including IL-6, which may result in CRP release. Frequent responses to aversive interpersonal interactions may result in heightened noradrenergic drive in hostile individuals and thus result in increased production of pro-inflammatory cytokines and CRP.

Episodic Factors and C-Reactive Protein: Exhaustion and Depression

Prolonged emotional challenges may result in general distress, exhaustion, and depression. These stress-related conditions wax and wane with the intensity of the environmental challenges and the success of an individual's coping strategies. The predictive value of these conditions for cardiovascular events is strongest in the first 2 years after assessment. Because of the transient nature of these conditions and their stronger predictive value for adverse events within 2 years following assessment, these factors are referred to as episodic psychological risk factors.

Episodes of prolonged distress have been associated with markers of immunosuppression. The psychoneuroimmunology literature generally categorizes the immunosuppressive correlates of distress-related conditions along with the long-term immunological consequences of depressive disorders and other conditions characterized by negative affect (e.g., bereavement, separation, and daily hassles). Based on the Cardiovascular Health Study, our group has documented significantly elevated CRP levels among exhausted men (6.82 ± 2.10 mg l^{-1}) versus nonexhausted men (3.05 ± 0.16 mg l^{-1}; $p = 0.007$) aged over 65 years. The association for women was less strong, but still statistically significant when adjusting for co-variates including age, gender, race, diabetes mellitus, smoking status, and systolic blood pressure. Elevated CRP levels in depression, exhaustion, and other markers of prolonged distress have been consistently reported in the literature, with only a few exceptions (3/30 reviewed articles).

The mechanisms accounting for the associations between exhaustion and depression with CRP include biological pathways involving the central and autonomic nervous systems, and adverse health behaviors (e.g., overweight status and smoking). Prolonged distress commonly results in norepinephrine released from the locus coeruleus as well as hypothalamic corticotropin-releasing hormone (CRH), which are the main effectors of what Selye has described as the general adaptation response. The most common finding in depression, especially melancholia, involves activation of the CRH system and hence elevated cortisol levels. The clinical nature of depression (i.e., melancholic depression versus atypical depression and exhaustion) may influence the association between depressive symptoms and immune system parameters. CRH is elevated in typical depression, and acts as the main regulatory hormone in the acute-stress response, resulting in the release of pro-inflammatory cytokines, as well as a wide range of other immune system responses. These effects may be less strong or even reversed in atypical depression and exhaustion.

The autonomic nervous system also plays an important role in the acute-phase reaction, and parasympathetic outflow inhibits macrophage activation via the cholinergic anti-inflammatory pathway. Exhaustion and depression are associated with decreased parasympathetic nervous system activity, which may thus contribute to elevations in pro-inflammatory cytokines and elevated CRP.

The neuroimmunological responses to prolonged distress generally occur in the context of health behavior-mediated physical changes, particularly being overweight, affecting multiple metabolic processes. Thus, an overall imbalance of normal homeostatic function may be characteristic of episodic risk factors, resulting in prolonged CRP elevations.

Acute Psychological Factors and C-Reactive Protein

Acute psychological factors relevant to cardiovascular disease involve responses to acute mental or emotional challenges, such as outbursts of anger. These acute psychological factors can act as triggers of myocardial infarction by inducing cardiac ischemia and promoting plaque rupture and thrombus formation in advanced stages of coronary artery disease. There is increasing interest in the role of acute stress-induced inflammatory responses in relation to cardiovascular disease risk.

Some evidence suggests that acute mental challenge tasks induce elevations in CRP in individuals with inflammation-related conditions. However, in healthy individuals the results have been largely negative. One study examined CRP 45 min and 2 h postmental stress in healthy individuals, without significant CRP elevations. The optimal timing of CRP reactivity is an issue of current debate. Studies have demonstrated an immediate response in patients with cardiac problems and individuals with rheumatic arthritis (<5 min poststress).

A few methodological issues are relevant to the acute CRP response. Acute psychological distress elicits increases in arterial blood pressure and changes in blood rheology, including decreases in plasma volume and increases in blood viscosity. CRP is a relatively small molecule, but when plasma volume decreases in response to mental challenge, CRP does not readily pass into the interstitial space because of its molecular structure. Therefore, studies examining the acute CRP response need to adjust for changes in plasma volume. CRP levels at baseline are also highly correlated with levels obtained during mental stress (r values of >0.85), which results in statistical significance of very small absolute changes from baseline. Of note is that IL-6 responses tend to be unrelated to CRP responses, which suggests that mechanisms other than hepatic release may play a role in the acute CRP response. These may include endothelial cells and other tissues, and the local release could possibly be mediated by circulating neurohormones. However, acute CRP responses may not be as important when compared with other acute responses of the immune system relevant to cardiovascular disease (e.g., IL-6, shift in lymphocyte distribution towards increased CD8+ and decreased CD4+). The timing of IL-6 should theoretically precede hepatic CRP release, and current data do not support such a pathway. Storage of biologically active signals can cause an immediate physiological effect, but the translation from messenger ribonucleic acid (mRNA) to protein takes several hours. Acute increases in circulating CRP are therefore not likely to reflect production of newly synthesized protein by tissues such as vascular endothelial cells or adherent leukocytes.

Conclusion and Future Directions

CRP is a critical component of the innate immune system, providing early defense against infectious agents and other pathogens. Substantial individual differences have been observed in CRP levels in the range below clinical inflammation (i.e., CRP levels <10 mg l^{-1}). Psychological factors are associated with elevated CRP levels, and distress-related inflammatory processes may therefore partially account for the relationship between psychosocial factors and adverse cardiovascular health outcomes. Evidence for elevated CRP levels is strongest for episodic risk factors such as depression and exhaustion. These conditions reflect the consequences of prolonged psychological distress, and elevated CRP levels in these conditions have a plausible biobehavioral explanation. Evidence for chronic psychosocial factors is also consistent, with the strongest support for low SES as predictor of elevated CRP. Acute CRP responses have been documented in patients with rheumatic arthritis and coronary disease, but the acute effects are small and probably do not reflect an increase in CRP secretion but rather a redistribution of CRP.

Further studies are needed to document the relative importance of catecholamines and hypothalamic pituitary adrenal axis hormones in elevated CRP levels. These studies need to be conducted in the context of important behavioral concomitants of inflammation, particularly assessments of adipose tissue because metabolic imbalance may be a common explanatory factor. In addition, prolonged stress may lead to increased allostatic load which may further promote the cascade of distress and elevated inflammatory markers.

Many of the psychological factors mentioned above are interrelated, which partially results from the currently available measurement tools but may also reflect a general stress-related psychological factor. Such a general prolonged distress factor could account for increased levels of pro-inflammatory markers. More research is needed to identify potentially common environmental and/or genetic factors for vulnerability for stress-related psychological traits and high levels of inflammatory parameters.

Minor CRP elevations are associated with a diverse range of conditions. Current research suggests that the stimulus for CRP production involves a mild degree of tissue stress or injury, suggesting the presence of challenged cells, rather than a subsequent inflammatory response to these cellular challenges. Nonetheless, CRP has potentially pragmatic utility for cardiovascular-risk stratification, and further improvements in the assessment of inflammatory processes will contribute to a better understanding of the biopsychosocial factors involved in cardiovascular and other inflammation-related disorders.

Acknowledgments

Supported in part by a grant from the NIH (HL066149).

Further Reading

Casas, J. P., Shah, T., Cooper, J., et al. (2006). Insight into the nature of the CRP-coronary event association using Mendelian randomization. *International Journal of Epidemiology* **35**, 922–931.

Cesari, M., Penninx, B. W., Newman, A. B., et al. (2003). Inflammatory markers and onset of cardiovascular events: results from the Health ABC study. *Circulation* **108**, 2317–2322.

Danesh, J., Wheeler, J. G., Hirschfield, G. M., et al. (2004). C-reactive protein and other circulating markers of inflammation in the prediction of coronary heart disease. *New England Journal of Medicine* **350**, 1387–1397.

Kop, W. J. and Cohen, N. (2007). Psychoneuroimmunological pathways involved in acute coronary syndromes. In: Ader, R. (ed.) *Psychoneuroimmunology*, pp. 921–943. Amsterdam, Boston: Academic Press.

Kop, W. J., Gottdiener, J. S., Tangen, C. M., et al. (2002). Inflammation and coagulation factors in persons >65 years of age with symptoms of depression but without evidence of myocardial ischemia. *American Journal of Cardiology* **89**, 419–424.

Kushner, I., Rzewnicki, D. and Samols, D. (2006). What does minor elevation of C-reactive protein signify? *American Journal of Medicine* **119**, e17–28.

Miller, G. E., Freedland, K. E., Carney, R. M., et al. (2003). Pathways linking depression, adiposity, and inflammatory markers in healthy young adults. *Brain Behavior and Immunity* **17**, 276–285.

Owen, N., Poulton, T., Hay, F. C., et al. (2003). Socioeconomic status, C-reactive protein, immune factors, and responses to acute mental stress. *Brain Behavior and Immunity* **17**, 286–295.

Ridker, P. M., Rifai, N., Rose, L., et al. (2002). Comparison of C-reactive protein and low-density lipoprotein cholesterol levels in the prediction of first cardiovascular events. *New England Journal of Medicine* **347**, 1557–1565.

Roberts, W. L. (2004). CDC/AHA workshop on markers of inflammation and cardiovascular disease: application to clinical and public health practice: laboratory tests available to assess inflammation–performance and standardization: a background paper. *Circulation* **110**, e572–e576.

Rozanski, A., Blumenthal, J. A. and Kaplan, J. (1999). Impact of psychological factors on the pathogenesis of cardiovascular disease and implications for therapy. *Circulation* **99**, 2192–2217.

Segerstrom, S. C. and Miller, G. E. (2004). Psychological stress and the human immune system: a meta-analytic study of 30 years of inquiry. *Psychological Bulletin* **130**, 601–630.

Steptoe, A., Willemsen, G., Owen, N., et al. (2001). Acute mental stress elicits delayed increases in circulating inflammatory cytokine levels. *Clinical Science* **101**, 185–192.

Suarez, E. C. (2004). C-reactive protein is associated with psychological risk factors of cardiovascular disease in apparently healthy adults. *Psychosomatic Medicine* **66**, 684–691.

Cytokines, Chronic Stress, and Fatigue

S Jain and P J Mills
University of California San Diego,
San Diego, CA, USA

Glossary

Cancer-related fatigue — A persistent feeling of tiredness, weakness, or lack of energy related to cancer and/or its treatment; it is more severe than general fatigue and interferes with regular functioning and quality of life.

Chronic fatigue syndrome (CFS) — A complex syndrome of unknown etiology marked by persistent fatigue that lasts for over 6 months and interferes with daily functioning.

C-reactive protein (CRP) — An acute-phase protein that is produced by the liver during inflammation. CRP increases in response to the cytokine interleukin-6. Elevated CRP levels are currently considered the strongest prognostic indicator of increased risk for stroke as well as for myocardial infarction and death from coronary events. Recent studies indicate that elevated CRP is associated with cognitive decline.

Cytokines — A diverse group of potent, low-molecular-weight proteins and glycoproteins that mediate important physiological processes within the immune system as well as the nervous and endocrine systems. Major types of cytokines include the interleukins (ILs), tumor necrosis factors (TNF), and interferons (IFNs).

Fatigue — A persistent feeling of tiredness, weakness, or lack of energy. There are many components of fatigue, including physiological (such as flulike symptoms and anemia), psychological (including depression), cognitive (including memory and attention problems), and chronobiological (such as circadian rhythms disorders and sleep disruption).

Multiple sclerosis (MS) — An autoimmune disorder characterized by the degeneration of myelin in the central nervous system, leading to muscle weakness, cognitive disorientation, and fatigue.

Soluble cytokine receptors — Biologically active receptors that circulate in the extracellular matrix. Soluble cytokine receptors may function as antagonists (i.e., inhibiting the effects of a cytokine by binding to it and blocking it from attaching to its cell-bound receptor) or agonists (i.e., promoting the effects of a cytokine by binding to it and forming a complex that binds to a different receptor subunit that initiates signal transduction).

Vascular endothelial growth factor (VEGF) — An important cytokine that is produced by the endothelial cells. It is an angiogenic cytokine, meaning it supports the formation of new blood vessels, including those for tumors.

Vital exhaustion — A syndrome marked by persistent fatigue, often stemming from an inability to cope with one or more chronic stressors, and implicated as an independent risk factor for negative cardiovascular events.

Cytokines: Description and Classification

Description

Cytokines are potent immunotransmitters that play a pivotal role in immune system response and communication with other physiological systems, both to maintain homeostasis and to respond appropriately to infection and injury. The functions of cytokines are diverse: They assist in the development and proliferation of immune cell subsets, promotion of inflammatory as well as noninflammatory processes, and alteration of neurochemical and neuroendocrine processes that affect overall physiology and behavior. Cytokines may be thought of as similar to neurotransmitters and hormones in that they are mediators of specific physiological responses, rely on receptor–ligand interactions, and have self (autocrine), local (paracrine), and distal (endocrine) effects.

In addition to their multiple effects within the immune system, cytokines also have extensive bidirectional communication with the central nervous system (CNS) and hypothalamic-pituitary-adrenal (HPA) axis. Probably due to this communication, cytokines are correlated with a number of psychological states, including chronic stress and fatigue.

Classification

There are major families of cytokines. The interleukins (ILs) are a large class of cytokines that promote cell-to-cell interactions and the stimulation of humoral or cell-mediated immune responses. The tumor necrosis factors (TNFs) include a host of cytokines characterized by several molecules, such as TNF-α and TNF-β and soluble TNF receptor-I (sTNFRI) and TNF receptor-II (sTNFRII). The activation of the TNF family promotes a variety of cell functions related to inflammation as well as immune organ development and maintenance, including cell proliferation and adhesion, cell differentiation, apoptosis, and cell survival. The interferons (IFNs) play an important role immunosurveillance, antiviral, and antitumor effects. IFN-α and IFN-β inhibit virus replication in infected cells, and IFN-γ stimulates major histocompatability complex (MHC) presentation on antigen-presenting cells, aiding in the recognition and lysing of foreign cells. In addition, INFs initiate cascades of cytokine responses, which result in a further immune activation.

Soluble receptors of cytokines are formed either by the cleavage of portions of transmembrane protein complexes, thereby becoming part of the extracellular matrix, or by translation from alternatively spliced mRNAs. They can serve as both antagonists or agonists. Examples of soluble cytokine antagonists include IL-1 receptor antagonist (IL-1Ra) and TNFRI receptor antagonist. Examples of soluble cytokine agonists include IL-6 receptor (IL-6R). In certain situations, some cytokine receptors may function as agonists or antagonists, depending on their isoforms (e.g., TNFRII).

Because of their notable variability in structure and function, there have been many attempts to classify cytokines. A classification system that has proven useful for stress and behavioral medicine researchers is the classification of cytokines as either pro-inflammatory or anti-inflammatory. Pro-inflammatory cytokines, which include IL-1, IL-2, IL-6, TNF-α, and IFN-γ, promote a variety of cell functions that stimulate and enhance inflammation through various methods, including promoting the differentiation of cytotoxic T cells, enhancing increased vascular permeability and cellular adhesion and migration to tissues, and stimulating the release of acute-phase proteins from the liver. These inflammatory immune responses are often described as T-helper-1 (Th1) responses, referring to the T-helper cell subset that generally produces cytokines that initiate inflammatory processes.

Anti-inflammatory cytokines, which include IL-3, IL-4, IL-5, IL-10, and IL-13, are sometimes described as immunosuppressors due to their ability to inhibit the Th1-mediated inflammatory response (often via direct antagonism of Th1-secreted inflammatory cytokines). However, these cytokines themselves promote certain increases in immune response, most notably increased overall production of antibodies and increased eosinophil and mast cell production. Often called the T-helper-2 (Th2) response, these cascades of cytokine-induced immune activation support allergic reactions. It is important to note that some cytokines support both pro- and anti-inflammatory effects depending on the situation (e.g., IL-6 and IL-8), thus rendering the nomenclature of cytokines as either pro-inflammatory or anti-inflammatory less that perfect. IL-6 is also classified as a myokine because it is produced by contracting skeletal muscle and plays an important role in the anti-inflammatory effects of acute exercise.

Cytokines: Central Nervous System and Endocrine Interactions

Cytokines and the Central Nervous System

It is well understood that cytokines are secreted by certain classes of brain cells, including microglial cells and astrocytes. The endogenous expression of cytokines and their receptors have been found in the hypothalamus, basal ganglia, cerebellum, circumventricular sites, and brain-stem nuclei. Included in the considerably large list of brain-active cytokines are IFN-α and IFN-γ; TNF-α and TNF-β; and IL-1, -2, -3, -4, -5, -6, -8, -10, and -12. Studies involving the systematic administration of cytokines in some of the brain regions previously mentioned indicate that cytokines promote the release of neurotransmitters, including norepinephrine, dopamine, and serotonin. Thus, in addition to their immunoprotective effects (such as the regulation of infiltrating leukocytes during times of infection) within the brain, cytokines may promote neurochemical cascades that directly affect mood and behavior. In addition, elevated pro-inflammatory cytokines may also be associated with neurodegenerative disorders; for example, increased IL-6, TNF-α, and IL-1β have been found in patients with Parkinson's disease.

Cytokines also affect the CNS via peripheral mechanisms. Although cytokines are too large to effectively cross the blood–brain barrier, there are several posited indirect mechanisms of action. One hypothesis is that cytokines enter the brain via passive transport in areas where the blood–brain barrier is not present (e.g., circumventricular sites). Another is that cytokines might bind to cerebral vascular endothelium, facilitating the release of active second messengers such as nitric oxide. Yet another hypothesis is that cytokines might be transported across the blood–brain-barrier via carrier-mediated transport. Finally, it has been posited that cytokines might affect the CNS indirectly via the stimulation of peripheral afferent nerve terminals, via the vagus.

Cytokines and the Hypothalamic-Pituitary-Adrenal Axis

The HPA is part of the neuroendocrine system that is responsible for the cortical as well as adrenal release of hormones in response to stress. Considerable progress has been made in understanding the complex interactions between cytokines and the HPA. Briefly, it is now well understood that complex and dynamic interactive communication exists between cytokines and the HPA and that the regulation of cytokine release, as well as HPA responses to immune insults, are governed in part by positive and negative feedback loops between the two systems. In particular, pro-inflammatory cytokines have been shown to stimulate HPA stress responses, whereas Th2 cytokines can inhibit this activation. For example, pro-inflammatory cytokines appear to activate corticotropin releasing hormone (CRH) and arginine vasopressin neurons in the parvocellular paraventricular nucleus within the hypothalamus. This activation results in a downstream HPA cascade in which CRH is released from the hypothalamus, promoting the release of adrenocorticotropic hormone (ACTH) from the anterior pituitary gland and resulting in release of the glucocorticoids corticosterone and cortisol from the adrenal cortex. There are several postulated mechanisms of action for how this cascade is initiated by pro-inflammatory cytokines, some of which involve mediating effects of cytokines on the HPA via afferent vagal fiber activity.

In addition to their effects on the anterior pituitary and adrenal cortex via CRH release from the hypothalamus, pro-inflammatory cytokines may also affect the anterior pituitary and adrenal cortex directly, resulting in similar end-organ effects (release of corticosterone from the adrenal cortex). For example, IL-6 is synthesized and released within the human adrenal gland itself, promoting glucocorticoid release. The multitude of sites of action allows pro-inflammatory cytokines several pathways of promoting a similar end-organ response so that even if higher-level actions of cytokines on hypothalamic or anterior pituitary structures are inhibited (e.g., via antagonism by a Th2 cytokine such as IL-10), some level of glucocorticoid release into the circulation is preserved. In turn, glucocorticoid actions on cytokines help to maintain homeostasis via negative feedback loops. For example, cortisol inhibits cellular synthesis and release of pro-inflammatory cytokines, thus acting to preserve homeostasis in the system. However, the effects of glucocorticoids on maintaining this homeostasis are dampened in cases of chronic stress, possibly due to the ability of the pro-inflammatory cytokines to promote receptor desensitization, downregulation, or prevalence of negative isoforms of the glucocorticoid receptor, causing decreased glucocorticoid sensitivity or glucocorticoid resistance. Thus, cytokines are intimately intertwined with HPA responses, providing a potent influence on stress responses and appearing to play a very active role in HPA modulations during chronic stress and fatigue.

Cytokine Measurement

When we examine cytokines in biological fluids, there are two broad categories for methods of measurement. Immunoassays measure the prevalence of cytokines or their soluble receptors by using either radioisotope-tagged antibodies (i.e., radioimmunoassays, RIAs), or enzyme-linked antibodies (i.e., enzyme-linked immunosorbant assays, ELISAs) that are specific for certain peptides that are part of the cytokine structure. The strengths of immunoassays in general are their ease of use and relatively low cost, combined with a relatively high specificity due to the use of monoclonal antibodies. However, these methods are not immune to methodological problems, and they do not provide information on functionality of the cytokine. Bioassays measure cytokine functionality as indexed by specific biological responses such as chemotaxis (movement through a chemical diffusion gradient), proliferation (increase in numbers of the particular cell line), cytotoxicity (ability of cells to kill pathogens), expression of cell surface molecules, or subsequent release of specific proteins. Bioassays thus give the researcher information not simply about soluble cytokine levels, but also about some aspect of their functionality. Although they are very sensitive tests, they are generally less specific, less reliable, and more time-consuming than immunoassays.

Other, newer methods also exist for examining whole cells' capacities to produce and release cytokines. Two such notable methods are flow cytometry and enzyme-linked immunospot (ELISPOT), which measure the abilities of single cells to produce or release cytokines, respectively. Most studies discussed in this article relied on ELISA methods for measuring basal (resting) levels of circulating cytokines in peripheral blood, although some studies examined cytokines after stimulating immune cells with a mitogen known to enhance cytokine release (e.g., lipopolysaccharide, LPS).

Cytokines and Chronic Stress

A few studies have examined the effects of chronic stressors on cytokines in humans. Most studies have been conducted with Alzheimer caregivers and the diagnosis of vital exhaustion. Interestingly, chronic stress appears to be associated with immunosuppresion in Alzheimer caregivers but associated with pro-inflammatory activity in vital exhaustion.

Chronic Stress Studies with Alzheimer's Disease Caregivers

An early study examining chronic stress and wound healing in Alzheimer caregivers compared to matched controls showed a decrease in IL-1 mRNA secretion in response to LPS stimulation of peripheral blood leukocytes in Alzheimer's caregivers. Significantly, this may have contributed to slower wound healing in this group. Another study reported lower IL-1β and IL-2 responses to virus-specific stimulation for Alzheimer caregivers than for controls. Alzheimer caregivers have also shown increased intracellular IL-10 (but no change in INF-γ or IL-2) levels in T-helper and T-cytotoxic cells compared to controls, with the difference between these groups being significantly greater for younger subjects. A recent longitudinal study, in which IL-6 levels for Alzheimer's caregivers and controls were tracked over 6 years, showed an almost fourfold rate of increase of IL-6 levels in Alzheimer's caregivers compared to matched controls. This result was consistent even for caregivers whose spouses had died during the 6-year period. Another study examining IL-6 associations with aging and chronic stress in women indicated that Alzheimer's caregivers showed significantly higher levels of IL-6 compared to age-matched women who were experiencing moderate forms of stress (i.e., moving), as well as compared to older and younger control subjects. These findings suggest that chronic stress associated with Alzheimer's caregiving in the elderly promotes increases in Th2 cytokines and the inhibition of Th1 cytokines. The findings also suggest pathways by which caregiving in the elderly leads to significantly increased risk for deleterious health outcomes even well after the death of the spouse being cared for.

Chronic Stress Studies with Vital Exhaustion

Vital exhaustion has been implicated as an independent risk factor for negative cardiovascular events, such as first stroke and myocardial infarction. Vital exhaustion in women has been linked to elevated circulating TNF-α levels. A study comparing vitally exhausted middle-age males with controls indicated that vital exhaustion was associated with increased levels of IL-6, IL-1Ra, and IL-10 levels, as well as increased procoagulant activity. Similarly, a recent study examining vital versus nonvital exhaustion in male industrial workers showed decreased glucocorticoid sensitivity for highly exhausted men, both by dexamethasone inhibition of LPS-stimulated IL-6 release and by the median inhibitory concentration (IC_{50}; a measure of glucocorticoid sensitivity that is independent of absolute cytokine release). In addition, vitally exhausted workers showed significantly increased resting levels of CRP. Together, the findings suggest that chronic stress-related fatigue in otherwise healthy women and men may be associated with a shift toward a pro-inflammatory profile. These findings are important because they point to some of the linkages between stress-related fatigue in vital exhaustion and the risk of coronary events. Longitudinal studies in this area are needed to elucidate the direction of relationship between elevations in pro-inflammatory cytokines and vital exhaustion.

Cytokines and Fatigue in Clinical Disorders

As already indicated, cytokines have been shown to be associated with fatigue in otherwise healthy individuals. However, alterations in cytokines have also been examined in the context of several clinical disorders marked by persistent fatigue, such as cancer, chronic fatigue syndrome, and multiple sclerosis.

Cytokines and Fatigue in Cancer

Fatigue is one of the most frequent complaints of cancer patients, with studies showing 40–75% of patients reporting feeling tired and weak, and with rates up to 95% during chemotherapy and/or radiotherapy treatment. Much of the fatigue that cancer patients experience is probably attributable to cytokines that are elevated either by the cellular damage from the cancer itself or by its treatment. Although high levels of certain endogenous cytokines (e.g., TNF-α) are associated with tumor genesis and growth, paradoxically, the exogenous administration of pro-inflammatory cytokines attenuate cancer growth and thus are often used in cancer treatment. This exogenous administration of cytokines for the treatment of cancer often elicits sickness behavior, a syndrome characterized by flulike symptoms including fatigue and depression. In addition, treatments such as chemotherapy and radiation therapy are associated with elevations in pro-inflammatory cytokines (such as IL-1Ra, IL-6, and TNF-α), which, in turn, are associated with elevations in fatigue. We have shown that circulating levels of VEGF are elevated in response to chemotherapy for breast cancer and that these elevated levels are associated with the significantly increased feelings of fatigue and poorer quality of life that result from chemotherapy. Elevations in cytokines may also persist along with fatigue well after treatment. For example, significantly higher serum levels of IL-1Ra and sTNFRII have been found among breast cancer survivors who report a high level of fatigue compared to low-fatigue breast cancer patients, independent of depression.

In addition, sleep loss, a common correlate of fatigue, is associated with elevations in pro-inflammatory cytokines. For example, pro-inflammatory cytokines such as IL-6 and TNF-α are fatigue-inducing cytokines that are elevated during the day in disorders of excessive daytime sleepiness and in healthy subjects following sleep deprivation. Thus, evidence for the interaction between cytokines and cancer-related fatigue suggests that higher levels of endogenous or exogenous pro-inflammatory cytokines predict higher fatigue. However, higher levels of fatigue pretreatment may predict poorer outcomes related to treatment as well. For example, our group has found that breast cancer patients with high fatigue prior to chemotherapy experience poorer sleep in response to chemotherapy (both subjectively and objectively) compared to those with lower fatigue prior to chemotherapy. Whether these alterations in sleep patterns for high-fatigue patients are associated with alterations in cytokine responses to chemotherapy remains to be elucidated.

Cytokines and Fatigue in Multiple Sclerosis

The immune profile of multiple sclerosis (MS) appears to be characterized by self-reactive T cells, as well as an relative elevation in pro-inflammatory or Th1 cytokines such as IL-2, TNF-α, and IFN-γ compared to anti-inflammatory cytokines such as IL-4 and IL-10. Fatigue is a common complaint in MS, with over one-third of patients reporting significant fatigue. Although the specific etiology of fatigue in these patients remains to be completely understood, a few studies have reported significant associations with fatigue and IL-1 and TNF-α in MS patients. One study has also reported positive associations with CRP and fatigue in MS patients. Several studies have also related fatigue to HPA axis dysregulation. Most studies have reported HPA axis hyperactivity in MS, with a handful of studies reporting significant associations with HPA axis hyperactivity and fatigue. Many researchers in this field suggest that a potential mechanism of fatigue in MS patients stems from elevations in pro-inflammatory cytokines (such as IL-1 and IL-6), which impair in glucocorticoid receptor signaling, driving HPA axis hyperreactivity, which leads to feelings of fatigue. However, this theory remains to be tested.

Cytokines and Fatigue in Chronic Fatigue Syndrome

The immune profile in CFS is complex and mechanisms that are linked to the particular experience of fatigue in these patients are yet to be understood. Common symptoms in CFS include decreased natural killer (NK) cell cytotoxic activity and lymphocyte proliferation, and increased allergic and autoimmune activities. Such a profile is consistent with a relative elevation in Th2 versus Th1 cellular activity; however, findings in the literature cannot yet confirm this contention. For example, findings on basal cytokine levels have been mixed; whereas several studies report elevations in IL-1α and IL-1β for CFS patients versus controls, a similar number of studies have reported no differences. Similar equivocal results have been reported for levels in TNF-α, TNF-β, IL-6, and IL-2 for CFS patients versus controls, and findings on HPA dysregulation are also mixed. Heterogeneity in findings is probably due to study differences in methodology as well as the ranges of patient symptoms and comorbidities studied.

With respect to fatigue ratings and cytokines in CFS, very little work has systematically looked at the relations between fatigue ratings and circulating cytokine levels. However, a recent study reports significant associations with fatigue ratings and LPS-stimulated levels of TNF-α and IL-6 compared to control subjects, who showed significant associations with fatigue and stimulated levels of IL-6 but not of TNF-α.

Cytokines and Fatigue in Clinical Disorders: Summary

Studies examining the relation of cytokines and fatigue in clinical populations are burgeoning, with more studies needed to confirm the preliminary results. However, a common thread in studies with cancer, MS, and CFS appears to be a consistent association with pro-inflammatory cytokines with reports of fatigue in these patients. However, the immunological profile in each of these disorders is quite complex, and future studies will need to be more specific in their assessment of disease stage/severity as well as other potential covariates (including depression) before these preliminary results can be confirmed.

In addition, given the preliminary findings on HPA dysregulation and fatigue, as well as the close interaction of cytokines with the HPA axis, future studies should examine in detail the interactions with potential elevations in pro-inflammatory cytokines and glucocorticoid sensitivity. The use of structural equation modeling methods combined with a careful assessment of data should shed light on proposed theories of cytokine-induced dysregulation of HPA axis activity and its relation to fatigue.

Chronic Stress, Fatigue, and Cytokines: Relevance for Disease Processes

There is a possibility that the chronic prevalence of fatigue in otherwise healthy individuals may also increase their risk for cardiovascular disorders via a cytokine-mediated response. We already mentioned that vital exhaustion is characterized by a generalized increased inflammatory profile. Not surprisingly, individuals who experience vital exhaustion also report a general lack of energy and some symptoms of depression, such as hopelessness. A relatively recent large-scale study indicated that vital exhaustion was independently associated with a twofold risk of mortality from coronary heart disease in older men. In addition, a recent study reports that vital exhaustion is a significant independent risk indicator for first stroke in middle-age men and women, implying that this state of persistent and excessive fatigue (and its negative effects) is not necessarily a consequence of existing cardiovascular disorders. Given that elevations in IL-6 as well CRP are associated with greater risk of peripheral vascular disease, myocardial infarction, and stroke and that elevations in these inflammatory markers are found in patients with vital exhaustion, it is not unreasonable to suspect that chronic elevations in inflammation associated with vital exhaustion lead over time to an increased risk for deleterious cardiovascular events. Longitudinal studies with younger, chronically stressed men and women will help to elucidate the potential effects of persistent stress and fatigue on glucocorticoid resistance, cytokine balance, and subsequent immune response over time.

Obviously, alterations in cytokines that are associated with chronic stress and fatigue affect more than cardiovascular disease progression. Increases in pro-inflammatory cytokines associated with chronic stress and fatigue may directly exacerbate disease progression for disorders such as rheumatoid arthritis, MS, and diabetes, which are already characterized by increased pro-inflammatory activity. What remains uncertain is whether persistent fatigue in clinical populations may affect tolerance for other therapies. For example, it will be important to better understand whether patients with higher fatigue (and higher inflammation) respond more poorly to inflammation-inducing treatments such as INF treatment, chemotherapy, and radiation, both in terms of poorer physiological tolerance or response to treatment and in terms of the psychological ramifications of treatment, such as increased depression. To date, there are very few studies that have examined such potential differential psychological and physiological responses with respect to fatigue. These studies will be very important because they may identify a potential need to ameliorate fatigue in some patients either before or during treatment to enhance psychological and physiological responses to treatment.

Conclusion

Cytokines have emerged as not only important mediators of immune function but also as immunotransmitters that have widely varying and far-reaching effects on other physiological systems, including the CNS and HPA. Imbalances in cytokines and their effects on psychosocial and physiological functioning are reflected in numerous populations of relevance to chronic stress and fatigue, including (but not limited to) cancer, cardiovascular disorders, MS, and CFS. In addition, because of their far-reaching effects, it is becoming clearer that cytokines play an important role in the psychophysiological states of chronic stress and fatigue. It is our hope that continued rigorous research in these areas will further elucidate the linkages between cytokines and these psychological states, as well as identifying effective behavioral and/or pharmacological interventions aimed at relieving the associated symptomatology.

Further Reading

Banks, R. E. (2000). Measurement of cytokines in clinical samples using immunoassays: problems and pitfalls. *Critical Reviews in Clinical Laboratory Science* **37**(2), 131–182.

Gottschalk, M., Kumpfel, T., Flachenecker, P., et al. (2005). Fatigue and regulation of the hypothalamo-pituitary-adrenal axis in multiple sclerosis. *Archives of Neurology* **62**(2), 277–280.

John, C. D. and Buckingham, J. C. (2003). Cytokines: regulation of the hypothalamo-pituitary-adrenocortical axis. *Current Opinions in Pharmacology* **3**(1), 78–84.

Kurzrock, R. (2001). The role of cytokines in cancer-related fatigue. *Cancer* **92**(6S), 1684–1688.

Lipman, A. J. and Lawrence, D. P. (2004). The management of fatigue in cancer patients. *Oncology* **18**(12), 1527–1535.

Mills, P. J., Parker, B., Dimsdale, J. E., et al. (2005). The relationship between fatigue and quality of life and inflammation during anthracycline-based chemotherapy in breast cancer. *Biological Psychology* **69**, 85–96.

Patarca, R. (2001). Cytokines and chronic fatigue syndrome. *Annals of the New York Academy of Sciences* **933**, 185–200.

Vollmer-Conna, U., Fazou, C., Cameron, B., et al. (2004). Production of pro-inflammatory cytokines correlates with the symptoms of acute sickness behaviour in humans. *Psychology and Medicine* **34**(7), 1289–1297.

Dermatological Conditions

M A Gupta
University of Western Ontario and Mediprobe Research Inc., London, Canada

Glossary

Alopecia areata An immunologically mediated disorder that results in hair loss; it may present in three degrees of severity: (1) single or multiple patches of well-demarcated hair loss, often on the scalp; (2) total or near total loss of scalp hair (termed alopecia totalis); and (3) generalized loss of body hair (termed alopecia universalis). Alopecia areata may occur at any age; the peak incidence is during the third to fifth decades.

Atopic dermatitis A chronically relapsing disorder, marked by periods of exacerbations and remission, characterized by a rash manifesting from patches of red irritated skin and raised papules to areas where the skin is thickened, with accentuation of the skin markings, usually due to repeated scratching. In any one individual, the skin lesions can vary; itching is a central feature of the disorder and some patients may present with dry scaly skin. It appears in early infancy, childhood, and adolescence, frequently associated with elevated serum immunoglobulin E levels and a family history of atopic dermatitis, allergic rhinitis, and asthma; also called atopic eczema.

Hyperhidrosis An increased, above normal sweat production.

Pruritus Itching; this symptom is the predominant feature of inflammatory skin diseases; however, it may be a symptom of a wide range of disorders, from dry skin to an occult cancer. Repeated scratching and rubbing can lead to thickening of the skin with accentuated skin markings and a clinical entity known as lichen simplex chronicus.

Psoriasis A chronic relapsing disorder characterized by skin lesions of variable appearance. The skin lesions often present as raised circular plaques with redness and scales on the elbows, knees, and the scalp behind the ears; however, the lesions may be generalized and affect the entire body or may be localized to just the palms and soles. Pitting of the nails is often associated with psoriasis. Itching and the shedding of the skin scales are some of the most bothersome symptoms.

Rosacea A chronic disorder of the face, often the nose, characterized by redness and superficial blood vessels, with or without papules. It is a disorder of adults, usually

	between ages 30 and 50 years. The onset of rosacea is insidious.
Urticaria	Hives that present as circumscribed, typically itchy, red evanescent areas of swelling. The individual lesions arrive suddenly and rarely persist for longer than 48 h; however, they may continue to recur for indefinite periods. Immunological factors such as allergies play a central role in acute urticaria; however, in the majority of cases of chronic urticaria (i.e., when the lesions are present beyond 6–8 weeks) the underlying cause is not determined.

Overview of Stress and Dermatology

Psychosocial stress has long been recognized as being associated with the onset and/or exacerbation of a wide range of dermatological disorders. Most of the literature on stress and skin disease refers to atopic dermatitis or atopic eczema and psoriasis. The term stress has been used to address three major areas in dermatology: (1) major stressful life events such as the death of a loved one, divorce, or loss of livelihood; (2) stress resulting from the social stigma associated with a cosmetically disfiguring skin disorder such as psoriasis or interpersonal stress resulting from having to provide care to someone with a chronic and recurring disorder such as childhood eczema, which in turn may have an adverse impact on the course of a stress-reactive skin disorder; and (3) traumatic life events that represent situations that overwhelm the coping capacity of the individual – unlike commonly experienced situations (such as simple bereavement), traumatic events such as maternal neglect, severe emotional abuse, and sexual abuse generally are events that are outside the range of normal human experience and are significantly distressing to almost everyone.

Stress may influence dermatological symptoms in three major situations: (1) in primary stress-reactive skin disorders, such as psoriasis, atopic dermatitis or eczema, urticaria, acne, and alopecia areata, in which neuroendocrine and psychoneuroimmunological factors are believed to play an important role; (2) in disorders that represent an accentuated physiological response such as hyperhidrosis (or excessive perspiration) and blushing; and (3) in skin disorders, such as dermatitis artefacta, neurotic excoriations, or trichotillomania, that are secondary to an underlying psychiatric condition such as obsessive-compulsive disorder, posttraumatic stress disorder, or major depressive disorder. Nutritional deficiencies encountered in eating disorders such as anorexia nervosa and sometimes bulimia nervosa can result in diffuse hair loss or alopecia. Stress exacerbates the dermatological symptoms by aggravating the underlying psychiatric disorder.

Various neurobiological factors have been implicated in stress-mediated skin disorders. Stress-induced analgesia is observed in animals faced with inescapable stressors. Fear activates the secretion of endogenous opioid peptides, and this effect is blocked by naloxone in animal models. This may be a factor in itching, scratching and self-injury that occur during extremely stressful situations.

Psychosocial stress has been associated with the activation of the hypothalamic-pituitary-adrenocortical (HPA) axis and the sympathetic and adrenomedullary (SAM) system. Stressful emotional experiences disturb the regulation of the HPA and the SAM systems; that is, in the face of stress, physiological systems may operate at higher levels, resulting in higher glucocorticoid levels, or lower levels than normal. Recent studies have shown that psychological stress, such as examination-related stress, is associated with derangements in the epidermal (most superficial layer of the skin) permeability barrier function and that the alterations were proportional to the severity of the stressor. It has been proposed that this is mediated by increased endogenous glucocorticoids. Both psoriasis and atopic dermatitis demonstrate increased transepidermal water loss and deterioration of barrier function. Higher anxiety levels in acne patients have been associated with high blood catecholamine levels, which decreased with the treatment of the acne, suggesting that the anxiety in acne is associated with significant physiological stress for the patient and activation of the SAM system.

It has further been observed that there is increased responsiveness of the HPA axis in response to a heel prick stressor in newborns with a family history of atopy or elevated levels of cord blood immunoglobulin E (IgE). Patients with atopic dermatitis also show elevated eosinophil counts and elevated IgE expression in response to stress. Atopic patients with serum IgE levels greater than 100 IU ml^{-1} demonstrated significantly higher levels of excitability and less adequate coping with stress than did patients with lower IgE levels. IgE is considered to be important in atopic dermatitis because it mediates hypersensitivity reactions by stimulating mast cells and basophils.

Chronic stress may induce a state of hyporesponsiveness of the HPA axis whereby glucocorticoid secretion is decreased, leading to an increased secretion of mediators of inflammation such as the cytokines, which are normally regulated by cortisol. Animal data show that a blunted responsiveness of the HPA axis to stress is closely linked to an increased susceptibility to inflammatory disease. Stress-induced hyporesponsiveness of the HPA system has also been proposed to be a factor in some chronic inflammatory dermatoses such as atopic dermatitis.

Role of Stress over the Life Cycle

The interface between psychosocial stress and dermatological disorders begins early in the life cycle and persists throughout adult life because of the role of the skin as a vital organ of communication. The role of stress in dermatological disorders therefore has to be assessed from a developmental perspective. The skin plays an integral role as an organ of communication right from birth because the skin is the primary organ of attachment. The newborn infant's initial physical experience is largely tactile, and the child requires secure holding and hugging to develop physically, neurologically and psychosocially. Psychosocial stressors, such as maternal deprivation, neglect, or abuse during early life and the lack of adequate tactile nurturance in institutions such as orphanages, can impact a child's entire body, and the sequelae of such types of stressors are often manifested in a wide range of dermatological symptoms. Spitz observed that the lack of a nurturing mother–child relationship in an institutional setting was associated with the development of certain syndromes such as rocking, fecal play, and infantile eczema. In this institutionalized population, 15% of the infants had infantile eczema compared with a 2–3% prevalence in the general population. A child's need to be held and physically nurtured may be neglected in cases in which he or she has a severe skin disease; alternatively a child's chronic recurring skin disorder may place inordinate stress on the caregiver and affect his or her capacity to nurture the child. In some instances, this interpersonal stress may in turn have an adverse impact on stress-reactive skin conditions such as eczema in a vicious cycle.

The onset of a cosmetically disfiguring skin disorder during adolescence often renders the patient very vulnerable to stress because he or she is also dealing with emerging hormonal and physical changes of puberty, body-image issues, and dealing with other developmental tasks of adolescence such as peer pressure, dating, and career choice. Adolescence is also associated with a high incidence of mood disorders such as major depressive disorder. The peak incidence of acne is during adolescence. In addition to the rise in the level of androgens that is the primary trigger for acne, the psychosocial stresses of this life stage can also contribute to flare-ups of the acne. Therefore, psychosocial stress may contribute to flare-up of acne and the acne in turn may result in significant stress for the patient. It is important to recognize that the adolescent patient may be especially vulnerable and may react to even relatively minor acne with a serious psychiatric disorder such as major depression and suicidal ideation. Alternatively, there have been incidences of violent acting out by adolescents who were having difficulty coping with the psychosocial, particularly peer-related, stresses associated with disfiguring acne. In young adulthood and later life, the emergence of stress-reactive disorders such as psoriasis may have a significant impact on the patient's social and occupational functioning, and the stress resulting from the stigmatization may in turn cause flare-ups of the psoriasis.

The Role of Stress in a Wide Range of Dermatological Symptoms

Some general stress-related factors may play a role in a wide range of skin disorders.

Pruritus or Itching

Pruritus is a feature of a wide range of skin disorders to varying degrees, including the common disorders that are exacerbated by psychological stress such as psoriasis, atopic dermatitis, and urticaria. Pruritus has been reported to be exacerbated by stress in up to 86% of cases in large surveys. Stress may also increase scratching behavior, which in turn can trigger the itch–scratch cycle and, in some instances, cause further flare-ups of the underlying skin condition, such as atopic dermatitis. Pruritus may further be a source of significant distress for the patient; it is often rated as the most bothersome feature of the skin disorder and has been associated with suicide. Stress-induced scratching and itching may lead to the development of conditions such as lichen simplex chronicus, in which the superficial layer of the skin thickens as a result of repetitive scratching.

Disease-Related Stress

The impact of a skin disorder on quality of life, especially due to the cosmetic disfigurement and social stigma that are typically associated with a wide range of skin disorders, can be a source of significant stress for the patient. In some chronic stress-reactive dermatoses such as psoriasis and atopic dermatitis, this disease-related stress may in turn cause the underlying skin condition to flare up and may become an important confounding factor.

Stress-Related Self-Injury/Manipulation of the Skin

When faced with stressful situations, patients may pick at minor irregularities or existing lesions in their skin, scratch themselves excessively, or pluck their hair. Injury to the skin may exacerbate a primary skin condition such as psoriasis secondary to the Koebner phenomenon or may cause flare-ups of acne as a result of the underlying inflammatory process.

The skin is frequently the focus of tension-reducing behaviors, both because of its easy access and because of the primary role of the skin in early attachment. Attachment-related trauma occurs when there is abuse or neglect in early life, and this is often associated with self-injury to the body, especially the skin. Posttraumatic stress disorder (PTSD) associated with a history of sexual, physical, and/or emotional abuse results in a dysregulation of internal emotional states. The PTSD patients may excessively manipulate their skin or hair in a attempt to regulate their affect. The tension-reducing behavior and self-injury may manifest as the self-induced dermatological conditions such as neurotic excoriations, dermatitis artefacta, neurodermatitis, and trichotillomania. In cases in which high levels of stress and dissociation are present, patients may not even recall self-inducing their lesions as a result of dissociative amnesia and may be mistaken as malingerers.

Stress and Some Specific Dermatological Disorders

Acne

Emotionally stressful events such as examinations are known to exacerbate acne; furthermore, increasing stress has been shown to be correlated with an increase in acne severity. The stress resulting from the impact of acne on the quality of life of the patient is comparable to chronic disorders such as diabetes and asthma, and it often does not correlate with the clinical severity of acne – even mild acne may be associated with significant stress.

Acne excoriee is a condition that results from repetitive picking and excoriation of the acne lesions. A stress-related syndrome that is often underrecognized in acne excoriee is PTSD, usually secondary to abuse and/or neglect during early life; patients with PTSD often injure themselves, and this can manifest as recurrent acne excoriee. In some of these patients, the problems caused by the recurrent self-excoriation are more problematic than the primary acne lesions that were excoriated. Some PTSD patients dissociate when excoriating themselves and may not have full recollection of the times when they excoriated their acne lesions.

Alopecia Areata

Psychosocial stress has been reported to play a role in the onset and exacerbation of alopecia areata; however, this association is less robust. Various studies indicate a lack of a direct relationship between stress and the severity of alopecia areata, suggesting stress may be a factor that just triggers the onset of the disease process. One study reported mental stress within 3 months before the onset of alopecia areata by 23% of 114 patients surveyed, and an additional 22% reported suffering from stress that was not related to the appearance of the alopecia. In one study of 52 patients, all patients reported "a very unhappy or stressful life," whereas in another study only 6.7% of 178 patients reported a severely disturbing event 6 months before the onset of symptoms. One study reported that patients whose alopecia areata is stress-reactive may suffer from depressive illness.

Atopic Dermatitis or Atopic Eczema

Stressful life events may precede the onset of atopic dermatitis or eczema in up to 70% of cases. Itching is a central feature of atopic dermatitis. Disease-related stress, interpersonal stress, and stress resulting from the family environment are important predictors of symptom severity in atopic dermatitis. Atopic patients have been shown to scratch more readily in response to an itch stimulus, suggesting that they develop a conditioned scratch response more readily than controls. Perceived itch may be enhanced in atopic patients in response to mental stress. The scratching can trigger the itch–scratch cycle, which can become a problem in cases of nocturnal itching and scratching. Some earlier studies reported high psychophysiological reactivity in atopic patients; however, this has not been supported by more recent studies that carried out psychophysiological measures such as blood pressure, heart rate, and skin conductance.

Hyperhidrosis or Excessive Perspiration

Hyperhidrosis has been associated with stress in up to 100% of cases. Over 25% of patients with social phobia or social anxiety disorder, in which the patients experience heightened stress and physiological arousal in social situations, report hyperhidrosis to be a significantly distressing symptom.

Psoriasis

Various studies have reported an association between stress and psoriasis. A study that retrospectively examined the role of stress in the onset of a wide range of skin conditions reported that patients with psoriasis were more likely to report that a stressful experience predated the onset and exacerbation of their condition than patients with other skin diseases. In a study of 132 psoriasis patients, 39% recalled a significant stressful life event (e.g., interpersonal stress within the family, death or hospitalization of close relatives, accidents, sexual assault, and examinations) within 1 month before the first episode of psoriasis, in contrast to 10% of patients with conditions that are generally not associated with stress. A stressful life event was reported 1 month before the onset of psoriasis in 72% of 179 patients with psoriasis. In a survey of 245 children with psoriasis, stress was observed to be a provocative factor among 90% of the children. The severity of the stressor does not typically correlate with the time to onset or the exacerbation of psoriasis, possibly because of considerable individual variation in coping skills and the importance of the emotional meaning rather than the absolute intensity of the life event. PTSD has been associated with a long-term impact on physical health and a wide range of disorders affecting the immune system, including psoriasis. A recent study of 2490 Vietnam war veterans reported an adjusted odds ratio of 4.7 (95%, CI 1.9–11.7) for psoriasis among veterans with comorbid PTSD. The autonomic dsyregulation associated with PTSD may be an underlying perpetuating factor in patients with recurring or treatment-resistant psoriasis.

Rosacea

Factors such as overwhelming life stress, an anxious and immature personality associated with excessive feelings of guilt and shame, and social anxiety secondary to easy blushing have all been implicated in rosacea. Psychological stress has been implicated as a factor among 20–94% of patients with rosacea.

Urticaria

Increased mental tension and fatigue have been spontaneously reported as the main exacerbating or precipitating factors by 77% of 43 patients. Out of 100 patients with chronic urticaria and/or angioedema, 51% reported that stressful life situations were associated with the onset of symptoms, compared with 8% of surgical controls. Earthquakes and other catastrophic life events have been associated with the onset of urticaria. There have been case reports of patients with PTSD secondary to severe physical abuse, who developed linear urticarial lesions in the same region of the body where they had experienced the beatings in their early life.

Further Reading

Boscarino, J. A. (2004). Posttraumatic stress disorder and physical illness. Results from clinical and epidemiologic studies. *Annals of the New York Academy of Sciences* **1032**, 141–153.

Buske-Kirschbaum, A. and Hellhammer, D. H. (2003). Endocrine and immune responses to stress in chronic inflammatory skin disorders. *Annals of the New York Academy of Sciences* **992**, 231–240.

Garg, A., Chren, M., Sands, L. P., et al. (2001). Psychological stress perturbs epidermal permeability barrier homeostasis: implications for the pathogenesis of stress-associated skin disorders. *Archives of Dermatology* **137**, 53–59.

Gavenda, A. (ed.) (2005). Psychocutaneous disease. *Dermatologic Clinics* **23**, 4.

Griesemer, R. D. (1978). Emotionally triggered disease in a dermatological practice. *Psychiatric Annals* **8**, 49–56.

Gupta, M. A. and Gupta, A. K. (1996). Psychodermatology: an update. *Journal of the American Academy of Dermatology* **34**, 1030–1046.

Gupta, M. A. and Gupta, A. K. (2003). Psychiatric and psychological co-morbidity in patients with dermatologic disorders. *American Journal of Clinical Dermatology* **4**, 833–842.

Koblenzer, C. S. (1987). *Psychocutaneous disease.* Orlando, FL: Grune & Stratton.

Koo, J. Y. M. and Lee, C. S. (eds.) (2003). *Psychocutaneous medicine.* New York: Marcel Dekker Inc.

Panconesi, E. (ed.) (1984). Stress and skin diseases: psychosomatic dermatology. *Clinics in Dermatology* **2**(4).

Spitz, R. A. (1965). *The first year of life: a psychoanalytic study of normal and deviant development of object relations.* New York: International Universities Press.

Ulceration, Gastric

R Murison and A M Milde
University of Bergen, Bergen, Norway

This is a revised version of the article by R Murison, Encyclopedia of Stress First Edition, volume 3, pp 631–633, © 2000, Elsevier Inc.

Glossary

Analgesia	Insensibility to painful stimuli.
Corticotropin releasing hormone	A hormone released from the hypothalamus which leads to secretion of cortisol from the adrenal cortex into the circulation.
Dopamine	A catecholamine neurotransmitter.
Gastric acid	Hydrochloric acid secreted by cells in the stomach.
Helicobacter pylori (H. pylori)	A gram-negative bacterium found in the majority of patients with peptic ulcer.
Immunomodulation	Changes in the function of the body's immune defence system.
Ischemia	Localized oxygen deficit as a result of obstruction of the blood supply or vasoconstriction.
Lactobacillus	A bacterium found particularly in dairy produce and meat.
Limbic	Referring to several phylogenetically old brain structures thought to be central to emotionality and learning.
Mucosa	The mucous membrane lining the stomach and intestines.
Pepsinogen	The precursor of pepsin, found in the stomach mucosa.
Peptic ulcer	An ulcer involving the mucosa, submucosa, and muscular layers of the stomach, or duodenum, due in part at least to the action of gastric juices.
Rumen	The part of the stomach lacking acid-producing glands.
Spontaneously hypertensive rats	A specially bred strain of rats with high susceptibility to develop high blood pressure.
Sympathetic	The part of the autonomic nervous system which prepares the organism for the fight/flight response.
Vagotomy	Severing of the vagus nerve.
Vagus nerve	The tenth cranial nerve forming an important part of the parasympathetic system.

Background

Ulcerations of the stomach, typically manifested as nonpenetrating erosions of the gastric mucosa, are found following stress in many mammalian species (mice, rats, horses, primates, swine, reindeer, and dogs, among others). The condition is therefore considered to be a reflection of fundamental common psychobiological processes activated by stress. Although there are significant exceptions, most psychobiological studies have focused on the rat because of the extensive pool of knowledge of behavior and central nervous system (CNS) function in that species. The ulcerations are found in both the rumen and the glandular areas of the stomach. The former appear to be the result of food deprivation procedures, whereas the latter are sensitive to psychological factors (stress). The ulcerations are typically bleeding erosions of the superficial gastric mucosa along the ridges of the gastric folds. Prolonged application of the stressor may cause full-blown ulcers, with the erosions reaching through the muscularis mucosa. Given a respite from the stressor and other potential ulcerogenic factors, however, the ulcerations typically heal within a few days.

Controversy surrounds the homologous condition in humans. Earlier, gastric ulcerations in rodents and monkeys were used as models of peptic ulcer in humans, even though the location of ulcer in humans is more typically the duodenum. Later, gastric ulcerations were regarded as homologous to the acute stress ulcers seen after burn injuries or traumatic surgery in humans. Since the discovery of the role of *Helicobacter pylori* in peptic ulcers in humans, it has been surmised that ulcerations in animals are homologous to the erosive prepyloric changes of the gastric mucosa reported in subgroups of patients diagnosed with functional dyspepsia. However, there is much more to the story.

Psychological Influences on Development of Ulceration

In the wild, ulcerations are observed in animals (both rodents and primates) following social defeat. In both wild and domestic animals, ulcerations have been reported in connection with the stress of transport and confinement. In the laboratory, ulcerations are produced by a wide variety of stressors in animals – electric shock, restraint, cold, activity stress, social stress, or combinations of these – with the purpose of exploring the role of psychological factors that may modulate the incidence and/or severity of the mucosal injury. Consciousness is a modulating, if not necessary, condition for the development of ulcerations.

Ulcerations played a key role in Selye's description of the general adaptation syndrome and constituted one of the elements of this nonspecific response to diverse nocuous agents, together with shrinkage of the thymus and enlargement of the adrenal glands.

Acute Effects

To identify the psychological factors in ulceration (and other stress-related phenomena), many have employed the triadic design. Animals are tested in triplets. One animal (the executive) is subjected to a physical stressor (most commonly electric shock) that can be escaped from or avoided by instrumental responses. The second (yoked) animal is wired to the first such that the same physical stress is experienced but there is no possibility of avoidance or escape. The third (control) animal is subjected to the same apparatus conditions as the first two but not to the stressor. By comparing the amount of ulceration between the first two animals, the psychological and physical components of the stressor can be identified.

The Executive Monkey studies with monkeys, by Brady and his colleagues, were based on a triadic design, and indicated that the executive was more vulnerable to ulceration than its yoked partner. These results were widely accepted at the time, but their interpretation was later questioned. In contrast to the Brady results, Weiss reported that executive rats developed less ulceration than their yoked partners. These inconsistencies between the monkey and rat results have been attributed to the particular group-assignment procedures and experimental parameters used by Brady rather than to species differences.

Later, Weiss demonstrated that ulceration in rats was attenuated by providing the animals with predictability for shock and was exacerbated by either increasing the response requirements (effort) required to maintain instrumental control or by introducing a component of psychological conflict. Weiss's model predicts ulceration as a function of the effort required to maintain instrumental control over a stressor and an inverse function of the feedback provided by such control. Successful coping behaviors (high feedback) ameliorate ulceration, but greater workload (effort) will increase ulceration. This model has played an important role in the development of recent theories concerning the relationships among stress, coping, and ill health in humans. Between- and within-strain studies have led to the notion that more emotional animals are more vulnerable to ulcerations than less emotional conspecifics. For example, spontaneously hypertensive rats are less vulnerable than the more emotional Wistar–Kyoto strain. Potential biological markers for vulnerability to ulceration include plasma levels of pepsinogen (also in humans) and dopaminergic function. Genetic factors certainly play a role in vulnerability to ulceration, but these are modulated by early life experiences and previous experiences of coping/noncoping, which also modulate dopaminergic function.

Proactive Effects

A number of experimenters have investigated proactive effects of one or more stressor exposures on vulnerability to ulceration under later exposure to either the same or a different stressor. Rats previously subjected to the stress of whole-body restraint generally develop less ulceration under later restraint, whereas previous exposure to an activity wheel primes the animal for later activity-stress ulceration. Using heterogeneous stress experiences, rats subjected to the same shock stress parameters that are used to induce learned helplessness (a putative model for human depression) develop greater amounts of ulceration under a later radically different type of stressor, restraint in water. This phenomenon is mediated by opioid mechanisms in the same way that stress-induced analgesia and stress-induced immunomodulation are also invoked by these same shock parameters. Previous experience with escapable shock, on the other hand, has proactive protective effects against later ulceration, although the mechanisms of this phenomenon remain unexplored. More recent studies have complemented these earlier reports in showing that prior experience with seminaturalistic coping responses is protective against later ulcerogenesis. Similarly, prior experience with uncontrollable shocks, but in which safety signals are provided at the end of each shock, also reduces vulnerability under later stress.

Early weaning of rats (at day 16) leads to a drastic increase in vulnerability to ulceration during a limited period later on (22–40 days). Although later studies indicated that this effect was due more to nutritional and thermoregulatory influences than to psychobiological phenomena, recent reports suggest that such very early manipulations have profound long-term effects on dopaminergic system function, which is known to play an important role in ulceration.

Mechanisms

Peripheral Mechanisms

The peripheral mechanisms of ulceration were originally believed to be limited to increased levels of vagally mediated gastric acid secretion, and vagotomy does reduce ulceration. Although the old saying "no acid – no ulcer" still holds, recent approaches have focused on combinations of changes in gastric motility, gastric blood flow, and sympathetic tone. A common view is that enhanced vagally mediated acid secretion and reduced gastric blood flow represent key aggressive factors, whereas the protective factors include prostaglandin-mediated secretion of mucous, secretion of bicarbonate, and maintenance of an adequate blood supply.

The development of ulceration appears to be greatest in the period immediately following an acute stress. This has led to the concept of ulceration as a poststress or rebound phenomenon, whereby gastric acid secretion is inhibited during the application of a strong stressor (although certain stressors may increase secretion). A concurrent strong sympathetically mediated constriction of the mucosal blood vessels increases the risk for local ischemia, and slow rhythmic contractions may cause further physical damage. On release from the inhibitory (sympathetic) influence of the acute stressor, gastric acid levels are rapidly elevated, leaving a vulnerable mucosa open to damage.

Interactions between stress and bacterial flora The role of bacterial flora is now under intensive study since the discovery that ulcer disease in humans is related to the presence of *H. pylori*. Animal psychobiological models for *Helicobacter* infection have been hindered by the fact that most behavioral studies of ulceration have been performed in rats, whereas the models for infection have largely been limited to mice, ferrets, and gerbils. It remains unclear whether bacterial flora play any part in either ulceration in animals or erosive prepyloric erosions in humans. Germ-free animals do develop stress gastric ulcerations, although to a lesser extent than normal animals, and antibiotic treatment accelerates the healing of the ulceration. From the human data, it is apparent that factors additional to *H. pylori* are involved in gastric pathology, and it remains to be clarified to what extent stress, either alone or in combination with bacterial factors, is involved. Recent results also suggest that the relationship between the bacterial population of gut and ulceration is two way: The induction of ulceration in animals by the direct application of acetic acid to the stomach lining dramatically changes the predominant bacterial species, which then return to normal as the ulceration heals. In particular, *Lactobacillus* seems to be protective and enhances the healing process. Consistent with these animal data, a small-scale study in humans has shown that *H. pylori*, although present in all patients with duodenal ulceration with a duration greater than 6 months, was not present in patients with a shorter history, suggesting that the infection is not so much a cause as a factor producing chronicity. On the other hand, a recent study of patients admitted to intensive care units shows that *H. pylori* infection was more frequent in patients exhibiting upper gastrointestinal bleeding than in patients who were not bleeding. Thus, the controversy concerning the role of *H. pylori* remains unresolved.

Central and Neuroendocrine Influences

Studies of the central mechanisms of ulcerations have focused on limbic structures, in particular the amygdala (with its close association with the vagus nerve), the septum, and the hippocampus. The stimulation of the amygdala elicits ulceration, whereas lesions of the central nucleus of the amygdala attenuate their formation. The stimulation of the dorsolateral septum reduces the amount of ulceration induced by cold-restraint stress. Lesions of the hippocampus, in particular the ventral hippocampus, exacerbate ulceration, presumably acting through the amygdala-vagal pathways.

Studies of centrally acting peptides show that corticotropin releasing hormone (CRH) has a potent protective effect when applied directly in the central amygdala. When injected peripherally, CRH protects against stress ulceration in young, but not old, rats (in old rats, the effect is exacerbatory). CRH acts through sympathetic pathways to inhibit gastric acid secretion while at the same time stimulating bicarbonate production and inhibiting slow gastric contractions. Tests of the CRH type-1 receptor antagonist antalarmin demonstrate a potent anti-ulcerogenic effect, but the glucocorticoid/progesterone antagonist RU-38486 significantly potentiates the formation of stress-induced gastric erosions. The role of the CRH system in ulcerogenesis remains unclear and peripheral corticosterone may play an important role in cytoprotection during stress.

Thyrotropin releasing hormone (TRH) acts as a potent ulcerogenic agent and is stimulated by cold. TRH promotes both gastric acid secretion and the slow gastric contractions associated with the development of ulcerations induced by cold restraint stress. The main site of action for TRH appears to be the dorsal motor nucleus of the vagus, although a number of hypothalamic nuclei and the amygdala are also implicated.

Adrenalectomy increases the incidence of ulceration, and there is little support for the earlier notion that corticosterone plays any causal role in ulcerogenesis. Rather, the events likely to activate the pathogenic mechanisms for ulceration are also the kind of events that activate the hypothalamic-pituitary-adrenal axis.

Of the centrally acting neurotransmitters, most attention has been paid to dopamine and in particular to the D1 and D2 receptors. In line with the observation that schizophrenics rarely develop ulcers, whereas untreated Parkinson's patients are at high risk, numerous studies have provided evidence that central dopamine is protective against ulceration. A more complex picture has now become apparent because results suggest that the stimulation of dopamine D1 receptors inhibits ulceration whereas stimulation of dopamine D2 receptors has a pro-ulcerogenic effect. Within-strain comparisons of rats rated as high emotional versus low emotional reveal that the former are more vulnerable to stress ulcerations than the latter, as well as having lower levels of dopamine in the amygdala. A similar difference between these two types of animal was observed with respect to ethanol-induced ulcerations. Rats differing in their sensitivity to the dopaminergic agonist apomorphine are differentially susceptible to ulcerations and recover at different rates, and experience with shock parameters demonstrated to increase vulnerability to ulceration change their apomorphine sensitivity accordingly. Recent evidence also suggests that the dopamine content of the gastric mucosa is important in cell proliferation of the gastric mucosa. These and other data suggest that vulnerability profiles of animals to ulcerations are manifest at both the central and peripheral levels.

Future Directions

Studies on the etiology of stress gastric ulceration have become reduced in number since the experience that *H. pylori* eradication is the most effective treatment for human peptic ulcer. However, the bacterial risk factor and the effectiveness of treatment do not in themselves account for either historical or contemporary links between stress and ulcerogenesis. Recent developments in psychoneuroimmunology offer opportunities to study how host factors (including CNS-mediated immunomodulation) may interact with pathophysiological agents, both bacterial and others, in causing and maintaining gastric mucosal changes. Specifically, stress-related failures of immune defenses may provide a window of opportunity for *H. pylori* to cause problems.

Further Reading

Boulos, P. B., Botha, A., Hobsley, M., et al. (2002). Possible absence of *Helicobacter pylori* in the early stages of duodenal ulceration. *Quarterly Journal of Medicine* **95**, 749–752.

Degen, S. B., Geven, E. J., Sluyter, F., et al. (2003). Apomorphine-susceptible and apomorphine-unsusceptible Wistar rats differ in their recovery from stress-induced ulcers. *Life Sciences* **72**, 1117–1124.

Desai, J. K., Goyal, R. K. and Parmar, N. S. (1999). Characterization of dopamine receptor subtypes involved in experimentally induced gastric and duodenal ulcers in rats. *Journal of Pharmacy and Pharmacology* **51**, 187–192.

Elliott, S. N., Buret, A., McKnight, W., et al. (1998). Bacteria rapidly colonize and modulate healing of gastric ulcers in rats. *American Journal of Physiology* **275**, G425–G432.

Filaretova, L., Podvigina, T., Bagaeva, T., et al. (2001). Gastroprotective action of glucocorticoids during the formation and the healing of indomethacin-induced gastric erosions in rats. *Journal of Physiology* (Paris) **95**, 201–208.

Gabry, K. E., Chrousos, G. P., Rice, K. C., et al. (2002). Marked suppression of gastric ulcerogenesis and intestinal responses to stress by a novel class of drugs. *Molecular Psychiatry* **7**, 433, 474–483.

Glavin, G. B., Murison, R., Overmier, J. B., et al. (1991). The neurobiology of stress ulcers. *Brain Research Reviews* **16**, 301–343.

Levenstein, S. (2000). The very model of a modern etiology: a biopsychosocial view of peptic ulcer. *Psychosomatic Medicine* **62**, 176–185.

Maury, E., Tankovic, J., Ebel, A., et al. (2005). An observational study of upper gastrointestinal bleeding in intensive care units: is *Helicobacter pylori* the culprit? *Critical Care Medicine* **33**, 1513–1518.

Murison, R. (2001). Is there a role for psychology in ulcer disease? *Integrative Physiological and Behavioral Science* **36**, 75–83.

Overmier, J. B. and Murison, R. (2000). Anxiety and helplessness in the face of stress predisposes, precipitates, and sustains gastric ulceration. *Behavioral Brain Research* **110**, 161–174.

Sapolsky, R. M. (2004). *Why zebras don't get ulcers* (3rd edn.). New York: Henry Holt.

Szabo, S. (1979). Dopamine disorder in duodenal ulceration. *Lancet* **2**(8148), 880–882.

Weiner, H. (1991). From simplicity to complexity (1950–1990): the case of peptic ulceration. I: Human studies. *Psychosomatic Medicine* **53**, 467–490.

Weiner, H. (1991). From simplicity to complexity (1950–1990): the case of peptic ulceration. II: Animal studies. *Psychosomatic Medicine* **53**, 491–516.

V. PSYCHOSOCIAL

Stress, Beneficial Effects of

S Joseph
University of Nottingham, Nottingham, UK
P A Linley
University of Leicester, Leicester UK

Glossary

Adversarial growth — Increased psychological functioning and personal development following exposure to a stressful and traumatic event; also called posttraumatic growth or stress-related growth.

Assumptive world — Cognitive schemata about the self and world that determine how meaning is perceived.

A number of literatures, religions, and philosophies throughout human history have conveyed the idea that there are benefits to be found in suffering. However, it is only relatively recently that the topic of benefit finding following stress and trauma has become a research focus. Initially there was some debate over the validity of the concept of benefit finding, with some commentators questioning whether it was anything more than positive illusion and self-deception. But there is now convincing evidence that people often experience benefits following stress and trauma. These benefits have been variously labeled adversarial growth, benefit finding, flourishing, heightened existential awareness, perceived benefits, positive by-products, positive changes, positive meaning, posttraumatic growth, quantum change, self-renewal, stress-related growth, thriving, and transformational coping. These terms have been used interchangeably to refer not just to recovery following stressful and traumatic events but to how events can sometimes serve as a springboard to a higher level of psychological functioning.

Types of Benefit

Three broad interrelated dimensions of benefit finding have been discussed. First, relationships are enhanced in some way; for example, people now value their friends and family more and feel an increased compassion and altruism toward others. Second, people change their views of themselves in some way; for example, they have a greater sense of personal resiliency, wisdom, and strength, perhaps coupled with a greater acceptance of their vulnerabilities and limitations. Third, people report changes in life philosophy; for example, they find a fresh appreciation for each new day and renegotiate what really matters in the full realization that their life is finite, including possibly changing their spiritual beliefs. Various psychometric self-report instruments have been developed with which to assess positive changes and personal growth following adversity: the Changes in Outlook Questionnaire, the Perceived Benefit Scale, the Posttraumatic Growth Inventory, the Stress-Related Growth Scale, and the Thriving Scale. The development of these instruments has led to further empirical investigation.

Prevalence

Prevalence varies among studies due to samples, contexts, and methodological issues, but it is expected that anywhere between 30 and 70% of people may experience some form of benefit following traumatic events, although the benefits are not usually reported in the immediate aftermath but at some later time. Also, the benefits are likely to coexist with psychological distress; the experience of benefits is not mutually exclusive with other more negative psychological consequences.

Etiological Factors

Studies have reported benefits following a range of stressful and traumatic events, for example, bereavements; accidents and disasters; chronic and life-threatening illnesses; sexual, physical, and emotional abuse in childhood; sexual assaults; and wars and conflicts. Research has also begun to document the correlates and predictors of growth, with evidence pointing to the importance of stress-appraisal, coping, and personality variables, with the more optimistic, self-efficacious, extraverted, and stable people, who use more spiritual, accepting, emotionally expressive, and emotionally focused forms of coping, being more likely to report benefits. Social support is thought to be important too.

Theoretical Developments

Tedeschi and Calhoun's functional-descriptive model shows how traumatic events serve as seismic challenges to the pretrauma schema by shattering prior goals, beliefs, and ways of managing emotional distress. When these schemas are shattered in this way, this leads to ruminative activity as people try to make sense of what has happened and to deal with their emotional reactions to the trauma. In the initial stages, this ruminative activity is more automatic than deliberate. Although distressing, automatic ruminative activity is indicative of cognitive activity that is directed at rebuilding the pretrauma schema. This ruminative process is influenced by social support networks, which provide sources of comfort and relief, as well as being influenced by new coping behaviors and available options for the construction of new posttrauma schemas. Successful coping at this stage facilitates disengagement from goals that are now unreachable and from beliefs that are no longer tenable in the post-trauma environment, together with decreased emotional distress. As successful coping aids adaptation, the initial ruminative activity that was characterized by its automatic nature shifts toward a more effortful ruminative activity. This effortful ruminative activity is characterized by narrative development, part of which may be the search for meaning.

Introducing a metatheoretical perspective, Joseph and Linley proposed that human beings are active, growth-oriented organisms. The theory proposes that individuals are intrinsically motivated to cognitively accommodate their psychological experiences and thus find benefit. The confrontation with a stressful and traumatic event has a shattering effect on the person's assumptive world. When the social environment is able to provide for the basic human needs of autonomy, competence, and relatedness, then models of the self and world transform to accommodate the new trauma-related information. When the social environment does not provide support for these basic human needs, the process of accommodation is thwarted and benefits are less likely to be experienced.

Similarly, but from a biopsychosocial-evolutionary perspective, Christopher regarded growth, rather than pathology, as the normal outcome of the traumatic stress response. Reviewing and synthesizing the trauma literature, Christopher articulated seven interconnected theoretical conclusions:

1. Stress is best understood as a prerational form of biopsychological feedback.
2. The normal outcome of traumatic stress is growth.
3. Any resultant psychopathology is a function of a maladaptive modulation of the stress response.
4. Trauma transforms individuals on the biological as well as psychological levels.
5. Biological processes underlying stress response are universal, but there are specific dynamics that are a function of the individual.
6. Biological changes can occur even if there are no psychological changes.
7. Rationality is humanity's evolutionary newest and most sophisticated stress-reduction mechanism.

Clinical Applications

The interest in benefit finding can be seen as part of the wider positive psychology movement. Positive psychology is seen as a balance to mainstream psychology, which has been for too long overly concerned with the negative aspects of human experience. Research in positive psychology is now beginning to focus on its applications, and the study of benefit finding promises to have important applications for clinical, counseling, and health psychologists, who when working with clients who have experienced stressful and traumatic events need not be concerned only with helping to alleviate distress but also with helping to facilitate more positive functioning.

The importance of this avenue of investigation is seen in the seminal work of Affleck and colleagues, who found that perceived benefits at 7 weeks following a heart attack significantly predicted less chance of heart attack recurrence and lower general health morbidity at an 8-year follow-up. Experimental studies to test whether the principles of growth might somehow be introduced as part of a clinical intervention are encouraging. For example, Stanton and colleagues randomly assigned breast cancer patients to one of two groups, one group to write about the facts of the cancer experience and the other to write about positive thoughts and feelings regarding the experience. It was found that those assigned to write about their positive experiences had significantly fewer medical appointments for cancer-related morbidities 3 months later.

Clinicians should be aware of the potential for positive change in their clients following stress and trauma. But it must also be recognized that adversity does not lead to positive change for everyone. Therefore, therapists need to be careful not to inadvertently imply that patients have in some way failed by not making more of their experience or that there is anything inherently positive in their experiences. Personal growth after trauma should be viewed as originating not from the event, but from within the patients themselves through the process of their struggle with the event and its aftermath.

See Also the Following Articles

Caregivers, Stress and; Religion and Stress.

Further Reading

Affleck, G., Tennen, H., Croog, S., et al. (1987). Causal attribution, perceived benefits, and morbidity after a heart attack: an 8-year study. *Journal of Consulting and Clinical Psychology* 55, 29–35.

Calhoun, L. G. and Tedeschi, R. G. (1999). *Facilitating posttraumatic growth: a clinician's guide*. Mahwah, NJ: Lawrence Erlbaum.
Christopher, M. (2004). A broader view of trauma: a biopsychosocial-evolutionary view of the role of the traumatic stress response in the emergence of pathology and/or growth. *Clinical Psychology Review* **24**, 75–98.
Cordova, M. J., Cunningham, L. L. C., Carlson, C. R., et al. (2001). Posttraumatic growth following breast cancer: a controlled comparison study. *Health Psychology* **20**, 176–185.
Frazier, P., Tashiro, T., Berman, M., et al. (2004). Correlates of levels and patterns of positive life changes following sexual assault. *Journal of Consulting and Clinical Psychology* **72**, 19–30.
Joseph, S. and Linley, P. A. (2005). Positive adjustment to threatening events: an organismic valuing theory of growth through adversity. *Review of General Psychology* **9**, 262–280.
Linley, P. A. and Joseph, S. (2004). Positive change following trauma and adversity: a review. *Journal of Traumatic Stress* **17**, 11–21.
O'Leary, V. E., Alday, C. S. and Ickovics, J. R. (1998). Models of life change and posttraumatic growth. In: Tedeschi, R. G., Park, C. L. & Calhoun, L. G. (eds.) *Posttraumatic growth: positive changes in the aftermath of crisis*, pp. 127–151. Mahwah, NJ: Lawrence Erlbaum.
Park, C. L., Cohen, L. H. and Murch, R. (1996). Assessment and prediction of stress-related growth. *Journal of Personality* **64**, 71–105.
Seligman, M. E. P. and Csikszentmihalyi, M. (2000). Positive psychology: an introduction. *American Psychologist* **55**, 5–14.
Stanton, A. L., Danoff-Burg, S., Sworowski, L. A., et al. (2002). Randomized controlled trial of written emotional expression and benefit finding in breast cancer patients. *Journal of Clinical Oncology* **20**, 4160–4168.
Tedeschi, R. G. and Calhoun, L. G. (2004). A clinical approach to posttraumatic growth. In: Linley, P. A. & Joseph, S. (eds.) *Positive psychology in practice*, pp. 405–419. Hoboken, NJ: John Wiley.
Tedeschi, R. G. and Calhoun, L. G. (2004). Posttraumatic growth: conceptual foundations and empirical evidence. *Psychological Inquiry* **15**, 1–18.
Tedeschi, R. G., Park, C. L. and Calhoun, L. G. (eds.) (1998). *Posttraumatic growth: positive changes in the aftermath of crisis*. Mahwah, NJ: Lawrence Erlbaum.
Tennen, H. and Affleck, G. (2002). Benefit-finding and benefit-reminding. In: Snyder, C. R. & Lopez, S. J. (eds.) *Handbook of positive psychology*, pp. 584–597. New York: Oxford University Press.

Psychosocial Factors and Stress

J Siegrist
University of Duesseldorf, Duesseldorf, Germany

This is a revised version of the article by J Siegrist, Encyclopedia of Stress First Edition, volume 3, pp 299–303, © 2000, Elsevier Inc.

Glossary

Self-efficacy — Personal beliefs about one's ability to master challenges.
Self-esteem — Firm feelings and beliefs about one's own worth as a person (influenced strongly by experience on how significant others react toward one's self early in life).
Social anomie — Lack of social rules and orientations in a social group, often associated with feelings of anxiety or helplessness.
Social capital — Patterns of cooperative social exchange in neighborhood and community life characterized by mutual commitment and trust.
Social role — Set of expectations or norms (duties, options) directed toward people who hold important social positions (e.g., family role, work role).
Type A behavior — Complex of behaviors and emotions defined by excessive striving, competitiveness, hostility, and impatience.

General Background

In evolutionary terms, the development of the human brain, particularly its neocortical structures, has critically advanced the species' capacity to cope with environmental challenges and threats. As a consequence, inherited biobehavioral patterns of response to threats to the integrity, survival, and reproduction of the organism have become more variable and complex compared to those of the nonhuman primates. Increasingly, these patterns of response depend on the appraisal of stimulus properties and available opportunities for successful agency and are modulated by prior experience, learned skills, and interpersonal support. This may hold true for responses to natural and man-made disasters and for chronically demanding socioenvironmental conditions. However, in all these instances, a person's sense of the control over the challenge and over his or her actions in dealing with it must be considered a crucial variable that triggers the quality and intensity of stressful experience. Stressful experience is defined as the experience of a mismatch between the demands put on an individual in a challenging situation and his or her ability to meet the situation with adequate responses. At the level of emotional reactions, this mismatch is likely to elicit feelings of anxiety, irritation, anger, disappointment, or even helplessness and despair. These emotions are often paralleled by sustained neuronal and neuroendocrine activation due to the existence of powerful neuronal circuits that link neocortical information processing with mesolimbic and brain stem activity.

Humans are particularly vulnerable to the distress-enhancing effects of socioenvironmental challenges and threats because the preservation of a person's self relies so heavily on his or her social surrounding. In human infancy, attachment behavior, which develops through reciprocal exchange with a caregiver, is essential for survival and normal psychological functioning. Later in childhood and adolescence, a person's social identity emerges from recurrent exchange with significant others. Moreover, in adult life, core social roles, such as the work role and the family and marital role, serve to link the individual person with a structured, goal-oriented social environment. Thus, important life domains that matter most for the individual person are inherently social in a cooperative or competitive sense.

Placed in this context, human health and well-being are closely related to successful self-regulation in a conducive social environment, and a stressful experience is likely to result from failed opportunities for successful agency, goal achievement, and reward experience in interpersonal exchange. The question then is what analytical concepts have been developed by the social and behavioral sciences to identify relevant socioenvironmental and personal triggers of recurrent stressful experience. The term psychosocial factor is used as a summary label to characterize the still-heterogeneous state of the art in this field. In other words, scientific progress has not yet resulted in a universally accepted taxonomy of stress-eliciting or stress-buffering social and personal (psychological) conditions.

This article presents a brief overview of some of the major concepts of identifying psychosocial influences on stress and health. The two main procedures mediating this association are (1) enhanced neuronal/neuroendocrine/neuroimmune activation and (2) initiation of health-damaging behaviors.

There are multiple ways in which social and personal factors interact in influencing health and disease. It is useful to think of a stream of events where the most distal parts, the upstream factors, relate to the society at large or its main institutions (the macrosocial influences) and where the most proximal parts, the downstream factors, concern an individual's close or immediate social surroundings (the microsocial influences) and his or her personal ways of coping with the environment. In the following section, the discussion of psychosocial factors starts with the more distal parts of this stream and then proceeds to more proximal phenomena, including person characteristics. Finally, special attention is given to concepts that focus explicitly on the interaction between person and environment.

Overview of Psychosocial Factors Influencing Stress and Health

Macrosocial and Microsocial Factors

Every human society is characterized by a set of social values, norms, and institutions that are instrumental for the survival and growth of its members. If these values and norms lose their validity and meaning, or if society's patterns of social exchange become unpredictable and unstable, individuals tend to suffer from states of social anomie (lack of rules and orientations). A number of epidemiological investigations have explored the adverse effects on health produced by sociocultural instability, rapid social change, or a high level of social anomie. A majority of these studies found evidence of elevated risks of subsequent physical and mental illness.

One type of study was conducted in native societies that, after a long period of social stability, experienced rapid sociocultural transformation. As a consequence, less solidarity was witnessed among group members, and more deviant behavior, including violence, crime, and disruption of social ties, occurred. Equally distressing, the internalized cultural canon, which had been developed over many generations, broke down. Essential beliefs and ways of interpreting life were lost or fragmented. Under these conditions, cardiovascular risk factors, particularly hypertension, and coronary heart disease manifestation became more prevalent.

Similar observations were made by investigators who followed migrant populations from their original places to new sociocultural environments. Interestingly, migrants who were able to maintain strong social ties with their traditional groups in the new environment were more likely to be protected against subsequent health risks compared to migrants who deprived themselves from these traditional bonds. This observation led to the conclusion that a stable social network and a particular quality of social exchange, termed social support, may act as a protective resource in coping with stressful circumstances. Social support is defined as the experience of, or access to, social relationships that offer mutual understanding and trust and that recurrently elicit positive emotions.

There is now convincing evidence that negative health effects result from social separation and social isolation, either due to loss of a loved one or due to poor opportunities for developing or maintaining relationships. Again, under these conditions, social support is less likely to be experienced and thus a strong psychosocial resource against stress is lacking.

While close social ties and social support denote downstream phenomena close to the intimate experiences made by individual persons, the more distal, macrostructural conditions of participating in the social fabric were shown to affect health as well. In particular, disinvestment in social capital was found to exert strong effects on morbidity and mortality at the level of whole populations. The term disinvestment in social capital describes a decline in reciprocal social exchange in neighborhood and community life, including a lack of solidarity and trust. For instance, when an area has a higher level of poverty, less investments are made into shared resources of community life, and hostile encounters or competitive struggles are more frequent.

Disinvestment in social capital is one of several health-adverse developments resulting from widening social inequalities. The demonstration of an inverse social gradient of morbidity and mortality within and between populations in a large number of advanced societies must be considered one of the most consistent and important findings of modern social epidemiology: the lower a person's socioeconomic status (in terms of educational attainment, income, and occupational standing), the higher his or her risk of poor health. These differentials are substantial. For instance, mean life expectancy in countries such as Finland or the United Kingdom is shortened by 5 to 6 years among members of the lowest as compared to the highest socioeconomic status group. It is important to note that these social differentials in health are spread across the whole of the society rather than being concentrated on a deprived group at the bottom of the society. So what are the causes of relative social deprivation in health?

Research repeatedly came to the conclusion that access to or quality of health care is not the main cause, as might be expected. Rather, unhealthy behaviors and exposure to stressful material and psychosocial environments, including lack of appropriate resources, must be considered the main determinants of social inequalities in health in advanced societies. These latter conditions include poor living and working conditions, threats to, or experience of, unemployment and income loss, and unstable social networks. Under these circumstances of relative social deprivation, feelings of anger, disapproval, and hopelessness are more frequent, intense, and long-lasting, thus aggravating the burden of stressful experience (see later).

Person Characteristics

Clearly, not every individual reacts to stressful environments in the same way. On the one hand, specific genetic or psychosocial factors may protect a person from adverse effects on health even under highly demanding circumstances. On the other hand, a person's threshold of susceptibility may be very low, thus predisposing him or her to illness onset under conditions of moderate stress. With the introduction of methods of molecular medicine into epidemiological studies, important advances in identifying people at elevated risk of disease were achieved. For instance, combining sociological information on stressful life events with genetic information on specific polymorphisms of the serotonin transporter receptor gene was shown to improve the prediction of early onset of depression in young adults.

One direction of research has focused on psychological traits that predispose an individual to spend high levels of energy. This pattern is functional if demands or threats are faced. However, in less demanding contexts, this may harm the organism by recurrent excessive physiological activation. Originally, researchers were interested in so-called type A behavior, a complex of behaviors and emotions defined by excessive striving, competitiveness, hostility, and impatience. Type A individuals were identified on the basis of specific psychomotor and speech characteristics, such as unrest, hectic, inability to relax, loud speech, and intrusive behaviors. As can be expected from a stress physiological perspective, excessive sympathoadrenergic arousal predisposes these individuals to cardiovascular dysfunction and disease.

Today, however, refined concepts following this direction of research are more successful in predicting future cardiovascular risk. One such concept concentrates on cognitive and affective components of hostility. The former include negative beliefs about people and negative attitudes toward others, such as cynicism and mistrust, whereas the latter focuses on a frequent and intense experience of anger. A high level of hostility was found to promote health-adverse behaviors such as smoking and alcohol use in adolescence and young adulthood. Moreover, increased sympathetic function in combination with decreased parasympathetic function was observed. This observation could explain at least part of the direct statistical associations between hostility and coronary heart disease incidence that have been reported from several studies.

A similar approach emphasizes cognitive-motivational mechanisms of excessive energy spending. People characterized by overcommitment when facing demands tend to misjudge (e.g., underestimate) challenging stimuli and to expose themselves to multiple obligations. This may be due to their strong desire to control or dominate their environment, to exceed others, and to experience approval. For instance, workaholic behavior in occupational contexts can be interpreted in this context (see later). After a period of continued overcommitment, these individuals are susceptible to a state of vital exhaustion and psychophysiological breakdown, particularly when confronted with loss of control and failure. Overcommitment has been identified as a cardiovascular risk factor in epidemiological and experimental investigations.

A second line of research demonstrates adverse health effects of passive behaviors and associated low levels of energy spending. Importantly, inhibition or withdrawal of activity due to depressive mood and cognitions of helplessness and lack of self-esteem was found not only in reaction to but also preceding any experience of severe threat or loss. Some investigations conclude that individuals characterized by these psychological traits are at elevated risk of suffering from reduced immunocompetence and its pathophysiological consequences. Thus, over- and underactivation of a person's potential of vital energy in relation to self-regulating processes affect health at more fundamental, cellular and subcellular, levels, e.g., by increasing endogeneous oxidation and decreasing DNA repair capacity.

Although these behavioral patterns are influenced, to some extent, by genetic predisposition, evidence indicates that socioenvironmental factors have a strong impact on gene expression via methylation of DNA. Again, combining research on epigenetic processes with sociobehavioral research has promise for advancing the frontiers of knowledge.

In conclusion, distinct personal traits have been identified that must be considered psychological risk factors or protective factors. Protective factors include a sense of mastery and self-efficacy (i.e., positive beliefs about one's agency) and favorable self-esteem, often paralleled by optimism and trust. Risk factors, as evidenced earlier, include overactive behaviors such as hostility, overcommitment, and excessive striving. These traits carry the risk of precipitating feelings of frustration and helplessness and triggering states of vital exhaustion. Moreover, risk factors include those cognitive, motivational, and affective traits that predispose individuals to withdraw from activity, to experience low levels of personal control and self-esteem, and to suffer from depressive mood and negative attributional style.

Person–Environment Interaction

Traditionally, the disciplines of medical sociology and social epidemiology have emphasized the role of socioenvironmental factors in health and disease, whereas medical psychology and psychosomatic medicine have stressed the importance of personality factors. Therefore, despite the obvious need for a more comprehensive analysis, few attempts were made to combine the two disciplinary approaches. Of these attempts, two developments deserve special attention.

First, in a period of declining impact of psychoanalytic thinking on etiological research, new interest emerged in understanding how socioenvironmental and personal factors interact in promoting health and triggering disease in a life course perspective. For instance, birth cohort studies demonstrate that adverse social circumstances of parents at the time of their children's birth increase the risk of premature mortality in children's later life. Explanations for this refer to elevated vulnerability during pregnancy and experience of cumulative cognitive, behavioral, and social disadvantage during childhood.

Among early psychological risk factors, a disturbed pattern of attachment between mother and child in infancy was shown to be of particular significance for later well-being. However, favorable social circumstances in childhood can compensate for these deficits to some extent by promoting children's resilience.

A second line of extensive research on how person and environment interact in producing stress-related disease has been concerned with the impact of working life on health. In contemporary societies, the work role still defines one of the crucial social roles in adulthood with powerful effects on successful or unsuccessful self-regulation. The adverse effects of job loss and related social isolation on health were mentioned earlier. Additional findings demonstrate that among low-status members of the workforce, stressful, health-damaging jobs in terms of a combination of high demands and low control are more prevalent. In this context, the model of effort–reward imbalance at work is of interest, as it explicitly combines situational and person characteristics.

This model claims that lack of reciprocity between costs spent and gains obtained at work (high-cost/

low-gain conditions) defines a state of emotional distress with special propensity to autonomic arousal and neuroendocrine stress response. Effort at work is spent as part of a socially organized exchange process to which society contributes in terms of rewards (money, esteem, and career opportunities). An imbalance between effort and reward is maintained if no alternative choice is available in the labor market. Moreover, people characterized by a high level of overcommitment and related cognitive distortion of demand appraisal (see earlier discussion) are equally prone to experience an effort–reward imbalance. Prospective epidemiological studies documented that stressful work in terms of high effort, low reward, and low control doubles the risk of incident fatal or nonfatal cardiovascular disease. In addition, onset of depression is more likely to occur.

Implications for Intervention

This article documents a solid body of research on the role of distinct psychosocial factors in triggering stress-related disease (risk factors) and in promoting health (protective factors). It highlights that both upstream (macrosocial) and downstream (microsocial and personal) factors are important in explaining elevated risk of morbidity and mortality. Finally, a combined approach focusing on person–environment interaction, including analyses of epigenetic processes, holds special promise for advancing scientific understanding and its consequences for prevention.

At all levels discussed so far, implications for intervention are obvious. At the macrostructural level, however, it is difficult to imagine how a reduction in the amount of relative social deprivation can be achieved. Policy measures such as limitations in income inequality, labor market regulations, and allocation of means to improve social capital can hardly be realized on the basis of anticipated health gain.

A more realistic approach toward intervention concerns the mesosocial level. For instance, several theory-based concepts of workplace health promotion have been implemented and evaluated. Reductions in blood pressure, heart rate variability, and levels of stress hormones and atherogenic lipids are examples of favorable health outcomes following task reorganization with enlarged decision latitude, improved social support, and improved leadership skills of superiors.

Similarly, more comprehensive intervention programs at the level of community, neighborhood, or school are being developed. Some of these programs pay special attention to sustained health gain in socially deprived groups or in high-risk groups. Examples are early-childhood family education programs, preschool programs, and adolescent health promotion activities. Improving successful parenting in socially deprived families was found to strengthen children's cognitive and emotional development.

Finally, an obvious level of intervention concerns the microsocial and personal level. Several behavioral intervention techniques have been developed and tested in both primary and secondary prevention. These include stress management, promotion of self-control and self-efficacy, personal empowerment, and an increase in social skills and coping effectiveness. These techniques proved to be particularly successful in reducing health-adverse behaviors such as unhealthy diet, smoking, alcohol, and drug consumption. In addition, the provision of social support and the formation of self-help groups are instrumental in reinforcing newly acquired attitudes, motivations, and behaviors. In summary, a rich potential of interpersonal and behavioral intervention approaches is now available that supplements traditional biomedical treatment techniques and that provides new opportunities for primary and secondary prevention. It is important to emphasize that this potential is based on scientific evidence obtained from pioneering research on psychosocial factors, stress, and health.

See Also the Following Articles

Hostility.

Further Reading

Antoniou, A. S. G. and Cooper, C. L. (eds.) (2005). *Research companion to organizational health psychology.* Cheltenham, UK: Edward Elgar.

Bandura, A. (1997). *Self efficacy: the exercise of control.* New York: Freeman.

Berkman, L. and Kawachi, I. (2000). *Social epidemiology.* Oxford, UK: Oxford University Press.

Caspi, A., Sugden, K., Moffitt, T. E., et al. (2003). Influence of life stress on depression. Moderation by a polymorphism in the 5-HTT-gene. *Science* **301**, 386–389.

Marmot, M. and Wilkinson, R. (eds.) (2005). *Social determinants of health.* Oxford, UK: Oxford University Press.

Orth-Gomer, K. and Schneiderman, N. (eds.) (1996). *Behavioral medicine approaches to cardiovascular disease prevention.* Mahwah, NJ: Erlbaum.

Siegrist, J. and Marmot, M. (eds.) (2006). *Social inequalities in health: new evidence and policy implications.* Oxford, UK: Oxford University Press.

Turner, J. R., Cardon, L. R. and Hewitt, J. K. (eds.) (1995). *Behavior genetic approaches in behavioral medicine.* New York: Plenum Press.

Weiner, H. (1992). *Perturbing the organism: the biology of stressful experience.* Chicago, IL: University of Chicago Press.

Quality of Life

S M Skevington
University of Bath, Bath, UK

Glossary

Subjective	Personal.
Objective	Detached from personal views.
Observable	Visible.
Perceptions	Views.
Functioning	What a person is capable of doing.
Encephalograph (EEG)	Measured electrical changes in brain waves.
Eustress	Positive or "good" stress.

The Concept of Quality of Life

Quality of life (QoL) has become a key goal of contemporary health care. It is often confused with standard-of-living. However, standard-of-living refers to the possession of wealth or material goods. Although a certain number of square feet of living space in United States, or oxen owned in Ethiopia, makes a tangible difference in people's lives, it does not necessarily bring greater happiness or well-being; we can observe this in lottery winners. International figures on annual income per capita collected by the World Bank show that once income exceeds a critical level – $13,000 in 1995 – the close relationship between subjective well-being and income becomes increasingly loose and dissipated. Furthermore, in the world's richest countries standard-of-living increases do not appear to make a significant difference to people's QoL, a finding that is highly perplexing for policy makers.

A consensus about how to define and measure QoL is still widely debated. In the 1970s, its definitions contained terminological similarities to definitions of stress. At a time when stress was seen as a phenomenon that exceeded people's resources, in order to provide a good QoL these resources needed to be adequate in terms of satisfying people's wants, needs, and capacities. Since then, definitions have placed greater emphasis on people's subjective perceptions of the important features of their life and, in particular, explored the varied meanings ascribed to these experiences. The ways in which people interpret life's events (e.g., as stressful or pleasant) affects how they see their QoL. Wenger et al. (1984) defined QOL as "an individual's perceptions of his or her functioning and well-being in different domains of life." Judgments about QoL are now seen as a rich interplay and balance between how people see their internal state, such as the tension in muscles or happiness, and the external events that impinge on them from their environment, such as changing jobs or being bereaved.

Assessment of Quality of Life

The history of QoL assessment measures shows that some of the earliest versions were designed by clinicians for their own use in distributing health-care resources, for example the assessment of Quality Adjusted Life Years (QALYS). This approach excluded a systematic assessment of patients' views, with the assumption that clinicians held a reasonably accurate view of their patients' QoL. However, research has consistently shown that QoL judgments by clinicians and other observers (e.g., spouses or caregivers) often correlate weakly with the views held by the patients about their own QoL. Such proxy information is therefore unreliable, and this is particularly apparent in the case of dementia or stroke, in which the patients' own perceptions can be difficult or impossible to obtain. This discrepancy arises from the observation that many aspects of QoL are simply not open to inspection but are hidden from view like the submerged parts of an iceberg. Furthermore, when measures have limited their contents to subjective reports of observable behaviors such as mobility and activities of daily living, it has resulted in the assessment of a constricted rather than holistic concept of QoL, due to the exclusion of important but invisible QoL issues such as spirituality and social relationships.

The need for QoL assessment in health has been driven by the problem-solving demands of clinical practice. The aim was to better understand the patient's priorities in order to deliver appropriate care. However, this approach may have provided an unduly negative view of QoL. Patients expect to report their problems during a consultation and to do this succinctly. In these time-limited conditions, they are unlikely to also discuss the positive qualities of life such as the pleasure they get from playing with children, listening to Mozart, or seeing a dewdrop on a leaf. Consequently, many measures have tended to focus on assessing symptoms and dysfunctional aspects of life to the exclusion of the good life. This not only gives health professionals the view that the QoL of their patients is worse than it is, but it also causes the patients who complete the questionnaire to report feeling miserable after focusing unduly on the bad things instead of a more balanced life. Even highly disabled, chronic-pain patients entering a pain management program after many surgical and pharmacological treatments report that chronic pain affects only half the important qualities of life when a range of positive and negative issues are presented for evaluation. The good life was acknowledged by Aristotle and several eighteenth-century philosophers, but has only recently been endorsed again as pertinent to outcomes measurements in health care. Hence, more recent definitions of QoL have sought to emphasize a positive orientation: "The essential characteristics of life, which in the general public is often interpreted as the positive values of life, or the good parts of life, or the total existence of an individual, group or society" (Lindstrom, 1992).

The Example of Sleep as a Quality of Life

Another debate concerns the type of information that constitutes the best measure of QoL, and here sleep provides a suitable example. Researchers have assessed sleep-related QoL by tracing electroencephalograph (EEG) waves, considering this to be an objective indicator. Others assess the timing of sleep and wakening, insomnia patterns, medication use, and so forth, in looking at people's objective perceptions of their sleep. However, we can argue that information derived from either of these channels of inquiry tells us only indirectly about people's QoL. These types of information require further interpretation by the researchers, and their own assumptions may lead them to draw an erroneous conclusion. Would the people you know see your QoL as good or bad if you told them you slept 3 h a night? What about 12 h a night? Without additional information about whether that sleep was refreshing, it is not possible to draw an accurate conclusion. For this reason the most reliable way to avoid this pitfall is to ask subjective QoL questions such as whether people find their sleep to be refreshing or not. Conclusions about these qualities cannot, therefore, be deduced; direct questioning about the meaning of events is required. Like stressful life events (e.g., divorce), it is the interpretation that matters. Although all these three types of information are themselves valuable and can be used together to form a fuller picture, we contend that QoL is best measured as a subjective phenomenon and that the use of the term should be restricted to this type of information.

The World Health Organisation Definition

Questions have been raised about whether QoL is a global phenomenon or just a Western concept. Although culture has sometimes been included in QoL models, it is usually seen as extraneous and additional, rather than taking a central role in explaining the diverse ways in which different cultural groups interpret QoL. Concerned to understand QoL relating to global health, the World Health Organisation views culture as a "lens" through which people interpret the experiences that affect their QoL. It defines QoL as "an individual's perception of their position in life, in the context of the culture and value systems in which they live, and in relation to their goals, expectations, standards, and concerns" (World Health Organisation Quality of Life Group, 1994: 43). This unusual definition also implies that comparisons are used in helping to make decisions about QoL; that in evaluating their own QoL, people consider how far they have achieved their goals, expectations, and standards, in addition to considering problematic concerns.

Dimensions of Quality of Life

So what does a good QoL consist of, and is there consensus about whether these dimensions are universal? Many hundreds of QoL questionnaires have included the two broad components of physical and mental health identified by Descartes as essential. However, physical health is operationalized in some assessments in terms of symptoms; adding symptoms does not give a clear view of people's QoL because, paradoxically, patients with many symptoms often report a relatively good QoL and, conversely, those with very few symptoms report it to be poor. Measures also often include estimates of independence or functional status, such as mobility, activities of daily living, and so on. Physicians have traditionally favored those QoL dimensions for which they can independently inspect corroborating evidence alongside the subjective reports. Some issues such as spirituality have largely been ignored as being too difficult to measure and/or irrelevant to health and health care.

The universality of QoL and its dimensions have been addressed by the World Health Organisation Quality of Life (WHOQOL) Group, which has confirmed that physical, psychological, independence, social relations, environmental and spiritual dimensions are important in a wide range of cultures and settings and to sick and well people. Within these broad domains, the group confirms 25 detailed aspects (facets) of QoL that are reliable and valid internationally. A series of novel procedures was used by the WHOQOL Group to create several multilingual instruments and a short version – the WHOQOL-Bref – is now available in over 50 different languages. In addition to the main measures, add-on modules of extra questions have recently become available to support work on spirituality, human immunodeficiency virus (HIV)/acquired immunodeficiency syndrome (AIDS), older adults, and pain. The WHOQOL results provide support for the view that there is broad recognition and universal agreement about a concept called QoL, even though it may not be labeled as such, and that there are cultural variations in the relative importance of the dimensions included, as well as in how these issues themselves are expressed.

Uses of Quality of Life Assessments

QoL assessments are used for monitoring outcomes (e.g., after policy change). In particular, they are valued widely as a suitable outcome measure in randomized controlled clinical trials. Although outcomes are the main focus here, it is worth noting that QoL can also be investigated as a process. Because psychometric measures are designed to tap into outcomes, the results from these instruments provide merely a snapshot of QoL at one time in an ever-adjusting process. Different theories and techniques may be needed to investigate how and when QoL changes over time and precisely which factors (e.g., stress and eustress) affect positive and negative changes.

Further Reading

Coen, R. F. (1999). Individual quality of life and assessment by carers or 'proxy' respondents. In: Joyce, C. R. B., O'Boyle, C. A. & & McGee, H. (eds.) *Individul quality of life: approaches to coceptualization anassessment*, pp. 185–196. Amsterdam: Harwood Academic.

Inglehardt, R. and Klingemann, H. D. (2000). Genes, culture, democracy and happiness. In: Diener, E. & & Suh, E. M. (eds.) *Culture subjective well-being*, pp. 185–218. Cambridge, MA: MIT Press.

Layard, R. (2005). *Happiness: lessons from a new science.* London: Penguin Books.

Lindstrom, B. (1992). Quality of life – a model for evaluating health for all: conceptual considerations and policy implications. *Sozial und Preventivmedizin* **37**, 301–306.

Shin, D. C. and Johnson, D. M. (1978). Avowed happiness as an overall assessment of quality of life. *Social Indicators Research* 5, 475–492.

Skevington, S. M. (2002). Advancing cross-cultural research on quality of life: observations drawn from the WHOQOL development. *Quality of Life Research* **11**, 135–144.

Skevington, S. M., Lotfy, M. and O'Connell, K. A. (2004). The World Health Organisation's WHOQOL-BREF Quality of Life assessment: psychometric properties and results of the international field trial – a report from the WHOQOL Group. *Quality of Life Research* **13**, 299–310.

Skevington, S. M., Sartorius, N., Amir, M., et al. (2004). Developing methods for assessing quality of life in different cultural settings: the history of the WHOQOL instruments. *Social Psychiatry and Psychiatric Epidemiology* **39**, 1–8.

Skevington, S. M. and Wright, A. (2001). Changes in the quality of life of patients receiving anti-depressant medication in primary care: validating the WHOQOL-100. *British Journal of Psychiatry* **178**, 261–267.

Staquet, M. J., Hayes, R. D. and Fayers, P. M. (1998). *Quality of life assessment in clinical trials: methods and practice.* Oxford: Oxford University Press.

Wenger, N. K., Mattson, M. E., Furberg, C. D., et al. (1984). Assessment of quality of life in clinical trials of cardiovascular therapies. *American Journal of Cardiology* **54**, 908–913.

World Health Organisation Quality of Life Group (1994). The development of the World Health Organisation Quality of Life assessment instrument (The WHOQOL). In: Orley, J. & & Kuyken, W. (eds.). *Quality of life assessment: international perspectives*, pp. 41–60. Berlin: Springer-Verlag.

World Health Organisation Quality of Life Group (1995). The World Health Organisation Quality of Life assessment (WHOQOL): position paper from the World Health Organisation. *Social Science & Medicine* **41**, 1403–1409.

World Health Organisation Quality of Life Group (1998). The World Health Organization Quality of Life assessment (WHOQOL): development and general psychometric properties. *Social Science & Medicine* **46**, 1569–1585.

Aggression

E F Coccaro and E C Manning
University of Chicago, Chicago, IL, USA

This is a revised version of the article by E F Coccaro, Encyclopedia of Stress First Edition, volume 1, pp 95–99, © 2000, Elsevier Inc.

Glossary

Antisocial behavior — Behavior in which the rights of others are violated; includes behavior that provides grounds for arrest, deceitfulness, failure to honor obligations, lack of remorse, and irritability and aggressiveness against people and property (i.e., vandalism).

Criminal behavior — Behavior in which a crime is committed, usually behavior that is identified by the criminal justice system.

Delinquent behavior — Antisocial behavior seen in children and adolescents, including aggression and other dysfunctional behaviors (e.g., school truancy).

Epidemiological survey — A study in which a representative sample of a population of individuals is studied to estimate the number of individuals

	from that general population that have a certain condition or diagnosis.
Functional magnetic resonance imaging (fMRI)	fMRI is the abbreviation for functional magnetic resonance imaging. fMRI allows imaging of brain-related activity in response to human subjects involved in cognitive or emotional tasks.
Genetic studies	Studies that are designed to estimate whether a condition or disorder has an underlying genetic component. These include family studies, which can show whether a condition runs in families; twin studies, which can show whether a condition is more likely to occur in identical than in fraternal twins and therefore must have a genetic component; and adoption studies, which can show the separate and interactive contributions of environmental and genetic factors.
Heritability estimate	A mathematical estimate of the magnitude of the importance of the role of genetic factors in a condition or disorder.
Neurochemistry	The aspect of biological functioning related to chemicals that transmit neuronal signals from one nerve to another.
Norepinephrine (NE)	NE is the abbreviation for norepinephrine, one of the main monoamines in the brain. NE is widely distributed in the brain and is involved in mediating a variety of brain and behavioral functions including, but not limited to, arousal.
Problem solving	The ability to find solutions to everyday types of problems.
Psychosocial influences	Potential influences on behavior (or on conditions/disorders) that are not apparently due to genetic or biological factors.
Serotonin (5-hydrotryptamine, 5-HT)	5-HT is the abbreviation for serotonin, one of the main monoamines in the brain. 5-HT is widely distributed and is involved in mediating a variety of brain and behavioral functions including, but not limited to, behavioral inhibition.
Transgenerational studies	Studies comparing different generations (e.g., grandparents, parents, and offspring).
Violent behavior	Behavior in which physical aggression in some form is present.

Types of Aggression

Aggression can be defined as intentional act committed by an individual that has the potential to result in the physical or emotional harm of a person or of an object. Although aggression is typically thought of as constituting a physical assault, acts of aggression also include verbal outbursts in which the individual's voice is used to convey anger in an uncontrolled manner. Broadly speaking, aggression can be subdivided into two types: impulsive aggression and premeditated or nonimpulsive aggression. Aggression is impulsive when the aggressive act is unplanned or in response to an aversive stimulus, generally uncontrolled, and committed without the expectation of achieving a tangible objective. By contrast, premeditated aggression is controlled, involves planning, and is associated with an expectation of reaching a specific goal such as, for example, the intimidation of the victim. Although acts of impulsive aggression can sometimes be criminal in nature, premeditated aggression is more likely to occur in the context of other criminal behavior. Because impulsive, rather than premeditated, aggression appears to be associated with specific biological and pharmacological response characteristics, this review focuses on impulsive aggression.

Epidemiology of Aggression

Despite the clinical importance of impulsive aggression, there is very little epidemiological data specifically regarding impulsive aggressive behavior. Existing epidemiological data exclusively refer to homicide and physical assault (i.e., aggression in general). Currently, the age-adjusted rate for homicide in the United States, based on vital statistics records, is 0.01%. Epidemiologic survey data find that approximately 25% of all males report a history of some physical fighting since 18 years of age, a rate that is twice as high as is found in adult females. Accordingly, approximately 10–15% of the general population report that they have engaged in physical fighting as an adult. This proportion translates into at least 25.0–37.5 million individuals in the United States alone. Although we cannot know what proportion of homicides or physical assault were impulsive in nature, it is likely that a substantial proportion represent impulsive aggressive acts.

Genetics of Aggression

Data from twin, adoption, and family studies support the hypothesis that aggression is under significant, if variable, genetic influence. The differences seen in these results are due, most likely, to the fact that different studies examined aggression in different ways using differing assessment measures. Specifically, aggression has been examined in these types of studies by using categories that more or less reflect aggression (such as delinquent behavior, antisocial behavior, criminal behavior, and violent behavior) in populations with psychiatric diagnoses or by using scales that more or less reflect the severity of aggression in the general population or in university students. In clinical populations, genetic influences appear to underlie both delinquent behavior and antisocial behavior. In general populations, heritability estimates for measures of aggression range from substantial in children to moderately substantial in adults (44–72%) to apparently nonexistent in adolescents. Most noteworthy is the observation that the aggression measures with the greatest heritability estimates reflect anger and hostility and/or anger, impulsiveness, and irritability. These are the type of behavioral traits that appear to be associated with impulsive aggressive behaviors and that, in turn, have been shown to be strongly correlated with biological factors and with psychopharmacological responses to treatment with anti-aggressive agents.

Psychosocial Factors in Aggression

The most important psychosocial factors involved in the development of aggression appear to be low socioeconomic status (SES), ineffective parenting style, physical punishment during childhood, and exposure to aggression in- and outside the family. Factors involved in maintaining aggression appear to be the poor development of problem-solving skills, a bias to attribute hostile intent to others, and a deficiency in appropriately detecting environmental and social cues.

Low Socioeconomic Status and Parenting Style

Low SES has been linked to the development of aggression in numerous studies. However, it is likely that low SES exerts its effect on aggression through more relevant behavioral factors such as being raised in a criminally violent family and exposure to gang activity and violence. The stress associated with poverty is associated with negative parental interactions and, consequently, parental irritability, a factor that was associated with aggressiveness in children. More specifically, marital problems in low-SES families has been linked to aggression in children. In addition, an association between lack of maternal responsiveness (and poor child rearing) in low-SES homes and aggressiveness has also been reported, a finding consistent with earlier reports showing that nonnurturing parents tend to have aggressive children. A critical predictor in this regard appears to be the lack of favorable warmth toward the children. This factor appears to be associated with the impairment of effective parenting so that children in these families do not fully internalize the difference between right and wrong.

Exposure to Violence

Exposure to violence both inside and outside the home has also been linked to aggression. Physical punishment and child abuse has also been associated with the development of aggression in children. In transgenerational studies, parents who behaved aggressively toward their children had aggressive children who, in turn, raised similarly aggressive children. Harsh discipline and child abuse (regardless of SES) appears to specifically predict the development of impulsive, but not nonimpulsive, aggressive behavior in children. Witnessing aggression has also been associated with the development and instigation of aggression, and it is likely that the presence of aggressive environmental cues may increase the immediate risk of aggression in susceptible individuals.

Deficiency in Problem Solving

A deficiency in problem-solving skills has been noted to be involved in the maintenance of aggression in impulsive aggressive children in particular. Impulsive aggressive children tend to have interpersonal problems and often get rejected by their peers. Although aggressiveness may appear to be a prime reason for peer rejection, cognitive factors may also play a role in this regard. Specifically, aggressive children tend to attribute hostile intent to others with whom they are interacting. It is important to note that the attribution of hostile intent to others may act as the provocation for an aggressive encounter. This hostile attribution is specific to their own interactions; these children do not attribute hostile intentions to other children with whom they are not interacting. The tendency of aggressive children to attribute hostile intent to others may be related to the observation that aggressive children, specifically impulsive aggressive children, have difficulty reading relevant social cues. For example, impulsive, but not nonimpulsive, aggressive children have been found to incorrectly label a visual cue (i.e., a sad face is identified as reflecting another emotion).

It is important to recognize, however, that these various psychosocial factors demonstrate a variable association with aggressive behavior. Like genetic factors, psychosocial factors can only predict aggressiveness as a probabilistic function of who may become aggressive given the presence of other factors. Clues to understanding this finding may be found in examining the role of biology in aggressive behavior.

Biology of Aggression

Among the constitutional/developmental biological factors possibly involved in aggression, the most studied factors relate to brain neurochemistry, specifically to monoamines such as serotonin (5-HT) and other centrally acting neurotransmitters.

Serotonin

The evidence for a role of brain 5-HT in human aggression is especially strong. In fact, the inverse relationship between impulsive aggressive behavior is the most consistent of all findings in biological psychiatry. Various measures reflecting brain 5-HT function have been shown to correlate inversely with life history, self-report questionnaire, and laboratory measures of aggression. Most notable is the replicated observation that evidence of reduced central 5-HT is present in impulsive, but not premeditated, aggressive subjects. This indicates that impulsive aggressive behavior can be distinguished biologically from nonimpulsive aggression and, accordingly, is a valid subtype of human aggressive behavior. An inverse relationship between 5-HT and aggression is reported in most, although not all, studies. However, when studies are at variance with this basic finding, issues related to sample populations probably account for the differences in reported findings.

Nonserotonin Systems

Catecholamines and vasopressin Although there are less data available to support the role of non-5-HT brain systems and modulators in human impulsive aggression, there are limited data suggesting a facilitatory role for catecholamines (i.e., dopamine and NE) and vasopressin in impulsive aggressive behavior. The relationship of catecholamines and vasopressin to aggression and serotonin, specifically, is noteworthy. In the case of the catecholamines, the typically inverse relationship between aggression and 5-HT may not be seen when catecholamine system function is reduced. Accordingly, correlations between measures of 5-HT and aggression are generally absent in depressed subjects, who typically demonstrate diminished NE system function. In the case of central vasopressin and aggression, 5-HT appears to be inversely related to both central vasopressin and aggression in both animal and human subjects. In human subjects, the relationship between central vasopressin and aggression is present even after vasopressin's relationship with 5-HT is accounted for. In animal studies, both central vasopressin activity and aggression can be suppressed by treatment with selective serotonin reuptake inhibitor (SSRI) agents.

Testosterone and cholesterol In addition to non-5-HT central neurotransmitters, at least two peripheral substances appear to have a relationship with aggression. Based on data from both animal and human studies, testosterone appears to have a facilitatory relationship with aggression. The relationship among testosterone, aggression, and 5-HT is less clear, although chronic testosterone exposure appears to downregulate central 5-HT receptors in some studies.

Another peripheral, although centrally active, substance that appears to influence aggressive behavior is cholesterol. Over the past decade, data from a variety of studies suggest that a reduction in circulating levels of cholesterol may be associated with an increase in aggressive behavior in both human and animal subjects. Although a link to 5-HT has not been conclusively demonstrated in human subjects, studies in nonhuman primates clearly demonstrate that a reduction in circulating cholesterol levels is associated with a reduction in measures that reflect central 5-HT function.

Localization of Biological Abnormalities

Reductions in cerebrospinal fluid (CSF) levels of neurotransmitter metabolites (e.g., 5-HIAA) suggest a central location for alterations in biological systems. However, CSF metabolites cannot reflect abnormalities in specific locations. Abnormalities in hormonal responses to pharmaco-challenge agents do suggest an abnormality in the hypothalamus (a part of the limbic system involved in the regulation of emotion and behavior) of impulsive aggressive individuals. Recent clinical neuroscience and brain-imaging studies have reported data suggesting the hypofunction of parts of the prefrontal cortex and relative hyperfunction of deeper subcortical structures. For example, fluorodeoxyglucose positron emission tomography (FDG-PET) scan data demonstrate lower metabolic rates bilaterally in the lateral and medial areas of the prefrontal cortex of impulsive, but not premeditated, murderers than in normal controls. In contrast, the metabolic rates of subcortical structures (e.g., hippocampus, amygdala, thalamus, and midbrain) in the right hemisphere were found to be elevated in both impulsive and premeditated murderers compared with normal controls. More recent data from fMRI studies suggest a dysfunction of the amygdala-orbital prefrontal cortex such that there is greater activation of the amygdala and less activation of the orbital frontal prefrontal cortex. Because prefrontal structures are thought to regulate inhibition and subcortical structures, such as amygdala, are thought to regulate arousal, these data suggest that impulsive aggressive individuals have, compared to normal controls, less prefrontal inhibition in the context of greater subcortical emotional drive. Premeditated aggressive individuals, by contrast have normal prefrontal inhibition but greater subcortical emotional drive. These data, in addition to the neurotransmitter-specific data already discussed, suggest that aggression in impulsive aggressive individuals can be treated by strategies that increase prefrontal inhibitory mechanisms and reduce subcortical facilitatory mechanisms.

Psychopharmacology of Aggression

As might be expected from the results of the biological study of aggression, several psychopharmacological agents appear to have anti- or pro-aggressive effects. The classes of agents shown to have anti-aggressive effects in double-blind, placebo-controlled trials include mood stabilizers (e.g., lithium), 5-HT uptake inhibitors (e.g., fluoxetine), anticonvulsants (e.g., diphenhydantoin, carbamazepine, and depakote), and NE beta-blockers (e.g., propanolol and nadolol). The classes of agents that may have pro-aggressive effects include tricylic antidepressants (e.g., amitriptyline), benzodiazapines (e.g., alprazolam), and stimulant and hallucinatory drugs of abuse (e.g., amphetamines, cocaine, and phencyclidine). The most notable findings from the relatively small literature of the double-blind, placebo-controlled, clinical trials of anti-aggressive agents is that their anti-aggressive efficacy is limited to the impulsive, and not the nonimpulsive, aggressive individual. This indicates that psychopharmacology at this time may have little to offer society in the management of criminally motivated aggression. It remains to be seen, however, what the effect of treatment using agents that possibly dampen the function of deeper subcortical structures might be in a group of nonimpulsively aggressive individuals. A second potentially important finding is emerging evidence of a differential psychopharmacology in this area so that some subjects may respond to some agents but not others. In our recent studies with fluoxetine, we noted an inverse relationship between pretreatment 5-HT function and anti-aggressive response to fluoxetine. Moreover, most fluoxetine nonresponders appeared to respond to treatment with divalproate, and the latter drug has also been shown to have anti-aggressive activity in selected impulsive aggressive patients with personality disorder. Given, the differential biology of impulsive aggression, it is likely that multiple strategies may be effective in impulsive aggressive individuals, depending on their own individual neurobiological substrate.

See Also the Following Articles

Domestic Violence.

Further Reading

Barratt, E. S., Stanford, M. S., Felthous, A. R., et al. (1997). The effects of phenytoin on impulsive and premeditated aggression: a controlled study. *Journal of Clinical Psychopharmacology* **17**, 341–349.

Best, M., Williams, J. M. and Coccaro, E. F. (2002). Evidence for a dysfunctional prefrontal circuit in patients with an impulsive aggressive disorder. *Proceedings of the National Academy of Sciences USA* **99**, 8448–8453.

Coccaro, E. F. (1998). Central neurotransmitter function in human aggression. In: Maes, M. & Coccaro, E. (eds.) *Neurobiology and clinical views on aggression and impulsivity*, pp. 143–168. New York: John Wiley & Sons.

Coccaro, E. F. (2003). Intermittent explosive disorder. In: Coccaro, E. F. (ed.) *Aggression, psychiatric treatment and assessment*, pp. 149–166. New York: Marcel Dekker.

Coccaro, E. F. and Kavoussi, R. J. (1997). Fluoxetine and impulsive aggressive behavior in personality disordered subjects. *Archives of General Psychiatry* **54**, 1081–1088.

Coccaro, E. F., Siever, L. J., Klar, H. M., et al. (1989). Serotonergic studies in affective and personality disorder: correlates with suicidal and impulsive aggressive behavior. *Archives of General Psychiatry* **46**, 587–599.

Cowdry, R. W. and Gardner, D. L. (1988). Pharmacotherapy of borderline personality disorder: alprazolam, carbamazepine, trifluroperazine, and trancypromine. *Archives of General Psychiatry* **45**, 111–119.

Dodge, K. A., Lochman, J. E., Harnish, J. D., et al. (1997). Reactive and proactive aggression in school children and psychiatrically impaired chronically assaultive youth. *Journal of Abnormal Psychology* **106**, 37–51.

Hollander, E., Tracy, K. A., Swann, A. C., et al. (2003). Divalproex in the treatment of impulsive aggression: efficacy in Cluster B personality disorders. *Neuropsychopharmacology* **28**, 1186–1197.

Huesmann, L. R., Leonard, E., Lefkowitz, M., et al. (1984). Stability of aggression over time and generations. *Developmental Psychopathology* **20**, 1120–1134.

Kavoussi, R. K. and Coccaro, E. F. (1998). Divalproex sodium for impulsive aggressive behavior in patients with personality disorder. *Journal of Clinical Psychiatry* **59**, 676–680.

Linnoila, M., Virkkunen, M., Scheinin, M., et al. (1983). Low cerebrospinal fluid 5-hydroxyindolacetic acid concentration differentiates impulsive from nonimpulsive violent behavior. *Life Sciences* **33**, 2609–2614.

Miles, C. G. (1997). Genetic and environmental architecture of human aggression. *Journal of Personality and Social Psychology* **72**, 207–217.

Raine, A., Meloy, J. R., Bihrle, S., et al. (1998). Reduced prefrontal and increased subcortical brain functioning assessed using positron emission tomography in predatory and affective murderers. *Behavioral Sciences & the Law* **16**, 319–332.

Virkkunen, M., Rawlings, R., Tokola, R., et al. (1994). CSF biochemistries, glucose metabolism, and diurnal activity rhythms in alcoholic, violent offenders, fire setters, and healthy volunteers. *Archives of General Psychiatry* **51**, 20–27.

Anger

R W Novaco
University of California, Irvine, CA, USA

This is a revised version of the article by R W Novaco, Encyclopedia of Stress First Edition, volume 1, pp 188–194, © 2000, Elsevier Inc.

Glossary

Aggression Behavior intended to cause psychological or physical harm to someone or to a surrogate target. The behavior may be verbal or physical, direct or indirect.

Anger A negatively toned emotion, subjectively experienced as an aroused state of antagonism toward someone or something perceived to be the source of an aversive event.

Anger reactivity Responding to aversive, threatening, or other stressful stimuli with anger reactions characterized by automaticity of engagement, high intensity, and short latency.

Cathartic effect The lowering of the probability of aggression as a function of the direct expression of aggression toward an anger instigator. The lowering of arousal associated with such catharsis is more or less immediate and can be reversed by re-instigation.

Escalation of provocation Incremental increases in the probability of anger and aggression, occurring as reciprocally heightened antagonism in an interpersonal exchange.

Excitation transfer The carryover of undissipated arousal, originating from some prior source, to a new situation having a new source of arousal, which then heightens the probability of aggression toward that new and more proximate source.

Hostility An attitudinal disposition of antagonism toward another person or social system. It represents a predisposition to respond with aggression under conditions of perceived threat.

Inhibition A restraining influence on anger expression. The restraint many be associated with either external or internal factors.

Anger and Stress

Anger is a negatively toned emotion, subjectively experienced as an aroused state of antagonism toward someone or something perceived to be the source of an aversive event. It is triggered or provoked situationally by events that are perceived to constitute deliberate harm-doing by an instigator toward oneself or toward those to whom one is endeared. Provocations usually take the form of insults, unfair treatments, or intended thwartings. Anger is prototypically experienced as a justified response to some wrong that has been done. While anger is situationally triggered by acute, proximal occurrences, it is shaped and facilitated contextually by conditions affecting the cognitive, arousal, and behavioral systems that comprise anger reactions. Anger activation is centrally linked to threat perceptions and survival responding.

As a normal human emotion, anger has considerable adaptive value, although there are sociocultural variations in the acceptability of its expression and the form that such expression takes. In the face of adversity, it can mobilize psychological resources, energize behaviors for corrective action, and facilitate perseverance. Anger serves as a guardian to self-esteem, operates as a means of communicating negative sentiment, potentiates the ability to redress grievances, and boosts determination to overcome obstacles to our happiness and aspirations. Akin to aggressive behavior, anger has functional value for survival.

Despite having multiple adaptive functions, anger also has maladaptive effects on personal and social well-being. Generally, strong physiological arousal impairs the processing of information and lessens cognitive control of behavior. Because heightened physiological arousal is a core component of anger, people are not cognitively proficient when they become angry. Also, because the activation of anger is accompanied by aggressive impulses, anger can motivate harm toward other people, which in turn can produce undesirable consequences for the angered person, from direct retaliation, loss of supportive relationships, or social censure. An angry person is not optimally alert, thoughtful, empathic, prudent, or physically healthy. Being a turbulent emotion ubiquitous in everyday life, anger is now known to be substantially associated with stress-related cardiovascular disorders, both coronary heart disease and essential hypertension. Anger is also a symptom of posttraumatic stress disorder (PTSD), and it has high relevance to the PTSD derivative of violent crime victimization and especially to combat or war zone exposure.

The Experience and Expression of Anger

There is a duality of psychosocial images associated with anger experience and anger expression. The emotional state is depicted as eruptive, destructive, unbridled, savage, venomous, burning, and consuming but also as energizing, empowering, justifying, signifying, rectifying, and relieving. The metaphors, on the one hand, connote something pressing for expression and utilization, but on the other, imply something requiring containment and control. This duality in psychosocial imagery reflects conflicting intuitions about anger, its expression, and its consequences that abound in ordinary language and are reflected in both scholarly literature and artistic works from the classical period to contemporary times. This Janus-faced character of anger foils attempts to understand it and to therapeutically intervene with recurrently angry individuals.

The facial and skeletal musculature are strongly affected by anger, mobilized by a mixture of adrenaline and noradrenaline hormonal secretions. The face becomes flushed, and the brow muscles move inward and downward, fixing a hard stare on the target. The nostrils flare, and the jaw tends toward clenching. This is an innate pattern of facial expression that can be observed in toddlers. Tension in the skeletal musculature, including raising of the arms and adopting a squared-off stance, are preparatory actions for attack and defense. The muscle tension provides a sense of strength and self-assurance. An impulse to strike out accompanies this subjective feeling of potency. From an evolutionary perspective, our perceptual system has been shaped to detect angry faces rapidly, especially those of angry males.

When people report anger experiences, they most typically give accounts of things that have happened to them. For the most part, they describe events physically and temporally proximate to their anger arousal. As a rule, they provide accounts of provocations ascribed to events in the immediate situation of the anger experience. This fosters the illusion that anger has a discrete external cause. The provocation sources are ordinarily identified as the aversive and deliberate behavior of others; thus, anger is portrayed in the telling as being something about which anger is quite fitting. People are very much inclined to attribute the causes of their anger to the personal, stable, and controllable aspects of another person's behavior.

However, the response to the question "What has made you angry?" hinges on self-observational proficiencies and is often based on intuitions. Precisely because getting angry involves a loss in self-monitoring capacity, people are neither good nor objective observers when they are angry. When inspecting any particular episode, the immediate causes of the anger are readily identifiable. Far less commonly do people disaggregate their anger experiences into multi-causal origins, some of which may be prior, remote events and ambient circumstances, rather than acute, proximal events. Anger experiences are embedded or nested within an environmental-temporal context. Disturbances that may not have involved anger at the outset leave residues that are not readily recognized but that operate as a lingering backdrop for focal provocations.

Anger is inherently a disposition to respond aggressively, but aggression is not an automatic consequence of anger because aggressive behavior is regulated by inhibitory control mechanisms, engaged by internal and external cues. In this regard, physical constraints, expectations of punishment or retaliation, empathy, consideration of consequences, and prosocial values operate as regulatory controls on aggression. While the experience of anger creates a readiness to respond with aggression, that disposition may be otherwise directed, suppressed, or reconstituted. Thus, the expression of anger is differentiated from its experience.

One aspect of anger that influences the probability of aggression is its degree of intensity. The higher the level of arousal, the stronger the motivation for aggression and the greater the likelihood that inhibitory controls will be overridden. Strong arousal not only impels action, but also impairs cognitive processing of aggression-mitigating information. A person in a state of high anger arousal is perceptually biased toward the confirmation of threat, is less able to attend to threat-discounting elements of the situation, and is not so capable of re-appraising provocation cues as benign. Because anger and aggression occur in a dynamic interactional context, the occurrence of aggression will, in turn, influence the level of anger. Thus, anger reactivity can be seen as a mode of responding characterized by automaticity, high intensity, and short latency.

Important forms of the dynamic interrelation of anger and aggression are the escalation of provocation and the cathartic effect. Escalation involves increases away from equilibrium, whereby succeeding events intensify their own precursors. In the case of anger and aggression, escalation refers to incremental change in their respective probabilities, occurring as reciprocally heightened antagonism in an interpersonal exchange. Anger-elicited aggression may evoke further anger in response, progressively generating justification for retaliation. In contrast, when physical aggression is deployed by an angry person against the anger instigator and there is no retaliation, anger arousal and further aggression are diminished. This is called the cathartic effect – its conditions should not be confused (as they often are) with those involving aggression by non-angry people, vicarious or observed aggression, or aggression not received by the anger instigator. However, the arousal-reducing effect of aggression carried out by angry people against those who have made them angry is reinforcing of aggressive behavior. This means that when anger is reinstated by a new provocation, the likelihood of aggressive behavior is increased. The cathartic expression of anger, whether through destructive aggression or through verbal communication intended to be constructive, can be understood as an organismic action to restore equilibrium.

An alternative to the deliberate expression of anger is suppression, which is largely a product of inhibitory controls. Anger suppression can be functional in promoting interpersonal or social conciliation. For example, when there is a high probability of impending violence, it is prudent to restrain anger expression to diminish the likelihood of triggering a physical assault. Whether in a domestic, occupational, or street context, anger is adaptively muffled when physical retaliation can be expected or when a cool head is needed to solve a problem. In the short term, suppressing even the verbalization of anger not only may be beneficial interpersonally, but also may lead to more regulated physiological reactivity levels. However, recurrent deployment of anger suppression as a stress-coping style will most likely have deleterious effects on cardiovascular health, as has been found for essential hypertension.

Because anger and aggression are thought to be differentially socialized for males and females, the question of gender differences in the experience and expression of anger arises. It has generally been found that the anger of women is comparable to that of men from the standpoint of experienced intensity. However, the style of anger expression varies by gender, especially according to the context of anger activation and its anticipated consequences. Males are more likely to be angered in a public place or by impersonal triggers, whereas females are more likely to be angered at home or by being let down by someone close to them. Females are more likely to become angered by verbal aggression and insensitive/condescending behavior, and males are more likely to be angered by behavior causing physical harm. Men, when angered, are more inclined to use physical aggression than women, who in turn are more likely to fear aggressive retaliation.

Anger Physiology

A defining condition of anger is physiological arousal, the activation of which has evolutionary roots. For our prehistoric ancestors, when a threat to survival or survival resources was detected, it was advantageous to be mobilized to respond energetically and to sustain effort. The flight-or-fight response refers to this hard-wired physiological mechanism that gets instantaneously triggered to engage survival behavior, to focus attention on the survival threat, and to enable the organism to not succumb to pain. Anger is the emotional complement of the organismic preparation for attack, which also entails the orchestration of signals of attack readiness so as to ward off opponents or to coerce compliance.

The arousal of anger is marked by physiological activation in the cardiovascular, endocrine, and limbic systems, as well as other autonomic and central nervous system areas, and by tension in the skeletal musculature. The autonomic signature of anger corresponds to a mixture of adrenaline and noradrenaline. Autonomic system arousal, especially cardiovascular, has been commonly observed in conjunction with anger by scholars from the classical age (such as Seneca, Aristotle, and Plutarch) to the early behavioral scientists of the nineteenth and twentieth centuries (especially Charles Darwin, William James, G. Stanley Hall, and Walter B. Cannon). Laboratory research has reliably found anger arousal to entail increases in both systolic and diastolic blood pressure and, to a somewhat lesser extent, heart rate. It is differentiated from fear by a stronger increase in diastolic pressure, in muscle electrical activity (measured by electromyogram recordings), and in total peripheral resistance. Associated with this cardiovascular activation is facial flushing, which is often reported by people reflecting on their anger experience and also is measured by face temperature. Indeed, in terms of psychosocial imagery, there is no better metaphor for anger than hot fluid in a container.

Autonomic arousal is primarily engaged through adrenomedullary and adrenocortical hormonal activity. The secretion by the adrenal medulla of the catecholamines adrenaline and noradrenaline and by the adrenal cortex of glucocorticoids provides a sympathetic system effect that mobilizes the body for immediate action (e.g., the release of glucose, stored in the liver and muscles as glycogen). In anger, the catecholamine activation is more strongly noradrenaline than adrenaline (the reverse being the case for fear). The adrenocortical effects, which have longer duration than the adrenomedullary ones, are mediated by secretions of the pituitary gland, which also influences testosterone levels. The pituitary-adrenocortical and pituitary-gonadal systems are thought to affect readiness or potentiation for anger responding.

The central nervous system structure that has been identified in anger activation is the amygdala, the almond-shaped limbic system component located deep in the temporal lobe. The amygdala is the key site for aversive motivational system. Activation in the corticomedial amygdala is associated with anger and attack priming. Anger has also been linked with left-prefrontal cortical activity, which has typically been associated with positive affect and approach motivation. The central nervous system neurotransmitter serotonin, which is also present in blood platelets, affects anger potentiation, as low levels of this hormone are associated with irritable mood. Serotonin imbalances are related to deficits in the modulation of emotion. While serotonin and other neurotransmitters (noradrenaline and dopamine) are involved in anger activation, the neural structures and circuitry in anger dysregulation remain to be disentangled.

These various physiological mechanisms thus pertain not only to the intensity of anger arousal but also to its duration. Arousal activation eventually decays to baseline levels, but recovery time may be prolonged by exposure to new arousal sources or by rumination. The potency of a provocation may be heightened by the carryover of undissipated excitation from a prior arousal source, which may not have been anger specific (i.e., an otherwise stressful circumstance, such as exposure to bad news, work pressure, or traffic congestion). This excitation transfer of arousal residues facilitates anger, augments its intensity, amplifies blood pressure, and raises the probability of aggression. Residual arousal from unresolved anger events can transfer to future conflicts and further intensify anger reactivity to instigating events. In turn, unexpressed anger is associated with exaggerated and more prolonged cardiovascular responses to a variety of stressful stimuli.

In this regard, a stress framework is highly useful. It is unquestionably the case that physiological arousal is activated by exposure to commonly identified stressors, such as noise, crowding, difficult tasks, and high-pressure job environments filled with time demands or exposure to abrasive interactions. Both acute and prolonged exposure to such conditions may induce physiological activation that decays slowly. Therefore, when someone experiences an event that pulls for the cognitive label anger and this event occurs concurrently with already elevated arousal, the anger system is then more easily engaged.

Cognition, Anger, and Threat

Humans have elaborate neurocognitive systems for detecting threat. We have a neural architecture (especially the limbic system) specialized for the processing of emotion and emotion–cognition interactions, and the amygdala is centrally involved in detecting events as threats. In parallel, higher level cognitive reasoning elaborates this information, in what are termed appraisal processes. The perception of threat is conjoined with sympathetic nervous system activation of autonomic arousal components, such as heart rate, blood pressure, and respiration increases, that prepare the body for emergency action.

In addition to potentiating action, anger in such states of mobilization has adaptive value as a source of information. To others, it communicates perceived wrongdoing, threat of aggression, or intent of reprisal. Such information exchange prior to aggression can facilitate social and interpersonal negotiations toward conflict resolution. For the self, it serves as information for prioritizing and decision making. The intensity of anger, for example, can help focus and maintain attention on relevant goals and help one estimate progress toward those goals. When pressed to make a decision, anger serves as a summary affective cue that can be processed without need for elaborate analysis.

To get angry about something, one must pay attention to it. Anger is often the result of selective attention to cues having high provocation value. A principal function of cognitive systems is to guide behavior, and attention itself is guided by integrated cognitive structures, known as schemas, that incorporate rules about environment–behavior relationships. What receives attention is a product of the cognitive network that assigns meaning to events and the complex stimuli that configure them. Expectations guide attentional search for cues relevant to particular needs or goals. Once a repertoire of anger schemas has been developed, events (e.g., being asked a question by someone) and their characteristics (e.g., the way the question was asked, when it was asked, or who asked it) are encoded or interpreted as having meaning in accord with the pre-existing schema. Because of their survival function, the threat-sensing aspect of anger schemas carries urgent priority and can pre-empt other information processing.

Since the writings of the Stoic philosophers of the classical period, anger has been understood to be strongly determined by personal interpretations of events. The concept of appraisal is that of interpretation, judgment, or meaning embedded in the perception of something – not as a cognitive event occurring after that something has happened. The appraisal of provocation is in the seeing or hearing. Appraisal, though, is an ongoing process, so various reappraisals of experience will occur and will correspondingly affect whether or not the probability of aggression is lessened, maintained, or intensified. Rumination about provoking circumstances will of course extend or re-vivify anger reactions. In addition, the occurrence of certain thoughts can prime semantically related ideas that are part of an anger schema.

Perceived malevolence is one of the most common forms of anger-inducing appraisal. When another person's behavior is interpreted as intending to be harmful to oneself, anger and aggression schemas are activated. In turn, receiving information about mitigating circumstances (e.g., learning that the person was fatigued and working overtime) can defuse the appraisal of personal attack and promote a benign reappraisal. Perceiving malevolence pulls for anger by involving the important theme of justification, which includes the externalization of blame. When harm or injustice has been done, the social norms of retaliation and retribution are engaged. Indeed, one view of anger is that it is a socially constituted syndrome or a transitory social role governed by social rules. Thus, its meaning and function would be determined by the social systems in which it occurs and of which it is an integral part.

Justification is a core theme with regard to the activation of anger and aggression, being rooted in ancient religious texts, such as the Bible and the Koran, as well as classical mythologies about deities and historical accounts of the behavior of ancient rulers. Correspondingly, anger and physical aggression are often viewed as ways of applying a legitimate punitive response for transgression or as ways of correcting injustice. Frequently, however, an embellished justification serves the exoneration of blame for destructive outcomes of expressed anger.

As people monitor their physical and social environment for threats to their resources or self-esteem, they operate with expectations about how events and the behavior of others will unfold. When opposition, anger, or antagonism is expected, this can lead to selective perception of situational cues in line with an aggressive script, a cognitive programming that guides behavior. Anger arousal provides energy and justification for aggressive script enactment.

Anger Dyscontrol and Regulation

Anger is a highly functional human emotion, and it is one to be appreciated as a rich part of cultural life, but the survival value of the aggression-enabling function of anger is an archaic remnant with rare contemporary necessity. The challenges presented by civilized society are predominantly psychological, rather than physical, thus attenuating anger's adaptive worth. Effective coping with the demands of modern life requires understanding complex information, problem solving, and prudent action, not energized rapid responding. Even in emergency situations, anger requires regulation. Contrary to intuitions, anger can be detrimental to survival in a physical threat crisis. It is counterproductive for energy conservation in a prolonged fight, for monitoring additional threat elements and hazards, and for effective strategy selection in circumstances in which survival threat lingers and/or remains obscure. The regulation of the intensity and duration of anger arousal is pivotal to its merit or utility.

While the physiological components of anger, such as increased blood flow, may be adaptive for survival in a short-term danger episode, the byproducts of recurrent engagement of anger are hazardous in the long term. Unregulated anger commonly has been found to be associated with physical and psychological health impairments. In the realm of physical health, chronic anger has been established as having detrimental effects most centrally on the cardiovascular system, and these are related to mortality. Persons high in generalized hostility who are reactively angry are at considerable risk for coronary heart disease. When such persons are confronted with a stressful demand, they have strong cardiovascular responses in blood pressure, neurohormonal secretions, and cholesterol. A hostile, cynical, and distrusting outlook also necessitates high vigilance for thwarting and malevolence, resulting in prolonged neurohormonal activation conducive to atherosclerosis.

In addition to these pathogenic effects for a personality style that is overly expressive of anger, the coronary system is also impaired by recurrently suppressed anger and has long been identified as a causal variable in the etiology of essential hypertension. People who have difficulties expressing anger tend to be at risk for chronically elevated blood pressure, as mediated by high plasma renin activity and noradrenaline. The suppression of anger has been robustly correlated to elevated blood pressure in laboratory studies and to sustained hypertension in field studies. Also, studies using ambulatory recorders of blood pressure have found that persons who are high in hostility and who have a tendency to inhibit the expression of that hostility have greater cardiovascular reactivity to provocation events, as well as elevated resting blood pressure.

With regard to psychological well-being, anger occurs in conjunction with a wide range of psychiatrically classified disorders, including a variety of impulse control dysfunctions, mood disorders, personality disorders, and forms of schizophrenia, especially paranoid schizophrenia. In addition, the activation of anger has long been recognized as a feature of clinical disorders that result from trauma, such as dissociative disorders, brain damage syndromes, and, especially, PTSD. Anger also appears in mental state disturbances produced by general medical conditions, such as dementia, substance abuse disorders, and neurological dysfunctions resulting from perinatal difficulties.

Among hospitalized psychiatric patients in long-term care in both civil commitment and forensic institutions, anger is a salient problem, as identified by both clinical staff and the patients themselves. Importantly, it is linked to assaultive behavior by psychiatric patients both inside and outside such facilities. Such patients typically have traumatic life histories, replete with experiences of abandonment and rejection, as well as economic and psychological impoverishment. For them, anger becomes entrenched as a mode of reactance to stressful or aversive experiences, and it is a significant aspect of their resistance to treatment. Chronically angry people are reluctant to surrender the anger-aggression system that they have found useful to engage and because they discount the costs of its engagement. Psychiatric hospital staff, especially those on acute admissions units and in long-term institutions, have very stressful occupations as a result of the anger episodes of the patients in their care. Posttraumatic stress disorder commonly occurs among staff who have been victims of assault by patients.

Anger Treatment

In the treatment of anger disorders, cognitive-behavioral therapy (CBT) approaches have been found to be effective with a wide range of clinical populations. CBT approaches incorporate many elements of behavior therapy, such as training in self-monitoring, relaxation, and social skills, but also centrally seek to modify cognitive structures and the way in which a person processes information about social situations. They strongly emphasize self-regulation, cognitive flexibility in appraising situations, arousal control, and learning prosocial values and scripts. By making extensive use of therapist modeling and client rehearsal, anger proneness is modified by first motivating client engagement and then restructuring cognitive schemas, increasing capacity to regulate arousal and facilitating the use of constructive coping behaviors.

A misleading aspect of the notion of anger management is that it implies that treatment is centrally about what to do when one gets angry. Instead, a very significant objective of anger treatment is about how to not get angry in the first place – hence the priority given to regulatory controls for anger experience or activation. The parameters or state markers for anger activation that receive attention in CBT anger treatment are reactivity (frequency on onset and how easily anger is triggered), latency (how rapidly activated), intensity (how strongly engaged), and duration (persistence of arousal). Treatment aims to minimize anger reactivity, intensity, and duration and to moderate anger expression to reduce the costs of anger dyscontrol.

To facilitate anger regulation, anger treatment procedures strive to disconnect anger from the threat system. This is done first through the provision of safety, patience, and psychological space for reflection, exploration, and choice. The client's view of anger is normalized, to obviate worries about being a bad or unworthy person. The therapist acknowledges the legitimacy of the client's feelings, affirming his or her self-worth. Building trust in the therapeutic relationship is pivotal. As self-regulation hinges on knowledge, education about anger and discovery of the client's personal anger patterns or anger signature is facilitated. Much is done to augment self-monitoring and to encourage the moderation of anger intensity. As tension or strain may surface in the course of treatment, the therapist models and reinforces non-anger alternative responding so as to build replacements for the automatized angry reactions that had been the client's default coping style.

One CBT approach to anger treatment that has received significant support for its efficacy is called stress inoculation (SI). In this treatment approach, anger provocation is simulated by therapeutically paced exposure to anger incidents created in imaginal visualization and in role play. The progressively graduated exposure, directed by the therapist, involves a hierarchy of anger incidents produced by the collaborative work of client and therapist. This graduated, hierarchical exposure, done in conjunction with the teaching of stress coping skills, is the basis for the inoculation metaphor.

The SI approach to anger treatment involves the following key components: (1) client education about anger, stress, and aggression; (2) self-monitoring of anger frequency, intensity, and situational triggers; (3) construction of a personal anger provocation hierarchy, created from the self-monitoring data and used for the practice and testing of anger coping skills; (4) arousal reduction techniques of progressive muscle relaxation, breathing-focused relaxation, and guided imagery training; (5) cognitive restructuring by altering attentional focus, modifying appraisals, and using self-instruction; (6) training behavioral coping in communication and respectful assertiveness as modeled and rehearsed with the therapist; and (7) practicing the cognitive, arousal regulatory, and behavioral coping skills while visualizing and role playing progressively more intense anger-arousing scenes from the personal hierarchies.

See Also the Following Articles

Aggression; Hostility.

Further Reading

Averill, J. R. (1982). *Anger and aggression: an essay on emotion.* New York: Springer-Verlag.

Berkowitz, L. (1993). *Aggression: its causes, consequences, and control.* New York: McGraw Hill.

Chesney, M. and Rosenman, R. H. (1985). *Anger and hostility in cardiovascular and behavioral disorders.* Washington, D.C.: Hemisphere.

Follette, V. M., Rusek, J. I. and Abueg, F. R. (1998). *Cognitive behavioral therapies for trauma.* New York: Guilford.

Friedman, H. (1992). *Hostility, coping, and health.* Washington, D.C.: American Psychological Association.

Johnson, E. H., Gentry, W. D. and Julius, S. (1992). *Personality, elevated blood pressure, and essential hypertension.* Washington, D.C.: Hemisphere.

Lazarus, R. S. (1991). *Emotion and adaptation.* Oxford, UK: Oxford University Press.

Ortony, A., Clore, G. L. and Collins, A. (1988). *The cognitive structure of emotions.* New York: Cambridge University Press.

Philippot, P. and Feldman, R. S. (2004). *The regulation of emotion.* Mahwah, NJ: Erlbaum.

Potegal, M. and Knutson, J. F. (1994). *The dynamics of aggression: biological and social processes in dyads and groups.* Hillsdale, NJ: Erlbaum.

Siegman, A. W. and Smith, T. W. (eds.) (1994). *Anger, hostility, and the heart.* Hillsdale, NJ: Erlbaum.

Taylor, J. L. and Novaco, R. W. (2005). *Anger treatment for people with developmental disabilities.* Chicester, UK: Wiley.

Hostility

L H Powell and K Williams
Rush University Medical Center, Chicago, IL, USA

This is a revised version of the article by L H Powell, Encyclopedia of Stress First Edition, volume 2, pp 407–412, © 2000, Elsevier Inc.

Glossary

Anger	An unpleasant emotion, ranging in intensity from irritation or annoyance to fury or rage, that is an emotional expression of hostility.
Cynicism	A component of hostility characterized by the belief that others are motivated by selfish concerns.
Hostile interactional style	A style of interaction characterized by the tendency to challenge, evade questions, and become easily irritated.
Hostility	A general cognitive personality trait including a devaluation of others' worth and motives, an expectation of wrong-doing in others, an oppositional approach to others, and a desire to see others harmed.
Mistrust	A component of hostility characterized by the belief that others are likely to be provoking and hurtful.
Type A behavior pattern	The early conceptualization of coronary-prone behavior that featured two key components: excessive time urgency and free-floating hostility.

History of the Concept

In the 1960s, the concept of the type A behavior pattern was introduced by cardiologists Meyer Friedman and Ray Rosenman to describe individuals who possessed excessive time urgency and free-floating hostility and who, by virtue of this behavior pattern, were believed to be coronary-prone. This conceptualization fostered hundreds of investigations in the 1970s and 1980s aimed at replicating early associations with coronary disease, refining its measurement, and understanding its physiological underpinnings. In 1980, a classic paper was published by Williams and his colleagues that suggested that the hostility component of the type A behavior pattern was its toxic core (**Figure 1**). Angiography patients were divided by gender, type A behavior, and hostility, and these classifications were related to occlusive disease. For both males and females, hostility was a better predictor of $\geq 75\%$ occlusion than type A behavior. This seminal investigation was subsequently replicated in a large number of studies using a variety of subjects and study designs and resulted in a shift in thinking away from type A behavior toward hostility as a key coronary-prone behavior.

Conceptualization

Hostility is a negative attitude toward others consisting of enmity, denigration, and ill will. It is a stable personality trait with stability coefficients of 0.85

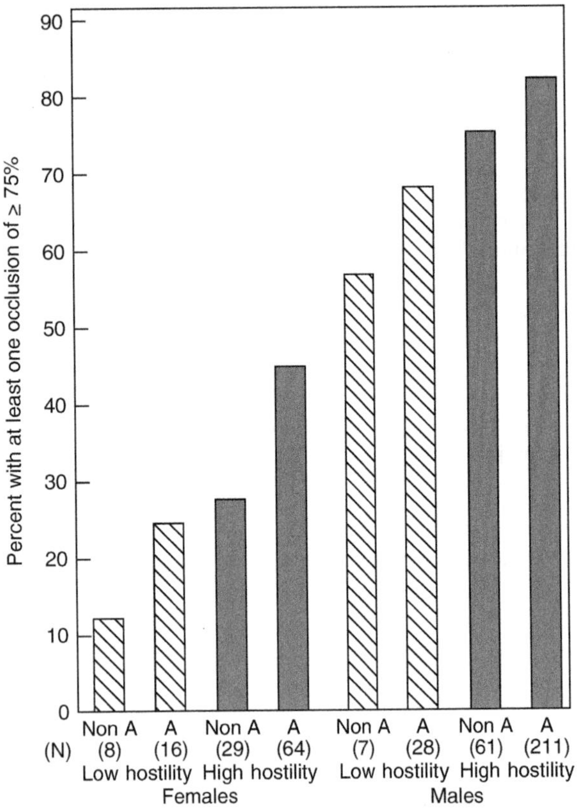

Figure 1 Relation of type A behavior pattern, hostility, and gender to presence of significant coronary occlusions. From Williams, R. B., et al. (1980). *Psychosomatic Medicine* **42,** 539–549, with permission.

over 1 or 4 years, 0.67 over 5 years, and 0.40 over 24 years. Hostility appears to be a multidimensional trait with from two to four factor analyzed components. There is general agreement that the two key components are cynicism, or the belief that others are motivated by selfish concerns, and mistrust, or the belief that others are likely to be provoking and hurtful. Other components include such things as a hostile attributional style, which is the tendency to construe the actions of others as involving aggressive intent, and a hostile interactional style characterized by the tendency to challenge others, evade questions, and become easily irritated. Smith has argued for a transactional view of hostility, which includes aspects of both the person and the environment. When both hostility and social support are considered jointly, three distinct components emerge: (1) nonhostile and high socially supported healthy individuals, (2) highly hostile and low socially supported submissive individuals, and (3) highly hostile and high socially supported aggressive individuals.

Although hostility is often linked to the risk factors of anger and aggression, it is distinct from them in that it refers to a cognitive personality trait. Anger is an emotion that includes reactions ranging from mild irritation to intense anger and can be a transitory feeling state or an enduring predisposition. Aggression is a behavior defined as attacking or hurtful actions toward others, whether the harm is physical or verbal. Correlations among these characteristics are moderate, suggesting that they are related, but nonetheless distinct.

Studies that have examined the sociodemographic correlates of hostility have found that it increases with age, is higher in men than in women, is higher in minorities than in Caucasians, and is higher in individuals of lower than in those of higher socioeconomic status. Moreover, there is consistent evidence that hostility is associated with smoking, elevated body mass index, and heavy alcohol consumption. Since these correlates are, in themselves, risk factors for disease, they can serve as confounders for any association between hostility and disease. Confounding in this case would be making the mistake that the true association is between hostility and coronary disease, when in fact the true association is actually between one or more of these established coronary risk factors (which are linked to hostility) and coronary disease. It is important to control for these potential confounders in the design or analysis of studies assessing the health impact of hostility.

Assessment

There are three popular assessment measures of hostility, all of which have subscales. Two of these are self-report questionnaires and the third is a behavioral rating. **Table 1** presents selected items from these scales.

The Cook-Medley Hostility Scale

The Cook-Medley Hostility Scale is a subscale of the Minnesota Multiphasic Personality Inventory (MMPI) that is composed of 52 true–false items. Several factor analyses of this scale have produced slightly different solutions ranging from two to four factors. The two-factor solution includes the components of cynicism and mistrust/hostile attributions. The four-factor solution includes the components of cynicism, mistrust/hostile attributions, hostile affect, and aggressive responding. Studies of hostility as a risk factor have used the entire scale, the cynicism subscale, or the Abbreviated Cook-Medley (ACM) with the four subscales. The major limitation of the Cook-Medley scale is that it correlates consistently with depression and anxiety, characteristics that may be outside of the conceptual domain of hostility.

Table 1 Selected items from the most popular hostility assessment scales

SELF-REPORT QUESTIONNAIRES	
Cook-Medley Hostility Scale: Mark each item as "true" or "false"	
Cynicism	I think most people would lie to get ahead
	Most people are honest chiefly through fear of being caught
Mistrust/hostile attributions	It is safer to trust nobody
	I tend to be on guard with people who are somewhat more friendly than I had expected
Hostile affect	Some of my family have habits that bother and annoy me very much
Aggressive responding	I have at times had to be rough with people who were rude or annoying
Buss-Durkee Hostility Inventory: Mark each item as "true" or "false"	
Expressed hostility	I lose my temper easily but get over it
	When people yell, I yell back
	I raise my voice when arguing
Experiential hostility	I don't seem to get what's coming to me (resentment)
	I know that people tend to talk about me behind my back (suspicion)
	My motto is "Never trust strangers" (mistrust)
BEHAVIORAL RATINGS	
Interpersonal Hostility Assessment Technique: Behavioral ratings from a structured interview, based upon style of interaction	
Direct challenges	Direct or explicit challenge of the question or the interviewer
Indirect challenges	Implication that the answer was obvious or the interviewer was stupid for having asked it
Hostile withholding or evasion	Avoidance or refusal to answer a question, associated hostile tone and intent not to answer
Irritation	Irritated tone, impatience, exasperation with the interview or interviewer, aroused reliving of negative events, condescension or snide remarks, harsh generalizations, punched words with angry emphasis

The Buss-Durkee Hostility Inventory

The Buss-Durkee Hostility Inventory is composed of 66 true–false items that are grouped into seven subscales: assault, indirect hostility, irritability, negativism, resentment, suspicion, and verbal hostility. In factor analytic studies, it has been consistently shown to assess two correlated dimensions, expressive hostility and experiential hostility. Expressive hostility assesses verbal and physical aggressiveness and is more highly correlated with antagonism than with neuroticism. Experiential hostility assesses the subjective experience of resentment, suspicion, mistrust, and irritation and is more highly correlated with neuroticism than with antagonism.

The Interpersonal Hostility Assessment Technique (IHAT)

The IHAT is an evolution of the structured interview for type A behavior in which the focus is on behavioral ratings of a hostile interpersonal style. It provides more objective criteria for assessing hostility than the subjective judgments that have characterized past interview ratings. Four types of hostile behaviors are rated from type A interview scripts, including direct challenges to the interviewer, indirect challenges to the interviewer, irritation, and hostile withholding of information or evasion. IHAT ratings have been correlated ($r = 0.32$) with potential for hostility ratings from the structured interview for type A behavior and have been shown to be stable over a 4-year period ($r = 0.69$).

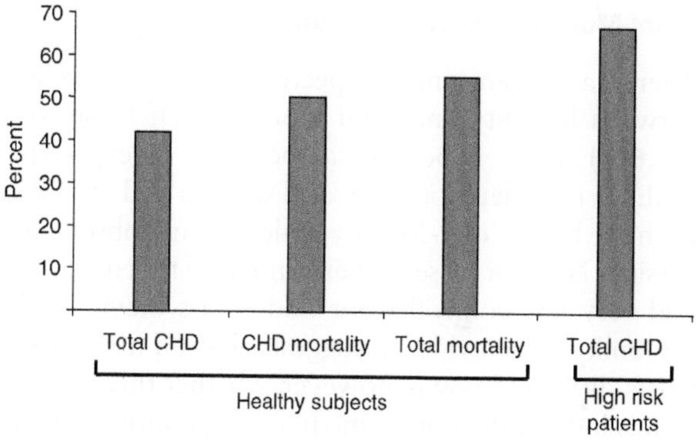

Figure 2 Percentage of prospective studies that have found a positive link between hostility and physical health.

Link to Physical Disease in Longitudinal Studies

Figure 2 summarizes the longitudinal studies that have examined a link between hostility and physical disease. Approximately half of all longitudinal studies have found the expected association.

Coronary Heart Disease in Healthy Subjects

To date there have been 12 longitudinal studies that have examined the role of hostility on the incidence of coronary heart disease (coronary mortality or myocardial infarction), six longitudinal studies that have examined the role of hostility on coronary heart disease (CHD) mortality, and two longitudinal studies that have examined the role of hostility on subclinical cardiovascular disease. Positive associations were found in five (41.7%) of the CHD studies, three (50%) of the CHD mortality studies, and two (100%) of the subclinical cardiovascular disease studies. Evidence exists that hostility is equally predictive in men and women, older and younger subjects, African American and Caucasian subjects, and the total scale and the abbreviated subscales.

Since hostility is embedded in a behavioral complex of other risk factors for coronary disease that includes lower education, higher body mass index, current smoking, and heavy alcohol consumption, these risk factors must be controlled for in multivariate analyses to avoid the problem of confounding. When the prospective studies that showed significant associations were examined for the adequacy of their control for these confounders, none of the studies controlled for all of these factors and most controlled only one or two of them. In one study, direct adjustment for these potential confounders eliminated a prior positive association. This suggests that any link between hostility and CHD may not be independent of standard risk factors but instead may be mediated by them.

Total Mortality in Healthy Subjects

There have been nine prospective studies of the link between hostility and total mortality. Of these, five (55.6%) found a positive association. The positive findings included both men and women and included both the total Cook-Medley scale and an abbreviated version. None of these studies controlled for education, and very few controlled for body mass index. Thus, the bulk of the evidence suggests that an association exists. It is not known, however, whether this association is independent of, or mediated by, established risk factors.

Coronary Heart Disease in High-Risk Subjects

There have been nine prospective studies of hostility and clinical CHD outcomes in patients with evidence of existing coronary disease. Of these, six (66.5%) found a positive association. These studies are characterized by inadequate control for confounding, with one exception. In a study of postmenopausal women with existing CHD from the Heart and Estrogen/Progestin Replacement Study (HERS) cohort, both the total Cook-Medley scale and the cynicism subscale predicted total CHD events after excellent controls for demographic and CHD risk factor confounders in multivariate analyses. Thus, the evidence is slightly stronger that an association, which is independent of the risk incurred by established risk factors, exists between hostility and CHD in high-risk patients than in their healthy counterparts.

Mechanisms of Association

There are three key mechanisms by which hostility may be associated with physical disease. The first is a direct mechanism whereby hostility triggers neuroendocrine pathogenic mechanisms for physical disease. The second is an indirect association whereby hostility fosters elevations in established risk factors and these risk factors increase risk for physical disease. The third suggests that hostility is embedded in a constellation of psychosocial risk factors, which together increase the psychosocial burden and, concomitantly, the risk of physical disease. Literature on potential mechanisms is growing rapidly, particularly evidence for a direct physiological link between hostility and disease.

Physiological

There is consistent evidence that hostility exerts a direct effect on CHD and total mortality through the mechanisms of amplified cardiovascular reactivity and neuroendocrine responses to stressors. Evidence exists for an association between hostility and such pathophysiological mechanisms as heart rate and blood pressure reactivity, increased platelet aggregation, vasoconstriction of atherosclerotic arteries, silent ischemia, decreased ejection fraction, decreased threshold for ventricular fibrillation, and decreased heart rate variability. There also is evidence that hostility activates the sympathetic branch, and/or suppresses the parasympathetic branch, of the autonomic nervous system, mediated through epinephrine, norepinephrine, testosterone, and serotonin. Recent research suggests other possible physiological mechanisms involving the metabolic syndrome and inflammatory processes. Hostility has been associated with the metabolic syndrome of high levels of plasma lipids, insulin resistance, visceral body fat, and elevated blood pressure. Hostility has also been associated with inflammatory processes, specifically pro-inflammatory cytokines, tumor necrosis factor-α, and interleukin-6.

Health Behaviors

Evidence is accumulating that hostility is associated with smoking, heavy alcohol consumption, a sedentary lifestyle, obesity and overweight, elevated blood pressure, and lowered HDL cholesterol. Moreover, hostile individuals may be more likely to ignore health warnings and fail to comply with medical regimens. Two studies exist that have directly tested this model by examining the association between hostility and CHD before and after adjusting for established risk factors. One found that the association was maintained after adjustment; the other found that the association was eliminated. Thus, there is evidence from one study to support this mechanism.

Psychosocial Vulnerability

Hostile individuals not only may be hostile but also may have other psychosocial characteristics that have been observed to be coronary prone, including depression, anxiety, low social support, and/or general distress. Correlations between measures of hostility and these other psychosocial risk factors are between 0.25 and 0.30. Thus, it may not be the hostility alone but the overall adverse psychosocial risk factor profile that is associated with physical disease. For example, one study found that general distress was a better predictor than hostility of 6-month recurrence in patients with myocardial infarction. Another study found that although hostility is related to lower social support, when it is available, it provides fewer physiological benefits to hostile persons.

Intervention

Intervention for hostility can take one of two forms. Pharmacological interventions focus on blocking the impact of key physiological mechanisms on cardiac targets. Behavioral interventions focus on altering the cognitive, behavioral, and emotional concomitants of hostility as a way to reduce the frequency and intensity with which the physiological pathways are mobilized.

Pharmacological

β-adrenergic blocking drugs block the impact of increased sympathetic tone on the heart, triggered by hostility, and thereby reduce the hemodynamic response that may lead to plaque disruption. With this therapy, hostile individuals may construe the stressor as threatening, but the concomitant sympathetic arousal has little, if any, impact on heart rate or blood pressure. Aspirin has antiplatelet properties and thus may prevent sympathetically induced platelet aggregation that leads to thrombus formation. Estrogen therapy in women with existing coronary disease does not weaken the ability of hostility to predict recurrent coronary events.

Behavioral

Effective behavioral interventions for hostility must begin with the development of sensitivity to signs and symptoms of hostility in the individual him- or herself. This is a difficult task because hostility tends to be well rationalized, based upon real or perceived insults from the social environment. Interventions are most effective when they focus on the development of skills and competencies in all of the domains of hostility. Relaxation therapies help the individual to develop the skill to switch from sympathetic arousal to parasympathetic relaxation. Assertiveness training can help individuals to replace hostile interactional styles with less arousing and more effective alternatives. Cognitive therapy can help individuals to identify cognitions, such as blaming others, that are associated with arousal and to replace them with alternatives that are more rational and less arousing. The development of efficacy in controlling emotional arousal in response to environmental challenges has the effect of improving self-esteem, improving interpersonal effectiveness, and producing more positive feedback from the social environment. Progressively, as skills develop, the enhanced interpersonal effectiveness can challenge core cynical and mistrusting beliefs.

See Also the Following Articles

Aggression; Anger.

Further Reading

Barefoot, J. C., Dodge, K. A., Peterson, B. L., Dahlstrom, W. G. and Williams, R. B., Jr. (1989). The Cook-Medley hostility scale: item content and ability to predict survival. *Psychosomatic Medicine* **51**, 46–57.

Buss, A. H. and Durkee, A. (1957). An inventory for assessing different kinds of hostility. *Journal of Consulting Psychology* **21**, 343–349.

Chaput, L. A., Adams, S. H., Simon, J. A., Blumenthal, R. S., Vittinghoff, E., Lin, F., et al. (2002). Hostility predicts recurrent events among postmenopausal women with coronary heart disease. *American Journal of Epidemiology* **156**, 1092–1099.

Cook, W. W. and Medley, D. M. (1954). Proposed hostility and pharisaic virtue scales for the MMPI. *Journal of Applied Psychology* **38**, 414–418.

Haney, T. L., Maynard, K. E., Houseworth, S. J., et al. (1996). Interpersonal hostility assessment technique: description and validation against the criterion of coronary artery disease. *Journal of Personal Assessment* **66**, 386–401.

McEwen, B. S. and Stellar, E. (1993). Stress and the individual. Mechanisms leading to disease. *Archives of Internal Medicine* **153**, 2093–2101.

Miller, T. Q., Smith, T. W., Turner, C. W., Guijarro, M. L. and Hallet, A. J. (1996). A meta-analytic review of research on hostility and physical health. *Psychiatric Bulletin* **119**, 322–348.

Siegman, A. W. and Smith, T. W. (1994). *Anger, hostility, and the heart.* Hillsdale, NJ: Lawrence Erlbaum.

Smith, T. W., Glazer, K., Ruiz, J. M. and Gallo, L. C. (2004). Hostility, anger, aggressiveness, and coronary heart

disease: an interpersonal perspective on personality, emotion, and health. *Journal of Personality* 72, 1217–1270.
Suarez, E. C. (2003). Joint effect of hostility and severity of depressive symptoms on plasma interleukin-6 concentration. *Psychosomatic Medicine* 65, 523–527.
Suls, J. and Wan, C. K. (1993). The relationship between trait hostility and cardiovascular reactivity: a quantitative review and analysis. *Psychophysiology* 30, 615–626.
Williams, R. and Williams, V. (1993). *Anger kills. Seventeen strategies for controlling the hostility that can harm your health.* New York: Times Books, Random House.

Violence

E K Englander
Bridgewater State College, Bridgewater, MA, USA

This is a revised version of the article by E K Englander, Encyclopedia of Stress First Edition, volume 3, pp 662–668, © 2000, Elsevier Inc.

Glossary

Adoption studies	Research wherein a child with one set of biological parents and a different set of psychological parents is studied.
Biological environmental influences	Events that affect a person biologically but are not encoded into the person's DNA.
Concordance rates	The frequency with which one twin is diagnosed with an illness, when his or her twin is also diagnosed with the same illness.
Cortisol	The hormone that regulates the body's reaction to stress.
Genetic influences	The biological blueprints for behavior that are contained in a person's chromosomes.
Imitation	A theory that states that children may learn to be violent by imitating an adult's aggression.
Minimal brain dysfunction or minimal brain damage	Very low levels of brain dysfunction, theoretically affecting behavior, emotions, learning, or memory.
Neurotransmitters	Chemicals secreted by the brain, some of which have been linked to aggression.
Paranoid misperceptions	Attitudes or belief systems that misinterpret ambiguous circumstances as signs of danger when none actually exists.
Resilient state	The state in which a person is likely to resist developing a disorder.
Serotonin	One of the monoamines, low levels of which have been implicated as related to aggression.
Testosterone	One of the androgens. A male sex hormone that is associated with aggression.
Vulnerable state	The state in which a person is likely to develop a disorder.

Violent crimes can be as baffling as they are repelling. In England, two 10-year-old boys lured a 2-year-old away from his mother at a shopping mall; they took him down to the local railroad tracks, where they beat him to death and left his body to be run over by a train. In the United States, a group of teenagers shot and killed a man whose car they were stealing – even though the man had willingly handed over his car keys and was not resisting the theft in any way. In Massachusetts, a group of young teenage schoolgirls planned to murder their English teacher because she was too strict.

To understand the causes of violence, it is not always enough to understand the external circumstances that often drive other types of criminal behavior. It is true that violence sometimes results from factors such as an individual's desire for financial gain or an individual's repeated exposure to violent behavior in his or her social environments. Sometimes, however, violence also happens in an apparently motiveless fashion. Violence is never truly without motive, but the motives may be so complex and elusive that the violence appears motiveless. In all cases, but particularly in cases of violence that appear to have no motive, internal or individual factors may be critical for understanding the cause of such behavior. A variety of different biological and psychological influences and mechanisms have been considered over the years. This article summarizes them and attempts to construct a more comprehensive model of the causes of violent behavior.

Types of Biological Influences

There exists a mistaken tendency to use the terms biological and genetic interchangeably. In fact, genetic influences are only one type of biological influences on behavior. There are (at least) two different types of biological influences: genetic influences and biological environmental influences. Genetic influences refer to the blueprints for behavior that are contained in a person's chromosomes. Chromosomes contain deoxyribonucleic acid (DNA), the genetic material a person inherits from his or her biological parents, which is referred to as their genotype. Biological environmental influences, unlike genetic influences, are events that affect a person biologically but that are not encoded into the person's DNA. For example, consider a head injury from a car accident, which subsequently changes the victim's personality. The head injury is unmistakably a biological environmental influence. No genotype determines that someone will have a car accident; however, such an accident, and its accompanying head injury, can still have an important biological effect on the person's behavior.

Although learning is clearly related to violent behavior, learning theories alone cannot fully explain violence in human beings. As an example, consider the principle of imitation. It states that children may learn to be violent by imitating an adult's aggression. According to this principle, one would expect that children who grow up watching violent parents would be violent themselves. As the theory predicts, a higher proportion of children who witness violent parents are violent, in comparison to other children; however, despite their higher risk, many children of violent parents do not, in fact, behave aggressively as adults. Some children who are exposed to violent psychosocial environments do become violent; many other children who are similarly exposed do not. This fact has led researchers to coin the terms resilient and invincible to describe children who survive and cope well despite terrible circumstances.

What makes one child resilient and another child vulnerable? Researchers have identified a variety of differences, including biological differences, that distinguish resilient and vulnerable children. It is important to note that such biological differences do not entirely explain why one child is vulnerable and another is resilient; rather, biology appears to be an important part of the determination. It is reasonable to assume that different biological influences will play different roles in the determination of vulnerability and resiliency.

One important area that researchers have studied focuses on minimal brain damage. Also called minimal brain dysfunction, minimal brain damage does not look like major brain damage. A person with minimal brain dysfunction will not have obvious brain damage; however, minimal dysfunction may affect behavior, emotions, learning, or memory – that is, the more subtle (or higher) functions of the brain. For example, although major brain damage might result in severe mental retardation, minor brain dysfunction might result in a learning disability that would not necessarily affect intelligence in any way (e.g., dyslexia). It has been repeatedly demonstrated that minimal brain dysfunction is related to problems such as learning disorders and hyperactivity. Those relationships emerged as a rationale for studying a link between minimal brain dysfunction and violence, but how to study such a link is somewhat controversial in the field. Some researchers have examined violent individuals to see if they have high levels of minor physical anomalies, while others have given aggressive and violent men neuropsychological examinations. Still other psychologists have combed through the medical histories of violent individuals, seeking unusually high levels of brain injury in their histories. Although different researchers have taken different tacks, their findings have been consistent. However one chooses to measure minimal brain dysfunction, a host of research suggests that it is indeed related to persistent aggression and violence. Further, although both major and minor brain damage may cause violence, the weight of the evidence suggests that the most important type of brain dysfunction in people who are chronically violent and criminal is minimal brain dysfunction. Although it is almost certain that most people with minimal brain dysfunction will never be violent, a noticeably high number of repeat violent offenders show some level of brain dysfunction (usually minimal).

Neurotransmitters

There are many different types of neurotransmitters, and they tend to specialize in function. How much, or how little, of any particular neurotransmitter chemical is in your brain is an important determinant of many types of behavior. Both biology and psychosocial environment affect the levels of different neurotransmitters, and thus affect behavior. A logical question, therefore, is whether violent behavior is related (at least in part) to the level of certain neurotransmitters in the brains of violent people.

Monoamine neurotransmitters have been most significantly linked to aggression. Of the monoamines, low levels of serotonin have been implicated most strongly in recent research. Several studies have found consistent relationships between reduced serotonin activity and aggression and hostility in both boys and men. As is often the case in such research, the relationship was strongest among males, regardless of their age. This set of studies is interesting because it establishes such relationships among psychiatrically well patients as well as among behaviorally disordered individuals.

Hormones

Two hormones have been the focus of most research on aggression and criminality: testosterone and cortisol. Testosterone is one of the male sex hormones, called androgens. Both males and females secrete androgens, but males secrete a much greater quantity than females. Androgens are frequently cited as an important cause of aggressive behavior, particularly intermale aggression. This area of study is not completely consistent, however, and while some research points to aggression and dominance/hostility as being related to testosterone, other research fails to find that dominance/hostility measures are related to sex hormones. Some research notes a testosterone–aggression relationship in both males and females; other research finds it only for males. To muddy the waters even further, researchers who follow those experiments involving reduced testosterone functioning do not note that this is a clearly effective means of stopping aggression. In addition, psychosocial researchers suggest that high testosterone might result in kids being treated differently socially, since high testosterone is associated with being bigger and stronger. Androgens, therefore, have been implicated, but not strongly, in the cause of aggression.

A second hormone that has been implicated more recently is cortisol. Cortisol is the hormone that regulates the body's reaction to stress. It is involved with the immune system and with sex hormones as well. A few studies have linked low levels of cortisol with a tendency to be aggressive. Although this should be characterized as an exploratory area of research, it is interesting to note that low cortisol has even been found in females with conduct disorders.

Genetics

The majority of researchers agree that violence does not appear to be a behavioral tendency that is transmitted via a simple, directly acting gene. In any case, it is clear that if genetic bases for aggression and violence exist, they are clearly mutable and changeable by a person's psychological environment; the old idea that genetics determines one's behavior absolutely is clearly mistaken.

The case for genetics as a cause of aggression and adult criminal violence has to be pieced together from a number of different areas of study. First, we know that children with violent parents do have a higher tendency to be violent themselves. Second, data from twin studies show the same trend.

Twin studies are natural genetic laboratories; they are studies that typically compare identical (monozygotic) to fraternal (dizygotic) twins. Identical twins are the only human beings alive who are genetically identical. Some psychological disorders have much higher concordance rates for monozygotic twins. For example, schizophrenia has a concordance rate of 50%; if one identical twin has schizophrenia, then there is a 50% chance that the other twin will also have schizophrenia. Similar, and even higher, rates of concordance for aggressive behavior have been noted among twin pairs.

Despite these family studies finding a reasonably strong genetic link for aggression, some clarification is important. Specifically, the field needs to make the critical distinction between biological heredity versus family psychology. Parents provide a psychological, as well as a biological, environment for their children. Likewise, twin studies fail to tease apart the effects of psychosocial environment and genetics. In addition to sharing genes, twins also often share an environment that treats them similarly.

For this reason, adoption studies (in which a child has one set of biological parents and a different set of psychological parents) may do a better job of teasing apart heredity and psychological environment. Earlier classic studies, which examined children prospectively in long-term studies, found that children seemed to follow their adoptive parents' behavior, rather than their genetic parents (suggesting a stronger link with psychological environment than genetics). More recent research has also found that biological siblings had a higher concordance for aggression, in comparison to adoptive siblings.

Both family studies and adoption studies suggest a definite degree of heritability for aggression, but there is a third body of research that is relevant here: studies that examine the heritability of childhood precursors of violence in adulthood. This body of research examines childhood disorders that are highly related to violence and studies whether these childhood disorders are heritable. For example, attention-deficit/hyperactivity disorder and conduct disorders are both childhood disorders with strong ties to adult violence, and both disorders appear to be at least partially heritable. The heritability of a disorder such as violence may therefore proceed through the pathways of other, co-existing disorders, or, alternatively, some childhood disorders may be precursors to adult violence in a child who has inherited that behavioral tendency.

In summary, much of the data on the genetic basis of violence is suggestive of a significant, but not total or direct, heritability.

Hostile Interpretation of Ambiguous Events, or Cognitive Distortions

In 1996, a 17-year-old boy attacked a total stranger, unprovoked, with an ax. He knocked on the man's door, and when it was opened he attempted to attack before he was driven off by his intended victim. His defense in court? That he was mentally deranged and unusually paranoid due to late-stage Lyme disease.

Before he became ill, this boy apparently had no behavioral problems, but his Lyme disease caused him to develop the unusual, but not unheard of, symptom of paranoid delusional misperceptions.

Cases this like are certainly rare. But are paranoid misperceptions rare among violent individuals? One theory suggests that such biased misperceptions may in fact help explain why some people are violent. Indeed, as the theory goes, under certain circumstances, aggression may be a normal and adaptive response. This may particularly be the case when an individual is faced with hostile or threatening forces, and violence is perceived as a necessary response. Given that a hostile environment might provoke an aggressive response in almost anyone, some researchers have investigated the possibility that violent individuals are not people who inappropriately choose violence; rather, they are people who inappropriately perceive hostility in situations where most people would not. That is, perhaps it is not the response that is skewed, but the perception of the environment.

How do aggressive children perceive the environment, and are their perceptions uniform? Studies find that aggressive children have two perceptual tendencies that nonaggressive children lack. Aggressive children are more likely to believe that other people had hostile intentions, and they are more likely to evaluate the results of aggression positively. Classic research has identified this thought pattern and has found that hostile biases were particularly characteristic of reactive-aggressive children. Researchers have similarly found that aggressive boys are significantly better at recognizing aggressively slanted comments. Studies have noted that children with memories that emphasize hostility process information in a more negatively biased way and are more likely to develop stable negative cognitive biases and stably aggressive behavior.

This line of study sheds some light on why it may be so difficult to treat violent offenders. Trying to teach such offenders to be nonviolent may in fact be trying to teach them to react nonviolently to what they perceive to be intensely threatening situations. For example, imagine that you are standing in a field holding a gun, and an elephant is charging toward you in a rage at full speed with his tusks aimed right at you. Trying to teach violent offenders to be nonviolent might be like trying to teach them not to shoot that elephant, even though there is every indication that that elephant is deadly.

Other research has examined different types of violent offenders and has found cognitive misinterpretations and biases that appear to be specific to the type of offense. For example, rather than making general, nonspecific hostile misinterpretations, adults who commit child abuse tend to misinterpret children's behavior. Specifically, they tend to regard children's misbehaviors as more intentional than they really are – possibly paving the way to righteous anger and abuse. Sexually aggressive men, rather than suffering from blanket distortions, may differ from other men primarily in their distortion of women's communications. It seems clear that a wide variety of cognitive misperceptions seems to pave the way for a variety of different types of aggressive and violent behavior, and may help explain the difficulty of effectively treating such behavior.

Summary

Strong evidence exists to support the theory that individual differences can affect a person's risk for developing chronically violent behavior. These risks appear to interact with psychosocially learned factors and may differ significantly from individual to individual. The mechanism by which these associated risk factors contribute to violence is less well established. Research has identified heritability, hormones, minimal brain dysfunction, and biased cognitive misperceptions as likely areas of dysfunction related to violence and aggression. Future research will focus on effective prevention efforts and a better understanding of how risk factors influence individuals' behaviors.

Acknowledgments

This article was adapted, with permission, from *Understanding Violence* (Lawrence Erlbaum & Associates, Inc., 2003).

See Also the Following Articles

Aggression.

Further Reading

Crick, N. and Dodge, K. (1996). Social information-processing mechanisms in reactive and proactive aggression. *Child Development* 67(3), 993–1003.

Englander, E. K. (2003). *Understanding violence* (2nd edn.). Mahwah, N.J.: Lawrence Erlbaum Publishers, Inc.

Mednick, S. A., Gabrielli, W. F. and Hutchings, B. (1984). Genetic influences in criminal convictions: evidence from an adoption cohort. *Science* 234, 891–894.

Werner, E. E. and Smith, R. S. (1982). *Vulnerable but invincible: a study of resilient children.* New York: McGraw-Hill.

Antisocial Disorders

K Pajer
The Ohio State University, Columbus, OH, USA

This is a revised version of the article by K Pajer, Encyclopedia of Stress First Edition, volume 1, pp 222–225, © 2000, Elsevier Inc.

Glossary

Antisocial personality disorder (ASPD)	Personality disorder characterized by frequent violation of social and legal norms, grandiose thoughts, arrogance, manipulative behavior, superficial charm, lack of attachment to others, little empathy, and an absence of guilt. Synonyms are sociopathy, psychopathy, and dyssocial personality.
Conduct disorder (CD)	Behavior disorder of childhood and adolescence characterized by truancy, stealing, running away, fighting, vandalism, fire setting, sexual assault, or other illegal activities.
Continuity	A term used in developmental psychopathology to refer to behaviors that continue from one stage of life to another, e.g., from adolescence to adulthood.
Desistance	A term used by criminologists to describe the cessation of criminal activity in a person who has previously committed illegal acts.
Developmental psychopathology	A field of study that focuses on the development and longitudinal course of psychiatric disorders across the life cycle.
Discontinuity	A term from the field of developmental psychopathology referring to behaviors that do not persist from one life stage to another.
Escalation	A term used in criminology to describe an increase in the frequency of illegal acts or an increase in the severity of such behavior over time.

Definition

Clinical Example

A.W. is a 40-year-old male who was released from prison 6 months ago. This was his second prison term; both terms had been served for burglary. A.W. was first sent to prison for 3 years when he was 25 years old. He had been working as a security system installer. He would install an alarm system and then return later and rob the house. A.W. proudly says that he robbed more than 800 houses in a 3-year period. After he served his first sentence, he learned how to open safes. He did several large jobs in houses and businesses before getting caught and sent back to prison for 10 years.

A.W. has a history of violence, consisting of fights in bars and on the street with other men, and fighting with his wife and girlfriends. His family believes he may have murdered his first wife and successfully hidden the body, but this has never been proven. A.W. openly admits that he initiates violence because he is bored or irritated. He himself was a childhood victim of severe violence perpetrated by his alcoholic father, who would also attack A.W.'s mother. He reports that he was beat many times with his father's hands and fists, as well as with a belt, board, and electrical cord. He suffered multiple episodes of head trauma. A.W. started fighting peers when he was 12 and hit his father for the first time when he was 14.

School was not easy for A.W., and he had numerous learning problems. He left school in the seventh grade at the age of 15 and joined the Army, using his dead brother's Social Security number. Testing in the Army revealed that he was bright and actually was functioning on a 12th grade level, but he got into so many fights that he eventually received a dishonorable discharge.

A.W.'s health is not good. He suffered his first grand mal seizure while in prison 10 years ago. He now has them regularly, despite medication. He has chronic bronchitis and hypertension. He used to drink heavily, but stopped 10 years ago when put back into prison, and reports that he will not drink again. He denies any drug use other than early experimentation with marijuana.

There have been several long-term female relationships in A.W.'s life, although he has had multiple brief liaisons. He has seven children, born to three different women. His first wife disappeared after the birth of their second child, and it was widely known that A.W. was angry because he thought she was seeing another man. He has had two other important relationships, and both these women have complained that he was physically abusive. He denies being abusive to his children, but has not been home enough to actually parent them. He reports sadness about that, as four of his children are in foster care.

Classification of Antisocial Disorders

The adult syndrome of antisocial personality disorder (ASPD) was first described by Harvey Cleckley in his famous book *The Mask of Insanity.* Cleckley's original characterization of interpersonal, behavioral, and affective deviance has remained the core of subsequent diagnostic criteria. As exemplified by A.W.'s history, people with this disorder are narcissistic, superficially charming, manipulative, often aggressive, and short-tempered; have multiple, unstable relationships; lack empathy and guilt; and display irresponsible behavior, often with overt criminality. The *Diagnostic and Statistical Manual*, 4th edition (DSM-IV) has defined ASPD as a persistent pattern of behavior that does not take into account the rights of others or that seeks to do overt harm to others. Criteria include an inability to maintain a stable relationship or employment, irresponsible behavior such as avoidance of financial obligations or parenting duties, cruel behavior toward animals or humans, and repeated arrests (or illegal activities, even if not caught). The *International Classification of Diseases,*10th edition (ICD-10) has similar criteria for dissocial personality. Most adults with ASPD began to display deviant behavior in childhood or adolescence. Youths with three or more of the following symptoms by age 13 are classified in the DSM-IV as having conduct disorder (CD): stealing with or without confrontation with the victim, running away, acts of cruelty or bullying, fighting, truancy, forcing someone into sexual relations, carrying or using a weapon, vandalism, and arrests.

Psychiatric diagnoses are traditionally made through clinical interviews, interviewer-rated symptom questionnaires, or self-report questionnaires. Each of these methods is difficult to use with the person who has antisocial personality features. These patients are rarely suffering or complaining of symptoms. In fact, in a brief interaction such as an examination, they may be quite charming and engaging. They are often puzzled as to why a psychiatric evaluation has been requested and usually blame others for their actions. Self-report inventories are problematic because of the high rate of lying in this population. The two most frequently used methods of assessment are highly structured interviews that follow strict diagnostic criteria such as those found in DSM-IV or the Hare Psychopathy Checklist (PCL). Filling out the PCL requires the use of multiple sources of information, rather than just using a clinical interview.

Epidemiology

The estimated prevalence of CD in prepubertal children is between 2 and 8% for boys and is less than 2% for girls. The gender gap narrows in adolescence and rates increase, with 3–12% of boys meeting criteria for the diagnosis compared to 8–10% of girls. CD is more common in urban areas than in suburban or rural neighborhoods, but poverty is a consistent correlate.

From 5 to 15% of the general adult population may meet criteria for this disorder; in the prison populations, the estimates range from 20 to 80%. ASPD is also much more common in adult males than in females.

Development and Course

In general, most of the studies on the development and course of antisocial disorders have studied males, although more studies are now including antisocial females. The majority of the studies have also used delinquent or criminal populations, so it is often difficult to generalize findings to nonincarcerated populations.

Biological Factors

There are several major lines of research into the biological factors that may underlie antisocial behaviors. One hypothesis is that CD or ASPD is caused by a general hypoarousal of the stress response system, producing a lack of response to stimuli that would normally provoke stress, fear, or pain. Numerous studies of men and boys with antisocial behavior demonstrate that their autonomic arousal, as measured by changes in skin conductance, heart rate, or blood pressure, is blunted in response to stimuli such as psychological threat, noise, or pain. The few studies conducted in girls have also reported blunted responses. The hypothalamic-pituitary-adrenocortical (HPA) axis also appears to be hypoactive in both the circadian secretion of cortisol and the response to psychological stimuli. These findings have been reported for boys, girls, and men who have antisocial behavior.

This lack of response would lead people with antisocial disorders to pursue excessive stimulation, manifested by sensation-seeking and risk-taking behaviors. Furthermore, they would be unable to learn from aversive consequences or punishment because their stress response would not be robust enough. Studies of heart rate, skin conductance, electroencephalogram (EEG) changes, and basal cortisol levels in subjects with antisocial behavior all support a theory of hypoarousal. Some of these characteristics in childhood and adolescence have been reported to predict adult sociopathy. Indicators of hypoarousal also differentiated between sociopathic and nonsociopathic subjects in a group of men whose fathers were all incarcerated, implying that the abnormalities in arousal may have a genetic basis.

A second line of research on putative biological mechanisms for sociopathy stems from neuropsychological and neuroimaging studies. Both types of data indicate that antisocial behavior is associated with abnormalities in the prefrontal and frontotemporal areas of the brain. These areas of the brain are responsible for the executive functions of the brain: impulse control, evaluation and integration of new data, and regulation of emotional tone and motivation. Abnormalities in these brain areas could lead to a pattern of sociopathic behavior by reducing the ability to delay gratification, decreasing the ability to learn new behaviors in response to past mistakes, and producing intense emotional states such as rage on an unpredictable basis.

Neurotransmitter function and gonadal hormonal influences on aggressive and impulsive behaviors in subjects with sociopathy have also been investigated. The findings in both domains are somewhat contradictory, but this may be due to methodological differences between studies.

In general, decreased serotonin neurotransmission in the central nervous system appears to be associated with aggression, although some researchers suggest that the link may actually be between low serotonin and impulsivity. Testosterone levels appear to be higher in some groups of violent males, but the relationship seems to be a reflection more of dominance than of pathological aggression.

Stress

The association between stress and antisocial behavior is complex and poorly understood. Many adults and children with antisocial behavior have histories of early exposure to adverse environmental circumstances. Similarly, longitudinal studies of young children demonstrate that many of them who experience obstetrical complications, early abuse or neglect, or repeated traumatizing events develop antisocial behavior by adolescence. This is particularly true for boys.

However, both adults and children with antisocial behavior report far lower subjective stress about these events than most people experience. The stress response system hypoactivity described previously is at odds with what we know from previous clinical and animal studies about exposure to adverse events. In these studies, the resulting stress response system dysfunction is most often characterized by either normal or increased resting function accompanied by hyperreactive and prolonged responses to stimuli. These physiological changes are usually accompanied by a heightened subjective experience of distress in humans. A chronically aroused state such as this can be associated with significant physical and psychiatric morbidity (e.g., hypertension, osteoporosis, dementia, depression). Therefore, one current theory is that stress response system hypoactivity in people with antisocial behavior may be protective, allowing them to survive in very difficult environments.

Childhood Risk Factors

Several risk factors present in childhood are associated with adult sociopathy. One of the most consistent findings, whether measured retrospectively or prospectively, is exposure to inconsistent and harsh parental discipline. The severity of the punishments can range from frequent verbal shaming to overt physical abuse, but the key prognostic factor appears to be the unpredictability of the hostile parental behaviors.

Children who have attentional problems with hyperactivity seem to be at particularly high risk of developing antisocial behavior. These studies have reported the same results for boys and girls. If the child also has a low IQ and one antisocial parent, then early sociopathic behavior is quite likely.

Developmental Paths

The course or path of childhood and adolescent antisocial behavior varies from person to person, but the continuity between this type of behavior and adult sociopathy is one of the most robust findings in clinical psychiatric research. Children who begin to display antisocial behavior prepubertally appear to be at the highest risk for severe sociopathy and progression to overt adult criminality.

Both childhood and adolescent-onset CD may progress through levels of increasing severity and frequency of the behaviors, a process known as escalation. Escalation is associated with an early onset of antisocial behavior, a history of family sociopathy, violence and aggressive behaviors, social marginalization in childhood, school failure, attention deficit and hyperactivity symptoms, and continued association with deviant peers. The behaviors may also simply cease in adolescence or early adulthood (desistence). Desistence is associated with a later onset of sociopathic behavior, an absence of aggression, a strong family structure, and early school and social success. The course of the disorder may also change when a person becomes involved with drugs or alcohol.

The majority of data on developmental paths have come from studies of males. Although less is known about females, a comprehensive review of the existing literature reported that girls with CD also appear to be at an increased risk for adult sociopathy. Additionally, many of these girls develop other psychiatric disorders and have a great deal of difficulty functioning as mothers or employees. Fewer girls progress to overt criminality when compared to boys, but many remain aggressive and destructive toward family members (e.g., their children or spouses).

Researchers are in disagreement about whether a subgroup of girls exists analogous to the subgroup of boys with early-onset antisocial behavior and a particularly severe and intractable course.

Prevention and Treatment

As discussed earlier, antisocial behaviors often begin in childhood or adolescence. Once established, they are very difficult to treat. As a result, researchers in the past two decades have begun to study the effectiveness of prevention. Some innovative prevention programs have reported surprisingly good results.

Although the programs differ somewhat, they have one common feature. All of them provide services to the child in every domain of his or her life. The programs often focus on mothers identified to be at risk for producing antisocial children and work to improve maternal physical and psychological health during pregnancy or following delivery. Didactic parenting training, coupled with close supervision by a visiting nurse, has also been helpful. Helping the mothers to establish their own support systems and showing them how to negotiate through the intricacies of the medical, welfare, and mental health systems has also been effective. The second type of preventive program focuses on assisting at-risk children in learning social skills in preschool and the community and early recognition and treatment of comorbid disorders such as attentional problems. Prevention programs that focus on whole communities of children or teens at risk have also had some success. These interventions usually occur in selected schools and consist of improving self-esteem through academic achievement or increasing prosocial behavior with game-based activities and rewards.

Standard psychiatric or psychological treatments are not very useful with patients who have antisocial disorders. The most effective treatment strategies are multimodal. Interventions that combine individual cognitive-behavioral psychotherapy, pharmacotherapy for aggression or hyperactivity, parenting training, school supervision, and anger management skills (often for the entire family) have the highest rates of success.

Once a youth has committed an illegal act and is arrested, or adjudicated delinquent, it is much harder for him or her to receive treatment rather than punishment. Data suggest that employing multimodal treatment programs, in combination with a compensation process, to atone for the offense and psychiatric treatment of comorbid disorders works better than incarceration at promoting desistence.

The same treatment dilemma exists for adults with ASPD. Those who do not engage in criminal behavior rarely present for treatment unless they are in the midst of a crisis such as a divorce. The personality characteristics of these patients make them poor candidates for psychotherapy. They may be noncompliant with any type of long-term treatment because they are only temporarily motivated to reduce the discomfort produced by the crisis. Adults with ASPD who have committed crimes do present for treatment while incarcerated, but this is usually because of comorbid psychiatric disorders such as depression. Pharmacological treatment of these comorbid problems or specific problematic behaviors such as aggression is possible, but the underlying pattern of sociopathic behavior is rarely altered.

See Also the Following Articles

Aggression; Child Abuse.

Further Reading

Cleckley, H. (1976). *The mask of sanity. An attempt to clarify some issues about the so-called psychopathic personality.* St. Louis, MO: The C. V. Mosby Company.

Ehrensaft, M. K., Moffitt, T. E. and Caspi, A. (2004). Clinically abusive relationships in an unselected birth cohort: men's and women's participation and developmental antecedents. *Journal of Abnormal Psychology* **113**, 258–270.

Farrington, D. P., Loeber, R., Yin, Y., et al. (2002). Are within-individual causes of delinquency the same as between-individual causes? *Criminal Behaviour and Mental Health* **12**, 53–68.

Hare, R. D., Hart, S. D. and Harpur, T. J. (1991). Psychopathy and the DSM-IV criteria for antisocial personality disorder. *Journal of Abnormal Psychology* **100**, 391–398.

Kazdin, A. E. (2002). Family and parenting interventions for conduct disorder and delinquency: a meta-analysis of randomized controlled trials. *Journal of Pediatrics* **141**, 738.

Laub, J. H. and Sampson, R. J. (2003). *Shared beginnings, divergent lives. Delinquent boys to age 70.* Cambridge, MA: Harvard University Press.

Lilienfeld, S. O. (1998). Methodological advances and developments in the assessment of psychopathy. *Behaviour Research and Therapy* **36**, 99–125.

Loeber, R., Stouthamer-Loeber, M., Farrington, D. P., et al. (2002). Three longitudinal studies of children's development in Pittsburgh: the Developmental Trends Study, the Pittsburgh Youth Study, and the Pittsburgh Girls Study. *Criminal Behaviour and Mental Health* **12**, 1–23.

Morgan, A. B. and Lilienfeld, S. O. (2000). A meta-analytic review of the relation between antisocial behavior and neuropsychological measures of executive function. *Clinical Psychology Review* **20**, 113–136.

Pajer, K. (1998). What happens to "bad" girls? A review of the adult outcomes of antisocial adolescent girls. *American Journal of Psychiatry* **155**, 862–870.
Pajer, K., Gardner, W., Rubin, R., et al. (2001). Decreased cortisol levels in adolescent girls with conduct disorder. *Archives of General Psychiatry* **58**, 297–302.
Raine, A. (2002). Biosocial studies of antisocial and violent behavior in children and adults: a review. *Journal of Abnormal Child Psychology* **30**, 311–326.
Silverthorn, P. and Frick, P. J. (1999). Developmental pathways to antisocial behavior: The delayed-onset pathway in girls. *Development and Psychopathology* **11**, 101–126.

Domestic Violence

B Donohue, H Hill and T Maier-Paarlberg
University of Nevada at Las Vegas, Las Vegas, NV, USA

This is a revised version of the article by T Maier-Paarlberg and B Donohue, Encyclopedia of Stress First Edition, volume 1, pp 734–738, © 2000, Elsevier Inc.

Glossary

Domestic violence Any act of maltreatment occurring in the home environment of the victim perpetrated by a person who assumes the role of a caregiver or who is in an established relationship with the victim.

Neglect The omission of appropriate caretaking functions that leads to a lack of self-preservation and growth in the dependent individual.

Physical abuse A harmful act carried out on an individual with the intention of causing physical pain or injury.

Sexual abuse Illegal, nonconsensual, or socially inappropriate contact or exposure of genitalia.

Verbal/ emotional/ mental abuse The use of derogatory statements that cause the victim psychological pain or feelings of devaluation.

Description

Domestic violence includes all aspects of abuse and neglect that are perpetrated within the victim's home environment by a person who assumes the role of a caregiver or who is in an established relationship with the victim. Abuse and neglect have been around since the beginning of civilization; however, various forms of abuse have only recently been defined and studied extensively. Although definitions of abuse vary considerably, neglect and three types of abuse (physical abuse, sexual abuse, and psychological/mental/emotional/verbal abuse) have consistently been recognized in the domestic violence literature. This article provides an overview of domestic violence, including its risk factors, its prevalence, and a delineation of neglect and abuse.

Neglect

In general, neglect refers to the omission of appropriate caretaking functions that results in harm to the dependent individual. Victims of neglect are therefore dependent on a guardian or caregiver for self-preservation and growth. Most often, victims of neglect include children, adults who evidence severe mental or physical disabilities (e.g., mental retardation and Parkinson's disease), and elderly people with medical complications or other problems associated with old age. Prevalence studies consistently indicate that neglect is the most frequently occurring form of maltreatment. For instance, the National Clearinghouse on Child Abuse and Neglect reported that an estimated 906,000 children were determined to be victims of child abuse in 2003 and that, of those claims, more than 60% experienced neglect. Although risk factors are varied, they most often include substance abuse, physical disabilities, social isolation, psychiatric illness, social isolation, stress, poor parenting skills, and unrealistic expectations of the child's development. People of lower economic status appear to be overrepresented in abuse samples, perhaps because abuse is more common for these individuals but also because they may be reported and charged with abuse more often due to reasons associated with poverty (e.g., relatively inadequate representation by legal counsel). Incidents of neglect include interfering with (or delaying) medical protocol, leaving small children unattended for extended periods of time in potentially dangerous situations (e.g., being left in an automobile while the caregiver drinks alcohol inside a bar), restricting or failing to provide sufficient nutrients or shelter, failing to repair home hazards (e.g., exposed electrical wires and broken steps), exposing victim to toxins or bacteria (e.g., failing to clean dog feces from the kitchen floor where an infant crawls), failing to provide adequate affection, and restricting children from attending school. Indicators of neglect include dirty and unkempt bodies, rotten teeth, clothes that are too small or are in need of repair, and untidy and disheveled home environments.

Psychological Abuse

Psychological abuse, also known as verbal, mental, or emotional abuse, typically refers to derogatory statements that cause harm to or interfere with the psychological adjustment of the victim. These statements are most often attacks on the victim's competence ("You can't do anything right; you're just a big dummy") or character (e.g., "You're a lazy, unpopular, good for nothing"). Psychological abuse is usually associated with obscenities, negative voice tones, exploitation, encouraging corruption and delinquent behavior, excessive teasing, harmful threats, ridicule, or derogatory statements about the victim or people whom the victim likes. There do not appear to be significant gender differences regarding the prevalence of psychological abuse because studies have consistently indicated that the vast majority of the population has experienced some level of psychological abuse from an adult family member in their lifetime. Interestingly, people often underestimate the severity of psychological abuse relative to other forms of maltreatment because its consequences are subtle and there are few, if any, legal sanctions that mitigate against its use. Nevertheless, severe consequences of verbal abuse have been found, including depression, antisocial behaviors, low self-esteem, intellectual deficits, academic difficulties, health problems, shyness, problem-solving deficits, anxiety, and difficulties with conflict resolution and other social skills. Moreover, psychological abuse is often a precursor of physical abuse by the perpetrator and of retaliatory aggression by the victim.

Physical Abuse

Physical abuse is usually defined as any harmful act carried out on an individual with the intention of causing pain or injury (e.g., kicking, spanking severe enough to cause bruises, whipping with an extension cord, punching, biting, or threatening with a knife or a gun). Victims are usually people who are emotionally or financially dependent on the perpetrator (e.g., spouses, lovers, children, or the elderly). Although neglect is estimated to be the most frequently occurring form of maltreatment, physical abuse has probably received greater attention in the scientific literature. According to a 1998 Commonwealth Fund Survey, approximately 3 million women are physically abused each year by their intimate companions, sometimes resulting in fatalities. In 2003, the Bureau of Justice Statistics Crime data indicated that, on average, more than three women are murdered by their husbands or boyfriends each day in the United States. Approximately one-half of the adult victims of physical abuse retaliate with physical violence of their own due to self-defense or escalation of violence, lending support to the notion that physical abuse in adults is often reciprocal. Indeed, males in dependent relationships also suffer from physical abuse; however, it is relatively less often reported to authorities and the maltreatment is usually not as severe. Interestingly, the prevalence rates of physical abuse among homosexual adult relationships approximate those of heterosexual adult relationships.

Children are prime targets for physical abuse. Indeed, estimates of physical-abuse victimization in children are usually around 30%. The perpetrators of child physical abuse are often of lower economic status, substance abusers, single parents, socially isolated, and depressed; evince inadequate coping skills; and report a history of being maltreated as a child. Other risk factors include low birth weight, physical and mental disabilities, immaturity, child noncompliance and misconduct, impulsiveness, deficits in family cohesion, family conflict, history of abuse, limited positive interactions, unrealistic expectations and negative perceptions of children, inconsistent parenting styles, lack of familiarity with the developmental norms of children, stress, lack of empathy, and antisocial personality. The number of studies conducted with elderly victims of physical abuse and other forms of maltreatment has recently increased, more so than in other age groups. Although this increased attention is due to multiple factors, several are fairly obvious. The human life span has increased, resulting in more elderly individuals who are living with age-associated medical problems and physical limitations. Changes in health care, among other factors, have forced older adults to reside with family who are often ill-equipped to tolerate the added stress associated with their care, which often results in frustration for both the victim and perpetrator. A recent study of nursing home residents revealed that aggression from residents toward the staff was the strongest predictor of elder abuse. Investigations of the risk factors for elderly abuse are consonant with those of other age groups.

Sexual Abuse

Sexual abuse is generally defined as any illegal, nonconsensual, or inappropriate contact or exposure of genitalia, including sexual humiliation. However, legal definitions of sexual abuse vary considerably. For instance, some agencies (i.e., Federal Bureau of Investigation) have defined rape as attempted or completed vaginal intercourse with a female by force and against her will, whereas states have adopted unique qualifiers for this term, such as gender neutrality; anal or oral penetration; insertion of objects; and being unable to give sexual consent because of mental illness, mental retardation, or intoxication. Other common patterns of sexual abuse include, but are not limited to, being forced to observe or perform pornography and fondling or kissing the genitalia of a child or nonconsenting adult. Approximately 10% of marriages have involved rape without physical violence, and estimates from the National Clearinghouse on Child Abuse and Neglect have indicated that as much as 10% of reported abuse cases in the United States involved inappropriate sexual contact or exposure. Sexual abuse victimization may occur as early as infancy, and it is characteristically progressive; approximately half of sexually abused children will continue to be abused until they leave the abusive home. The perpetrators of domestic sexual abuse are very often in-laws, foster parents, nonrelatives, older siblings, or cousins, but they may also include other relatives living in the home of the victim. The majority of perpetrators of sexual abuse are male. However, female perpetrators may be more common than studies suggest, perhaps because their abuse is not reported more often than that of males. A large percentage of rapes in college populations are committed by someone the victim knows. Factors that have been found to influence sexual abuse include neurological disorders, particularly frontal lobe abnormalities; sexual abuse of or repeated witnessing of pornography by the perpetrator during childhood; mental illness; substance abuse; and dysfunctional family systems.

Consequences

The consequences of abuse and neglect are, as might be inferred, extremely debilitating for the victim, and these negative consequences inevitably affect close relatives and friends of the victim. Consequences that have been identified include low self-worth, anxiety and mood disorders, problems maintaining pleasant functional relationships, problems in toileting, antisocial conduct and maltreatment of others, suicide, poor social and coping skills, problems in school or employment, substance abuse, and personality disorders. Malnutrition is a hallmark of neglect. Sexual abuse victims may demonstrate inappropriate or promiscuous sexual activity, including prostitution and other illegal sexual undertakings. A particular concern is the recapitulation of abuse because, more often than not, the victim becomes a perpetrator with the passage of time.

Remediation Strategies

Professionals (i.e., teachers, police officers, ministers, and health-care workers) are mandated in most states to report suspected incidents of domestic violence. Familiarity with the risk factors and consequences of domestic violence are of great assistance in the identification of abuse. However, professionals are often not trained, or able, to recognize abuse, particularly because victims are motivated to deny or minimize assaultive behaviors because their perpetrators are usually people whom they often love, fear, or respect. Moreover, once identified, domestic violence is difficult to remediate. Initial strategies focus on assessing the victim's environment to determine if it is (1) safe for the victim to remain in the home with the perpetrator, (2) necessary to remove the victim from the home (to live with other relative, in a foster-care home, or in a shelter), or (3) necessary to mandate that the perpetrator leave the home. The separation of the victim from the perpetrator is certainly the safest strategy for terminating the abuse. However, this approach is often not possible because relatives are frequently unavailable and shelters and foster-care homes usually operate with inadequate funding, causing them to sometimes be full, dangerous, or overcrowded. Moreover, familial separation is marked with changes that bring about stress (e.g., new school placements, feelings of abandonment and rejection, and financial losses). Therefore, separation is typically sought only when cases of maltreatment are severe (e.g., sexual abuse or repeated instances of physical abuse). Adult victims and perpetrators of domestic violence are usually forced to fund their own therapy. However, state child protective service agencies will provide psychologically based intervention for child victims and relevant family members at no cost, when indicated. Interventions may be focused on reunifying and improving the function of the existing family system or facilitating a comfortable and healthy transition for the victim without the perpetrator. Therapy is ordinarily mandated by the legal system for child victims and their perpetrators when the goal is family reunification.

Of the interventions that have been evaluated, the cognitive-behavioral and stress-reduction strategies appear to be most promising. Cognitive-behavioral interventions most often include the recognition of the early signs of abuse, learning strategies to improve safety and prevent the escalation of abuse, restructuring faulty cognitions and beliefs about the abuse (e.g., victims may blame themselves for abuse; perpetrators might think the role of a woman is to serve her spouse), learning to improve appropriate social/assertion skills, anger-management skills training, contingency contracting (obtaining rewards that are contingent on behavioral improvement, e.g., good grades in school, compliance to the directives of parents, and making statements of affection), learning to eliminate home hazards and improve home beautification, behavioral substance-abuse counseling (e.g., controlling urges to use substances, restructuring the environment so that drug use is less likely, and contingency contracting), vocational skills training, learning positive parenting techniques (e.g., reinforcing the child for desired behaviors, positive practice, and learning about child development and nutrition), marital counseling, multisystemic family therapy, and communication skills training. Stress-management strategies include bringing children to day care or babysitters to allow the caregiver a relaxing break at home, learning problem-solving and coping skills, attending Parents Anonymous groups (an organization established to support the victims and perpetrators of abuse), planning pleasant activities with the family, and encouraging/facilitating participation in community groups (e.g., church and boys' and girls' clubs).

Historical Perspectives

Perceptions of domestic violence have changed markedly throughout history and across cultures. Indeed, it was not until the past century that laws were initiated to protect children and wives from being beaten by their parents and husbands; for instance, as recently as 1968 many states did not mandate professionals to report their knowledge of abusive treatment to abuse registries. Nevertheless, there have been radical improvements in public sentiment and the legal system regarding the eradication of domestic violence. In ancient times, individuals with mental and physical disabilities were scorned or killed to rid the state and parents of the economic burden of caring for them. Although the treatment of children and women improved somewhat in most societies during the Middle Ages, neglect, ridicule, slavery, and harsh physical punishment continued. It is also interesting to note that children in nineteenth-century industrialized nations were forced to work up to 14 h a day in hazardous conditions.

The improvements in the rights of children and women were partially a result of humanitarians who wrote books about the injustice of domestic violence. For instance, during the Renaissance Thomas Phaire wrote a book addressing the problems of children called *The Book of Chyldren,* and in the late 1600s and early 1700s Locke and Rousseau wrote books that mentioned issues pertaining to the development of children. Erin Pizzey's 1974 book *Scream Quietly or the Neighbors Will Hear* was one of the first manuscripts in the literature that specifically addressed remediation procedures for spousal abuse.

National organizations, governmental meetings, and activists also influenced the passing of laws protecting against domestic violence. The Society for the Prevention of Cruelty to Children in the late 1800s was formed to protect rights and welfare of children. In 1909, President Theodore Roosevelt organized the first meeting in the White House on children's welfare, which supported the Children's Bureau in 1912 to protect the welfare and rights of children. Pizzey was responsible for developing the first refuge for female victims of spousal abuse in England in 1971; the first refuge for women and their children in the United States was initiated by the Women's Advocates in 1972.

Although domestic violence continues today at relatively high rates, research and public opinion and protection laws against domestic violence are at their highest level of sophistication. Indeed, all 50 states currently require professionals to report suspected instances of child maltreatment, and most states have explicitly allocated significant funding to programs for the prevention and treatment of domestic violence. Indeed, law enforcement personnel now routinely receive specialized training for managing situations involving domestic violence, including victim-sensitivity training. Violence treatment programs have also become increasingly more evidence-based while addressing contemporary issues such as violence among same-sex couples, date rape, violence prevention within school settings, and comorbid conditions (e.g., substance abuse).

See Also the Following Articles

Aggression; Caregivers, Stress and; Child Abuse; Male Partner Violence; Marital Conflict; Sexual Assault.

Further Reading

Bergen, R. (ed.) (1998). *Issues in intimate violence.* Thousand Oaks, CA: Sage.

Donohue, B., Ammerman, R. T. and Zelis, K. (1998). Child physical abuse and neglect. In: Watson, T. S. & Gresham F. M. (eds.) *Handbook of child behavioral therapy*, pp. 183–202. New York: Plenum.

Feindler, E. L., Rathus, J. H. and Silver, L. B. (2003). *Assessment of family violence: a handbook for researchers and practitioners.* Washington, DC: American Psychological Association.

Lutzker, J. R. (2006). *Preventing violence: research and evidence-based intervention strategies.* Washington, DC: American Psychological Association.

Child Abuse

C C Swenson and L Saldana
Medical University of South Carolina, Charleston, SC, USA

This is a revised version of the article by C C Swenson and C E Ezzel, Encyclopedia of Stress First Edition, volume 1, pp 438–441, © 2000, Elsevier Inc.

Glossary

Factitious disorder by proxy — Disorder that occurs when adults deliberately produce or feign physical or psychological symptoms in a child under their care with the presumed motivation a psychological need to assume the sick role.

Failure to thrive — In infancy this is indicated by a growth delay with postural signs (poor muscle tone, persistence of infantile postures) and behavioral signs (unresponsive, minimal smiling, few vocalizations) and may be a result of child neglect.

Multisystemic therapy for child abuse and neglect (MST-CAN) — An ecological treatment model that takes into account all of the etiological factors related to a problem behavior and treats those factors through changes in the family and social ecology. The delivery of treatment is generally in the home and at times convenient for families, with 24 hours a day, 7 days a week on-call coverage for crises. This treatment is an adaptation of standard MST that has established efficacy with deep-end delinquents. MST-CAN, developed at the Medical University of South Carolina, has been shown to be effective with physically abused children and their families.

Parent–child interaction therapy (PCIT) — A short-term early intervention approach in which young children and their parents are provided with direct coaching in interactions during play or specific tasks. PCIT is appropriate for young children demonstrating externalizing and internalizing behavior problems. PCIT has recently been established as effective with physically abused children and their families in a clinical trial at the University of Oklahoma Health Sciences Center.

Reinforcement-based intensive outpatient therapy (RBT) — A treatment model developed at Johns Hopkins University and applied to mothers with heroin or cocaine addiction. The model provides intensive treatment and focuses on skills needed to become abstinent, monitoring of substance use, abstinence-contingent housing, prosocial recreational activities, social skills, and employment counseling.

Shaken baby syndrome — An injury to the brain of an infant that results from vigorous shaking. Shaken baby syndrome is a form of physical abuse and often results in death to the child.

Child Physical Abuse

Child physical abuse is defined as physical injury to a child under age 18 by an adult. Acts of physical abuse may vary from hitting that leaves bruising to actions that involve welts, cuts, bites, broken bones, burns, poisoning, and internal injures to soft tissue and organs. In special cases, termed factitious disorder by proxy, adults inflict injury or induce illness in a child under their care, present the child for medical care, and feign no knowledge of the etiology.

Epidemiology

According to reports from state agencies, nearly 3 million children are abused and neglected annually. Among those reported for suspicions of abuse, roughly 25% are investigated for physical abuse. In a congressionally mandated prevalence study of child abuse and neglect called the Third National Incidence Study, a broader sample of cases that extended beyond child protection reports was included. Of the 2 815 600 abused or neglected youth, 22% were physically abused.

Etiology

The complexity of child abuse and neglect is highlighted in the literature, showing that multiple risk factors relate to whether physical abuse will occur. These risk factors include (1) parent factors such as history of abuse, substance abuse, deficits in knowledge of child development, depression, poor impulse control, negative perception of the child, and neuropsychological dysfunction; (2) child factors such as age, aggression, noncompliance, and delayed development; (3) family factors such as high conflict, spouse or partner abuse, and single marital status; (4) social network factors such as social isolation, low use of community resources, and limited involvement in community activities; and (5) community factors such as economic disadvantage, instability, poor organization, and high resource need coupled with low resources available for child care. Although each of the systems noted above (i.e. family, community) is part of every child's life, the particular risk factors within each system will differ from family to family. For example, in one family, substance abuse, child aggression, and isolation from social networks may be the key factors driving the abuse. In another family, partner violence, child developmental delay, living in an unstable neighborhood, and low parenting skills may be the driving risk factors.

Medical and Mental Health Effects

Physical abuse injuries range from mild (e.g., bruises) to severe (e.g., broken bones, gunshot wound) and account for 10% of injuries among children who present for emergency room care. Physical injuries that might be mild for an older child can be fatal for an infant. For example, when babies are shaken, the resulting damage to the brain can leave children severely developmentally delayed but may also result in death. This act against infants is termed shaken baby syndrome. Some children do not need medical care following physical abuse, but an assessment of potential injury is always a safe bet. Mental health effects of child physical abuse vary by the child, experience, and context of the abuse. These effects generally occur in five domains: (1) aggression and behavioral dysfunction toward peers and adults; (2) poor interpersonal relations and social competence such as social skills deficits, poor social problem solving, and peer rejection; (3) trauma-related emotional symptoms such as depression, posttraumatic stress disorder (PTSD), anxiety, and suicidality; (4) developmental deficits in relationship skills including anxious attachment in very young children, low frustration tolerance, and difficulty managing conflict; and, (5) cognitive and neuropsychological impairment such as receptive and expressive language difficulties and low performance in math and reading. In addition, physical abuse places children at risk of long-term mental health difficulties in adulthood such as substance abuse, violent crime, depression, and relationship problems.

Treatment Approaches

In a number of practice settings, physically abused children participate in individual treatment and parents go to parenting groups. The literature on physical abuse indicates that behavioral parent training has empirical support with this population for reducing parental aggression toward children. However, the problem of child abuse and neglect is so complex that individual child treatment or parent training alone will not resolve the risk factors that have led to the abuse in the first place. Since 1996, advances have been made in research regarding the treatment of physically abused children and their families. Through randomized clinical trials, three treatments are showing promise: parent–child interaction therapy (PCIT), trauma-focused cognitive-behavioral therapy (CBT), and multisystemic therapy for child abuse and neglect (MST-CAN). All three are treatments that address parent and child risk factors. This characteristic is important in that past research has focused on treatment of the parent or child only. Given the multidetermined etiology that relates to physical abuse, the importance of continued evaluation of comprehensive treatments and dissemination of effective treatments is paramount. Parental substance abuse has become a major factor in child abuse and neglect reports and out-of-home placement. Treatments that successfully address substance abuse and child abuse are sorely needed.

Child Neglect

Despite inconsistencies in state definitions, generally neglect is defined as physical (refusal or delay in seeking health care; inadequate supervision, hygiene, nutrition, and safety), emotional (failure to provide adequate attention, warmth, and affection and/or exposure to substance abuse or violence), and/or educational (failure to promote education or school attendance and inattention to special education needs) omissions in parenting. Recent evidence suggests that these neglectful behaviors fall into three distinct categories: physical, psychological, and environmental neglect. Child neglect has been grossly underresearched in the United States, leading to the phrase neglect of neglect. Throughout the literature, child abuse and neglect often are grouped together despite the clear distinction between acts of commission and those of omission. Whereas many people think of child abuse when considering child maltreatment, child neglect is in fact more prevalent, costly, and detrimental.

Epidemiology

Of the 896 000 indicated child maltreatment cases in the United States in 2002, over 60% of those children were exposed to neglect. The number of youths who experience child neglect has more than doubled since the mid-1980s, an increase more than eight times greater than the rise in children's population. Moreover, prevalence studies suggest that approximately 45% of child maltreatment fatalities are the result of neglect, with 1 400 deaths recorded in 2002. These figures likely provide a gross underestimate of the incidence of child neglect in our country, as acts of omission are far more difficult to identify than those of commission. Studies from the general population suggest that as many as 2 million children are endangered by neglect.

Etiology

As with child physical abuse, the factors related to neglectful parenting practices are multidetermined. Evidence suggests that risk factors include (1) parent factors such as mental illness, low cognitive functioning, substance abuse, and a history of child maltreatment; (2) family factors such as domestic violence, social isolation, high levels of family stress, and poverty; (3) child factors such as child physical disability or chronic illness; and (4) community factors such as impoverished neighborhoods, acceptance among community members of low monitoring or low school attendance, and poor community cohesion.

Although the etiology of neglectful parenting is multifaceted, of particular note is the influence of substance abuse. There appears to be an association between the staggering increase in neglectful parenting practices and the increase in identified substance abuse among child welfare cases. Children whose parents abuse substances are more than four times as likely to be neglected as those who are not abusing substances, and parental substance abuse is more often a factor in reports of child neglect than other forms of child maltreatment. Parental substance abuse, which is identified in up to 79% of child protection cases, not only is one of the strongest risk factors for abuse and neglect, but also is the deciding factor in the majority of cases in which children are taken into custody and placed out of the home.

Medical and Mental Health Effects of Child Neglect

The medical and mental health effects of neglect on the child are dependent on the nature of the neglectful parenting practices. Potential consequences are immense and can cause deleterious physiological and emotional stress on the child and family. Compared to other forms of maltreatment, child neglect has been associated with the most profound developmental and cognitive delays and has the greatest risk of enduring effects. Children who are neglected often evidence language and academic deficits, inadequate social skills, poor growth development including nonorganic failure to thrive, medical problems, and poor attachments and interpersonal relationships. Moreover, those who are neglected by substance-abusing mothers are at increased risk for conduct problems including delinquency, substance abuse, and maltreatment of their own children. The most severe forms of neglect, however, result in child fatality.

Treatment Approaches

There is a dearth of controlled clinical trials with sufficient power to examine outcomes with regard to neglect. Despite these deficits in the literature, there is evidence to suggest that an ecological approach to treatment is beneficial with neglectful families. Across studies, results suggest that neglectful parents benefit from skills training including improved problem solving, reducing safety hazards, increasing hygienic and home cleaning practices, and improving child nutrition and intellectual stimulation. Further, studies have demonstrated positive parental response to protocols targeting improving adaptive attachment styles, affective relationships, and recognition of children's emotional needs. Despite these advances in treatment approaches with neglectful parents, there is a strong need for evidenced-based practice in this area. In particular, an urgent need exists for treatment models to address co-occurring substance abuse and child abuse and neglect. At present, the majority of treatments address the two problems independently. Work has begun in Connecticut on a project known as Building Stronger Families. This project involves the integration of MST-CAN and reinforcement-based therapy. The latter has established efficacy with serious substance abuse.

See Also the Following Articles

Child Sexual Abuse; Childhood Stress; Child Physical Abuse.

Further Reading

Chaffin, M., Silovsky, J. F., Funderburk, B., et al. (2004). Parent–child interaction therapy with physically abusive parents: efficacy for reducing future abuse reports. *Journal of Consulting and Clinical Psychology* 72, 500–510.

Donohue, B. (2004). Coexisting child neglect and drug abuse in young mothers. *Behavior Modification* **28**, 206–233.
Dubowitz, H. (1999). *Neglected children: research, practice, and policy.* Thousand Oaks, CA: Sage.
Gaudin, J. (1993). *Child neglect: a guide for intervention.* Washington, D.C: U.S. Department of Health and Human Services.
Gruber, K., Chutuape, M. A. and Stitzer, M. L. (2000). Reinforcement-based intensive outpatient treatment for inner city opiate abusers: a short-term evaluation. *Drug and Alcohol Dependence* **57**, 211–223.
Kolko, D. J. and Swenson, C. C. (2002). *Assessing and treating physically abused children and their families: a cognitive behavioral approach.* Thousand Oaks, CA: Sage Publications.
National Clearinghouse on Child Abuse and Neglect (2004). *Child maltreatment 2002: summary of key findings.* Washington, D.C: U.S. Department of Health and Human Services.
Sedlak, A. J. and Broadhurst, D. D. (1996). *Executive summary of the Third National Incidence Study of Child Abuse and Neglect.* Washington, D.C: U.S. Department of Health and Human Services.
Swenson, C. C., Saldana, L., Joyner, C. D. and Henggeler, S. W. (in press). *Ecological treatment for parent to child violence. Interventions for children exposed to violence.* New Brunswick, NJ: Johnson & Johnson.

Child Physical Abuse

C C Swenson
Medical University of South Carolina, Charleston, SC, USA

Glossary

Child physical abuse Involves physical behavior by an adult toward a child that results in injury to the child. Signs of physical abuse may include bruises, welts, cuts, broken bones, skull fractures, burns, poisoning, internal injuries of soft tissue and organs, and injuries to the bone and tissue joints of a child under the age of 18 years

Multisystemic therapy for child abuse and neglect (MST-CAN) An adaptation of multisystemic therapy for delinquency that involves treatment of the entire family through interventions targeting multiple risk factors. Treatment is delivered in the home and at times convenient for families, with 24 hours a day, 7 days a week on-call coverage for crises. This model, developed at the Medical University of South Carolina, is applied to families who have come under the guidance of child protection due to physical abuse.

Munchausen by proxy syndrome (MBPS) A form of child abuse in which a parent fabricates or produces illness in a child and/or creates physical signs that persistently result in unnecessary medical treatment.

Parent–child interaction therapy (PCIT) A short-term intervention currently applied to young children and their parents. The method involves direct coaching of parents in interactions during play or specific tasks. Through a recent clinical trial conducted at the University of Oklahoma Health Sciences Center, PCIT was established as effective for treating young physically abused children.

Shaken baby syndrome Applies to infants who undergo vigorous shaking that leads to acceleration–deceleration injuries to the brain. These infants generally present at less than 1 year of age with seizures, vomiting, lethargy or bradycardia, hypotension, respiratory irregularities, coma, or death.

Child physical abuse is a major public health problem that generally involves acts of physical violence by a parent or carer toward a child. Because physically abusive acts range greatly in intensity and duration, the subsequent mental health consequences vary widely. Treatment must involve the child, parent, and entire family.

Prevalence

Data regarding the prevalence of child physical abuse (CPA) in the United States are gathered from child protection agencies and through national surveys. These data indicate that annually, nearly 3 million children are abused and neglected. Among those reported for suspicions of abuse, roughly 25% are investigated for physical abuse. In an evaluation of reporting practices of professionals, the National Center on Child Abuse and Neglect (NCCAN) conducted a series of National Incidence Studies of Child Abuse and Neglect. They found that approximately 2.3/1000 children are physically abused. The 1995 Gallup poll estimated the rate of CPA to be 49/1000 children, more than five times the NCCAN report.

Etiology

The etiological factors related to CPA are multiple and complex. They range across many different systems (e.g., parent, child, family) and vary by individual families. Current research has not established what factors cause physical abuse. At best, the understanding of etiology involves factors that correlate with physical abuse, also called risk factors. These risk factors are specific to the child, parent, family, and community.

The children most at risk of physical abuse are those who (1) are younger, (2) have developmental delays, (3) have other special needs such as chronic medical conditions, and (4) exhibit noncompliant behavior. A number of parent factors increase the risk of physical abuse. First is childhood abuse history. Roughly one-third of adults who were physically abused as children go on to abuse their own children. Second, certain cognitive factors increase the parent's risk of harm to the child. Parents who view their child in a negative light, distort beliefs about the reasons why children act as they do (e.g., he cries to make me upset), expect the child to be responsible for the parent's welfare, and have unrealistic expectations beyond age and skill capability are at greater risk of abusing their child. Parents who physically abuse are more likely to show emotional difficulties such as difficulty regulating emotions, including irritability, sadness, anxiety, explosiveness, hostility, anger, and perceptions that life is more stressful. They are more likely to show deficits in positive parenting. Psychiatric difficulties such as depression and posttraumatic stress disorder may make general problem solving difficult and hamper an individual's capacity to regulate emotions and parent in a nonphysical way. Parental substance abuse, in particular, is a factor that places parents at significant risk of abusing their children and is a major factor in the decision to remove children from their families and place them in state custody. Family factors that increase the risk of physical abuse include a volatile home environment in which there is domestic violence, limited psychosocial resources, and general family stressors such as frequent moves or family dissolution. Existing research has identified economic disadvantage, instability and isolation, and neighborhood burden as factors that increase the risk of child maltreatment. The latter factor, neighborhood burden, refers to greater childcare need with fewer resources.

Mental Health Effects

Mental health difficulties related to CPA include those that occur in the short term and those that persist. It should be noted that some physically abused children will not experience mental health problems. Others will experience problems that dissipate with time or with intervention, and yet others will experience problems that endure into adulthood and result in patterns of behavior and coping that disrupt the management of behavior, emotions, and relationships.

Risk and Buffering Factors

In part, the emergence and persistence of symptomatology relate to factors specific to the event, cultural and community context, family, and individual characteristics. Such factors may potentiate a negative or a buffering effect. In relationship to the event, exposure to multiple incidents of maltreatment increases vulnerability for the development of mental health problems, such as substance abuse, severe suicidal behavior, and emotional problems. In fact, as the number and type of traumatic events accumulate, the outcomes (i.e., internalizing and externalizing disorders) appear to worsen. In addition, chronicity of physical punishment during childhood also has been associated with delinquent behavior, symptoms of depression, suicidal thoughts, and alcohol abuse later in life.

Factors specific to the child, such as gender (e.g., girls are at risk of internalizing disorders; boys are at risk of externalizing) or developmental disabilities may place him or her at risk of psychiatric symptomatology. In families, greater maternal stress and poor conflict management are associated with severity of functional impairment. The combination of low family cohesion and high family conflict are common risk factors for aggression and substance abuse problems. Social and family support and placing responsibility on the adult who abused rather than the child relate to more positive mental health outcomes.

Short-Term Effects

Multiple effects have been associated with the occurrence of CPA. Behavioral and emotional difficulties include externalizing problems, such as aggression, and internalizing problems, such as anxiety or depression. Social and relationship difficulties include poor peer and adult relations that are exacerbated by difficulty managing conflict and low confidence in regulating negative mood. Cognitive and neuropsychological impairment is typically shown through skills deficits in expressive and receptive language, reading comprehension, and auditory attention. More severe forms of physical abuse result in risk of death. These include shaken baby syndrome and Munchausen's by proxy. In the latter, parents have been shown to conduct behaviors such as smothering to create a medical problem that then wins them attention.

Long-Term Effects

The potential long-term impact of CPA falls into three categories: aggression, substance abuse, and emotional problems. Aggression is expressed toward peers, family members, and dating partners and may include violent crimes or physical abuse of one's own child. CPA is associated with substance use, more lifetime treatment, and a more severe course of substance abuse later in adulthood. For adults, a history of CPA has been found to relate to a host of emotional difficulties, including somatization, anxiety, depression, hostility, paranoid ideation, psychosis, dissociation, and self-injurious and suicidal behavior.

Treatment Approaches

Treatments for the effects of CPA are those that are directed toward child, parent, or family symptomatology and comprehensive approaches that address all persons involved or impacted. Most studies targeting child symptoms have been with preschoolers who are in a day treatment program or receiving instruction in peer relations and have shown success in increasing social skills and peer relations. One cognitive-behavioral group therapy study with school-age physically abused children found reductions on self-report measures of posttraumatic stress disorder, general anxiety, depression, and anger symptoms but no improvement on social competence and externalizing behaviors, potentially highlighting the need to include carers in treatment. In a small number of studies, parent training has been shown to decrease abusive behaviors in parents. More comprehensive models, such as cognitive-behavioral treatment with parent and child, parent–child interaction therapy, and multisystemic therapy for child abuse and neglect, are showing promise for reducing child symptoms, adult risk factors related to CPA, and re-abuse. Importantly, recent comprehensive pilot programs such as the Building Stronger Families program being implemented by the Connecticut Department of Children and Families are targeting risk factors within the family and ecology with an intensive focus on parental substance abuse.

See Also the Following Articles

Childhood Stress; Domestic Violence.

Further Reading

Borrego, J., Urquiza, A. J., Rasmussen, R. A. and Zebell, N. (1999). Parent-child interaction therapy with a family at high risk for physical abuse. *Child Maltreatment* **4**, 331–342.

Chaffin, M., Kelleher, K. and Hollenberg, J. (1996). Onset of physical abuse and neglect: psychiatric, substance abuse, and social risk factors from prospective community data. *Child Abuse & Neglect* **20**, 191–203.

Chaffin, M., Silovsky, J. F., Funderburk, B., et al. (2004). Parent-child interaction therapy with physically abusive parents: efficacy for reducing future abuse reports. *Journal of Consulting and Clinical Psychology* **72**, 500–510.

Chapman, D., Whitfield, C., Felitti, V., Dube, S., Edwards, V. and Anda, R. (2004). Adverse childhood experiences and the risk of depressive disorders in adulthood. *Journal of Affective Disorders* **82**, 217–225.

Chasnoff, I. J. and Lowder, L. A. (1999). Parental alcohol and drug use and risk for child maltreatment: a timely approach to intervention. In: Dubowitz, H. (ed.) *Neglected children: research, practice, and policy*, pp. 132–155. Thousand Oaks, CA: Sage.

Finkelhor, D. and Dziuba-Leatherman, J. (1994). Children as victims of violence: a national survey. *Pediatrics* **94**, 413–420.

Hien, D. and Honeyman, T. (2000). A closer look at the drug abuse-maternal aggression link. *Journal of Interpersonal Violence* **15**, 503–522.

Kolko, D. J. (1996). Individual cognitive behavioral treatment and family therapy for physically abused children and their offending parents: a comparison of clinical outcomes. *Child Maltreatment* **1**, 322–342.

Kolko, D. J. and Swenson, C. C. (2002). *Assessing and treating physically abused children and their families: a cognitive behavioral approach.* Thousand Oaks, CA: Sage.

Meyers, J. E. B., Berliner, L., Briere, J., Hendrix, C. T., Jenny, C. and Reid, T. A. (2002). *The APSAC handbook on child maltreatment* (2nd edn., pp. 205–232). Thousand Oaks, CA: Sage.

Swenson, C. C. and Brown, E. J. (1999). Cognitive-behavioral group treatment for physically abused children. *Cognitive and Behavioral Practice* **6**, 212–220.

Swenson, C. C. and Chaffin, M. (2006). Beyond psychotherapy: treating abused children by changing their social ecology. *Aggression and Violent Behavior* **11**, 120–137.

Swenson, C. C., Randall, J., Henggeler, S. W. and Ward, D. (2000). Outcomes and costs of an interagency partnership to serve maltreated children in state custody. *Children's Services: Social Policy, Research, and Practice* 3, 191–209.

Swenson, C. C., Saldana, L., Joyner, C. D. and Henggeler, S. W. (2006). Ecological treatment for parent to child violence. In: Lieberman, A. & DeMartino, R. (eds.) *Interventions for children exposed to violence*, pp. 155–185. New Brunswick, NJ: Johnson & Johnson Pediatric Institute.

Swenson, C. C., Brown, E. J. and Lutzker, J. R. (in press). Issues of maltreatment and abuse. In: Freeman A. & Reinecke, M. (eds.) *Personality disorders in childhood and adolescence.*

Child Sexual Abuse

J A Cohen
Drexel University College of Medicine, Philadelphia, PA, USA

This is a revised version of the article by J A Cohen, Encyclopedia of Stress First Edition, volume 1, pp 450–453, © 2000, Elsevier Inc.

Definition and Epidemiology

Child sexual abuse is not a clinical disorder or diagnosis in itself. It is, rather, a variety of events or experiences to which there may be a wide range of behavioral and emotional responses. In this sense, sexual abuse is best conceptualized as a life stressor rather than as a distinct clinical entity. The legal definition of child sexual abuse varies from state to state, and there is little consensus regarding what acts constitute sexual abuse among mental health-care providers. A common operational definition of sexual abuse is sexual exploitation involving physical contact between a child and another person. Exploitation implies an inequality of power between the child and the abuser, on the basis of age, physical size, and/or the nature of the emotional relationship. Physical contact includes anal, genital, oral, or breast contact. The definition obviously encompasses a number of different behaviors; sexual abuse is therefore not a unitary phenomenon.

It is difficult to know the exact incidence and prevalence of sexual abuse in our society because most sexual abuse is not reported immediately, and sometimes it is never reported. The Third National Incidence Study on Child Abuse and Neglect estimated that more than 300 000 children were sexually abused in the United States in 1993. However, this study includes only reported cases of sexual abuse. This is probably an underestimation of the frequency of sexual abuse, as there is evidence that only about one-fifth of true abuse cases are actually reported. Although sexual abuse occurs across religious, racial, and socioeconomic lines, several factors may put children at higher risk for sexual abuse. There is some controversy over the relationship between social class and child sexual abuse. Some researchers have found that reported cases of sexual abuse have come predominantly from families in the lower socioeconomic levels of society, but other studies have not supported this relationship. It is likely that this apparent relationship is due to a reporting bias because economically disadvantaged families are more likely to be scrutinized by social service agencies.

Symptomatology

There is also a great deal of variability in the behavioral, emotional, and social consequences of child sexual abuse. As a group, sexually abused children have been found to manifest significantly more behavioral and emotional difficulties than do nonabused children. Some researchers have found significant levels of self-reported depression in these children, while others have not. A significant number of these children and adolescents exhibit posttraumatic stress disorder (PTSD) and other anxiety symptoms. Recent, well designed studies which have controlled for factors such as genetics and family environment variables have demonstrated that child sexual abuse significantly increases risk for adverse psychological outcomes including depression, suicide attempts, substance abuse, anxiety, and subsequent sexual assault (Brent et al., 2002; Nelson et al., 2002).

Certain clinical issues appear to be common to most sexually abused children. These include feeling different or damaged compared to other children; feeling responsible for the abuse; feeling angry, fearful, or sad; taking on inappropriate behaviors and roles (including sexual ones); and losing trust in others. Briere's research on the Trauma Symptom Checklist for Children (TSCC) provided empirical support for these difficulties. The factor analysis of the TSCC demonstrated six discrete symptom fields: difficulties with sexual concerns, dissociation, anger, posttraumatic stress, depression, and anxiety symptoms.

Finkelhor discussed four traumagenic dynamics of sexual abuse, which included traumatic sexualization, stigmatization, powerlessness, and betrayal. The Children's Attributions and Perceptions Scale (CAPS) measures issues parallel to these traumagenic dynamics, in addition to measuring attributions about the sexual abuse. This study demonstrated that feeling different from peers (stigmatization), personal attribution for negative events, impaired trust (betrayal), and decreased perceived credibility (one aspect of powerlessness) were significant issues for sexually abused children compared to a normal control group. Wolfe et al. developed an instrument, The Children's Impact of Traumatic Events Scale (CITES) to measure abuse-specific thoughts and attributions. Factor analyses revealed distinct issues including attributions, betrayal, guilt, helplessness, intrusive thoughts, sexualization, and stigmatization. Thus, there is strong empirical evidence that sexually abused children have clinical issues and difficulties specific to sexual abuse, which can be measured by newly developed standardized instruments.

Friedrich demonstrated that sexually abused children exhibit significantly higher rates of sexually inappropriate behavior than nonabused populations. These may arise as a result of learning inappropriate behaviors through the abusive experience or from the fact that children with preexisting sexually inappropriate behavior are more likely to be targeted as victims of sexual abuse. However, there may be other, non-abuse-related reasons for children to exhibit sexually inappropriate behaviors. These behaviors are therefore not diagnostic of the sexual abuse. It is also important to note that the majority of sexually abused children do not exhibit sexually inappropriate behaviors.

It should be clear from this discussion that there is no such entity as a child sexual abuse syndrome. That is, there is no characteristic presentation that clinically distinguishes sexually abused children from non-sexually abused children. Rather, sexual abuse may result in a variety of clinical presentations. Sexual abuse therefore cannot be diagnosed by the clinical features present at evaluation. Such a determination depends on careful history taking and interviews with the child and significant others.

Assessment

Because child sexual abuse is an event (or events) rather than a clinical syndrome, and psychological responses to this experience differ considerably, one would expect psychiatric diagnoses in sexually abused children to also vary considerably. This has been documented in the literature. McLeer et al. evaluated psychiatric diagnoses in sexually abused and non-sexually abused children referred for outpatient pediatric assessment, using the Schedule for Affective Disorders and Schizophrenia for School-Age Children (K-SADS). The only significant difference in diagnoses between the two groups was the higher prevalence of PTSD in the sexually abused (42.3%) compared to the non-sexually abused (8.7%) children. In other diagnostic categories, there were no significant differences.

The process of determining accurate *Diagnostic and Statistical Manual of Mental Disorders,* 4th edition (DSM-IV) psychiatric diagnoses in sexually abused children is similar to that used in nonabused populations. The issue of determining whether or not a particular child has experienced sexual abuse is a complex medical, psychiatric, and legal process, which is beyond the scope of the present article. In addition to determining DSM-IV diagnosis, there are several special areas of concern related to the sexual abuse experience that should also be addressed when assessing sexually abused children. These include possible legal involvement, child protective services interventions, medical issues related to the abuse, and other abuse-related issues of the child and family. Factors such as the type of sexual abuse experienced, how long it was going on, whether the parent(s) or other siblings also experienced sexual abuse, and the identity of the perpetrator may have direct effects on the child's and/or family's emotional reactions, attitudes, and concerns about the abuse. Some families may be most upset because the abuse involved actual intercourse, whereas to other families this may be less important than the fact that the abuse was perpetrated by a trusted family member. This information is helpful in determining appropriate therapeutic interventions.

The child's and family's perceptions of why the sexual abuse occurred are also important. Does the family blame the perpetrator, the child, the parents, or some combination? The child's symptoms may be more closely related to these attributions than to the specific details of the abuse itself. Specifically, children who blame themselves rather than the perpetrator may be more likely to feel guilt, shame, or poor self-esteem; children who blame the abuse on the unpredictability of the world may have more difficulty with fear and anxiety symptoms. Similarly, parents who blame the abuse in part on the child's behavior or appearance may be less likely to be supportive of the child, or even less likely to view the experience as abuse.

The parent's emotional reaction to their child's sexual abuse also has an effect on child symptomatology. Low levels of maternal support and maternal depression correlate with greater behavioral and emotional symptoms in sexually abused children. Higher levels of parental distress related to the child's sexual abuse have also been found to predict higher levels of behavioral problems in the child.

Because of the complex legal and child protective issues involved in cases of child sexual abuse, it is essential for the clinician to clearly define his or her role in the case. There are many differences between treatment and forensic roles, and these should be kept separate and distinct as much as possible. It is regarded as a conflict of interest to evaluate a child for credibility of sexual abuse allegations or to evaluate a child and parents for custody determination following sexual abuse, and then to provide ongoing treatment for that child or family.

Treatment

Several randomized controlled treatment studies for sexually abused children have been published since 1990. At this time, trauma-focused cognitive-behavioral therapy (TF-CBT) has the strongest empirical support for treating this population. TF-CBT is a hybrid treatment model incorporating cognitive-behavioral principles with trauma-sensitive interventions along with family and developmental theory. TF-CBT includes the following treatment components, summarized by the acronym "PRACTICE:" Parenting skills (psychoeducation); Relaxation skills; Affective modulation skills; Cognitive coping skills; Trauma narrative and cognitive processing of the sexual abuse or other traumatic experiences; In vivo desensitization to trauma reminders; Conjoint child-parent treatment sessions; and Enhancing safety and future developmental trajectory.

Deblinger et al. evaluated the effectiveness of TF-CBT in decreasing PTSD and other psychological difficulties in 100 sexually abused children. Subjects were randomly assigned to one of four treatment conditions: child treatment only, mother treatment only, mother and child treatment, or usual community care. Children who received the TF-CBT treatment exhibited significantly fewer PTSD symptoms than children who did not receive this treatment. Children whose mothers received TF-CBT exhibited fewer externalizing symptoms and depressive symptoms compared to children whose parents did not receive TF-CBT.

Cohen and Mannarino compared TF-CBT to nondirective supportive therapy (NST) provided during individual sessions to sexually abused preschoolers and their primary caretakers. Children receiving TF-CBT showed more symptomatic improvement than those receiving NST. This differential treatment response was particularly strong with regard to children's sexually inappropriate behavior. Follow-up assessments indicated that these treatment group differences were sustained over the course of 12 months. This study also evaluated the impact of several child and family factors on treatment outcome. The strongest predictor of outcome was the parent's emotional reaction to the sexual abuse. Specifically, higher levels of parental distress at pretreatment strongly predicted higher levels of the child's post-treatment symptomatology.

In a parallel study for sexually abused children aged 8–14 years, TF-CBT was superior to NST in improving depressive symptoms and social competency. At 12 month follow-up, TF-CBT completers experienced a significantly greater improvement in PTSD and dissociation than noncompleters. Intent-to-treat analyses indicated significant group × time effects in favor of the TF-CBT group on measures of depression, anxiety, and sexual problems. In these older children, a higher level of parental support was a strong predictor of positive treatment outcome.

In a large multisite study, Cohen et al. randomly assigned 229 8- to 14-year-old sexually abused children who had experienced multiple traumas. Over 90% of this cohort met full criteria for PTSD diagnosis at pretreatment. Childred were randomly "assigned" to TF-CBT or to child-centered therapy (CCT) along with their nonoffending caretaking parent. This study demonstrated that even for these multiply traumatized children, TF-CBT was superior to CCT with regard to improvement in PTSD, depression, anxiety, shame, behavior problems, and abuse-related attributions. Parents receiving TF-CBT also experienced significantly greater improvement in their own depressive symptoms and positive parenting than those receiving CCT. Thus, there is evidence that trauma-focused CBT interventions are efficacious in decreasing symptomatology in multiply traumatized sexually abused children. All of the above studies also lend support to the importance of including nonoffending parents in treatment. More research is needed to further assess the efficacy of CBT and other potentially effective interventions and to clarify whatcomponents of these treatments may be most effective for which subgroups of children. Such TF-CBT treatment interventions may be provided either individually or in a group setting.

Other CBT-related approaches have been developed and are currently being tested for adolescents experiencing chronic PTSD related to sexual abuse. For example, the SPARCS (Structured Psychotherapy for Adolescents Recovering from Chronic Stress) and STAIR (Skills Training in Affective and Interpersonal Regulation) models show promise in this regard.

Other approaches to treating sexually abused children have received less empirical evaluation. One study has evaluated the efficacy of psychodynamic therapy for this population. Trowell and colleagues randomly assigned sexually abused children to 18 sessions of psychoeducation groups or 30 sessions of individual psychoanalytic therapy. The psychoanalytic group experienced greater improvement in PTSD symptoms, but the design of this study makes it difficult to determine whether this differential response was due to treatment type (psychoanalytic vs. psychoeducation), modality (individual vs. group), or dosage (30 sessions vs. 18). There are probably many efficacious therapeutic techniques for sexually abused children. Follow-up studies have indicated that many sexually abused children recover fully from this stressful experience and do not suffer ongoing negative sequelae. Hopefully, future research will more clearly elucidate which treatment approaches are most likely to result in this positive outcome.

See Also the Following Articles

Child Abuse; Child Physical Abuse.

Further Reading

Brent, D. A., Oquendo, M., Birmaher, B., et al. (2002). Familial pathways to early-onset suicide attempts: Risk for suicidal behavior in offspring of mood-disordered suicide attempters. *Archives of General Psychiatry* **59**, 801–807.

Briere, J. (1995). *The Trauma Symptom Checklist for Children.* Odessa, FL: Psychological Assessment Resources.

Cohen, J. A. and Mannarino, A. P. (1993). A treatment model for sexually abused preschool children. *Journal of Interpersonal Violence* 8(1), 115–131.

Cohen, J. A. and Mannarino, A. P. (1996). A treatment outcome study for sexually abused preschool children: initial findings. *Journal of the American Academy of Child and Adolescent Psychiatry* 35(1), 42–60.

Cohen, J. A. and Mannarino, A. P. (1998). Interventions for sexually abused children: initial treatment outcome findings. *Child Maltreatment* 3(1), 17–26.

Cohen, J. A., Deblinger, E., Mannarino, A. P. and Steer, R. (2004). A multisite, randomized controlled trial for sexually abused children with PTSD symptoms. *Journal of the American Academy of Child and Adolescent Psychiatry* **43**, 393–402.

Cohen, J. A., Mannarino, A. P. and Knudsen, K. (2005). Treating sexually abused children: one year follow-up of a randomized controlled trial. *Child Abuse and Neglect.*

Cohen, J. A., Mannarino, A. P. and Deblinger, E. (2006). *Treating trauma and traumatic grief in children and adolescents.* New York: Guilford Press.

Deblinger, E. and Heflin, A. H. (1996). *Treating sexually abused children and their nonoffending parents: a cognitive behavioral approach.* Sage: Newbury Park, CA.

Deblinger, E., Lippmann, J. and Steer, R. (1996). Sexually abused children suffering posttraumatic stress symptoms: initial treatment outcome findings. *Child Maltreatment* **1**(4), 104–114.

Finkelhor, D. (1987). The trauma of child sexual abuse: two models. *Journal of Interpersonal Violence* **2**(4), 348–366.

Finkelhor, D. and Barron, L. (1986). Risk factors for sexual abuse. *Journal of Interpersonal Violence* **1**(1), 43–71.

Friedrich, W. N. (1998). *The Child Sexual Behavior Inventory.* Odessa, FL: Psychological Assessment Resources.

Mannarino, A. P. and Cohen, J. A. (1996). Family related variables and psychological symptom formation in sexually abused girls. *Journal of Child Sex Abuse* **5**(1), 105–119.

McLeer, S. V., Callaghan, M., Henry, D. and Wallen, J. (1994). Psychiatric disorders in sexually abused children. *Journal of the American Academy of Child and Adolescent Psychiatry* **33**(3), 313–319.

Nelson, E. C., Heath, A. C., Madden, P. A. F., et al. (2002). Association between self-reported childhood sexual abuse and adverse psychosocial outcomes. *Archives of General Psychiatry* **59**, 139–145.

Trowell, J., Kolvin, I., Weeramanthri, T., Sadowski, H., Berelowitz, M., Glasser, D. and Leitch, I. (2002). Psychotherapy for sexually abused girls: psychopathological outcome findings and patterns of change. *British Journal of Psychiatry* **160**, 234–247.

Wolfe, V. V., Gentile, C. and Wolfe, D. A. (1989). The impact of child sexual abuse on children: a PTSD formulation. *Behavioral Therapy* **20**, 215–228.

Childhood Stress

S Sandberg
University College London, London, UK

This is a revised version of the article by S Sandberg, Encyclopedia of Stress First Edition, volume 1, pp 442–449, © 2000, Elsevier Inc.

Glossary

Contextual threat — The level of threat caused or implied by the life event to an average child of the same age, sex, and biographical characteristics as the child in question.

Life event — Any event or circumstance occurring in the life of a child that may have the potential to alter his or her present state of mental or physical health.

Limbic kindling — A psychophysiological process in which the limbic system (a border between the new and the old brain, forming a circuit primarily concerned with emotions, memory, olfaction, and neuroendocrine control) receives electrical stimulation resulting in increased responsiveness to low levels of stimulation over time. In this way, repeated traumatization, as in child abuse, or a trauma followed by intrusive memories could kindle limbic nuclei, leading to behavioral changes.

Ongoing process in which the delineation of a beginning and end stage is not

Long-term psychosocial experience	always possible. The experience may be adverse (e.g., parents' marital disharmony or financial hardship), desirable or hedonically positive (e.g., a rewarding hobby), or socially required for normal development or for protection against negative experiences (e.g., supportive relationship with a parent or having a close friend).
Modifier	A variable, aspect, or characteristic that exerts modifier effects on risk. If the risk is intensified, then the variable carries a vulnerability effect; if the risk is diminished, then the variable carries a protective effect. A vulnerability/protective factor is a moderator and is demonstrated statistically with a significant interaction effect.
Negative life event	A life event exerting a particular undesirable impact on the child.
Positive life event	A life event that is hedonically positive, enhances self-esteem, or has a beneficial effect on the child's life circumstances.
Risk factor	A variable that negatively influences outcome regardless of the presence or absence of adversity.
Stress, stressor, and stress reaction	A form of stimulus, an inferred inner state, and an observable response reaction, respectively.

Definitions of Stress

Stress, Stressor, and Stress Reaction

Child stress can be defined as any intrusion (stressor) into children's normal physical or psychosocial life experiences that acutely or chronically unbalances physiological or psychological equilibrium, threatens security or safety, or distorts physical or psychological growth and development and the psychophysiological consequences (stress reaction) of such an intrusion or distortion.

Harmful vs. Beneficial Stress

The traditional view of stress as a significant discrepancy between the demands of a situation and the organism's capacity to respond, resulting in detrimental consequences, implies that all stress is harmful. However, as far as children are concerned, the opposite is sometimes true. Mild stressors are often benign and sometimes even growth promoting.

Additive and Synergistic Stress

Apart from their individual effects, stressors can also act additively and synergistically. For example, deprivation and malnutrition can each compound fetal alcohol effects. Even the same cause can stress the child through two or more different mechanisms. Thus, maternal alcoholism can stress the fetal brain chemically and then psychologically stress the newborn infant through maternal unavailability, neglect, or abuse. Poverty can stress the child through malnutrition, inadequate environmental stimulation, and poor parenting due to worry, preoccupation, and discouragement.

Measurement of Stress

Chronic Stress

There exist a variety of questionnaire and interview instruments for the assessment of chronic stress in children, usually stemming from enduring adverse circumstances such as environmental or socioeconomic deprivation, parental unemployment or illness, and family discord or criminality. Also, the two widely used diagnostic classification systems, the *Diagnostic and Statistical Manual of Mental Disorders,* 4th edition (DSM-IV) and the *International Classification of Diseases* (ICD-10), contain a separate axis for systematic measurement of stressors of likely relevance for children's health.

Life Events

Questionnaire measures The first-generation measures of stress in childhood were based on the questionnaire format to provide overall scores of degree of life change. The assumption was that change per se, not necessarily the unpleasant nature of the experience, was stressful for children. In parallel with these overall approaches, numerous studies of specific life events such as family breakup, bereavement, and disasters such as floods, earthquakes, or hijacking were carried out.

Interview measures

The meaning of life experiences The realization that it was necessary to take into account the social context of life events in order to assess their meaning and hence their stressful quality constituted perhaps the most significant conceptual advance. The clear implication of this advance was that interviews rather than questionnaire approaches were needed for adequate assessment of life events.

Undesirability, cognitive appraisal, and independence A major reappraisal of psychosocial stress research involved the emphasis on the need to differentiate between desirable and undesirable life changes and to highlight the role of cognitive appraisal of the events. The distinction between life events that could have been brought about by the person's own actions and those that are independent of behavior constitutes another conceptual advance.

This distinction is especially important when considering stressful life events as causal agents for psychiatric disorders.

Contextual threat The concept of contextual threat has represented a decisive step in the assessment of children's life events. In determining the stressful quality of life events, it is necessary to take into account their social context, i.e., their meaning to an individual. For example, it is unreasonable to treat moving as a unitary event. The effects would be very different for a child who moved within the same neighborhood and maintained the same school and friends compared to one whose new home was in another town, or even another country, resulting in loss of friends, surroundings, and school. To understand this difference, interviews rather than questionnaire approaches are needed.

The assessment is usually made separately for short-term (based on immediate impact), and long-term (the likely impact occurring some 10 days later) threat. In addition, it has become customary to conceptualize the overall rating of contextual threat as being made up of one or more components that vary somewhat depending on the instrument used. These components commonly include the following: loss of an attachment figure (e.g., losing a parent or a close friend), loss of a valued idea (a major disappointment, letdown, or humiliation), risk of loss of attachment figure (the threat of losing someone close), physical jeopardy (being in physical danger due to accident, etc.), trauma as witness (being witness to an unpleasant or frightening incident), and psychological challenge (the event involving the subject in a new role or with new responsibilities).

Some life events encountered by children rate high on contextual threat because they cause a major alteration in the life circumstances (e.g., the death of a parent). In other events, the threat is primarily cognitive. This means that the event may not result in any actual change in the external environment, but instead drastically changes the child's perception of an aspect of him- or herself, or of other people or things in a way that presents a threat to the child's self-esteem (e.g., severe humiliation) or reduces his or her perceived sense of security (e.g., a parent threatening to abandon the child). Life events may also involve a combination of real life change and cognitively mediated threat (e.g., the parents' marital separation).

Effects of Stress

Developmental Interferences

Physical development The ill effects of compromised prenatal, perinatal, and early postnatal care on the child's development and well-being have long been recognized. For example, in the multiple associations between prematurity, illness, and outcome, environmental factors are known to play a central role. Likewise, children suffering from the non-organic failure to thrive syndrome frequently exhibit a complex entanglement of caloric and protein intake, touch, and the release of growth hormone.

Neurodevelopment

Neuroanatomy Stress can also influence the development of the brain. To develop properly, undifferentiated neuronal systems are dependent on environmental cues such as neurochemical and hormonal factors. These processes in turn are dependent on the child's sensory experiences. A narrow window appears to exist during which specific experiences are required for the optimal development of the brain. After birth, brain development mainly consists of an ongoing process of wiring and rewiring. Early experiences can, for example, cause the final number of synapses to increase or decrease. Infants confined to their cots and with little opportunity to explore or experiment, and who are rarely spoken to, may fail to develop neural pathways that facilitate later learning.

Neurotransmitters and hormones play a major role in neuronal migration, differentiation, and synaptic proliferation. Massive increases in catecholamine activity caused by severe or prolonged stressors are expected to have a significant impact on brain development. The hippocampus is a likely target for the effects of early stress because neurogenesis in this area continues into postnatal life. The amygdaloid nuclei are critically involved in the formation of emotional memory and in stress-induced memory enhancement. Repeated trauma may lead to limbic kindling. Thus, during critical periods in early childhood, experiences can organize brain systems; nurture may become nature. This would also suggest that it is more appropriate to speak of early childhood malleability than resilience.

Primate research has presented strong evidence that chronic unpredictable stress during pregnancy may have long-lasting effects on brain activity and behavior of the offspring. Furthermore, prenatal stress appears to be capable of affecting the neurobiology of the neonate so that its responses to common events and stimuli are markedly altered. These effects on brain mechanisms are more likely to be diffuse, rather than specific. As a consequence, the neonate may, for example, be more fussy and difficult, affecting how the caregiver is able to cope. Thus, prenatal stress appears to set the infant's neurobiology into a state in which vital attachments are hard to achieve and adverse experiences are more likely. The adverse experiences can in turn result in further neurobiological deflection of development.

Prenatal effects on fetal neurobiological development may also be easily confused with genetic predisposition. It therefore remains a challenge to determine how prenatal environment contributes to persisting and traitlike organization of neurobiological systems. This, in turn, would markedly further our understanding of how genetic and postnatal environmental factors play a role in the expression of developmental psychopathology, for example.

Neurophysiology When a child is exposed to a strong stressor, a series of interactive, complicated neurophysiological reactions take place in the brain, the autonomic system, the hypothalamus-pituitary-adrenocortical axis, and the immunosystem, with concomitant release of stress hormones. Neurophysiological activation during acute stress is usually rapid and reversible. As such, it has an adaptive purpose. Following severe prolonged or repeated stress, however, these changes may no longer be reversible, and become maladaptive. One explanation for this is that the organisms have not yet evolved mechanisms to deal adaptively with chronic stress. Stress-induced sensitization may also occur, with the systems underlying the stress response becoming more sensitive to future adverse experiences. Children growing up in a persistently threatening environment develop stress response systems in midbrain and brain stem that are overreactive and hypersensitive. This development may be highly adaptive, but only as long as the child remains in a violent, chaotic environment. Profound cognitive disturbances can accompany this process.

Some young children, especially girls, however, react in the opposite way by freezing rather than by becoming visibly anxious or hyperactive. Flooding of adrenocortical hormones during periods of acute stress may also have negative consequences on memory and the anatomical substrates of memory.

Trauma response Traumatic events impact structures in the central nervous system – though the exact mechanism of this remains unknown at present. Structures underlying cognitive, affective, sensory, integrative, regulatory, neuroendocrine, and motor functions are coordinated in the life threat response. This may lead neuronal networks, excited during a life-threatening event, to become identified for later potentiation, forming the basis for permanent registration in memory.

In younger children whose brains are maturing in use-dependent interaction with their environment, aspects of such memory states may become lifelong traits. It has been suggested, for example, that children using a dissociative adaptive defense in an acute response to trauma would later demonstrate primarily dissociative or somatic symptoms. On the other hand, children who primarily use hyperarousal adaptation to an acute stressor would be more likely to develop chronic hyperarousal symptoms, such as startle response, anxiety, motor hyperactivity, sleep disturbance, or tachycardia.

Psychological development

Cognitive development Persistent environmental stress and deprivation can significantly impair the development of the child's cognitive abilities, including attention skills, memory, and language as well as intellectual capabilities. Conversely, a child's level of cognitive development is an important determinant of how he or she will deal with trauma. Ability to label and express feelings, to receive reality-based feedback, and to incorporate the experience into a narrative are relevant developmental achievements.

Emotional development Because a child's most pressing emotional needs change over time, a particular trauma may have more influence during one stage of development than during another. The cognitive interpretation of the same trauma may also be different depending on the child's developmental level.

Effects on Physical Health

Numerous studies in the fields of pediatrics and psychosomatic medicine have shown that children with increased psychosocial stress are significantly more likely to experience illness and hospitalization as well as use health services more frequently than other children. Stress as a precipitating and/or provoking factor has been implicated for asthma, appendicitis, rheumatoid arthritis, and leukemia, for example. High levels of psychosocial stress have also been shown to predict greater morbidity in children who already have a chronic disease. For example, recent studies on children with asthma have demonstrated time-related associations between exposure to stress and acute worsening of symptoms.

The role of stress in viral infections has been the focus of research in more recent years. Well-controlled prospective and experimental studies have shown that adverse life events and other stressful experiences significantly increase a person's susceptibility to acute and recurrent respiratory infections. One likely explanation for this association is that stress compromises the body's immune responses, with individual differences in susceptibility possibly being accounted for by differences in psychobiological reactivity. It is acknowledged, for example, that the immune system and the central nervous system form a bidirectional communication network. In this network, pro-inflammatory cytokines play a critical role.

Effects on Mental Health

A range of research strategies have demonstrated beyond all reasonable doubt that psychosocial factors exercise causal effects on children's psychosocial functioning. They also have contributed in a major way to the multifactorial causation of psychiatric disorders in childhood. In this respect, the main risk stems from chronic psychosocial adversity such as unhappy family life, parental psychopathology (including substance abuse and criminality), and parental stress caused by poverty or unemployment, or being a victim of bullying or other victimization. Acutely stressful life events, especially those that carry long-term threat to the psychological security of the child, add to the risk caused by chronic stressors, and in some instances constitute sufficient risk in their own right. Negative life events that are associated with chronic psychosocial adversity, rather than those that arise out of the blue, have also been shown to provoke an onset of psychiatric disorder, particularly depression, in children. Their main effect, however, appears to be to determine the timing of a new episode of disorder in a child already at risk due to chronic stress or made vulnerable through lack of emotional support.

Reasons for Individual Differences

Personal vulnerability Compared with adults, far less work has been carried out to examine the importance of personal vulnerability to stressful experiences in children. The role of close, supportive relationships, however, has received support. Thus, difficulties in the child's own friendships as well as their mother's lack of confiding relationships have been shown to predict depression and other emotional disorders. Likewise, the overall risk of psychiatric disorder in the presence of severely negative life events is significantly enhanced in children lacking a confiding relationship with a parent or a close adult relative.

Exposure to stressful experiences The very large individual differences in children experiencing stress and adversity are acknowledged. A variety of explanations are likely to apply. First, some stressful life events represent chance or acts of fate, including natural and man-made disasters such as war, floods, earthquakes, and shipping accidents. Second, stressful life events can also be a function of structural factors in the society, making negative experiences much more likely in some segments of the population than in others. In children, the effect of low social class on stressful life events appears to be an indirect one, via chronic psychosocial adversities such as family ill health and interparental conflicts, which in turn increase the likelihood of acute negative events. Likewise, family poverty is associated with multiple risk factors for children. Many of these risks are mediated via parental responses to such pressures. Being poor is linked with chronic psychological distress in parents, thus impeding effective parenting through harsh discipline, inconsistency, lack of monitoring, family conflict, and multiple changes in family configuration. Third, many of the stressful life events occurring to children are a function of their parents' behavior in one way or another. This is the case with divorce, abuse, and a parent being arrested, for example. Such stressful, family-dependent life events tend to be rooted in parental psychopathology, substance abuse, or criminality.

Genetic factors are also implicated as bases of individual differences in environmental risk exposure – a phenomenon known as gene–environment correlation. The parents who pass their genes to their children are usually the same parents who provide the rearing experience. For example, antisocial adults are much more likely than other people to provide negative rearing environments to their children. Antisocial behavior in one or both parents in turn predicts a much increased rate of marital breakdown and negative parent–child interactions and, hence, life events that are stressful to children. Gene–environment correlation can also lead to environmental risk that impinges differently on the children.

Susceptibility There are large individual differences in children's responses to stressful life experiences. A major reason for this may lie in the crucial importance of the personal meaning of the particular experience involved. In addition, previous experiences are likely to color a person's reaction to a new experience. Stressful life events can be strengthening as well as weakening; they can steel as well as sensitize. Other factors determining individual differences are the child's age, sex, temperament, locus of control, and family support.

Several other explanations may account for the individual differences. One of these is gene–environment interaction, a concept introduced more recently. In this case, the vulnerability to stress is viewed as being genetically determined rather than acquired through experience.

Mechanisms

Additivity of stressful experiences There is no doubt that a single major life event such bereavement or kidnapping can be quite sufficient on its own to provoke psychiatric disorder. However, it also appears that there is a cumulative effect when several major life events occur together during a short period of time. Likewise, the multiplicative effect of the co-occurrence of several chronic adversities has been demonstrated in children.

Potentiation of stress Chronic adverse circumstances such as unhappy family life; parental psychopathology, substance abuse, or criminality; economic hardship; or stressors in the school environment all in themselves increase the risk of child psychiatric disorder. Their presence also makes it more likely that acute stressful events will occur, often stemming directly from the ongoing adversity. Discord leading to divorce or criminality resulting in jail sentence, from the child's point of view, both involve separation from a parent. Apart from increasing the likelihood of stressful life events to occur, chronic adversity is also apt to potentiate their adverse effects.

Vulnerability and protective mechanisms There also exist complex vulnerability and protective mechanisms, i.e., those that increase and those that decrease stress effects. These include interactions, not just main effects. Such mechanisms need to be considered in relation to the child's individual characteristics as well as to their experiential properties.

A moderator is a variable that influences the strength or the direction of a relationship between a predictor variable and a criterion variable. An example is a finding that in the context of a child's chronic physical illness, family stress is negatively associated with child psychological adjustment. When the nature of the association is further examined, it may turn out that the effect is stronger (or weaker) in the presence of other contextual variables. For example, the strength or the direction of the relationship between stress and adjustment may depend on the type of coping used by the family. That is, a significant association may emerge only when a parent (or child) copes in a maladaptive manner.

A protective factor either ameliorates negative outcomes or promotes adaptive functioning. The protective factor serves its protective role only in the context of adversity; a protective factor does not operate in conditions of low adversity. Conversely, a vulnerability factor is a moderator that increases the chances for negative (maladaptive) outcomes in the presence of adversity. Similar to a protective factor, a vulnerability factor operates only in the context of adversity.

Mediating mechanisms There are a number of mechanisms through which psychosocial stressors lead to child disorder. Some acute life events bring about lasting adverse alterations in life circumstances. Examples include bereavement and parental divorce. Thus, for a child, the ill effects arising from the loss of a parent are highly dependent on whether the loss is associated with family discord or leads to serious impairment in parenting. Loss that does not have these adverse sequelae may be painful at the time, but usually remains of limited significance as a causal factor for persisting disorder.

Stress may also be associated with loss that is only in the person's mind. The mechanism of cognitive threat is a likely possibility. Young children, for example, appraise their situation and contemplate their life circumstances in ways that differ from those typical of adults.

Recurrent hospital admission is a known stressor in young children, with the key mediating mechanism being the disturbed parent–child relationship engendered by the child's behavior upon the return home. A comparable situation is the birth of a sibling. Here the disturbance of the prior parent–child relationship is more important, suggesting that the main stress for the child may reside in the parental reaction rather than in the child's response to the event as such.

Chain events With children, it is also important to consider mediating mechanisms in long-term consequences, i.e., how adverse early experiences influence later psychosocial functioning. The sequelae frequently depend on chain events that involve a number of different links reflecting separate psychological processes. These include learned maladaptive emotional responses, self-perpetuating behavior patterns or habits, lowered self-esteem influencing the ability to deal with future experiences, poor coping skills, internal working models of insecure relationships, or behavior that serves to shape later environments or increase the individual's exposure to stressful life events.

Positive experiences as protectors Compared with the volume of research that has been carried out on the effects of negative experiences on children's health, studies examining the role of positive life experiences are lacking. Furthermore, the meager evidence available so far fails to support the notion that hedonically positive events and life situations would have an ameliorating effect on psychiatric risk. The situation, however, may be different with regard to somatic manifestations of illness. Positive life events have been shown to offset the increased risk for new asthma exacerbations associated with severely negative life events.

Beneficial stress There are both beneficial and harmful stress experiences. The distinction is likely to lie in the child's temperamental qualities and in how the particular past experience has been coped with. This has implications for prevention. It is possible that successful prevention only partly lies in the avoidance of stressors, but largely lies in helping children to overcome negative experiences. The overcoming of stress can be strengthening, ensuring that children encounter stressors at times and in ways that make it more likely that they will come out on top with a sense of accomplishment rather than with feelings of fear and humiliation.

Turning points Turning points in development is another issue likely to affect long-term sequelae of childhood stress. A turning point refers to an experience either internal (as with puberty) or external (as with dropping out of school) that carries with it the potential for enduring change because the experience either closes doors or opens up opportunities, or because it is associated with a lasting alteration in life circumstances. Most turning points concern very ordinary life experiences, but, in each case, the particular individual circumstances are crucial. Therefore, life events need to be conceived of not just in terms of their threat features, but also in terms of their effects on the person's social group and life opportunities.

Specificity of stressors vs. specificity of outcome It is conceivable that specific associations between particular stressors and particular outcomes are mediated by psychological, biological, or social processes and the specific nature of the stressor. Little evidence of this, however, exists so far. This may be because until recently very few studies testing full specificity designs (i.e., specific stressors linked to specific outcomes, via specific mediators, in the context of specific moderators) have been carried out in children. Across the various stressors such as exposure to poverty, illness, marital conflict, divorce, violence, or abuse, the only consistent evidence appears to be in relation to sexual abuse. Sexual abuse has been found to be associated specifically with internalizing problems, posttraumatic stress disorder, and sexual acting out.

The lack of specificity may have several explanations, including significant rates of co-occurrence and comorbidity of psychopathology in childhood, the lack of a well-established taxonomy of stressors, and the fact that specific characteristics and environmental contexts of the child moderate the associations between stressor and outcome in unique ways. Particular stressors may also be linked with particular outcomes only in the presence of particular moderating and mediating processes. Furthermore, stressors categorized by type may include a variety of stressors that are different in nature. It is known, for example, that poverty is associated with a range of additional stressful experiences, which include conflict (e.g., exposure to violence, physical abuse, divorce/marital conflict) and stressors involving loss (e.g., deaths, separations, disasters).

See Also the Following Articles

Child Abuse; Child Sexual Abuse; Child Physical Abuse.

Further Reading

Arnold, L. E. (1990). *Childhood stress.* New York: Wiley.

Friedman, R. J. and Chase-Lansdale, P. L. (2002). Chronic adversities. In: Rutter, M. & Taylor, E. (eds.) *Child and adolescent psychiatry* (4th edn., pp. 261–276). Oxford: Blackwell Science.

Goodyer, I. (1990). *Life experiences, development and psychopathology.* Chichester, UK: Wiley.

Grossman, A. W., Churchhill, J. D., McKinney, B. C., et al. (2003). Experience effects on brain development: possible contributions to psychopathology. *Journal of Child Psychology and Psychiatry* **44**, 33–63.

Maier, S. F. (2003). Bi-directional immune-brain communication: implications for understanding stress, pain, and cognition. *Brain, Behavior and Immunity* **17**, 69–85.

McMahon, S. D., Grant, K. E., Compas, B. E., Thurm, A. E. and Ey, S. (2003). Stress and psychopathology in children and adolescents: is there evidence of specificity? *Journal of Child Psychology and Psychiatry* **44**, 107–133.

Perry, B. D. (1996). *Maltreated children. brain development and the next generation.* New York: Norton.

Sandberg, S. and Rutter, M. (2002). The role of acute life stresses. In: Rutter, M. & Taylor, E. (eds.) *Child and adolescent psychiatry* (4th edn., pp. 287–298). Oxford: Blackwell Science.

Sandberg, S., Jarvenpaa, S., Penttinen, A., Paton, J. Y. and McCann, D. C. (2004). Asthma exacerbations in children immediately following stressful life events: a Cox's hierarchical regression. *Thorax* **59**, 1046–1051.

Sandberg, S., Paton, J. Y., Ahola, S., McCann, D. C., McGuinness, D., et al. (2000). The role of acute and chronic stress in asthma attacks in children. *Lancet* **356**, 982–987.

Shea, A., Walsh, C., MacMillan, H. and Steiner, M. (2004). Child maltreatment and HPA axis dysregulation: relationship to major depressive disorder and post traumatic disorder in females. *Psychoneuroendocrinology* **30**, 162–178.

Marital Status and Health Problems

I M A Joung
Erasmus University, Rotterdam, Netherlands

This article is reproduced from Encyclopedia of Stress First Edition, volume 2, pp 685–691, © 2000, Elsevier Inc.

Glossary

Determinants of health	Factors associated with health and illness, such as socioeconomic status and alcohol consumption.
Intermediary factors	Determinants of health through which marital status affects health outcomes.
Unmarried	People who have never been married, are divorced, or are widowed.
Selection	The theory about health differences between marital status groups in which it is assumed that health affects marital status.
Social causation	The theory about health differences between marital status groups in which it is assumed that marital status affects health.

Marital status is associated with all kinds of health outcomes: both subjective health states (illness, e.g., self-perceived health) and objective health states (disease, e.g., clinically diagnosed conditions), both mental and physical health, and both morbidity and mortality. Health differences between marital status groups are generally assumed to result from both an effect of health on marital status (selection) and an effect of marital status on health (social causation). Marital status affects health through several intermediary factors; of these, psychosocial factors, especially psychosocial stress, occupy a central position.

Health Differences among Marital Status Groups

The general pattern for health differences among marital status groups is that married people have the fewest health problems, followed by never-married and widowed people, whereas divorced people have the most health problems. This ranking is found both among men and women; however, the differences among the marital status groups are generally larger among men than among women.

In most studies in which separated people are distinguished as a separate group, it is found that they have as many as or even more health problems than divorced people. However, in many studies on health differences among marital status groups, separated people have not been treated as a separate marital status category but have been grouped with either divorced or married people.

In many Western countries, nonmarital cohabitation is of increasing importance. The few studies that have addressed health differences between married people and people living in consensual unions have found either no health differences or that the health of people in consensual unions compared somewhat unfavorably with that of married people but favorably with that of the unmarried, noncohabitating people. The remainder of this article focuses on health differences among married, never-married, divorced, and widowed people.

Mortality

Mortality differences among marital status groups were described in the nineteenth century. For instance, in 1853 William Farr examined age-specific mortality rates for never-married, married, and widowed people living in France. He found that the mortality rates of married men and women compared favorably to those of never-married and widowed men and women. For example, at the ages 40–50 mortality rates were 17.7, 10.3, and 20.1 per 1000 for never-married, married, and widowed men, respectively. Since then numerous researchers in many countries have looked at mortality differences among marital status groups. A considerable number of studies have been performed on this subject in the last decades. The results from these studies indicate very consistently that married people have lower mortality rates than unmarried people.

The sizes of the mortality differences between married and unmarried groups and the rankings of the mortality rates of the three unmarried groups have changed over time. For instance, in the Netherlands in the period of 1869–1872, the differences in total mortality between married and never-married women were rather small, and under the age of 40 never-married women actually had lower mortality rates than married women. This was mainly due to the high childbirth mortality rate among married women. In the following decades, the differences in total mortality between married and never = married women increased as, childbirth mortality rate, among others, decreased.

The relationship between marital status and mortality also shows some differences between countries. Hu and Goldman explored mortality differences between marital status groups in 16 industrialized countries for the period of 1950–1980. They found that, for the majority of countries, divorced men experienced the highest mortality rates among men and that, in about half of the countries, the same pattern existed for women. Generally, the mortality rates of divorced men and women were 2–2.5 and 1.5–2 times, respectively, those of their married counterparts. In Japan, however, the mortality rate of never-married men was as high as the rate of divorced men and never-married women had much higher mortality rates than divorced women. Also, mortality rate differences between the never married and married in Japan far exceeded the largest mortality rate differences by marital status in the other countries (being more than three times that of the married group).

The differences in total mortality rates among marital status groups are more or less mirrored in the differences in rates for specific causes of death. For the majority of causes of death, the largest differences are found between the rates for divorced and married people. In general, never-married and widowed people have higher rates of cause-specific mortality than married people, alternately occupying the position of the group with the second highest mortality rate. In comparison with the differences found for the total mortality rate, the relative size of the differences in the rates of mortality due to cardiovascular diseases and cancer is somewhat smaller, but it is considerably larger for the mortality rates due to external causes of death (e.g., accident and suicide). **Table 1** shows the age-adjusted relative risks of divorced men and women compared to married men and women for total mortality and mortality from a number of specific causes of death.

Morbidity

More recently, differences in morbidity, short-term disability, and health-care use among marital status groups have been studied. Morbidity differences largely have patterns similar to mortality rate differences: married people have the lowest rates, divorced people have the highest rates, and never-married and widowed people have rates in between. The size of the differences among marital status groups is generally larger for indicators of subjective health (e.g., self-perceived general health and subjective health complaints) than for indicators of objective health (e.g., chronic diseases) and is larger for mental than for physical health.

Morbidity differentials are by and large reflected in the patterns for health-care use and short-term disability. Widowed and divorced people have higher rates for physician contacts, hospital admissions, and use of medicines and report more bed days and days of restricted activity than married people. Never-married people, however, seem to have a lower health-care use and less bed disability days than married people, despite their higher morbidity rates.

Table 1 Relative risks of divorced men and women compared to their married counterparts in the Netherlands, 1986–1990[a]

	Divorced men	*Divorced women*
Total mortality	1.6	1.5[b]
Cardiovascular diseases	1.5	1.4
Cancer	1.2	1.3
External causes	3.8	3.0
Infective diseases	2.2	2.1
Cirrhosis of the liver (with mention of alcohol)	9.1	6.0
Diabetes mellitus	2.2	1.4

[a]*Source*: Statistics Netherlands.
[b]For example, a relative risks of 1.5 means that the mortality rate of divorced women is 1.5 times that of married women.

Theories about the Explanation

Several explanations have been suggested for the association between marital status and health. First, it has been put forward that the association might be due to data errors and thus be an artifact. Although data errors might explain part of the association between marital status and health found in earlier studies, more recent studies have shown convincingly that there are genuine health differences among marital status groups. Other explanations that have been proposed can be grouped into two main theories: selection theory and social causation theory. According to selection theory, the relatively good health of married people is the result of the selection of healthy people into and unhealthy people out of the married state. According to social causation theory, marriage has a health-promoting or a health-protective effect, whereas the unmarried state has adverse health effects. Thus, in selection theory, health status precedes marital status; in social causation theory, marital status precedes health status. A graphic representation of these explanations is shown in **Figure 1**. In order to establish whether or to what extent health differences precede differences in marital status or vice versa, longitudinal data are required. Selection theory and social causation theory are not mutually exclusive, and it is generally accepted that a combination of selective and causal factors are responsible for the observed health patterns in marital status groups.

Selection on Health and Determinants of Health

According to selection theory, the relatively good health of married people is the result of the selection

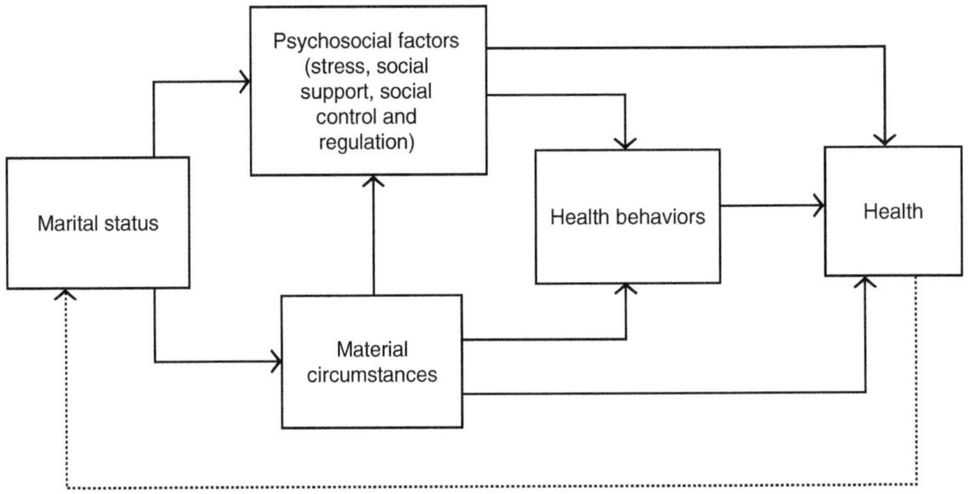

Figure 1 A representation of the explanations for health differences among marital status groups. →, social causation; ⇢, selection.

of healthy people into and unhealthy people out of the married state, thus increasing the relative amount of unhealthy people in the unmarried states. A distinction can be made between direct selection and indirect selection. In direct selection, health itself is the selection criterion; in indirect selection, the determinants of health are the selection criteria.

The process of selection could occur with regard to first marriages as well as other marital transitions (divorce, bereavement, and remarriage) and could cause the health differences by marital status in several ways. Selection in partner choice is the most straightforward mechanism: unhealthy people may be less attractive marriage partners and thus may either not be chosen or, if illness develops during marriage, might be discarded as marriage partners. Selection may also operate through assortive mating, the fact that people generally tend to marry partners with traits that they themselves possess, such as physical attractiveness. Assortive mating could also includes health status and does not so much influence whether a person marries as whom the person marries. If, indeed, unhealthy people are more likely to marry unhealthy others, we could find that unhealthy married people are more likely to become widowed because their unhealthy partner is at greater risk of mortality. In addition, it is conceivable that relationships in which both partners are unhealthy are more stressful and therefore more prone to dissolution. Finally, with regard to the transition from the married to the widowed state, selection may also operate through processes independent of partner choice due to health considerations, for instance, through both spouses developing health problems after marriage for reasons such as a joint unfavorable environment (e.g., shared material deprivation or unhealthy behaviors). In this case, the health differences between married and widowed people are not caused by the conditions of widowhood itself (social causation) but are, instead, based in already existing health differences between those who will become widowed and those who will remain married (selection).

Direct Selection

It has been demonstrated in several longitudinal studies that direct selection is operative in marital transitions. However, the evidence is still partial and sometimes inconsistent. There are indications that the presence of disease decreases the marriage probabilities of never-married people and increases the divorce probabilities of married people. It has also been found that direct selection might be able to explain a considerable part of the health differences among marital status groups. However, other studies have been unable to demonstrate selection effects, and sometimes even evidence for adverse selection was found (i.e., that healthier people were less likely to marry).

Indirect Selection

As stated earlier, selection may operate not only through the exclusion of unhealthy people from marriage (direct selection) but also through selection on a wide range of determinants of health (indirect selection). The determinants of health that may operate in this way are, for instance, socioeconomic status, physical appearance (e.g., body length and obesity), and health-related habits (e.g., alcohol consumption). Research has demonstrated that indirect selection is indeed operative in marital transitions and that its direction is mostly, but not always, in accordance with the health differences observed among marital status groups. Adverse selection occurs, for instance, with regard to educational level among women – people with a higher educational level have more favorable health outcomes than those with a lower educational level, but women with a high educational level are overrepresented among never-married and divorced women.

Social Causation, Intermediary Factors, and Biological Pathways

According to social causation theory, health depends on marital status. Marital status may, on the one hand, affect the etiology of health problems: the married state may prevent people from becoming ill, whereas the unmarried state may be the cause of a decline in resistance to diseases. Marital status may, on the other hand, once health problems have developed, affect the course and outcome of the disease. Ample evidence from longitudinal studies shows that differences in marital status are associated with subsequent health differences; thus social causation mechanisms explain (part of the) health differences among marital status groups. The effect of marital status on health is not assumed to be a direct effect but to be intermediated by psychosocial factors (e.g., stress and social relationships), material circumstances (e.g., financial situation and housing conditions), and health behaviors (e.g., smoking and alcohol consumption).

Psychosocial Factors

Psychosocial stress is related causally to illness and mortality. Lazarus and Folkman defined psychosocial stress as "a particular relationship between the person and the environment that is appraised by the individual as taxing or exceeding his or her resources and endangering his or her well-being." Psychosocial stress varies among marital status groups. First, bereavement and divorce are stressful life events in themselves. On the social readjustment rating scale of Holmes and Rahe, a scale of 43 life events ordered on the basis of the assumed intensity and length of time necessary to accommodate to the life event, bereavement and divorce rank first and second, respectively. Understandingly, the loss of a beloved person is an important source of stress itself. Feelings of failure, lowered self-esteem, and sense of incompetence, which are often experienced by divorced people, also evoke stress. Furthermore, the many concurrent changes in the lives of bereaved or divorced people, such as lowered income, change in parental responsibilities, forced move to other housing, or the loss of familiar activities and habit systems, also contribute highly to the total amount of stress experienced.

Second, the differences in psychosocial stress among marital status groups are also caused by mechanisms other than the stressful character of the event of bereavement or divorce. Negative societal attitudes toward the marital status a person occupies can be a source of stress. Although societal attitudes toward alternatives to marriage have become more liberal in recent years, prejudices and stereotyped images of never-married people and divorced people still exist. Uncertainty about social roles is also a source of stress, and certainty about social roles differs according to marital status. Marriage provides people with clear and socially acceptable roles, whereas divorce lacks clearly defined norms.

Other psychosocial factors may also contribute to the effect of marital status on health. Several aspects of social relationships are associated with health status and differ among the marital status groups. First, social integration (the existence and quantity of social relationships) is related directly to health. Psychological and sociobiological theories suggest that the mere presence of, or sense of relatedness with, another organism may promote health through relatively direct motivational, emotional, or neuroendocrinal effects. Married people are, on average, more socially integrated for several reasons: they have at least one social tie in their spouse; their children constitute additional social ties, which most never-married people lack; and their social network is expanded with the social ties of their spouse. Consequently, the loss of a spouse also means a break in the social network.

Second, social support (the functional nature or quality of social relationships) has been found to be related directly and indirectly to health. With regard to the latter, social support is assumed to buffer the negative health effects of stress, thus modifying the relationship between stress and health. In this case, social support has no beneficial effect on the health of people who experience little stress, but the beneficial effects of social support increase with increasing stress. Social support is the aid that is transmitted between social network members. An distinction is often made between emotional and instrumental support. Emotional support includes expressions of affection, admiration, respect, or affirmation; instrumental support is the provision of advice, information, or more practical assistance. The availability and quality of social support differ by marital status. Partner relationships are, in general, more supportive than are other types of relationships. This also means that in cases of bereavement or divorce an important provider of social support is lost.

Finally, differences in social relationships among marital status groups result in differences in social regulation and control. Married people experience more social control; wives, in particular, try to influence their spouses' health behaviors. Furthermore, married people have a more regulated life, which facilitates health-promoting behaviors such as proper sleep, diet, and exercise; the moderate use of alcohol; the adherence to medical regiment; and seeking appropriate medical care.

Material Circumstances

Differences in material resources among marital status groups constitute another intermediary of the relationship between marital status and health. People who share a household profit from economies of scale in the purchasing and use of housing and other goods and services. In addition, changes in marital status are often associated with large changes in material resources. Bereavement and divorce are, especially among women, often accompanied by a decline of their financial situation and, consequently, a deterioration in other structural living circumstances (e.g., housing). This is most obvious in situations in which the husband is the sole wage earner. However, even in cases of double incomes the wife is likely to be worse off financially after divorce or bereavement. Women are generally married to men of a higher or equivalent educational level, and in many countries men earn on average more than women of an equivalent educational level earn. The fact that the material situation of women generally deteriorates after a divorce does not necessarily imply that men gain materially from divorce. In a divorce, possessions are divided between the former spouses, the ex-husband might be obliged to pay alimony, and economies of scale are lost. This might put divorced men in a materially disadvantaged position compared to married men. Widowed women are generally better off financially than divorced women, even with comparable levels of household income, because divorced women lose their house and must divide assets with their ex-husband, whereas widowed women more often keep the family home and other financial assets intact.

Health Behaviors

Differences in health behaviors among marital status groups are also seen as an intermediary of the association between marital status and health. Marriage often has a deterrent effect on negative health behaviors, such as smoking, excessive alcohol consumption, substance use, and other risk-taking behavior, and marriage promotes an orderly lifestyle. Differences in sexual and reproductive behavior among the marital status groups have been mentioned as explanations for differences in mortality rates from several malignant neoplasms – the excessive mortality rate among never-married women from breast cancer, uterine cancer, and ovarian cancer; the higher mortality rate among divorced women from cervical cancer; and the lower mortality rate among never-married men from prostate cancer.

Finally, differences in the use of health services among marital groups have been mentioned (e.g., married people are more inclined to use preventive health services) and in compliance with required prolonged treatment (married people are more willing to undertake the required treatments for diabetes mellitus and tuberculosis).

Interrelationships between Intermediary Factors

Psychosocial factors, material circumstances, and health behaviors have been mentioned as possible intermediary factors in the effects of marriage on health. However, the effects of marriage on health through intermediary factors cannot be viewed as three independent pathways. Several interrelationships could exist among the three intermediary factors. In the conceptual model of these interrelationships is shown in **Figure 1**, marital status is not assumed to have a direct effect on health behavior but to influence health behavior only indirectly through psychosocial factors and material conditions.

Psychosocial factors may have direct health effects or may operate through an effect on health behaviors. Unmarried people experience higher levels of psychosocial stress. Cigarette smoking and alcohol consumption are palliative coping responses to psychosocial stress. In addition, social support is important in health behavior changes; partner support, for instance, is beneficial to smoking-cessation maintenance. Finally, the more regulated life of married people facilitates healthy behaviors, and married people attempt to influence the health behaviors of their spouses.

Also, the material circumstances associated with marital status may have direct health effects, increase psychosocial stress, or operate through changes in health behaviors. With regard to the latter, unhealthy eating habits and a lack of recreation possibilities could, in part, be determined by an individual's financial position.

Evidence from several studies shows that psychosocial factors, material circumstances, and health behaviors act separately as intermediary factors in the relationship between marital status and health. The relative importance of these three groups of intermediary factors has been addressed only recently. Tentative results suggest that psychosocial factors are the most important intermediary factor in health differences between marital status groups among men, whereas material circumstances constitute the major intermediary factor of health differences among women.

Pathways of Intermediary Factors to Health

The effects of health behaviors such as smoking, alcohol consumption, obesity, and lack of physical activity on health are relatively well known. For instance, smoking is, in the long term, associated with cardiovascular diseases, chronic obstructive lung diseases, and many malignant neoplasms such as cancer of the lung, bronchus, trachea, larynx, pancreas, and bladder. Excessive alcohol consumption is associated with diseases of the liver, stomach, and central nervous system and is related to external causes of death, such as traffic accidents and suicide. Obesity and lack of physical exercise are both associated with cardiovascular diseases and conditions of the locomotor system; obesity is also associated with the development of non-insulin-dependent diabetes mellitus.

There is also a considerable amount of research on the relationship between psychosocial stress and health. Stress may cause direct physiological changes in the endocrine, immune, and autonomic nervous systems. Evidence shows that these physiological changes increase susceptibility to infectious diseases, cancer, and cardiovascular diseases. It has also been suggested that marital status, mediated by psychosocial stress, enhances susceptibility to diseases in general rather than having specific etiological effects. This theory of generalized susceptibility might explain why marital status is associated with many apparently different causes of disease and death.

The direct links between social relationships and health are more speculative. Evidence suggests that biological and psychological mechanisms are involved. A variety of studies of animals and humans suggest that the mere presence of, and especially affectionate physical contact with, another similar or nonthreatening organism reduces cardiovascular and other forms of physiological reactivity. The psychological mechanisms are related to, but partially independent of, the biological mechanisms and might, for instance, be affective in nature (if there is a basic human need for relationships or attachments, people will feel better psychologically when that need is fulfilled, with physiological consequences).

The direct health effects of material circumstances (i.e., health effects not mediated by psychosocial stress or health behaviors) are also of a more speculative nature. In previous centuries, poverty might have been the cause of starvation, death from hypothermia, or increased susceptibility to infectious diseases because of undernourishment. However, the contribution of these causes of death to overall mortality are minimal in current Western societies. However, it is conceivable that unfavorable material circumstances still increase risks for respiratory infections or the transmission of infectious agents through effects on living conditions (damp houses, presence of fungal mold, and crowding). The results of studies on this subject are inconclusive, however. The health effects of material circumstances are presumably mediated mainly by changes in psychosocial stress and, to a lesser extent, by changes in health behaviors.

A final comment with regard to the social causation theory is that we should keep in mind that marital relationships are not always health enhancing. Marital relationships may also have negative health effects, whereas divorce may have positive health effects. Marital problems are a source of stress, and social control in an environment in which hazardous health behaviors are valued could have unfavorable consequences. With regard to the positive health effects of divorce, it has, for instance, been found that people improve their health after divorce, depending on the stress of the marriage. In addition, several studies have reported that unhappily married people are less healthy than divorced people and happy married people. On the average, however, marriage is associated favorably with intermediary factors and with health.

See Also the Following Articles

Marital Conflict; Psychosocial Factors and Stress.

Further Reading

Burman, B. and Margolin, G. (1992). Analysis of the association between marital relationships and health problems: an interactional perspective. *Psychological Bulletin* **112**, 39–63.

Joung, I. M. A. (1996). *Marital status and health: descriptive and explanatory studies.* Alblasserdam, Netherlands: Haveka.

Joung, J. M. A., van de Mheen, H., Stronks, K., et al. (1998). A longitudinal study of health selection in marital transitions. *Social Science & Medicine* **46**, 425–435.

Joung, I. M. A., Stronks, K., van de Mheen, H., et al. (1997). Contribution of psychosocial factors, material circumstances and health behaviours to marital status differences in self-reported health. *Journal of Marriage and the Family* **59**, 476–490.

Stroebe, W. and Stroebe, M. S. (1987). *Bereavement and health.* New York: Cambridge University Press.

Waldron, I., Weis, C. C. and Hughes, M. E. (1997). Marital status effects on health: are there differences between never married women and divorced and separated women? *Social Science & Medicine* **45**, 1387–1397.

Marital Conflict

P T McFarland and A Christensen
University of California, Los Angeles, Los Angeles, CA, USA

This is a revised version of the article by P T McFarland and A Christensen, Encyclopedia of Stress First Edition, volume 2, pp 682–684, © 2000, Elsevier Inc.

Glossary

Demand–withdraw interaction	A pattern of interaction in which one member of a couple attempts to engage in the discussion of relationship issues and pressures, nags, demands, or criticizes the other while the other member attempts to avoid such discussions and becomes silent, withdraws, or acts defensively.
Process of conflict	The interaction that takes place around a conflict of interest.
Psychoneuro-immunology	The study of the interactions among the psychological, neurological, and immunological systems.
Structure of conflict	The conflict of interest between spouses; the incompatibility of needs, desires, or preferences that characterize a couple's struggle.

What Is Conflict?

Conflict in marital relationships is normal and inevitable. Indeed, conflict occurs to a much greater extent in marriage than in any other long-term relationship. Although some theorists have suggested that conflict may serve constructive or functional purposes, such as allowing for the disclosure of feelings and the creative resolution of problems, the focus in the marital literature has generally been on the destructive or dysfunctional consequences of conflict.

An important distinction is made in the marital literature between the structure of conflict and the process of conflict. The structure of conflict refers to the conflict of interest between the spouses, that is, the incompatibility of needs, desires, or preferences that characterize the couple's struggle. The process of conflict refers to the actual interaction that occurs between the spouses regarding the conflict of interest. It is important to note that a particular conflict of interest may give rise to a variety of conflictual processes. Couples may engage in overt conflict about the issue, or they may choose to avoid discussion about the issue altogether. Some theorists suggest that the decision to engage or to avoid is determined by spouses' beliefs about the likelihood that their efforts at resolving the conflict will be successful. Others have suggested that factors such as commitment to the relationship and negative feelings about the partner may also influence engagement or avoidance in conflict.

What Happens During Conflict?

Assuming that the management of conflict affects the quality and stability of the relationship, marital researchers have focused more of their attention on the process of conflict than on the structure of conflict. Researchers often study marital conflict by having couples discuss a conflict of interest in a laboratory setting for a predetermined amount of time (typically 10–15 min) while the resulting interaction is audiotaped or videotaped. Trained observers then code the problem-solving interaction for categories or dimensions of interest. Although the same type of discussion leads to more intense negative affect at home than it does in the laboratory, the observational research paradigm described does produce interactions that are similar to those experienced by couples in naturalistic settings.

One of the objectives of marital research has been to identify conflict behaviors that are associated with relationship satisfaction and thus differentiate between distressed and nondistressed couples. Although a number of differences have been identified, there are a few consistent findings across studies. First, distressed couples display higher rates of negative behaviors during conflictual interactions than nondistressed couples. These negative behaviors include criticism, complaints, hostility, defensiveness, denial of responsibility, and withdrawal. Second, compared to nondistressed spouses, distressed spouses exhibit greater reciprocity of negative behavior. That is, when a distressed spouse behaves in a negative manner, the other spouse tends to respond in kind, which escalates the conflict and leads to a cycle of negativity that is difficult to break. Third, nondistressed couples display higher rates of positive behaviors, such as approval and humor, during conflictual interactions than distressed couples. Similar to this cross-sectional research, longitudinal research has also demonstrated the deleterious effect of negative interactions on future satisfaction and stability.

A pattern of conflictual interaction that has received much empirical attention and has been found to be highly correlated with marital dissatisfaction is the demand–withdraw interaction pattern. In this pattern, one spouse (the demander) attempts to engage in the discussion of relationship issues and pressures, nags, demands, or criticizes the other while the other spouse (the withdrawer) attempts to avoid such discussions and becomes silent, withdraws, or acts defensively. Although both self-report and observational studies have demonstrated a gender linkage in roles in this pattern, with wives generally in the role of demander and husbands generally in the role of withdrawer, this gender effect is moderated by the specific issue that is being discussed. Specifically, the gender linkage in roles is apparent during discussions in which wives' issues are being addressed, but this linkage is not apparent during discussions in which husbands' issues are being addressed. Also, the pattern often occurs when a structural conflict of interest exists between partners whereby the partners have a differential investment in change on an issue. The spouse who desires a change that can only be achieved through the cooperation of the other (e.g., spending more time together) will generally take on a demanding role during discussion, whereas the spouse who seeks no change or change that can be achieved unilaterally (e.g., spending less time together) will generally take on the withdrawing role because discussion will only create an argument or undesired change.

In addition to studying overt behavior, marital researchers have also examined covert factors that may impact marital conflict and satisfaction, such as affective processes and perceptual differences between spouses. One area that has received much attention in the marital literature concerns the attributions that spouses make in accounting for events that occur in marriage. There is accumulating evidence indicating that attributions for negative events can promote conflict, such as when negative partner behavior is attributed to the selfish intent of the partner. Such attributions have been found to be related to less effective problem-solving behavior and to higher rates of negative behavior during problem-solving tasks. Moreover, research has demonstrated that attributions for negative partner behavior affect a spouse's own behavior toward the partner.

Recent years have seen a growing emphasis on the application of social psychological theories to the study of marital conflict. Attachment theory is one such theory that has been the focus of increased attention in marital conflict research. Attachment theory asserts that mental models of the self and other develop in the context of early parent–child interactions and that these models influence the communications and reactions of spouses to partner behaviors. Research findings generally suggest that spouses with secure attachment styles are more likely to compromise when dealing with conflict, whereas those with insecure attachment styles tend to employ less productive approaches to marital conflict.

What Are the Consequences of Conflict?

Conflict not only has an effect on the marital relationship itself, but it can also affect the health of individual partners. A growing body of research documents the association between marital conflict and the physical and mental well-being of spouses. Although married people tend to be healthier than those who are not married, marital conflict has been linked to an increase in physical illnesses such as rheumatoid arthritis and cardiac problems. Marital conflict also increases the risk for mental disorders. The association between marital conflict and depression is well established, as is the association between marital conflict and the physical and psychological abuse of spouses. Some of the most compelling data relating marital conflict to mental disorders are seen in the strong linkage between marital conflict and substance abuse.

The link between marital discord and poorer health outcomes has been systematically explored over the past decade. Negative and hostile behaviors during marital conflict are associated with various physiological effects in spouses, such as elevations in blood pressure and heart rate and changes in endocrine and immune functioning. Across studies, these negative physiological effects are more severe and persistent for wives than for husbands. Research in the field of psychoneuroimmunology suggests that there are negative long-term health consequences for spouses who are unable to physiologically recover from marital conflicts or cannot adapt physiologically to repeated conflicts.

In addition to its negative effects on spouses, marital conflict is related to problems in family functioning, including parenting and sibling relationships. Moreover, research has demonstrated the effects of marital conflict on the parent–child relationship, such as attachment difficulties and parent–child conflict, and to a wide range of adjustment problems in children, including internalizing problems such as depression and anxiety and externalizing problems such as aggression, delinquency, and conduct disorders. Exposure to frequent and severe marital conflict, such as physical aggression, seems to be particularly disturbing for children.

Not only is marital conflict itself a stressor, but other life stressors can affect marital conflict. For example, greater work demands among air traffic controllers and unemployment in blue-collar workers have been shown to be associated with more negative marital interactions. Stressful events may increase conflict by diminishing the capacity of spouses to provide support to one another, even as it increases their need for support. Such events may also affect marital interactions by giving rise to new conflicts of interest or by exacerbating old ones.

See Also the Following Articles

Marital Status and Health Problems.

Further Reading

Aubry, T., Tefft, B. and Kingsbury, N. (1990). Behavioral and psychological consequences of unemployment in blue-collar couples. *Journal of Community Psychology* **18**, 99–109.

Beach, S. R. H., Fincham, F. D. and Katz, J. (1998). Marital therapy in the treatment of depression: toward a third generation of therapy and research. *Clinical Psychology Review* **18**, 635–661.

Bradbury, T. N. and Fincham, F. D. (1992). Attributions and behavior in marital interaction. *Journal of Personality and Social Psychology* **63**, 613–628.

Burman, B. and Margolin, G. (1992). Analysis of the association between marital relationships and health problems: an interactional perspective. *Psychological Bulletin* **112**, 39–63.

Christensen, A. and Heavey, C. L. (1990). Gender and social structure in the demand/withdraw pattern of marital conflict. *Journal of Personality and Social Psychology* **59**, 73–81.

Cummings, E. M. and Davies, P. T. (2002). Effects of marital conflict on children: recent advances and emerging themes in process-oriented research. *Journal of Child Psychology and Psychiatry* **43**, 31–63.

Ewart, C. K., Taylor, C. B., Kraemer, H. C., et al. (1991). High blood pressure and marital discord: not being nasty matters more than being nice. *Health Psychology* **10**, 155–163.

Gottman, J. M. (1979). *Marital interaction: experimental investigations.* New York: Academic Press.

Grych, J. H. and Fincham, F. D. (1990). Marital conflict and children's adjustment: a cognitive-contextual framework. *Psychological Bulletin* **108**, 267–290.

Halford, W. K. and Markman, H. J. (eds.) (1997). *Clinical handbook of marriage and couples intervention.* London: John Wiley.

Hazan, C. and Shaver, P. R. (1994). Attachment as an organizational framework for research on close relationships. *Psychological Inquiry* **5**, 1–22.

Kiecolt-Glaser, J. K., Malarkey, W. B., Chee, M. A., et al. (1993). Negative behavior during marital conflict is associated with immunological down-regulation. *Psychosomatic Medicine* **55**, 395–409.

Kiecolt-Glaser, J. K., Glaser, R., Cacioppo, J. T., et al. (1997). Marital conflict in older adults: endocrinological and immunological correlates. *Psychosomatic Medicine* **59**, 339–349.

Repetti, R. L. (1989). Effects of daily workload on subsequent behavior during marital interaction: the roles of social withdrawal and spouse support. *Journal of Personality and Social Psychology* **57**, 651–659.

Robles, T. F. and Kiecolt-Glaser, J. K. (2003). The physiology of marriage: pathways to health. *Physiology and Behavior* **79**, 409–416.

Divorce, Children of

K N Hipke
Wisconsin Psychiatric Institute and Clinics, Madison, WI, USA
S A Wolchik and I N Sandler
Arizona State University, Tempe, AZ, USA

This is a revised version of the article by K N Hipke, I N Sandler and S A Wolchik, Encyclopedia of Stress First Edition, volume 1, pp 730–733, © 2000, Elsevier Inc.

Glossary

Effect size — A statistical indicator, expressed in standard deviation units, of the magnitude of the relation between two variables.

Externalizing — A constellation of psychological symptoms indicative of acting-out behavior, such as aggression and conduct problems.

Internalizing — A constellation of psychological symptoms experienced internally, such as depression and anxiety.

Meta-analysis — A quantitative method of literature review in which measures of central tendency (e.g., the mean) and variation are obtained for outcomes examined across multiple studies.

Moderator — A variable that affects the direction and/or strength of the relation between an independent or predictor variable (e.g., divorce) and a dependent or criterion variable (children's mental health problems).

Divorce-Related Stressors

Parental divorce has become a common experience for children, particularly in the United States, where divorce is more common than in any other developed country. The rate of divorce in the United States has increased over the course of the twentieth century, with a particularly rapid rise beginning in the decades of the 1960s and 1970s followed by a modest decline at the close of the century. Currently, close to half of all marriages end in divorce, affecting approximately 1.5 million children a year. Although divorce rates vary among families of different demographic profiles, between 30 and 40% of all children are expected to live in a divorced, single-parent home by the age of 16.

Parental divorce is not a singular event. Rather, it marks a multitude of potential stressful changes and disruptions in children's social and physical environments that occur before, during, and after parental separation. For example, interparental conflict often begins many months and/or years prior to separation, can escalate around separation and/or divorce, and can continue well after separation as parents negotiate new parenting-related issues such as child custody, visitation arrangements, and child support. As in the case of interparental conflict, many of the stressful changes and experiences faced by children from divorced families occur in the family domain, involve interpersonal loss and/or conflict, and are not easily controllable by children.

Several of these changes occur in children's relationships with parents. Despite an increasing emphasis on joint custody in many states, over 80% of children from divorced families still reside primarily with their mothers. Consequently, parental separation often means the loss of daily contact with fathers. Moreover, for most children contact with noncustodial fathers becomes increasingly infrequent over time. Children with continued father involvement may face the challenge of residing in two households, with different rules and discipline practices. The quality of relationship between fathers and children may also change following divorce, as fathers try to adapt to a parenting role when they do not reside with their children. Considerable research indicates that a positive relationship, including warm and supportive interactions as well as appropriate discipline, is an important factor affecting children's well-being following divorce.

Children's relationships with their mothers also change. Custodial mothers report high levels of stress as they negotiate the dual task of adjusting to the dissolution of marriage as well as to a new lifestyle with increased responsibilities. Juggling single parenthood, work-related demands, legal matters, and the re-negotiation of social relationships places custodial mothers at increased risk for psychological distress and physical illness. Maternal stress and distress, in turn, have been linked to disruptions in parenting behavior. Following divorce, many custodial mothers are less supportive, affectionate, and consistent in their discipline practices and engage in more conflict with children.

Many newly divorced families also face financial stress. Both mothers and fathers may experience a decline in standard of living following divorce. Income loss can result in potentially stressful changes for children, including moving to a different home, changing neighborhoods, and changing schools. While these transitions involve the loss of material possessions, children also face the loss of friends, teachers, and other important members of their social support networks.

When asked about the various changes that arise following divorce, children, parents, and clinicians who work with children from divorced families agreed that the most stressful experiences children face occur in the nuclear family domain. These include being blamed for the divorce, verbal and/or physical interparental conflict, and derogation of one parent by another. Other experiences perceived as highly stressful by children include derogation of parents by relatives or neighbors, having to give up possessions, and maternal psychological distress.

For many children, parental divorce is the first of several family transitions, each of which brings a new set of stressful changes. Forty percent of divorced couples remarry before their youngest child reaches age 18. Given that remarriages are also more likely than first marriages to end in divorce, a sizeable number of children face multiple family transitions over the course of their childhood. Although remarriage can improve the financial and emotional support provided to parents, it requires complex family reconfiguration. For children, this includes the addition of a stepparent, as well as other stepkin relations such as stepsiblings, grandparents, and other extended family members. When additional children are born into the family following remarriage, half-sibling relationships are created. The incorporation of new family members alters family dynamics, including relationships with biological parents. In addition, children may face physical transitions such as an additional residential move or sharing of a room with other children.

Mental Health Consequences

The findings from five decades of empirical research have consistently demonstrated that children from divorced families are at increased risk for adjustment or mental health problems relative to children from continuously married families. When this body of literature is summarized using meta-analysis, the effect sizes are small to moderate, with the largest group difference occurring in the domain of externalizing problems or conduct problems. Children from divorced homes, on average, engage in more misbehavior, are more aggressive, and/or have higher rates of delinquency. Children from divorced homes also show greater difficulties in the areas of psychological adjustment (i.e., depression, anxiety, happiness), social adjustment, self-concept, and school achievement.

The small to moderate effect sizes have caused some researchers to question the significance of parental divorce as a risk factor for adjustment problems. However, there are several reasons why divorce should be considered an important risk factor with significant population-level implications. First, given the high prevalence of divorce in society, small to moderate effects on child maladjustment have a substantial impact on population rates of problem outcomes for children from divorced families. Second, trends in studies from the 1990s show that effect sizes have increased from the 1980s. Third, a sizeable subset of children from divorced families have significant mental health problems. Approximately 20–35% of children from divorced families experience clinically significant mental health problems, a rate at least twice that of children from two-parent families. Fourth, adolescents from divorced homes engage in more high-risk behavior with potentially long-ranging consequences. Adolescents from divorced homes are more likely than those from two-parent homes, for example, to drop out of school, become sexually active or pregnant at an earlier age, and use drugs or alcohol.

Finally, the effects of divorce for many children and adolescents are not transitory. Longitudinal studies indicate that children from divorced families are at elevated risk for difficulties several years after parental separation, with problems continuing throughout adulthood. Across studies, adults who experienced divorce in childhood or adolescence have been found to function more poorly on a range of indicators including depression, life satisfaction, marital quality, educational attainment, income, occupational prestige, and health outcomes such as illness and mortality. Adults who experienced divorce as children or adolescents are also more likely to divorce themselves. Researchers have speculated that these long-term consequences are the result of disruptions in normal development during childhood and adolescence.

Risk and Resilience

Although children from divorced families are at elevated risk for adjustment problems, there is tremendous variability in response. The majority of children in divorced families show no adverse effects relative to children raised by continuously married families. Thus, research on children from divorced families has shifted over time from examining the mental health and adjustment consequences of divorce toward understanding why some children are more adversely affected by divorce than others. Researchers have identified several risk and protective factors that act as moderators between divorce and children's mental health, including stress, parent–child relationships, and child characteristics.

Exposure to Stressors

Greater exposure to stressful divorce-related stressors is associated with increased mental health problems among children. The frequency of divorce-related changes faced by children and families, as assessed by divorce events checklists, relates positively to difficulties in the domains of internalizing and externalizing symptoms, self-concept, and social and academic competence. Children exposed to more divorce-related stressors also show maladaptive cognitions, including a reduced sense of their ability to affect their environments.

Studies have also examined the relations between specific types of divorce stressors and children's mental health. More limited post-divorce economic resources have been consistently related to increased maladjustment. Exposure to interparental conflict is one of the most potent determinants of children's post-divorce adjustment problems. A positive association between intense marital conflict and child mental health problems has been well documented. Researchers increasingly believe that children in families marked by intense, chronic marital conflict and/or violence may be better off in the long run if their parents divorce and the degree of conflict is reduced (although a decrease in conflict does not always occur). Interestingly, in divorcing families in which overt conflict was very low or absent prior to separation, children are also at risk for poor adjustment, perhaps due to the unexpected nature of the dissolution. In either scenario, post-divorce conflict that involves putting a child in the middle by, for example, one parent denigrating the other parent or asking the child to carry hostile messages, is associated with higher levels of child depression and anxiety.

Parent–Child Relationships

The degree to which the quality of children's relationships with their parents is disrupted following divorce is predictive of adjustment problems. Children whose custodial mothers provide high levels of warmth, affection, and effective, consistent discipline following divorce exhibit fewer behavior problems, higher self-esteem, and better academic performance than children with low-quality mother–child relationships. Experimental research has shown that intervention-induced increases in maternal warmth and effective discipline mediate program effects to reduce children's mental health problems. Moreover, high-quality mother–child relationships serve as a buffer, mitigating the negative effects of divorce-related stressors on children's adjustment problems.

Because fathers are more likely to be noncustodial parents, research initially focused upon whether the amount of father–child contact affected children's adjustment after divorce. Findings from this line of research were inconclusive. It is now understood that it is the quality and not quantity of father–child contact that is important to divorce adaptation. High-quality father–child relationships are related to better child post-divorce adjustment than low-quality relationships.

Child Characteristics

Research examining the association between child demographics, such as age and gender, and post-divorce adjustment has revealed few consistent findings. Although some studies, particularly older studies or those examining conduct problems, indicate less advantageous outcomes for boys relative to girls, meta-analyses show that divorce is associated with a range of poor outcomes for both boys and girls. Similarly, while meta-analysis has also shown that children in middle childhood and adolescence appear to be more negatively impacted by divorce than preschoolers or college students, far fewer studies have examined divorce adjustment in these latter two age groups, making it difficult to draw firm conclusions regarding the effect of age on children's adaptation to divorce.

Recently, a body of literature has begun to emerge that shows that the manner in which children interpret and cope with divorce-related stressors has implications for their adjustment. Children who lack an internal sense of control over their environment or who have a tendency to interpret divorce-related stressors in a characteristically negative style or as threatening to their well-being are more likely to experience post-divorce adjustment problems. Also, children who use positive cognitive or behavioral coping strategies, such as active problem solving or positive cognitive restructuring, experience fewer psychological adjustment problems than children who employ avoidant coping strategies. Theoretically, researchers agree that the adaptive value of specific coping strategies depends on context. Children may benefit most, for example, by cognitively reframing a situation that is largely outside of their control, while problem solving may be an adaptive strategy for situations that are more controllable. There is also growing evidence that the effects of using appropriate coping strategies may be mediated by increasing children's sense of efficacy to deal with the problems they encounter in their lives.

Children's temperament, which theoretically modulates the expression of activity, emotionality, reactivity, and behavior, has also been implicated as important to children's post-divorce adjustment, although this area of research is currently small. Findings indicate, for example, that children rated as more emotionally reactive are at increased risk for maladjustment compared to children who are less reactive and that this effect may be mediated by leading to an increase in negative appraisals of the threat involved in stressful situations.

There is also evidence that the effects of parent and environmental factors are not independent of child factors, but rather are mediated through their effects on children's beliefs about their relations to the world and their ability to cope. For example, the effects of poor parenting quality on children's mental health appears to be partially mediated by increasing children's fears that they will not be cared for by anyone. Similarly, the effects of interparental conflict (a stressor over which children have little control) on children's mental health is in part mediated by decreasing children's coping efficacy beliefs.

Implications for Prevention

Efforts to facilitate adaptation to divorce and prevent maladjustment have focused on altering modifiable contextual, family, and/or child variables demonstrated to affect children's divorce adjustment. The most widely available preventive interventions are child-focused programs that are often provided in school settings. Such interventions generally seek to increase children's accurate understanding of divorce and teach new skills for coping with divorce-related stressors. Preventive programs that target custodial parents focus on teaching effective parenting skills to enhance the quality of parent–child relationships and help parents shield children from stressful experiences such as interparental conflict. Among programs that have been rigorously evaluated using experimental and/or quasi-experimental trials, results have been positive. Child-focused programs have been successful in improving child mental health outcomes, including internalizing and externalizing symptoms, with program effects still present at follow-up studies 1 to 2 years later. Similarly, prevention programs for custodial mothers have been successful in improving the quality of the mother–child relationship, effective discipline, and child mental health outcomes. Recent evidence shows that program effects last well into adolescence, leading to reductions in mental health problems, drug and alcohol use, school failure, and risky sexual behavior and improvements in academic performance and competence.

See Also the Following Articles

Adolescence; Childhood Stress; Marital Conflict; Marital Status and Health Problems.

Further Reading

Amato, P. R. (2000). The consequences of divorce for adults and children. *Journal of Marriage and the Family* **62**, 1269–1287.

Amato, P. R. (2001). Children of divorce in the 1990's: an update of the Amato and Keith (1991) meta-analysis. *Journal of Family Psychology* **15**, 355–370.

Amato, P. R. and Keith, B. (1991). Parental divorce and adult well-being: a meta-analysis. *Journal of Marriage and the Family* **53**, 43–58.

Grych, J. H. and Fincham, F. D. (1997). Children's adaptation to divorce: from description to explanation. In: Wolchik, S. A. & Sandler, I. N. (eds.) *Handbook of children's coping: linking theory and intervention.* New York: Plenum Press.

Haine, R. A., Sandler, I. N., Wolchik, S. A., Tein, J.-Y. and Dawson-McClure, S. R. (2003). Changing the legacy of divorce: evidence from prevention programs and future directions. *Family Relations* **52**, 397–405.

Hetherington, E. M., Bridges, M. and Isabella, G. M. (1998). What matters? What does not? Five perspectives on the association between marital transitions and children's adjustment. *American Psychologist* **53**, 167–184.

Kelly, J. B. and Emery, R. E. (2003). Children's adjustment following divorce: risk and resilience perspectives. *Family Relations* **52**, 352–362.

Pedro-Carroll, J. (2005). Fostering resilience in the aftermath of divorce: the role of evidence-based programs for children. *Family Court Review* **43**, 52–63.

Sandler, I. N., Wolchik, S. A., Davis, C., Haine, R. and Ayers, T. (2003). Correlational and experimental study of resilience in children of divorce and parentally bereaved children. In: Luthar, S. L. (ed.) *Resilience and vulnerability. Adaptation in the context of childhood adversities.* Cambridge, UK: Cambridge University Press.

Wolchik, S. A., Sandler, I. N., Millsap, R. E., et al. (2002). Six-year follow-up of a randomized, controlled trial of preventive interventions for children of divorce. *Journal of the American Medical Association* **288**, 1874–1881.

Wolchik, S. A., Sandler, I. N., Winslow, E. and Smith-Daniels, V. (2005). Programs for promoting parenting residential parents: moving from efficacy to effectiveness. *Family Court Review* **43**, 65–80.

Incest

A P Mannarino
Allegheny General Hospital, Pittsburgh, PA, USA

This is a revised version of the article by A P Mannarino, Encyclopedia of Stress First Edition, volume 2, pp 554–557, © 2000, Elsevier Inc.

Glossary

Incest	A type of sexual abuse in which the abuser is a family member.
Nonoffending parent	The nonabusive parent, who typically has custody of the child.
Perpetrator	The family member who abuses the child.
Posttraumatic stress disorder (PTSD)	A stress disorder that includes three categories of psychiatric symptoms in response to a traumatic life event.
Sexual abuse	Sexual exploitation involving physical contact between a child and another person.

Incest: Definition and Descriptive Characteristics

Sexual abuse can be defined as sexual exploitation involving physical contact between a child and another person. Exploitation implies an inequality of power between the child and the abuser on the basis of age, physical size, and/or the nature of the emotional relationship. There can also be noncontact sexual abuse, which includes exposing a child to pornography, taking photographs or videotaping a child for sexual purposes, or sexual exploitation through the Internet.

Incest is a type of sexual abuse in which the abuser is a family member. The abuser may be a parent, stepparent, grandparent, older sibling, or other close relative. Sociological surveys by Finkelhor and others have suggested that 25–30% of all girls and 10–15% of all boys are sexually abused by the age of 18. The proportion of sexual abuse that is incestuous in nature is not absolutely known, but in clinical studies it seems to account for approximately one-half of all reported cases.

Incest is not limited to sexual intercourse. It also includes oral or anal intercourse, fondling of the breasts or genitals, and sexualized, inappropriate kissing. The empirical literature suggests that approximately 50% of incest cases involve oral, anal, or vaginal intercourse while the other half involve genital fondling. Violence is not typically perpetrated against a child victim as part of an act of incest, although threats of violence are common. A child may be coerced to participate in a sexual experience through the promise of rewards or the threat of punishment. In some families, children who are sexually abused may also be physically abused or witness domestic violence.

Children may be victimized by incest at any age. Despite the public misconception that only girls are victimized, boys may also be subjected to an incestuous relationship. The great majority of perpetrators of incest are male, with statistics suggesting that males account for 90% or more of reported cases. The severity of incest can vary from one episode of genital touching to hundreds of episodes of sexual abuse, including intercourse, which may extend over many years. Although incest is commonly reported across all socioeconomic classes, studies by Finkelhor have demonstrated that poor children are more vulnerable to this type of victimization.

Diagnosis

In the nomenclature of the American Psychiatric Association (*Diagnostic and Statistical Manual,* 4th edn.-TR), sexual abuse or incest is not usually considered to be a primary diagnosis (axis I) but is classified as a psychosocial stressor (axis IV) that may contribute to the primary diagnosis. (However, in situations in which the sexual abuse of the child is the primary focus of clinical attention, it can be coded on axis I.) Children who are victimized by incest do not manifest a unitary syndrome of traits, characteristics, or symptoms. Although, as a group, incest victims display more emotional and behavioral symptoms than normal children, these problems are typically diverse in nature. Moreover, approximately 30% of all incest victims are asymptomatic. Sexual preoccupation or sexualized behaviors are more common in incest victims than nonvictims, but the latter group may exhibit these problems as well. Overall, the general conclusion is that incest cannot be diagnosed based solely on the symptom presentation.

On medical examination, less than 20% of all incest victims display significant clinical findings. Even in cases in which the victim has been vaginally or anally penetrated, significant physical findings may not be present. Accordingly, the absence of significant physical findings does not mean that incest has not occurred.

Determining that incest has occurred is a complex legal and clinical problem. With very young children, they may engage in sexualized behaviors and only disclose alleged abuse after being questioned by the nonoffending parent. Older children may disclose the alleged victimization to a friend, relative, teacher, or other trusted adult. In the great majority of incest cases, the alleged perpetrator initially denies the victimization. In the absence of significant medical findings or a perpetrator confession, it is ultimately very difficult to prove that incest has occurred.

Interviewing the alleged victim is the most frequent method used to determine whether incest has been perpetrated. The nonoffending parent typically provides background data and information about what the child has previously disclosed. If the alleged perpetrator is a parent, he or she may also be interviewed; however, it is recommended that this be done at a separate time from the alleged victim. Most experts recommend that a comprehensive evaluation, including interviews with both parents, be conducted when incest is disclosed in the context of divorce or custody issues.

Over the past 15 years, many concerns have been generated regarding the procedures used to interview alleged sexual abuse and incest victims. Questions have been raised about children's memory and their ability to recall accurately what allegedly occurred. Laboratory research related to this issue has provided mixed results, with some studies suggesting that children do accurately recall the core features of significant events and other studies indicating that children can produce inaccurate information, particularly in response to repetitive or coercive-like questions. In this regard, criticism sometimes has been directed at child protective service workers, mental health consultants, and other investigative interviewers for allegedly pressuring children to make abuse disclosures or for using inappropriate interviewing techniques (i.e., leading questions). Unfortunately, with the exception of some highly publicized cases, it is impossible to know how often investigations of sexual abuse and incest have been contaminated by improper interview strategies.

In light of the significant issues related to interview methods, some professional guidelines have been promulgated to address this problem. For example, the American Professional Society on the Abuse of Children has developed guidelines for the evaluation of suspected sexual abuse in children, and the American Academy of Child and Adolescent Psychiatry has established practice parameters for the forensic evaluation of children and adolescents who may have been physically or sexually abused. Although it is impossible to know to what degree investigative interviewers are aware of and follow these guidelines, in the past few years there seem to be fewer concerns about inappropriate interviewing procedures.

The Psychological Impact of Incest

As mentioned earlier, children who have been victimized through an incestuous relationship may display a variety of emotional and/or behavioral difficulties subsequent to disclosure. Despite the diversity of the symptom presentation of this population, a number of studies have reported that 20–50% of sexual abuse and incest victims meet full or partial criteria for PTSD. The symptoms of PTSD fall into three categories: re-experiencing symptoms (i.e., intrusive thoughts, nightmares, and flashbacks), avoidance symptoms (i.e., avoid thoughts or feelings about the trauma, emotional detachment, and inability to recall important aspects of the trauma), and symptoms of increased arousal (i.e., sleep disturbance, hypervigilance, and difficulty concentrating). Other psychiatric sequelae of incest may include clinical depression, other anxiety disorders, low self-esteem, sexually reactive behaviors, and, for adolescents, substance abuse problems.

Recent studies have suggested that the frequency and severity of psychiatric symptoms in sexual abuse and incest victims may be mediated by their attributions and perceptions related to the victimization. Thus, victims who feel different from other children, who blame themselves for the abuse, who feel that others do not believe what they say, or have a decreased amount of interpersonal trust are at higher risk for more serious symptomatology. In particular, children who feel that they are to blame for the victimization are more vulnerable to experiencing depressive disorders.

Legal proceedings may also have an impact on outcome. There is some evidence that when legal proceedings are delayed, emotional/behavioral symptoms in sexual abuse victims tend to increase. Also, when children have to testify in court and are subjected to a very hostile cross-examination or are required to testify multiple times, psychiatric symptomatology appears to worsen.

The psychological impact of being victimized by an incestuous relationship may be moderated by several factors. A number of major studies have demonstrated that emotional support of the victim from the nonoffending parent, which includes not blaming the child for the victimization, has a highly beneficial effect and is correlated with fewer psychiatric symptoms in the victim. Also, as we would anticipate, many nonoffending parents have highly intense emotional reactions to their child's disclosure of incest. These emotional reactions may include anxiety, guilt, anger, and shame. Recent empirical investigations have shown that, when nonoffending parents are able, over time, to resolve their emotional upset related to their child's victimization, this correlates with a reduction in the frequency and severity of the child's emotional and behavioral symptoms.

Treatment of Incest Victims

The treatment of incest may involve a variety of interventions, including individual and/or group therapy for the child victim, supportive therapy with the nonoffending parent, counseling for the perpetrator, and family therapy. Space does not permit a discussion of perpetrator treatment, except to say that most incest perpetrators initially deny victimizing the child and/or minimize its impact and typically require long-term therapy to address their difficulty in taking responsibility for the abuse, cognitive distortions, and issues related to potential relapse.

With the increased attention to and reporting of sexual abuse over the past two decades in the United States, a proliferation of clinical programs has occurred that focus on victim treatment. Unfortunately, the efficacy of the interventions offered in most of these programs has not been investigated. Nonetheless, there is now strong empirical evidence that Trauma-Focused Cognitive Behavioral Therapy (TF-CBT) is an efficacious treatment for sexual abuse and incest victims. Specifically, TF-CBT has been found to be superior to nondirective supportive therapy in reducing PTSD, depressive symptoms, shame, and general behavioral difficulties in the victimized child and parental distress and depressive symptoms in the nonoffending caretaker. This pattern of results has been replicated in a large multisite study of sexual abuse victims, most of whom had also been subjected to other traumatic events.

There are a number of core components of TF-CBT. These include psychoeducation, stress reduction strategies (e.g., relaxation training), creating a trauma narrative, cognitive processing to address inappropriate attributions (i.e, self-blame), and the development of safety and other coping skills.

Work with the nonoffending parent is an essential component of TF-CBT for sexual abuse and incest victims. Critical interventions with the nonoffending parents include addressing their attributions about the sexual abuse, enhancing their support of the victimized child, and behavioral management strategies.

In some treatment programs for incest families, family therapy is the intervention of choice. This is true even though family treatment has not been widely investigated empirically as a potentially effective therapeutic strategy for incestuous families. Family therapy for incest is based on the belief that family dynamics either contribute to the occurrence of the incestuous situation, help maintain the secrecy of the incestuous relationship, or can be changed to prevent future episodes of victimization. The perpetrator of the abuse may be included in family treatment, especially if there is a possibility of family reunification. However, the inclusion of the perpetrator in family sessions would typically occur only after the perpetrator has experienced extensive individual and/or group treatment and has been willing to accept total responsibility for the victimization.

See Also the Following Articles

Child Sexual Abuse; Sexual Assault.

Further Reading

American Academy of Child and Adolescent Psychiatry (1997). Practice parameters for the forensic evaluation of children and adolescents who may have been physically or sexually abused. *Journal of the American Academy of Child and Adolescent Psychiatry* **36**, 432–442.

American Professional Society on the Abuse of Children (1990). *Guidelines for psychosocial evaluation of suspected sexual abuse in young children.* Chicago: Author.

American Psychiatric Association (2000). *Diagnostic and statistical manual* (4th edn.). Washington, DC: American Psychiatric Press.

Bruck, M. and Ceci, S. J. (1998). Reliability and credibility of young children's reports: From research to policy and practice. *American Psychologist* **53**, 136–151.

Cohen, J. A., Deblinger, E. and Mannarino, A. P. (2005). Trauma-focused cognitive behavioral therapy for sexually abused children. In: Hibbs, E. & Jensen, P. (eds.) *Psychosocial treatments for child and adolescent disorders: empirically-based strategies for clinical practice.* (2nd edn., pp. 743–765). Washington, DC: American Psychological Association.

Cohen, J. A., Deblinger, E., Mannarino, et al. (2004). A multisite, randomized controlled trial for sexually abused children with PTSD symptoms. *Journal of the American Academy of Child and Adolescent Psychiatry* **43**, 393–402.

Cohen, J. A. and Mannarino, A. P. (1996). A treatment outcome study for sexually abused preschool children: initial findings. *Journal of the American Academy of Child and Adolescent Psychiatry* **35**, 42–50.

Deblinger, E., Lippman, J. and Steer, R. (1996). Sexually abused children suffering PTSD symptoms: initial treatment outcome findings. *Child Maltreatment* **1**, 310–321.

Finkelhor, D. and Baron, L. (1986). Risk factors for child sexual abuse. *Journal of Interpersonal Violence* **1**, 43–71.

Mannarino, A. P. and Cohen, J. A. (1996). Abuse-related attributions and perceptions, general attributions, and locus of control in sexually abused girls. *Journal of Interpersonal Violence* **11**, 162–180.

Runyan, D. K., Hunter, W. M. and Everson, M. D. (1992). Impact of legal intervention on sexually abused children. *Journal of Pediatrics* **113**, 647–653.

Saywitz, K. J., Goodman, G. S. and Lyon, T. D. (2002). Interviewing children in and out of court: current research and practice implications. In: Myers, J. E. B., Berliner, L., Briere, J., Hendrix, C. T., Tenny, C. & Reid, T. A. (eds.) *The APSAC handbook on child maltreatmen* (2nd edn., pp. 349–377). Thousand Oaks, CA: Sage.

Saywitz, K. J., Mannarino, A. P., Berliner, L., et al. (2000). Treatment for sexually abused children and adolescents. *American Psychologist* **55**, 1040–1049.

Elder Abuse

C P Holstege
University of Virginia, Charlottesville, VA, USA
H Holstege
Calvin College, Grand Rapids, MI, USA

This is a revised version of the article by C P Holstege and H Holstege, Encyclopedia of Stress First Edition, volume 2, pp 19–22, © 2000, Elsevier Inc.

Glossary

Domestic elder abuse — The abuse of an elderly person by someone closely associated within that elder's home or by somebody in the home of the person caring for that elder.

Elder abandonment — The desertion or willful forsaking of an elder by any person having the care or custody of that elder under circumstances in which a reasonable person would continue to provide care.

Elder neglect — The failure of a caregiver to fulfill his or her obligation or duty to care for an elder.

Elder self-abuse — A neglectful or abusive behavior by an elder that is dangerous to his or her own safety or health.

Financial elder abuse — Any theft or misuse of an elder's financial funds, property, or other resources by a person in a position of trust with an elder.

Institutional elder abuse — The abuse that occurs by paid staff in establishments designated to care

	for the elderly, including foster homes, group homes, and nursing homes.
Physical elder abuse	The willful infliction of physical force against an elder that results in tangible injury, pain, or impairment by a person who cares for or has custody of or who stands in a position of trust with that elder.
Psychological elder abuse	The deliberate infliction of mental or emotional suffering upon an elder by use of insults, humiliation, intimidation, threats, or other verbal or nonverbal abusive conduct.
Sexual elder abuse	The nonconsensual sexual contact of an elderly person.

Demographics of Elder Abuse

In the United States, the National Center on Elder Abuse reported that nearly 400 000 adult/elder abuse reports were investigated by Adult Protective Services in 2000. Of these, 48.5% were substantiated by Adult Protective Services. The majority of reports involved the domestic setting (60.7%), with only 8.3% occurring in the institutional setting. Perpetrators were most commonly family members (61.7%), especially spouses or intimate partners (30.2%) and adult children (17.6%). Evidence points toward the validity of the iceberg theory of elder abuse, which states that only the most visible types of elder abuse and neglect are reported to official sources (e.g., Adult Protective Services) and that a large number of other incidents are unidentified and unreported.

Characteristics of the Abused

Women are disproportionately victimized, representing two-thirds of the victims of physical abuse, three-fourths of the incidents of psychological abuse, and greater than 90% of the cases of financial abuse. Elderly living alone have lower rates of abuse than elderly living with other persons. Increasing age is associated with a higher incidence of abuse and neglect. Elderly in poor health are nearly four times more likely to be abused than comparably aged elderly in good health. The elderly who are widowed, divorced, or never married are less likely to be abused.

Characteristics of the Abuser

Men are slightly more likely than women to abuse elders. Approximately 90% of alleged elder abusers are related to their victims. The majority of perpetrators of elder abuse are either the elder's spouse or adult children. Since families are frequently the primary caregivers for elderly relatives in domestic settings, the fact that family members are the primary perpetrators of elder abuse is not surprising. Most elder abusers are younger than their victims. This fact is most striking in the area of financial abuse, where nearly half of the abusers are 40 years old or younger.

Theories about the Cause of Elder Abuse

Numerous studies have examined the possible etiologies of elder abuse. Although the causes of most cases of elder abuse are multifactorial, six widely accepted theories have been reported in the literature.

Psychopathology in the Abuser

The psychopathology of the abuser theory focuses on the abuser's mental derangement as the primary cause of elder abuse. Specific conditions, such as psychiatric illness, alcohol and drug addiction, dementia, and mental retardation, lead to inadequacy in the abuser. As a result, the abuser is unable to positively relate to the elder. This subsequently leads to the abuse. Approximately 30% of abusers have documented psychiatric illness, and nearly 40% have a history of substance abuse.

Transgenerational Violence

According to the transgenerational violence theory, the abuser learns abusive behavior from other family members, and this dysfunctional behavior is passed from one generation to the next. A cycle of violence then ensues. For these families, violence is perceived as a normal behavior pattern. For example, a person who was abused as child becomes the abuser when his or her parents become elderly and more dependent. Child, spouse, and elder abuse may be seen in these extended families.

Caregiver Stress

The caregiver stress theory emphasizes the stress of the abuser as the predominant factor that leads to elder mistreatment. The obligations associated with providing care for the elderly may place overwhelming demands on providers. Frequent falls, wandering, incontinence, disrobing, and verbal abuse by elders are examples of occurrences that place undue stress upon the caregiver. External stresses upon the caregiver (e.g., unemployment, personal illness, and financial hardship) may lead to his or her lashing out at the elder in frustration. A good relationship between the caregiver and the care recipient prior to illness and disability has been shown to minimize stress, even in the face of heavy caregiver demands.

The Web of Dependency

The web of dependency theory suggests that the frailty of an elder in and of itself is a cause for abuse and neglect. Increasing physical and mental impairment in the elder leads to an increasing dependency on a caregiver for the activities of daily living. As the caregiver's obligations increase, the burden and stress on him or her is also increased. As a result of this increased dependency, abuse occurs. Greater impairment and subsequent dependency of the elder may also diminish his or her ability to defend him- or herself from abuse or to escape the situation.

Caregiving Context

The caregiving context theory places emphasis on the situation of the caregiving. Elderly who are socially isolated are more prone to be abused. Families in which abuse occurs remain secluded to avoid detection. Elderly who share living space with their caregiver are also more prone to be abused. Tensions and daily conflicts are more difficult to avoid when the parties live together.

The Sociocultural Climate

Cultural and ethnic diversity may influence the prevalence of abuse. In cultures in which elders are highly esteemed or in which a strong value is placed on family responsibility, caring for an elder member of the family is expected. Failure to fulfill this caregiver role may cause shame and frustration. Cultural sanctions against revealing family problems to outsiders may subsequently prevent families from seeking help. If a family has relocated to a foreign country, adaptation to that culture may create additional stress and conflict as to how to care for their elders.

Institutional Abuse

Abuse occurs not only in domestic settings, but also in institutions such as nursing homes, mental institutions, and adult foster homes. At least half of all nursing home patients suffer from some form of dementia or mental illness. This group of patients is more prone to be abused and is less likely to report the abuse. In institutional settings, physical elder abuse has been reported to occur in one-third of patients, with psychological abuse occurring in up to 80% of elders. The causes for this abuse in institutions are multifactorial. The lack of understanding of the cause of the elder's behavior, dissatisfaction among the institution's staff, patient–staff conflict, and burnout among staff have been sited as causes for institutional elder abuse. Education of the staff is the most important factor to decrease elder abuse in institutions. In addition, more psychiatric services need to be provided for elders residing within institutions.

Signs and Symptoms of Elder Abuse

The signs and symptoms of elder abuse can range from subtle to grossly apparent. Professionals who routinely work with the elderly are typically not well trained in evaluating signs and symptoms of elder abuse. As a result of this lack of training, an underreporting of abuse has been clearly documented. Possible signs and symptoms of elder abuse are demonstrated in **Table 1**. Elder abandonment also occurs and can manifest as the desertion of an elder at a hospital,

Table 1 Possible signs of elder abuse and neglect

Physical abuse	*Physical neglect*	*Sexual abuse*	*Emotional abuse*
Bruises	Consistent hunger	Difficulty walking	**Habit disorder**
Unexplained	Poor hygiene	Difficulty sitting	Sucking
In various stages of healing	Inappropriate dress	Genitalia itching/pain	Biting
In regular patterns	Soiled clothing	Bruised/bloody genitalia	Rocking
In shape of the article used	Weight loss	Bruises around breasts	**Conduct disorder**
Bite marks	Dehydration	Vaginal bleeding/tears	Antisocial
In an unusual location	Urine burns	Anal tears/bruising	Destructive
Burns	Pressure sores	Stained/bloody underwear	**Neurotic traits**
In the shape of cigarette/cigar	Over- or undermedication	Sexually transmitted diseases	Sleep disorders
Immersion burns	Hypothermia		Speech disorders
Patterned burns (e.g., from an iron)	Lice		Inhibition of play
Rope burns	Lack of functional aids,		**Psychoneurotie reaction**
Caustic burns	e.g., glasses, dentures,		Hysteria
Fractures	hearing aids, walking aids		Obsession
Unexplained			Compulsion
In various stages of healing			Phobias
Multiple			Hypochondria
Spiral			
Lacerations			
Unexplained			
In an unusual location			
Internal injuries			

Table 2 Signs of financial or material exploitation

Abrupt changes in a will or other financial documents
Inclusion of additional names on an elder's bank signature card
Unauthorized withdrawal of funds from an elder's financial account
Unexplained disappearance of money or other valuables
Forging of an elder's signature for financial transactions
Sudden appearance of previously uninvolved relatives claiming rights to an elder's possessions
Sudden transfer of the elder's assets to another individual
Unnecessary services being rendered by an elder (such as unnecessary home improvements)
Unpaid bills or inability to purchase basic provisions despite availability of adequate financial resources
Sudden changes in a financial account or the banking practice of an elder
Elder's report of financial exploitation

nursing facility, shopping center, or other public location. Financial or material exploitation can manifest in a number of ways, with examples given in **Table 2**. Self-neglect is difficult to determine, and, depending on where the elder lives, specific laws exist pertaining to when the elder's self rights become superseded by the government. Signs of self-neglect include unsanitary living conditions (e.g., animal or insect infestation, no functioning toilet, fecal or urine smell), hazardous living quarters (e.g., improper wiring, no heat or running water), inappropriate or inadequate clothing, lack of necessary medical aids (e.g., eyeglasses, hearing aids, dentures), grossly inadequate housing or homelessness, poor personal hygiene, and improperly attended medical conditions. Social workers, the medical profession, law enforcement, and the general public must be educated to increase awareness and thereby decrease the occurrence of elder mistreatment.

See Also the Following Articles

Caregivers, Stress and; Child Abuse.

Further Reading

Jones, J. S., Holstege, C. P. and Holstege, H. (1997). Elder abuse and neglect: understanding the causes and potential risk factors. *American Journal of Emergency Medicine* **15**, 579–583.

Kosberg, J. I. and Jordan, L. G. (1995). *Elder abuse: international and cross-cultural perspectives.* Binghamton, NY: Hawthorne Press.

Lachs, M. S. and Pillemer, K. (2004). Elder abuse. *Lancet* **364**(9441), 1263–1272.

Riekse, R. J. and Holstege, H. (1996). *Growing older in America.* New York: McGraw-Hill.

Relevant Website

http://www.elderabusecenter.org – National Center on Elder Abuse (NCEA), U.S. Administration on Aging 2005.

Male Partner Violence

M Ingram, N P Yuan and M P Koss
University of Arizona, Tucson, AZ, USA

This is a revised version of the article by M P Koss and M Ingram, Encyclopedia of Stress First Edition, volume 2, pp 676–681, © 2000, Elsevier Inc.

Glossary

Physical abuse — Physical violence directed toward an intimate partner including pushing, slapping, punching, kicking, choking, assault with a weapon, tying down, and restraining; threats of bodily harm and threats of violence directed at the woman's children; and behaviors liable to cause fear of physical safety such as leaving a woman in a dangerous place, driving fast and recklessly to frighten her, and refusing to help when she is sick or injured.

Psychological abuse — Abusive behaviors whose damage is primarily emotional including physical and social isolation, extreme jealousy, possessiveness, and removing access to communication or transportation; deprivation, degradation, and humiliation; emotional distress inflicted through threats to harm companion animals or livestock; and intimidation, intense criticizing, insulting, belittling, and ridiculing.

Sexual assault — Forced sexual acts or sexual degradation, such as coercing a woman to perform sexual acts against her will; hurting her during sex or assaulting her genitals, including using objects intravaginally, orally, or anally; pursuing sex when she is not fully conscious or otherwise unable to consent; insisting on sex without protection against pregnancy or sexually transmitted diseases; and forcing her to have sex with others either privately or while being observed by the partner; often part of violent relationships.

Stalking A pattern of repeated harassing or threatening behavior including following a woman, appearing at her home or place of business, making harassing phone calls, leaving written messages or objects, and vandalizing her property, even in the absence of threat of serious harm.

Male partner violence is broadly defined to be inclusive of the various types of behaviors that are used to coerce, control, and demean women. According to a report on intimate partner violence by the U.S. Department of Justice, 20% of all nonfatal violence against women in 2001 was committed by current or former spouses or boyfriends, whereas intimate partners committed 3% of nonfatal violence against men. Women are at a greater risk of assault, including rape and homicide, by a husband, ex-husband, boyfriend, or ex-boyfriend than they are by an acquaintance or stranger. Some methodologies generate data showing equal rates of intimate partner violence by men and by women; however, women are more likely to sustain minor or serious injuries. Violence within an abusive relationship is characterized as a recurrent experience when a woman is repeatedly placed in physical danger or controlled by the threat or use of force. Specifically included in these definitions, along with physical assault, are sexual assault, battering, threats, intimidation designed to obtain power and control by inducing fear in the victim, and stalking. The United Nations, the American Medical Association, and the American Psychological Association Presidential Task Force on Violence and the Family have established definitions of violence that recognize a pattern of physical, sexual, and/or psychological acts aimed at harming, intimidating, or coercing someone who is or was involved in an intimate relationship with the perpetrator.

Prevalence

Over the past 25 years, researchers have documented that violence by male intimates is one of the most prevalent and serious threats to the well-being of women in the United States and internationally. The landmark 1998 National Violence Against Women survey (NVAW), consisting of telephone interviews with 16,000 men and women, found that 25% of the women surveyed had been raped and/or physically assaulted in their lifetime by a current or former spouse, cohabiting partner, or date. The National Crime Victimization Survey (NCVS), an annual general survey of crime, indicated that the rate of intimate partner violence against women dropped by 49% between 1993 and 2001 but that the rate in 2001 was still high. There was an estimated 691,710 nonfatal incidents of violence committed by current or former spouses, boyfriends, or girlfriends, and the victims were primarily women (85%). These estimates, however, must be understood in the context of the limitations of the methods used to obtain them. National estimates based on telephone surveys are likely to be conservative due to the exclusion of the homeless, those too poor to own a telephone, people with limited English, recent immigrants who may be fearful of the government, and women whose partners control their ability to freely receive calls. Household-based samples mean that several living situations are missed in which women may be at high risk for violence including prisons, psychiatric hospitals, military settings, and colleges. These and other differences in methods contribute to substantial variation in estimate size across surveys.

Physical Assault

The NVAW documented that 22% of women were physically assaulted by current or former intimate partners during their lifetime. The majority of assaults were relatively minor, involving pushing, grabbing, and shoving. Few incidents involved more extreme forms of aggression, such as kicking or beating, threatening with a knife or gun, or using a weapon.

Sexual Assault

NVAW have shown that more than 7% of women report being raped by a current or former intimate partner in their lifetime. Those subjected to physical abuse are especially vulnerable to sexual abuse, with 26% to 52% of physically abused women reporting also being raped. Men who are both physically and sexually abusive are consistently found to perpetrate the most violent and severe assaults on their partners, with the majority of victims being repeatedly assaulted during the course of the relationship. Women who are victims of both physical and sexual violence are also at greater risk for abuse during pregnancy as well as at greater risk of homicide.

Psychological Abuse

Emotional abuse is generally concomitant with physical or sexual assault. In a recent study of primary-care patients, all women who were physically abused also reported emotional abuse in that relationship. The Canadian Centre for Justice Statistics National Survey on Violence Against Women included questions on jealousy, limiting contact with family or friends, belittling and insulting female partners, preventing access to family income, and insisting on knowing a partner's whereabouts at all times. Approximately one-third of ever-married women in Canada reported that their current or previous partner was emotionally abusive in at least one of these five ways. In the majority of cases, emotional abuse was concomitant with physical or sexual abuse; only 18% of women who experienced emotional abuse reported no physical violence by a partner.

Stalking

Stalking by male partners also threatens the health of women. Based on a definition that includes experiencing fear, approximately 5% of women (compared to about 1% of men) have been stalked by a current or former intimate partner in their lifetime, according to the NVAW. Among women who were stalked by a former or current partner, 81% were also physically assaulted and 31% were sexually assaulted by the same man. Stalking frequently escalates among women who have left their abusive partners. The likelihood of being stalked by a male partner increases with the duration of time that the woman has been separated from the abusive relationship.

Risk Factors

Various factors increase the likelihood that a woman will be assaulted by a male partner. Research has identified several demographic risk factors. They include being younger in age; being single, divorced, or separated; having lower income; and having less education. In addition, ethnic minorities report higher rates of male partner violence compared to Whites. The NVAW indicated that American Indians/Alaska Native women had the highest rates, followed by African Americans. White and Hispanic women reported similar rates and Asian/Pacific Islanders reported the lowest rates of victimization by an intimate partner. These differences may reflect, in part, socioeconomic differences. However, researchers have found that differences in risk exist even after controlling for such variables. It is of note that studies consisting of only Native American samples have shown that some tribes have higher rates of partner violence, whereas others do not. Immigrant women experiencing partner violence are also a vulnerable population because they are often isolated in a foreign country, in constant fear of deportation, and feel at the mercy of their spouse to gain legal status. A history of childhood physical abuse, alcohol-related problems, drug use, and certain personality characteristics also increase the likelihood that women will be assaulted by a male partner. Certain characteristics of the male partner also increase the risk of victimization, including childhood exposure to intimate partner violence, partner alcohol-related problems, and emotionally abusive and controlling behaviors.

Psychological Impact

Victims of male partner violence are subject to physical, emotional, and perhaps sexual violence over an extended period of time. The impact on a woman's mental health is thus not derived solely from specific acts of violence but rather from the stress of living with recurrent, escalating, and unpredictable attacks. Not surprisingly, the severity and frequency of violence is associated with an increase in mental health symptoms, and symptoms have been shown to decrease when a woman is free from the abuse.

Posttraumatic Stress Disorder

Posttraumatic stress disorder (PTSD), as defined in the Diagnostic and Statistical Manual of Mental Disorders, fourth edition, has become the predominant diagnosis used to describe the various symptoms of psychological trauma exhibited by partner violence victims, with intensity of exposure being the primary etiological variable for PTSD. Rates of PTSD among abused women range from 31 to 84%. The occurrence of sexual assault in marriage is associated with greater trauma, more severe depression, and lower self-esteem than is found among victims of physical abuse alone. The most common symptoms of the disorder among abused women are nightmares, intrusive memories of abuse, avoidance of reminders of the abuse, and anxiety symptoms. Victims may also exhibit cognitive symptoms such as difficulty concentrating, problems with memory, and anger.

There is concern within the mental health profession and among victim advocates regarding the constructive use of PTSD as a diagnostic tool. PTSD pathologizes the victim's response to violence rather than focus the source of the trauma. In treating the symptoms of PTSD, the causal role of violence is neglected, placing victims at risk of misdiagnosis, inappropriate medication, and even possible further abuse. In addition, the victim may perceive the diagnosis as evidence of her own inadequacy rather than as condemnation of the violent behavior being perpetrated on her. Research has shown that access to both social support and victim advocacy services leads to a reduction in PTSD symptoms among abused women.

Depression

Prior to the introduction of PTSD, depression was the preferred diagnosis for victims of partner violence. Today, depression continues to be prevalent among victims of intimate partner violence with rates varying between 39 and 83%. Women are more likely to be diagnosed with either depression or PTSD, and an investigation of the co-occurrence in physically abused women found that only 17% met the criteria of both. Depression is more likely among victims when psychological and sexual abuse occur within a physically violent relationship. Having low levels of social support has also been associated with depressive symptoms among victims.

Although it is imperative to investigate, document, and respond to the impact of trauma on the mental health of victims, the attempt to diagnose a woman trapped in a violent relationship with a mental disorder may be counterproductive.

Other Psychiatric Disorders

Victims of male partner violence are at greater risk of alcohol abuse and illicit drug use than nonabused women. Although partner violence may involve alcohol consumption by the female victim, or by the perpetrator and victim, increased alcohol use and illicit drug use by women frequently follows victimization. Compared to nonvictims, victims are also at higher risk for exhibiting eating disorders and more likely to report attempted suicide.

Physical Impact

Researchers and health-care providers worldwide single out partner violence as a major public health threat to women. The most severe physical outcome is death. Approximately 30% of murders of women that occurred between 1976 and 1996 were committed by male partners. The majority of these women were abused by a partner prior to being killed. Female victims also experience high rates of short-term and long-term health consequences. Children are also often affected because of prenatal or postnatal exposure to violence. Therefore, it is not surprising that women with a history of partner abuse demonstrate increased health-care use. Female victims of partner violence seek care for violence-related injuries, general health problems, and mental health problems.

Acute Injuries

Male partner violence is the largest single cause of injury to women requiring emergency medical treatment. Estimates of emergency department visits by women due to partner assault are between 13 and 25%. In a Bureau of Justice Statistics report on violence-related injuries treated in hospital emergency departments, only 14% of the injuries treated in women were inflicted by strangers compared to 29% in men. Physically abused women experience injuries to multiple parts of the body, including injuries to the face, head, neck, throat, breast, chest, and abdomen. Battered women are more likely to have abrasions and contusions or pains for which no physiological cause can be discovered. Fractures, dislocations, and lacerations occur with about equal frequency in abused and nonabused women. One of the most troublesome aspects of male partner violence is the recurrent and often escalating nature of the abuse. Women who frequently present for medical treatment of trauma are likely to have been treated previously for injuries from abuse. Victims of partner violence have on average seven treatment episodes in the emergency service compared to two among nonbattered women. The pattern of escalation is also evident in homicide rates. In one study, 14% of the women who were killed had been in the health-care system for violence-related injuries. Approximately 47% had received health-care services for some type of problem during the year before they were killed.

Chronic Health Problems

Women of all ages with a history of past or current partner abuse are disproportionately represented among women receiving a variety of services in primary-care settings. The injuries, emotional stress, and fear associated with male partner violence can contribute to the development of chronic health problems. They include chronic pain (e.g., headaches and back pain) and central nervous system symptoms, such as fainting and seizures. Women who have been abused report higher rates of gastrointestinal symptoms and functional gastrointestinal disorders, such as irritable bowel syndrome and nonulcer dyspepsia, compared to other women. These disorders have no known pathogenesis or established treatment and are the most common chronic gastrointestinal conditions seen in primary care, as well as the most common reason for referral to gastroenterologists. In various clinical samples, between 44 and 67% of all female gastroenterology patients report a history of sexual violation, and between 32 and 48% of female patients had experienced severe physical trauma in childhood or adulthood. Gynecological problems are also long-lasting outcomes of male partner violence. Symptoms and conditions include HIV infection, other sexually-transmitted diseases, vaginal bleeding or infections, decreased sexual desire, genital irritation, painful intercourse, chronic pelvic pain, and urinary tract infections. The likelihood of having a gynecological problem is three times greater among women who are abused by spouses.

Birth Outcomes

Because young women in their most active childbearing years are at highest risk for abuse, abuse during pregnancy deserves special mention. Women who are abused and pregnant are more likely to engage in poor maternal health behavior. They frequently delay prenatal care. Compared to nonabused women, women who are abused are twice as likely to delay prenatal care until the third trimester. Pregnant women who are abused report higher levels of alcohol, tobacco, and drug use than other pregnant women. Pregnancy complications may include preterm labor, low birth weight, spontaneous abortion, anemia, and infections. It is also important to mention the effects of intimate partner violence on children. Children who observe violence against their mothers are at higher risk of emotional, behavioral, physiological, cognitive, and social problems.

Prevention

Primary Prevention

The aim of primary prevention, as applied in public health, is the reduction of the risk of obtaining a disease or health condition. Specific to male partner violence, primary prevention focuses on learning not to use violence. Primary prevention strategies include changing social norms promoting violence against women, changing male roles, promoting the status of women, and increasing the public's awareness of the problem of male partner violence. Other approaches focus on training to improve relationship, conflict resolution, and anger management skills.

Secondary Prevention

Secondary prevention occurs when an individual has a disease or health condition, but health consequences have not yet developed. One approach for partner violence is to conduct violence screening in health-care settings and non-health-care settings, such as workplaces, schools, and military bases. Intimate partner violence screening facilitates early identification and treatment referrals for female victims. Specific to perpetrators, secondary prevention efforts include training to deescalate aggression and counseling and hotlines for violent partners.

Intervention

The response to male partner violence must include effective interventions, not only in specific cases of victimization but in communities and from a societal perspective. Beyond providing victim services, communities need to develop a coordinated response across different types of agencies, and public policy needs to counter the systemic issues related to male partner violence.

Mental Health Services

Mental health clinicians have the potential to play a vital role in assisting the recovery process for survivors of partner violence. However, to avoid retraumatizing the survivors, clinical services must focus on providing specific interventions to counter the impact of trauma rather than on the mental disorders of the victim. For a woman living in a violent situation, mental health practitioners should prioritize her physical safety and assisting her to access victim services as a first step in addressing mental health concerns. Key to this process is assisting women to identify and develop formal and informal support networks that will help facilitate situational realities associated with both living in or leaving a violent relationship. For this to be feasible, strong linkages need to be fostered between clinical services and women's services, such as advocacy centers, domestic violence shelters, and rape crisis organizations. Additional resources are also needed to ensure that women who are using victim services, for example, those living in shelters, are able to access appropriate clinical services.

Coordinated Community Response

Mental health services should also be addressed within the framework of implementing a coordinated community response to partner violence. The development of coordinated community response is an outgrowth of the efforts of women's advocates to make reforms within the often-fragmented criminal justice system. The objective of the coordinated community response is to ensure that components of the system work together to form a consistent and systematic response that shifts responsibility away from victims and holds perpetrators of violence responsible for their behavior. Women's safety is considered of primary importance. Within this framework, emphasis is placed on batterer rehabilitation programs and support and advocacy for victims, but not specifically on the provision of clinical services for women suffering from trauma. Accessibility to immediate, appropriate clinical services could serve to avert the escalation of trauma symptoms.

Public Policy and Advocacy

Examples of proactive public policy are demonstrated in the Violence Against Women Act (VAWA) of 1994, which sponsored legislation to support increased police personnel, higher levels of prosecution, more severe penalties for perpetrators, and extended victim services. VAWA also recognized that immigration law placed abused women at risk and provided relief by giving abused immigrant women the means to establish lawful permanent residence without the help of a spouse. VAWA 2000 strengthened protections for battered immigrant women, sexual assault survivors, and victims of dating violence. Appropriate interpretation and enforcement of mandatory arrest laws is another area of public-policy intervention that should be pursued. Coupled with an advocacy agenda is the need for a public health response. This perspective, emphasizing the establishment of screening protocol, early interventions, and multiple approaches to prevention, offers hope of reducing the incidence of partner violence and minimizing its effects.

Conclusion

Women's Advocates Incorporated calculated in 2002 that intimate partner violence costs the U.S. economy $12.6 billion on an annual basis in legal services, direct medical care, policing, lost productivity, and victim services. Efforts have been made in the past decade to address this issue through initiatives such as mandatory arrest and sentencing laws within the criminal justice system and the development and implementation of screening protocols by health and social service organizations. However, the fact that thousands of women are injured or killed each year by an intimate partner indicates the need for social norms to be addressed. There is much to be done in terms of creating a comprehensive systematic response to male partner violence both in the United States and internationally, and the lack of such response contributes to the perception of societal support or even encouragement of violence. Although victims and perpetrators must both have access to appropriate intervention, the prevention of male partner violence is of paramount importance and requires action on a multiple levels.

See Also the Following Articles

Marital Conflict; Sexual Assault; Violence.

Further Reading

Campbell, J. C. (2002). Health consequences of intimate partner violence. *Lancet* **359**, 1331–1336.

Coker, A. L. (2004). Primary prevention of intimate partner violence for women's health: a response to Plichta. *Journal of Interpersonal Violence* **19**, 1324–1334.

Crowell, N. A. and Burgess, A. W. (eds.) (1996). *Understanding violence against women, Panel on Research on Violence against Women, Committee on Law and Justice, Commission on Behavioral and Social Sciences and Education, National Research Council,* Washington, DC: National Academy Press.

Field, C. A. and Caetano, R. (2004). Ethnic differences in intimate partner violence in the U.S. general population: the role of alcohol use and socioeconomic status. *Trauma, Violence, & Abuse* **5**, 303–317.

Humphreys, C. and Stephens, J. (2004). Domestic violence and the politics of trauma. *Women's Studies International Forum* **27**(5–6), 449–570.

Koss, M. P., Goodman, L. A., Browne, A., Fitzgerald, L. F., Keita, G. P. and Russo, N. F. (1994). *No safe haven: violence against women at home, work, and in the community.* Washington, DC: American Psychological Association Press.

Koss, M. P., Bailey, J. A., Yuan, N. P., et al. (2003). Depression and PTSD in survivors of male violence: research and training initiatives to facilitate recovery. *Psychology of Women Quarterly* **27**, 130–142.

Max, W., Rice, D. P., Finkelstein, E., et al. (2004). The economic toll of intimate partner violence against women in the United States. *Violence & Victims* **19**, 259–272.

Plichta, S. B. (2004). Intimate partner violence and physical health consequences: policy and practice implications. *Journal of Interpersonal Violence* **19**, 1296–1323.

Rennison, C. M. (2003). *Intimate partner violence, 1993–2001.* Washington, DC: Bureau of Justice Statistics, Crime Data Brief, National Institute of Justice.

Tjaden, P. and Thoennes, N. (2000). *Extent, nature, and consequences of intimate partner violence.* Washington, DC: Office of Justice Programs, National Institute of Justice, U.S. Department of Justice.

Violence Against Women Act of 1994. (1994). Pub. L. No. 103–322, Title IV, 108 Sat. 1902. Washington, DC: Government Printing Office.

Waters, H., Hyder, A., Rajkotia, Y., Basu, S., Rehwinkel, J. and Butchart, A. (2004). *The economic dimensions of interpersonal violence.* Geneva: World Health Organization.

Sexual Assault

N C Feeny and T J Linares
Case Western Reserve University, Cleveland, OH, USA
E B Foa
University of Pennsylvania, Philadelphia, PA, USA

This is a revised version of the article by N C Feeny and E B Foa, Encyclopedia of Stress First Edition, volume 3, pp 435–439, © 2000, Elsevier Inc.

Glossary

Arousal — A cluster of PTSD symptoms that includes concentration problems, anger, exaggerated startle response, sleep disturbance, and being overly alert.

Avoidance — A cluster of PTSD symptoms including behavioral and psychic avoidance, such as avoidance of thoughts, feelings, and reminders of the trauma; emotional numbing; loss of interest in activities; feeling disconnected from others; psychogenic amnesia; and a sense of foreshortened future.

Diagnostic and Statistical Manual of Mental Disorders, 4th edition (DSM-IV) — A reference manual used by mental health professionals that includes descriptions and diagnostic criteria for psychiatric disorders.

Posttraumatic stress disorder (PTSD) — An anxiety disorder that develops in response to a traumatic event and is characterized by three clusters of symptoms re-experiencing, avoidance, and arousal. PTSD is diagnosed after a 1-month period of sustained symptoms following the traumatic event.

Prevalence — How widespread a disorder or an event (e.g., sexual assault) is at a given time.

Re-experiencing — A cluster of PTSD symptoms that includes experiencing the trauma in the form of nightmares, flashbacks, intrusive distressing thoughts, or becoming intensely emotionally upset or having physiological arousal upon exposure to reminders of the trauma.

Trauma — An event experienced or witnessed, in which an individual is subjected to the threat of death, injury, or physical integrity, and during which an individual feels terrified, horrified, or helpless.

Prevalence of Traumatic Events and Sexual Assault

Estimates of exposure to traumatic events vary, but on the whole, they are quite high. Several studies have examined rates of traumatic experiences in the general population. In a nationally representative sample of approximately 6000 people, ages 15–54, 60% of men and 51% of women reported experiencing at least one traumatic event in their lifetime. Similar findings emerged from a second study using a large, racially diverse sample; 74% of men and 65% of women reported experiencing at least one traumatic event. Somewhat lower prevalence was found in a sample of young adult health maintenance organization (HMO) members ($n = 1007$): 43% of men and 39% of women reported a traumatic experience in their lifetime. This discrepancy may be accounted for by differences in the samples; members of an HMO may be of higher socioeconomic status than the general population, which may have shielded them from a high-risk level of exposure to trauma. Studies examining rates of trauma exposure internationally have found similarly high levels of exposure. In a large sample of four cities in Mexico, 76% of the participants reported at least one traumatic event in their lifetime, and the majority of the participants experienced multiple versus single traumas.

Another large epidemiological study examined rate of exposure to traumatic events among a representative sample of 4000 women. Consistent with other results, almost 70% of women reported having experienced a traumatic event during their lifetime. In addition to these high rates of single trauma exposure, prevalence data have shown women to be at high risk for experiencing multiple episodes of violence throughout their lives.

Women are more likely than men to experience the traumas of rape and sexual assault. In the literature, rape is typically considered oral or vaginal penetration, while sexual assault is a more broad term that encompasses the use of pressure and coercion to force sexual contact. Lifetime prevalence estimates of rape and sexual assault among women vary widely across studies, ranging from 2 to almost 30%. Among adult women, several studies estimated prevalence of completed rape to be 20%. Others, however, have documented much lower rates, ranging from 2 to 14%.

In an epidemiological study of 4008 women, the prevalence of completed rape was 13%; other types of sexual assault were reported by 14% of the sample. Prevalence of childhood sexual abuse is similarly high. In a nationally representative sample of 2626 adults, almost one-third (27%) of the women reported a history of sexual abuse (e.g., being touched, grabbed, kissed, shown genitals) during childhood. Of these women who reported childhood sexual abuse, 49%

(13% of the entire sample) reported actual or attempted intercourse. Among adolescents, one study found that 43% of the sample had experienced a traumatic event, of which rape accounted for 2% of the traumas. Further, female adolescents were significantly more likely to report a completed rape than males, which highlights young women's risk for sexual assault. International samples also report similar levels of sexual assault in women. Of the types of trauma reported by women in the Mexico study, nearly 15% reported some type of sexual assault (10.5% sexual molestation, 3.9% sexual assault). Since sexual assault is less likely to be reported to the police than other crimes, it is safe to assume that the rates mentioned above are an underestimation of the actual prevalence of sexual assault.

Psychological Sequelae of Sexual Assault

Posttraumatic Stress Disorder (PTSD)

Sexual assault is associated with a variety of psychological difficulties. Among the most common are symptoms of posttraumatic stress, a set of psychological and physical symptoms that follow a traumatic experience. In some cases, these symptoms persist beyond the immediate aftermath of the trauma and develop into posttraumatic stress disorder (PTSD), an anxiety disorder that includes symptoms of arousal, avoidance, and re-experiencing, which lasts for more than 1 month and causes significant impairment in social or occupational functioning. This disorder affects from 1 to 12% of the general population and close to 25% of those exposed to a traumatic event. Women appear to be twice as likely to develop PTSD as men (10% of women vs. 5% of men).

Retrospective and prospective studies show female victims of sexual assault to be at particular risk for developing PTSD. For example, Norris examined the impact of 10 common traumatic events (e.g., robbery, assault, disaster) in a large, racially diverse sample. Of all the traumatic events surveyed, sexual assault yielded the highest rate of PTSD (14% lifetime). Similarly, Resnick et al. found that 12% of rape victims had current PTSD compared to 3% of victims of nonviolent traumas. Using a national sample of 1500 women, rape and sexual assault led to the highest lifetime (39%) and current (13%) rates of PTSD. In a community sample of 400 adult females, of women who had experienced a completed rape, 57% met lifetime diagnostic criteria and 17% met criteria for current PTSD. Lower rates (37% lifetime and 11% current) were found in females who had experienced a nonsexual assault.

Two prospective assessment studies have examined the prevalence of PTSD following sexual or nonsexual assault. In a study of female rape victims, 94% of the women met symptom criteria for PTSD within 2 weeks following the assault. Three months after the sexual assault, rates of PTSD had declined considerably; however, 47% continued to meet PTSD criteria. Women who did not meet criteria for PTSD 3 months after the assault showed a steady reduction in symptoms over the 12 weeks of assessment. Minimal symptom improvement was seen for those women who continued to meet PTSD criteria 3 months after the trauma. Follow-up assessments conducted 6 and 9 months after the assault revealed that 42% of women continued to meet criteria for PTSD at each time point. In a second study, Riggs et al. found that 90% of rape victims and 62% of nonsexual assault victims met symptom criteria for PTSD within 2 weeks of an assault. At the 1-month assessment, the rate was 60% for rape and 44% for nonsexual assault survivors. At 3 months, the rate had dropped to 51 and 21% for rape and nonsexual assault survivors, respectively. Similar findings have been shown in adolescents, with those who experienced a sexual assault being seven times more likely to meet PTSD criteria compared to all other reported trauma types. These results, taken together, suggest that sexual assault is more likely to produce PTSD than other simple assaults.

Prevalence of other Psychological Reactions

Reactions to sexual assault other than PTSD are also common. Anxiety, anger, depression, substance abuse, and dissociation occur with high frequency and are discussed in the following sections.

Anxiety Anxiety and fear are among the most common reactions to sexual assault, but are often discussed under the rubric of PTSD. After an assault, women are often quite afraid of rape- and assault-related situations and also experience general anxiety at high levels. Such fears have been documented to last up to 16 years postassault. Indeed, in one study, only 23% of sexual assault victims did not show elevated fear 1 year after the assault. Although victims' fearfulness declined over time, they remained more fearful than nonvictimized controls 1 year after the assault. Thus, fear and anxiety levels remain elevated in many victims of sexual violence long after the assault.

Anger

Elevated anger levels are often seen among sexually assaulted women compared to nonvictimized controls. In a prospective study of 116 rape and other crime victims and 50 matched nonvictimized controls, Riggs et al. found that level of anger was related to aspects of the assault such as the use of a weapon and the victim's response to the attack. In addition, elevated anger levels were related to PTSD symptoms 1 month after the assault. Similarly, Feeny et al. found anger levels 1 month after an assault to be predictive of PTSD symptom severity at 3 months postassault. The authors hypothesized that anger interferes with recovery by preventing emotional processing of the traumatic event.

Depression Depression is another common reaction to sexual assault, although some evidence suggests that it is less persistent than fear and anxiety. In a study of psychological reactions to rape, Frank and Stewart found that almost half of their sample was diagnosed with major depression; however, over 3 months' time, these symptoms declined considerably. Retrospective examinations of depression among trauma victims, however, suggest more enduring symptoms. For example, one study found that an average of almost 22 years postassault, rape victims were more depressed than nonvictims.

In the North Carolina catchment area study, the lifetime prevalence rate of depression was significantly related to sexual assault: women who had been sexually assaulted were more than twice as likely to manifest a major depressive episode as women who had not been sexually assaulted. In addition, comorbidity of PTSD and depression is high: 48% of those who met lifetime criteria for PTSD also met lifetime criteria for depression, and 43% evidenced current comorbidity of the two disorders. In a sample seeking treatment for PTSD, 63% met criteria for current major depression. These results suggest that depression should be routinely assessed in victims of trauma who are seeking treatment.

Substance abuse Female assault victims, particularly those who develop PTSD, are also at risk for substance abuse. In a national probability sample of women, crime victims (sexual and nonsexual assault) were at increased risk of developing an alcohol use disorder, independent of their PTSD status. Moreover, those diagnosed with PTSD were 3 times more likely to have serious alcohol problems than those without the disorder and 14 times more likely than those without a history of criminal victimization. In the North Carolina catchment area study, lifetime prevalence of substance (alcohol and drugs) abuse and dependence was significantly related to the presence of sexual assault. In a recent longitudinal study, recent and past assault were associated with two to three times the risk of alcohol abuse in women, even after controlling for past alcohol use, age, race, and education.

Additionally, the prevalence of PTSD in patients enrolled in a substance abuse treatment program ranges from 12 to 34%, and prevalence rates are significantly higher among women, ranging from 33 to 59%. Among psychiatric outpatients, the rate of victimization among alcoholic women was higher than among nonalcoholic women, suggesting a specific link between early victimization and later alcohol abuse among adult women. In summary, being a victim of a trauma appears to substantially increase the risk of developing a substance use disorder and vice versa: substance abuse seems to increase the likelihood of victimization.

Dissociation The construct of dissociation typically focuses on three clinical entities: alterations in memory (e.g., aspects of the trauma not consciously accessible), in identity (e.g., disengagement between self and environment), and in consciousness. Dissociation has been conceptualized to reflect emotional disengagement from trauma memories, which has been thought to hinder recovery. Indeed, several studies suggest that dissociation does hinder the processing of the traumatic event and subsequent natural recovery process. Trauma victims with PTSD exhibit more dissociative symptoms than those without PTSD. Moreover, if dissociation is present during or immediately after a trauma it is predictive of later psychopathology. Similarly, acute stress disorder, which emphasizes dissociative symptoms, has been found to be predictive of later posttrauma symptoms. The role of dissociation in promoting emotional disengagement needs further exploration in studies that evaluate risk factors in trauma exposed individuals.

Treatment of Sexual Assault-Related PTSD

Several cognitive behavioral treatment (CBT) programs have been developed to treat PTSD related to sexual assault, including exposure therapy, stress inoculation training (SIT), cognitive therapy (CT), eye movement desensitization and reprocessing (EMDR), and cognitive processing therapy (CPT). In this section, outcome studies, which evaluate the efficacy of these treatments with assault victims, are reviewed.

Recent studies examining the use of CBT with female sexual and physical assault victims have utilized well-controlled designs, and all but one utilized many of the methodological gold standards proposed by Foa and Meadows, including presence of PTSD diagnosis, assessment of PTSD severity, reliable and valid measures of related psychopathology, randomization to treatment conditions, and presence of control or comparison groups.

Prolonged exposure (PE) is an exposure therapy program that involves confrontation aimed at ameliorating PTSD, which typically includes mentally reliving the traumatic event repeatedly and *in vivo* confrontation with trauma-related situations, which evoke fear but are not objectively dangerous. In the first controlled study of exposure for rape-related PTSD, the efficacy of PE, SIT, supportive counseling (SC), and a wait-list control was compared for female victims of sexual assault. PTSD symptoms were assessed at pretreatment, posttreatment, and follow-up evaluations with psychometrically sound interviews and self-report measures administered by trained clinicians who were blind to treatment assignment. PE and SIT showed significant pre-post reductions on re-experiencing and avoidance clusters of PTSD, while SC and wait list did not. Also, at the end of treatment 50% of patients in SIT and 40% of those in PE no longer met criteria for PTSD; in contrast, only 10% of SC patients and none in the wait list no longer met diagnostic criteria. At follow-up, patients in the PE group tended to show further reduction in PTSD symptoms, whereas patients in SIT and SC did not show further improvement.

In a second study, Foa et al. obtained further support for the efficacy of a modified PE in treating rape-related PTSD. This study compared the efficacy of PE to SIT, a combination of both treatments (PE/SIT), and a wait-list condition. All active treatments resulted in substantial symptom reduction and were superior to the wait-list condition in ameliorating PTSD and related symptoms. PE was superior to the other treatments: it effected a greater reduction of anxiety and depression and resulted in fewer dropouts than SIT and PE/SIT. In addition, the number of patients who achieved good end-state functioning tended to be larger for the PE group than for the SIT and PE/SIT groups. In a third study, Foa et al. examined the efficacy of PE relative to a program that includes PE and cognitive restructuring (PE/CR). Results indicated that PE and PE/CR were superior to wait list at posttreatment on measures of PTSD and depression, with these gains maintained at follow-up. The addition of the cognitive restructuring component did not appear to enhance treatment outcomes; as with most posttreatment outcomes, PE and PE/CR did not differ from one another. Additionally, no differences in outcome were found among patients who were treated by experienced or recently trained counselors, suggesting that PE could be easily disseminated into community settings.

EMDR is a form of exposure accompanied by saccadic eye movements that has been the focus of considerable controversy due to initial claims of remarkable success in only a single session. Of the number of studies evaluating the efficacy of EMDR, only a few utilized well-controlled designs and thus yielded interpretable results. One well-controlled study evaluated the efficacy of EMDR relative to a wait-list control condition for PTSD in female rape victims. Three sessions of EMDR resulted in greater improvement for PTSD symptoms (57% reduction in independently evaluated PTSD at posttreatment and 71% in self-reported PTSD at follow-up), relative to the wait-list condition (10% reduction at posttreatment). However, in contrast to other controlled studies, one therapist conducted all treatments, and therefore the contribution of therapist and treatment effects were confounded. A more recent study comparing PE and EMDR found that both treatment groups had significant reductions in PTSD symptoms at posttreatment. At 6-month follow-up, PE resulted in more adaptive scores on a number of anxiety and depression measures than those seen for participants who received EMDR. This study provides further support for the use of exposure techniques in the treatment of sexual assault.

Another recent study compared EMDR, PE, and relaxation training. This study found that PE effected the largest reductions in symptoms of re-experiencing and avoidance compared to EMDR and relaxation training and also effected the quickest reduction in avoidance symptoms. This study reported that EMDR and relaxation training did not differ from each other in efficacy or speed of change. Additionally, recent meta-analyses have found no evidence that the use of eye movements, integral to this treatment, have any effect on treatment outcomes. Thus, the use of the exposure techniques, which are a part of this treatment protocol, appears to account for the treatment outcomes using EMDR.

CPT is a program that was developed specifically for use with rape victims and includes cognitive restructuring and an exposure variant (i.e., writing the traumatic memories and reading the account aloud to the therapist). In a quasi-experimental design, CPT was compared to a naturally occurring wait-list control group. Overall, women who received CPT improved significantly from pre- to posttreatment (about 50% reduction in PTSD symptoms), whereas the wait-list group did not show significant improvement. In a second study, Resnick et al. compared the efficacy of a 12-session CPT, a 9-session PE, and a wait-list control in rape victims with chronic PTSD. After 9 weeks of PE and 12 of CPT, both treatments were highly effective in reducing PTSD symptoms. At follow-up assessments 3 and 9 months posttreatment, treatment gains were maintained.

A treatment specifically designed for women who experienced childhood sexual abuse has also been investigated; it is similar to CPT in that it is a combination treatment utilizing exposure and cognitive components. This treatment consists of skills training in affect and interpersonal regulation followed by a modified PE protocol (STAIR-modified PE). In a controlled study, relative to a wait-list condition, participants receiving STAIR-modified PE showed significant improvement in symptoms of PTSD, as well as improvements in affect regulation. This study provided evidence for the use of CBT procedures with childhood abuse survivors; however, future studies should compare the usefulness of the addition of the skills training as compared to PE alone, as previous studies utilizing PE have not found beneficial effects of adding components beyond exposure techniques.

In summary, the CBT program that has received the most empirical support in controlled studies is PE, and its efficacy in reducing PTSD symptoms is at least as high as that of comparison CBT programs. Additionally, recent evidence suggests that it can be successfully used in community settings. Thus, at present, PE is the recommended psychosocial treatment choice.

Predictors of PTSD

As is apparent from the results reviewed previously, not all women who have been sexually assaulted develop chronic PTSD; thus the identification of factors that are involved in hindering recovery has been the focus of much investigation. Foa and Riggs proposed to classify predictors into three categories: pretrauma, trauma, and posttrauma variables. In terms of pretrauma variables, it appears that poor psychological functioning prior to the trauma renders the individual vulnerable to developing chronic disturbances posttrauma. In addition, a prior history of traumatic events in child- or adulthood intensifies the response to subsequent trauma. Factors related to the trauma itself, including trauma severity, also appear to predict the development of PTSD, as well as posttrauma variables such as social support.

In a prospective study of 277 female assault victims, Amir et al. tested a predictive model of PTSD that included all three domains thought to be relevant to the prediction of PTSD. Several variables emerged as significant predictors at 1 and 3 months postassault: trauma history, trauma severity, cognitions and complex emotions, basic emotions, and early PTSD symptoms. Trauma history had an impact on cognitions and emotions, which, in turn, influenced PTSD symptom severity 4 and 12 weeks after the assault. Trauma severity influenced PTSD symptoms 2 weeks after the assault.

Recent meta-analyses provide additional information regarding the predictors of PTSD. One meta-analysis found that the effects of predictors varied based on the sample under investigation; however, three variables were consistently significant predictors of PTSD: psychiatric history, childhood abuse, and family psychiatric history. Also, the largest effect sizes were found with predictors that were at or around the time of the trauma (e.g., social support following trauma). A second meta-analysis reviewed 476 studies that investigated PTSD predictors. Of the reviewed studies, 68 evaluated several of the hypothesized major predictors of PTSD, which include prior trauma, prior psychological adjustment, family history of psychopathology, perceived life threat, posttrauma social support, emotional response to trauma, and dissociation to trauma. Of these predictors, dissociation at the time of the trauma was the largest predictor of later developing PTSD. Indeed, the predictors with the largest effect sizes were those that were related more proximally to the trauma itself (e.g., dissociation and emotional response), similar to the finding in the Brewin et al. analyses. These results underscore the complexity of the mechanisms underlying the development of PTSD.

Conclusion

The majority of people in the United States are exposed to at least one traumatic experience in their lifetime; however, only a minority develop long-lasting psychological difficulties, including chronic PTSD. Importantly, not all traumas are equal in causing the development of PTSD; traumas inflicted by another person, especially sexual assaults, are particularly prone to produce lasting disturbances. Once established, PTSD is unlikely to remit unless treated. The most empirically validated type of therapy for this disorder is CBT, and among the various CBT programs, PE has gained the most empirical support.

See Also the Following Articles

Anger.

Further Reading

American Psychiatric Association (1994). *Diagnostic and statistical manual of mental health disorders* (4th edn.). Washington, D.C.: American Psychiatric Association.

Davidson, J. and Foa, E. B. (eds.) (1993). *Posttraumatic stress disorder: DSM-IV and beyond.* Washington D.C.: American Psychiatric Press.
Foa, E. B. and Rothbaum, B. O. (1998). *Treating the trauma of rape.* New York: Guilford Press.
Foa, E. B., Dancu, C. V., Hembree, E. A., Jaycox, L. H., Meadows, E. A. and Street, G. P. (1999). A comparison of exposure therapy, stress inoculation training, and their combination for reducing posttraumatic stress disorder in female assault victims. *Journal of Consulting and Clinical Psychology* **67**(2), 194–200.
Kessler, R. C., Sonnega, A., Bromet, E., Hughes, M. and Nelson, C. B. (1995). Posttraumatic stress disorder in the national comorbidity survey. *Archives of General Psychiatry* **52**, 1048–1060.
Resnick, H. S., Kilpatrick, D. G., Dansky, B. S., Saunders, B. E. and Best, C. L. (1993). Prevalence of civilian trauma and posttraumatic stress disorder in a representative national sample of women. *Journal of Consulting and Clinical Psychology* **61**(6), 984–991.

Sexual Offenders

F M Saleh
University of Massachusetts Medical School, Worcester, MA USA
H M Malin
Institute for Advanced Study of Human Sexuality, San Francisco, CA, USA

Glossary

Ephebophilia — A paraphilia in which the object of sexual attraction is a pubescent youth (child or adolescent), but not yet a fully sexually mature person, of either sex; also called hebephilia.

Paraphilia — Recurrent, intense sexual urges and fantasies, sometimes accompanied by sexually driven behaviors, occurring over a period of at least 6 months, involving one or more of the following: (1) a nonconsenting partner (e.g., children or a rape victim), (2) an object or body part (e.g., fur or feet), or (3) a sensory/emotional state (e.g., pain or humiliation) not typically associated with the archetypal sexual-response cycle. Paraphilias may be obligatory, in which case they are necessary components for completing the sexual-response cycle, or nonobligatory, in which case they may sometimes be incorporated in the sexual-response cycle but are not always essential for its completion. Paraphilias may be either pathological on nonpathological depending on the degree to which they impair the paraphile's social functioning and emotional well-being. They may be dangerous (such as lust murder or autoasphyxiophilia) or benign (such as transvestic fetishism or foot partialism) depending on their potential for lethality or adverse physical or social impact on self or others.

Pedophilia — A paraphilia involving sexual arousal to a prepubescent child or children of either sex.

Perversion — Once a psychiatric term roughly equivalent in meaning to paraphilia; now generally a pejorative term used by nonprofessionals to describe "kinky" sex or other expressions of sexuality (e.g., homosexual behavior) of which they disapprove.

Phenomenology — In the study of paraphilias or other psychiatric phenomena, the scientific method in which the phenomena experienced by the individual, as measured by observation and/or self-report, are described and classified rather than explained or interpreted.

Sex offender — A legal term denoting an individual who has broken a law governing the conduct of sexual behavior; the term is usually reserved for individuals who have been convicted of a crime involving sexual behavior.

Sexual-response cycle — The sequence of stages and events typically occurring in the progression of sexual activity from the beginning of sexual arousal to orgasm and resolution. Based on work by Masters and Johnson and amplified by other sexologists, the sexual-response cycle is sometimes arbitrarily divided into five stages or phases: (1) desire phase (sometimes called libido or drive); (2) excitement phase (sometimes called arousal), in which sexual arousal normally builds; (3) plateau (the point of highest arousal sustainable short of triggering orgasm); (4) orgasm (or climax); and (5) resolution (sometimes called the refractory period), in which arousal returns to prebaseline desire and during which an additional stimulus does not immediately lead to a repetition of the cycle.

General Considerations

It is universally assumed to be axiomatic that victims of sexual assault in its various manifestations suffer from the stress of their experiences to one degree or another. However, little or no scientific investigation has been conducted that sheds light on the relationship of stress to the experience of having been sexually victimized. Among important unstudied and, therefore, unanswerable questions are: What experiences are most likely to cause toxic stress, who is at greatest risk for developing stress-induced sequelae, and what factors might protect against or mitigate the adverse consequences of stress resulting from sexual victimization? It may be concluded, however, that those who work with and care for the sexually victimized are highly sensitized to the importance of stress-related components of sexual assault, whether the assault takes the form of uninvited genital exposure or rape with the threat of death.

The situation with respect to sex offenders is roughly equivalent, although there is the added variable that cultures typically do not concern themselves much with the impact of stress on sex offenders, who are generally regarded as willful evildoers and not as psychiatrically ill. In this article, it is not our intent to explore to any great degree the ongoing controversy of whether sex offenders are criminals or patients and the degree to which the psychiatric impairment in some sex offenders may influence culpability for their offending behavior.

The question of whether individuals who engage in illegal paraphilia-driven behaviors should be considered as having diminished criminal culpability given their psychiatric diagnosis is controversial and complex. Over a century ago, the eminent British psychiatrist Henry Maudsley expressed concern that society often fails to even consider such a possibility. He wrote, "If the law cannot adjust the measure of punishment to the actual degree of responsibility . . . that is no reason why we should shut our eyes to the facts; it is still our duty to place them on the record, in the confident assurance that a time will come when men will be more able to deal more wisely with them."

By definition, however, sex offenders are criminals with offenses ranging from misdemeanors to felonies. The term sex offender is strictly a legal term. There is no psychiatric diagnosis of sex offender, although there is some overlap between psychiatry and the law in that some individuals who have diagnosable psychiatric illness do commit sex offenses. Some sex offenders, including but not limited to those with paraphilias, may be more likely than others to commit sex offenses as a result of their psychiatric syndromes. Although severe comorbid psychiatric conditions may mitigate social response (e.g., the punishment may be less severe for an exhibitionist responding to command hallucinations), sex offenders are generally assumed to have adequate volitional control over their offending behaviors and are, thus, expected to conform their behavior to the expectations of society. Those who do not are likely to feel the full measure of retribution social systems are capable of bringing to bear in dealing with them. That response, inevitably, induces toxic stress.

Indeed, with the diminishing emphasis on rehabilitation and the ascendancy of retribution in American penology, punishment is meted out with the specific intention of subjecting sex offenders to pain, suffering, and the attendant stress the retributive penal philosophy guarantees. The response of society to sex offenses is deliberately and systematically to induce intensive stress in the offender by prescribing a continuum of ever harsher punishment ranging, at minimum, from humiliation and social opprobrium to often-lengthy prison sentences and, occasionally, death. These stressors are intentionally inflicted with full knowledge of the adverse consequences of the stress they engender.

The underlying philosophy of retributive penology appears to be threefold. First, it is axiomatic that in serious offenses, retribution by the state is both appropriate and desirable because the state itself and the social values it defends are directly aggrieved by the crime. Second, it is axiomatic that the state has the duty to punish on behalf of individuals more specifically aggrieved by the crime, to bring miscreants to justice as their proxy, which prevents the degeneration of retribution into vengeance, which, in turn, risks sowing the seeds of vendetta and the further destabilization of society. Finally, retributive penology is motivated by the premise that institutionalized punishment promotes deterrence by example. That is, not only is the offender punished but those who would follow in his criminal footsteps, witnessing his punishment, will be deterred from committing similar crimes. In some cases, there is a bonus – a sex offender incarcerated for life or executed for his crimes will not himself recidivate. We mention, parenthetically, an observation first made by John Money that certain paraphilias are the only mental illnesses deemed to merit the death penalty rather than psychiatric treatment in some jurisdictions.

With respect to perpetrators of sex offenses, the authors are not aware of any peer-reviewed research or literature directly addressing the issue of stress in the offender, although it seems equally axiomatic that both victims and offenders may experience toxic stress when the sex offending takes place. There have been limited studies of stress in prison populations, which may provide leads for research in this area. It is thought, for example, that inmates or corrections officers with a certain psychological makeup or privileged position are immunized against the stress of the prison setting to a greater degree than other inmates or corrections officers in the same setting.

Part of the difficulty in assessing the impact of stress on both victims and sex offenders is that neither is a homogeneous group. In this article, we raise some issues relevant to stress in sex offenders and leave to others the parallel task of defining stress-related issues in the victims of sex offenses.

Definitional Considerations

Sex Offender

As we have pointed out, the term sex offense is a legal term. What constitutes a sex offense differs from jurisdiction to jurisdiction. As we pointed out in the preceding section, sex offenders are not a homogeneous group, with the sole exception of the fact that they have broken some law governing sexual behavior in a given culture or jurisdiction. It is sometimes not well understood that cross-cultural as well as intracultural considerations must be taken into account in defining sex offenses as well stress with respect to atypical sexual urges, fantasies, and behaviors.

For example, in some jurisdictions in the United States and in similarly less sexually tolerant foreign cultures, certain sexual behaviors such as premarital or extra-marital sexual contact, homosexual acts, cross-dressing, and heterosexual oral-genital or anal sexual contact are sex crimes and their practitioners are thus sex offenders. In virtually all cultures and jurisdictions, some sexual behaviors such as sexual contact with children (although the age of majority varies widely) are crimes and the individuals who engage in them are sex offenders as well.

Whether or not such criminal behaviors always, or even usually, engender stress depends on myriad considerations, including the degree of enforcement of the laws prohibiting the behavior, potential punishments, and whether individuals who engage in them find their own behavior personally acceptable (ego-syntonic) or unacceptable (ego-dystonic). Just as sex offenders are not a homogeneous group, the resultant stress from sex offending is not homogeneous.

Perhaps the only constant in the term sex offense and its equivalents in other cultures is that it is a legal construct. As such, it is not necessarily congruent with psychiatric or psychological views of these acts. Indeed, the differences between legal and psychiatric conceptualizations of sexual behaviors often leads to considerable dissonance and clouds the social debate about what should be done about sex offenders; they can lead to violent culture clashes, complicating considerably our understanding of stress as it relates to sex offending.

Phenomenology

Phenomenology, as we use the term here, is the personal, internal experience of the sexual fantasy or behavior without respect to explanations for the behavior itself. Phenomenology, which has its roots in existential philosophy and, by extension, existential psychology, concerns itself with a scientific approach based on the phenomena themselves (here sexual drives, feelings, and motivated behaviors), without attempting to further explain them, as, for example, a psychodynamic approach might do. It also fails to embrace *in toto* the tenets and conventions of behaviorism. This theoretical approach has profound implications for treatment of "sex offenders."

Phenomenology is premised on the concept that behavior is determined by the way a person perceives reality rather than on some external objective reality. Thus, phenomenology does not rely on attempts to explain or interpret in order to classify sex offending. Nor does it rely overly much on changing behaviors themselves with the expectation that changing behaviors will change behavior. As a theory of psychology, phenomenology draws heavily on the tenets of existential psychology, which posits that psychology should concern itself with the organism's own experience of existence in the world. It draws heavily on the philosophical work of Karl Jaspers and the psychological application of that work by existential theorists such as Medart Boss, Ludwig Binswanger, and Viktor Frankl.

Paraphilias

Sex offenses and sex offenders are often classified as paraphilic or nonparaphilic.

The term, paraphilia, (from Greek *para-* beside + *philos* love) is an English translation of a term first proposed by Wilhelm Stekel in his book *Sexual Aberrations,* which first appeared in English about 1925. Reportedly, Stekel believed that a new term with less pejorative connotations than perversion (from Latin for turning around) would be helpful in examining and ameliorating these mental illnesses. Freud used the term, but it was not in widespread use in the psychiatric literature until the 1950s.

The *Diagnostic and Statistical Manual* (4th edn., text revision, DSM-IV-TR) of the American Psychiatric Association proposes that the "essential features of a paraphilia are recurrent, sexually arousing fantasies, sexual urges or behaviors generally involving 1) non-human objects, 2) the suffering or humiliation of oneself or one's partner, or 3) children or other non-consenting persons, that occur over a period of at least 6 months" (Criterion A; 2000: 566). DSM-IV-TR suggests that for some individuals "paraphilic fantasies or stimuli are obligatory for erotic arousal and are always included in sexual activity." For other individuals, paraphilic "preferences appear only episodically (e.g., during periods of stress)" (2000: 566). Criterion B for paraphilias, according to the DSM-IV-TR, is that they "must cause clinically significant impairment in social, occupational or other important area of functioning" (2000: 566). Thus, the DSM-IV-TR definition of paraphilia is at variance with the definition that we proposed previously, in that behavior alone is sufficient to make a diagnosis. We insist on a definition of paraphilia that presupposes motivated behavior that is sexually driven by recurrent, intense sexual urges and fantasies.

As an example, consider the variety of motivations driving the behavior of genital exposure:

- Preparing to bathe, dress, urinate, or otherwise engage in the gamut of biologically or socially based needs ordinarily considered to be nonsexual.
- Engaging in nude sunbathing, swimming, or other nonsexual recreational pursuits alone or with consenting others in lawful locations.
- Permitting a genital examination or other procedure for medical reasons.
- Engaging in sexual behavior with oneself or with consenting others.
- Attempting to attract the attention of nonconsenting people with or without the intention to initiate sexual contact.
- Attempting to shock, embarrass, humiliate, punish, frighten, or harass a nonconsenting person.
- Engaging in a social or cultural protest or making a political statement.
- Responding to a dare, exposing oneself as a penalty in a game or as a requirement for consensual initiation into social group.
- Engaging in a marginally socially accepted behavior, such as streaking or flashing, or participating exposed in a parade, festival, or other activity in which others are likely to do the same thing.
- Modeling for sculpture, painting, photography, or other artistic endeavors such as making films or participating in theatrical performances, either for remuneration or for altruistic reasons.
- Stripping for remuneration at a club or prenuptial party.
- Being sexually assaulted or intimidated into exposing oneself.
- Submitting to a lawful strip search.
- Preparing to commit a sexual assault on a nonconsenting person.
- Exposing oneself secondary to disinhibition caused by exogenous substances.
- Exposing oneself in response to command hallucinations.
- Exposing oneself secondary to dementia or traumatic brain insult.

Surely, most of these instances of genital exposure cannot be considered paraphilic. Some are prosocial, whereas some are antisocial. Some have negative or neutral erotosexual valence, whereas some are highly erotic. Paraphilic behavior, influencing as it does the sexual-response cycle, is by definition erotosexual. Yet only a subset of the exposing behaviors listed here that have positive erotosexual valence might be motivated by recurrent, intense sexual urges and fantasies outside some presumptive or defined norm. Only those that satisfy this criterion can be considered paraphilic.

Etiology There is no known etiology of paraphilias, but some investigators believe there are associations between paraphilias and other life experiences. The most common association reported is between paraphilias and early childhood experiences. Theories change and track dominant schools of psychological thought. For example, when psychodynamic theory was the predominant psychiatric theory, fur fetishism was explained as a sequella of the birth experience, in which an infant became fixated on the pubic hair of the mother during childhood. In the light of present-day understanding, such an explanation seems unlikely. However, more satisfying explanations have not yet been forthcoming.

More recently, various researchers have postulated a relationship between the development of paraphilias and childhood physical or sexual abuse. Such theories have led to concepts such as the cycle of abuse, in which it is postulated that the abused becomes the abuser by some mechanism as yet not clearly delineated. There is currently considerable debate about the proposition that such abuse may have occurred in preverbal children and the memories recovered many years later. Empirical studies have not been kind to the cycle of abuse construct, although it is at the foundation of a number of still widely used treatment regimens.

Although a good statistical correlation between having been abused as a child and perpetrating abuse as an adult has not been demonstrated, in some sexually abusive individuals there is a considerable history of childhood sexual, physical, and/or emotional abuse or neglect. The recalled or sometimes corroborated sexual biographies of a great many paraphilic individuals contain experiences in which the patient's paraphilia seems closely linked to these experiences. For example, individuals who received frequent spankings, enemas, or even highly embarrassing physical examinations as children have sometimes reported that as adults these unpleasant experiences have become highly pleasurable with positive erotic valence and may be incorporated as obligatory or nonobligatory paraphilic components of their sexual-response cycle. One possible explanation for this transformation may be the mechanism of opponent process theory of acquired motivation proposed by Richard Solomon and his colleagues, in which, like skydiving, an intensely fear-laden experience gradually becomes highly pleasurable, sought-after exhilarating activity. Other investigators have suggested that paraphilias are reinforced by masturbation to deviant fantasies. Unfortunately, all these ideas, as well as others, await solid empirical evidence. At this point, we can say with certainty only that the genesis of paraphilias remains largely unknown.

Prevalence There are in excess of 50 named paraphilias in the sexological literature. Some appear to be quite rare, whereas others, especially in their nonobligatory form, seem relatively common. The paraphilias most frequently coming to the attention of clinicians are pedophilia (which typically includes ephebophilia, although they are different paraphilias), voyeurism, and exhibitionism, according to DSM-IV-TR. This is hardly surprising, given that acting on these paraphilias is illegal in most jurisdictions, and individuals acting on these paraphilias are the most likely to seek clinical treatment, typically mandated by the judiciary. Given the distribution of pornographic materials with legal paraphilic content, for example, films and magazines devoted to transvestic fetishism, leather fetishism, or the milder forms of sadism and masochism, we might speculate that these paraphilias are among the more common. Yet sadism and masochism are relatively infrequently seen in clinical practice.

Erotic materials depicting other kinds of paraphilias, for example zoophilia, are typically suppressed. And although zoophilia is illegal in most jurisdictions, it seems to be less aggressively prosecuted, even when it comes to the attention of the authorities, than, say, sexual behavior involving children. It is difficult to extrapolate from any available data the prevalence of a given paraphilia or an all-inclusive prevalence of paraphilias in the American culture. DSM-IV-TR reports that, except for sexual masochism, with a sex ratio of 20 males to each female, paraphilias are almost never diagnosed in females. DSM-IV-TR further reports that approximately half of all individuals with paraphilia seen in clinics are married.

Treatment of Sex Offenders

In practice, the treatment of sex offenders may depend less on careful differential diagnosis than on the convictions that the treatment provider holds about sex offenders. Treatment providers with a behavioral view rely more heavily on psychological treatments designed to change behaviors than do treatment providers who subscribe to a more medical model approach. These providers tend to use more pharmacologically based interventions than their behaviorist colleagues. The authors rely on an approach that takes advantage of an appropriate mix of interventions, following a careful differential diagnosis.

Psychological Treatments

The various psychological therapies, whether individual or group therapies, are designed to change behaviors through a variety of strategies including challenging patients' distorted thought and belief patterns (cognitive behavioral therapy), developing strategies to anticipate and resist deviant sexual cravings (relapse prevention), and replacing maladaptive behaviors with more functional behaviors (behavioral therapy). More traditional psychodynamic and psychoanalytic psychotherapy treatment modalities have been largely abandoned in the treatment of sex offenders because of their lack of demonstrated efficacy despite decades of attempts.

Behavior therapy Behavioral therapy is guided by learning theory, specifically social learning theory. In contrast to psychodynamic therapies, behavior therapies are primarily concerned with the aberrant behavior itself and not its underlying cause. That is, behavior therapy aims to decrease and extinguish deviant sexual arousal through a set of techniques, such as systematic desensitization, aversion therapy, biofeedback, minimal arousal conditioning with aversive conditioning, and covert sensitization. (Masturbatory satiation, a form of arousal reconditioning, is no longer widely used.)

Covert sensitization, a form of aversion therapy, has been widely used in the treatment of paraphilic patients. It is postulated that the pairing of deviant sexual fantasies with the mental image of its humiliating consequences (i.e., the aversive experience) will dissuade a patient from acting out sexually. In covert sensitization, deviant arousal or excitement is paired with a visualized distressing thought or fantasy. To give an example, a voyeur will be asked to imagine being taking into custody as soon as he begins to contemplate peeping into other people's windows.

In contrast to the aversive behavioral therapies, operant conditioning methods use positive reinforcers. For example, positive olfactory conditioning employs pleasant aromas with nondeviant sexual stimuli.

Cognitive-behavioral therapy Cognitive-behavioral therapy hypothesizes that paraphilias are maintained by distorted cognitions and reinforced by masturbation to inappropriate fantasy. The aim of cognitive therapy is to change maladaptive thoughts and beliefs through techniques such as cognitive restructuring and thought stopping and to eliminate reinforcers that maintain distorted cognitions. The technique of cognitive restructuring teaches patients to identify, challenge, and ultimately replace erroneous (i.e., distorted) beliefs with adaptive and pro-social cognitions. Thought stopping is a technique that aims to decrease the frequency and duration of deviant sexual thoughts.

More often than not, a combination of one or more of these therapies is used. Victim empathy training has traditionally been an important component of all behavioral treatment and involves helping a patient take on the perspective of his victim(s). In addition, assertiveness and a variety of social skills training programs have been deemed to be important components in treatment programs, although recent research seems to indicate that empathy or social skills training have little or no impact on sexual recidivism in treated populations.

Relapse prevention A relapse is a recurrence of undesirable behavior after a period that has been free of the undesirable behavior. The term "relapse" is not synonymous with "recidivism" which indicates re-arrest for an illegal behavior. The objective of relapse prevention is to help a patient maintain behavioral changes. In order to reduce the risk of inappropriate sexual behavior, patients are taught to identify their deviant cycle and to develop strategies to implement when the cycle is triggered.

Group therapy Group psychotherapy is a widely accepted treatment modality used in the treatment of paraphilic and nonparaphilic sex offenders. It incorporates relapse prevention and cognitive-behavioral techniques, as well as empathy and social skills training. Group therapy creates a supportive milieu that is conducive to frank discussion and that provides guidance regarding effective relapse prevention strategies. It also encourages the development of a social support network and of healthy adult relationships. One of the primary advantages of group therapy over individual therapy is that it allows patients to be challenged by members of the group rather than by the therapist. This is important given that patients may respond and be more willing to change if challenged by one of their peers.

Effectiveness of psychological treatments The effectiveness of the psychological treatments in treating paraphilias is difficult to assess. One measure of treatment success has traditionally been recidivism. Some studies have concluded that these treatments have positive effects; other studies have found minimal or no effect with behavioral therapies. The interpretation of these studies may be confounded by a number of variables such as non-standardized treatment delivery or heterogeneous populations. Also, studies of the treatment of sex offenders generally do not differentiate paraphilic from nonparaphilic offenders.

Nor is it clear that treatment delivered in one setting, say a prison, generalizes to another setting, such as the community. State-dependent learning, for example, may impact psychological treatments that depend on a psycho-educational approach. Relapse prevention, a widely used psychological treatment modality, may be less effective than previously believed. In one randomized clinical trial that compared the reoffense rates of patients in an inpatient relapse prevention treatment program with the reoffense rates in two untreated prison control groups, no significant differences among the three groups in rates of sexual or violent reoffending over an 8-year follow-up period were found.

Biological Treatments

The authors believe that with certain patients, for example those with dangerous paraphilias or those at acute risk of victimizing someone, pharmacological intervention should be the treatment option of first resort. Biologically based treatments should also be made available to paraphilic patients if, for example, cravings for deviant sexual activities become overpowering or when specific symptoms are not responsive to less invasive treatment modalities (e.g., behavioral therapy).

Surgery Among the biologically based treatments, we must differentiate between surgical and pharmacological interventions. Stereotaxic hypothalamotomy is only of historical interest. On the other hand, the orchiectomy (surgical removal of the gonads) data are particularly relevant in that they provide the basis for our understanding of the benefits of the currently used testosterone-lowering agents. Orchiectomy consistently lowers the rate of recidivism. Orchiectomy has been rendered largely unnecessary with the advent of the pharmacological treatment.

Pharmacotherapy For ethical and medical reasons, randomized, double-blind, placebo-controlled pharmacological treatment studies cannot be conducted with symptomatic paraphilic patients who reside in the community. Such studies could only be justified on patients with relatively innocuous paraphilias. Nevertheless, the number of medications used to treat paraphilias has been steadily increasing. These medications can be divided into two general classes: those that act by lowering available androgens (e.g., progesterone derivatives and the gonadotropin releasing hormone analogs) and those that do not directly reduce androgen activity but reduce libido and/or sexual function as a side effect (e.g., some serotonin reuptake inhibitors). As with all pharmacological treatments, the choice of which medication to use is primarily based on the patient's presenting symptoms, his or her concomitant psychiatric/neurological disorders, and the results of the psychosexual and medical workup. A regrettable shortcoming of pharmacotherapy, however, is that it does not selectively reduce the risk for sex offending without generally impairing overall sexual functioning.

Concluding Remarks

There are a number of studies in the literature suggesting that treatment can be helpful, particularly in paraphilic samples. One such study reported rates of recidivism following treatment in a primarily paraphilic sample that were well below the rates reported in the world literature for comparable untreated cases. In another, a meta-analysis that reviewed data from 43 studies examining the sex offense recidivism rate for mixed sex offenders without differentiating between paraphilic and nonparaphilic patients found that recidivism, on average, was approximately 12% lower for treatment groups than for nontreatment groups.

Measuring treatment effectiveness presents significant problems. Recidivism, defined as some subset of involvement with the criminal justice system during or after the completion of treatment, is the most commonly used end point for determining treatment effectiveness in sex offenders. But not all paraphiles are sex offenders and not all sex offenders are paraphiles. Clearly, it is not possible to use recidivism as a measure of treatment efficacy with patients whose paraphilias are not illegal. Defining recidivism and dealing with important but largely unknown variables such as the base rate for reoffending and other methodological impediments greatly influence the interpretation of the available data and are central to answering questions about which treatment modalities work and which do not.

Sex offenses are prevalent and those motivated by paraphilia-driven phenomenology often constitute significant psychiatric disorders. Other, nonparaphilic sex crimes may have their roots in serious psychopathology as well. All too frequently, patients manifesting these conditions are simply ostracized, stigmatized, and punished when what is called for is enlightened psychiatric care.

Ignoring phenomenology and defining even observable manifestations of human sexuality in purely behavioral terms can only lead to egregious errors. Nowhere is this more apparent than in the arena of sex offender treatment. The phrase itself seems to us to be misleading, if not an oxymoron. With or without civil commitment statutes, clinicians are often called on to treat sex offenders. For example, a phenenomenological view of rape implies that rape is not a monolithic sex offense but a highly variable one. Rape may be an opportunistic act, carried out by an individual without a sense of conscience. It may be the result of command hallucinations. It may also be paraphilic. It seems reasonable to assume, as in all psychiatric treatment, that how we approach the treatment of a rapist, or for that matter any sex offender, must depend to some degree on differential diagnosis, which, in turn, depends on the phenomenology underlying the behavior.

See Also the Following Articles

Antisocial Disorders; Sexual Assault.

Further Reading

Abel, G. G., Mittleman, M., Becker, J. V., et al. (1988). Predicting childmolesters' response to treatment. *Annals of the New York Academy of Sciences* **528**, 223–224.

American Psychiatric Association (2000). *Diagnostic and statistical manual of mental disorders* (4th edn., text rev.). Washington, DC: American Psychiatric Association.

Berlin, F. S. (1989). The paraphilias and depo-provera: some medical, ethical and legal considerations. *Bulletin of the American Academy of Psychiatry and the Law* **17**(3), 233–239.

Berlin, F. and Malin, H. (1991). Media distortion of the public's perception of recidivism and psychiatric rehabilitation. *American Journal of Psychiatry* **148**(11), 1572–1576.

Bradford, J. M. W. (2000). The treatment of sexual deviation using a pharmacological approach. *Journal of Sex Research* 37(3), 248–257.

Freund, K. (1980). Therapeutic sex drive reduction. *Acta Psychiatrica Scandinavica* **62**(supplement 287), 1–39.
Frost, J. J. and Mayberg, H. S. (1986). Alteration in brain opiate receptor binding in man following arousal using C-11 carfentanil and positive emission tomography. *Journal of Nuclear Medicine* **27**, 1027 (abstract of presentation at the 33rd annual meeting of the Society of Nuclear Medicine).
Greenberg, D. M., Bradford, J. M. W., Curry, S., et al. (1996). A comparison of treatment of paraphilias with three serotonin reuptake inhibitors: a retrospective study. *Bulletin of the American Academy of Psychiatry and the Law* **24**(4), 525–532.
Hanson, R. K., Gordon, A., Harris, A. J., et al. (2002). First report of the collaborative outcome data project on the effectiveness of psychological treatment for sex offenders. *Sex Abuse* **14**(2), 169–194.
Krafft-Ebing, R. von. (1965). *Psychopathia sexualis (1886).* New York: G. P. Putnam's Sons.
Langelüddecke, A. (1963). *Die Entmannung von Sittlichkeitsverbrechern in Deutchland.* Berlin: DeGruyter.
Laws, D. R., Hudson, S. M. and Ward, T. (2000). *Remaking relapse prevention with sex offenders: a sourcebook.* Thousand Oaks, CA: Sage.
Marshall, D. R. and Laws, W. L. (2003). A brief history of behavioral and cognitive behavioral approaches to sexual offenders. Part 1: Early developments. *Sexual Abuse: A Journal of Research and Treatment* **15**(2), 93–120.
Money, J. (1985). *The destroying angel.* Buffalo, NY: Prometheus Books.
Money, J. (1986). *Venuses penuses: sexology, sexosophy and exigency theory.* Buffalo, NY: Prometheus Books.
Moser, C. (2002). Are any of the paraphilias in the DSM mental disorders? *Sexual Behavior* **31**(6), 490–491.
Murphy, W. D. and Carich, M. S. (2001). Cognitive distortions and restructuring in sexual abuser treatment. In: Carich, M. S. & Stephens, E. M. (eds.). *Handbook for sexual abuser assessment and treatment*, pp. 65–75. Brandon, VT: Safer Society Press.
Ortman, J. (1980). The treatment of sexual offenders: castration and antihormone therapy. *International Journal of Law and Psychiatry* **3**, 443–451.
Quinsey, V. L., Harris, G. T., Rice, M. E., et al. (1993). Assessing treatment efficacy in outcome studies of sex offenders. *Journal of Interpersonal Violence* **8**, 512–523.
Rosler, A. and Witztum, E. (1998). Treatment of men with paraphilia with a long acting analogue of gonadotropin-releasing hormone. *New England Journal of Medicine* **338**, 416–465.
Saleh, F. M. and Berlin, F. S. (2003). Sex hormones, neurotransmitters and psychopharmacological treatments in men with paraphilic disorders. *Journal Child Sexual Abuse* **12**(3–4), 53–74.
Saleh, F. M. and Guidry, L. L. (2003). Psychosocial and biological treatment considerations for the paraphilic and nonparaphilic sex offender. *Journal of the American Academy of Psychiatry and the Law* **31**, 486–493.
Saleh, F. M., Niel, T. and Fishman, M. (2004). Treatment of paraphilia in young adults with leuprolide acetate: a preliminary case report series. *Journal of Forensic Sciences* **49**(6), 2–6.
Stürup, G. K. (1968). Treatment of sexual offenders in Herstedvester, Denmark: the rapist. *Acta Psychiatrica Scandinavica* **44**, 5–63.

Adolescence

G N Swanson
Allegheny General Hospital, Pittsburgh, PA, USA

This is a revised version of the article by G N Swanson, Encyclopedia of Stress First Edition, volume 1, pp 32–41, © 2000, Elsevier Inc.

Glossary

Adolescence — A stage of life from puberty to adulthood usually thought of as occurring between the ages of 12 and 19 years. It is characterized by marked physical, psychological, and social change. The developmental task of adolescence is the change from dependence to independence.

Identity — A central aspect of the healthy personality, consisting of an inner awareness of continuity of self and an ability to identify with others, share in their goals, and participate in society.

Puberty — A normal growth process that begins in early adolescence, lasts 2–4 years, and leads to sexual and physical maturity.

Resiliency — The ability to overcome or adapt to stress by maintaining developmental progress and adequate social and academic functioning.

Introduction

Adolescence has been characterized as a challenging stage of life, defined by the psychological task of identity formation. Adolescents develop better coping skills as they mature both as a consequence of their cognitive and emotional development and because of the changes they experience. Teenagers generally respond successfully to many common stressors, such as puberty, school demands, family changes, and peer relations. Unusual stressors may lead to some difficulties, especially in those who are more vulnerable.

Traumatic stressors, although not universally harmful, often impinge on the emotional wellbeing of teenagers and may leave lasting scars. An adolescent's ability to cope with stressors depends on a number of factors, including family support, cognitive development, previous experiences, and their own unique temperament.

Normal Adolescence

The discrete stage of adolescence has been recognized for only a short period of time. It seems to have come about in Western society as a consequence of the Industrial Revolution, when social changes necessitated the prolongation of childhood. Children, who had previously been able to enter the adult world at an early age, did not have the skills or abilities to perform adult work. Child labor laws were passed, and public schools were established. Families were also better able to financially provide for children for a longer period of time. The transition from childhood to adulthood lengthened, encompassing most of the second decade of life. Indeed, many teenagers nowadays maintain their dependency on their parents during college, thereby extending this transition even further. Puberty is often identified as the starting point of adolescence, although this can normally start as early as 9 or 10 years of age. The endpoint has been less well defined, as there are differences in the legal age of adulthood (18–21 years), and the criteria of independence, the completion of school, starting a new family, and getting a job are even more variable.

Adolescence is often thought of as a period of rebellion, marked by conflicts with parents as a child grows to be an adult. Anna Freud, G. Stanley Hall, and others characterized this stage of life as a time of storm and stress. Psychoanalysts believed that it was an indication of pathology if these stormy relations did not occur. Erik Erikson believed that the psychological task of this stage of life is the development of identity. Specifically, he thought that the adolescent would commit to a core set of values and assume a sex role and career plan. Failure to complete this task would result in identity diffusion, leading to further difficulties in adulthood. Adolescence was the period of an identity crisis, which led to considerable emotional turmoil.

However, Offer and associates have shown that the vast majority (~80%) of adolescents do not experience significant emotional distress. Instead, these teenagers manage the transition to adulthood smoothly, without experiencing a severe identity crisis. They have a positive self-image and are not afraid of the physical changes associated with puberty. They do not report significant conflicts with their parents and have positive feelings toward their families. They are confident, optimistic about the future, and are willing to work hard in order to reach a goal.

However, a significant minority (~20%) of teenagers reports difficulties in these areas. They report that they feel emotionally empty and overwhelmed by life's problems. They feel much less able to control the world around them. These adolescents also report that they are much less able to talk with their parents about their problems. They appear to be more vulnerable to stressors and may exhibit more behavioral and emotional problems as a result. It seems that the stereotype of the moody, confused, and rebellious teenager is more applicable to this smaller group than to most adolescents.

Considerable cognitive development occurs during adolescence. Early adolescents become very self-conscious, which leads to a tendency to be more egocentric. They tend to believe that the thoughts and feelings that they have are unique. Furthermore, they do not seem to recognize that their peers are going through the same situation. In time, older teenagers become better able to empathize, to think abstractly, and to be introspective. They are able to consider possibilities and to imagine other realities. This leads them to become more philosophical, and to question the rules and realities of their lives in an attempt to gain a clearer understanding of the world. These cognitive abilities lead them to question their identity and to see themselves as individuals with some control over who and what they will be.

These changes become manifest in the adolescents' social environment. In particular, the family becomes less influential, while peer groups become more so. Adolescents begin to establish and exercise independence from parental controls. They learn to negotiate, although some conflicts arise. They spend more time with their friends than they did in childhood. They often imitate influential peers and adults. They try on different hats to see what they might look like, in order to establish an identity of their own. However, although they may dress like their friends or listen to music that their parents abhor, they often retain similar values and beliefs as their parents.

Adolescents tend to get better at coping with stress as they get older. They learn skills over time, utilizing their individual temperament and modeling parental coping strategies. Early in adolescence, teenagers tend to reactive defensively, denying problems, and thinking wishfully. They misinterpret situations, making mis-attributions to others, and overlooking information that would help them to see things more clearly. They also tend to either under- or overestimate both potential risks and their ability to handle them.

They may vent their frustration or anxiety in open emotional outbursts or they may withdraw and try to keep their feelings hidden. They seek solace and support from others, but do not readily ask for or listen to advice. As they develop, they become better able to appraise problems themselves. They try to change the stressful situation and to negotiate solutions. They learn that communication skills, the art of compromise, and assertiveness are more effective responses than are emotional outbursts or withdrawal. They learn how much of their feelings they need to reveal and become more adept at managing their emotions. They also become better at reading social cues and reacting appropriately. They think about ways to deal with problems and discuss potential solutions with others. Successful responses to stress lead to more success, although at times they may revert to previous, less effective strategies, usually in an impulsive fashion. Over time, most adolescents develop the skills necessary to cope with stress effectively, although some do not.

Common Stressors

Adolescents face a variety of challenges as a normal part of their lives. These include the physical and sexual changes associated with puberty; the demands of school; the desire to initiate and maintain friendships, both platonic and romantic; the need to start working and to make a career choice; and the gradual development of independence from the family. All of these changes can be stressful, but most teenagers report that they do not feel overwhelmed or unable to deal with them. Regardless of gender, socioeconomic status, or race, teenagers identify their most important concerns as career, school performance, and college plans. Many worry about violence, theft, and work. Some report concerns about peer conflicts and parental expectations. Teens are least worried about drugs and alcohol. Boys are more concerned about sexuality and extracurricular activities, while girls are more concerned about their appearance.

Puberty

Puberty, as the starting point for adolescence, is often thought of as very stressful. The physical changes are obvious, as is an increased sexual interest. Parents and teachers often attribute all behavioral changes to raging hormones, but the fact is that there are other social, and psychological factors that must be considered as well. Nevertheless, there is a biological effect of puberty on cognitive, social, and emotional development as well. In particular, the timing of puberty can be stressful and does seem to have an impact on academic and psychosocial functioning. Boys appear to benefit academically and socially if they reach puberty early, although they often end up having a shorter stature than their later-developing peers. Early in adolescence, girls seem to have a better body image and are more popular if they develop early. However, as a group, they do not seem to do as well academically. Furthermore, by the time adolescence ends, later developing girls have a better body image than girls who reached puberty earlier do.

This may be related to the fact that girls with a later onset of puberty are more slender, which more closely fits with current cultural standards of attractiveness. More importantly, girls who reach puberty later have had a longer time to anticipate and adapt to these changes and as a result seem better able to cognitively process and cope with pubertal changes when they do occur. Finally, puberty may be most stressful when it is very early or very late, as this leads the adolescent to be markedly different from other peers. This information coincides with Offer's reports that most adolescents are comfortable with, and not distressed by, the changes of puberty, as most adolescents will enter puberty at about the same time as their peers and experience it as a normative process.

Peer Relationships

Peer relationships take on much more importance during adolescence. Teenagers expand their social relationships, looking to increase their connections with others. Girls in general seem to develop a capacity for intimacy sooner than boys do. Most teenagers believe they can make friends easily and that they can tell their friends intimate details about themselves. Early adolescents are very interested in being popular and want to fit in with a popular same-sex peer group. There is a degree of stress associated with this, especially if a young teenager wants to belong to a group, yet does not. Most are able to find a group, however, and do not find establishing friendships difficult. These peer groups are often very supportive and discourage deviant behavior.

In middle adolescence, boys and girls begin to mix. Romance and dating become extremely important. Once again, teenagers report some stress during this phase, as they grapple with the new social skills required to establish romantic relationships. However, most report that they believe they are interesting to members of the opposite sex and believe that they are capable of finding a romantic partner.

Dating usually begins between the ages of 12 and 16 years. Adolescents may face some peer pressure to date and may be dropped from a particular group if they do not do so. Similarly, they may feel pressure to engage in a similar level of sexual activity as their peers. The pressure to conform to a perceived peer norm, which is in conflict with cultural, religious, family, or individual values, seems to be the most stressful aspect of romantic relationships. There are many similarities between adult and adolescent love relationships.

However, adolescent relationships are notably more transient, with strong feelings that do not usually lead to enduring intimacy or self-disclosure. Cognitive development as adolescence progresses helps teenagers to better cope with relationship changes. Gay adolescents are especially vulnerable to stress, due to feelings of isolation from peers and family and to difficulty integrating homosexuality into their identity.

Parents of teenagers frequently describe family life as stressful, due to the ongoing development of adolescent independence. This reflects a change in family roles, which parents may perceive as more difficult than adolescents do. Early adolescence is marked by considerable variation in roles, as the adolescent vacillates between asserting independence and maintaining dependency. There is some anxiety associated with becoming independent, felt by both parent and child. As they become older, most teenagers are confident about their ability to make decisions and try to demonstrate this to their parents. However, although they are in the process of individuating, they neither sever their emotional attachments to their parents nor become free of their parents' influences. Adolescents appear to be less distressed when parents utilize an authoritative parenting style which encourages and supports independence. Parents provide limits and controls with explanations, while allowing the adolescent to express their views. Nevertheless, tensions are still present as negotiations proceed and opposing needs are balanced.

Race and Culture

Racial and cultural issues pose interesting challenges, particularly for the adolescent. A child forms both gender and ethnic identities around the ages of 3–5 years. Children become familiar with cultural differences and history long before puberty begins. However, it is in adolescence that teenagers make a conscious commitment to be a member of their culture. They will generally embrace the values of their culture, which may not be the same as the dominant culture. This may lead to stress, especially if they have frequent interactions with peers of other cultures. They also can understand the abstract concepts of racism and inequality. They may be more likely to experience these as they leave their family and have more contact with peers and adults from other walks of life. Nonwhite adolescents are twice as likely as their white peers to be funneled into the juvenile justice system rather than the mental health system when they have a problem with the law. They are also more likely to identify their main stressors as environmental ones (such as living in a dangerous neighborhood) rather than more personal ones. Most teenagers come to terms with their ethnic identity and with negative stereotypes and prejudices. They are able to accept themselves and their place within both society and their own ethnic culture. Those that do not do so have more difficulty with self-image and psychological adjustment. Adolescents who immigrate to a new country face additional stress, as they become more dependent on their families at a time when they are trying to develop independence. If they do push to be more independent, they may be more likely to join an inappropriate peer group.

Academics and School

School situations and academic demands are yet other common stressors that teenagers confront. The transition to middle school and the transition to high school are both major life events. Most teenagers report a combination of eagerness and apprehension as they move up to a bigger school with more challenging assignments, more complicated schedules, and more competent upper classmen. Middle schools represent a challenge as they are more impersonal and may require independence than early adolescents are capable of. Most middle-school students have not mastered the social skills needed for this setting, although they may learn them quickly if provided with opportunities to succeed in small groups.

High schools offer more extracurricular activities, which provide opportunities to join in new peer groups, but the many choices may be overwhelming and confusing, and some adolescents may end up feeling excluded. Grades become more meaningful, especially for those planning on college. Parental expectations, Scholastic Amplitude Test (SAT) scores, and college applications create tension, as does the search for a job after graduation.

Work

Most teenagers express a desire to work and feel satisfaction in a job well done. Earning money helps older adolescents become more independent and enables them to practice some of the skills they will need as adults. However, trying to balance a part-time job with school demands, sports, and social activities is often difficult. Adolescents who work are less invested in school, spending less time on homework and missing classes more often than peers who do not work. They usually work in low-paying jobs and have little authority or opportunity to advance. Those who work the most hours tend to have the lowest grades. However, part-time work has also been associated with better self-esteem and a sense of responsibility in adolescents. Teenagers cope with the stress of work best if they can balance the time they work with their other priorities. Working raises other issues, as adolescents may be overwhelmed with the choices they have.

Establishing a life goal is a daunting task for adolescents. Many are reluctant to commit to a specific career path, as this means eliminating other possibilities. This lack of commitment may be interpreted as a lack of motivation by parents, leading to conflicts. Adolescents also have many misconceptions and cognitive distortions about themselves and the careers they are considering. Accurate information and a frank discussion of their strengths and weaknesses are important. The support of a mentoring adult is often very helpful, as is providing the perspective that any choice is not etched in stone. This issue is also one that tends to extend adolescence most often, as it is commonly the last one resolved.

Unusual Stressors

Some teenagers face more unusual challenges. These can include family problems, such as mental or physical illness; drug or alcohol abuse; parental separation or divorce; social problems, such as poverty and violence; and individual problems, such as pregnancy, serious illness, and school failure. In some instances, teens may experience traumas such as abuse or the death of a loved one. Adolescents with adequate cognitive abilities, emotional development, and supportive families seem better able to cope with these problems successfully. Teenagers who have experienced multiple stressors, have a previous history of psychopathology, or have little parental support are much more vulnerable.

Parent with Medical/Psychiatric Illness

Adolescents who are raised in homes where a parent has a serious medical or psychiatric illness have the ability to understand the illness better than younger children and may have more questions as a result. They are also more likely to exhibit anger and acting out behaviors. This may occur because of the conflict involved between the family's needs for help from the adolescent and the adolescent's needs to become more independent. Younger children may be more likely to avoid discussion of the parent's illness and to experience intrusive thoughts and feelings, while adolescents are more likely to exhibit symptoms of anxiety and depression. This is particularly true of teenage girls whose mothers have cancer. Parental coping skills play a part in how adolescents respond to parental illness. Parents who are less anxious and depressed have a positive effect on their children. There are some important differences to be considered when a family member has a severe mental illness as opposed to a physical illness. Parents with mental illness are much less likely to be in treatment, which means that professional education and advice are much less forthcoming. There is considerable stigma associated with mental illnesses (although some physical illnesses carry a stigma, such as HIV infection). Adolescents may therefore be much less likely to seek peer or adult support as a result. Teenagers are at a higher risk for depression and other mood disorders when their parents have a chronic mental illness, but studies have not been able to separate genetic influences from psychosocial effects on children and adolescents. Finally, parental conflicts, divorce, and inconsistent parenting practices often are present in families where a parent has a severe mental illness. These multiple risk factors compound the stress on an adolescent, more so than in families where a parent has a severe physical illness. Adolescents who cope best when parents have a serious medical or psychiatric illness share several characteristics. They tend to be actively involved in school, church, work, and other outside activities. They have a close relationship with a supportive adult. They also understand that they are not responsible for their parents' illness. Their families are more cohesive, flexible, and are able to maintain family rituals. Finally, their families effectively communicate information and feelings about the parental illness and are able to make plans for the future.

Parental Alcohol Abuse

The effects of parental alcohol abuse have also been studied, although more attention has been paid to younger children in alcoholic families. Adolescents raised in alcoholic families have been found to have a higher risk of conduct disorder, substance abuse, sexual acting-out, physical and sexual abuse, and academic problems. They also have more difficulties in their peer relationships and are more likely to have romantic relationships with adolescents with substance abuse problems themselves. Some adolescents may take on a more adult role within the family in an attempt to maintain family functioning, while others may disengage. Boys seem to have a higher risk of problems than girls do. Teenagers who cope effectively with parental alcoholism tend to have healthy and supportive relationships with adults outside of the family. Families that are able to maintain family rituals (e.g., such as holiday celebrations, family dinners, and church attendance) have teenagers that are more resilient in the face of parental substance abuse.

Adolescents with an easy temperament, at least average intelligence, and an internal locus of control are also more resilient. Not all teenagers from alcoholic homes require treatment, although parents with alcoholism should be referred for treatment. However, it is not clear what effect, if any, parental recovery has on adolescents who are already exhibiting problems. Alateen, a self-help program for adolescents from alcoholic families in the USA and Canada, has been effective in providing information and improving mood and self-esteem for teenagers. Group, individual, and family therapy have been helpful. All interventions should provide education regarding the adolescent's increased risk of substance abuse in an attempt at prevention.

Parental Marital Conflict and Divorce

Parental conflict and divorce is a fairly common, but nonetheless major, stressor in today's culture. Most research on separation and divorce has focused on younger children. Studies with adolescents suggest that they too may have difficulty adjusting to this stressor. In addition, children who experience divorce may not manifest problems until adolescence. It is important to remember that most children and adolescents do adapt to divorce and are able to function effectively as adults. Younger adolescents whose parents divorce are more likely to be noncompliant and aggressive and to have problems with substance abuse than are adolescents in nondivorced families. Gender differences have been reported. Adolescent girls from divorced families have had more problems with self-esteem and promiscuity, while adolescent boys have a higher incidence of substance abuse. Both boys and girls have lower academic achievement, but teenage boys are also likely to drop out of school if their parents have divorced and they are living with their mother. Girls are at a greater risk of dropping out if they live with their remarried mother and stepfather. These findings appear to hold even when factors such as race and socioeconomic status are controlled for. Conflict between divorced mothers and their adolescent daughters is common, possibly connected to the teenage girls' tendency to increased sexual acting out. Adolescent boys have a higher risk of disengaging from their family and to engage in delinquent behavior with peers. This may be related to the absence and lack of influence of the noncustodial father, which is all too common in divorce. Many factors mediate adolescents' responses to divorce. An authoritative custodial parent seems to be the most important factor, as the parent is able to provide the understanding and support needed while maintaining an authority position in the family. Generally, teenagers are better able to cognitively process and understand the reasons for parental divorce than younger children are. However, those who have limited insight, poor problem solving skills, and a history of temperamental difficulty are more vulnerable to experiencing problems with the divorce. The degree of conflict between parents and the amount of contact with each parent are also important. Depression and delinquency have been connected to prolonged parental conflict.

Poverty and Violence

Sociocultural stressors such as poverty and violence have long been recognized as stressful for children and adolescents. However, it is very difficult to disentangle the specific effects these stressors have from each other as well as from other associated risk factors, such as parenting styles and other environmental stressors. Approximately 20% of American children live in poverty – the highest rate for any Western industrialized country. Black children are twice as likely to experience poverty as white children are. Length of time spent in poverty varies, although around 90% of poor children spend less than 5 years in poverty. Contrary to popular belief, poverty is more common in rural rather than urban areas.

Adolescents who experience poverty have a higher rate of delinquency, depression, and poor self-image. They may also incorporate the idea of poverty into their identity rather than to see it as a temporary external condition. Again, parental responses and styles have a marked effect on adolescent coping strategies. Families living in poverty are more likely to utilize inconsistent, punitive, and authoritarian parenting styles, which leads to increased stress and conflict. In contrast, poor but supportive parents, who have a positive outlook on the future, have less distressed teenagers. Teenagers are also able to recognize when they live in less desirable neighborhoods and are well aware of the risks of violence. Living with this chronic stress is difficult and can have a marked effect on their outlook on the future. They may be more fatalistic and experience more posttraumatic stress disorder (PTSD) symptoms as a result of their exposure to violence. Anecdotes abound, both describing those who have problems and those who have been resilient. However, at this time there are no systematic studies that have assessed these issues.

Pregnancy

Some teenagers face significant individual stressors, such as pregnancy, serious illness, or school failure. These teenagers already tend to be at a higher risk for other stressors, as outlined above. However, considerable study has been given to these issues. Teenage girls who get pregnant are less prepared than their adult counterparts to raise children. They know less about infants and are more distressed by the pregnancy. Around 40% choose abortion, while 45% choose to keep their child. The other 15% either miscarry or choose adoption. Teenage mothers are less responsive to the needs of their babies than are adults. However, longitudinal studies have shown that a majority of teenage mothers complete high school and hold regular employment thereafter. Most support themselves and their children, although they are on welfare at times. They do not end up having more children than peers who have children later. Most importantly, the majority seems to cope effectively over the long run.

In contrast, teenage girls who ultimately choose abortion report considerable psychological distress during the time of pregnancy. This seems to fade somewhat after the abortion. However, studies of women who have undergone abortion indicate that most negative reactions and distress occur in those who are young, unmarried, previously nulliparous, and who delay the procedure until the second trimester. Adolescents are much more likely to fit into this profile and so appear to be at a higher risk for psychological sequelas as a result of the abortion. The debate about the psychological effects of abortion is unresolved, as this particular group remains difficult to study due to the many other stressors that they face.

Serious Illness

It is estimated that 5–10% of teenagers face a serious illness during adolescence. Adolescents who suffer from serious illnesses struggle with a variety of issues. Early adolescents tend to try to deny the existence of their illness, using avoidant coping strategies. These problems are more likely to occur in families where there is little cohesiveness. This often leads to treatment noncompliance and more problems with the illness itself. Conversely, chronic or serious illnesses may impair normal adolescent development.

This seems to be due to the fact that the illness and treatment requirements make the adolescent more dependent on his parents. They in turn may be more unwilling to let the teenager be more independent. Adolescents may also incorporate their illness into their identity. In some situations, such as diabetes, these may be unavoidable due to the nature of the illness. For those who have cancer, however, this may be more problematic. Adolescents with a history of cancer are not more likely to be depressed, but they are more likely to have somatic complaints and preoccupations and to be distrusting of their bodies. They also tend to have greater difficulties in romantic relationships. Misattributions and misunderstandings about their illness and its prognosis should be addressed when present. Parents and adolescents often need much more education and support than they receive. Efforts should be made to help adolescents understand both their illness and treatment, and information should be made readily available to them. This should occur in a stepwise fashion, allowing teenagers some time to adjust to changes and react to them emotionally and intellectually.

Dropping Out of School

Approximately 10–15% of adolescents drop out of school. Often, they have parents or siblings who have done the same. Parental attitudes about education have a great impact on academic performance, even in adolescence. Adolescents whose home lives are already distressed or whose fathers are absent are much more likely to drop out. Those who have already failed a class or who have been held back a grade are at greater risk as well. Many are working, and many have children. Teenagers find dropping out is very stressful and would recommend against it. Job opportunities are limited and they are often unable to function independently. Successful prevention requires strong cooperation between parents and schools, providing the support and guidance necessary to vulnerable teenagers.

Peer Victimization

Several forms of adolescent victimization have been recognized, including bullying, sexual harassment, and interpersonal violence and emotional abuse in dating relationships. Research is limited, but most adolescents have had some limited experiences of victimization. There may be significant differences based on gender, socioeconomic status, and racial and ethnic groups. Those teenagers who complain of significant levels of psychological distress tend to have been targeted on multiple occasions, and in several forms of victimization. They also feel less of a sense of school belonging. In addition, adolescents who have experienced bullying are more likely to have self blaming attributions than those who have not been clinicians and school personnel should be carefully assessing for the occurrence of victimization in multiple areas if a teenager reports experiencing any one form of victimization.

Trauma Trauma often leads to emotional and behavioral changes. Most studies on trauma have looked at younger children, children and adolescents together, or at adolescents who were traumatized as children. However, adolescents can be abused physically, sexually, emotionally, or in combination. Due in part to their increasing independence and to their cognitive and emotional development, adolescents are less likely than are children to be abused by family members. However, they are more likely to be the victims of rape, assault, or robbery than younger children or adults. There are some gender differences in adolescents, as girls are more likely to experience sexual trauma, while boys are more likely to witness the injury or death of another. Catastrophic life events also may occur, including the death of a parent, sibling, or peer due to illness, accident, violence, disaster, or terrorism. Although age-based differences in stress reaction have received research attention, findings have been inconsistent, due in large part to the lack of normative and pretrauma psychological functioning data.

Teenagers who have been abused may come to attention for incidents that have just recently occurred and been disclosed or may have occurred many years earlier. The length of time since the occurrence of abuse or trauma does not mitigate the severity of symptoms or the need for treatment. It is also not clear if abuse or trauma at an earlier or later age leads to more problems. Adolescents are less likely to be abused than are young children. However, many adolescent victims of abuse have been abused as children. Therefore, teenagers who present with physical or sexual abuse may have a lengthy history of abuse and may have more difficulty as a result.

Multiple neurotransmitter systems are involved in the response to traumatic stress, and chronic stress has been associated with long-term changes in neuronal function in structure. A comprehensive study by De Bellis et al. demonstrated alterations in biological stress systems and adverse influences on brain development in maltreated children and adolescents with PTSD. Increased levels of catecholaminergic neurotransmitters and steroid hormones during traumatic experiences could negatively affect brain development. Causal relationships have not yet been established, however, and it is unclear how traumatic stress specifically affects the still developing adolescent brain.

Abuse Teenagers who have been sexually abused are less likely to show unusual sexual behaviors or preoccupations than are young children. Abused teens also are more likely than children to disclose purposefully, usually out of anger toward the perpetrator. Adolescents are also more likely to have their reports substantiated. However, because they are older, victimized adolescents may be blamed, just as women who are victims of domestic violence are often blamed for not seeking help or leaving an abusive situation. In addition, adolescents who are physically abused may be seen as provoking a parent, thereby earning physical discipline. This is particularly true in teenagers who have a history of physical aggression, threats, delinquent behavior, noncompliance, and/or defiance. The juvenile justice system is more likely to be involved in these situations and may be less cognizant of the possibility of abuse than either mental health or child protective services.

When evaluating adolescents who have been abused, it is important to be sensitive and to allow them some control over what, when, and how much they disclose. Teenagers will often want to avoid talking about the issue and to minimize the effects it has had on them. Recognition and support for their attempts to cope with the abuse should be provided, in keeping with their psychological development, especially their need to be independent and successful. In addition, it may be helpful to separate the problem from their identity as a person. Hecht et al. suggest a statement such as, "I've talked with a lot of people your age who have been through sexual abuse. We talk about the effects it has had on them. Everyone's different, but I want to find out if some of the things that have bothered other young people have bothered you. I'd also like to find out what sorts of things you have done that seem to help the most." It is also important to understand the adolescent's attributions about the abuse. As adolescents are more independent and society holds them more responsible for their actions, they may be more likely to blame themselves.

Furthermore, teens may want to maintain the idea that they have control over what happens to them, in keeping with their developmental stage. At the same time, adolescents will often fear disclosure to their peers, perhaps believing that they will be stigmatized or that their peers will hold them responsible.

Nevertheless, having the support and understanding of a peer is often very helpful. In assessing an adolescent who has been abused, it is important to obtain a complete history as well as to address possible PTSD symptoms. In addition, any problems with aggression, impulsivity, social skills, attention span, academic performance, depression, anxiety, substance abuse, and delinquency should be explored. Abused adolescents are also at a higher risk for eating disorders, sleep problems, and self-injurious behavior.

Treatment interventions should be individualized, but may include sexual education, information about PTSD symptoms and abuse, and, perhaps most importantly, an attempt to work out with the adolescent an explanation as to why the abuse happened. Group and individual therapies have both been utilized with success. Treatment interventions should address both the needs of parents and the adolescent. Social skills, problem-solving, and cognitive treatments have been effective with adolescents, but family interventions in particular seem to help maintain progress over the long term. Court-mandated treatment helps to keep abusive parents in treatment.

Death Adolescents rarely experience the death of a parent, sibling, or of a close friend. Furthermore, studies of children who have lost a parent usually group younger children with adolescents. As a result, unique characteristics of adolescent bereavement are difficult to identify. Adolescents are able to conceptualize death abstractly. This allows them to consider religious and philosophical issues and may lead to more uncertainty than in younger children. Adolescents who have never experienced a death have a difficult time adjusting to this change. Adolescents who have experienced the death of a parent are at a higher risk for delinquency, anxiety and depressive symptoms, somatic complaints, and PTSD symptoms. Adolescents who have experienced a disaster are more likely to experience PTSD symptoms if they lost a loved one (parent, friend, or classmate) in the event. However, displacement from home, community, and school also contributes to these problems.

Teenage boys who lose a father are at a higher risk for behavioral and emotional problems as are early adolescents. Sudden deaths are clearly more difficult to cope with than deaths that occur after a protracted illness, as adolescents have a chance to prepare emotionally and intellectually for the event. However, a strong and supportive surviving parent can offer some protection. Once again, teens that can confide in an another adult (such as a relative, teacher, or neighbor) seem to cope better, as they are able to talk about their dead parent openly. It is important to remember that subsequent events, such as graduation, making a sports team, dating, or getting a job, may reopen grief feelings and should be considered as additional stressors. Nevertheless, the majority of adolescents appear to cope effectively with the death of a parent. The death of a peer is also a rare event. Studies in this area have been limited and have primarily focused on peers who commit suicide. In these instances, adolescents have exhibited depressive symptoms, but have not had an increase in suicide attempts.

See Also the Following Articles

Childhood Stress; Divorce, Children of.

Further Reading

Cobb, N. (1995). *Adolescence – Continuity, Conformity and Change* (2nd edn.). Mountain View, CA: Mayfield.

Cohen, J., Mannarino, A. and Deblinger, E. (2006). *Treating traumatic stress and grief in children: a clinician's guide*. New York: Guilford Press.

De Bellis, M., Baum, A. S., Birmaher, B., et al. (1999). Developmental traumatology. Part I Biological stress systems and Part II brain development. *Biological Psychiatry* **45**, 1259–1284.

Eth, S. and Pvnoos, R. (1985). Developmental perspectives on psychic trauma in childhood. In: Figley, C. (ed.) *Trauma and its wake*. New York: Brunner/Mazel.

Haggerty, R., Sherrod, L. R., Garmezy, N., et al. (eds.) (1996). *Stress, risk and resilience in children and adolescents*. Cambridge: Cambridge University Press.

Hecht, D., Chaffin, M., Bonner, B. L., et al. (2002). Treating sexually abused adolescents. In: Myers, J., Berliner, L., Briere, J., et al. (eds.) *The APSAC handbook on child maltreatment*. Thousand Oaks, CA: Sage.

Hersen, M., Thomas, J. and Ammerman, R. (2006). *Comprehensive handbook of personality and psychopathology – child psychopathology* (Vol. 3). New York: Wiley.

Kendall-Tackett, K. and Giacomoni, S. (2005). *Child victimization*. Kingston, NJ: Civic Research Institute.

LaGreca, A., Silverman, W. K., Venberg, E. M., et al. (2002). *Helping children cope with disasters and terrorism*. Washington DC: American Psychological Association.

Lewis, M. (2002). *Child and adolescent psychiatry – a comprehensive textbook*. Baltimore, MD: Williams & Wilkins.

Offer, D., Ostrov, E., Howard, K. and Atkinson, R. (1990). Normality and adolescence. *Psychiatric Clinics of North America* **13**, 377–388.

Saigh, P. and Bremner, J. D. (1999). *Posttraumatic stress disorder: a comprehensive textbook*. Boston, MA: Allyn and Bacon.

Youngblade, L. and Belsky, J. (1990). Social and emotional consequences of child maltreatment. In: Ammerman, R. & Hersen, M. (eds.) *Children at risk*. New York: Plenum.

Premenstrual Dysphoric Disorder

S Nowakowski
San Diego State University/University of California, San Diego, CA, USA
P Haynes
University of Arizona, Tucson, AZ, USA
B L Parry
University of California, San Diego, CA, USA

This is a revised version of the article by P Haynes and B L Parry, Encyclopedia of Stress First Edition, volume 3, pp 201–207, © 2000, Elsevier Inc.

Glossary

Circadian oscillator — A pacemaker located in the superchiasmatic nucleus of the hypothalamus with an output that repeats about once per day.

Dysphoric mood — A symptom of depression; feeling sad, despondent, discouraged, unhappy, anxious, or irritable.

Entrainment — The process by which the circadian oscillator becomes synchronized with the external environment.

Follicular phase — Also called the proliferative phase or estrogenic phase, the follicular phase of the menstrual cycle lasts from the first day of menstruation until ovulation. As assessed by the secretion of luteinizing hormone (LH), gonadotropin-releasing hormone (GnRH) is secreted from the hypothalamus in a pulsatile manner at a frequency of once per 90 min during the early follicular phase and increasing to once per 60–70 min. Follicle-stimulating hormone (FSH) is secreted by the anterior pituitary, and its concentrations in plasma increase from the first day of the cycle. The rise in FSH levels can be attributed to a decrease in progesterone and estrogen levels at the end of the previous cycle and the subsequent removal of inhibition of FSH by these ovarian hormones. FSH stimulates the development of 15–20 follicles each month and stimulates ovarian follicular secretion of estradiol. Estrogen levels peak toward the end of the follicular phase of the menstrual cycle, at which point estrogen exerts positive feedback on the hypothalamic-pituitary-gonadotrope system, thereby triggering the preovulatory LH surge.

Luteal phase — Approximately the second half of the menstrual cycle occurring after ovulation during which there is a decrease in frequency and increase in amplitude of time, ovarian steroid, and pulsatile release LH (and presumably GnRH) secretion. The luteal cells of the corpus luteum produce progesterone, the plasma levels of which peak by the middle of the luteal phase (days 20–22). By day 28, the corpus luteum has regressed with a consequent decrease in the output of estrogen and progesterone. The latter causes local ischemia and subsequent necrosis of the endometrium (i.e., menstrual flow).

Zeitgeber — German for time giver; a regular, external cue that synchronizes the internal clock to environmental cues; light is the most powerful zeitgebers in humans.

Premenstrual dysphoric disorder (PMDD) is a clearly defined syndrome that is often referred to as premenstrual syndrome (PMS) among the nonmedical population. As delineated in the *Diagnostic and Statistical Manual,* 4th edition (DSM-IV-TR), five symptoms are required to make the diagnosis of PMDD, and at least one symptom must be a moderate to severe mood symptom (see **Table 1**). The criteria for PMDD are more stringent and delineate increased specificity and severity of premenstrual symptoms with an emphasis on affective symptoms (see **Table 1**). The criteria for PMDD are stringent and delineate increased specificity and severity of premenstrual symptoms with an emphasis on affective symptoms (see **Table 1**). Symptoms typically begin in the late luteal (premenstrual) phase of the menstrual cycle, which is associated with declining estrogen and progesterone levels from the degenerating corpus luteum. Premenstrual symptoms typically remit within the first few days of the follicular phase, when estrogen levels increase as a result of follicular growth. The diagnosis of PMDD requires documentation of luteal phase timing of symptoms and a symptom-free interval from approximately day 4 of menses to the onset of ovulation. The National Institute of Mental Health Premenstrual Syndrome Workshop (1983) specified that a 30% change in symptom severity during the luteal phase is required for a PMDD diagnosis. In addition, a diagnostic requirement is that symptoms must cause functional impairment.

Diagnostic Issues

R. T. Frank first identified physical, psychological, and behavioral changes corresponding to monthly

Table 1 Diagnostic criteria for premenstrual dysphoric disorder

A. In most menstrual cycles during the past year, at least five of the following symptoms must have been present most of the time during the last week of the luteal phase and disappear within a week after the onset of menstruation. At least one of the symptoms must be one of the first four.

1. Feeling sad, hopeless, or self-deprecating
2. Feeling tense, anxious or on edge
3. Marked lability of mood interspersed with frequent tearfulness or increased sensitivity to rejection
4. Persistent irritability, anger, and increased interpersonal conflicts
5. Decreased interest in usual activities
6. Difficulty concentrating
7. Feeling fatigued, lethargic, or lacking in energy
8. Marked changes in appetite, which may be associated with binge eating or craving certain foods
9. Hypersomnia or insomnia
10. A subjective feeling of being overwhelmed or out of control
11. Physical symptoms such as breast tenderness or swelling, headaches, or sensations of bloating or weight gain

B. The symptoms must cause an obvious and marked impairment in the ability to function socially or occupationally.

C. The symptoms may be superimposed on another disorder but are not merely an exacerbation of the symptoms of another disorder, such as major depression, panic disorder, dysthymia, or a personality disorder.

D. Criteria A, B, C, and D must be confirmed by prospective daily self-ratings during at least two consecutive symptomatic cycles. (The diagnosis may be made provisionally prior to this confirmation.)

From the American Psychiatric Association (2000). *Diagnostic and Statistical Manual of Mental Disorders,* 4th edition, text revision. Washington, D.C.: American Psychiatric Association, with permission.

changes in reproductive hormones in 1931. However, public awareness of the concurrent change in mood with phases of the menstrual cycle has increased dramatically over the past two decades. The media has disseminated a wide body of information shaping a societal notion of what is popularly termed premenstrual syndrome (PMS). Definitions for PMS have varied widely. Typically, PMS refers to a large number of symptoms, including irritability, tension, fatigue, dysphoria, distractibility, impaired motor coordination, changes in eating and sleeping, and libido changes, which occur in the late luteal phase and remit after the beginning of menstruation. Up to 90% of women experience some premenstrual symptoms, and 50% of women may experience many symptoms together, thus comprising a syndrome.

Many women experience mood disruptions or physical complaints during the late luteal phase. For this reason, the PMDD diagnosis has been controversial among psychiatrists, psychologists, gynecologists, and sociologists. One reason for the ambiguity may be the failure to distinguish normal from pathological premenstrual mood disturbance. Unlike other psychiatric syndromes, the remission and relapse of premenstrual symptoms is connected to a physiological process, the menstrual cycle. Every woman does not experience a pathological premenstrual mood disorder, however. Furthermore, there are discrepant views in defining depression as a categorical versus spectrum illness. Depression can be defined as a discrete, all-or-none variable or on a continuum of symptom severity. Thus, the differentiation between the normal and pathological is important in terms of investigative research, interdisciplinary discourse, as well as treatment.

Premenstrual criteria were included in the appendix of DSM-III-R as late luteal phase dysphoric disorder (LLPDD), and they are currently included as PMDD in the appendix of the DSM-IV-TR as a depressive disorder, not otherwise specified. Some researchers have postulated that moving PMDD into the depressive disorders not otherwise specified section of the DSM-IV has reinforced the view that PMDD is depression, rather than a unique disorder. Moreover, the treatment of PMDD with selective serotonin reuptake inhibitors (SSRIs) may be treating symptoms of depression rather than the etiological disturbance; thus, treatment may provide little information on the nature of the disorder and raises the problem of comorbidity with other mood disturbances (e.g., major depressive disorder).

Besides emotional distress, the disturbance must cause impairment in occupational or social functioning. Also, the mood disturbances must begin during the late luteal phase and remit at the follicular phase; this trend of mood fluctuation must occur over at least two consecutive cycles. Because retrospective ratings may not be accurate due to an expectation bias, premenstrual trends must be documented by daily mood ratings. In the United States, approximately 3–5% of women are thought to experience symptoms that meet criteria for PMDD. Even with the DSM-IV-established criteria, debate over defining criteria of PMDD is ongoing. The requirement of absence of symptoms postmenstrually may be unreasonably conservative, and the criterion for premenstrual interference in daily activities contributes little to the diagnosis of PMDD. Poor classification proves to be particularly problematic because, over time, untreated PMDD becomes progressively more severe, and episodes of dysphoria extend in duration. For this reason, women diagnosed with PMDD are vulnerable to developing major depressive disorder at a later date.

Etiology

Various disciplines conceptualize the etiological basis of premenstrual mood disturbance. Biological theorists maintain that premenstrual symptoms originate from the biological reactivity or sensitivity to reproductive hormones. Psychological theorists suggest that premenstrual symptoms arise from the maladaptive response of the individual to the environment. Social theorists assert that the social, patriarchal environment elicits symptoms. Regardless of the etiological model, hormonal changes associated with the menstrual cycle are likely to serve as contributory factors to mood disruption.

Biomedical Model

Investigators and clinicians have recognized the spectrum of premenstrual mood: symptoms ranging from mild to severe. Those with severe symptoms have a decreased ability to function effectively and meet criteria for PMDD. Rather than psychosomatic origins, researchers have investigated physiological underpinnings to the disorder that are expressed in mood and behavior, that is, conceptualized as a somato-psychic illness.

Estrogen and progesterone Research in this area began with the hypothesis that the absolute amount of estrogen (E2) and progesterone (P4), e.g., P4 deficiency, E2 excess, were responsible for mood disturbances. Inconsistencies in research findings have called this hypothesis into question. The rate of hormonal change, however, may play an important role in the pathogenesis of the disorder. Schmidt and colleagues examined the role of E2 and P4 by testing the effects of ovarian suppression with leuprolide, an agonist analog of gonadotropin-releasing hormone, versus placebo in women with and without PMS. The authors found that leuprolide caused a significant decrease in symptom scores for women with PMS compared with placebo treatment. In a subsequent phase of the study, Schmidt and colleagues administered a conjunct hormone therapy (leuprolide plus estradiol or progesterone) to the women with PMS whose symptoms responded to ovarian suppression, which resulted in a significant recurrence of symptoms. Thus, baseline levels of gonadal steroids or changes in hormone levels triggered a change in mood in women sensitive to mood instability. This study suggests that the occurrence of PMS symptoms may represent an abnormal response to normal hormonal changes. In addition, it suggests that E2 and P4 variations likely exert their influence on mood indirectly rather than directly. The central nervous system (CNS) is thus a nontraditional target for sex steroids.

Other neuroendocrine variables Research also suggests that abnormal fluctuations in thyroid, cortisol, prolactin, mineralocorticoids, prostaglandins (PGs), and endogenous opiates correspond to mood changes during the menstrual cycle. In addition, women with PMDD have a brief, transient, heightened cortisol response to ovine (o) corticotropin-releasing hormone (CRH) stimulation, blunted cortisol responses to serotonergic agonists in the late luteal phase, and lower evening plasma cortisol levels. Alterations in phase but not amplitude measures of cortisol have been found in women with PMDD during the menstrual cycle. These findings suggest a physiological dysfunction between the hypothalamic-pituitary-adrenocortical (HPA) and the hypothalamic-pituitary-ovarian (HPO) axis for women with PMDD. This relationship may be complex and include a variety of other systems in its interaction.

Neurotransmitters Current research suggests that neurotransmitter abnormalities in PMDD are similar to those implicated in major depressive disorder. Specifically, PMDD patients have been differentiated from normal control patients by deficiencies in the serotonergic system. Investigators have found that women with PMDD have reduced platelet uptake of serotonin 1 week before menstruation, low whole blood serotonin during the last 10 days of the menstrual cycle, and an abnormal response to tryptophan loading in the late luteal phase. SSRIs (e.g., fluoxetine, sertraline, paroxetine, fluvoxamine) have been found to be efficacious in the treatment of PMDD. The efficacy of this pharmacological class is further evidenced by the FDA approval of fluoxetine and sertraline for PMDD. Recent work has shown that fluoxetine, citalopram, clomipramine, and sertraline can be effective if administered intermittently during the luteal phase. Further work is necessary to corroborate these findings. This medication regimen may be preferable to some women who do not wish to take chronic medication for a periodic condition. Women on a luteal dosing schedule generally reach response rates of 65%, with some women experiencing no significant benefits. This response rate may be reduced by nonadherence with a luteal phase dosing regimen.

In addition to serotonin, norepinephrine has been examined as another neurotransmitter that might contribute to PMDD. However, trials comparing fluoxetine to bupropion, sertraline to desipramine, and paroxetine to maprotiline demonstrate that augmenting noradrenergic activity alone is not effective for the treatment of PMDD.

Circadian rhythms Besides antidepressant medication, sleep and light therapies also have been found to be beneficial in reducing symptoms. The efficacy of these treatments is based on a chronobiological hypothesis of depression. Chronobiological investigations indicate that people with major depressive disorder may have disruptions in the internal regulation of rapid eye movement (REM) sleep propensity, temperature, cortisol, and melatonin, which occur throughout the 24-h daily cycle. Furthermore, the oscillator regulating these circadian rhythms may be desynchronized with the sleep–wake cycle. External cues, such as bright light, play an important role in the modulation and synchronization of these circadian rhythms. For example, exposure to 500 lux of light acutely suppresses melatonin secretion, a marker for circadian phase position. Light also shifts circadian rhythms and melatonin. Research indicates that patients with affective illness may be supersensitive to the suppressive effects of light on melatonin secretion, possibly due to inadequate exposure to daytime light; they may have altered amplitude of melatonin secretion and body temperature.

There may be differences between men and women in the regulation or expression of circadian rhythms. Compared with men, menstruating women have a shorter free-running period (i.e., length of time of a rhythm in an environment free of external cues, such as light), longer sleep duration, and lower amplitude in body temperature that varies with phases of the menstrual cycle. These findings suggest that reproductive hormones (including testosterone) affect circadian rhythm amplitude and synchronization. Indeed, comparative studies in rodents show that estrogen advances and progesterone delays circadian rhythms. Estrogen also appears to enhance synchronization between the oscillators.

Thus, fluctuations of menstrual cycle hormones may alter circadian rhythmicity. Instability of circadian rhythms resulting from changing reproductive hormonal levels may increase the risk for depression in some women. Chronobiological hypotheses contend that disrupted circadian rhythmicity is a factor contributing to depression. Women with PMDD have been reported to have decreased melatonin amplitudes, higher nocturnal body temperatures, and disturbances in the timing and amplitude of prolactin and thyroid-stimulating hormone (TSH) secretion. Also, the offset and duration of the melatonin rhythm may be disturbed and show an abnormal response to light. Light and sleep therapies may relieve PMDD symptoms by helping to realign underlying circadian clocks.

Psychological Model

In this model, women experiencing pathological premenstrual symptoms are distinguished from healthy women on the basis of the way they perceive or react to the environment. Therefore, treatment of PMDD is often directed toward physical activity, psychotherapy, relaxation training, support groups, and stress management.

One psychological model has studied PMDD from a state-dependent learning perspective, while biological markers tend to be trait dependent. Compared with healthy subjects, women with menstrually related mood disorders report more negative life events and greater distress associated with those events only in the late luteal phase of the cycle. Thus, symptoms are conceptualized as occurring in an experiential state, such as the late luteal phase, which is characterized by affective and cognitive components. In support of the state-dependent model, women with severe premenstrual symptoms were more likely to use emotionally based coping techniques (i.e., catharsis) in the premenstrual phase than other strategies, such as cognitive reappraisal. Also during this phase, women with premenstrual dysphoria may be more likely than healthy controls to seek social support when perceiving daily stressors as uncontrollable.

Other findings fail to support the state-dependent hypothesis. Woods and colleagues suggested that a general stressful life context predicts premenstrual symptoms more than stress experienced during a particular menstrual cycle phase. A stressful milieu was a large predictor of perimenstrual symptoms and especially negative affect. Major life stressors play an important role in the development of depressive symptoms; however, the cumulative effect of daily stressors may be more influential in the generation of global premenstrual symptoms.

Type of stressor may also affect the manifestation of symptoms. For example, some research indicates that women with premenstrual dysphoria experience negative interpersonal interactions. Kuczmierczyk, Labrum, and Johnson found that women with PMDD perceive their work and especially their family lives as more stressful. Increased conflict and less self-sufficiency and assertiveness were noted in family environments of PMDD patients, which suggest that enmeshed and rigid family structures may have a role in the development of PMDD. These types of family structures have been previously implicated in other somatization processes.

In addition to disturbances in mood, women with PMDD may experience physical and cognitive changes. Cognitive deficits in major depression have been well documented and often include disturbances in attention, forgetfulness, psychomotor retardation, and proneness to confusion. In some cases, these cognitive disturbances may be secondary to mood disturbances. However, in the case of PMDD, the role reproductive hormone fluctuation may have on memory and cognitive functioning recently has been the focus of several studies. In healthy women without psychiatric illness, performance on neuropsychological tests has been found to vary with the monthly fluctuation in reproductive hormones. High levels of E2, as experienced in the late follicular phase, may elevate performance on automatization abilities, perceptual motor speed, mental arithmetic, and verbal memory. Lower levels of E2, as experienced during the menstrual phase, may be associated with higher performance on visuospatial tasks. The majority of these effects have been subtle and were not able to be replicated; this effect may be due to difficulties in documentation and measurement of ovulation, plasma hormone levels, mood symptoms, and individual variation in cycle length. Furthermore, cyclic performance changes are minor and are unlikely to interfere with normal functioning.

Social Model

From the earliest times, various facets of women's personalities, capabilities, and moods have been attributed to menstruation. Instability, resulting from women's reproductive cycles, has been used to justify denying women equal access to education and employment. One feminist model maintains that premenstrual syndrome pathologizes a naturally occurring phenomenon. Theorists state that high prevalence rates of premenstrual symptoms support this assumption and that the distinction of a separate pathological disorder is a spurious dichotomy. Based on historical comparisons of PMS and hysteria, writers have suggested that the use of a biological explanation for this disorder may legitimize societal prejudices. Furthermore, social theorists state that the medical model may pathologize normal biological processes and oversimplify women's feelings, problems, and conflicts through the diagnosis of PMDD. In fact, medical investigations have revealed that increases in cyclicity can be viewed as adaptive because it leads to homeostasis, stabilization, and longevity in life. Thus, it is the diagnosis of PMDD that leads to the medicalization of women's experiences of the menstrual cycle and not the cycle-related changes themselves. It is suggested that PMDD is a socially constructed disorder rather than a psychiatric disorder.

Since Western society is a contributory factor in this model, research on the prevalence of PMDD in other cultures is of importance in understanding the universality of symptoms. A limited number of studies have examined symptoms of PMDD in non-Western societies. This research has been plagued by a number of important methodological concerns and questionable validity of instruments that have been translated for use in populations other than those in which they were developed. In addition, the sociopolitical position of women in other cultures and their societal beliefs and expectations about menstruation are difficult to quantify and thus have not been taken into account. Despite these difficulties, cross-cultural studies are of interest in considering the relative importance of biological versus sociological factors in the etiology of PMDD. Investigative studies have indicated a widespread variance in the type and severity of premenstrual symptoms experienced, which supports the interpretation of normal cyclical change. Eriksen found that women in developing countries tended to report shifts in mood associated with the onset of menstruation or throughout the menstrual cycle. Several studies have found reports of higher rates of somatic than affective symptoms in populations outside the United States, suggesting that culture may influence the symptoms that women notice, as well as the symptoms they determine to be problematic during the premenstrual period. As a result of these observed cross-cultural differences, menstrual socialization has been proposed as a determinant of premenstrual complaints. These findings suggest that PMDD is a culture-bound syndrome specific to Western cultures in which most women have been socialized to have negative expectations about menstruation. More specifically, it is argued that North American culture and media perpetuate the idea that the premenstrual period will be associated with negative affect and mood instability, causing women to interpret normal physiological changes that are essentially neutral in nature to have negative connotations.

Emergence of a Biopsychosocial Model

Since the relatively recent invention of radioimmunoassays, biomedical research has clearly dominated the area of PMDD. Because PMDD symptoms are associated with hormonal fluctuations, cultural and psychological phenomena associated with the disorder have often been ignored in scientific research, which has resulted in a poor integration of the findings. In the field of depression and other mood disorders, multidimensional theoretical models have emerged and contributed greatly to understanding the experience of depression for an individual. In addition, exploring the interaction of biological, psychological, and social processes has expanded the range of treatment options and provided individuals who suffer from depression effective alternatives to medication. For similar reasons, an integrative approach could greatly benefit research and clinical work in the area of premenstrual mood disturbances. A two-phase approach to encompass a comprehensive biopsychosocial perspective is recommended, with the first phase emphasizing self-monitoring through charting, stress management, and dietary and exercise programs. In addition, cognitive-behavioral coping strategies and reattribution training may help alleviate symptoms. The second phase consists of a pharmacological approach to mitigate biological aspects contributing to PMDD.

In the area of affective illness, a social zeitgeber theory of mood disturbance has been one unifying hypothesis linking biological and psychosocial models. Social zeitgebers are personal relationships, social demands, or tasks that entrain biological rhythms. Similar to the effect of light, social events are external regulators that synchronize circadian rhythms. For instance, marriage, birth of a child, divorce, and loss of a job are social events that disrupt natural mealtimes, sleeping times, and times of activity, which affect the stability of biological rhythms. In individuals predisposed to affective disruption, disturbances in the biological clock may develop into a state of ongoing desynchronization as observed in major depression. Social rhythm disruptions also have been implicated in the onset of manic episodes. Ehlers and colleagues suggested that both interpersonal psychotherapy and cognitive-behavioral therapy, two empirically supported treatments for depression, address the regularity of social routine. In addition, they state that the model is likely to be influenced by personality factors, gender, social support, coping, genetic/familial loading, and past treatment experience.

Adoption of the social zeitgeber model for premenstrual mood disturbances may potentially elucidate the interaction of important psychosocial and biological etiological variables. Socially, women may be particularly prone to respond more dramatically to interpersonal conflicts because they may rely on social zeitgebers, or social relationships, more than men. Some feminist models may explain this perspective. For instance, Carol Gilligan proposed that women may view relationships in terms of interconnections and caring, and men may view relationships in terms of hierarchy and power. Developmental research has documented that girls may be more likely to engage in prosocial behavior than boys. On self-report measures, women are often more empathetic and nurturing than men. The emphasis that women may place on connection with others possibly serves as a vulnerability to a mood disturbance; interpersonal disruptions may have a greater impact on women than on men. Animal and human studies have also shown that responses to social interactions can lead to fluctuations in whole blood serotonin levels. Therefore, women may be able to regulate serotonin function by seeking appropriately rewarding social interactions; the inability to seek or receive the social interactions could lead to further physiological dysregulation via circadian rhythm disruption and/or reduction of serotonin, manifesting as symptoms of PMDD.

At the same time, this increased need for social support may be more adaptive in the long term; women may cope with stress, such as job loss or a death, better than men. Therefore, the increased variation in mood may be more adaptive by enhancing the mechanism of homeostasis, thus protecting women against other types of long-standing illness and increasing longevity.

These correlations between behavior and neuroendocrinology have also been explored within a framework of functional hypothalamic amenorrhea. For some time, researchers have noted that psychosocial variables, such as exercise, personality traits, and environmental stress, have the potential to induce ovarian acyclicity by inhibiting the release of gonadotropin-releasing hormone (GnRH) through mediating variables, such as CRH, endogenous opioids, dopamine, and TSH. Further work in this area potentially could elucidate important somato-psychic interactions, which are key to understanding the etiology of PMDD.

The biological, psychological, and social approaches to PMDD taken independently do not take into account the more complex relationships that formulate the disorder. Practically, it may be useful to examine PMDD through a single pathway that focuses on main effects and a linear relationship. However, lack of attention to the cluster of influences and their dynamic relations may oversimplify pathways as to how individuals develop severe premenstrual disturbances. Increasingly, the biopsychosocial model of PMDD is being examined to generate a more comprehensive model. Although great strides have been made in the past decade in increasing our understanding of PMDD, we must continue to supplement current approaches with research that focuses on more complex interactions among various factors. This future direction can only be accomplished through the continued interdisciplinary effort on a multivariate, biopsychosocial approach to PMDD.

Further Reading

Blak, F., Salkovskis, P., Gath, D., et al. (1998). Cognitive therapy for premenstrual syndrome: a controlled study. *Journal of Psychosomatic Research* **45**(4), 307–318.

Dimmock, P. W., Wyatt, K. M., Jones, P. W., et al. (2000). Efficacy of selective serotonin-reuptake inhibitors in premenstrual syndrome: a systematic review. *Lancet (North American Edition)* **356**, 1131–1136.

Endicott, J. (2000). History, evaluation and diagnosis of premenstrual dysphoric disorder. *Jounral of Clinical Psychiatry* **61**(12), 5–8.

Eriksson, E., Andersch, B., Ho, H. P., et al. (2002). Diagnosis and treatment of premenstrual dysphoria. *Journal of Clinical Psychiatry* **63**(7), 16–23.

Halbreich, U., Bergeron, R., Yonkers, K. A., et al. (2002). Efficacy of intermittent, luteal phase sertraline treatment of premenstrual dysphoric disorder. *Obstetrics & Gynecology* **100**(6), 1219–1229.

Parry, B. L. (2001). The role of central serotonergic dysfunction in the aetiology of premenstrual dysphoric disorder: therapeutic implications. *CNS Drugs* **15**(4), 277–285.

Parry, B. L. and Berga, S. L. (2002). Premenstrual dysphoric disorder. In: Arnold, A. P., Etgen, A. M., Fahrbach, S. E. & Rubin, R. T. (eds.) *Hormones, brain, and behavior* (vol. 5, chap. 99) pp. 531–552. New York: Academic Press/Elsevier Science.

Parry, B. L., Berga, S. L., Mostofi, N., et al. (1989). Morning vs. evening light treatment of late luteal phase dysphoric disorder. *American Journal of Psychiatry* **146**, 1215–1217.

Ross, L. E. and Steiner, M. (2003). A biopsychosocial approach to premenstrual dysphoric disorder. *Psychiatric Clinics of North America* **26**, 259–546.

Schmidt, P. J., Nieman, L. K., Danaceau, M. A., et al. (1998). Differential behavioral effects of gonadal steroids in women with and in those without premenstrual syndrome. *The New England Journal of Medicine* **338**, 209–216.

Caregivers, Stress and

S H Zarit
Pennsylvania State University, University Park, PA, USA
K Bottigi and J E Gaugler
University of Minnesota, Minneapolis, USA

This is a revised version of the article by S H Zarit and J E Gaugler, Encyclopedia of Stress First Edition, volume 1, pp 404–407, © 2000, Elsevier Inc.

Glossary

Burden — The emotional, psychological, physical, and financial challenges assumed by caregivers.

Caregiver — Person who provides informal (i.e., unpaid) assistance provided to a disabled individual, such as an adult child providing help to an elderly parent with Alzheimer's disease or an associated dementia.

Objective burden — The disruptions and degree of changes caregivers experience in various life domains.

Stress process model — A multidimensional framework that examines the proliferation or spread of stress from care-related dimensions to other life domains to global indicators of well-being.

Subjective appraisals/burden — Emotional reactions to stressors, such as fatigue or feelings of being trapped.

Wear and tear hypothesis — Posits that the longer a caregiver remains in her or his role, the more likely it is that negative outcomes will occur.

With increasing longevity and improvements in medical treatment for a range of chronic diseases, more people are surviving to advanced ages. Although most older people are healthy and independent, a significant minority suffer from a variety of physical, cognitive, and psychiatric disabilities that require regular ongoing care and supervision. Despite the visibility of nursing homes and other institutions, families provide the largest part of informal (i.e., unpaid) long-term care assistance to disabled older adults in the United States, and a major emphasis of public care policy is to keep older adults in community settings and under the care of families or other informal providers in order to reduce the need for nursing home care.

Families have always cared for their elders, but changes in contemporary society have placed increasing strains on their resources to provide assistance. Elders are living longer after the onset of disabilities, and many suffer from severe chronic disabilities that necessitate extensive care. With women increasingly employed outside the home, the role of caregiver falls either on a spouse, who may have his or her own age-related limitations, or on a daughter or daughter-in-law, who must balance the multiple roles of worker, homemaker, caregiver, and, in some cases, mother to her own young children. It is not surprising, then, that much of the emphasis in research on caregiving has focused on the stressors and emotional strains of informal care. Early research focused on correlates of burden, or the emotional, psychological, physical, and financial challenges assumed by caregivers, as well as caregivers' subjective appraisals of how task performance affects their lives. However, the past two decades have seen the development of sophisticated conceptual models to capture the longitudinal dynamics of family care, as well as the development of psychosocial interventions to alleviate negative outcomes in informal long-term care systems.

Caregiving Burden

Early research on family caregivers to older adults suffering from chronic illnesses such as Alzheimer's disease often attempted to correlate contextual variables (e.g., duration of care, relationship of caregiver to care recipient) and care demands (e.g., severity of behavior problems, intensity of cognitive impairment, extent of activities of daily life [ADL] dependencies) with unidimensional constructs representing burden. Burden was often operationalized as the caregiver's subjective experience of care demands. Subsequent research suggested that burden was a multidimensional construct, with objective and subjective components. Objective indices of burden reflect the disruptions and degree of changes caregivers experience in various life domains, while subjective burden refers to caregivers' emotional reactions to care demands. Studies that incorporate this conceptualization of burden have found that different factors are associated with objective and subjective burden, underscoring the theoretical usefulness in approaching the demands of caregiving as multifaceted.

Other research has moved beyond the caregiver's subjective experience to consider the physiological effects of stress. The chronic stress of caregiving has been found to increase a caregiver's risk for health problems. This increased risk of illness is attributable to an overproduction of stress hormones and/or a decline in the use of preventative health measures by the caregiver, such as having annual physical exams, exercising, and having a healthy diet. Research examining caregiving at other points in the life span suggests that the burdens associated with informal care provision to a chronically ill care recipient can have negative implications at the cellular level, including shortened telomere length, reduced telomerase activity, and increased oxidative stress.

The Stress Process

With the greater concern given to the multidimensionality of caregiving stress and the various factors that account for such outcomes, conceptual models were developed to capture the process of informal long-term care. Perhaps the most noteworthy model is the stress process model (SPM), which is largely grounded in sociological perspectives of stress. Specifically, this approach suggests that the occurrence of some environmental demand that is potentially harmful (primary objective stressor) has an immediate impact on the caregiver's life (primary subjective stressor), for example, leading to feelings of overload or to the loss of valued aspects of the relationship with the other person. This immediate impact may proliferate into other areas of life (secondary role strains), for instance, interfering with employment or creating conflict in the family, and thereby increase the likelihood of poor adaptation (e.g., negative mental or physical health outcomes). Conversely, resources such as social support and coping skills can contain the primary stressors, limiting their impact on other roles and relationships and on well-being. Although this model was developed specifically for caregivers of Alzheimer's patients, its grounding in general sociological theory makes it potentially applicable to caregivers of older adults with other kinds of disabilities and impairments.

Longitudinal Effects of Caregiving

Much of the literature on caregiving is cross-sectional, that is, a one-time snapshot of the caregiver's situation. Many of these studies have attempted to explore the wear and tear hypothesis, which posits that the longer a caregiver remains in her or his role, the more likely it is that negative outcomes, such as caregiver distress or even care recipient institutionalization, will occur. Longitudinal studies, however, make it possible to examine the dynamic interplay of stressors and adaptation. These studies support more complex views of the longitudinal progression of caregiving than that suggested by the wear and tear hypothesis. Several panel studies of dementia caregiving have found an adaptation effect, in which caregivers who remain in the role report decreases in negative emotional and psychological outcomes, such as burden and depression. These studies have supported counter hypotheses that emphasize the ability of families to tolerate once stressful situations or to adapt to and successfully manage chronic caregiving demands and stressors.

Other analyses have examined various transition points that can occur in informal long-term care, such as onset, institutionalization, and bereavement. While few analyses consider onset of informal care responsibilities, recent research suggests that individuals who experienced less abrupt entries into their caregiving roles are more likely to delay nursing home placement as well as indicate decreases in emotional distress and depression over time. Such findings imply that how people assume care responsibilities or manage problems early in their careers has important longitudinal implications, particularly in chronic diseases.

Given the potential public and private costs of nursing home placement, a number of studies have examined the influence of caregiving indicators (e.g., stress, sociodemographic context) on institutionalization. Several indicators have been identified as potential triggers of nursing home placement. Caregiving stressors (such as feelings of overload or feeling trapped by caregiving responsibilities), depression, or impaired subjective health appear likely to expedite placement and, in some instances, appear more likely to trigger institutionalization than functional indicators of the older care recipient. Other promising work in this area has emphasized that institutionalization is not an endpoint in caregiving. Caregivers remain involved in care and various dimensions of emotional distress and psychological well-being are relatively stable after nursing home placement. Similar studies have emphasized the complex progression of stress and depression of informal caregivers prior to and following bereavement.

Psychosocial Interventions for Caregivers

A major emphasis in the field has been the development of programs, services, and other interventions designed to relieve the stress of caregivers. Increasingly, these interventions have used stress theory to identify modifiable features of the stress process that can lead to improved outcomes. The most successful interventions with caregivers have been multidimensional, addressing several dimensions of the stress process. Another common component of these interventions has been inclusion of the wider family network in treatment, usually through one or two family meetings. Help from families may be particularly useful, since it is flexible and personal. Family level interventions can also address conflict and misunderstandings about the nature of the elder's disease or how care is being provided. Outcomes of these interventions have included reduced subjective burden, lower negative appraisals of the elder's behavior, decreased depression, and delayed institutionalization. Some of these effects have been found to persist or even increase for 3 years or more beyond the intervention period. Interventions designed to reduce depressive behaviors for elders with comorbid depression and dementia have also been found to have corresponding benefits for caregivers' own feelings of depression and subjective burden.

Another way of addressing the stress on family caregivers is by initiating formal, paid help. A variety of services are available to elders and their families, including care management, in-home respite, and adult day services. The impact of these programs on caregivers' stress and well-being has been mixed. It is often the case, however, that caregivers included in these studies have received only low levels of assistance. In the one study that controlled for amount of exposure to the intervention, caregivers who used adult day services on a regular basis for 3 months or more experienced decreased overload, emotional strain, and depressive symptoms compared to a control group. This issue of therapeutic exposure is particularly relevant for caregiving research. Caregivers who are faced with multiple, chronic, and severe stressors are not likely to gain much benefit from brief or unfocused interventions.

Further Reading

Epel, E. S., Blackburn, E. H., Lin, J., et al. (2004). Accelerated telomere shortening in response to life stress. *Proceedings of the National Academy of Sciences of the United States of America* **101**, 17312–17315.

Gaugler, J. E., Kane, R. L., Kane, R. A., Clay, T. and Newcomer, R. (2003). Predicting institutionalization of cognitively impaired older people: utilizing dynamic predictors of change. *The Gerontologist* **43**, 219–229.

Gaugler, J. E., Zarit, S. H. and Pearlin, L. I. (2003). The onset of dementia caregiving and its longitudinal implications. *Psychology and Aging* **18**, 171–180.

Mittelman, M. S., Roth, D. L., Coon, D. W. and Haley, W. E. (2004). Sustained benefit of supportive intervention for depressive symptoms in caregivers of patients with Alzheimer's disease. *American Journal of Psychiatry* **161**, 850–856.

Montgomery, R. J. V., Gonyea, J. G. and Hooyman, N. R. (1985). Caregiving and the experience of subjective and objective burden. *Family Relations* **34**, 19–26.

Pearlin, L. I., Mullan, J. T., Semple, S. J. and Skaff, M. M. (1990). Caregiving and the stress process: an overview of concepts and their measures. *The Gerontologist* **30**, 583–594.

Pinquart, M. and Sorensen, S. (2003). Associations of stressors and uplifts of caregiving with caregiver burden and depressive mood: A meta-analysis. *Journal of Gerontology* **58B**(2), P112–P128.

Roth, D., Haley, W., Owen, J., Clay, O. and Goode, K. (2001). Latent growth models of the longitudinal effects of dementia caregiving: a comparison of African-American and White family caregivers. *Psychology and Aging* **16**, 427–436.

Schulz, R., Mendelsohn, A. B., Haley, W. E., et al. (2003). End-of-life care and the effects of bereavement on family caregivers of persons with dementia. *New England Journal of Medicine* **349**, 1936–1942.

Schulz, R., Belle, S. H., Czaja, S. J., et al. (2004). Long-term care placement of dementia patients and caregiver health and well-being. *Journal of the American Medical Association* **292**, 961–967.

Sorensen, S., Pinquart, M., Habil, X. and Duberstein, P. (2002). How effective are interventions with caregivers? An updated meta-analysis. *The Gerontologist* **42**, 356–372.

Vitaliano, P. P., Zhang, J. and Scanlan, J. M. (2003). Is caregiving hazardous to one's physical health? A meta-analysis. *Psychological Bulletin* **129**, 946–972.

Zarit, S. H. and Leitsch, S. A. (2001). Developing and evaluating community based intervention programs for Alzheimer's patients and their caregivers. *Aging and Mental Health* **5**(Supplement), S84–S98.

Zarit, S. H., Reever, K. E. and Bach-Peterson, J. (1980). Relatives of the impaired elderly: correlates of feelings of burden. *The Gerontologist* **20**(6), 649–655.

Zarit, S. H., Stephens, M. A. P., Townsend, A. and Greene, R. (1998). Stress reduction for family caregivers: Effects of day care use. *Journal of Gerontology: Social Sciences* **53B**, S267–S277.

Childbirth and Stress

S Ayers and E Ford
University of Sussex, Brighton, UK

Glossary

Baby blues	A short period of mood swings and emotional reactivity in the 2 weeks following childbirth.
Epidural anesthesia	Analgesia injected into the space around the spinal cord to block pain in the abdomen.
Episiotomy	A cut made to the woman's perineum to help the baby be delivered.
Intrapartum	During labor.
Oxytocin	A hormone used to induce labor and stimulate contractions of the uterus.
Parity	Number of live children born to a woman.
Polymorphic (cycloid) psychosis	Psychosis with rapidly changing and variable psychotic symptoms and emotional states as a cardinal feature.
Postnatal depression	Depressive disorder in women in the year following childbirth.
Postpartum	After childbirth.
Prophylaxis	Measures taken to prevent a disease.
Puerperal	Pertaining to childbirth.

Introduction

Childbirth is an intense event that involves extreme physical stress and carries emotional, cognitive, social, and cultural significance. Physically, women have to cope with acute changes as the uterus contracts, the cervix dilates, and the baby and placenta are delivered. General responses to stress such as release of endorphins, epinephrine, and catecholamines have been shown in laboring women, as well as increases in cardiac output and blood pressure. Emotionally, labor and the birth of the baby usually involve intense positive and negative emotions. Cognitive demands are also placed on the woman as she copes with the events of birth. Interpersonal dynamics between the woman and her birth partner and medical attendants can be supportive or can increase stress levels if birth attendants are perceived as unhelpful or dismissive. Finally, birth and motherhood are associated with many cultural expectations and perceived norms. In Western societies, for example, birth is highly medicalized, yet often emphasis is placed on women trying to achieve a so-called natural birth with minimal intervention or pain relief.

Childbirth is therefore an intense acute stressor that many women go through. It also enables the study of the interaction between pre-event and event factors in perceived stress and the effect of this on physical and psychological outcomes. This is consistent with the diathesis stress approach to health outcome, in which pre-existing vulnerability (physical, psychological, and social) interacts with event characteristics to determine outcomes. However, the classification of childbirth as an acute stressor is rather artificial, and the impact of childbirth must be placed in the context of previous adjustment to pregnancy and postnatal adjustment to motherhood and a new baby, both of which are also potentially stressful and difficult.

Research into the role of psychosocial factors in birth outcome has generally established that psychosocial factors are important in physical outcomes, such as morbidity and mortality, and psychological outcomes, such as maternal satisfaction and psychopathology. The postnatal period is associated with a number of psychological problems that are seen as specific to childbirth, namely, the baby blues, postnatal depression, and puerperal psychosis. However, it is still debated whether childbirth has specific effects that distinguish postnatal psychopathology from psychopathology occurring at other times. More recently, childbirth has also been linked with posttraumatic stress disorder.

The experience of birth and the outcome of birth are therefore influenced by multiple psychosocial factors. The importance of these factors varies for different outcomes and between individuals. For example, a woman with a history of psychological problems may have a high vulnerability to postnatal psychopathology, so other factors during and after birth may not be as important as they are for a woman with no previous history of psychological problems. This is one of the challenges of research in this area, and it is therefore an area characterized by conflicting findings. It is thus important to consider methodological quality of studies and weight of evidence when drawing conclusions. This article provides a brief overview of some of the current research and understanding of psychosocial factors that are important in three broad areas of birth outcome: physical outcome, maternal satisfaction, and psychopathology; then it looks generally at what conclusions can be drawn regarding childbirth and stress.

Physical Outcome

The physical outcome of birth includes complications during birth, type of labor and delivery, and complications with the infant. As in other areas of health, low socioeconomic status is associated with increased complications of birth (e.g., pre-term labor) and maternal and infant morbidity (e.g., low birth weight) and mortality. It is hypothesized that the effect of low socioeconomic status is due to material deprivation but is mediated by psychosocial factors such as level of education, access to information, a lack of social support, and negative life events. These in turn may lead to stress, anxiety, lowered self-esteem, and depression, with cognitive problems such as dysfunctional attitudes, which result in a set of maladaptive coping strategies such as learned helplessness and risk taking.

It is well established that the physical outcome of birth can be affected by psychosocial factors during pregnancy and birth such as support or anxiety. In the literature, continuous support during labor has received the most attention. A series of experimental studies has been carried out in countries where it is usual for women to give birth without a birth companion. These studies compare women allocated a doula during birth to women who have no birth companion. A doula is a layperson (usually female) trained in supporting laboring women, but not medically qualified. A review of 15 doula studies involving over 12 000 women showed that women with the continuous support of a birth companion used less analgesia during birth, were less likely to have an operative birth, and were less likely to report dissatisfaction with their birth experiences. In general, continuous support during birth was associated with greater benefits when the provider was not a member of the hospital staff, when the support began early in labor, and in settings in which epidural analgesia was not routinely available.

A number of explanations have been put forward for why support in labor has such a powerful effect on birth outcome, and these typically focus on biological or psychological mechanisms. From a biological perspective it has been hypothesized that the complicated neuroendocrinal control of labor and birth can be disrupted by stress in various ways, reducing the efficacy of the birthing process. For example, it has been posited that labor pain leads to a strong stress response, resulting in increased autonomic activity, uncoordinated uterine contractions, and abnormal fetal heart rate, which all impede the progress of labor. Whether this effect is a direct result of the pain or is mediated by stress or anxiety is not established.

Psychological explanations suggest that support in labor improves outcomes by increasing women's feelings of control and competence, decreasing the stress response, and thereby reducing the necessity for medical interventions. Emotional support may also reduce fear and anxiety and their associated effects.

Maternal Satisfaction

Research looking at maternal satisfaction has largely focused on women's satisfaction with the birth generally and has not looked at specific elements such as satisfaction with coping, birth outcome, and health-care provision. The main factors during birth that have been examined in relation to maternal satisfaction are support during birth, pain relief, perceived control, and levels of intervention during birth. For example, as previously discussed, continuous support during labor is associated with increased maternal satisfaction, as is continuity of care. It was found that women assigned to a one-to-one midwifery care model, who were cared for by the same caregivers throughout their pregnancy and birth, reported significantly more satisfaction with their experience than women assigned to obstetrician-led care who met different caregivers at each visit, without any difference in clinical outcome.

Most research on satisfaction with the birth experience has focused on pain relief, in the belief that if the pain is controlled or alleviated the experience of giving birth will be more positive. This appears to be the case, with studies showing that women who receive more effective pain relief rate their experience as more satisfying. However, most studies have shown that satisfaction is high overall, regardless of pain relief received, suggesting that many other factors are also important. A woman's expectation of the pain may play a role, with research showing that women who expect more pain are likely to be more satisfied afterward. Furthermore, if women expect to be able to give birth without pain relief, they report a decline in satisfaction if they did have to use analgesia, notably epidural anesthesia.

Other factors associated with maternal satisfaction are personal control, having expectations met, and social class. Extensive medical interventions (electronic fetal monitors, episiotomies, perineal shaves, and enemas) are negatively correlated with maternal satisfaction. However, active management of labor (e.g., early rupturing of membranes, vaginal assessments, and early use of oxytocin for slow progress) does not affect women's satisfaction overall compared to routine management.

A systematic review concluded that expectations, support, the quality of the caregiver–patient relationship, and involvement in decision making (control) are the most important factors in determining maternal satisfaction. Secondary factors are pain, socioeconomic status, preparation for birth, interventions, and continuity of care.

Psychopathology

Baby Blues

The baby blues are a period of emotional lability and overreactivity that appears in the first 2 weeks following birth. The blues do not seem to be part of a continuum with postpartum depression or puerperal psychosis, and sadness and depression are not typical features. Instead, women seem to exhibit mood fluctuations such as elation, hostility, tearfulness, and general lability of affect. Some women who experience severe blues will go on to develop postnatal depression. The blues affect between 26 and 85% of women, the variability in figures being due to the fact that the baby blues are not classified as a psychiatric disorder and therefore not uniformly defined.

Several competing theories have been proposed to account for the blues, most notably a hormonal/biological account, suggesting that the large fluctuations in hormones following delivery are responsible. The changes in concentrations of hormones such as estrogen, progesterone, and cortisol are hypothesized to cause a neurotransmitter imbalance, which is expressed by widely fluctuating moods. It has been suggested that this could be evolutionarily adaptive, as this excessive emotionality separates the mother from her usual concerns and makes her available solely for the baby, facilitating mother–baby bonding. Historically, it may also have been responsible for promoting some of the rituals that surround the birth of a baby, such as extensive periods of confinement and good support for the mother. However, there is no consistent evidence linking changes in hormone levels with fluctuating postnatal mood. Other theories suggest that psychosocial factors are important. While demographic factors such as age and race are not predictive of the baby blues, in the West the blues have been associated with economic insecurity and lack of social support. It has also been proposed that it may be a grief reaction in women who have been disappointed with pregnancy and birth events and outcome, and has been shown to be correlated to pessimism in late pregnancy.

The baby blues appear to be time limited and require no specific treatment other than support. However, the blues should be distinguished from depression and sadness in the immediate postpartum period, which is predictive of postnatal depression later.

Postnatal Depression

Postnatal depression (PND) is the most well known of postpartum psychiatric disorders. Between 10 and 20% of women are believed to suffer from it during the first year after birth. However, the disease still remains underdiagnosed and undertreated. Recently, controlled studies have shown there is no significant difference between postnatal women and appropriate female controls in the incidence of depression. Therefore, postnatal women are no more at risk of developing depression than at other times in their lives. However, it is argued that PND has a greater psychosocial impact than depression at other times in a woman's life, as it can cause considerable strain in relationships and family life, affect the mother–infant relationship, and possibly also affect the infant's development. Currently self-report scales are used to screen for depression in postnatal women. These screening tools can be a useful measure for identifying women at risk, although patients who score above threshold on screening questionnaires are heterogeneous and may be suffering from anxiety, obsessive, or posttraumatic stress disorders.

Like the baby blues, postnatal depression has also been postulated to be a result of a hormone imbalance in the period following birth. A large drop in levels of estrogen and progesterone occurs after birth, suggesting that postpartum mood changes can be explained by the effect of the withdrawal of these hormones. This has been supported by studies in which women were administered these hormones in the postpartum period, resulting in alleviation of the depression. A further hypothesis is that hormonal changes trigger pathological mechanisms at the neurotransmitter level, resulting in depression. However, many studies measuring levels of hormones in women after birth have found no differences in hormone concentrations between women with and without depression, suggesting that the link between hormone levels and depression is weak if not nonexistent.

It has been argued that because prevalence of PND is no greater than depression in women in general, PND should be seen as primarily a psychosocial disorder. Studies have shown associations with previous depression and other psychiatric illness, stressful life events, and disturbed relationships. Other predictors include high parity, stress in pregnancy, social isolation, material deprivation, and low social support. A history of depression, and depression during pregnancy, appear to be some of the strongest predictors of PND. Furthermore, genetic factors have been shown to explain 25–38% of the variance. The psychosocial model would suggest that good social support following childbirth would protect women from depression, and studies seem to bear this out. If, as suggested, prevalence of depression postnatally is not greater than prevalence in women of childbearing age in general, and if PND is related to similar factors to depression in nonpostnatal women, it may be hypothesized that PND is not a separate illness from depression in general.

Puerperal Psychosis

Puerperal psychosis (PP) is a rare disorder occurring in about one woman in a thousand following childbirth. It generally takes the form of mania, severe depression (with delusions, confusion, or stupor), or acute polymorphic (cycloid) psychosis. It does not overlap completely with bipolar mood disorder, although there is evidence of a link between the two, especially as the majority of patients presenting with a severe postpartum psychiatric disorder appear to have a cycloid psychosis. It has been proposed that PP may be one of a spectrum of bipolar disorders. In susceptible women, childbirth, abortion, and even menstruation can trigger bipolar episodes. However, other researchers propose that PP has a pattern of symptoms unlike any other psychiatric disorder; for example, patients exhibit a high rate of disorientation, confusion, and depersonalization. Hallucinations appear in about half of patients with PP, suggesting an overlap with schizophrenia, and mania is not as pronounced in postpartum patients as in those with a diagnosis of bipolar disorder. Thus, some argue that PP is a separate disorder from other psychoses.

Puerperal psychosis appears to be highly heritable, with 10–25% of relatives of women with PP having some kind of severe psychiatric disorder. It also tends to recur, with a chance of about 1 in 4 in each pregnancy. It can be treated safely with newer neuroleptic drugs. In certain circumstances electroconvulsive therapy can be useful, and lithium has been explored as a prophylaxis.

Postnatal Posttraumatic Stress Disorder

Posttraumatic stress disorder (PTSD) is characterized by three types of symptoms: re-experiencing (flashbacks, nightmares), avoidance (of reminders of the stressor, emotional numbing), and hyperarousal (insomnia, difficulties concentrating). There is converging evidence that approximately one-third of women appraise their birth experience as traumatic and 1–2% of women will develop PTSD after childbirth. Case studies suggest that the disorder might result in an impaired mother–baby relationship, sexual dysfunction, and fear of subsequent childbirth (tokophobia), although this has not yet been confirmed by quantitative research.

Studies of factors associated with postnatal PTSD suggest an interaction between prenatal factors, birth experience, and postnatal factors. The type of delivery appears to be important, with women who undergo operative deliveries more at risk of postnatal PTSD. However, this is not a consistent finding. Indeed, one study noted that the majority of women with PTSD had an obstetrically normal vaginal delivery. Thus, in common with PTSD following other events, there is unlikely to be a direct relationship between the severity of birth and PTSD. Other labor and birth characteristics variously associated with rating birth as traumatic are medical intervention, pain in first stage, a long labor, feelings of powerlessness, and receiving inadequate information. PTSD has been associated with feelings of fear for self and baby during labor and birth. It has also been found that low control, higher trait anxiety, and greater fear were associated with symptoms of PTSD.

Several prenatal vulnerability factors have been investigated, and those that emerge as important are a history of trauma or psychological problems and possibly trait anxiety. Dysfunctional attitudes are predictive of postpartum depressive symptoms, and it has been hypothesized that there are cognitive vulnerabilities to PTSD as well, although this has not yet been examined in relation to postnatal PTSD. Postnatally, social and professional support in the period after birth may be a protective factor, and aftercare trauma services might be useful. Several studies have analyzed the effectiveness of debriefing services with a midwife or doctor following birth in preventing PTSD, but results have been inconsistent.

Conclusion

The association between different psychosocial factors and the outcomes discussed in this article demonstrates the complexity of this field. In summary, physical outcomes are associated with socioeconomic status and continuous support in labor. Maternal satisfaction is associated with expectations, support in labor, the quality of caregiving in labor, and involvement in decision making. Postnatal depression is associated with previous history of depression or other psychiatric illness, additional stressors, and low social support. Puerperal psychosis is associated with a personal history or family history of psychiatric illness. Postnatal PTSD is associated with a history of trauma and psychiatric illness, type of delivery, and life threat.

Models of the interaction between prenatal, birth, and postnatal factors therefore tend to be complex psychosocial models. However, it could be argued that models specific to childbirth are not necessary, as, in many cases, the determinants of postnatal psychopathology are similar to psychopathology at other times. For example, the finding that postnatal depression is associated with previous depression, additional stressors, and low social support is similar to research findings regarding vulnerability to depression generally. Equally, the finding that there is no dose–response relationship between the obstetric severity of birth and postnatal PTSD is comparable to research into PTSD following other events. This etiological similarity between postnatal psychopathology and psychopathology at other times implies that stress and coping processes similar to those in other types of life events act to determine the outcome of childbirth. Therefore, childbirth can be used as a research paradigm with which to study stress processes and outcomes that generalize to other acute life events. As such, it may also help us better understand the complexity of stress processes.

Further Reading

Ayers, S. (2004). Delivery as a traumatic event: prevalence, risk factors, screening and treatment. *Clinical Obstetrics and Gynecology* **47**(3), 552–567.

Brockington, I. (2004). Postpartum psychiatric disorders. *The Lancet* **363**, 303–310.

Brownridge, P. (1995). The nature and consequences of childbirth pain. *European Journal of Obstetrics and Gynaecology and Reproductive Biology* **59**(supplement), S9–S15.

Clement, S. and Page, L. (eds.) (1998). *Psychological perspectives on pregnancy and childbirth.* Edinburgh, UK: Churchill Livingston.

Elliott, S. A. (2006). Postnatal depression. In: Ayers, A., Baum, A., Newman, S., McManus, C., Wallston, K., Weinman, J. & West, R. (eds.) *Cambridge handbook of psychology, health and medicine* (2nd edn.). Cambridge, UK: Cambridge University Press.

Goodman, P., Mackay, M., et al. (2004). Factors related to childbirth satisfaction. *Journal of Advanced Nursing* **46**(2), 212–219.

Hodnett, E., Gates, S., et al. (2003). Continuous support for women during childbirth. *The Cochrane Database of Systematic Reviews* **3**, CD003766.

Hodnett, E. D. (2002). Pain and women's satisfaction with the experience of childbirth: a systematic review. *American Journal of Obstetrics and Gynecology* **186**(5, part 2), S160–S172.

Kyman, W. (1991). Maternal satisfaction with the birth experience. *Journal of Social Behaviour and Personality* **6**(1), 57–70.

Quine, L. and Steadman, L. (2006). Pregnancy and childbirth. In: Ayers, A., Baum, A., Newman, S., McManus,

C., Wallston, K., Weinman, J. & West, R. (eds.) *Cambridge handbook of psychology, health and medicine* (2nd edn.). Cambridge, UK: Cambridge University Press.

Robertson, E., Grace, S., et al. (2004). Antenatal risk factors for postpartum depression: a synthesis of recent literature. *General Hospital Psychiatry* **26**(4), 289–295.

Rutter, D. R. and Quine, L. (1990). Inequalities in pregnancy outcome: A review of psychosocial and behavioural mediators. *Social Science and Medicine* **30**(5), 553–568.

Slade, P., MacPherson, S., et al. (1993). Expectations, experiences and satisfaction with labour. *British Journal of Clinical Psychology* **32**, 469–483.

Stanton, A. L., Lobel, M., Sears, S. and DeLuca, R. S. (2002). Psychosocial aspects of selected issues in women's reproductive health: current status and future directions. *Journal of Consulting and Clinical Psychology* **70**(3), 751–770.

Coping Skills

A DeLongis and E Puterman
University of British Columbia, Vancouver, BC, Canada

This is a revised version of the article by A DeLongis and M Preece, Encyclopedia of Stress First Edition, volume 1, pp 532–540, © 2000, Elsevier Inc.

Glossary

Cognitive reappraisal	A form of coping that focuses on changing one's attitudes and beliefs toward a stressful situation.
Coping	Cognitive and behavioral efforts to manage stress.
Emotion-focused coping	Attempts to manage one's emotions during stressful periods.
Problem-focused coping	Attempts to directly change a stressful situation.
Relationship-focused coping	Attempts to manage one's social relationships during stressful periods.

Coping describes cognitive and behavioral responses to a stressful situation. These responses are determined by the interaction between the characteristics of the person and characteristics of the situation. When these responses are particularly effective in reducing strain, due to the expertise with which they are selected and employed, we could say these responses are particularly skillful. When an individual experiences a stressor that threatens to overwhelm current personal resources, such as a chronic illness, an intervention that emphasizes coping skills training can be helpful. However, there is no one coping skill that, once learned, becomes a magic bullet, effective with all kinds of stress. An important part of being a skilled coper is being able to match a stressful situation with the most effective strategy that is appropriate for the given context. Given this, flexibility in coping appears to be a key aspect of effective stress management.

Stress and Coping

Everyone experiences stress at times during his or her life. However, what is extremely stressful to one individual may not be at all stressful to another. How a situation is evaluated, or appraised, is an important determinant of the degree of stress experienced by the individual. Coping is loosely defined as the things we think and actions we take to ameliorate the negative aspects of a stressful situation. How we manage stress is critical because overwhelming stress can cause psychological distress as well as have both short- and long-term negative consequences for physical health. The ability to cope successfully with a stressful situation depends on a number of factors. Primary among these are the resources one brings to the stressful situation. These resources include one's personality, age, financial assets, education, previous experiences, social support, and physical and mental health. Both resources and subjective appraisals are important determinants of the degree of stress experienced by the individual. If a situation is not appraised as taxing one's resources or ability to cope, it may not be experienced as stress at all. Features of the situation, such as the desirability, controllability, and severity of the stressor, are important in shaping coping responses. Certainly there are many types of stressors that are a tremendous strain for almost any individual.

We review here ways of coping with stress. Reviewing the entire literature on effective and maladaptive coping across a multitude of stressors is beyond the scope of this article. Here we focus primarily on chronic illness, which has been the center of a great deal of research. At some point in their lives, all individuals must cope with chronic illness, either personally or through a significant other. Finally, we review evidence-based coping skills interventions.

Ways of Coping

Problem-focused coping Problem solving is a strategy that quickly comes to mind as an effective way of attempting to remedy a negative situation. Defining the problem, generating alternative solutions, comparing these alternatives in terms of their likely costs and benefits, selecting a likely solution, coming up with a plan, and then acting on it are steps that most of us take when we determine a situation to be one that we can do something about. These strategies primarily involve changing aspects of the situation. Other problem-focused coping strategies may be geared toward changing ourselves, such as learning new skills and procedures, thereby increasing one's coping resources.

Many problem-focused coping strategies that can be enumerated as applicable in specific situations do not generalize broadly across all types of stressors. For example, problem-focused strategies used to cope with chronic pain may not be useful for coping with a pressing deadline at work. Even in situations in which problem-focused strategies could be used to great effect, if the individual perceives the level of threat to be very high, it may be impossible for such strategies to be employed effectively. Excessive threat has been found to have negative effects on cognitive functioning and on the capacity for information processing. A common example of this often occurs in a physician's office, when patients are given bad news about their health. At such times, patients may have difficulty comprehending any additional information about treatment and prognosis that the physician may wish to convey. This phenomenon is due to a reduction in cognitive functioning brought about by the patient's experience of feelings of threat or harm.

Another important determinant of problem-focused coping is the individual's perception of the situation as one that is amenable to change. In a study of middle-age people coping with stressful encounters, Lazarus and colleagues found that people adapted better to stress when they used more problem-focused coping for an encounter that the person felt could be manipulated. However, if the encounter was judged as one requiring acceptance, more emphasis was put on emotion-focused coping.

Emotion-focused coping The primary goal of emotion-focused coping is to lessen emotional distress. Some of the ways this may be achieved are through avoidance, distancing, and wishful thinking. Another approach may be to minimize the threat of the situation, for example, via cognitive reappraisal. Cognitive reappraisals involve changing the meaning of the situation without changing it objectively. For example, a stressed person may focus on how much worse things could be, perhaps by comparing him- or herself to others less fortunate. Noting how much better one's situation is than the situation of others is called "engaging in downward social comparisons." There are also emotion-focused strategies directed toward diverting attention from the problem, such as engaging in physical exercise, meditating, having a drink, expressing one's anger, or seeking emotional support. Similar to problem-focused coping, a coping response that is helpful in one situation may be harmful in another. For example, denying the severity of chronic heart disease may be beneficial right after diagnosis to alleviate anxiety and anger, but it is problematic during rehabilitation.

Relationship-focused coping Recently, attention has also been directed toward the ways that people attempt to maintain their important social relationships during periods of stress. People in enduring relationships cannot concern themselves only with the situation they are facing, but must also consider the implications for their partner and for the relationship. This focus on relationships during stressful episodes may be particularly important when a loved one has a chronic illness or disability. For example, O'Brien and DeLongis pointed out the usefulness of empathic coping by caregivers of Alzheimer's patients. Other types of relationship-focused coping involve providing support and attempting to compromise when there is a disagreement. Not all attempts to manage relationships during stressful periods have positive effects. Coyne has found that emotional overinvolvement can have serious negative consequences on the health of family members.

Although some people are more skilled at coping with stress than are others, it is impossible to identify a set of coping strategies that can be called "good" ways of coping. The context in which the stressful situation occurs, the type of problem, the other people involved, and the personality characteristics of the individual are only some of the factors that affect how to best deal with the situation. Further, two people might use identical strategies with different degrees of success, depending on how skillfully the strategy is implemented. However, researchers have pinpointed some general ways of coping that appear to be either adaptive or maladaptive in particular types of situations. A major type of stressor is chronic illness, but differing types of illnesses require different coping skills.

Chronic Illness

Due to medical and technological advances, acute illnesses have given way to increases in chronic illnesses as the primary cause of death in advanced countries. Given the improvements in treatment of chronic illnesses, people who adhere to medical advice can often live relatively normal lives for a long time after diagnosis. It is therefore important to understand how successful adherence and coping with illness can aid in adaptation.

Adherence

Ajzen and Fishbein identified two factors that predict someone's intention to adhere to medical recommendations for a chronic illness, in particular, and to any health behavior, in general. First, a person's attitudes toward the behavior, determined by the extent the person values the outcome of the behavior, predict the person's intentions. Second, this intention is predicted by the perception that important people in the person's life value the behavior and the extent he or she cares about what these people think. Although these factors predict intention well, they fare less well in predicting actual adherence to medical regimens and recommendations for adaptation to chronic illness. People may intend to perform a health behavior but might not if they are not able or ready.

Adhering to health recommendations is often strikingly low, particularly for lifestyle-change recommendations associated with chronic illness. Rates of adherence are influenced by the experience of side effects, treatment complexity (e.g., one pill a day at dinner versus a handful at different times per day, as in some cases of HIV treatment), the quality and quantity of support received from both the health professionals and important others, and cultural norms. Furthermore, some people avoid recommendations from health professionals and do not adhere to a prescribed regimen, and still others may deny that they are at risk as a way of coping with the stress associated with being ill. These methods of coping may have negative consequences for illness progression. Other people may actively cope by strictly sticking to the medical regimen.

Coping with Chronic Illnesses

When confronted with illness, people's physical and psychological worlds often become disrupted. People with chronic illness face potential mental and physical health problems and disruptions in social functioning. Those with chronic illnesses are challenged by having to alter their self-perception, to integrate the concept of being chronically ill into their lives, and to find meaning in their illness and lives. People who find positive meaning in their illnesses and accept the physical, mental, and social changes that occur with a chronic illness adjust better to illnesses than those who do not. In the following sections, we review four major health problems that impact individuals and thus receive increased attention and research: cancer, chronic heart disease, HIV disease, and chronic pain.

Coping with cancer The question of whether psychological factors, such as coping strategies, affect cancer development has intrigued researchers for years. Some research has suggested that a "fighting spirit," or coping by fighting angrily against the diagnosis, may be associated with living longer with cancer, whereas passively accepting ("stoic acceptance") of the disease and feeling hopeless may predict poorer courses. Under some circumstances, people who minimize or deny the illness's impact on their lives and continue on with daily activities also have longer survival rates. In contrast, repressing negative emotions may be linked with speedier cancer progression. Although the jury is out on whether social support and coping effect initiation, disease course, and mortality rates among cancer patients, research clearly indicates that how people psychologically cope with the illness and whether support is received affect the psychological well-being, adjustment, and quality of life of cancer patients. The benefits of psychological interventions are apparent in the emotional lives of cancer patients, even though claims of extending patient's lives may be premature.

Coping with Chronic Heart Disease

Reacting to stress with anxiety and anger has been linked to the development of chronic heart disease (CHD), especially in men. In addition, during the first stage of recovery following a heart attack, coping responses that involve denial and that may serve to reduce anxiety and anger toward the illness appear to be more beneficial than are more active coping strategies. During the first stage of the disease, supportive interventions are often most useful. However, after a patient's discharge from a coronary care unit, more active coping strategies are important. For example, interventions that focus on stress management, as well as educational interventions that emphasize lifestyle changes and compliance with medical advice are important in increasing both health and well-being. Good nutrition and exercise are critical factors in preventing CHD as well as in recovery from a heart attack, and many preventive interventions are focused on changing these health-related behaviors.

Coping with human immunodeficiency virus disease The course of human immunodeficiency virus (HIV) disease often begins with an acute, flulike illness, but then remits into an asymptomatic stage that could last between 2 and 10 years. People with HIV may then cycle among (1) chronic infections, (2) symptoms that lead to a diagnosis of acquired immune deficiency syndrome (AIDS), and (3) back into an asymptomatic stage, depending on the effectiveness of the antiretroviral medications and other factors. The risk of continuously cycling through these stages and the fears associated with them may cause severe distress for those affected by HIV.

When people learn of a positive HIV antibody test result, they usually react with increased psychological distress. Blaming oneself for the illness, denying the reality that one has contracted and is living with HIV, and holding onto false hope have been associated with poor psychological adjustment to HIV disease and lower levels of CD4 cells, markers of immune functioning. On the other hand, those who find meaning and who create positive experiences in their lives tend to fare better psychologically. Finally, active coping strategies that promote taking care of one's health, getting information about the illness, seeking support, and adhering to medication have all been associated with better psychological and physical outcomes for people with HIV.

Psychological interventions for people with HIV disease range from encouraging people to seek out information regarding their illness to helping them weigh the pros and cons of disclosure and drug adherence. Therapists can also help patients plan their drug-adherence schedules and teach them coping skills to deal with potential side effects. As well, psychological interventions may promote psychological adaptation to the illness and help people find meaning in their experience with HIV.

Coping with chronic pain Pain is considered chronic when the symptoms have lasted for a period longer than 6 months. Common types of chronic pain are lower back pain; joint pain as a result of rheumatoid arthritis or osteoarthritis; headaches; pain resulting from chronic illnesses, such as HIV disease and cancer; and various myofascial pain syndromes, usually associated with diffuse musculoskeletal pain. Research has demonstrated that psychosocial factors, such as social support, coping, and patients' beliefs, predict approximately half of the variation of long-term disability resulting from chronic pain.

Most coping efforts are directed toward two main goals: (1) prevention or reduction of pain and (2) maximization of quality of life despite pain. A host of factors, such as the nature of the pain, the expectation of relief, and the specific situation, influences the effectiveness of a particular coping strategy. However, there are consistent findings that point to a relationship between particular classes of coping strategies and the degree of impairment.

Catastrophizing is a cognitive process that includes negative self-statements and excessively negative beliefs about the future. Pain patients may express such things to themselves or to others, saying, "This pain will never go away" or "I can't cope with this pain anymore." Catastrophizing and avoiding activities related to illness-specific exercises and social-leisure activities have been found to be associated with poor outcomes. The diversity of these outcomes is remarkable: increased pain and disability, greater use of the health care system and medication, limited activities, and depressive symptoms in patients with chronic pain.

Probably the most adaptive method of coping with chronic pain involves behaviors or cognitions that divert the person's attention from the pain and toward some more positive experience. Distracting oneself with other activities such as socializing, reading, and painting reduces emphasis on the experience of pain and has beneficial effects on mood as well. Activities requiring a focus of attention tend to reduce the activation of the sympathetic nervous system, leading to further reductions in pain intensity. Guided relaxation, or transformational imagery techniques, in addition to reducing pain, can also serve to increase feelings of self-efficacy.

Structured Coping Programs: Learning How to Cope Effectively

Coping interventions often focus on learning to appraise stressful contexts more adaptively and then to cope more effectively with the demands of these contexts. In other words, reducing the experience of stressors as threatening and adjusting the sense of control people have over the stressors are key to adaptive coping. We review here three evidence-based coping skills interventions designed for patients with chronic illnesses: coping effectiveness training (CET), cognitive-behavioral therapy (CBT), and mindfulness-based therapies.

Coping Effectiveness Training Program

Folkman, Chesney, and colleagues developed a group-based coping intervention at the Center for AIDS Prevention Studies at the University of California at San Francisco. This intervention follows closely

Lazarus's model of stress and coping. The intervention focuses on helping individuals to change their appraisals, improve their coping skills, and obtain beneficial social support when needed. Although this intervention has been tested with HIV-positive men, it is designed to apply to a broad range of stressful contexts and has been applied to various chronic problems, such as spinal cord injury.

First, participants learn to distinguish between global and specific stressful situations. It is much easier to feel in control of a specific stressor (e.g., fears associated with receiving HIV antibody test results) than a vague, complex, global condition (e.g., coping with AIDS more generally). Second, participants learn to distinguish between those aspects of specific stressors that are changeable (e.g., finding ways to spend time while waiting for lab results) and those that are unchangeable (e.g., the lab results per se).

Emotion- and problem-focused coping strategies are then evaluated as possible methods of coping with the unchangeable and changeable situations, respectively. Strategies developed and practiced include cognitively reframing the situation as less stressful, selectively attending to positive aspects and distancing oneself from distressing aspects of the situation, asking for information, and using humor to diminish the negative impact of the situation. They also consider maladaptive forms of emotion-focused coping, such as smoking, drug use, and overeating, and the resulting negative impact associated with these strategies. Various decision-making strategies are taught, including ways to evaluate the probable outcomes of different approaches to a problem. Participants are also trained in communication skills, such as listening, communicating, and negotiating.

CET also has a component to help people obtain the social support they need from others. Support is considered to be informational, emotional, or tangible, and participants are taught to identify those members of their social network who are most able to provide the specific type of support required and how to best enlist their aid.

Cognitive-Behavioral Therapy

Many people who have a chronic illness or psychological problem see themselves as incapable of changing their situation. CBT directly challenges people to alter the way they think about themselves, the way they behave, and the way they deal with problems and their illnesses. The theoretical underpinning behind these therapies is that cognitions, behaviors, and emotions are intricately interconnected and that altering one affects and alters the other two.

CBT is a structured, evidence-based intervention that combines two effective forms of therapy: behavioral and cognitive therapy. Treatment usually begins with a behavioral component, breaking long-term goals or problems into small steps that can easily be taken by an individual. For example, a person with debilitating chronic back pain who wants to be able to work again may be encouraged to break down the goal into a shorter-term goal, such as being able to go for a 10-min walk again. In such a way, the person is encouraged to drop the overwhelmingly large long-term goal for simpler smaller goals that are manageable and attainable. Asking a patient to engage in activities, such as exercise and social activities, has the added benefit of getting the person active again and challenges the person's thinking that he or she cannot do anything. Accordingly, the person's self-efficacy can be slowly and incrementally heightened.

The cognitive component of CBT aids patients in coming to understand how their patterns of thinking might cause psychological problems. Maladaptive ways of experiencing oneself and situations can cause and enhance the psychological problems associated with mental or physical illness. Therapy and homework are designed to heighten the awareness of behaviors, feelings, and thoughts associated with specific stressors, situations, or conditions. Then, the person is encouraged to evaluate the pros and cons of his or her attitudes and beliefs regarding the stressor and to offer positive interpretations or cognitive reappraisals of situations with the intention of challenging the negative thought pattern. The patient, therefore, learns to actively seek new ways of perceiving or appraising situations that are less damaging to their psychological and physical well-being.

Mindfulness-Based Therapies

Over the past 2 decades, we have seen growing interest in incorporating mindfulness-based approaches into therapies for such conditions as chronic pain, stress, depression relapses, and CHD, to name a few. The goals of these therapies are to teach people how to manage everyday stress and pain and take responsibility for their well-being. Mindfulness involves moment-by-moment awareness of what a person is experiencing, such as paying close attention to breathing, noises, sensations in the body, inner feelings and thoughts, and our reactions to specific situations. Mindful awareness involves meditation exercises and is often coupled with stretching to help attain a mindful state. The person observes the moment-by-moment sensations, cognitions, and emotions without judging whether they are bad or good, important or trivial, or sick or healthy (nonjudgmental observation). The person is encouraged to recognize and accept his or her limits and body, as opposed to pushing and pulling at his or her physical and psychological limits. The goal is for the person to experience a new relationship with the mental or physical condition instead of doing the same old catastrophizing, avoiding, or other maladaptive coping strategy.

Mindfulness-based approaches have been applied to various physical and emotional problems and have received empirical support. Questions have been raised, however, regarding the methodology employed in studies designed to evaluate the therapies. Others consider mindfulness-based therapies as an alternative to more traditional approaches that involve learning skills that directly manipulate the stressor, negative thoughts, or feelings.

Summary

There are a number of factors that determine whether an individual can cope effectively with a particular stressor. An important first step is to appraise the situation in a positive yet realistic manner. Further, breaking up a global stressor into those aspects that can be changed and those that must be accepted can facilitate the identification of potential coping strategies. Practicing new coping strategies, considering the possible consequences of several different approaches, and obtaining support from others can result in a reduction in the negative consequences of stress. For those situations that threaten to overwhelm an individual's current resources, coping interventions that provide support, information, and skills training can be effective.

Acknowledgments

Anita DeLongis's research is supported by the Social Science and Humanities Research Council of Canada. Eli Puterman's research is supported by the Social Science and Humanities Research Council of Canada and the Michael Smith Foundation for Health Research in British Columbia.

See Also the Following Articles

Caregivers, Stress and; Psychosocial Factors and Stress.

Further Reading

Ajzen, I. and Fishbein, M. (2000). The prediction of behavior from attitudinal and normative variables. In: Higgins, E. T. & Kruglanski, A. W. (eds.) *Motivational science: social and personality perspectives*, pp. 177–190. New York: Psychology Press.

Baer, R. A. (2003). Mindfulness training as a clinical intervention: a conceptual and empirical review. *Clinical Psychology: Science and Practice* **10**, 125–143.

Baum, A., Revenson, T. A. and Singer, J. E. (eds.) (2001). *Handbook of health psychology.* Mahwah, NJ: Lawrence Erlbaum.

Chesney, M., Chambers, A., Taylor, D. B., et al. (2003). Coping effectiveness training for men living with HIV: results from a randomized clinical trial testing a group-based intervention. *Psychosomatic Medicine* **65**, 1038–1046.

Craig, K. D. (2005). Emotions and psychobiology. In: McMahon, S. & Koltzenburg, M. (eds.) *Melzack and Wall's Textbook of pain* (5th edn.). pp. 231–239. Edinburgh: Elsevier/Churchill Livingstone.

DeLongis, A. and Holtzman, S. (2005). Coping in context: the role of personality and social relationships. *Special issue on daily process methodology. Journal of Personality* 73, 1–24.

Folkman, S., Lazarus, R. S., Dunkel-Schetter, C., et al. (2000). The dynamics of a stressful encounter. In: Higgins, E. T. & Kruglanski, A. W. (eds.) *Motivational science: social and personality perspectives*, pp. 111–127. Philadelphia: Psychology Press.

Garssen, B. (2004). Psychological factors and cancer development: evidence after 30 years of research. *Clinical Psychology Reviews* **24**, 315–338.

Revenson, T. A., Kayser, K. and Bodenmann, G. (eds.) (2005). *Couples coping with stress: emerging perspectives on dyadic coping.* Washington, DC: American Psychological Association.

Teasdale, J. D. (2004). Mindfulness-based cognitive therapy. In: Yiend, J. (ed.) *Cognition, emotion and psychopathology: theoretical, empirical and clinical directions*, pp. 270–289. New York: Cambridge University Press.

Turk, D. C. and Okifuji, A. (2002). Psychological factors in chronic pain: evolution and revolution. *Journal of Consulting and Clinical Psychology* **70**, 678–690.

Homosexuality, Stress and

J Drescher
New York, NY, USA

Glossary

Being in the closet	Psychological and behavioral activities intended to keep one's homosexuality a secret.
Coming out	Admitting one's homosexuality to oneself or revealing it to others.
Dissociation	A psychological mechanism that allows individuals to keep unwanted or anxiety-producing information out of their awareness.
External homophobia	The irrational fear and hatred that heterosexuals feel toward gay people.
Gay bashing	Physical violence directed at people because they are gay.
Gender beliefs	Cultural ideas about what constitutes the essential qualities of men and women.
Gender identity	An individual's psychological sense of being either a man or a woman.
Heterosexism	A belief system that naturalizes and idealizes heterosexuality and either dismisses or ignores a gay subjectivity.
Internal/internalized homophobia	The self-loathing gay people feel for themselves.
Moral condemnations of homosexuality	Beliefs that regard homosexual acts as intrinsically harmful to the individual, to the individual's spirit, and to the social fabric.
Outing	The unwanted revelation of an individual's homosexuality to others by a third party.
Sexual orientation	A person's attraction to members of either the same sex (homosexual), the other sex (heterosexual), or to both sexes (bisexual).
Sodomy laws	Legislation that criminalizes homosexual behavior, ruled unconstitutional by the United States in 2003 by the Supreme Court.

Throughout the life cycle, gay, lesbian, and bisexual (GLB) individuals experience significant stressors that are a consequence of society's antihomosexual attitudes. Some of those attitudes and the stresses they engender are discussed here.

Heterosexism

Those with GLB identities are routinely stressed by cultural expectations that each individual have a heterosexual identity. This is known as heterosexism, a belief system that naturalizes and idealizes heterosexuality and either dismisses or ignores a gay subjectivity.

Heterosexism does not necessarily imply malice or ill will toward GLB individuals; idealizing oneself does not necessarily require denigrating those who are different. However, heterosexist ideology typically frames its antihomosexual arguments in terms of the normal, the natural, or the traditional. Such arguments, sometimes implicitly and at other times explicitly, tend to equate identities that are not conventionally heterosexual with immorality and can rationalize condemnations of same-sex feelings and behaviors. Heterosexist attitudes are pervasive in many cultures, and they inevitably place gay people in the awkward and often stressful position of either (1) keeping their homosexuality a secret (being in the closet) or (2) having to reveal they are gay (coming out) to disprove cultural myths and assumptions about homosexuality. The most dramatic example of this stressful dilemma can be seen in the U.S. military's Don't Ask, Don't Tell policy, under which either revealing oneself to be gay or being found out to be gay can lead to a discharge.

In Western culture, most books, plays, movies, and print and television ads contain naturalized depictions of heterosexuality. "Boy meets girl, boy loses girl, boy gets girl" are the common elements of a heterosexist script. Heterosexism renders gay lives so invisible that at the time of writing this chapter, there is enormous media attention and controversy over *Brokeback Mountain,* a film in which the two male leads fall in love. Many heterosexual people have openly stated either their reluctance or opposition to seeing two men kiss on the silver screen.

Common expressions of heterosexism include valuing heterosexual relationships above homosexual ones, unquestioned opposition to gay parenting regardless of a gay parent's actual qualities as a parent, and the belief that lesbians and gay men are unsuited to teach small children, to serve in government, or to practice medicine. Heterosexist assumptions lead to separating men and women from one another in locker rooms. Yet gay teenagers may be stressed by having to hide any possible arousal they may experience on seeing naked peers in the locker room's ostensibly asexual environment. Similarly, a heterosexist world may make it difficult for elderly gay couples to openly live together in either retirement communities or assisted living programs.

A decade ago, marriage was implicitly assumed to be a ritual reserved for heterosexual couples. As a result of lawsuits initiated by gay couples in the 1990s and following the 2003 decision to allow same-sex marriage in Massachusetts, many other states rewrote their constitutions to specifically state that marriage should only be between a man and a woman. The stated impetus for these constitutional changes is often termed the "defense of marriage." Yet laws ostensibly written to preserve heterosexual relations inevitably create stress for gay couples and their families. The U.S. General Accounting Office has computed over 1000 rights, privileges, and benefits accrued through marriage. Consequently, the heterosexist denial of legal marriage to long-term, committed gay couples adds to the latter's stress by denying them and their families basic needs, including clearly defined inheritance rights, pension benefits, survivor death benefits, custody rights in cases of divorce, and health benefits, just to name a few. A growing literature also indicates increased psychological resilience in those who marry; denying legal marriage to same-sex couples denies them marriage's psychological benefits as well.

Gender Beliefs and Gender Stress

Any discussion of antihomosexual stressors necessitates some discussion of both scientific and popular heterosexist beliefs about gender and sexuality. Modern sexology distinguishes a person's gender identity, or the sense that one is a man or a woman, from the person's sexual orientation, whether one is attracted to members of the same sex (homosexual), the other sex (heterosexual), or to both sexes (bisexual). However, the general culture uses conventional heterosexuality as an organizing frame of reference and frequently conflates the categories of gender identity and sexual orientation. These common but mistaken gender beliefs include the notion that an attraction to men is a female trait or that gay men feel and act like girls. Although such mundane gender beliefs can be stressful because they misrepresent GLB people, GLB individuals are not alone in having to contend with them. Gender beliefs also include ideas about the kind of shoes men should wear (construction boots rather than spike heels) and the kind of career a woman should choose (becoming a nurse rather than a doctor). In other words, gender beliefs are not confined to the realm of sexuality; they concern themselves with many aspects of day-to-day life.

Gender beliefs play an important role in the development of gender identity. One may be born with an anatomical gender, but one's psychological gender is a later acquisition that has both cognitive and affective elements. How one's gender identity actually develops is not precisely known, although empirical data suggest it is a long and complex process. Clinical work shows that a person's sense of being a man or a woman can involve processes that are entirely dependent on attitudes from the external environment over extended periods of time. Children must learn a psychological construct of gender that is based not solely on anatomy but also on myriad cultural and familial clues (e.g., boys like to play ball or girls are made of sugar and spice). Consequently, the meanings of, for example, aggression in girls or a lack of athletic interests in boys can be internalized along a family or cultural model that codes these attributes as gender-specific. From this developmental perspective, a gender identity can be thought of as the accretion of experiences or interactions with the external and internalized gender-coding environment. That is to say, a person's gender is an activity occurring in a relational matrix.

For children who grow up to be heterosexuals, conformity to conventional gender beliefs and norms can sometimes offer a sense of comfort. However, gender beliefs can be stressful to heterosexuals as well. Real men and real women are powerful cultural ideals against which all men and women may unfavorably compare themselves. However, GLB individuals must contend with the dissonance created by early same-sex attractions and their learned cultural beliefs about the relationship between homosexuality and gender. Consequently, in some children who grow up to be gay, their developing gender beliefs about the meanings of their homoerotic feelings may lead them to question their own gender identities.

Seen from this perspective, children who grow up to be gay may be gender stressed. This is a process that can occur over a protracted period of time as early homoerotic feelings become linked to other gender-nonconforming interests and as these children come to realize that they are failing to meet the cultural and social expectations of their assigned gender. This is commonly seen in gay men who were effeminate boys, often denigrated for being sissies. However, even gay men who were more conventionally masculine as children recall gender stresses in their attempts to integrate their same-sex feelings into a male identity. Sometimes gender stress can lead to gender confusion. Clinically, gender confusion can be expressed as "If I am attracted to boys, I must be like a girl." But it might also include responses such as "I am depraved," "I will be alone," or "I have sinned." These are common and stressful gender beliefs associated with transgressing gender boundaries.

Homophobia

George Weinberg is generally credited with coining the term homophobia. He defines external homophobia as the irrational fear and hatred that heterosexuals feel toward gay people and internal (or internalized) homophobia as the self-loathing gay people feel for themselves. Weinberg suggests several origins of homophobia: the religious motive, the secret fear of being homosexual, repressed envy, and the threat to values. In fact, plethysmographic studies demonstrate that in some men, homophobic attitudes may defend against unwanted homoerotic feelings.

Weinberg's early work has been followed by an ever-expanding literature devoted to studying intolerance of homosexuality. Other factors thought to contribute to homophobic attitudes include (1) rare contact with GLB people, (2) a lack of homosexual experiences of one's own, (3) perceiving that one's own community does not accept homosexuality, (4) living in communities where homosexuality is unacceptable, (5) being older, (6) being less educated, (7) identifying oneself as religious or as belonging to a conservative religion, (8) being less permissive about sexuality in general, and (9) expressing high levels of authoritarianism.

In 1954, the U.S. Supreme Court ruled in *Brown v. The Board of Education* that racial segregation was unconstitutional. In support of that decision, the justices cited the psychological literature of the time that demonstrated how stressful and harmful racism was to the self-esteem of black children. Just as one cannot grow up black in America without internalizing racism, one cannot grow up gay without internalizing homophobic and other antihomosexual attitudes. Self-hatred is extremely stressful. In the clinical setting, internalized homophobia can present as low self-esteem, difficulty in sustaining relationships, estrangement from one's family of origin, work difficulties, or self-medication with drugs or alcohol to reduce stress-induced anxieties.

Homophobia is often expressed in the association of male homosexuality with effeminacy. Sissies of all ages are regularly targets of homophobia. The low social status accorded to sissies leads some parents, fearful that their children will grow up to be gay, to seek professional treatment to change the behaviors of their effeminate sons. However, when mental health professionals and parents join the social chorus of derision, presumably for a child's own good, being labeled effeminate at an early age can entail great stress and suffering.

Although some gay men are effeminate, assuming that all gay men are effeminate falls under the rubric of stereotyping. In addition to disdain for effeminacy, homophobia can be expressed in other stereotypes, clichés, or caricatures of sexual identities. Common stereotypes of gay men describe them as being sexually promiscuous or compulsive, having a talent for the arts, being mama's boys, or lacking in courage. Common stereotypes of gay women label them as being man-haters, tomboys, overly aggressive, or physically unattractive. Both gay men and women have been stereotyped as sexual predators or being fated to lead single lives of loneliness. Clinical experience has demonstrated that it is extremely stressful for GLB individuals to have to constantly prove to heterosexual families, friends, employers, and co-religionists – and sometimes to themselves – that these are just stereotypes.

Moral Condemnations of Homosexuality

People who morally condemn homosexuality regard homosexual acts as intrinsically harmful to the individual, to the individual's spirit, and to the social fabric. Those who morally condemn same-sex activities believe that the tradition of philosophical, legal, and religious opposition to homosexuality is, in and of itself, sufficient reason to forbid the open expression of homosexuality in the modern world. Although critics of these condemnations attribute them to homophobia, antihomosexuality stemming from moral beliefs is often more complex. For example, religious and secular social conservatives who morally condemn homosexuality claim they do so out of love or concern for something else. In today's culture wars, such individuals and groups actively and vocally oppose gay and lesbian civil rights at the municipal, state, and federal level. Their political activities, which arise from their moral condemnations, are an ongoing source of stress for the GLB community.

The most severe forms of moral condemnation are embodied in laws that criminalize homosexual behavior, once referred to as sodomy laws. In the mid-twentieth century, homosexuality was illegal in all 50 states. By 2003, only 13 states still had such laws. Although rarely enforced, they were often a source of stress for GLB populations. Selective enforcement of sodomy laws allowed antihomosexual law enforcement communities to harass and discriminate against gay citizens. Furthermore, it was routinely argued in states with sodomy laws that gay couples, as potential criminals, should not be allowed to adopt their foster children. Obviously, criminalizing the sexual behaviors felt to be part of one's normal sexuality is extremely stressful to those so charged. In 2003, however, the U.S. Supreme Court ruled in the case of *Lawrence and Garner v. Texas* that all state sodomy laws were unconstitutional.

Moral condemnations of homosexuality hampered the early public health response to the AIDS epidemic and, in the process, added significantly to the losses and stress of the GLB community. Initially – and incorrectly – perceiving AIDS to be primarily a disease of gay men, public health systems were unprepared to talk frankly about either homosexuality or the kind of sexual practices that transmitted the virus. In 1987, 6 years after the initial cases were identified, President Reagan first mentioned the word "AIDS." Although teaching safe sex practices to sexually active individuals was important in slowing the spread of the epidemic, moral disapproval of homosexuality made federal funding of such educational efforts illegal. Even though most global AIDS cases have been transmitted heterosexually, many still argue, usually in a condemnatory way, that homosexuality causes AIDS rather than unsafe sexual practices that spread the virus. After experiencing thousands of preventable deaths, it is not unsurprising that many in today's GLB community feel their own government does not value their lives.

In their more subtle forms, moral condemnations of homosexuality include an attitude known as love the sinner, hate the sin. In earlier historical eras, religious authorities condemned sodomites to eternal damnation, to prison, and sometimes even physical torture. However, science and medicine's redefinition of homosexuality, as well as the growing number of openly gay and lesbian voices, had an enormous impact on religious attitudes. Consequently, religious groups were forced to integrate the accumulating scientific data regarding the presumptive etiologies and naturalness of homosexuality.

Today's religious authorities find themselves having to contend with the spiritual needs of a growing number of gay people, as well as those of their families. Some religious denominations (i.e., Episcopalians and the United Church of Christ) have adopted an accepting model of homosexuality and openly embrace lesbian and gay worshipers. Some denominations even admit openly gay men and women as priests, rabbis, and ministers. However, acceptance has not been the majority approach.

Many religious authorities have instead chosen to embrace the homosexual but not the homosexuality. Contrary to mainstream scientific findings, antihomosexual religious authorities believe one chooses to be a homosexual despite the prohibitions against it – "choice" being a charged word in moral debates about homosexuality. In recent years, antihomosexual groups have been publicizing so-called sexual conversion or reparative therapies intended to change homosexuals. Rather than excluding gay people, they invite them back into the religious fold if they change their ways. However, the overstated claims surrounding conversion therapies have generated much interpersonal stress in many religious GLB individuals, particularly when family members pressure them to undergo the process. The public relations effort promoting these treatments is worrisome because (1) their efficacy is questionable, (2) the etiological theories on which they are based are not supported by current scientific research, (3) the practitioners of these treatments incorrectly label homosexuality as a mental disorder, (4) there is sparse documentation of the cure rates and when the rates are documented they are quite low (27–35%), (5) long-term results are rarely validated, (6) there are an increasing number of anecdotal reports that these treatments may cause harm, and (7) the false hopes raised in offering such treatments often delay individuals or their family members from accepting them as gay. In fact, the American Psychiatric Association has issued a position statement asking ethical practitioners to refrain from such practices and to do no harm.

Religious beliefs that disapprove of homosexuality constitute substantive, ongoing stressors in the lives of gay people, particularly for those who had strict, fundamentalist, or orthodox religious upbringings. Because they may no longer be participating in religious activities, they are often estranged from their communities where family, social, and religious activities are deeply intertwined. The social isolation that ensues from gay people's fear of moral condemnation can also be stressful.

Antigay Violence

In 1990 the federal government passed a law ordering a study of hate crimes, including attacks on gay men and women, the first time a federal civil rights law covered sexual orientation. In one common presentation of gay-bashing, gangs of young men descend on neighborhoods where gay people meet. Armed with bats, clubs, or other weapons, they attack anyone they believe to be gay.

Since the much-publicized beating to death of Matthew Shepard in 1998, there has been increased awareness and documentation of antigay violence and gay-bashing incidents. Publicized cases have also led to the open articulation of previously unspoken cultural beliefs, for example, the belief that violence is an excusable response to an unwanted sexual advance from a gay man. Termed the "gay panic defense," no court has yet accepted it as justification for antigay violence. Its underlying rationale is that gay victims are responsible for provoking the violence against them. Others, however, argue that antigay violence is the inevitable outgrowth of unexamined and unstated beliefs implicit in homophobia, heterosexism, and moral condemnation. They argue that not everyone can distinguish the sinner from the sin and that those who marginalize homosexuality are either directly or indirectly responsible for the brutality against gay men and women.

Leaving the unanswered question of antigay violence's origins aside, most GLB people have legitimate concerns about it. Holding one's partners hand in public or a chaste kiss may provoke a physical attack. Furthermore, antigay violence is believed to be an underreported phenomenon because its victims are often reluctant to come forward. Victims often blame themselves for being in the wrong place at the wrong time. Even gay people who have never been assaulted are sensitive to the ways in which members of the dominant culture, both in positions of authority or on its margins, can make threats and do as they please.

The Stress of Being in the Closet

In their developmental histories, gay men and lesbians often report periods of difficulty in acknowledging their homosexuality, both to themselves and to others. Children who grow up to be gay rarely receive family support in dealing with antihomosexual prejudices. On the contrary, beginning in childhood – and distinguishing them from racial and ethnic minorities – gay people are often subjected to the antihomosexual attitudes of their own families and communities. Consequently, gay men and lesbians may spend long periods of their lives unable to acknowledge their homosexuality, either to themselves or to others. Throughout childhood and the life cycle, even the suspicion of being gay can lead to teasing, ridicule, family censure, or even violence. Consequently, many gay people come to regard their homosexuality as an unpleasant fact they would rather not know about themselves, let alone admit to others; their homosexuality must be kept out of their awareness and separated from their public persona. The psychological means by which they accomplish this separation is called dissociation.

Dissociation, of course, is not limited to gay men and lesbians. Almost everyone is capable of pushing unwanted knowledge out of one's awareness. However, given some of the consequences of being openly gay – estrangement from family, loss of employment, loss of home, loss of child custody, loss of opportunity, loss of status and even blackmail – dissociation may seem a viable option for survival. Some closeted gay people can reflexively speak without revealing the gender of the person being discussed or without providing any gendered details of his or her personal life. Some closeted gay people marry and, on the surface, live their lives as if they were typical heterosexuals. Although some closeted gay men and women may not act on their homosexual feelings, others may develop secret sexual lives. In fact, through dissociation, a whole double life can be lived and yet never be acknowledged.

This psychological effort to solve one problem, however, creates others. It is stressful to continuously hide significant aspects of the self or to vigilantly separate aspects of the self from others. Constantly hiding creates difficulties in accurately assessing other people's perceptions of oneself as well as recognizing one's own strengths. Dissociation's impact on self-esteem can also make it difficult to feel one's actual accomplishments as reflections of one's own abilities. Hiding takes its toll, particularly because the psychological effort needed to maintain a double life often leads to errors in judgment that further add to one's stress. Maintaining a heterosexual identity while engaging in secret homosexual activity may inevitably lead a closeted individual into compromising situations.

Those who find this psychological split untenable may come out as either gay, lesbian, or bisexual. Coming out involves putting into words the feelings and ideas that previously had no acceptable form of open expression. Calling oneself gay or lesbian is an effort to reach some measure of self-acceptance. The process is not just about revealing oneself to others. It is a realization that previously unacceptable homosexual feelings or desires are actually part of one's self. Coming out is fraught with danger because of the social stigma attached to homosexuality due to antihomosexual attitudes in the culture. Given the difficulties associated with revealing a gay identity, it may seem a wonder that anyone comes out at all.

For some, coming out may be against their will, precipitated by an act of malice. In such cases of outing, a hidden homosexual identity is exposed by those seeking revenge, political advantage or financial gain. Fear of being outed is a major stressor in the lives of many closeted GLB individuals. However, those who come out of their own accord describe the experience positively, as "a switch being turned on," "coming home," or "discovering who I really am." For them, as stressful as it may be to come out, it may be even more stressful to stay in the closet.

Further Reading

Adams, H. E. (1996). Is homophobia associated with homosexual arousal? *Journal of Abnormal Psychology* **105**(3), 440–445.

Cabaj, R. P. and Stein, T. S. (eds.) (1996). *Textbook of homosexuality and mental health*. Washington, DC: American Psychiatric Press.

Drescher, J. (1998). *Psychoanalytic therapy and the gay man*. Hillsdale, NJ: The Analytic Press.

Drescher, J., Stein, T. S. and Byne, W. (2005). Homosexuality, gay and lesbian identities, and homosexual behavior. In: Sadock, B. & Sadock, V. (eds.) *Kaplan and Sadock's comprehensive textbook of psychiatry* (8th edn., pp. 1936–1965). Baltimore, MD: Williams and Wilkins.
Drescher, J. and Zucker, K. J. (2006). *Ex-gay research: analyzing the Spitzer study and its relation to science, religion, politics, and culture.* New York: The Haworth Press.
Herek, G. (1984). Beyond homophobia: a social psychological perspective on the attitudes toward lesbians and gay men. *Journal of Homosexuality* 10, 1–21. (Reprinted in DeCecco J. (ed.) (1985). *Bashers, baiters & bigots: homophobia in American society*, pp. 1–21. New York: Harrington Park Press.)
Hoffman, L. G., Hevesi, A. G., Lynch, P. E., et al. (2000). Homophobia: analysis of a "permissible" prejudice; a public forum of the American Psychoanalytic Association and the American Psychoanalytic Foundation. *Journal of Gay & Lesbian Psychotherapy* **4**(1), 5–53.
Kohlberg, L. (1966). A cognitive-developmental analysis of children's sex role concepts and attitudes. In: Maccoby, E. (ed.) *The development of sex differences*, pp. 82–172. Stanford, CA: Stanford University Press.
Shilts, R. (1987). *And the band played on: politics, people and the AIDS epidemic.* New York: St. Martin's Press.
Sullivan, A. (ed.) (1997). *Same-sex marriage: pro and con.* New York: Vintage Books.
Weinberg, G. (1972). *Society and the healthy homosexual.* New York: Anchor Books.

Impotence, Stress and

M R Gignac, G M Rooker and J K Cohen
Pittsburgh, PA, USA

This article is reproduced from Encyclopedia of Stress First Edition, volume 2, pp 547–550, © 2000, Elsevier Inc.

Glossary

Erectile dysfunction (ED)	Failure to obtain sufficient erectile rigidity of the penis to allow vaginal penetration, also known as impotence.
Erection	Tumescence or engorgement of the corporal bodies leading to elongation, widening, and rigidity of the penis.
Intrinsic/ extrinsic stress	Psychological forces a person experiences. Intrinsic stress, for example, could result from guilt over marital infidelity; extrinsic stress, for example, could result from the death of one's parents.
Libido	The desire to have sex.
Nocturnal erection	Normal physiological erection of the penis that occurs subconsciously during the rapid eye movement sleep cycle and, when present, is thought to exclude organic disease as a cause of erectile dysfunction.

Overview

The inability to obtain sufficient penile rigidity to allow vaginal penetration, regardless of the cause, is termed impotence or is perhaps better described as erectile dysfunction (ED). ED is an exceedingly common problem. In fact, nearly half of all men over the age of 40 suffer from some degree of ED at various times. ED is also strongly associated with advancing age. ED is commonly related to medical conditions as well as psychological disorders, and most physicians agree that in many cases there is significant overlap. Stress in the medical literature has been defined as physical or psychological forces experienced by a person. An example of a physical force leading to ED is severe vascular disease; this leads to failure of the physical erectile mechanism. A typical psychological stress leading to ED is depression, which may not only be the cause but also the result of ED. The role stress plays in the development of ED is significant and often difficult to define.

Physiology of Erection

Neurological and Psychological Aspects

The events that lead to normal penile erection are complex and involve psychological and physiological mechanisms. Volitional erection usually begins with psychological arousal. This involves all of the senses (sight, touch, smell, taste, and hearing) as well as imagination. The sensory input arrives to special areas of the conscious brain via afferent neural pathways. In the case of positive input, the signals are used to create the sensations and fantasy associated with sexual arousal. This process can be modulated by stress and hormonal imbalance. Next are the descending pathways from the brain, leading to erection centers in the spinal cord. From the spinal cord, the pathway leads to the paired cavernosal nerves running alongside the prostate (neurovascular bundles), which are responsible for the induction of erection. This series of neural connections can collectively be termed the efferent pathway. Stimulation of the genital organs sends signals to the spinal erection center, some of which are transmitted up to the brain and others of which lead to the reflex stimulation of the cavernosal nerves. Thus, three types of penile erection are thought to exist. Psychogenic erection is the result of conscious sensory input and fantasy. Reflexogenic erection occurs by a reflex pathway in the spinal cord initiated by genital stimulation. Finally, nocturnal erections occur by an as yet unknown mechanism.

Mechanical Aspects: Penile Hemodynamics

The physiological mechanics of penile erection are fairly well understood. Essentially, the efferent neural activation leads to a change in the blood flow pattern to the penis whereby more blood is trapped in the paired erectile bodies (corpora cavernosum). Thus, there is greater inflow compared to outflow, and the penis elongates, increases in diameter, and develops sufficient rigidity for vaginal penetration. This requires normally functioning arterial, cavernosal, and venous systems. It is obvious on the basis of our current understanding of sexual function that a complex interaction must occur between the psychological and physical aspects of erection and there are many potential areas in which stress can affect the outcome.

Erectile Dysfunction

For treatment purposes, clinicians commonly classify patients as having either organic or nonorganic causes of ED. This division roughly corresponds to physical and psychological causes, respectively.

Organic and Nonorganic Erectile Dysfunction

Organic causes of ED relate to specific malfunctions in the physiological mechanisms of erection, in other words, any pathological process that affects the afferent input, efferent output, or mechanics of erection. For example, multiple sclerosis can disrupt the afferent and efferent pathways, vascular disease or antihypertensive medications can interfere with the erectile hemodynamics, and diabetes may affect multiple physiological mechanisms.

Nonorganic ED refers to problems that cannot be explained easily by the failure of physiological mechanisms; it is also commonly referred to as psychogenic impotence. This type of ED has defied universally accepted classification; however, it has been subdivided into five major categories: type 1, anxiety, fear of failure (e.g., performance anxiety); type 2, depression; type 3, marital conflict, strained relationship; type 4, ignorance and misinformation, religious scruples (e.g., about normal anatomy or sexual function); and type 5, obsessive-compulsive personality (e.g., anhedonia).

Stress and Erectile Dysfunction

The role stress plays in the causation of ED has been difficult to study and therefore information is lacking. Several commonsense inferences can be made. First, the presence of ED, regardless of the cause, leads to psychological stress such as fear of underlying disease and loss of self-image. Second, intrinsic and extrinsic causes of psychological stress can lead to physiological changes altering the afferent and efferent pathways as well as the mechanical function of erection. For example, anxiety states can be associated with higher circulating levels of catecholamines and these neurotransmitters can affect the hemodynamics of the penis, causing failure of the normal erectile mechanism. This may explain some cases of ED due to performance anxiety. Finally, emotional tone can have a strong influence on how the senses are interpreted, potentially turning positive signals into inhibition of erection; thus, stress can diminish libido profoundly.

Evaluation and Treatment

History and Physical Examination

The evaluation of patients with ED has generally been performed by either urologists or psychiatrists. With changing attitudes toward sexuality and the advancement in the science of ED, many different types of doctors now possess the appropriate evaluation and management skills. Still, however, sexual dysfunction often remains overlooked in the treatment of many patients. The initial evaluation begins with a thorough history and physical examination. In cases in which psychological factors seem to predominate, the careful elucidation of the history is especially important and often is the only means by which the psychological stress can be discovered. The encounter is best suited to a quiet, comfortable examining room and the history taken with the patient fully clothed, followed by the physical examination. This allows the interaction to occur in a minimally intimidating format. Elements of the history that are relevant include a specific description of the degree of dysfunction, duration, circumstances associated with the onset, coexisting medical problems, loss of libido, past surgeries, injuries, medications, psychiatric problems, and temporal relationship to major life events. On occasion, it is informative to interview the partner separately. The physical examination should focus on signs of systemic disease;

thorough neurological evaluation; careful inspection of the genitalia, including rectal examination; and assessment for hormonal and vascular diseases.

Special Testing

On the basis of the initial interview, additional or second-line studies may be needed. These additional tests could include nocturnal penile tumescence (NPT) monitoring, injection cavernosometry and cavernosography, hormonal evaluation, and personality questionnaires.

Nocturnal penile tumescence monitoring The application of NPT monitoring is simple and can usually be performed at home by the patient. Either a one-time-use snap gauge device or an electronic monitor is applied to the penis at bedtime. The presence of normal nocturnal erections is considered proof that the mechanical aspects of penile erection are functioning appropriately. Both devices can measure the presence of an erection and, to some degree, the quality. The more sophisticated electronic monitor provides additional information, such as the number and duration of erections.

Injection cavernosometry and cavernosography Injection cavernosometry and cavernosography are invasive tests in which a vasoactive drug (e.g., prostaglandin) is injected directly into the body of the penis. The drugs work by stimulating the same hemodynamic changes as in normal erection. Before and after injection, pressures within the corporal bodies can be measured to determine an objective degree of tumescence, high-resolution ultrasound can be used to assess vascular changes, and intravenous contrast can be administered for the evaluation of venous leak. These tests are used to detect arterial (inflow) and venous (outflow) diseases.

Both NPT and injection testing are intended to evaluate the physiological mechanism of erection. The use of these tests is directed not only by the suspected diagnosis but also, and perhaps more important, by potential therapeutic alternatives. Stated differently, extensive physiological testing affects the choice of treatment options infrequently and therefore is indicated only in select cases.

Hormonal evaluation Suspicion of a hormonal imbalance needs to be confirmed by blood tests assessing the function of the pituitary (prolactin), thyroid (thyroid hormones T_3 and T_4 and thyrotropin), and testicle (testosterone). Common abnormalities causing decreased libido include hypogonadism and hypothyroidism. It is important to note that psychological stress can decrease libido without lowering testosterone or thyroid hormone levels. If testosterone is found to be low, then prolactin should be measured; a significant elevation of prolactin can indicate a pituitary problem.

Personality questionnaires Another second line type of testing that is seldom used by urologists and occasionally used by psychiatrists is personality questionnaires. Many have been developed (e.g., the Minnesota Multiphasic Personality Inventory), and they are intended to elicit information similar to a sexual history. The use of this technique may offer advantages in assessing the degree of psychological stress. Many clinicians feel that a detailed personal interview is equally effective, if not more so, and requires less interpretation skills than these instruments. This explains their infrequent use.

Treatment

For the successful management of ED, it is necessary to understand the degree to which both psychological and physiological factors are contributing. For instance, the successful correction of anxiety disorder is helpful, but ignoring concomitant vascular disease will result in treatment failure. Likewise, the placement of a penile prosthesis can restore an adequate erection, but if the patient has a depressed mood he may not be interested in having sex. Treatment is therefore directed toward both the correction of physiological malfunctions and behavioral modification. Furthermore, managing the physiological and psychological factors must be considered in the context of available treatment options. A precise cause can often be determined, particularly when physiological disease predominates, but cannot be precisely corrected given the current limitations in treatment. Thus, in most cases of ED, treatment is directed at the symptoms and not the specific cause.

Physiological treatments There are several approaches to the physiological treatment of ED. These options, from least to most invasive, include an external vacuum erection device (VED); medications in oral pill, intraurethral pellet, and intracavernosal injection; and surgical prosthesis placement. The VED works by creating negative pressure around the penis, thereby causing blood engorgement and erection. It is useful in all types of ED and leaves no permanent changes. Various medications have been used and all affect penile hemodynamics. Oral medications leave no permanent change and effectiveness depends on the cause of ED. Typically, injection therapy is considered most reliable, but it can ultimately lead to corporal fibrosis. Penile prostheses are mechanical devices that are surgically implanted to replace the cavernosal tissue. Implants come in a variety of types, including semirigid and inflatable. In general, treatment is offered from the simplest to the most invasive, depending on the patient's wishes and therapeutic effectiveness.

A major breakthrough in ED medicament treatment was provided by the discovery that phosphodiesterase 5 (PDE5) inhibitors were effective in helping to induce penile erection. PDE5 inhibitors increase the concentration of cyclic guanosine monophosphate in the corpus cavernosum: this results in smooth muscle relaxation (vasodilation) with consequent increased inflow of blood into the corpus cavernosum and penile erection. In 1998, the FDA approved a potent PDE5 inhibitor, sildenafil ("Viagra"), as an oral treatment for ED. Since then several clinical trials, including three independent double blind controlled trials in patients with erectile dysfunction, have demonstrated that sildenafil was significantly more effective than placebo in producing sustained improvements in confidence, self-esteem, and almost normal erectile function. Other effective PDE5 inhibitors, tadalafil ("Cialis") and vardenafil ("Levitra"), are now also available and widely used for the treatment of ED.

Psychological treatment Incorporated into any ED treatment plan must be a provision for the psychological component. This is particularly relevant for ED associated with stress and is probably most useful in patients without significant organic disease. First, any discovered psychological diagnosis, such as depression, should be treated appropriately. Second, sex therapy counseling should be used, not only to uncover functional problems but also to direct intervention and alter negative patterns of behavior. Sex counseling is usually performed by therapists specially trained in sex therapy. The session or sessions will probably require both partners to participate and may involve assignments and exercises to be performed at home. The goals of this intervention are to identify and correct behavioral patterns and to develop coping skills for sources of internal and external stress. In many cases of stress-associated ED, a combination of both physiological and psychological therapies are used.

Further Reading

Allen, J. R. (1987). Psychiatric treatment of erectile dysfunction. *Journal of the Oklahoma State Medical Association.* **80**, 19.

Althof, S. E., O'Leary, M. P., Cappelleri, J. C., Crowley, A. R., Tseng, L.-J. and Collins, S. (2006). Impact of erectile dysfunction on confidence, self-esteem and relationship satisfaction after 9 months of sildenafil citrate treatment. *The Journal of Urology* **175**, 2132–2137.

Blake, D. J. (1984). Issues in the psychiatric diagnosis and management of impotence. *Psychiatric Medicine* **2**, 109.

Hawton, K., Catalan, J. and Fagg, J. (1992). Sex therapy for erectile dysfunction: characteristics of couples, treatment outcome, and prognostic factors. *Archives of Sexual Behavior* **21**, 161.

Lue, T. F. (1998). Physiology of penile erection and pathophysiology of erectile dysfunction and priapism. In: Walsh, P. C., et al. (eds.) *Campbell's urology* (7th edn., pp. 1157–1179). Philadelphia: Saunders.

Tiefer, L. and Schuetz-Mueller, D. (1995). Psychological issues in diagnosis and treatment of erectile disorders. *Urologic Clinics of North America* **22**, 767.

Menopause and Stress

N E Avis
Wake Forest University School of Medicine, Winston-Salem, NC, USA

This is a revised version of the article by N E Avis, Encyclopedia of Stress First Edition, volume 2, pp 732–735, © 2000, Elsevier Inc.

Glossary

Menopause The permanent cessation of menses. The standard epidemiological definition of natural menopause is 12 consecutive months of amenorrhea, in the absence of surgery or other pathological or physiological cause (e.g., pregnancy, lactation, excessive exercise).

Perimenopause That period of time immediately prior to menopause when the endocrinological, biological, and clinical features of approaching menopause begin through the first year after the final menstrual period. It is characterized by increased variability in menstrual cycles, skipped menstrual cycles, and hormonal changes. Early perimenopause is defined as menses in the previous 3 months, but changes in regularity. Late perimenopause is defined as no menses in the previous 3 months, but menses in the preceding 11 months.

Premenstrual syndrome (PMS) A disorder characterized by a set of hormonal changes that trigger disruptive physical and emotional symptoms in a significant number of women for up to 2 weeks prior to menstruation.

Surgical menopause Menopause induced by a surgical procedure that stops menstruation. Women who have both ovaries or the uterus with or without removal of the ovaries are generally included in this category.

Menopause as a Stressful Life Event

Whether or not menopause is viewed as a stressful life event can be looked at in two ways: (1) women's attitudes toward menopause, and (2) women's affective responses to menopause.

Attitudes toward Menopause

Cross-cultural and anthropological studies provide evidence that the meaning of menopause varies greatly across cultures. How a society views menopause is influenced by how it views aging and women in general. Menopause is often viewed as a positive event in women's lives in non-Western cultures, where menopause removes constraints and prohibitions imposed upon menstruating women. In countries where women have low status or are not allowed to show sexuality (such as in India), menopause is seen positively, as it provides freedom to go out in public and do things usually forbidden to women. Among South Asian women, the end of childbearing and the menstrual cycle is welcomed. While social status is tied to motherhood, it is motherhood that is valued and not biological fertility itself.

Among both Mayan and Greek women, menopause is seen as a positive event, although for different reasons. Mayan women marry young, do not practice birth control, and spend most of their reproductive years either pregnant or lactating. Pregnancy is viewed as dangerous and stressful, and menopause frees women from restrictions and pregnancy. While Greek women attempt to curtail family size and often use abortion as a means of birth control, menopause also frees Greek women from taboos and restrictions. A postmenopausal Greek woman is allowed to participate fully in church activities, as she is no longer viewed as a sexual threat to the community. Both Mayan and Greek women report better sexual relationships with their husbands following menopause, as the fear of pregnancy is eliminated. In other cultures, women give menopause little thought. In Papago culture, menopause may be completely ignored, to the extent that the language contains no word for menopause. In Japan there is no word to describe hot flashes. As Lock points out, the lack of a Japanese word to describe hot flashes is remarkable in a language that is infinitely more sensitive than English in its ability to describe bodily states (e.g., there are more than 20 words to describe the state of the stomach).

In Western societies, women are valued for sexual attractiveness and do not face restrictions found in other cultures. Aging, especially among women, is not revered, but rather is viewed quite negatively. In these societies menopause takes on a very different meaning. Despite these negative societal views, women themselves do not hold such negative attitudes.

A review of research on women's attitudes toward menopause conducted across a wide range of populations and cultures shows that women consistently feel relief about the cessation of menses and do not agree that they become less sexually attractive following menopause. Women consistently report that they are glad to no longer deal with menstruation, accompanying PMS or menstrual cramps, fear of pregnancy, and purchase of feminine products. Thus, the end of menstruation, rather than bringing on a sense of psychological loss, is often met with relief. While women may feel a decrease in sexual desire or frequency, which they attribute to aging as much as to menopause, women overwhelmingly disagree with the statement that postmenopausal women are less feminine or attractive. Studies consistently show that postmenopausal women generally have a more positive view of menopause than premenopausal women. Thus, women's own attitudes toward menopause are not as negative as those of the medical profession or Western societies as a whole.

Women's Response to Menopause

Another way to examine whether menopause can be viewed as a stressful life event is to look at the impact of menopause on mental health. Earlier reports based on patient or clinic populations often perpetuated the perception that women become depressed and irritable and suffer a host of other symptoms during menopause. These studies, however, suffered from numerous methodological problems. First, such patient-based samples are highly biased. Fewer than half of menopausal women seek treatment, and those who do tend to report more stress in general and suffer more from clinical depression, anxiety, and psychological symptoms than nonpatient samples. Second, these studies often did not differentiate between women who experienced surgical and those who experienced natural menopause. Women who undergo surgical menopause have a very different experience of menopause, in that they experience more sudden hormonal changes, as well as a surgical procedure. A number of studies have found that women who have had a surgical menopause report more distress than women who experience a natural menopause. Finally, these studies often used menopausal checklists that asked women to check off symptoms that they experienced due to menopause. When asked in this way, women will check off any symptom they have that fits their beliefs about what women experience during menopause. This method thus perpetuates existing stereotypes of the menopause experience.

Cross-sectional epidemiological studies of community-based samples of women do not show consistent evidence of a relation between menopause and depression or other negative moods in the general population. More recently, several longitudinal studies have shown an increased risk of depressive symptoms during perimenopause. However, it is important to note that only a minority of women appear to experience an increase in negative mood or depression during perimenopause, and other factors, such as stress and socioeconomic factors, are more related to depressed mood than hormones or menopausal status. Longitudinal data suggest that prior depression is the primary factor related to depression during menopause. Studies have also found that women who report greater mood disturbances at menopause also report menstrual cycle or reproductive-related problems. These include previous or current premenstrual symptoms or complaints, dysmenorrhea, and postpartum depression. Researchers have also found that social circumstances and stress account for much of the mood effects during the menopause transition. Studies that have included measures of stress or life changes have typically found that social factors are highly related to mood, and often more so than menopause status.

Thus, for the majority of women, menopause does not appear to be a stressful life event. However, like other life events or changes, this does not mean that menopause is not stressful for some women. It has been hypothesized that women who find menopause stressful are those who see it as the end of reproduction or a sign of old age. Women with less education or knowledge about menopause generally have more negative attitudes, as do women who have more symptoms in general or worse mental health.

Impact of Stress on Menopause Symptomatology

Vasomotor symptoms (hot flashes/flushes and night sweats) are the primary symptoms associated with menopause. Estimates of the incidence of hot flashes from population studies in the United States and worldwide have ranged from 24 to 93%. Studies of menopause in different cultures reveal wide cultural variation in symptom reporting. For example, hot flashes are uncommon in Mayan women, and Japanese and Indonesian women report far fewer hot flashes than women in Western societies. Because women across cultures differ in terms of their diet, physical activity, number of pregnancies, use of contraception, as well as attitudes toward menopause, it has been difficult to assess the reason(s) for this variation. However, even within a culture, a high degree of variability of symptom reporting is found among women, suggesting considerable individual variation in symptom experience. What differentiates symptomatic from asymptomatic women is not well understood.

Women experiencing other sorts of stress are likely to notice or amplify menopausal symptoms, as they would any symptom. Epidemiological studies have shown greater vasomotor symptoms associated with less education, interpersonal stress, more general symptom reporting, and negative attitudes toward menopause. A relationship between stress and hot flashes has been shown in several correlational and treatment studies. One study has shown that laboratory-induced stressors correlate with women's objectively measured hot flashes. However, hot flashes did not concentrate around the actual stressor, suggesting that stress may potentiate (rather than cause) hot flashes by decreasing the threshold for the triggering of hot flashes at the hypothalamic level. Findings that women who report more symptoms premenopause also report more menopausal symptoms are consistent with the notion that some people have greater sensitivity to symptoms.

Thus, consistent with other research on stress and symptoms, there is some evidence that women experiencing stress for other reasons may have a tendency to notice or report greater menopausal symptoms. However, stress is only one of many factors that appear to impact menopausal symptoms.

Stress and Ovarian Function

Impact of Stress on Ovarian Function

Appropriate secretion of hypothalamic gonadotropin-releasing hormone (GnRH) is necessary for ovarian cyclicity. Decreased GnRH is a common cause of anovulation. Research in both humans and monkeys suggests that stress desynchronizes the GnRH neuronal network. High levels of stress have been shown to lead to altered menstrual function in premenopausal women. The impact of stress on perimenopausal women has not been well studied, but there is some evidence that marked increases in stress may alter menstrual cycles in the short term. It has also been hypothesized that high levels of stress may accelerate menopause. Recent research, however, has shown conflicting findings, with one study finding some evidence that stress accelerated menopausal age among women who were already experiencing irregular cycles or who were African-American, and another study finding that women who reported more psychological symptoms had a longer perimenopause.

Ovarian Function and Stress Responsivity

It has also been hypothesized that reproductive hormones influence the response to stress. Several researchers have examined the impact of ovarian function on reactivity to stress. These studies have largely examined cardiovascular reactivity in response to laboratory stresses among women in differing stages of ovarian functioning. While studies have shown greater responses among postmenopausal or surgically menopausal women as compared to premenopausal women, more recent research among women with experimentally suppressed ovarian function has not shown greater responses to stress. This remains an area of investigation.

Conclusions

Although menopause itself is a physiological event, a woman's response to menopause depends on cultural, behavioral, psychosocial, as well as physiological factors. How an individual woman responds to menopause is a complex interaction of physiology, her current life circumstances, attitudes/concerns about fertility, the culture in which she lives, and her history of responding to physiological changes/symptoms. On the whole, menopause is not a stressful event for most women. Concurrent stresses from other sources, however, may exacerbate a woman's response to menopausal symptoms.

See Also the Following Articles

Premenstrual Dysphoric Disorder.

Further Reading

Avis, N. E. (1996). Women's perceptions of the menopause. *European Menopause Journal* 3(2), 80–84.

Avis, N. E. (2000). Is menopause associated with mood disturbances? In: Lobo, R. A., Kelsey, J. & Marcus, R. (eds.) *Menopause: biology and pathobiology*, pp. 339–352. New York: Academic Press.

Avis, N. E., Crawford, S. L. and McKinlay, S. M. (1997). Psychosocial, behavioral, and health factors related to menopause symptomatology. *Women's Health: Research on Gender, Behavior, and Policy* 3(2), 103–120.

Barsom, S. H., Mansfield, P. K., Kock, P. B., Gierach, G. and West, S. G. (2004). Association between psychological stress and menstrual cycle characteristics in perimenopausal women. *Women's Health Issues* **14**, 235–241.

Berga, S. L. (1996). Stress and ovarian function. *The American Journal of Sports Medicine* **24**(6), S36–S37.

Berga, S. L. and Louks, T. L. (2005). The diagnosis and treatment of stress-induced anovulation. *Minerva Ginecologica* **57**, 45–54.

Beyene, Y. (1986). Cultural significance and physiological manifestations of menopause, a biocultural analysis. *Culture, Medicine & Psychiatry* **10**, 47–71.

Bromberger, J. T., Matthews, K. A., Kuller, L. H., et al. (1997). Prospective study of the determinants of age at menopause. *American Journal of Epidemiology* **145**, 124–133.

Freeman, E. W., Sammel, M. D., Liu, L., et al. (2004). Hormones and menopausal status as predictors of depression in women in transition to menopause. *Archives of General Psychiatry* **61**(1), 62–70.

Freeman, E. W., Sammel, M. D., Lin, H., et al. (2005). The role of anxiety and hormonal changes in menopausal hot flashes. *Menopause* **12**(3), 258–266.

Freeman, E. W., Sammel, M. D., Lin, H. and Nelson, D. B. (2006). Associations of hormones and menopausal status with depressed mood in women with no history of depression. *Archives of General Psychiatry* **63**(4), 375–382.

Gold, E. B., Colvin, A., Avis, N. E., et al. (2006). Longitudinal analysis of vasomotor symptoms and race/ethnicity across the menopausal transition: Study of Women's Health Across the Nation (SWAN). *American Journal of Public Health* 96(7), 1226–1235.

Kronenberg, F. (1990). Hot flashes: epidemiology and physiology. *Annals of the New York Academy of Sciences* **592**, 52–86.

Lock, M. (1986). Ambiguities of aging: Japanese experience and perceptions of menopause. *Culture, Medicine & Psychiatry* **10**, 23–46.

Nicol-Smith, L. (1996). Causality, menopause, and depression: a critical review of the literature. *British Journal of Medicine* **313**, 1229–1232.

Pearlstein, M. D., Rosen, K. and Stone, A. B. (1997). Mood disorders and menopause. *Endocrinology and Metabolism Clinics of North America* **26**(2), 279–294.

Shively, C. A., Watson, S. L., Williams, J. K., et al. (1998). Stress-menstrual cycle and cardiovascular disease. In: Orth-Gomer, K., Chesney, M. A. & Wenger, N. K. (eds.) *Women, stress, and heart disease.* Mahwah, NJ: Lawrence Erlbaum Associates, Inc.

Sommer, B., Avis, N., Meyer, P., et al. (1999). Attitudes toward menopause and aging across ethnic/racial groups. *Psychosomatic Medicine* **61**, 868–875.

Swartzman, L. C., Edelberg, R. and Kemmann, E. (1990). The menopausal hot flush: symptom reports and concomitant physiological changes. *Journal of Behavioral Medicine* 13(1), 15–31.

World Health Organization Scientific Group. (1996). Research on the menopause in the 1990's. *WHO Technical Services Report Series* 886.

Parenting, Stress of

K D Jennings
University of Pittsburgh, Pittsburgh, PA, USA
Laura J Dietz
University of Pittsburgh Medical Center, Pittsburgh, PA, USA

Glossary

Child temperament An enduring pattern of biological and physiological responses to the environment.

Coping Psychological processes that allow an individual to regulate negative emotions and behavior to adapt to stressful situations.

Daily hassles Normal or typical life experiences that increase negative affect and interpersonal distress by virtue of their high demands and low satisfaction.

Major life events Exceptional but time-limited life circumstances that produce stress in an individual by acutely increasing negative affect, interfering with daily functioning, and creating change in relationships and routines.

Parenting stress Pattern of adverse psychological and physiological reactions resulting from the demands of being a parent.

Self-efficacy An individual's perception of his or her competence in completing the tasks that define a particular domain.

Social support Interpersonal relationships that meet the emotional and instrumental needs of individuals experiencing distress.

Raising children is often a rewarding and positive experience, but it is also a challenging task that is inevitably stressful at times. Parenting requires a high level of effort and emotional involvement that can be overwhelming. It also involves a wide range of skills that must be used in a flexible manner. Parenting involves meeting the basic needs of children, socializing them to culturally appropriate rules of behavior, and promoting their self-esteem and emotional well-being. In the past 25 years, increasing attention has been paid to the stress of raising children and the effects of parenting stress on caregivers and families. Parenting stress has been defined as a pattern of adverse psychological and physiological reactions resulting from attempts to adapt to the demands of being a parent.

Why Parenting Can Be Stressful

Parenting Tasks

On a daily basis, parents must meet children's survival needs by providing them with shelter, food, clothing, and other necessities. They must ensure their physical safety by carefully monitoring their activities in different environments and by ensuring that proper medical attention is received. Parents must also meet their children's emotional needs by providing attention and affection in order to promote a healthy self concept and socioemotional development. Parents are also responsible for socializing children. They teach them how to adapt to their sociocultural environment by monitoring their behavior and reinforcing culturally appropriate responses. Parents also act as the primary models for regulating negative emotions and coping with distress in culturally specific ways. Parents actively help younger children cope with anger and disappointment by emotional scaffolding and redirecting attention. With older children, parents assist in problem solving and anticipating consequences prior to responding to a situation. Parents provide negative consequences to dissuade inappropriate anger responses such as aggression and prolonged displays of negative affect; in contrast, they praise and reward behaviors that are appropriate or polite. Finally, parents are responsible for introducing children to the larger community outside the family by providing opportunities for peer interaction, formal learning in school, and group activities. In all, parents are expected to carry out a wide variety of tasks that enable their children to successfully adapt to the demands of their sociocultural group and ultimately to become contributing members of their group.

Parenting Must Change as Children Develop

As children grow and develop, their needs and reliance on parents continually change. Being a parent is thus not a singular transition into a static role but rather a set of transitions within a dynamic role that is continually evolving to meet the changing needs of children. Furthermore, the role of being a parent requires synchrony between parents and children, and this synchrony falls largely on parents to achieve, especially when children are younger. Thus, children's developmental stages influence the amount of stress experienced by parents. For example, caring for a newborn is a time of high stress, particularly for the first-born child. In addition to the change in responsibilities and life style that occurs with the first child, newborns demand round-the-clock intensive caretaking. The preschool age has also been identified as stressful because parents must provide constant care and supervision while negotiating limits with their children as they begin to establish their independence. Other developmental stages provide their own set of challenges: entry into school, with exposure to and judgment by the larger community; adolescence, with increased demands for independence and a renegotiation of the parental role; and finally launching, facilitating the children's assumption of adult roles. Each developmental stage demands different characteristics of the parent; thus, parents differ on which stages they find easier or more difficult.

Parenting Must be Adapted to Children's Temperament and Special Needs

In addition to development, parents must adapt their interactions and interventions according to their child's individual temperament. There is not a single style of parenting that is ideal for every child. Instead, for example, parents must adapt their style to be more soothing for children with difficult temperaments who have problems regulating negative affect and more firm for children with temperaments that are high in novelty seeking. Children with more extreme temperaments or temperaments that differ from their parents can be experienced as more stressful. In addition, disabilities, developmental delays, chronic illnesses, or other special needs of children influence the level of stress experienced by parents. Such children typically require more physical care and more supervision; they also require that parents adjust to the loss of their perfect child and learn to cope with the medical and educational systems. Similarly, children with behavioral or emotional problems cause more stress for their parents.

Balancing Parenting with Other Roles

Parenting stress can also result from difficulty in balancing parenting responsibilities with other adult roles, particularly the roles of spouse and worker. For example, the transition to parenthood has been associated repeatedly with decreased marital satisfaction. The overwhelming, new responsibilities that come from the arrival of a newborn, combined with fatigue and the intense demands of caring for an infant, decrease the time and attention available for the marital relationship, which in turn may decrease marital satisfaction. Over time, parents must learn to balance the needs of all in the family, including the needs of their spouse and their own needs. Parents' difficulty in finding time and energy to meet their own needs is a major contributor to parenting stress.

Balancing work with parenting is another source of stress. Parents must make provisions for routine child care and also accommodate nonroutine events such as children's illnesses and school snow days. The rising demographic trend in first-world nations for dual-wage-earner families indicates that a high number of new mothers will continue to work outside of the home after a child is born. Thus, many families will be faced with the difficulties of balancing multiple roles.

Circumstances of Child Rearing

Specific circumstances of childrearing can exacerbate the level of stress experienced by parents. These circumstances include poverty, number of children, amount of social support, marital status, and physical or mental illness in parents. These stressors impede parents' efforts to care for their children. Thus, for example, single parents raising a number of children in poverty are likely to experience more stress than parents raising children in more favorable circumstances.

Types of Parenting Stress

Major Life Events

Early research on parenting stress focused on the consequences of major life events that increased emotional distress in parents and complicated normal parenting tasks. These major life events, such as death of a spouse, loss of employment, or divorce, were viewed as atypical of the everyday experience of parenting and were thought to increase parental distress and dysfunction and to impair effectiveness of meeting children's needs. Likewise, parenting stress was examined in relation to parenting children with a developmental disability, chronic physical illness, or an emotional disorder. This research did indeed indicate a link between major life events and various indices of parent, child, and family functioning. Parents who were coping with out-of-the-ordinary difficult circumstances reported reduced emotional well-being and increased psychopathology. They were also observed to have less optimal parenting skills. In turn, their children showed more psychopathology and lower social competence. However, a shortcoming of the major life events model is that it focuses on low-frequency events that cluster in high-risk populations with many problems. The life events model fails to capture the minor stress incurred by all parents in meeting the daily demands of childrearing.

Chronic Minor Stressors

Current research on stress in adults focuses on both major life events and the more mundane chronic stress stemming from meeting the demands of daily living. For parents, minor stressors are the daily hassles of meeting children's needs, including monitoring children's behavior, physically caring for children (i.e., feeding and cleaning), and balancing conflicting schedules of work and family life. Thus, the construct of minor stressors, or parenting hassles, refers to commonly occurring events in all families. Crnic and others argue that the chronic nature of these daily hassles of parenting may make them more likely to adversely affect family functioning than are major life events that occur infrequently. Furthermore, they argue that minor stress, or daily hassles, can provide a more universal model of the effects of stress on family functioning.

Perceived Stress

Stress resulting from daily hassles is largely a subjective experience. Some parents can cope with challenging aspects of parenting better than others. Accordingly, all parents do not experience the daily hassles of parenting in the same way. For example, coping with children's misbehavior is so stressful for some parents that changes occur in the parents' mood and level of anxiety; whereas for other parents these are merely transient annoyances of the day. Individual differences in perceptions of parenting stress reflect both biological and environmental influences. Adults bring to parenting different personality styles, different emotional resources, different coping skills, and different childhood experiences of being parented. Indeed, the best estimate of emotional well-being and functioning in parents is the level of well-being and functioning prior to becoming a parent, that is, prior to the birth of the first child. Personality styles most susceptible to experiencing stress are those marked by the prevalence of negative affect (i.e., moodiness and irritability) and trait anxiety (i.e., intolerance of uncertainty and intolerance of arousal). In addition, parents who as children experienced less positive relationships with their own parents and insecure attachments are more likely to perceive their experiences with their own children as less positive.

Critics of the minor stressors, or daily hassles, approach argue that the construct of daily hassles is inherently subjective, whereas major life events can be assessed more objectively. These critics argue that perceptions of minor hassles are confounded with the outcome measures of family functioning; for example, there is an overlap between perceiving parenting as burdensome and perceiving children's behavior as problematic. On the other hand, individual differences clearly exist in parents' ability to cope with the everyday challenges of parenting. And a large literature verifies that perceptions of events influence functioning.

Effects of Stress on Parents

Parental stress from both major life events and from daily hassles has been shown to negatively impact parents' emotional well-being, marital satisfaction, and parenting behavior.

Parental Mood and Emotional Well-Being

Parenting stress is associated with lower emotional well-being in parents. That is, parents who report more daily hassles in parenting and/or more major life events describe themselves as having less life satisfaction and more negative mood and emotional distress. There is some evidence that stress from daily hassles relates more strongly than does stress from major life events, but stress from each of these sources contributes to lower emotional well-being. In addition to the negative impact on their own emotional well-being, parents with high stress also report a less positive outlook on parenting and less satisfaction in the parental role. Furthermore, they tend to experience less pleasure in and enjoyment of their children. Not surprisingly, they report lower feelings of self-efficacy in the parenting role; that is, they feel less competent in carrying out their parental responsibilities and less confident that their efforts will have a positive impact on their children. For some parents, high levels of parenting stress contribute to psychological disorders, such as depression and anxiety. For example, mothers with higher parenting stress from low-birth-weight or medically ill infants are at higher risk for developing postpartum depression.

A bidirectional relationship exists between parenting stress and negative parental mood. Parenting stress can increase negative parental mood, but, conversely, negative mood may also increase perceptions of parenting stress. Parents with negative mood are more likely to attend to their children's negative behaviors, attribute negative intent to ambiguous behaviors, and have a decreased threshold for aversive behaviors.

Marital Satisfaction and Social Support

The stress of parenting can also affect the marital relationship. When parents feel competent in their abilities to care for their children and cope effectively with daily hassles of parenting, the marital relationship can be strengthened and serve as a solid foundation of the family. However, when high levels of parenting stress are experienced, parents often report lower levels of marital satisfaction. One reason for the decrease in marital satisfaction may be that parents who experience high levels of parenting stress have less time and emotional resources to devote to the marital relationship and to meeting their spouse's needs. Another reason may be that high levels of parenting stress increases the frequency of marital conflict and demonstrations of negative affect toward the spouse. Because the primary social support in parenting is typically the spouse, the decrease in marital satisfaction typically decreases the support a parent experiences in the role of parenting. However, others (such as grandparents) may increase the support that they provide so that a parent does not perceive a decrease in the overall support that he or she receive in the parental role.

Again bidirectional relationships occur. Parenting stress can impair marital satisfaction, but conversely, marital satisfaction can mitigate parenting stress. If parents work together, divide responsibilities, and support one another's efforts, the daily hassles of parenting are less stressful.

Parental Interactions with Children

Parenting stress can also have an adverse effect on parents' behavior toward their children. Parents who experience high levels of stress report more negative and coercive interactions with their children; similarly, they report using more authoritarian and power-assertive discipline strategies. They also describe themselves as less involved with their children. These disparate self-reports are suggestive of inconsistent management techniques. Indeed, high levels of stress have been associated with parents' reports of inconsistent disciplinary styles, that is, alternating between setting harsh and rigid limits for their children to being overly lax and permissive. Although much research has established that stressed parents report negatively on their parenting skills, it is less clear that their actual parenting skills are impaired. Research on observed parenting behaviors has been equivocal, although there is some evidence that mothers are more irritable with their children on days when they have experienced more minor stressors. Thus, parents who report higher levels of stress in caring for children may be less likely to initiate pleasurable interactions with the children and may be less able to use proactive disciplinary strategies.

Effects of Parenting Stress on Children

Parenting stress has repeatedly been found to relate to children's social competence and to behavior problems. Indeed, it is thought to be a primary contributor to the development of psychopathology in children. Again, however, much of this research is based on parental reports. Parents who report high stress describe their children as less socially competent and as having more behavior problems, both externalizing and internalizing problems. These parents also describe their children as exhibiting behaviors consistent with insecure attachments. Limited research using teacher reports and children's self-reports provides some support that parents' negative views may be accurate. Teachers rated the children of highly stressed parents as less socially competent, and children reported more adjustment problems when their parents were highly stressed.

How Might Parenting Stress Affect Children's Outcome?

Parenting stress negatively affects parents' interactions with their children, and the negative interactions, in turn, negatively impact child adjustment. In other words, parenting stress may lead to critical and negative parent–child interactions as well as inconsistent discipline; then these changes in parenting may have negative effects on the children's attachment, self-esteem, and behavior. Another way that parenting stress may affect children's outcome is through modeling affect and behavior regulation. Children observe how parents cope with frustrating situations and how they regulate negative emotions and impulsive behaviors. Parents who experience high parenting stress may model poor regulation of negative affect and more reactive behavioral responses to frustration. Finally, children may be directly experiencing some of the same factors that are causing stress in their parents, such as overcrowding.

Bidirectional effects occur in this arena as well. Parents are crucial in shaping children's behavior, but children also shape adults' parenting behavior. The bidirectional nature of parent–child interactions can create coercive relationships. In these relationships, parents' irritability and less-sensitive parenting fuel behavior problems in children, which evoke further punitive and negative parental behaviors. The cyclical interaction of parents' reactions to stressful circumstances and children's aversive behavior can reinforce a maladaptive pattern of interactions that can lead to chronic stress in the family environment and can place children at higher risk for delinquency.

Interventions for Parents and Children

With increased attention to the potentially harmful effects of stress on parents, the study of how to promote resiliency in parents has gained increasing attention. Social support and active coping skills have emerged as two primary areas of intervention for relieving parental stress. Social support has been related to decreases in self-reported parental stress. Being connected to others, sharing difficult experiences, and receiving help with the day-to-day care of children reduces parenting stress. Teaching parents strategies for coping with the daily hassles of parenting has also been shown to reduce stress in the parental role. Successful coping involves adapting to the daily hassles of parenting by anticipating problems and having a plan for actively addressing them. For some parents, coping may involve monitoring their children's behavior and environment in order to circumvent the escalation of problem behaviors; for others, it may involve establishing predictable daily routines for children and scheduling periods for taking time off, when another caregiver (e.g., spouse, grandparent, or babysitter) can provide respite care. Specific programs that teach effective parenting skills seem to reduce stress by increasing parents' confidence and efficacy in managing children's problem behaviors. Likewise, interventions that teach young children social problem-solving skills can also decrease parents' stress and increase positive parent–child exchanges. Finally, interventions to decrease parenting stress at the larger community level are also needed to support families with children. Systematic efforts to provide high-quality, affordable child care for working parents, job flexibility for balancing the demands of full-time employment and parenting, and community recreation programs for families will help reduce the burden of parenting and enhance parents' ability to care for their children.

Further Reading

Anthony, L. G., Anthony, B. J., Glanville, D. N., et al. (2005). The relationships between parenting stress, parenting behavior and preschoolers' social competence and behavior problems in the classroom. *Infant and Child Development* **14**, 133–154.

Belsky, J. (1984). The determinants of parenting. *Child Development* **55**, 83–96.

Crnic, K. A. and Acevedo, M. (1995). Everyday stresses and parenting. In: Bornstein, M. H. (ed.) *Handbook of parenting Vol. 4: Applied and practical parenting*, pp. 277–297. Mahwah, NJ: Lawrence Erlbaum.

Crnic, K. A., Gaze, C. and Hoffman, C. (2005). Cumulative parenting stress across the preschool period: relations to maternal parenting and child behavior at age 5. *Infant and Child Development* **14**, 117–132.

Crnic, K. A. and Greenberg, M. T. (1990). Minor parenting stresses with young children. *Child Development* **61**, 1628–1637.

Deater-Deckard, K. (1998). Parenting stress and child adjustment: some old hypotheses and new questions. *Clinical Psychology: Science and Practice* **5**, 314–332.

Deater-Deckard, K. (2004). *Parenting stress.* New Haven, CT: Yale University Press.

Deater-Deckard, K. (2005). Parenting stress and children's development: introduction to the special issue. *Infant and Child Development* **14**, 117–132.

Rodgers, A. Y. (1998). Multiple sources of stress and parenting behavior. *Children and Youth Services Review* **20**, 525–546.

Sepa, A., Frodi, A. and Ludvigsson, J. (2004). Psychosocial correlates of parenting stress, lack of support and lack of confidence/security. *Scandinavian Journal of Psychology* **45**, 169–179.

Prison

D L Whitehead and A Steptoe
University College London, London, UK

This is a revised version of the article by J Griffith and A Steptoe, Encyclopedia of Stress First Edition, volume 3, pp 241–246, © 2000, Elsevier Inc.

Glossary

Bullying	The act of repeatedly intimidating a weaker person by the real or threatened infliction of physical, verbal, or emotional abuse.
Role conflict	A form of social conflict that takes place when the person is forced to take on two different and incompatible roles at the same time.
Depersonalization	A feeling of detachment or estrangement from the self, in which the individual senses a loss of personal identity.
Punitive approach	The perspective on incarceration which reflects the belief that inflicting punishment on an individual will act as a deterrent and decrease the likelihood of the crime being repeated.
Rehabilitative approach	The perspective on incarceration which reflects the belief that an individual can be retrained to function appropriately in society through supportive educational programs in prison.

Scope of the Problem

In 2005, 714/100 000 U.S. residents were incarcerated in prisons and jails, a rate that had risen by 5.0% over the previous 5 years. Bureau of Justice statistics in the United States indicate that if current incarceration rates remain unchanged, an estimated 1 out of every 20 people (5.1%) will serve time in prison during his or her lifetime. U.S. incarceration rates are very much higher than in Europe, where there are wide variations between countries. Southern European countries have a relatively low rate of 80/100 000, compared with 184/100 000 in eastern and central Europe; rates in the United Kingdom fall in the middle, at 139/100 000 in 2005.

There is a very much higher incarceration rate among men than women, and more than 90% of convicts are men. However, one important change over recent years has been the rate of growth of the number of female inmates, which has outstripped that of men. The U.S. female prison population grew by 5.0% annually from 1999 to 2004, compared with a growth rate of 3.3% in the male population. Research has not kept pace with this change, and until recently most studies were conducted on the male inmate population. Overall, inmates are more likely to be young, single, and less well educated than the population at large. Ethnic minority groups are substantially overrepresented in the prison population. In 2004, 12.6% of Black American males in their late twenties were incarcerated, compared with 3.6% of Hispanic males and 1.7% of White males.

Imprisonment is one of the most stressful human experiences and figures high in all comparisons of negative life events. A combination of environmental and personal deprivation in unpleasant and often frightening circumstances can lead to the perception of extreme stress. Factors such as adherence to a strict daily routine, close living proximity, loss of control over life course, and loss of freedom have all been identified as causing psychological distress. Interpersonal relationships with prison officers and other inmates and the strain on relationships with friends and family are also causes of psychological disturbance. Associated factors such as financial hardship, coping with guilt, and dealing with aggressive fellow inmates can contribute to stress-related problems in prisoners.

Prison staff also report a range of stressors associated with the job. The main stressors are the maintenance of order and the risk of loss of control over hostile inmates, combined with the lack of support from supervisors and society. The difficulty in balancing the responsibility for the welfare of prisoners with the responsibility for security leads to conflicting work demands.

Prison Inmates

Sources of Stress

A number of studies have identified a range of stressors reported among inmates. These fall into several categories.

Personal relationships The separation from partner and family has been cited as one of the main stressors of serving time in prison. For female inmates, the separation from their children is particularly stressful. The majority of women in prison are mothers and many are also heads of households. The separation from their children has been found to be associated with a wide range of feelings such as guilt, anxiety about welfare of the children, and fear of losing close attachments to the children. This may be one reason why women have been found to suffer more emotional distress in prison than men.

The effects of separation are also evident from the finding that married men show higher levels of distress than single men. Being deprived of intimacy and worrying about the welfare of their family are also significant. The lack of confiding relationships and being denied meaningful contact with the opposite gender may create new anxieties regarding sexual identity. Coming to terms with such a mixture of emotions can pose a risk to mental health.

Establishing friendships within prison is an important aspect of adaptation. One study of young inmates found that social support and the ability to confide in friends in prison were major predictors of psychological well-being. The fear of rejection by other inmates and social isolation can cause heightened anxiety, especially in the initial stages of incarceration. However, in many cases such concerns are ill-founded because one study found that prisoners tend to receive more social support from other prisoners than they had anticipated.

Economic factors The loss of income associated with incarceration can be a major problem for prisoners and their families. Men who report financial hardship experience greater distress than those who are financially secure.

Prison environment Lack of privacy and crowding are serious problems within the prison environment. In many countries, prisons are filled beyond capacity. In the United Kingdom, for example, the Home Office released figures in 2005 that indicated a 106% occupancy rate across all prison service establishments. When personal space is threatened, angry or defensive reactions may result. Research has shown that men living in single cells report liking their accommodation more and perceive themselves having greater control than inmates living in multiple occupancy cells or dormitories. Violence is a serious concern for many inmates, and many have long-lasting fears of attack that may be associated with sustained neuroendocrine and autonomic activation. The rates of sexual and physical assault are difficult to estimate because much abuse goes unreported. Bullying and favoritism by staff are also found in many institutions.

Other aspects of the prison environment that can be sources of stress are noise levels, lack of control over lighting, physical discomfort arising from extremes of heat and cold, lack of contact with the natural environment, absence of intellectual stimulation, and constraints on physical activity.

One issue that is problematic is the pressure not to show evidence of distress. Often emotions associated with stress such as fear, grief, and depression are not admitted and are hidden from staff and other inmates. This hinders the analysis and solution of stress-related problems.

Time Course of Imprisonment

Certain sources of stress are more evident at different stages of imprisonment. Three phases of a prisoner's career have been identified.

Initial phase This is the most stressful period when the inmate first encounters prison life. First-time offenders are particularly vulnerable due to the loss of liberty and separation from friends and family. This stage is often characterized by feelings of denial followed by anxiety and depression, although other emotions such as shock, fear, isolation, grief, and anger are also reported frequently. The adjustment period typically lasts for the first 4–6 weeks of confinement. It is at this stage that many suicide attempts are made.

Middle phase During the middle stage of the sentence, the focus is on the prison community. Friendships are established, and some inmates experiment with drugs and gay sex. Mandatory drug testing has been introduced in many countries; despite efforts to prevent the importation and use of illegal drugs into prisons, the problem is common. In 2001, a UK prison survey found that 19% of inmates reported using cannabis in the previous month, and 13% reported using opiates. Although drug use is prevalent, a smaller proportion of inmates use drugs while in prison than did prior to incarceration.

Final phase Some convicts become preoccupied with their release in the final few weeks of their prison terms. Apprehension about cultural changes after long sentences is coupled with worry about the attitudes of friends and neighbors and the need to reestablish family relationships and reenter employment. Health and economic disparities that existed before incarceration are intensified following release, because access to jobs, health insurance, public housing and health benefits may be limited to ex-prisoners, particularly in the United States, and disproportionately in ethnic minority groups. Thus incarceration continues to exert effects leading to increased stress and poor health even after release.

Responses to the Stress of Prison Life

The stress experienced by prisoners has been measured in several ways: by self-report measures of mood, well-being, and mental health; by the incidence and prevalence of physical health outcomes, mental health outcomes, and physiological indicators of stress; and by the most powerful indicator of hopelessness and despair, suicide.

The investigation of the psychological state of inmates and stress-related effects in prisons faces a number of methodological challenges. First, assessing the impact of incarceration is complicated by limited knowledge about the prior health and well-being of inmates. Many studies of stress in prisons that use outcomes such as hospitalization for mental illness during incarceration are problematic in that incident psychopathology, that is, new onset mental illness, may be difficult to distinguish from prevalent psychopathology, which has been consistently demonstrated as having higher rates in prisoners. Longitudinal studies following prisoners from the first days of incarceration are the only way of studying the emergence of stress resulting from the prison environment rather than ongoing stress from psychosocial disadvantage or existing psychopathology that entails greater risk of conviction in the first place.

Second, the general population is a poor comparison group when assessing the relative prevalence of stress-related disorder in prisoners. Many individuals sent to prison have histories of psychological problems and drug abuse prior to sentencing. Inmates also tend to come from low-income families, to be unemployed, and to have limited education and therefore may have previously encountered negative life events, inadequate health care, and poor living conditions. Drug and alcohol problems frequently precede incarceration; a survey of convicts in state prisons in the United States indicated that 50% of those convicted of violent crimes were under the influence of drugs or alcohol at the time of the offense, and in 1993 drug offenders accounted for 61% of inmates in federal prisons. The high prevalence of some problems among inmates cannot, therefore, be attributed to the prison experience and is confounded by considerable preexisting psychosocial disadvantage in this group.

Nevertheless, anxiety, depression, and complaints of fatigue, sleeplessness, headache, and backache are common. In one study of female convicts, nearly half met the diagnostic criteria for posttraumatic stress disorder (PTSD), and major depression was more prevalent than in the general population. A study of a representative sample of imprisoned juvenile delinquents in California found that half experienced PTSD, with many having witnessed or been involved in traumatic violent episodes. The prevalence of infectious disease, sexually transmitted disease, and tuberculosis is also high compared with the general population. Substantial weight gain has been recorded among female inmates, resulting from the combination of the sedentary lifestyle and the availability of energy-dense high-fat foods. A recent British study investigating subjective health status in female inmates addressed the confounding by lower socioeconomic status in prisoners. Using a comparison group of women from lower-socioeconomic-status sectors of the community, a comparable level of physical health complaints and a greater level of mental health complaints were found in prisoners.

Blood pressure has been found to be elevated in prison inmates compared with matched controls and to increase with the duration of confinement and the degree of crowding in prison. One particularly impressive study used a quasi-experimental approach by measuring the blood pressure of male convicts assigned to individual cells, four-bed cells, and larger dormitories in a medium-security prison. Blood pressure increased to a greater extent in men who were transferred to multiple-occupancy cells and dormitories compared with those who were transferred to other individual cells.

However, a third methodological problem with studies of physiological stress markers is that prison studies have not kept pace with recent advances in measuring such markers as ambulatory blood pressure, cortisol, catecholamines, and inflammation. One notable exception is the Copenhagen Solitary Confinement study, which assessed changes in mood, orientation, and serum cortisol during the first 3 months and compared prisoners kept in solitary confinement (SC) with prisoners in shared cells. Although anxiety, depression, and morning cortisol levels were reduced over time in the non-SC group, such reductions did not occur in the SC group, indicating a lack of adaptation to the prison environment. Many physiological markers of stress are good prognostic indicators of health problems such as autoimmune and cardiovascular diseases, and therefore it may be fruitful to pursue this avenue.

International surveys have found that the suicide rate in prison is between 3 and 11 times greater than that of the general population, with a reported fivefold increase compared with the UK general male population from 1978 to 2003. Most suicides take place within the first few weeks of incarceration and are more common in crowded institutions than other prisons. High rates have been recorded among prisoners on remand and those convicted of murder and serving life sentences. Although suicide is most frequent in young males, self-harm is highly prevalent in female inmates, and recent UK Home Office statistics report a rate of 58.7%. Unlike the pattern in the general population, depression is not a common diagnosis at the time of death, although about one-third of male suicides had some form of psychiatric treatment in the past. Drug or alcohol dependence can be found in a substantial proportion of these cases.

There is also evidence for a European trend toward reinstitutionalization of those with mental health problems in recent years – but in prisons rather than in psychiatric hospitals. A systematic review of prevalence studies in Western countries in 2002 found an overall prevalence of 3.7% for psychotic disorders (10% for major depression), representing a two- to fourfold increase in mental illness compared with the general population. It is likely that U.S. prisons and jails hold up to twice as many individuals with mental illness than do state psychiatric hospitals; the prison system is not well equipped to support these individuals.

Characteristics of the Individual Convict

Some individuals adapt to incarceration better than others and survive even lengthy prison terms without experiencing high levels of distress. Older convicts tend to have more friends in prison, to have more contact with family and friends outside, and to report greater psychological well-being than younger individuals. A recent UK Home Office report, however, drew attention to the often overlooked but growing population of prisoners aged 60 and over. Although physical health problems in this cohort are often well provided for, psychiatric problems, in particular major depression, are not well treated. Political demand for longer sentencing for some crimes means that this older cohort will continue to provide an ongoing challenge for prison services. As noted earlier, higher levels of anxiety and depression are found in female than in male prisoners, although it is not clear whether this is a specific response to imprisonment or reflects the more general difference in distress found in the adult population at large. Members of ethnic and religious minorities suffer more than members of the majority because prejudice and cultural isolation are added to the other sources of stress present in prison.

In the United States, it has been noted that White prisoners are more likely to attempt and complete suicide than African American prisoners, but the reasons are poorly understood. One suggestion is that being raised in the tough conditions experienced by many African Americans makes adults more resilient to the pressures of prison life. Alternatively, because proportionately more Black than White Americans are incarcerated, they may come from a broader spectrum of society; White inmates may include a higher proportion of marginalized, psychologically vulnerable individuals.

Methods of Reducing Stress among Inmates

The management of stress in prison inmates involves several different levels of intervention. Medical and psychiatric services have an important role in preventing suicide and self-harm, in managing drug dependence, and in treating other psychiatric and neurological problems. Support is often hampered by the reluctance of inmates to divulge personal information to authorities or to reveal weakness. Training prison staff more generally in suicide prevention is also important. A recent public health initiative in Texas prisons led to improvements in health outcomes, and Telemedicine, allowing rapid access to telephone consultations for physical and mental health problems, proved to be a novel and effective way of delivering health care.

At a more general level, education, training, and other initiatives help build prisoners' self-esteem and confidence in their ability to adapt to civilian life after release. Increasing physical activity and exercise may also be beneficial. Studies have found that inmates who have a job detail or are on work-release programs show less evidence of stress than those who are not active.

Finally, changes at the institutional level may be warranted. It is likely that modifications of prison regimes in relation to aspects such as staff attitudes, privileges, training opportunities, and relocation of inmates to serve their terms near their families could play a key role in alleviating stress among inmates. However, the reality is that stress does not figure highly among the concerns of prison administrators or politicians, some of whom would argue that prison should be stressful.

Prison Staff

Sources of Stress

Research on prison staff members finds that many of the issues cited in the general literature on occupational stress are relevant for them as well. As with other jobs, factors such as work demands, role conflict, low control, and poor social support emerge as relevant. Thus, symptoms of psychological distress and job dissatisfaction are greater among correctional officers who report high work demands coupled with low control and low support from management and colleagues.

However, these problems are exacerbated by the peculiar requirements of working in prison. Prison officers cite the conflict of responsibilities in the job as an underlying source of stress and dissatisfaction. On the one hand, prison staff members are responsible for the welfare of inmates and for the maintenance of their physical and psychological well-being. On the other hand, they are required to maintain security and protect the public from the dangerous and sometimes violent convicts. The prison environment is often volatile, with a high risk of aggressive behavior from inmates. Confrontations with inmates and the threat of physical danger are cited as major sources of stress, irrespective of the age and gender of staff members. Ethnic minority prison officers have been found to experience lower stress levels, especially in the United States, where ethnic minorities are grossly overrepresented among inmates.

Some differences have been observed between new and long-serving staff. Newly appointed staff members report a lack of support from supervisors and a concern with lack of control over the working environment as particularly problematic. Those who have been working for longer periods are more troubled by the absence of support and respect from society and the lack of variation in the job. The combination of tedium associated with mundane day-to-day activities and the pressure to maintain vigilance in order to react quickly to high-risk incidents appears to be especially stressful.

Many prison officers believe that the responsibilities for security and the welfare of inmates are incompatible obligations. A recent meta-analysis of factors predicting work-related stress revealed an interesting effect of punitive versus rehabilitative attitudes – officers in the United States who endorsed rehabilitative attitudes experienced greater stress, whereas those in Canada with stronger punitive attitudes were more stressed. This suggests that when individuals' beliefs about their role are at odds with the ethos of the prison service in a particular country, stress and conflict are the result.

Outcomes of Stress

High rates of sick leave for both minor complaints (fatigue, headaches, and indigestion) and physical health problems (high blood pressure and peptic ulcers) occur among prison staff. In one study, the rates of coronary heart disease, hypertension, and ulcers were found to be greater among correctional officers than a comparable sample of police officers. The divorce rate in correctional officers is reported as being twice that of blue- and white-collar workers in general. Job dissatisfaction is coupled with the increased prevalence of divorce in this occupational group. The rates of sick leave are greater among staff members in maximum security prisons and in prisons with many drug users than in other correctional institutions.

There is a greater prevalence of psychological distress in prison officers. Much of the research has focused on burnout, with male and female staff members reporting similar high levels of depersonalization and emotional exhaustion. Self-reported anxiety and depression are also elevated compared with the general working population. Female officers are more likely to take sick leave than male officers, but this pattern may result from family demands rather than different levels of stress at work.

Methods of Reducing Stress in Prison Staff

It has been noted in the research literature that many prison officers do not perceive themselves to be stressed but, rather, see their colleagues as being stressed. Pressure not to show the effects of stress may be particularly evident in a male-dominated environment where there is fear that any sign of weakness will be exploited by the inmates. Admitting to feeling stressed may be interpreted as an inability to cope and therefore as not being strong enough for the job at hand. Alternatively, some prison officers may not be able to identify the personal effects of stress in themselves. This suggests that education about stress and how it can be managed may both benefit prison staff members directly and help them to identify the repercussions of stress in inmates.

A number of studies have found that exercise and fitness programs have positive effects. One investigation involving a 6-week strength and aerobic program showed reductions in body weight, skinfold thickness, and cholesterol levels, together with beneficial changes in smoking, alcohol consumption, sleep, nutritional habits, and stress tolerance.

Consultation and efforts to enhance social support at work have been found to counteract the effects of stress. Factors such as goal consensus among staff, a proactive management style, and increasing of decision latitude can be incorporated into the working environment.

Limitations and Conclusion

There are a number of limitations in the studies that have been carried out thus far about stress in prisons. Most have been cross-sectional in nature, identifying associations between aspects of prison experience and diminished well-being, and the causal sequence is uncertain. Longitudinal designs and data on inmates prior to imprisonment are important in the assessment of the impact of stressors because some apparent effects of incarceration may be the direct consequences of prior experience. The nature of the offense, family situation, and previous physical and mental health are all important factors that should be taken into account. Also, the civilian groups with which prisoners are compared in many studies may not be matched appropriately in terms of background characteristics.

The generalizability of results across populations is uncertain. The majority of studies have been conducted on White male adults and may not be relevant to women, ethnic minorities, and juveniles. This is not mere tokenism because it is apparent from the limited information available that the experience of prison is very different for people of different backgrounds and cultures. The applicability of findings to different prison systems must also be questioned. Justice systems in the United Kingdom and other European countries differ greatly from the U.S. system, and countries also vary in the extent to which individuals with serious psychiatric histories are found in prison. The application of management suggestions derived from one system must be reviewed carefully before their implementation elsewhere.

Nevertheless, the data do indicate that imprisonment is severely stressful for many inmates and that work within the prison system is also associated with higher rates of stress-related dysfunction than comparable jobs. Education and the implementation of specific stress-management programs may be beneficial to both groups and may help ensure that stress in prison is confined within tolerable limits.

Further Reading

Andersen, H. S. (2004). Mental health in prison populations: a review. *Acta Psychiatrica Scandinavica* **110**(supplement 424), 5–59.

Andersen, H. S., Sestoft, D., Lillebaek, T., et al. (2003). A longitudinal study of prisoners on remand: repeated measures of psychopathology in the initial phase of solitary versus nonsolitary confinement. *International Journal of Law and Psychiatry* **26**, 165–177.

Cooke, D. J., Baldwin, P. J. and Howison, J. (1993). *Psychology in prisons.* London: Routledge.

DeRosia, V. R. (1998). *Living inside prison walls: adjustment behavior.* Westport, CT: Praeger.

Hayes, L. M. and Blaauw, E. (eds.) (1997). *Special issue on prison suicide. Crisis: The Journal of Crisis Intervention and Suicide Prevention* **18**(4).

Dowden, C. and Tellier, C. (2004). Predicting work-related stress in correctional officers: a meta-analysis. *Journal of Criminal Justice* **32**, 31–47.

Lindquist, C. H. and Linquist, C. A. (1997). Gender differences in distress: mental health consequences of environmental stress among jail inmates. *Behavioral Sciences & the Law* **15**, 503–523.

Ostfeld, A. M., Kasl, S. V., D'Atri, D. A. and Fitzgerald, E. F. (1987). *Stress, crowding and blood pressure in prison.* Hillsdale, NJ: Lawrence Erlbaum.

Paulus, P. B. (1988). *Prison crowding: a psychological perspective.* New York: Springer-Verlag.

Religion and Stress

S Packer
New School for Social Research, New York, NY, USA

This is a revised version of the article by S Packer, Encyclopedia of Stress First Edition, volume 3, pp 348–355, © 2000, Elsevier Inc.

Glossary

Apocalyptic religion — A religion based on writings prophesying a cataclysmic time when evil forces are destroyed; includes millenarian religions that focus on the end of 1000-year period described in the Book of Revelation.

Cult — A pejorative term used to describe a new religious movement, especially one that is secretive, is socially isolated, is faddish, has unfamiliar rules and rituals, and uses coercive or manipulative or deceptive techniques used to win or keep new converts.

Prophetic religion — A religion that maintains that truth is revealed by prophecy; sometimes referred to as religions of revelation. Prophetic religions include Western monotheistic religions such as Judaism, Christianity, and Islam, as well as Zoroastrianism and Bahai.

Religion — A system of beliefs centered around the concept of a supernatural being or force.

Transcendent religion — A religion that teaches techniques for transcending or transforming the reality of the senses or that denies the existence or importance of mundane reality. Transcendent religions include many Eastern religions and some Western New Age beliefs.

Religion can be both a cause of stress and a cure for stress. Some go so far as to say that it is religion's ability to relieve the very stress that it induces that is partly responsible for its tenacious hold on its truest or newest believers. It has also been noted that religious sentiment and sectarianism rises during times of increased personal or societal stress. Because change and uncertainty are potent causes of stress, on a psychological, sociological, and physiological level, it is not surprising that some of history's most unusual religious movements have sprung up during the times of rapid social change and uncertainty. Individuals undergoing personal stress and lifestyle shifts are statistically more likely to get involved with unusual or innovative religious movements. Thus, adolescents who have recently left home, the newly divorced or bereaved or relocated, and prison inmates are especially susceptible to the appeal of new religions or radical religions. But charismatic religious groups or cults are not the only religious groups that gain momentum during times of stress; even the ranks of more garden-variety religions grow when the stresses of poverty, old age, war, illness, isolation, or impending death increase.

Religion as a Concept

Religion is anything but a single, all-embracing phenomenon. There are over 100,000 registered religions in the United States alone. The number of registered religions is increasing, not decreasing, and has been on the rise in the United States since the 1960s. The number of people who accept a personal spirituality, rather than a recognized religion, is rising even faster, to the point that spirituality is now a more politically correct and more all-embracing term that bypasses the conservative connotations of the word religion.

Even the meaning of the word religion is a source of contention. For the sake of simplicity, we define religion here as a system of beliefs centered around a supernatural being, power, or force. But, for the sake of accuracy, we must add that many well-respected definitions of religion that include systems of belief do not include a belief in the supernatural and that some well-known religions, such as Confucianism, are not concerned with a supernatural entity.

Given the large number of recognized religions in existence, it stands to reason that religions can differ dramatically from one another. Furthermore, some organized religions include far-flung sects and subsects that bear little superficial resemblance to the parent religion, and some (but certainly not all) religions host a wide variety of views on different issues. It may be tempting to think that religious beliefs, rites, customs, and concerns can be plotted out on a spreadsheet, so that different religions can be directly compared to one another. However, this straightforward approach of scientists leads to an inaccurate appreciation of the vagaries of religion and overlooks the fact that one religion stresses rites of worship, another concerns itself with right thinking, a third revolves around prayer or penitence, a fourth focuses on gender differences and reproduction issues, a fifth emphasizes the afterlife, and so forth. It is unlikely that each religion has something to say about every aspect of life (or death), even though each religion represents itself as the ultimate authority on human life.

Religion as a Cure for Stress

Both its fiercest critics and its most fervent advocates agree that religion (or at least some religions) can dampen psychological stress. Freud himself, that arch-enemy of religion, admitted as much in his seminal book on *The Future of an Illusion*. Personal testimonials and clergymen's sermons about religion's potential to relieve stress are too numerous to cite here. Religion is so commonly associated with stress that it is virtually a reflex to invoke it at moments of stress. Many images of religion and extreme stress spring to mind immediately, from foot-stomping spirituals of the segregation-era South to the footsteps of the death-row dweller listening to the last words of the seventy-first psalm to the prayers mumbled by chaplains for charging troops who face death on the front. We can even consider the fearlessness of the 9/11 suicide bombers who embraced their own death as (perverse) testimony to the power of faith.

Although not everyone finds relief in religion, there are some compelling sociological statistics supporting religion's overall ability to combat stress. It is well-established that people with strong personal religious beliefs and affiliations are less likely to commit suicide, which can be seen as the ultimate and most extreme response to stress. The fact that some Islamic extremists encouraged suicide missions, in spite of Islam's strong stance against suicide, is an aberration.

Philosophical Aspects

By positing the existence of a supernatural being who actively intervenes in the natural world and who has a plan for each individual human, religion provides an automatic antidote to the stress of being alone and awash in an unresponsive and uncaring universe. Philosophers and theologians alike note that existential angst and dread have plagued twentieth-century society, at least in the West. Ever since Nietzsche declared that "God is dead" as the nineteenth century ended, and as his own symptoms of neurosyphilis progressed, unwavering faith in the supernatural melted away and slowly but surely became the foremost source of stress. Only the lurking specter of a sudden nuclear holocaust overshadowed this stress. Pastoral pop psychologists tried to reverse the tide that Nietzsche set into motion. Best-selling books, such as Paul Tillich's *Man Is Not Alone,* played on Nietzsche's angst-inducing assertion in its title and appealed to this angst. Similarly, film titles and themes recapitulate the reflexive tendency to call on religion in times of crisis. For instance, the film *God is My Co-Pilot* appeared during World War II. More veiled religious themes bubble to the surface during other times of stress. When the Great Depression cast its shadow, *Lost Horizon* evoked legends of Shangri-La, where Tibetan monks and Christian missionaries fused good works and good karma and reinfused human souls. Then, as the twentieth century came to a close, and as second millennium neared – at the very same time that information technology zoomed ahead and rocked standard channels of communication – religious imagery once again resurfaced in secular guise, this time in the form of angels. New Age angels, which were retrieved from Renaissance-era paintings, appeared on postage stamps.

Psychological Aspects

Antidote to aloneness, abandonment, and dependency

When psychoanalysts try to explain why a belief in the supernatural relieves stress, they look for more personal, rather than societal, explanations. The consistently controversial Freud claimed that a belief in God substitutes for the presence of an all-protective, albeit sometimes punitive, parent. According to such theories, religion recreates the reassuring world of dependency that an infant enjoys. The oceanic feeling of connectedness with the universe that mystics describe could be a way to return to the peacefulness and protectiveness of the womb, where an umbilical cord delivered never-ending nourishment and where amniotic fluid buffered the baby from unkind blows from the world around. Religious redemption concepts that revolve around the return to Eden can be compared to psychoanalytic fantasies about the return to the womb.

More contemporary neo-Freudian psychoanalytic thinkers, such as Karl Winnicot, emphasized the importance of separation-individuation as the critical step in psychological growth. Unlike more orthodox Freudians, who viewed religious reassurance as a sign of psychological immaturity and as an obstacle to self-actualization, theorists such as Winnicot felt that religious belief functions as a useful transitional object, much like a baby blanket or a teddy bear. Both remind the child of the parent's perpetual presence and assuage a child's subjective stress of abandonment during the parents' absence. There are many, many more psychoanalytic theories about the ways that religion relieves stress, each unique and interesting in its own right and each as untestable by scientific techniques as the tenets of religion itself.

A more pragmatic and less theoretical take on religion as a surrogate dependency is found in the principles behind the Twelve-Step and Recovery Programs and Alcoholics Anonymous. These programs provide a strong social support system and also call on a Higher Power to relieve the psychological and physiological stress of alcohol withdrawal and as an aid in dealing with stresses that were previously ameliorated by addictions. Rather than admonishing their members for depending on this spiritual Higher Power, as more Freudian-influenced therapists did in the past, the Twelve-Step groups see spiritual dependency as far less harmful than chemical dependency. Such pro-spiritual approaches have gained increasing public and professional acceptance and have been adapted to the treatment of many other disorders.

Decreased sense of randomness and uncertainty

There are many other ways that religion relieves personal stress. Religion decreases the sense of randomness, uncertainty, and chaos in the world because it details the logic (or illogic) behind a world plan. It predicts or sometimes prophesies or, at the very least, attempts to explain those events that seem most inexplicable. In doing so, it creates a concept of stability that has been described as an ordered universe. Even religions that foretell the coming of adverse events in the future, such as an impending apocalypse, reincarnation, predestination, or bad karma, have the potential to offer partial relief from stress, simply because they help their members prepare themselves psychologically for adverse events. Providing explanations for events, even without providing a means for altering those events, is referred to as heuristics, and this is one of the most powerful psychological tools that religion possesses. Some critics of psychoanalysis say that its appeal also rests on its heuristic value and argue that unprovable psychoanalytic explanations provide reasons for behavior rather than remedies, in the same way that religion provides reasons for cosmic events and human nature.

Religions further relieve the stress of uncertainty by providing blueprints for behavior that can theoretically change the future. By prescribing prayer, penance, codes of charity, dietary laws, sacrificial rituals, or right thought, those religions reinstill a sense of personal control. More optimistic prophesies, and promises of paradise, confer hope and escape.

Cognitive coping techniques Above and beyond any theoretical parallels with psychoanalysis, many religions also provide specific cognitive techniques that are useful in coping with stress. For instance, the mere act of acknowledging and articulating the experience of stress can quell some distress. Long before Freud discovered his talking cure, religious prayers and petitions provided collective voices for stress and distress. Hebrew psalms that begin with words such as "From the depths I called out unto Thee" poeticize an acute sense of anguish, whereas Christian recreations of the crucifixion scene dramatize the ordeal of Christ on the cross. These words and images are especially appealing to people who do not have access to other avenues or expression, or who prefer to deflect their own subjective sense of distress by focusing on more universal, cosmic, or collective stresses.

Role models for stress endurance Religious lore offers as role models people who withstood extreme stress and either surmounted that stress, were valued because of their ability to endure stress, or went on to fulfill higher purposes because of those stresses. The Christ-figure is the consummate example of this sort, but it is hardly the only one. Biblical stories about Jonah being swallowed by a whale, Noah's ability to withstand a flood, Daniel's survival in the fiery lion's den, and Job's endurance of the loss of his family and his health all reassure believers that there is a relief for stress or, if there is no immediate relief, that there is a reason or perhaps even a reward in another life. The martyrdom of Christian saints before their beatification, the Buddhist *jataka* stories about Prince Shakyamuni's wandering as a mendicant monk before he achieved enlightenment as he sat under the Boddhi tree, and the image of the Israelite tribes wandering through the desert for 40 years before entering the Land of Israel and acquiring their status as the chosen people are other examples of the pivotal role that stress endurance plays in religious themes.

Consolation, devaluation, and dissociation Some religions provide such a sense of consolation that they have been dubbed the religions of consolation. Christianity's contention that the meek with inherit the Earth reassures people that their this-worldly stress and suffering will be relieved by other-worldly rewards. The promises of future paradise made by prophetic religions dull the pain of the present and appeal to the impoverished, the downtrodden, and the psychologically stressed. Some religions offer so much consolation for contemporary stress and distress that they devalue the material world completely by undermining its ultimate importance or by teaching that the real world is but a delusion and no different from a dream. Buddhism's belief that the material world is nothing more than a delusion, or *maya*, is an extreme example of such transcendent thinking. The Hindu yogin's aspiration to a waking state of dreamless sleep is another example of transcendence. Some psychotherapeutic techniques train patients to use similar techniques of detachment when confronted with stress-producing stimuli, although it cannot be overlooked that people who enter such dissociative states spontaneously and nonvolitionally develop serious difficulties in life.

Temporal and physical escapes from stress Even world-affirming religions, which affirm the importance of the material world, often offer temporary escape routes from daily stress. Religious holidays and religious services and other sacred times carve out stress-free time during the ordinary workweek and create an opportunity for rejuvenation. For those times when real-world stresses require even more relief than routine religious beliefs or rituals can confer, some religions offer physical as well as temporal retreats where food, clothing, and shelter are available, along with social support, structure, and spiritual exercises. Ashrams, yeshivas, monasteries, convents, and any number of other religious communities provide parallels to the retreats popular among certain Christian denominations. Such religious retreats not only legitimize the need for relief from stress, but also consecrate the choice to retreat from stress. Such religious retreats thereby provide participants with a renewed sense of self-worth, along with a sense of connectedness with others who share their belief system, and may even offer retraining in new vocations or avocations. Some retreats encourage members to contribute to society by doing good works or charity. The modern hospital movement evolved out of the monastic retreats in the Middle Ages, where people who originally sought relief for spiritual, physical, psychological ailments eventually provided care for others after their own recovery. In contrast, psychiatric rest cures and funny farms, which also offered retreats from the real world, stigmatize the participant, pathologize the process, and end social productivity. It is no wonder that religious retreats are often preferred over psychiatric treatment and that religion is often the first defense against stress.

Social Aspects

For some people, and for some religions, religion is a solitary matter and nothing but. For them, it is personal spirituality that matters most, with respect to stress relief and everything else. Although the title of William James's often-republished book is *The Varieties of Religious Experience,* in it James focused exclusively on religion that is experienced in solitude. Nevertheless, religion exists on a social as well as a personal level and acts to relieve social stress (or produce stress) on both levels as well. By providing a social support network through their communal services and activities, coupled with a sense of collective identity and purpose, religious organizations can directly combat the stress of loneliness, displacement, and *anomie* that Emil Durkheim implicated in his early sociological studies of suicide.

Some religions provide material benefits, such as charity, lodging, employment, social services, and subsidized medical care, which can counteract the intense stresses of economic hardship and ill health and can complement the psychological consolation inherent in religious theory. Religious bureaucracies also offer alternative, and much appreciated, channels for personal and political expression, particularly when access to legitimate political clout is closed. Moreover, organized religion can become powerful enough to challenge the existing political and economic powers and bring about lasting and legitimate social and legal change.

Studies of the conversion process are especially illustrative of the importance of social forces and religion. It often comes as a surprise to people who are ideologically committed to religion to learn that it is the social sway of a religious group that influences individuals to adopt new religious ideas rather than the other way around. In other words, rather than experiencing a life-changing epiphany before converting, similar to the epiphany that the Gospels attributed to Saul of Tarsus on the road to Damascus, converts to new religions are more likely to follow a socially paved path to new religious insights. They accept more and more of the ideas of the group as they gain greater and greater acceptance into that group and as they become more reliant on group members for social support. The process of conversion is more likely to be gradual than sudden; in most people, behavior changes incrementally rather than dramatically. Nor does everyone who gets involved with a new religious group remain committed to that group. Of the many factors that correlate with an individual's long-term involvement with a new religion, one of the most important factors revolves around the role of stress. The more stress relief that an individual experiences at the time of joining a new religious group, the more likely that person is to remain a member of that group. Furthermore, it is the stress that individuals experience when distancing themselves from such groups that typically compels them to return to those groups.

Because it is well known that people who are already in a state of stress stand to achieve the greatest degree of stress relief from a new religion, some such religions make it a point to stress their newest members. Techniques such as sleep deprivation, diet restriction, social isolation, overwork, enforced silence, sexual abstinence, or even physical or psychological threats make new recruits more receptive to the stress-relieving effects of the religion. Religions that rely on such insidious, quasi-coercive stress-inducing techniques are often denounced as cults and are disdained by nonmembers or former members. Such cultish religions predictably recruit in institutional settings, such as colleges, prisons, and retirement communities, where people are already in high stress states. Because such residents are pre-primed for proselytization, new religions have made major inroads in such places, at times to tragic ends.

It is the intense stress of prison life, rather than an earnest desire to reform or to atone their past acts, that propels some inmates to seek relief through religious conversion. Many ministries maintain an active presence in prisons because they recognize this potential. Sometimes, religious recruitment goes hand in hand with political indoctrination and can lead to involvement in militant religious factions. Many Black Muslims and Seven Percenters, including Malcolm X, traced their conversion to their incarceration. Yet, until 9/11 made the U.S. public more aware of this potential, there was little public opposition to religious recruitment in prisons. Most people assumed that religions strive to instill socially acceptable values that will substitute for criminal behavior, aid in rehabilitation and reentry into society, and thwart future incarceration. The recruitment of prisoners to a new religion was preferred over recruitment by antisocial prison gangs. However, in our post-9/11 world, we must consider the possibility that some extremist religions can instill antisocial attitudes and push some individuals into committing extreme acts.

In contrast, there has been a great public outcry about cult recruitment on college campuses, partly because some cultish religions have the opposite effect of prison-based cult religions. Rather than aiding the recruit's reentry into society, these cults isolate students from society and abort their attempts to achieve the status of other adults in society. Some cults cut off members' contact with families and friends, and cause severe stress in their relatives as a result. Although many legitimate religions were considered to be cults in their early stages – with Methodism being the most notable U.S. example – the mere fact that a small percentage of cults have been associated with mass suicide or homicide is enough to cause public concern and to stimulate psychiatric task forces to investigate these issues. The memories of 800 deaths in Jonestown, the loss of 19 lives in California's Heaven's Gate suicides, the subway poisonings by Japan's Aum Shinrikyo sect, and the murder of a Hare Krishna defector in North Carolina tend to overshadow studies that show the psychological benefits of conversion in some individuals.

Somatic Aspects

Stress is as much a physiological response as a psychological one. Some religious rites use physical means to achieve higher spiritual states and alleviate both psychological and physiological stress in the process. The muscle stretching systems of yoga, the breathing exercises of Zen, and the controlled movements of Tai Chi are just a few examples of Eastern-influenced mind–body methods that gained popularity in the West. Some of these methods are now taught in continuing education courses sponsored by the American Psychiatric Association.

Although it is impossible to verify the existence of higher spiritual states, it is possible to measure changes in heart rate, respiration, galvanic skin response (sweating), pupil size, secretions of stress hormones such as cortisol or gastric acid, brain waves (through an electroencephalogram, EEG), and muscle tension in people performing those spiritual exercises. Internist Harold Benson's studies of cardiovascular effects of Transcendental Meditation and Tibetan Buddhist chanting appear in juried medical journals and in his popular paperback, *The Relaxation Response*. Japanese psychiatrist Tomio Hirai correlated the EEG and electromyogram (EMG) effects of both Zen meditation and Hindu yoga with reports of spiritual and psychological states and published his results in the curious book *Zen Meditation and Psychotherapy*. These works represent serious research, but there have also been many hyperbolic claims about the benefits of Eastern (and Western) religious systems, leading some professionals to dismiss any and all claims reflexively and prematurely. Recent scientific studies confirming the correlation between stress relief and specific religious rites suggest that both an open mind – and an open eye – can help us to appreciate confirmed the mind–body benefits of religion and also to avoid misleading claims and cults.

Quite the opposite of the calming meditative techniques of Eastern religions are the ecstatic dances, shaking, quaking, rocking, and rolling movement of some sects, which inspired the names Holy Rollers, Ranters, Ravers, Quakers, Shaking Quakers, and Shakers. Such intense activity presumably relieves stress through the same mechanisms that jogging and exercise help more secular devotees. The Dionysian dances of Classical Greece, described in Euripides' play about the Bacchae, were but one of many recurring manifestations of frenzied religious dancing that serves a related function. Repetitive religious rituals in general are said to relieve stress as well.

Side Effects of Stress Relief

Religion's efficacy at relieving stress does not come without side effects. There are times when religion relieves stress so well that its practitioners are unaware of the demands of the real world and are unable to mount a defense against impending danger. Many social scientists have said that the religious devotion of African Americans shielded them from the pain and poverty of pre-Civil Rights America and delayed the adoption of more appropriate political tactics. Similarly, the Tibetan practice of sending one-third of its youth to Buddhist monasteries left the country defenseless against the Chinese invaders who destroyed temples, massacred monks and nuns, and sent their religious leaders into exile. Some secular Zionists claimed that the insulated and self-satisfied religious infrastructure of some eastern European Jewish communities obscured their awareness of the deadly fate that awaited Jews in Hitler's death camps. An analogous U.S. tragedy occurred when Native American warriors went into battle unarmed, believing that their Ghost Dance ritual would protect them from the guns and arrows of approaching armies. Marx and Engels blamed the mystical and occasionally bizarre religious belief of Russian orthodoxy and schismatics for numbing Russian reactions to the material exploitation by the capitalists and the Czars. This observation prompted Marx to coin his oft-quoted characterization of religion as "the opiate of the masses."

Religion as a Cause of Stress

As effective as religion can be at relieving stress, it can also produce stress. Threats of an afterlife full of hellfire and brimstone or of an impending apocalypse that will destroy the world are obvious stress-producers. On a more subtle level are the many moralistic demands and behavioral codes made by religion, which are often difficult to live up to and, thus, tend to leave some practitioners in a near-constant state of imperfection and incompleteness. Some practitioners adopt even more zealous beliefs and behavior in order to avoid that stress, in an ever spiraling pattern. Skeptics such as psychiatrist John Sargeant observed that some charismatic religions exploit this tandem stress relief–stress production effect when they proselytize and compared this push–pull effect of religion to behavioral conditioning, more nefarious methods of mind control and brainwashing, and even drug addiction.

For sure, religion-induced stress is not limited to perceived threats, nor is it confined to the personal psyche. In spite of its promises of eternal peace, organized religion has indeed injected some of the most realistic threats the world has ever witnessed. The Inquisition, the Crusades, and the wars of religion are but a few testimonies to reality-based stresses posed by religion in the past. Such stresses persist to the present day through suicide cults such as the California-based Heaven's Gate, Islamic terrorist attacks on the World Trade Center, the biological-weapon-wielding Aum Shinrikyo in Japan, the Hindu–Muslim–Sikh conflicts in an atomic-bomb-armed India, the religious-ethnic conflicts of the Balkans that set the stage for World War I, and right-ring religious assassinations in Jerusalem, to name just a few. Although some religions aspire to the day that "the lion will lie down with the lamb," that day has not yet arrived. Religion has been, and probably always will be, as intimately associated with the stress of war and violence as with the proverbial love and peace that it promises. Rising religious fundamentalism promises to produce more political and personal stresses for individuals and for the world at large. At the same time, the religions of reassurance will provide personal stress relief for individuals, creating a never-ending seesaw.

Religion as a Correlate of Stress

The correlation between the rapid rise of new and sometimes radical religious movements and the degree of social stress is nothing less than remarkable; it is cataloged in Norman Cohn's classic *Pursuit of the Millennium* and in his more recent *Chaos, Cosmos, and the World to Come.* A more recent book, *Radical Religion in America,* zeros in on extreme religious schisms that have arisen since 1970, during the times of high stress that followed the social turbulence of the 1960s. It is noteworthy that psychoanalysis, a once-esteemed and all-embracing psychiatric treatment that survives as a mere shadow of its former self, has also been accused of being a cult and of inducing a cultlike devotion that resembles religion more than science. Note that psychoanalysis's popularity peaked in the 1950s, during the times of high stress that followed World War II.

Further Reading

Cohn, N. (1993). *Cosmos, chaos, and the world to come.* New Haven, CT: Yale University Press.

Freud, S. (1961). The future of an illusion (1927). In: Strachey, J. (ed.) *Standard edition of the complete psychological works of Sigmund Freud* (vol. 21), pp. 3–56. New York: W. W. Norton.

Fuller, A. (1994). *Psychology & religion* (3rd edn.). Lanham, MD: Rowman and Littlefield.

Gallant, M. (ed.) (1989). *Cults and new religious movements.* Arlington, VA: American Psychiatric Association.

Girard, R. (1993). *Violence and the sacred.* Baltimore, MD: Johns Hopkins University Press.

Hirai, T. (1989). *Zen meditation & psychotherapy.* New York: Tokyo Publications.

James, W. (1982). *The varieties of religious experience.* New York: Penguin Books.

Kakar, S. (1982). *Shamans, mystics, and doctors.* Chicago: University of Chicago Press.

Kaplan, J. (1997). *Radical religion in America.* Syracuse, NY: Syracuse University Press.

Kinsley, D. (1996). *Health, healing, and religion.* Upper Saddle River: Prentice-Hall.

Klass, M. (1995). *Ordered universes.* Boulder, CO: Westview Press.

Meissner, W. W. (1984). *Psychoanalysis and religious experience.* New Haven, CT: Yale University.

Ostow, M. (ed.) (1982). *Judaism & psychoanalysis.* London: Karnac Books.

Packer, S. (1998). Jewish mystical movements and the European ergot epidemics. *Israel Journal of Psychiatry* 35, 227–241.

Paloutzian, R. (1996). *Invitation to the psychology of religion* (2nd edn.). Boston, MA: Allyn & Bacon.

Sargant, W. (1957). *Battle for the mind.* New York: Penguin Books.

Schumaker, J. F. (1992). *Religion and mental health.* New York: Oxford University Press.

Organ Transplantation, Stress of

M A Dew, A F DiMartini and R L Kormos
University of Pittsburgh School of Medicine and Medical Center, Pittsburgh, PA, USA

Glossary

Graft rejection The process by which the body's immune response system attacks the foreign organ or tissue.

Immunosuppression The suppression of the immune response by an agent such as a chemical or drug in order to enhance the body's acceptance of foreign organs or tissue.

Organ transplantation The process of removing an organ or tissue from one person's body and implanting it in another person's body.

Organ transplantation is increasingly often the procedure of choice for patients with end-stage diseases of the kidney, liver, heart, lung, pancreas, or intestines. Organ transplantation can significantly extend life, as well as dramatically improve the quality of individuals' lives. Yet each step in the transplantation process – encompassing the initial evaluation and wait for an organ, the transplant surgery, postsurgical recovery, and living permanently with the transplant – is also associated with significant stressors. These stressors include both acute events and chronic, ongoing health and psychosocial strains. Across the entire process, transplant patients face and must adapt to changing health and functional capacity, altered social relationships, new perceptions of self, and revised life goals and plans. An understanding of both the nature of such stressors and individuals' reactions to them is critical for three reasons. First, as transplantation becomes more common, it is imperative that patients and their families know what to expect during the transplant process and thereafter. Education regarding likely stressors as well as potential benefits of transplantation will increase the likelihood that organ recipients will achieve the best possible quality of life (QOL) in the months and years after transplant. Second, it is only through knowledge about the nature of transplant-related stressors that we will be able to develop and test appropriate stress reduction interventions for transplant recipients and their families. Third, knowledge regarding transplant-related stressors, and reactions to them, also has value for understanding similar reactions to the experience of other life-threatening chronic physical illnesses, their treatment, and their long-term outcomes.

Prevalence of Organ Transplantation

Although the potential benefits of solid organ transplantation were first realized in the 1950s, it was not until the advent of modern immunosuppression in the 1970s and 1980s that organ transplantation fully evolved from an experimental procedure to the standard of care for many end-stage diseases. Today, the greatest obstacle to receiving a transplant is the shortage of donor organs. As illustrated in **Figure 1**, the total number of individuals registered on the wait list for a transplant (including kidney, liver, heart, lung, heart-lung, pancreas, or intestines) far exceeds the number of transplants performed, and the gap continues to widen, despite the success of some social and governmental programs in increasing rates of donation. The lives of kidney transplant candidates can be maintained by dialysis during the wait for an organ. But for other solid organ candidates, for whom few or no such long-term alternative treatments exist, the consequence of the organ shortage is that a large proportion of them will die before a suitable organ becomes available.

In some areas of transplantation, living donor organs have helped to reduce waiting times and allow more candidates to receive transplants. For example, in the United States, living kidney donation – whether from a donor who is biologically or emotionally related to the recipient or from an anonymous, unrelated donor – is almost as prevalent as deceased donor transplantation. Living liver donation is also becoming a viable option for some patients. **Figure 2** shows the total numbers of deceased donor transplants (and living donor transplants, where applicable) that were performed for each type of organ transplant in 2004 in the United States. Overall, kidney transplantation (whether from deceased or living donors) is the most common type of transplant performed, followed by liver, heart, pancreas, and lung transplantation. Intestine and heart-lung transplants are the most rare. Similar distributions are reported in other countries.

As shown in **Figure 3**, survival rates following organ transplantation vary across organ type, but are good to excellent for many types of organs, especially in the early years after transplant. Kidney recipients, especially those with living donors, show the highest rates of survival. Even at 10 years posttransplant, 76% remain alive. Liver and heart recipients show slightly lower survival rates, but, even so, almost 75% survive at least 5 years posttransplant, and about 50% remain alive at 10 years

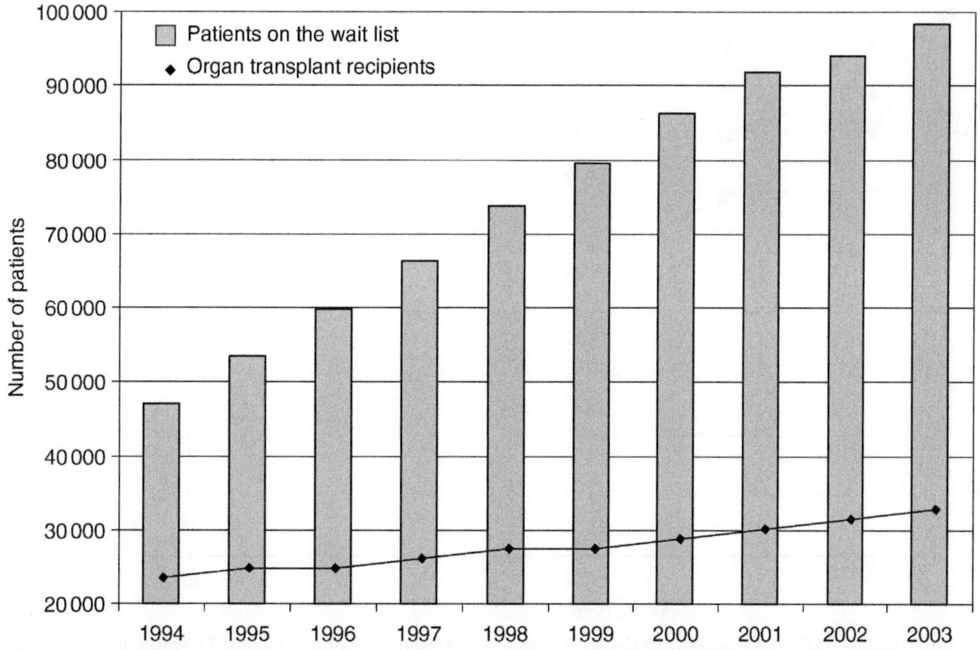

Figure 1 Combined United States and Eurotransplant statistics. From 2004 Annual Reports from United Network for Organ Sharing, Organ Procurement and Transplantation Network, which includes all United States data (www.optn.org), and Eurotransplant, which includes data from Austria, Belgium, Germany, Luxembourg, Netherlands, and Slovenia (www.eurotransplant.org).

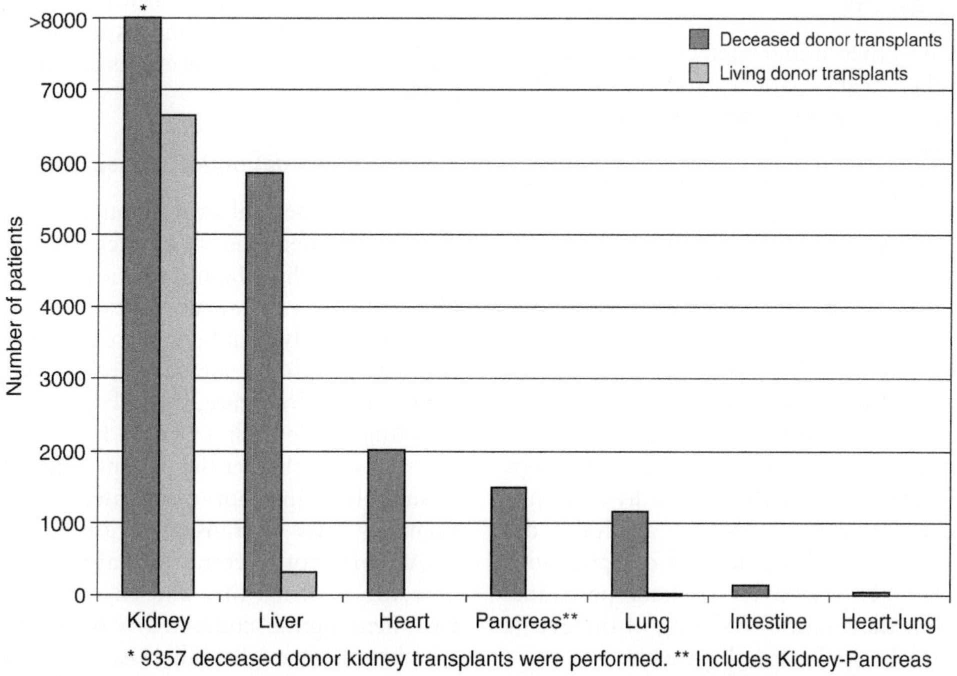

Figure 2 Numbers of deceased donor and living donor transplants of each organ type (including kidney-pancreas) in the United States in 2004; 9357 deceased donor kidney transplants were performed. From United Network for Organ Sharing, Organ Procurement and Transplantation Network (www.optn.org).

posttransplant. Survival rates for intestine and lung recipients remain substantially poorer, especially in the long-term. But even these rates have shown marked improvements in recent years. Given that annual mortality rates range up to 30% or more among candidates awaiting transplant, it is clear that transplantation provides a significant extension of life for many patients.

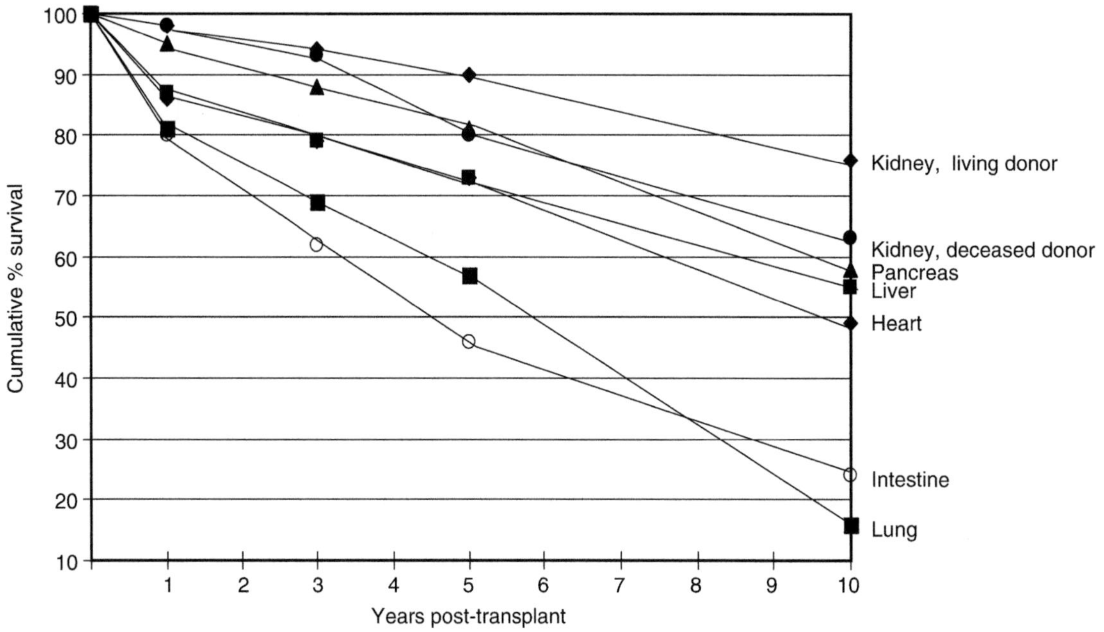

Figure 3 Patient survival, U.S. transplants, 1996–2003. From 2004 Annual Report, United Network for Organ Sharing, Organ Procurement and Transplantation Network.

The Transplantation Process for the Individual Patient

From the point of their initial contact and evaluation by the transplant team, patients and their families move through a relatively standard series of events and time periods associated with the transplant process. The typical time line is shown in **Figure 4**. The time line is punctuated by specific events that occur during the transplant process, and these events mark the onset and offset of important periods or stages, including the wait for a donor organ, the perioperative recovery period, the early posttransplant months, and the longer-term posttransplant years. The duration of each of these periods can vary considerably, depending on such factors as the rapidity with which end-stage organ disease develops in a given patient, the availability of a living donor (when living donation is possible) or a suitable deceased donor organ, and the medical complications that may occur perioperatively or later posttransplant. However, the essential ordering of the events and time periods is similar for all patients.

Figure 4 also lists the typical health and psychosocial issues that are associated with each time period. Some of these issues are unique to specific time periods (e.g., continued deterioration of the native organ's function during the waiting period, or early posttransplant physical rehabilitation). Others are present across almost all of the periods (e.g., changes in QOL), although the central elements of concern to patients and their families in these areas vary across time. Each of the sections below considers the stressors and related health and psychosocial issues that are relevant to the major events and the time periods in **Figure 4**.

The Initial Evaluation for Transplant

The formal medical evaluation for transplant candidacy is often the first occasion during which patients and their families seriously consider transplantation as a therapeutic option. For both patients and their family members, the evaluation may evoke conflicting feelings, including relief and the hope of having a healthy future, fears about surgical risks and adapting to life with an organ from another person, worry about whether the patient will be judged to be a suitable transplant candidate, worry about the financial costs of transplantation, concerns that an organ will not become available soon enough to save the patient's life, and eagerness to try a new treatment option combined with reservations as to whether there might still exist other seemingly less drastic medical interventions. For all of these reasons, studies of psychological distress among patients and family members conducted at the time of the evaluation typically find that many respondents' distress levels are high. Symptoms of anxiety and depression have been noted most frequently, and distress in these areas may reach the level of diagnosable disorder in some individuals.

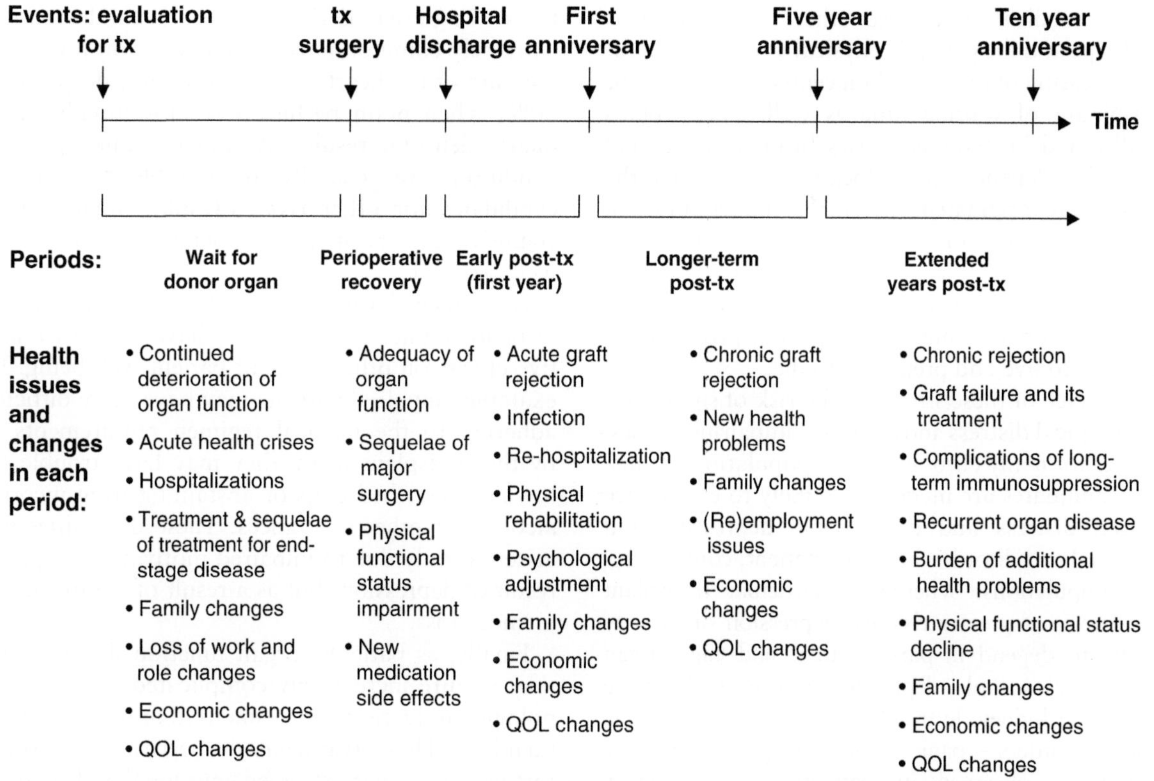

Figure 4 Organ transplant timeline: critical events, time periods, and health and psychosocial issues. Abbreviations: tx, transplantation; QOL, quality of life. Adapted from Dew, M. A. et al. (2002). Psychosocial aspects of transplantation. Reprinted with permission from Medscape Transplantation. © 2002, WebMD, Inc.

The evaluation for transplant is itself usually lengthy and complex because it is designed to assess all aspects of patients' medical and psychosocial status. Patients may be hospitalized during the several days of the evaluation in order to complete all required tests and procedures. An extensive array of medical and laboratory tests is required, and virtually all transplant programs consider patients' psychosocial and psychological histories. Although there is considerable variation across programs in the depth with which psychosocial history is probed, important elements that are usually evaluated to at least some degree include lifetime history and treatment of psychiatric disorder; lifetime history and current use of alcohol, nicotine, and other substances; current and past level of adherence to medical regimens; cognitive status and ability to understand what will be required for posttransplant care; social history including employment, financial circumstances, marital status, and availability of social supports from family and friends; personal views and expectations about the prospect of receiving a transplant; and personal strategies for coping with functional limitations due to health.

These psychosocial components are routinely assessed because patients' history and current status in these areas may influence their psychological adaptation to the wait for the transplant and to life after the transplant. However, these assessments often serve as important additional stressors to patients and families. They are stressful because of the personal nature of the questions as well as because the results may be used for decision making by the transplant team. Typically, these evaluations will contribute to judgments as to whether patients should be immediately listed as transplant candidates or whether they need to undergo additional interventions to improve their health status and adherence to the medical requirements set by the transplant team. For example, patients may be required to enroll in alcohol or smoking cessation programs before the transplant team will accept them onto the waiting list.

The Waiting Period

Many patients and their families perceive the waiting period to be the most psychologically stressful part of the transplant experience, due largely to patients' continued physical health deterioration and the inherent uncertainties about whether and when a suitable donor organ will become available. The duration of this period can vary from a few days (although brief waits are now rare) to several years, depending on the patient's medical status and other factors such as blood type and the patient's physical size. The geographical location of the transplant center can be a major determinant of waiting time as well, since organs are allocated in many countries through a regional system that depends on the location from which the donor organ originated. Given the uncertainties of obtaining a donor organ, plus the risks of the transplant surgery itself (especially as the patient's medical condition deteriorates), patients and their families are faced with the mutually opposing prospects of preparing to live and preparing to die.

In the face of these stressors, the risk of significant psychological distress and cognitive impairment rises. Thus, as for many chronic disease populations, transplant candidates are much more likely to experience elevated distress and diagnosable depressive and anxiety-related disorders than nonpatient, community-based populations. Whether a particular transplant candidate is at greater risk for depression or anxiety appears to depend in part on their end-stage organ disease. For example, depression appears to be more common in kidney, liver, and heart candidates, while anxiety disorders – panic disorder in particular – are more often observed in patients with end-stage lung disease.

In general, the longer a patient waits for a transplant, the greater the psychological toll on the patient and family. However, it is noteworthy that an extremely brief wait (e.g., in the case of patients who have very rapidly declining organ function and are fortuitously able to undergo transplantation very quickly) may have negative psychological consequences as well. For example, it has been found that levels of anxiety and rates of anxiety disorders in the first year after transplantation are higher in patients who wait for very brief periods of a few months or less, compared to those who wait for longer periods. It is thus possible that the waiting period – despite its central elements of uncertainty and its associated risk for psychological distress when the wait is prolonged – can provide important time for patients to adapt to the idea that they need a transplant. If they do not have time before the surgery to adjust to the prospect of transplantation, the immediate consequence may be greatly heightened distress as they attempt to adapt to the transplant experience in the early postsurgical period.

Neurocognitive impairments are common in transplant candidates. For example, hepatic encephalopathy is prevalent in liver candidates and ranges from mild cognitive deficits to delirium and coma. Even patients with chronic liver disease who do not have hepatic encephalopathy may have cognitive and behavioral abnormalities as results of more subtle derangements of metabolic and detoxification functions. Cognitive deficits in heart candidates are extremely common once cardiac ejection fraction (a measure of the heart's ability to pump) drops below 30%; when brain perfusion is substantially inadequate, delirium results. Although kidney patients' conditions are generally more stable compared to candidates for other types of solid organs, subtle cognitive deficits often occur when patients are not well dialyzed.

Continued elevations in psychological distress and/or neurocognitive changes may have their own negative effects on other areas of patient well-being. For example, impaired patients may have more difficulty adhering to the medical regimen requirements set by the transplant team: they may have trouble following prescribed diets or abstaining from nicotine, alcohol, or other substances. These difficulties may arise not only due to impaired motivation (e.g., as a result of depression) but as a result of confusion and memory loss.

Finally, as patients' organ function declines, they may require increasingly complicated medical technologies and treatment regimens in order to maintain their lives. These treatments also serve as stressors that further tax patients' strained emotional and cognitive resources. The strain may extend to the family as well. The patient's marriage and relationships with primary family caregivers (who are most often spouses of adult patients and parents of pediatric patients) are particularly vulnerable due to role changes within the family and changes in daily living activities and schedules. The financial ramifications of these changes – arising from medical expenses, the inability of the patient to work, and/or the need for key family members to take substantial time off from work – can further add to strain within the family.

The Surgery and the Perioperative Recovery Period

This phase of the transplant process is characterized by major, but often positive, physical and emotional transitions. With improvements in procedures and medical care in the immediate days posttransplant, hospital stays have been dramatically reduced. For example, patients who receive the most common types of transplant (kidney, liver, or heart) are frequently able to be discharged in 7 to 10 days. However, as with all major surgery, the possibility for medical complications exists, and this, plus the patient's physical status immediately prior to surgery, will affect the speed of perioperative recovery.

During the first few weeks after surgery, most patients and their families voice high levels of optimism about the patient's prospects for recovery. Their central concerns usually involve how well the new organ is functioning and the probable speed of the patient's physical rehabilitation. These concerns are sometimes heightened by the brief postsurgical hospital stays. Moreover, the short duration of the hospitalization is often perceived as stressful because patients and families typically receive many educational materials about life posttransplant during this time. (This information may have been provided before the transplant as well, but patients may have had difficulty absorbing it due to other stressors and/or cognitive impairment.) The positive feelings and optimism that often dominate after the surgery can interfere with educational efforts during the perioperative period because these feelings may lead patients and their families to be less able to accept and focus on information concerning potential complications, financial issues, and family difficulties that can arise posttransplant.

An additional source of stress arises from medication changes made in conjunction with the transplant. The immunosuppressants that transplant recipients will take for the remainder of their lives are introduced with the transplant, and they bring an extensive range of side effects. While some side effects abate with time, transplant patients – just like any other chronic disease population – will find that others appear to be permanent and unpleasant (e.g., tremor, altered body appearance, changes in sexual functioning, appetite changes). The new medications can also precipitate mood changes. For example, the introduction of corticosteroids can precipitate the onset or recurrences of mood or anxiety disorders. In addition, it is not uncommon for patients who were stabilized on psychotropic medications before transplant to have those medications abruptly discontinued after surgery. This can lead to rapid destabilization for patients, whose mood and/or anxiety disorders may quickly recur.

The First Year after the Transplant

For most patients, the first year posttransplant is a period of readjustment and rehabilitation, with gradual improvement in all domains of QOL, including physical, emotional, and social well-being. A frequent source of frustration for both patients and their families is the fact that the recovery process is generally considerably slower than they had expected. Moreover, important psychosocial elements of the transplant process may further prolong recovery and may also affect family members' well-being. These elements pertain to patients' need to (1) cope with common complications such as acute graft rejection episodes and infections, (2) alter their self-image from that of a critically ill or dying patient and resume a less illness-focused lifestyle, and (3) psychologically accept the fact that they have an organ from another person. Aside from these personal issues, patients may feel daunted by continuing financial issues related to the costs of the transplant, follow-up care, and medications. In addition, in terms of interpersonal relationships, both patients and family members can be dismayed that the same marital, parent–child, or other family-related difficulties that existed before (and/or during) the period of critical illness and transplant surgery continue after the patient returns home. In fact, the stress of the waiting period may have held some relationships together temporarily, and these may then dramatically decline after the transplant.

An additional area of difficulty for many patients is adherence to the complex posttransplant treatment regimen. Not only must patients take multiple medications, but they also must complete routine medical follow-up evaluations and laboratory tests, monitor vital signs at home (e.g., blood pressure, temperature), follow exercise and dietary requirements, and adhere to restrictions on smoking, alcohol, and other substance use. Just as for most chronic disease patients who must adhere to a complex regimen, transplant recipients' adherence tends to worsen with time. This worsening itself can be a source of frustration (as well as a health risk) for patients, who may become quite discouraged at their inability to refrain from long-standing habits (e.g., smoking) or maintain new ones (e.g., exercise).

A likely result of these many concerns is that the likelihood of experiencing high levels of emotional distress, as well as clinically significant episodes of depressive and anxiety-related disorders, is higher during the first year posttransplant than during subsequent years. For most patients, distress levels gradually abate over the course of the year, and some psychiatric disorders – for example, posttraumatic stress disorder (PTSD) related to the transplant – appear to rarely if ever recur in later years. Individuals with PTSD related to the transplant appear to be unable to come to terms with the transplant experience and may experience flashbacks, nightmares, and extreme distress when thinking about one or more of the stressors that occurred during the waiting period, the surgery, and/or the perioperative recovery period.

Not only can the elements that serve as posttransplant stressors exacerbate psychological distress, but also such distress can itself serve as a major source of strain that, in turn, contributes to the worsening of these other stressors. Thus, for example, episodes of depression and anxiety can lead to increased difficulties in adhering to the medical regimen, as well as affect the patient's ability to cope with new medical complications or the need for rehospitalizations.

There is evidence that, perhaps via these behavioral mechanisms, psychological distress can lead to poorer clinical outcomes and reduced survival rates after transplant.

The Longer-Term Years after the Transplant

By the end of the first year after transplant, most patients have achieved their maximal level of physical rehabilitation and have psychologically adjusted to the transplant experience. Most then embark on a multiyear period in which graft functioning remains high and the rate of serious or life-threatening medical complications is low. Acute graft rejection episodes may be rare or relatively infrequent, compared to the first year after transplant. Patients' QOL in the areas of physical, emotional, and social well-being is often high, and rates of rehospitalization for rejection, infections, etc., are low. Some patients will develop new health problems, including diabetes, hypertension, and kidney disease, often as a result of long-term immunosuppression use. Patients are also at greater risk for cancers due to these drugs. Generally, however, patients' level of functioning remains quite high during these years.

Focal issues for patients and their families during these years pertain to maintaining as high a level of QOL as possible and postponing the effects of any decline in graft function or other complications for as long as possible. Economic and financial concerns related to costs of medications and continuing health care can become more important as the years go by. Nevertheless, psychological distress related to the transplant experience and its medical or psychosocial sequelae is uncommon during these years. Instead, patients' mental health is much more likely to be influenced by the same sorts of acute life events and chronic life strains experienced by other community populations. Indeed, the fact that nontransplant life stressors assume increasing prominence as predictors of emotional difficulties during these years attests to the fact that the vast majority of patients – even those who had great psychological difficulty immediately posttransplant – eventually are able to incorporate the experience into their lives and go on to focus on other things.

The Very Extended Years after the Transplant

We know the least about the stressors and psychosocial outcomes experienced by transplant recipients and their families beyond the 5-year anniversary of the transplant. Even in the 1980s and early 1990s, survival rates were sufficiently poor beyond this point that most clinical and psychosocial research did not consider these later-term years. Currently, however, with large proportions of patients surviving even well beyond 10 years posttransplant, it is critical that the stressors, as well as the continued benefits, of transplantation be more carefully delineated.

Many of the complications that began but remained at low levels of severity in earlier years become symptomatic and can lead to major functional limitations beyond 5 years posttransplant. For example, chronic graft rejection, kidney disease that progresses to kidney failure, complications of diabetes, and cancers all increase in prevalence. In all types of organ transplant recipients, kidney failure, due to long-term immunosuppressant use, can precipitate the need for a kidney transplant. Many individuals who had originally received nonrenal transplants (i.e., liver, heart, lung) do not expect to eventually need another type of transplant, and learning that they now need a kidney transplant can reawaken the depression and anxiety that they experienced while awaiting their earlier transplants. Individuals who originally received kidney transplants can experience a profound sense of bereavement as their renal graft fails and they return to dialysis.

Recipients of nonrenal transplants may develop chronic rejection that is sufficiently severe that they require a retransplant with a new heart, liver, or pancreas. Retransplantation of nonrenal organs remains considerably less successful than first-time transplantation. Therefore, progressive graft failure for these individuals is likely to be associated with increasing psychological distress because treatment alternatives and the potential for good outcomes are poor.

In short, the accumulating medical burden experienced by all types of transplant recipients in the extended years posttransplant is likely to lead to decrements in all areas of well-being and QOL. Some of the health-related stressors and their likely sequelae will be similar to those experienced during the end-stage organ disease that necessitated the original transplant. Other stressors may be more similar to those experienced by other chronic disease and late-life populations as they approach the upper end of their life expectancies.

Interventions to Minimize Stressor Effects during the Transplant Process

Transplant programs have attempted a variety of strategies to help patients and their families cope with transplant-related stressors and/or to minimize the stressors' impact on patients' emotional well-being and QOL. These interventions have included educational, psychotherapeutic, and self-help support groups, patient-to-patient mentoring programs, and the provision of educational and referral materials

Table 1 Examples of interventions that have been evaluated for their ability to improve patient and family psychosocial outcomes during the organ transplantation process

Intervention	*Sample and study groups*	*Design*	*Key results*	*Reference*
Education classes (3x/week for 6 weeks) plus exercise and weight training sessions (2x/week for 6 weeks), compared to education alone. Education focused on lung disease, home health care, stress reduction techniques	Nine lung transplant candidates randomized to education plus exercise (n = 5) or education alone (n = 4)	Randomized controlled trial; assessments pre- and postintervention, no blinding	No significant between-group changes, but global QOL and physical functional status significantly improved in both groups. No other improvements in physical, emotional, or social well-being	Manzetti, J. D., Hoffman, L. A., Sereika, S. M., et al. (1994). Exercise, education, and quality of life in lung transplant candidates. *Journal of Heart and Lung Transplantation* **13**, 297–305
Telephone-based sessions (1x/week for 8 weeks) compared to usual care (medical management by transplant team). Telephone sessions were supportive counseling with cognitive-behavioral techniques to address stress, health, and coping	71 lung transplant candidates randomized to telephone (n = 36) or usual care (n = 35)	Randomized controlled trial; assessments pre- and postintervention; transplant team blinded to treatment assignment; assessors not blinded	Telephone group had lower somatic, anxiety, and depression symptoms and better global QOL, global mental health, and perceived social support postintervention, controlling for baseline levels. No group differences in physical functional QOL or perceived stress	Napolitano, M. A., Babyak, M. A., Palmer, S., et al. (2002). Effects of a telephone-based psychosocial intervention for patients awaiting lung transplantation. *Chest* **122**, 1176–1184
Individual compared to group psychotherapy (1x/week for 12 weeks). Each condition used systemic integrative psychotherapy, which focuses on patient understanding of problems and means to address them	89 kidney recipients randomized to individual (n = 49) or group therapy (n = 40). A control group receiving no treatment (n = 37) was also enrolled	Partially randomized trial, with the control group enrolled after all other subjects; assessment pre- and postintervention (or at similar intervals in controls), with 3-, 6-, 9-, and 12-month follow-up. No blinding	Both intervention groups showed significant reductions in depressive symptoms that were maintained through 1 year postintervention. Control group showed considerably lower depressive symptoms than intervention groups at baseline, and symptom levels rose over time. By the final assessment, symptom levels in the three groups were similar	Baines, L. S., Joseph, J. T. and Jindal, R. M. (2004). Prospective randomized study of individual and group psychotherapy versus controls in recipients of renal transplants. *Kidney International* **65**, 1937–1942
Psychosocial intervention (4 months exposure to Internet-based program) compared to usual care (medical management by transplant team). Internet intervention included components to address health education, stress management, psychological well-being, and medical compliance	60 heart recipients receiving either the intervention (n = 20) or usual care (n = 40). Each recipient's primary family caregiver was also enrolled	Controlled trial with historical comparison group (usual care); assessments pre- and postintervention (or at similar intervals in controls); transplant team blinded to intervention participation; assessors not blinded to intervention participation but blinded to study hypotheses	Intervention group patients had significantly improved depression and anxiety symptoms, and caregivers had significantly improved anxiety and anger symptoms, relative to the comparison group. Social functioning QOL significantly improved in intervention patients and caregivers (not assessed in comparison group). Patient medical compliance did not change, but the subgroup who used the component of the intervention focused on the medical regimen showed significant improvement in keeping clinic appointments, completing blood work, and following diet	Dew, M. A., Goycoolea, J. M., Harris, R. C., et al. (2004). An internet-based intervention to improve psychosocial outcomes in heart transplant recipients and family caregivers: development and evaluation. *Journal of Heart and Lung Transplantation,* **23**, 745–758

Mindfulness-based stress reduction program (1x/week for 8 weeks). Program consisted of training sessions and daily practice of meditation and gentle yoga techniques	20 transplant recipients (2 lung, 12 kidney, 5 kidney-pancreas, 1 pancreas)	Single-group trial; assessments pre- and postintervention and at 3 months follow-up; no blinding	Sleep, depressive symptoms, and overall mental health significantly improved pre- to postintervention. At 3-month follow-up, sleep improvement was maintained, but depressive symptoms had worsened. At 3-month follow-up, anxiety symptoms were improved from baseline. No changes in global QOL, physical functional QOL, or medical adherence	Gross, C. R., Kreitzer, M. J., Russas, V. et al. (2004). Mindfulness meditation to reduce symptoms after organ transplant: a pilot study. *Advances in Mind-body Medicine* **20**, 29–29
Telephone-based QOL therapy compared to telephone-based support therapy (1x/week for 8 to 12 weeks). QOL therapy used cognitive-behavioral strategies to address patient-identified problems in various QOL domains. Supportive therapy involved listening and providing information about the transplant experience	35 lung transplant candidates randomized to QOL therapy ($n = 17$) or supportive therapy ($n = 18$)	Randomized controlled trial; assessments pre- and 1-month, 3-month postintervention; transplant team blinded to treatment assignment	While the groups were equivalent at baseline, the QOL therapy group showed significantly better global QOL, lower mood disturbance, and a better relationship with spouse/partner at 1 month postintervention. QOL and mood improvements were maintained at 3-month postintervention	Rodrigue, J. R., Baz, M. A., Widows, M. R, et al. (2005). A randomized evaluation of quality-of-life therapy with patients awaiting lung transplantation. *American Journal of Transplantation* **5**, 2425–2432

using a variety of audiovisual formats. The effectiveness of the majority of these programs has not been empirically evaluated. A very small literature to date has tested psychosocial interventions that could be employed either face to face when organ candidates and recipients return to the medical center for care or by telephone or via the Internet. Examples of these interventions and study findings regarding improved patient and family psychosocial outcomes are listed in **Table 1**. More extensive intervention development and testing for effectiveness are critical needs in this field.

Acknowledgments

This article was supported in part by grant MH072718 from the National Institute of Mental Health, Rockville, MD, USA.

Further Reading

Cupples, S. A. and Ohler, L. (eds.) (2002). *Solid organ transplantation: a handbook for primary health care providers.* New York: Springer Publishing Co.

Dew, M. A., Switzer, G. E., DiMartini, A. F., et al. (2000). Psychosocial assessments and outcomes in organ transplantation. *Progress in Transplantation* **10**, 239–259.

Dew, M. A., Manzetti, J., Goycoolea, J. M., et al. (2002). Psychosocial aspects of transplantation. In: Smith, S. L. & & Ohler, L. (eds.) *Org transplantation: concepts, issues, practice anoutcomes,* chap. 8. New York: Medscape Transplantation, WebMD, Inc. (www.medscape.com/transplantationhome).

DiMartini, A. F., Dew, M. A. and Trzepacz, P. T. (2005). Organ transplantation. In: Levenson, J. L. (ed.) *The American Psychiatric Publishing textbook of psychosomatic medicine*, pp. 675–700. Washington, D.C.: The American Psychiatric Press, Inc.

Olbrisch, M. E., Benedict, S. M., Ashe, K. and Levenson, J. L. (2002). Psychological assessment and care of organ transplant patients. *Journal of Consulting and Clinical Psychology* **70**, 771–783.

Rodrigue, J. R. (ed.) (2001). *Biopsychosocial perspectives on transplantation.* New York: Kluwer.

Trzepacz, P. T. and DiMartini, A. F. (eds.) (2000). *The transplant patient: biological, psychiatric and ethical issues in organ transplantation.* Cambridge, UK: Cambridge University Press.

VI. SOCIOECONOMIC

Health and Socioeconomic Status

T Chandola and M Marmot
University College London, London, UK

This is a revised version of the article by M Marmot and A Feeney, Encyclopedia of Stress First Edition, volume 2, pp 313–321, © 2000, Elsevier Inc.

Glossary

Psychosocial factors Measurements of psychological phenomena that relate to specific social environments.

Social exclusion People or areas that suffer from a combination of linked problems such as poor health, unemployment, inadequate skills, low incomes, poor housing, high crime rates, lack of educational opportunities, and family breakdown.

Socioeconomic gradient The positive association between greater socioeconomic disadvantage and the amount of death, disability, and disease.

Socioeconomic status An individual's rank or status in a social hierarchy, usually evaluated with reference to a person's access to and consumption of goods, services, and knowledge in a society.

Socioeconomic Gradient in Health

The association between health and socioeconomic status results in the socioeconomic gradient in health. In rich countries, people who are more socioeconomically disadvantaged have poorer health and higher levels of chronic and infectious diseases. In poor countries, there is a similar socioeconomic gradient in infectious diseases and an emerging socioeconomic gradient in chronic diseases such as obesity.

These observed socioeconomic gradients are not simply a question of poverty. **Figure 1** shows the infant mortality rate by levels of wealth in some of the poorest countries in the world. There is a strong socioeconomic gradient in infant mortality, with richer people, in the poorest countries of the world, having much lower rates of infant mortality compared to poorer people. It is not just the poor who have high infant mortality rates. Those who are not poor, but also not rich, have higher infant mortality rates compared to the richest groups in poor countries.

Furthermore, within rich countries, there is a socioeconomic gradient in health even among relatively well-off sections of society. One of the most famous examples of this comes from the Whitehall and Whitehall II studies of British civil servants. In the original Whitehall study, which started in 1960, the initial finding after 5 years of follow-up was that coronary heart disease mortality was higher in the lower employment grades of the British civil service. After 25 years of follow-up, there was a similar finding of an inverse gradient in mortality: the lower the grade, the higher the mortality. Data from the more recent Whitehall II study (1985–2004) shows a similar inverse gradient in all-cause mortality. In **Figure 2**, as we proceed lower down the civil service hierarchy of jobs, the risks of mortality increase for all-cause, cardiovascular, and coronary heart disease deaths. It is not just the poor who suffer from higher levels of mortality and disease. Those who cannot be described as being in poverty, such as clerical British civil servants, have poorer health than the people at the top of the socioeconomic hierarchy.

Socioeconomic status (SES) refers to an individuals' rank or status in a social hierarchy, usually evaluated with reference to a person's access to and consumption of goods, services, and knowledge in a society. A number of different measures have been used as proxy indicators of SES, including income, educational level, and occupational prestige. Although they all display similar socioeconomic gradients in health and disease, it is important to distinguish between different measures of SES, as they may affect health through different mechanisms and pathways. For example, education is likely to have indirect effects on health through positive effects on occupation and income as well as on other factors influencing health, including health-related behaviors such as smoking and diet.

Furthermore, measurements of SES need to specify which period of life they are meant to represent. Socioeconomic disadvantage can accumulate over a lifetime, from early childhood, to school level education, to work experiences and living conditions, and on to retirement. Each of these periods of socioeconomic disadvantage can have independent effects on health later on in life. Because being disadvantaged at an earlier period increases the risk of being disadvantaged later in life, measures of SES across the life course are usually correlated with each other. However, a measure of SES in mid-life may not adequately capture the specific risks for poor health that arise from living in disadvantaged socioeconomic circumstances in childhood.

Any explanation of the association between SES and health has to take account of the socioeconomic gradient. This is not just a question about a divide

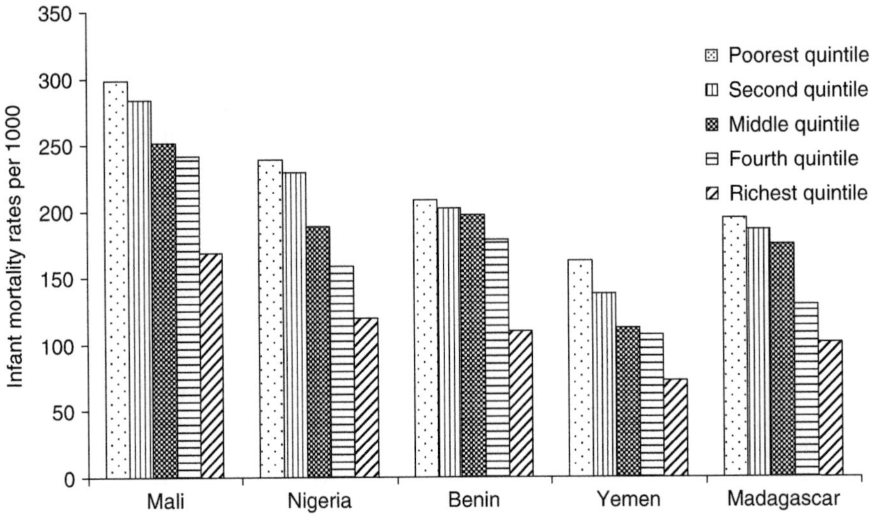

Figure 1 Infant mortality rates by wealth quintiles in Mali, Nigeria, Benin, Yemen and Madagascar. Data from Gwatkin et al. (2000).

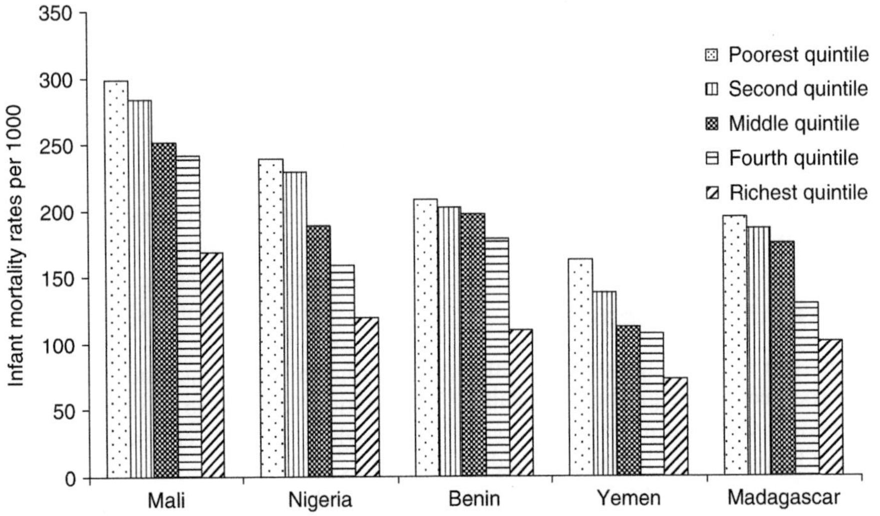

Figure 2 Percentage distribution of deaths by employment grade, adjusted for age and sex: Whitehall II cohort followed up for 19 years.

between those living in poverty and others. Explanations need to take account of the socioeconomic gradient in risk factors for disease and mortality and their distribution across the population. Furthermore, the challenge for explanations is not only to explain the socioeconomic gradient, but also to suggest how it is possible for everyone in the population to have the good health enjoyed by those at the top of the socioeconomic ranks. In order to progress toward eliminating socioeconomic gradients in health, we need to understand the causes of this gradient in health. For this, we need to have an appropriate model to describe how SES can get under our skin and affect health.

Model

It is not difficult to understand how poverty in the form of material deprivation – dirty water, poor nutrition, lack of medical care – can account for the poorer health and higher mortality of poor people. However, poverty alone cannot explain the socioeconomic gradient in health. First, dirty water, lack of calories, and poor medical care cannot account for why British civil servants who work in clerical jobs are over twice as likely to die compared to those in the top ranks of the civil service. Furthermore, the poverty-only model fails to take into account the fact that relief of such material deprivation is not simply a technical matter of providing clean water or better medical care – those resources are socially determined. Even among poorer sections of society, those who are relatively better off are more likely to take advantage of policy interventions to provide better material living conditions, thereby potentially perpetuating and increasing the socioeconomic gradient in health.

In order to reduce inequalities in health, we need to understand the mechanisms and pathways that link the socioeconomic circumstances to health. **Figure 3** presents a simplified model of how different causal factors link the social structure to cardiovascular disease outcomes. This helps us to understand the different mediators and pathways linking SES to health. This is not meant to be a complete model but a simplified representation. There are further causal factors that may be added to the model, and more causal arrows that may be drawn. This model, in particular, draws our attention to how potential causal factors in the work, social, living, and material environments relate to health behaviors or to more direct psychological processes that influence the psycho-neuro-endocrine-immune systems of the body.

This model helps us to understand how different causal factors interrelate, and it also provides a guide to potential points of intervention for reducing inequalities in health. For example, the metabolic syndrome is a risk factor for heart disease. Treatment of the metabolic syndrome through medical care may reduce heart disease, but may not reduce the socioeconomic gradient in heart disease if poorer people are less likely to have access to or get treated for the metabolic syndrome. Another potential point of intervention could be to change the health behaviors that influence the development of the metabolic syndrome. Getting more people to quit smoking may reduce the development of the syndrome, but telling people to quit smoking alone is not enough. The model suggests that there is a socioeconomic gradient in smoking that alerts us to the socioeconomic factors that underlie smoking behaviors. In order to reduce the socioeconomic gradient in the metabolic syndrome and consequently reduce heart disease, we need to understand the causes of the causes: the living, working, social, and material environmental

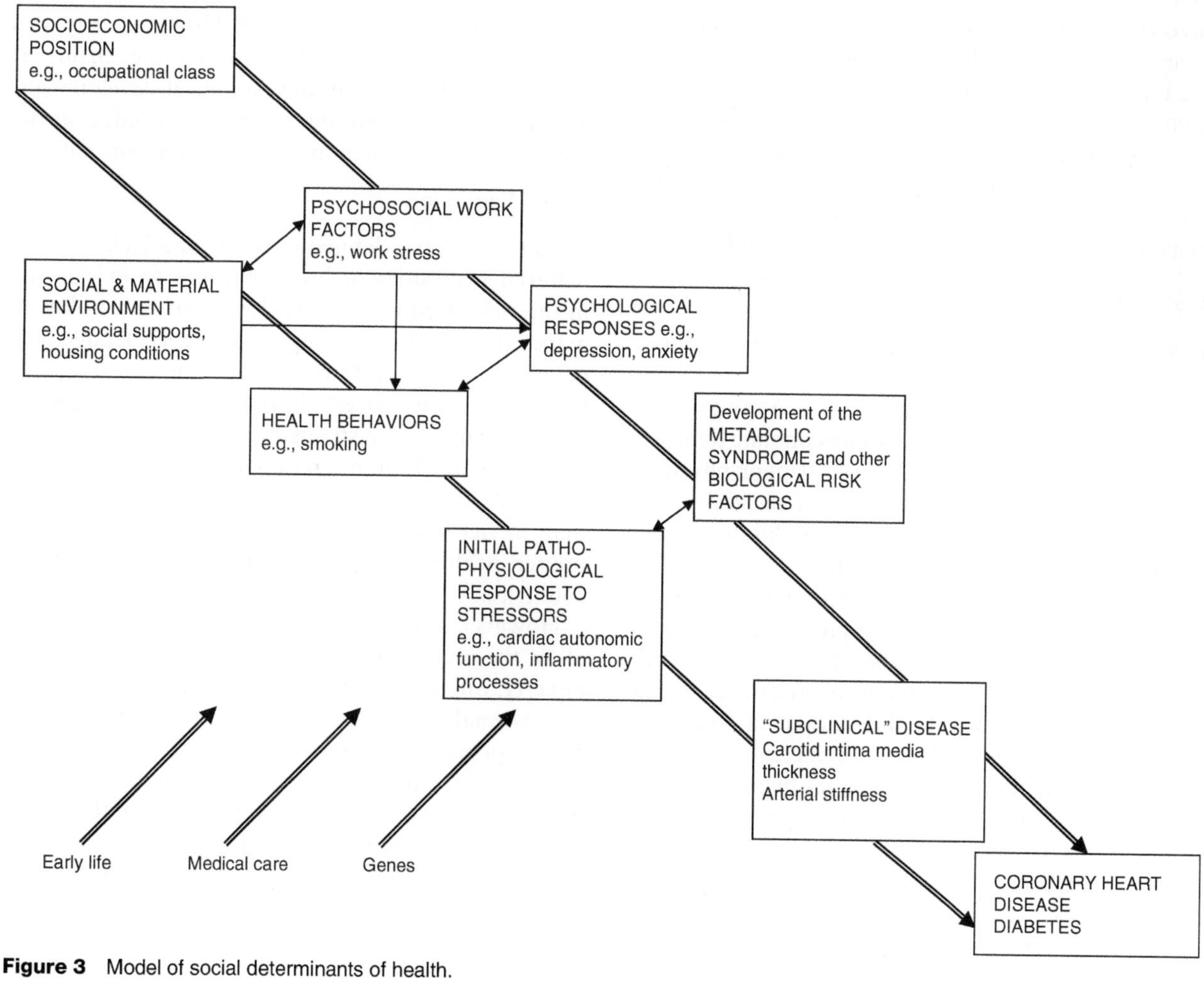

Figure 3 Model of social determinants of health.

contexts in which these health behaviors originate and operate. So if stressful work circumstances make it hard to give up smoking, we need to identify interventions that reduce stress at work. If being poor makes it hard to afford quitting smoking aids, then these aids need to be made freely available.

Explanations

The concept of multiple causal factors operating in conjunction with each other, as outlined in **Figure 3**, is not unique to the development of chronic diseases. Although the tubercle bacillus is the specific cause of tuberculosis, most people infected with the tubercle bacillus do not have clinical tuberculosis. Other factors, such as those associated with poverty and nutrition, influence susceptibility to the disease. In the case of tuberculosis, exposure to an infectious agent is not enough to cause a disease. The exposure, in conjunction with the socioeconomic circumstances, affects the development of the disease.

Similarly, we do not believe that the material, behavioral, psychosocial, and environmental causal factors outlined in **Figure 3** operate in isolation. The division of explanations of the socioeconomic gradient in health into these categories often dismisses the interrelationships and interactions between all of them. So instead, the following sections highlight some of the broad groups of factors related to the social determinants of health, all of which encompass different dimensions and combinations of material, behavioral, psychosocial, and environmental factors.

Early Life

Research from observational and intervention studies shows that the foundations of adult health are laid in early childhood and even before birth. Slow growth, poor emotional support, and socioeconomic deprivation in childhood increase the risk of poor physical, emotional, and cognitive functioning in adulthood. There is a strong patterning of these childhood risk factors for poor adult health by SES.

A number of factors associated with pregnancy, such as nutritional deficiencies during pregnancy, maternal stress, maternal smoking, misuse of drugs and alcohol, insufficient exercise, and inadequate prenatal care, can lead to less than optimal fetal development, low birth weight, and subsequently to an increased risk of heart disease in adulthood. A mother living in poorer socioeconomic circumstances is much more likely to experience some of these risk factors for poor fetal development compared to a mother living in better circumstances.

Infancy is a particularly important period of time for the development of integrated biological systems with long-term consequences for adult health. Research shows that biological systems in infancy are highly malleable through cognitive, emotional, and sensory inputs into the brain. Insecure emotional attachment and poor stimulation in infancy can lead to problematic behaviors in childhood, and adolescence as well as low educational attainment. This in turn increases the risk of social marginalization in adulthood and the ability to obtain employment or steady jobs. Furthermore, health-promoting behaviors in adulthood, such as exercise, healthy diet, and not smoking, are influenced by such parental behaviors in childhood.

It has been argued that parental poverty starts a chain of social and biological risk. Parental poverty increases the risk of poor fetal development, stimulation, and emotional and cognitive inputs in infancy. This leads to slow growth in childhood, poor behavior and educational attainment at school, leading to a raised risk of unemployment, low-status jobs, and lower SES. All of these links in the chain have consequences for physical and mental health in adulthood and old age – some of them indirectly, through influencing the risks further down the chain, others more directly influencing adult health. However, it is also possible to break the links between the chains at critical periods of social and biological development. This is the area where interventions on reducing the socioeconomic gradient in health need to concentrate.

Social Exclusion

Absolute poverty, defined in terms of a lack of basic material necessities of life, continues to exist, even in the richest countries. The long-term unemployed, many ethnic minority groups, guest workers, disabled people, refugees, and homeless people are at risk of living in absolute poverty in rich countries. Homeless people living on the streets have the highest rates of premature death. In poorer countries, the proportion of people living in absolute poverty is much larger than in richer countries, and this contributes to the poorer health in these countries relative to richer countries.

However, absolute poverty alone does not explain all of the socioeconomic gradient in health. Relative poverty, often defined as living on less than 60% of the national median income, affects a greater proportion of people in a population than absolute poverty. It could deny people access to decent housing and jobs, education, transport, and other vital factors for full participation in social life.

The stresses of living in absolute and relative poverty are particularly harmful during pregnancy, to babies, and to the elderly, when people are particularly vulnerable. People move in and out of poverty during their lives, so the number of people who experience poverty and social exclusion during their lifetime is far higher than the number of socially excluded people at any one time.

Furthermore, poverty and social exclusion increase the risk of social isolation, influencing divorce and separation, disability, illness, and addiction. Social isolation affects individuals and communities. Communities and neighborhoods that experience high levels of unemployment, deprivation, poor housing, and limited access to services often have far poorer health outcomes than would be expected by aggregating the number of poor people living in those communities. Social isolation in such communities is hard to escape from, as social exclusion and social isolation are intertwined, often forming a vicious cycle.

Unemployment

Unemployed people and their families have substantially increased risks of premature death and poorer physical and mental health compared to those with stable employment. People who are long-term unemployed, in particular, have much poorer health than the employed. The health effects of unemployment are linked to both its psychological consequences and the financial problems it brings.

The health effects start when people first feel that their jobs are threatened, even before they become unemployed and before any change in their financial circumstances. Job insecurity has been shown to increase the risk of anxiety and depression, sickness absence, smoking, lack of exercise, and heart disease. Unsatisfactory jobs can be just as harmful to health as unemployment; merely having a job will not always protect physical and mental health. As job insecurity grows, it can act as a chronic stressor whose pernicious effects on health increase with the length of exposure.

Disability and ill health increase the risk of unemployment. So the association between unemployment and health could be a result of prior ill health (or selection) or the effects of unemployment on health. There is evidence for both causal models. Any interventions aimed at reducing the association between unemployment and health need to take account of the risk of unemployment through ill health as well as the risk of ill health through unemployment.

Addiction

Alcohol dependence, illicit drug use, and cigarette smoking are all closely associated with socioeconomic disadvantage. Addictions to these substances may help alleviate some of the stressors associated with socioeconomic disadvantage, but in turn, they can generate further problems as well as have long-term consequences on biological systems.

Some of the transitional economies of Central and Eastern Europe experienced great social upheaval following the end of Communist governments at the end of the twentieth century. In these countries, deaths linked to alcohol use – such as accidents, violence, poisoning, injury, and suicide – rose sharply in the 1990s. Some have argued that this sudden increase in alcohol-related deaths was due to the changed socioeconomic circumstances in these countries. In the Whitehall II cohort, a stressful work environment, measured by an imbalance between effort and rewards at work, was found to be a risk factor for alcohol dependence in men.

Smoking is a well-established and important cause of ill health and premature death. Socioeconomic disadvantage is associated with high rates of smoking and very low rates of quitting. Furthermore, smoking is a major drain on poor people's incomes, thereby contributing to further financial deprivation as well as increasing risks of ill health. Simply increasing the price of cigarettes, to decrease the rates of smoking, may actually increase the socioeconomic gradient in smoking. Tackling addictions requires attention to the social determinants of these addictions.

Food

A good diet and adequate food supply are central for promoting health and well-being. Shortage of food and lack of variety cause malnutrition and deficiency diseases, which in turn are causes of other infectious and chronic diseases. While food deficiency occurs in poorer countries, in richer countries, excess food intake contributes to cardiovascular diseases, diabetes, cancer, and obesity. Furthermore, food poverty can exist side by side with food abundance. Some developing countries are experiencing the double burden of obesity and malnutrition-related diseases.

Economic growth and improvements in housing and sanitation resulted in an epidemiological transition from infectious to chronic diseases, as well as a nutritional transition. Diets have changed to overconsumption of energy-dense fats and sugars, producing more obesity. In rich countries, as well as some developing poor countries, obesity is becoming more common among the poor than the rich. The main dietary difference between socioeconomic groups is the sources of nutrients. The poor tend to substitute cheaper processed foods for fresh food, with much higher levels of energy-dense fats and sugars. People on low incomes are least able to obtain key nutrients from their diets.

The important public health issue is the availability and cost of healthful, nutritious food. Telling people they should eat healthfully is of little use when they do not have access to healthful food, either because they cannot afford it or because they live in food deserts where shops sell processed foods that are inexpensive but unhealthful.

Exercise

As mechanization has reduced the exercise involved in jobs, housework, and commuting, people need to find new ways of building physical activity and exercise into their lives. Regular exercise protects against heart disease and diabetes by limiting obesity. It also promotes a sense of well-being and can protect older people from depression.

There is a strong socioeconomic gradient in leisure-time physical activity – people from lower socioeconomic positions exercise less. This may be because they have less time to spend on exercise, they do not have access to leisure sports facilities, or they live in an environment that does not encourage walking or cycling.

Social Support

Supportive relationships are important emotional and practical resources that contribute to health. Social support may buffer the effects of negative events in a person's life, helping them to cope better with the effects of unemployment or disability. Alternatively, social support may directly contribute to a person's health by making him or her feel cared for, esteemed, and valued. Belonging to a social network and having mutual obligations have a powerful protective effect on health.

Social isolation, or the absence of social networks, is associated with increased rates of premature death and poor chances of survival after a heart attack. People who get less social and emotional support from others are more likely to have depression, poorer well-being, and higher levels of disability from chronic diseases. In addition, negative aspects of support from close relationships can lead to poor mental and physical health. Poverty can contribute to social isolation and negative social support.

Social cohesion, defined as the quality of social relationships and the existence of trust, mutual obligations, and respect in communities, helps to protect people and their health. Some argue that social inequalities tend to corrode good social relations and destroy social cohesion. Societies with high levels of income inequality tend to have less social cohesion and more violent crime. The breakdown of social relations, which is linked to greater inequality, reduces trust and increases levels of violence. Declines in social cohesion in some communities have also been linked to increases in rates of heart disease.

Stress

Disadvantaged social and psychological circumstances can cause long-term stress. Continuing anxiety, insecurity, low self-esteem, social isolation, and lack of control over work and home life have powerful effects on health. Such psychosocial risks accumulate during life and increase the chances of poor mental health and premature death. People in lower socioeconomic groups are more likely to experience these psychosocial stressors.

Psychosocial and other stressors activate hormones and the nervous system by triggering the fight-or-flight response: raising the heart rate, mobilizing stored energy, diverting blood to muscles, and increasing alertness. This stress response diverts energy and resources away from many physiological processes important to long-term health maintenance. While biological stress responses to acute stressors are healthy, both the cardiovascular and immune systems may be affected if there are repeated exposures to psychosocial stressors or if it goes on for too long. In the Whitehall II cohort, men from lower civil service grades had higher heart rates and lower heart rate variability, indicating poorer autonomic function (see **Figure 4**). In addition, those with low job control, an indicator of stress at work, were more likely to have impaired autonomic function.

Policy

Health policy was once thought to be about the provision and funding of medical care. This is now changing. While medical care can prolong survival and improve prognosis after some serious diseases, the socioeconomic conditions that make people ill in the first place are more important for the health of the population.

A review of policies in European countries identified several that took action on the social determinants of health, including policies on taxation, old age pensions, sickness benefits, maternity or child benefits, unemployment benefits, housing policies, labor markets, and community facilities. These policies may not be directly related to health, but the evidence suggests that they form part of the broader causes that indirectly influence health. The World Health Organization has set up an independent Commission on the Social Determinants of Health, with the mission to influence public policy, both national and global, to take into account the evidence on the social determinants of health and interventions and policies to address them.

Policies at all levels of government, and between national governments, need to take account of the evidence on the social determinants of health. Improving access to medical care is important for reducing the socioeconomic gradient in health. However, policies relating to poverty reduction, education, work stress, transport, unemployment, addiction, and social exclusion – policies that cut across the whole business of government – are also needed.

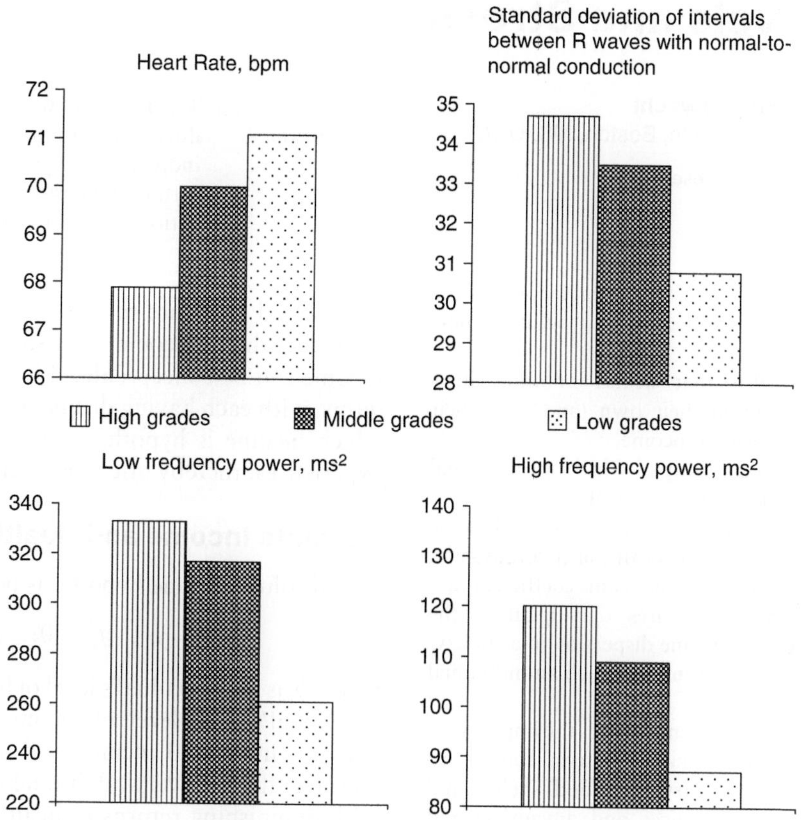

Figure 4 Heart rate variability by employment grade. Data from Hemingway et al. (2005).

The evidence suggests that telling individuals what they should do to improve their health does not reduce socioeconomic gradients in health. Understanding the causes of the causes implies emphasizing the social determinants of these health-promoting behaviors and recommending social, political, and economic interventions leading to healthier behaviors and healthier outcomes.

See Also the Following Articles

Economic Factors and Stress; Social Networks and Social Isolation.

Further Reading

Adler, N., Marmot, M. and McEwen, B. (eds.) (1999). *Socioeconomic status and health in industrial nations: social, psychological and biological pathways* (vol. 896). New York: New York Academy of Sciences.

Bartley, M. (2004). *Health inequality.* Cambridge: Polity Press.

Berkman, L. F. and Kawachi, I. (eds.) (2000). *Social epidemiology.* New York: Oxford University Press.

Brunner, E. J. (1997). Socioeconomic determinants of health: stress and the biology of inequality. *British Medical Journal* **314**, 1472–1476.

Gwatkin, D. R., Rustein, S., Johnson, K., Pande, R. and Wagstaff, A. (2000). *Socioeconomic differences in health, nutrition and population: health, nutrition and population discussion paper.* Washington, D.C.: World Bank.

Hemingway, H., Shipley, M., Brunner, E., Britton, A., Malik, M. and Marmot, M. G. (2005). Does autonomic function link social position to coronary risk? The Whitehall II Study. *Circulation* **111**, 3071–3077.

Krieger, N. (2001). A glossary for social epidemiology. *Journal of Epidemiology & Community Health* **55**, 693–700.

Kuh, D. and Ben-Shlomo, Y. (1997). *A life course approach to chronic disease epidemiology.* Oxford, UK: Oxford University Press.

Marmot, M. (2004). *The status syndrome.* New York: Henry Holt.

Marmot, M. (2005). Social determinants of health inequalities. *The Lancet* **365**(9464), 1099–1104.

Marmot, M. and Wilkinson, R. (eds.) (2006). *Social determinants of health,* (2nd edn.). Oxford: Oxford University Press.

Wilkinson, R. and Marmot, M. (eds.) (2003). *Social determinants of health: the solid facts,* (2nd edn.). Copenhagen: World Health Organisation.

Income Levels and Stress

S V Subramanian and I Kawachi
Harvard School of Public Health, Boston, MS, USA

Glossary

Absolute income The measure of the actual income of the individual; linked to the absolute income hypothesis.

Absolute income hypothesis The idea that health of individuals depends on their own (and only their own) level of income.

Comparative group The social group to which an individual compares him- or herself.

Income inequality The measure of the extent of income dispersion in a society or a community; measures such as Gini coefficient are summary measures that quantify the extent of income dispersion in a society.

Membership group The social group of which an individual feels a part.

Neomaterialist theory A theory that emphasizes the importance of access to tangible material conditions, both elementary (e.g., food, shelter, and access to services and amenities) and nonelementary (e.g., car and home ownership and access to telephones and the Internet).

Normative group The social group from which a person takes his or her standards or norms; this could be either the membership or the comparative group.

Pyschosocial effects The direct or indirect effects of stress stemming from either being lower on the socioeconomic hierarchy or living in conditions of relative socioeconomic disadvantage, which facilitates constant social comparisons.

Relative deprivation The condition in which individuals or groups subjectively perceive themselves to be unfairly disadvantaged compared to others who they perceive as having similar attributes and deserving similar rewards (typically their reference groups or groups to whom they typically compare themselves).

Relative income The measure of the income of the individual in relation to the incomes of others in the society or group in which the individual resides. It is linked to the relative income hypothesis.

Relative income hypothesis The idea that health depends not just on an individual's own level of income but also on the incomes of others in society.

Social comparison The metric that results from an individual's self-comparison of some other individual or group of individuals on certain dimension, such as income, education, and material possessions.

Differential exposure to stressors is one of the links through which income is associated with health. Income can be conceptualized in absolute or relative terms, with each having distinct mechanisms through which income is hypothesized to influence stressful experiences, thereby affecting health.

Absolute Income and Health

The absolute income hypothesis posits that:

$$h_i = f(y_i), \quad f_i' > 0, \quad f_i'' < 0 \tag{1}$$

where h_i is an individual's level of health, and y_i is that individual's own level of income. The relationship between individual income and individual health is concave; that is, every additional dollar is associated with diminishing returns to health. The relationship of individual income to health outcomes is often described as a gradient – at each level of income, individuals experience better health than those immediately below them. On the other hand, to describe the association between income and health as a gradient is possibly misleading because the relationship has been shown to be nonlinear; that is, there are diminishing returns to health improvement with additional rises in income. The concave relationship between income and health has been corroborated in numerous empirical demonstrations, in affluent countries as well as in poor countries. The absolute income hypothesis has been closely associated with the neomaterialist interpretation of the relationship between income and health, which posits that income matters for health because it confers on individuals the ability to purchase goods and services (e.g., health insurance, housing, and nutritious foods) that are necessary for maintaining health, even though the absolute income hypothesis could equally well have a psychosocial effect.

We can also posit a societal or community-level analog of the absolute income hypothesis, such that:

$$h_{ij} = f(Y_j, y_{ij}) \tag{2}$$

where the health of individual i in community j is now hypothesized to be a function of not just his or her own income (y_{ij}) but also of the average income level of the community (Y_j) in which the individual resides. Indeed, a neomaterialist interpretation of the absolute income hypothesis need not be restricted to the availability of income at the individual level; it can also reflect the presence or absence of collective infrastructure at a population or community level. Deprived communities (i.e., communities with high levels of absolute poverty) are less likely to have services and amenities (e.g., health clinics and supermarkets) that are essential for protecting and promoting the health of their residents. Even if an individual resident is not poor, his or her health may be detrimentally affected by living in such a community. A growing number of multilevel studies have now demonstrated that community poverty is linked to higher mortality, higher morbidity, and a more adverse pattern of health behaviors, even after taking into account individual incomes.

Relative Income and Health

In contrast to the absolute income hypothesis, the relative income hypothesis posits that:

$$h_i = f(y_i - y_r) \tag{3}$$

where health of an individual i is a function of the term $(y_i - y_r)$, which denotes the relative gap between an individual's income y_i and the income of some reference population y_r. The reference population could be the income of coworkers, neighbors, or the national population. The concept of relative deprivation was first rigorously formulated by Runciman. According to Runciman, "we can roughly say that A is relatively deprived of X when (i) he does not have X, (ii) he sees some other person or persons, which may include himself at some previous or expected time, as having X (whether or not this is or will be in fact the case), (iii) he wants X, and (iv) he sees it as feasible that he should have X" (Runciman, 1966: 10).

Runciman further conceptualizes the concept of relative deprivation in terms of magnitude, frequency and degree. "The magnitude of the relative deprivation is the extent of the difference between the desired situation and that of the person desiring it (as he sees it). The frequency of a relative deprivation is the proportion of a group who feel it. The degree of a relative deprivation is the intensity with which it is felt" p.10.

Runciman went on to elaborate three types of reference groups. The first is the membership group, of which an individual feels a part; the second is the normative group, "the group from which a person takes his standards" (Runciman, 1966: 12); and the third is the comparative group, which is the group to which an individual compares him- or herself. Significantly, these different sources of relative comparisons may well coincide, as in Runciman's example of members of the middle class who aspire to be aristocracy and who try to emulate the behavior of the upper class (the normative reference) as well as to attain their status (the comparative reference). Building on these sources of relative comparisons, he further proposed two forms of relative deprivation, depending on the source: egoistic deprivation (relative deprivation of an individual with respect to his or her own group) and fraternalistic deprivation (relative deprivation of an individual's own group compared to other groups in society).

Note that relative deprivation theory, as the phrase suggests, presumes that individuals typically make relative comparisons of themselves to those who are better off than they are and not to those who are worse off. The latter comparison is referred to as relative gratification or relative satisfaction. Indeed, relative deprivation measures happen to be correlated with relative satisfaction.

Although the theory of relative deprivation is quite sophisticated, the empirical identification of reference groups has proved tricky. Empirically, the relative income hypothesis has been operationalized using variations of equation (3), with an important operationalization provided by Yitzhaki, following Runciman's theory. Thus, for a person i with income y_i who is part of a reference group with N people, Yitzhaki's index is given as:

$$RD_i = (1/N)\sum_j (y_j - y_i), \quad \forall y_j > y_i \tag{4}$$

where the amount of relative deprivation (RD) for individual i is the sum of the incomes of j individuals who have incomes higher than that individual. The summation in equation (4), $\sum_j (y_j - y_i)$, is divided by the number of people in the reference group, N, making the measure invariant to size. If income is the object of relative comparison, then we can assess relative income deprivations by groups, based on, for instance, the state of residence, age group, race, educational attainment, gender, or occupation.

The British Whitehall Study of civil servants is frequently cited as evidence showing the health effects of relative deprivation (even though the study did not include any specific or explicit measures of relative deprivation). In that study, relatively lower-ranked civil servants were shown to have three times the mortality rate as the highest ranked civil servants, despite having access to the same National Health Service. Moreover, none of the subjects in the civil service cohort was deprived in an absolute sense; that is, they all had adequate nutrition, housing, and access to other material amenities. The mortality differential between civil service grades was thus attributed – at least in part – to the adverse psychosocial consequences of relative deprivation. Indeed, systematic tests suggest that people do take into account relative income position when making real-life decisions such as choosing between two earning schemes. For instance, Frank and Sunstein (2001) hypothesized two possible scenarios. In scenario A, the individual earns $110,000 per year and others earn $200,000; in scenario B, the individual earns $100,000 per year (less than in world A), but others earn only $85,000. Contrary to traditional economic perspective (wherein world A should be preferable because it offers higher absolute consumption), a substantial number of respondents opted for world B.

As we mentioned earlier, the absolute income hypothesis tends to be interpreted in materialist terms, whereas the relative income hypothesis tends to be interpreted in psychosocial terms. This dichotomy is unwarranted. For instance, the absolute income hypothesis is equally compatible with the psychosocial interpretation. That is, if lower income is associated with more stess (e.g., inability to pay the bills and to plan for the future), then an individual could end up with an income–health gradient even if no social comparison is taking place.

Analogously, the relative deprivation hypothesis could also be interpreted both ways (neomaterial as well as psychosocial). That is, an individual's social comparison to a reference group could be stressful (the psychosocial interpretation) or he or she may be unable to function in society because of limited access to material commodities (e.g., car ownership, Internet access, or air conditioning). For example, rising community living standards are often associated with an enlargement of the range of consumer goods that are necessary for an individual to function as a member of that community. Many consumer goods, such as central heating/air conditioning, telephone, and access to the Internet, have followed this trajectory, starting out as luxury goods and eventually ending up as necessities. Even if an individual is not deprived in any absolute sense (i.e., has adequate nutrition and housing), relative deprivation (compared to the standard basket of commodities that everyone else has access to) could adversely affect his or her health. In this sense, relative deprivation may affect health because it reflects the ability of affected individuals to access material goods and services that in turn promote well-being. This underscores the futility of distinguishing material from psychosocial effects of income – any effect of income on health could be simultaneously operating through material as well as psychosocial pathways.

Income Inequality and Health

The community-level analog of relative deprivation leads us to the idea of income inequality, which can be stated as:

$$h_{ij} = f(I_j, y_{ij}) \tag{5}$$

where I_j refers to summary measure of income distribution (e.g., the Gini coefficient) for community j in which the individual resides. Income inequality and relative deprivation are conceptually related because, as income inequality rises, those at the bottom end of the distribution become more relatively deprived. Various measures are available to quantify the extent of income inequality in a given community or society; of these, the Gini coefficient is frequently used. Algebraically, the Gini coefficient is defined as one-half of the arithmetic average of the absolute differences between all pairs of incomes in a population, the total then being normalized on the mean income. If incomes in a population are distributed completely equally, the Gini value is 0; and if one person has all the income (the condition of maximum inequality), the Gini is 1.0. The Gini coefficient can also be illustrated through the use of Lorenz curve (**Figure 1**). On the horizontal axis, the population (in this case, households) is sorted and ranked according to deciles of income, from the lowest-decile group to the top-decile group. The vertical axis then plots the proportion of the aggregate income within that community accruing to each group. Under conditions of perfect equality in the distribution of income (Gini = 0), each decile group

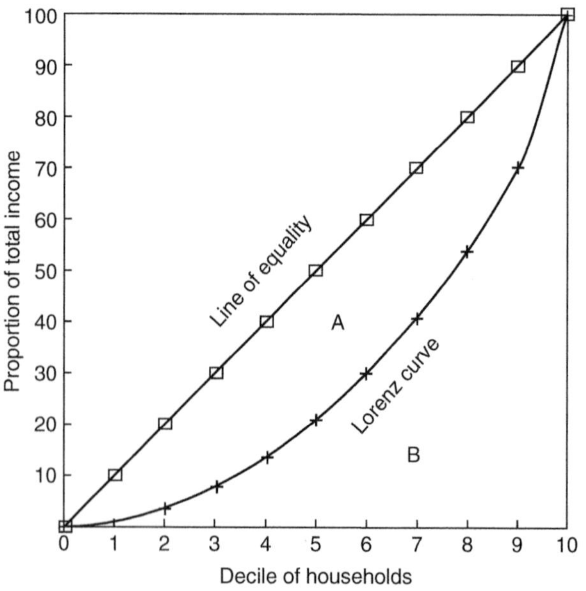

Figure 1 Lorenz curve.

would account for exactly 10 percent of the aggregate income and the Lorenz curve would follow the 45° line of equality. In reality, the Lorenz curve falls below the 45° line of equality because the bottom groups in the income distribution earn considerably less than their equal shares. In **Figure 1**, for instance, the bottom one-half of households accounts for just 20% of the aggregate income. The degree to which the Lorenz curve departs from the 45° line of equality is a measure of income inequality. As it turns out, the Gini coefficient is the ratio of the area between the Lorenz curve and the 45° line of equality (A) and the area of the triangle below the 45° line of equality (A + B).

There is some debate as to whether income inequality is a valid community analog of relative deprivation at the individual level. Some argue that Gini coefficient is the measure of relative deprivation. For instance, the relative deprivation curve that represents the gaps between an individual's income and the incomes of all individuals richer than him or her (as a proportion of mean income) turns out to be the Gini coefficient. Others have presented a generalization of Gini, the s-Ginis, that can be interpreted as indices of relative deprivation. Indeed, it has been stated that "the Gini coefficient may be interpreted as a transformation of an index of 'envy' evaluated through the comparison of the income of an individual and that of all other individuals richer than him/her"(Atkinson and Bourguignon, 2000: 43).

As mentioned earlier, the relationship between individual income and health status is concave, such that each additional dollar of income raises individual health by a decreasing amount. The concave relationship between income and health has important implications for the aggregate-level relationship between income distribution and average health achievement, as noted by Rodgers. As illustrated in **Figure 2**, in a hypothetical society consisting of

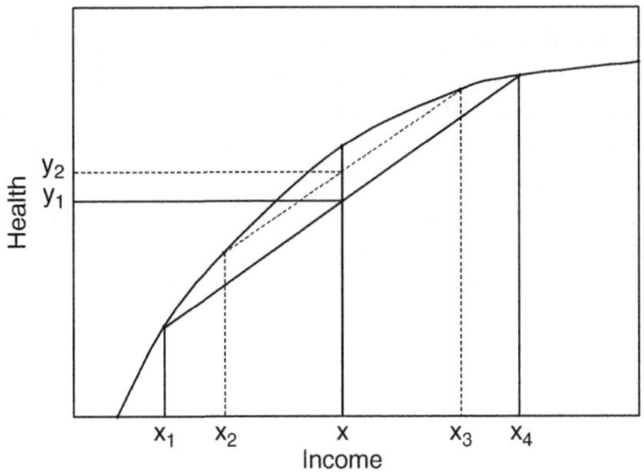

Figure 2 The individual-level relationship between income and health.

just two individuals – a rich one (with income x_4) and a poor one (with income x_1) – transferring a given amount of money (amount $x_4 - x_3$) from the rich person to the poor person will result in an improvement in average health (from y_1 to y_2) because the improvement in the health of the poor person more than offsets the loss in health of the rich person. Indeed, it is possible that, by transferring incomes from the relatively flat part of the income–health curve, there may be no loss in health for the wealthy person.

Consequently, researchers have posited that an aggregate relationship between the average health status of a society and the level of income inequality in a society could be observed if the individual-level relationship between income and health (within the society) is concave. That is, the aggregate relationship between income inequality and health may be observed simply due to the underlying concave functional form of the individual income–health relationship and assuming an x amount of transfer of money from rich to the poor. Indeed, such a transfer also implies a reduction in the income inequality level in that particularly society, and as such, the society with the narrower distribution of income will have a better average health status, all other things being equal. It is worth emphasizing that, if the relationship between income and health at the individual level is linear (not concave), then a transfer of income from the rich to the poor will reduce the level of income inequality but will not lead to improvements in the average health status of that society.

Occasionally, this expected relationship between income distribution and the average health status of a population (which is a direct function of the concave relationship between individual income and health) has been described as a statistical artifact of the concave relationship between individual income and health. The use of the term artifact is misleading here because it suggests that the potential for improving the health of the poor through income redistribution is a statistical illusion. Indeed, there is nothing artifactual about improving the health of the poor (and hence, average population health) through income and wealth redistribution – indeed the success of much philanthropy (e.g., donating money to provide vaccines to the world's poor) rests on the validity of this assumption.

In addition to the concavity effect just described, researchers have posited an additional contextual effect of income inequality on health. This is the hypothesis that the distribution of income in society, over and above individual incomes as well as societal average income, matters for population health such that individuals (regardless of their individual incomes) tend to have worse health in societies that are more unequal. Thus, income inequality *per se* may be damaging to public's health by causing a *downward shift* in the income–health curve. Thus, the income inequality hypothesis is viewed as an independent contextual effect akin to a social pollution effect.

Income and Health: The Role of Social Comparisons

Wilkinson argued that income inequality is harmful to health because it leads to invidious social comparisons among individuals in society and that these comparisons, in turn, may act as a stressor in the form of feelings of shame, anxiety, and social exclusion and, as such, impact physiological systems. The economist Juliet Schor described how widening inequalities have given rise to a culture of upward social comparisons (and the attendant frustration of aspirations). Thus, a mechanism linking income inequality to health involves psychosocial pathways that have adverse physiological consequences. Models of the direct effects of stress on physiological systems include allostatic load, which describes the wear and tear on the organism caused by exposure to daily adverse life circumstances. Stress may also affect health indirectly by leading to a more adverse profile of behaviors, such as smoking and excess drinking. This line of explanation links the community income inequality and individual health through individual relative deprivation (including those related to income). Researchers interested in adult health and mortality have argued that inequality worsens adult health through social comparison. They have argued that income inequality affects health because ranking low in the social hierarchy produces negative emotions such as shame and distrust that lead to worse health via neuroendocrine mechanisms and stress-induced behaviors such as smoking, excessive drinking, and drug use. Although the human body is remarkable in adapting to occasional bouts of stress, they have argued that cumulative exposures to stressors (such as chronic poverty, low socioeconomic status, and constant social comparisons) eventually result in strain on regulatory systems.

Although we have discussed here the role of social comparisons as a source of stress, there are other mechanisms that link income and health that can also be explained through stress-based explanations. For instance, a chronic exposure to unpredictable social and economic circumstances (associated with low income) can also be a source of stress in addition to inhibiting access to important material goods necessary to sustain desirable levels of well-being. The challenge for researchers on income and health is to elucidate the specific pathways through which the different conceptualizations of income may impact on health through differential types of stressors.

Acknowledgments

S. V. Subramanian is also supported by a National Institutes of Health/National Heart, Lung, Blood Institute Career Development Award (1 K25 HL081275).

See Also the Following Articles

Economic Factors and Stress; Health and Socioeconomic Status; Social Status and Stress.

Further Reading

Atkinson, A. B. and Bourguignon, F. (2000). Introduction: income distribution and economics. In: Atkinson, A. B. & Bourguignon, F. (ed.) *Handbook of income distribution*, (vol. 1), pp. 1–58. Amsterdam: Elsevier Science.

Deaton, A. (2003). Health, inequality, and economic development. *Journal of Economic Literature* **41**, 113–158.

Duclos, J.-Y. (2000). Gini indices and the redistribution of income. *International Tax and Public Finance* 7, 141–162.

Frank, R. H. and Sunstein, C. R. (2001). Cost-benefit analysis and relative position. *University of Chicago Law Review*, **68**: 323–374.

Kakwani, N. (1984). The relative deprivation curve and its applications. *Journal of Business and Economic Statistics* **2**, 384–394.

Kawachi, I. (2000). Income inequality and health. In: Berkman, L. F. & Kawachi, I. (ed.) *Social epidemiology*, pp. 76–94. New York: Oxford University Press.

Kawachi, I. and Kennedy, B. P. (2003). *The health of nations*. New York: The New Press.

Marmot, M. (2002). The influence of income on health: views of an epidemiologist. *Health Affairs* **21**(2), 31–46.

McEwen, B. S. and Seeman, T. S. (1999). Protective and damaging effects of mediators of stress: elaborating and testing the concepts of allostatis and allostatic load. *Annals of the New York Academy of Sciences* **896**, 30–47.

Rodgers, G. B. (1979). Income and inequality as determinants of mortality: an international cross-section analysis. *Population Studies* **33**, 343–351.

Runciman, W. G. (1966). *Relative deprivation and social justice*. London: Routledge.

Schor, J. B. (1998). *The overspent American*. New York: Basic Books.

Subramanian, S. V., Belli, P., and Kawachi, I. (2002). The macroeconomic determinants of health. *Annual Review of Public Health* **23**: 287–302.

Subramanian, S. V., and Kawachi, I. (2004). Income inequality and health: what have we learned so far. *Epidemiologic Reviews* **26**: 78–91.

Subramanian, S. V., and Kawachi, I. (2006). Whose health is affected by income inequality? A multilevel interaction analysis of contemporaneous and lagged affects of state income inequality on individual self-rated health in the United States. *Health and Place* **12**: 141–156.

Subramanian, S. V., Kawachi I. (2006). Being well doing well: on the importance of income for health. *International Journal of Social Welfare* **15**, S1: S13–S22.

Wagstaff, A. and van Doorslaer, E. (2000). Income inequality and health: what does the literature tell us? *Annual Review of Public Health* **21**, 543–567.

Wilkinson, R. G. (1996). *Unhealthy societies – the afflictions of inequality.* London: Routledge.

Wilkinson, R. G. (2005). *The impact of inequality.* New York: New Press.

Yitzhaki, S. (1979). Relative deprivation and the Gini coefficient. *Quarterly Journal of Economics* **93**(2), 321–324.

Job Insecurity: The Health Effects of a Psychosocial Work Stressor

J E Ferrie
University College London Medical School, London, UK
P Martikainen
University of Helsinki, Helsinki, Finland

Glossary

Downsizing The most common name given to the process whereby an organization reduces its workforce through natural wastage, early retirement, or redundancy.

Employment security While job security represents the ability to remain in a particular job, employment security represents the likelihood of being able to remain in paid employment, even if this is a succession of jobs.

Job insecurity In general terms, the discrepancy between the level of security a person experiences and the level he or she prefers. It can cover both the loss of any valued condition of employment and the threat of total job loss. The depth of the job insecurity experience is dependent on the perceived probability and perceived severity of the job loss. Job insecurity has a large subjective appraisal element that is highly context dependent, and the job insecurity experience may effect employees who do not lose their job as much as those who do. Job insecurity arising from the threat to a particular job may lead to loss of employment security if subsequent jobs prove hard to find. Job insecurity can be self-reported or externally attributed. The population in studies of self-reported job insecurity is composed of individuals who report their job as insecure. In studies of attributed job insecurity, the study population is deemed to be under threat of job loss by the researchers. Associations observed in studies of attributed job insecurity are likely to be underestimates, as the study population will contain respondents who do not perceive themselves to be under threat.

Primary labor market The highly regulated section of the labor market in which employees have traditionally enjoyed long-term, secure employment with many benefits, such as occupational pensions, maternity cover, etc.

Psychological contract Worker's beliefs regarding the terms and conditions of her or his employment. Fairness and good faith are implied in the psychological contract, and breaches have implications for the worker's trust in the organization, performance, and behavior.

Secondary labor market That section of the labor market in which wages are low and employment rights are few. Such employment is often seasonal, part-time, or temporary and is frequently used to buffer short-term changes in labor requirements.

Sickness presenteeism Describes the phenomenon that occurs when an employee, despite a level of ill health that should prompt rest and absence, still turns up at work.

Job Insecurity and the Labor Market

Over the past 25 years, large changes have taken place in the structure of the labor market in most industrialized countries. The major determinants of this restructuring have been deindustrialization, technological innovation, globalization, and a commitment to a free market economy, including the privatization of public services. There has been a marked shift from economies driven by manufacturing toward those dominated by employment in services. Technological innovation has allowed many routine functions largely to be replaced by electronic devices (such as cash dispensers), and global information systems have facilitated the rapid transfer of work to newly industrializing countries where labor is cheaper. This deindustrialization and technological change have generally been accompanied by the expansion and strengthening of the role of market forces. Many workers, who previously thought that they had a job for life, now feel much less secure, and job insecurity has become more widespread in all the countries belonging to the Organisation for Economic Co-operation and Development (OECD) since the mid-1980s. Like all social transformations, these changes have the potential to affect the health of individuals and populations.

The Job Insecurity Concept

Research during the major recessions of the 1930s and 1980s provided unequivocal evidence of the adverse effects of unemployment on health, particularly mental health. However, although it is a major determinant of unemployment, much less work has been done on job insecurity. This is partly because job insecurity did not excite attention until it affected white-collar workers in the 1990s and partly because it is less obvious that job insecurity could affect health, as, unlike unemployment, it involves no actual loss of income or status. However, some research has suggested that job insecurity may have detrimental consequences equal to those of job loss. This is consistent with the central proposition in stress research that anticipation of a stressful event provokes as much, if not more, anxiety than the event itself. For workers accustomed to long-term, secure employment, the threat of job loss involves a breach of the psychological contract and generates uncertainty, which, in addition to emotional reactions, can trigger changes in other psychosocial stressors, such as job involvement. The level of stress generated by job insecurity depends on the perceived probability and perceived severity of the threatened job loss. As job insecurity in the primary labor market has increased and research on psychosocial stressors has gained credence and prominence, interest in the effects of job insecurity has also developed.

Job security is a vital concern for both employees and their organizations. The general concept has been defined by Jean Hartley and colleagues as the discrepancy between the level of job security a person experiences and the level he or she prefers. Job insecurity can also be generated by deteriorating employment conditions and career opportunities, so some investigators have extended the concept to include loss of any valued condition of employment. These definitions encompass large numbers of workers who have insecure jobs, often seasonal, part-time, or temporary. For workers in this secondary labor market, job security is not part of the psychological contract and insecurity is an integral part of their work experience. However, widespread downsizing, privatization, outsourcing, mergers, and closures have led to the suggestion that job insecurity, even for employees in the primary labor market, is no longer a temporary break in an otherwise predictable work life pattern, but is becoming a structural feature of the new labor market. This new employment insecurity brings employees in the primary labor market closer to those in the secondary labor market.

The difficulty in studying the health effects of job insecurity among workers in the secondary labor market is working out whether poor health outcomes can be attributed to job insecurity and unemployment, or whether it is those already in poorer health who are selected into the secondary labor market. For this reason much of the published research has concentrated on workers in the primary labor market.

Job insecurity can be self-reported or externally attributed. Studies of self-reported job insecurity examine workers who say their job is insecure, while studies of attributed job insecurity examine workers deemed to be under threat of job loss because downsizings or workplace closures are expected or are taking place. There is a strong association between self-reported and attributed job insecurity. However, as stress levels are determined by the perceived probability and perceived severity of the job loss, self-reported job insecurity is generally considered to be the more potent stressor.

Mechanisms

Work examining potential explanations of any association between job insecurity and health remains patchy. Studies to date have implicated at least the following: pre-existing ill health; personal characteristics, such as pessimism; material factors, such as financial hardship; non-work psychosocial stressors, such as life events; other psychosocial and physical characteristics of the work environment, such as decreased job involvement; and health-related behavior (**Figure 1**).

The personal characteristics of pessimism, vigilance, neuroticism, mastery, and self-esteem have been found to explain part of the association between self-reported job insecurity and ill health

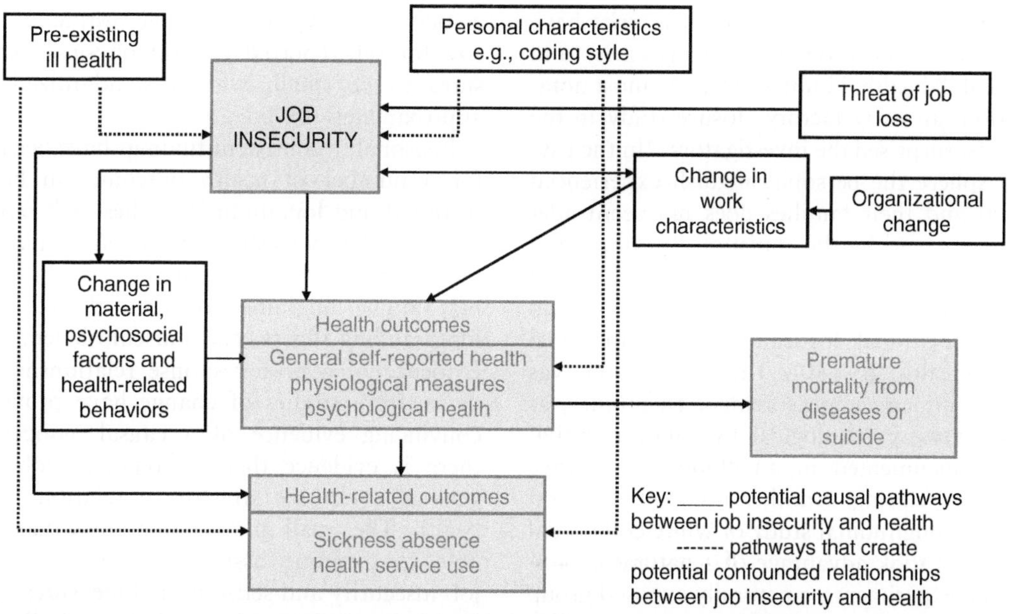

Figure 1 Possible pathways in the association between job insecurity and morbidity. Adapted from Ferrie, J. E., Shipley, M. S., Marmot, M. G., Martikainen, P., Stansfeld, S. and Davey Smith, G. (2001). Job insecurity in white-collar workers: towards an explanation of associations with health. *Journal of Occupational Health and Psychology* **6,** 26–42.

and health-related outcomes. One of the main explanations of associations between unemployment and health is loss of income. Although job insecurity involves no loss of income, pre-existing deprivation and fear of financial insecurity have been shown to explain part of the association between self-reported job insecurity and self-reported psychological and physical health outcomes. Much has also been made of the potential for job insecurity to interact with other material and psychosocial stressors outside work and to precipitate increases in smoking and drinking.

It seems obvious that organizational change, which involves a reduction in the size of the workforce, in addition to generating job insecurity, is likely to result in changes to other characteristics of the work environment. This has been examined in a number of studies on changes in other psychosocial work characteristics, in particular, loss of job satisfaction, job control, and social support at work. Other work has shown a synergistic adverse effect on health in workers with both high job insecurity and high job strain. Despite this work, much of the association between job insecurity and ill health remains unexplained and may be due either to direct effects of stress on the autoimmune system or to unobserved health-related selection.

Psychological Health

Most studies that have examined the effects of self-reported job insecurity on health have looked at psychological ill health as an outcome, often as the only outcome. Every study has documented consistent adverse effects on all measures of psychological health, although a combined analysis of the association between job insecurity and mental health outcomes in 37 study samples has estimated the effect size for self-reported psychological ill health to be medium rather than large, with a standardized effect of approximately 25%.

Good evidence for an association between job insecurity and poor psychological health has come from the observation of a dose–response relationship; that is, the higher the level of job insecurity, the greater the increase in psychological ill health. However, a dose–response relationship would be observed whether job insecurity increased psychological ill health or whether ill health increased the likelihood of reporting of job insecurity. In addition, self-reporting of both exposure (job insecurity) and outcome (psychological health) could contaminate the results if some participants have a tendency to report their situation, both work and health, in a negative light. Stronger evidence for the causal precedence of job insecurity comes from the study of change in job security. For example, it has been shown that, compared to employees whose jobs remain secure, psychological ill health increases among those who report a loss of job security. Studies that follow workers over time also show that self-reported job insecurity acts as a chronic stressor. This means that workers exposed to ongoing job insecurity experience the highest levels of psychological ill health.

Almost all studies of attributed job insecurity have documented an association between insecurity and psychological ill health. Findings from the most notable exception, an early factory closure study in the United States, surprised the investigators. "In the psychological sphere the personal anguish experienced by the men and their families does not seem adequately documented by the statistics" (Cobb, S and Kasl, S. V. (1977). Termination: the consequences of job loss. Cincinnati: DHEW-NIOSH Publication no. 77–224, National Institutes for Occupational Safety and Health, p. 180). The observation was attributed to imperfect measurement techniques, as numerous adverse psychological outcomes in individuals were documented in an eloquent narrative account of the closing. Another notable exception comes from a longitudinal study of white-collar civil servants, which took advantage of a natural experiment. In such experiments, a naturally exposed group is compared to an unexposed reference group. This means that there is no plausible selection process involved, and factors such as poor health or age are not influential in increasing the risk of job insecurity. Inferences about causality are strong under such conditions. In this particular natural experiment, well after the initial survey, one of the 20 departments in the study was unexpectedly sold to the private sector, a transfer of business in which most of the workforce lost their jobs. However, no effects on psychological health were seen in either sex in the run-up to the sale. A possible explanation of these seemingly contradictory findings recently emerged from a study that took advantage of a similar natural experiment in the Netherlands. One of the government agencies in the study was threatened with closure after the initial survey. Psychological ill health among employees in this agency was compared with that for employees in agencies unaffected by threat of closure, adjusting for ill health at baseline. Over the 13 months following the closure announcement, the number of new cases of psychological ill health in the closure group was significantly higher than in the nonclosure group. However, the increase in psychological distress among those working in the agency targeted, but who did not think they were at risk of job loss, was not significant; thus, self-reported rather than self-attributed job insecurity appeared to have been driving the association.

General Measures of Physical Health

Evidence is growing that self-reported job insecurity has adverse effects on self-reported general physical health measures, independent of effects on psychological health, although a combined analysis of the association in 19 study samples estimated the effect size for self-reported general physical health measures to be small, with a standardized effect of approximately 16%.

Reasonably consistent findings have been obtained for a number of health outcomes in both cross-sectional and longitudinal studies. Self-reported job insecurity has been shown to be associated with poor self-rated health, sleep disturbance, chronic insomnia, fatigue, migraine, colds and flu-like symptoms, longstanding illness, and musculoskeletal disorders. Evidence of a dose–response relationship and evidence from studies of change have provided more convincing evidence of a causal association, and there is evidence that self-reported job insecurity acts as a chronic stressor in relation to physical health. The small number of studies that have been able to examine associations between attributed job insecurity and self-reported measures of physical health have observed associations similar to those for self-reported job insecurity. However, there appears to be no evidence that attributed job insecurity acts as a chronic stressor, so it is possible that the finding for self-reported job insecurity may be due to a general tendency for negative reporting.

Very few studies have looked at the effect of either category of job insecurity on biomedical risk factors. There appears to be only two studies that have examined the association between self-reported job insecurity and blood pressure. Both studies found a significant increase in blood pressure compared with control workers who did not report job insecurity. Two studies of attributed job insecurity similarly found significant increases in blood pressure, but another two studies that examined a change in attributed security observed either no significant differences or effects in some groups but not others. Studies that have examined effects on body weight similarly report mixed findings, with no change as well as gain and loss in mean weight being observed. Resolution of these apparently divergent findings may lie in the observation that job insecurity has bidirectional effects on weight. A study of occupational factors and 5-year weight change among Danish men showed that job insecurity increased the likelihood of weight gain among obese men and weight loss among men who were lean.

Apart from two Scandinavian studies, there has been even less interest in biomedical risk factors other than blood pressure and body weight. Attributed job insecurity has been associated with nonsignificant increases in the stress hormone, cortisol, and in cholesterol in a mainly female blue-collar workforce, and levels of adrenal hormones have been shown to be raised among women at the bottom of the white-collar employment hierarchy. However, evidence on cholesterol from a longitudinal study of white-collar civil servants is mixed, and it remains uncertain what clinical relevance the observed changes in biomedical risk factors may have. Hardly any work has examined the effect of job insecurity on diagnosed diseases. Three studies have documented an association between self-reported job insecurity and various measures of coronary heart disease, and an association has been observed between attributed job insecurity and risk of ischemia (abnormal ECG or diagnosed angina) relative to unexposed employees. However, overall the evidence is limited. While the findings were indicative of adverse changes, these were modest and not significant after adjustment for major confounding somatic and behavioral coronary risk factors.

In part because job insecurity was rarely studied until the recession of the 1990s, there has been little research on the effect of job insecurity on mortality from diseases or suicide. Studies of self-reported job insecurity have not been documented, and there is no compelling evidence yet of an association between attributed job insecurity and premature death. Most work prior to the 1990s was a spin-off of studies of unemployment and health and found no significant differences between groups of workers exposed and unexposed to attributed job insecurity. More recently, a factory closure study in New Zealand examined mortality at the end of an 8-year follow-up as an outcome under the conditions of a natural experiment. The study found no statistically significant difference in the death rate for any cause between workers in the closing plant and in the control plant. This was by far the largest factory closure study to date, with nearly 2000 in both the study group and the control group. However, the number of deaths after 8 years was still relatively small, and instability in the sector, which led to the closing of the control plant by the end of the follow-up, may mean that these findings are minimum likely estimates of effects. Although temporary workers are generally considered to be part of the secondary labor market, recent work using Finnish data has looked at the effect on mortality of transfer from temporary to permanent employment. Moving from temporary to permanent employment is associated with a significantly lower risk of death, while remaining in temporary employment is associated with a significantly higher risk of death than being continuously in permanent employment. While moving the fittest temporary workers into permanent employment is likely to explain part of this effect, change in exposure to job insecurity may also contribute.

Consistent with the evidence of effects on psychological health, a review of eight studies of unemployment and suicide that used longitudinal data for individuals showed that in all but one there was greater job instability and occupational problems among suicides compared to nonsuicides. In the New Zealand factory closure study discussed previously, there was a significant, 2.5-fold increased risk of serious self-harm that led to hospitalization or death from suicide, and out of 46 men who lost their job during a U.S. factory closure, two committed suicide. Although this was 30 times the number expected, the number of people in the study population was too small to draw firm conclusions.

Health Outcomes of Interest to the Organization

A small number of studies have looked at the effect of self-reported job insecurity on safety at work. The main finding from this research is that job insecurity increases workplace injuries and accidents through detrimental effects on employee safety motivation and safety compliance. Both self-reported and attributed job insecurity have been associated with increases in short spells and medically certified spells of sickness absence from all causes, musculoskeletal disorders, and trauma. And a longitudinal study in Finland has shown that downsizing increases sickness absence more among low-income than high-income employees. In contrast to these findings, studies of British civil servants and Finnish workers on fixed-term contracts have shown that in some cases attributed job insecurity is associated with decreases in sickness absence, even when the workforce is known to have a higher level of ill health. This phenomenon is called sickness presenteeism and tends to occur when workers feel that being absent from work may increase their chance of redundancy. Unsurprisingly, sickness presenteeism appears to be more common among workers in the secondary labor market.

Job insecurity has also been widely studied in the organizational and managerial literature as a determinant of a number of outcomes that have adverse consequences for organizations, such as commitment, work effort, and productivity. Findings from the Netherlands have shown that not only is job insecurity a strong determinant of job change, but it is often the most valuable individuals that are most inclined to seek other job alternatives.

Effects beyond the Individual and the Workplace

A downstream effect of the stress caused by self-reported and attributed job insecurity is an increase in health service use: general practitioner (GP) consultations, hospital referrals, hospital attendance, and use of prescribed medicines, in particular, tranquilizers and antidepressants. However, as for sickness absence, effects can go either way, so there is also evidence that those with high levels of job insecurity may forgo a medical consultation or neglect care of themselves for fear of missing work. An in-depth study of effects on health service use also showed that these effects were not restricted to the workers themselves. GP consultations, hospital referrals, and attendance also increased significantly in the workers' families. Other effects on the family include increases in work–family conflict and tension in the home. Evidence of this spill-over confirms results from studies of both categories of job insecurity that have reported adverse effects on family members, family relationships and the behavior of children.

Who Experiences Job Insecurity: The Public Health Impact

Job insecurity is not evenly distributed throughout the working population. Along with unemployment, it falls more heavily on those with fewer skills, those with less education, and those at a disadvantage in the labor market such as immigrants and the disabled. Several studies have now demonstrated a strong inverse association between job insecurity and socioeconomic position, measured as occupational grade, social class, or education. This means that those at the top of the social hierarchy, however measured, are less likely to experience job insecurity than those at the bottom. Such inverse gradients have been demonstrated in specific occupational groups and in general population samples. There is also evidence that the effect of job insecurity on health is highest among those in the lowest socioeconomic group.

Studies of large companies or government employees – contexts in which most studies on the health effects of job insecurity have been carried out – may underestimate the extent of job insecurity in the general working population. A survey of a large sample of the working population in Taiwan found that job insecurity affected 50% of workers, and a study in Switzerland in 1997 showed that 10% of the working population reported a high level of job insecurity. These may be two extreme examples, but an OECD study showed that in 1996 experience of job insecurity was very common, with on average 67% of workers unable to agree strongly with the statement "my job is secure." With the experience of job insecurity being this common, any detrimental effects of job insecurity on health can have major repercussion on the health of the working population as a whole.

Summary

Unequivocal evidence of a causal association between job insecurity and health would require longitudinal studies, with information from a period of secure employment for those subsequently exposed to job insecurity, in addition to a well-matched control group who remained in secure employment. Such prerequisites mean that opportunities for ideal studies are rare. Consequently, although research interest in the health consequences of job insecurity has increased, strong evidence of a causal link between job insecurity and many health outcomes remains limited. Despite this, there is now firm evidence of a causal association between both self-reported and attributed job insecurity and all measures of psychological ill health, and evidence of an association with a number of self-reported physical health outcomes.

Self-reported and attributed job insecurity are associated with adverse changes in most biomedical risk factors that have been examined, but effects are mostly nonsignificant. There is an indication that attributed job insecurity is associated with an increase in heart disease, but no evidence yet of an association between job insecurity and death from diseases or suicide. Job insecurity has been shown to increase workplace injuries and accidents through detrimental effects on employee safety motivation and safety compliance. Most studies show that attributed job insecurity is accompanied by an increase in self-certified and medically certified sickness absence. However, lower rates of sickness absence as well as sickness presenteeism among temporary workers and employees facing imminent threat have also been demonstrated. Both self-reported and attributed job insecurity result in increased use of health services and medications among both those directly affected and their families.

It has been proposed that the effect of job insecurity on health may be mediated via changes in health-related behaviors. However, there is little evidence to support or refute this hypothesis. Although some studies have found the effect of job insecurity on health to be partially explained by other work characteristics such as job satisfaction, social support at work, and job control, much of the association between job insecurity and ill health remains unexplained and may be due either to direct effects of stress on the autoimmune system or to unobserved health-related selection.

Recent work has demonstrated a synergistic adverse effect on health in workers exposed to both high job insecurity and high job strain. In a context of downsizing and reliance on outsourced labor, perceptions of insecurity are likely to be widespread and, as fewer people do more, occur alongside increasing demands and perceptions of low control. If current trends continue, the number of employees exposed to both job insecurity and job strain will probably increase. Despite its limitations, existing research on the stress of job insecurity has much to contribute to policies that will improve the health of workers and their families and prevent adverse effects on the organizations that employ them.

See Also the Following Articles

Effort–Reward Imbalance Model; Unemployment, Stress, and; Workplace Stress.

Further Reading

Bartley, M. and Ferrie, J. E. (2001). Unemployment, job insecurity and health – glossary. *Journal of Epidemiology and Community Health* 55, 776–781.

Burchell, B., Day, D., Hudson, M., Ladipo, D., Mankelow, R., Nolan, J., et al. (1999). *Job insecurity and work intensification.* York: Joseph Rowntree Foundation.

Ferrie, J. E., Marmot, M. G., Griffiths, J. and Ziglio, E. (eds.) (1999). *Labour market changes and job insecurity: a challenge for social welfare and health promotion.* European Series No. 81. Copenhagen: World Health Organisation.

Hartley, J., Jacobson, D., Klandermans, B. and Van Vuuren, T. (1991). *Job insecurity: coping with jobs at risk.* London: Sage Publications Ltd.

Quinlan, M., Mayhew, C. and Bohle, E. (2001). The global expansion of precarious employment, work disorganisation, and consequences for occupational health: a review of recent research. *International Journal of Health Services* **31**, 335–414.

Platt, S., Pavis, S. and Akram, G. (1998). *Changing labour market conditions and health: a systematic literature review (1993–1998).* Dublin: European Foundation for the Improvement of Living and Working Conditions.

Effort–Reward Imbalance Model

J Siegrist
University of Duesseldorf, Duesseldorf, Germany

Glossary

Contract An agreement that defines a norm of equivalence by specifying obligations, benefits, rights, and duties in interpersonal exchange (e.g., work contract).

Overcommitment A motivational pattern of work-related striving toward high achievement that is associated with increased health risks in the long run.

Prediction error theory A theoretical model developed in neuroscience to predict neural activation and deactivation in relevant areas of the brain according to the principles of economy and learning.

Social reciprocity A fundamental principle of social exchange that guarantees equivalence of give and take between two individuals or parties.

Social role A set of expectations or norms (duties and options) directed toward people who hold important social positions (e.g., work role, family role, and volunteer role).

Theory

One of the important tasks of medical sociology consists in explaining how the social environment affects human health. Theoretical models are instrumental in identifying those aspects within the complex social reality that accounts for increased or reduced health risks in populations. These models are then translated into measures with the help of social science research methods that meet the criteria of adequate reliability and validity and are tested in the framework of epidemiological or experimental study designs.

One such model, labeled effort–reward imbalance, is concerned with adverse effects on health produced by the violation of one of the fundamental, evolutionarily stable principles of human societies – social reciprocity. According to this principle, any action or service provided by person A to person B that has some utility to B is expected to be returned by person B to A. Exchange expectancy does not implicate a full identity of the service in return, but it is essential that this activity meet some agreed-on standard of equivalence. To secure equivalence of return in crucial transactions, social contracts have been established as a universal societal institution. A contract defines a norm of equivalence by specifying obligations, benefits, rights, and duties in interpersonal exchange. Trade, work and employment, marriage, and intergenerational transfer are examples of contractual exchange. These contracts may vary considerably according to the specificity of their regulations, the sanctions expected in case of deviance, or the time frame of exchange. Yet, in all instances, contracts are instrumental in providing members of a society with a sense of security by creating trust. Trust is a mental state motivating people to engage in social exchange even if the trade-off is highly uncertain. Expectancy of reciprocity is the driving force of trust.

The principle of reciprocity not only is rooted in human evolution, but plays a significant role in ontogenesis as well. Research on attachment formation in infancy has demonstrated the importance of reciprocal exchange between infant and caregiver in early postnatal life as one of the preconditions of normal human development. For these reasons, breaking the norm of reciprocity in contractual exchange is expected to have adverse consequences for the health and well-being of disadvantaged people.

The model of effort–reward imbalance states that recurrent or long-lasting nonreciprocity in contractual exchange increases the risk of stress-related disorders in exposed people, due to the powerful role of this evolutionarily old grammar of interpersonal cooperation. This model has been developed and tested with regard to work and employment, and more recently has been expanded to less formalized types of contractual exchange, in particular marital or partnership relationship, exchange between parents and children, and voluntary work.

The principle of social reciprocity lies at the core of the employment contract, which defines distinct obligations or tasks to be performed in exchange for equitable rewards. Yet, according to the effort–reward imbalance model, nonsymmetric contractual exchange is expected to occur frequently under specific conditions (see **Figure 1**). In this case, high efforts spent at work are not reciprocated by equitable rewards in terms of money, esteem, and career opportunities, including job security. The model of effort–reward imbalance claims that lack of reciprocity between the costs and gains (i.e., high-cost, low-gain conditions) elicits strong negative emotions with a special propensity to sustained autonomic and neuroendocrine activation and their adverse long-term consequences for health.

There are three important conditions that increase the probability of recurrent effort–reward imbalance at work: dependency, strategic choice, and overcommitment. Dependency reflects the structural constraints observed in certain types of employment contracts (e.g., unskilled or semi-skilled workers and elderly employees) when no alternative choice in the labor market is available. In modern economies characterized by a globalized labor market and organizational downsizing, the lack of an alternative choice of workplace is relatively frequent.

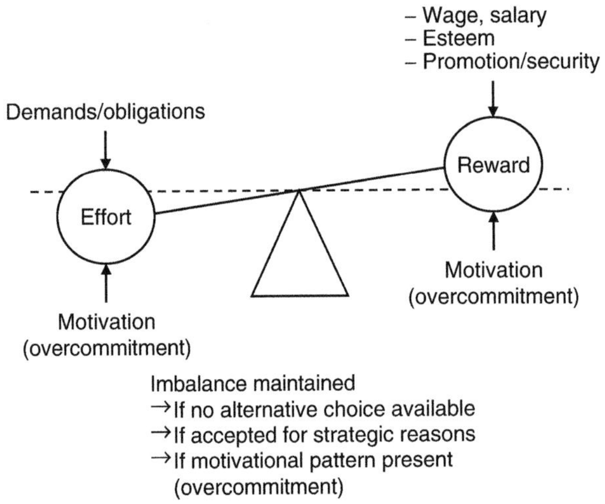

Figure 1 The model of effort–reward imbalance at work. Modified from Siegrist (1996).

In strategic choice, people accept high-cost, low-gain conditions of their employment for a certain time, often without being forced to do so, because they tend to improve their chances of career promotion and related rewards at a later stage. This pattern is frequently observed in early stages of professional careers and in jobs that are characterized by heavy competition.

The third condition, overcommitment, reflects the psychological reasons for a recurrent mismatch between efforts and rewards at work. People characterized by the motivational pattern of excessive work-related overcommitment may strive toward continuously high achievement because of their underlying need for approval and esteem at work. Although these excessive efforts often are not met by adequate rewards, overcommitted people tend to maintain their level of involvement. Work-related overcommitment is elicited and reinforced by a variety of job environments and is often experienced as self-rewarding over a period of years in occupational trajectories. However, in the long run, overcommitted people are susceptible to exhaustion and adaptive breakdown.

In summary, the model of effort–reward imbalance at work maintains that nonreciprocal contractual exchange is frequent under these structural and personal conditions, and that people experiencing dependency, strategic choice, or overcommitment, either separately or in combination, are at elevated risk of suffering from stress-related disorders.

Research Evidence

Several sources of information on the associations between nonreciprocal contractual exchange and health are available, such as data from cross-sectional and case-controlled studies, from prospective epidemiological observational investigations, from studies using ambulatory monitoring techniques or experimental designs, and from intervention trials. The prospective epidemiological observational study is considered a gold standard approach in this field because of its temporal sequence, its sample size, and the quantification of the subsequent disease risk following exposure.

Up to now, the model has been tested in approximately a dozen prospective epidemiological reports and, in addition, in many cross-sectional and case-controlled studies. Associations of either the full model or its main components with increased health risks were found in a majority of these studies. The relatively strongest and consistent effects concern cardiovascular diseases – effort–reward imbalance at work is associated with a doubling of risk over a mean 8-year observation period. In addition, nonreciprocity at work increases the probability of suffering from depression, psychosomatic symptoms, sickness absence, and poor self-rated health. With respect to health-adverse behaviors, and especially the intensity of daily cigarette smoking, alcohol dependence, and weight gain, associations with effort–reward imbalance at work were observed more consistently in men than in women. In addition to health-adverse effects, this type of chronic stress at work increases the likelihood of changing or giving up one's job, of retiring prematurely, and, according to first results, of deviating from regulations at work.

In summary, there is solid evidence indicating that failed reciprocity in a core social role, the work role, represents an independent risk factor for a variety of highly prevalent diseases. Moreover, it undermines work-related motivations and behaviors. Results are derived from a wide range of different occupations and professions, and they concern both genders, although, in general, the effects are stronger in men. In several studies, this imbalance was found to be more frequent among lower socioeconomic groups, and its effects on health are generally stronger in these groups.

So far, the bulk of evidence comes from investigations conducted in Europe, the United States, and Canada. Given the fact that the norm of contractual reciprocity is rooted in human evolution, we would expect recurrent violations of this norm to have similar effects on health across societies and cultures. According to recent studies, effort–reward imbalance at work is associated with several indicators of reduced health in Asian countries such as China, Taiwan, and Japan.

An additional line of research is devoted to the study of nonreciprocal exchange in marital or partnership relationships, in relationships between parents and children, and in other types of cooperative activities, such as voluntary work. The recurrent experience of effort–reward imbalance in these types of social exchange was found to reduce mental health and well-being in exposed people.

What are the neural and physiological correlates of the recurrent experience of effort–reward imbalance? Several studies investigated heart rate, heart rate variability, and blood pressure during work and nonwork days, using ambulatory monitoring techniques. In general, cardiovascular activity differed between employees scoring high on measures of effort–reward imbalance and those with low scores on these measures. One study, in addition, assessed salivary cortisol excretion and found a higher mean level in employees with high scores on the scale measuring work-related overcommitment.

The neural correlates of reward frustration are still poorly understood. Yet, in an investigation using functional magnetic resonance imaging with a monetary reward paradigm, neural activation in reward-sensitive prefrontal mesolimbic dopamine projection sites was not reduced when expected rewards were frustrated in otherwise healthy subjects with an extensive history of work-related effort–reward imbalance. This was different in subjects without chronic stress experience, in whom activation in these areas was reduced, as hypothesized by the prediction error theory.

Implications for Intervention

Measures to improve the balance between effort and reward and, hence, to improve reciprocity and contractual fairness at work can be implemented at three levels. The first level relates to the individual worker. Increasing awareness of failed reciprocity at work among employees, informing them about possible health effects, and providing cognitive-behavioral interventions in high-risk groups to reduce the intensity of stressful experiences (relaxation response, stress inoculation, self-instruction, and reducing high levels of overcommitment) are examples of this approach.

A related second level of health promotion at work, the interpersonal level, concerns training in leadership skills, the improvement in the handling of conflicts, or the improvement of communication and cooperation in everyday work settings. Providing appropriate esteem and recognition was shown to be an important component of the balance between effort and reward at work, and this target can be met by focused leadership training.

However, to produce a lasting impact, these human-relations measures need to be supplemented by evidence-based organizational and structural changes in the work environment. Such changes concern the division of work; its quantity and quality; work schedules and their flexibility; monetary incentives; tailored promotion opportunities, including investment in training and requalification on the job; and, most important, enhanced job security. The probability that these and related measures are realized will increase with available evidence of the economic benefits for companies and organizations that invest their increased efforts into health-promoting quality of work. Such measures are not limited to paid work, but may be extended to other types of contractual social exchange, in particular voluntary work. In conclusion, it remains to be seen how this new scientific evidence can be transferred into health-promoting policy measures that diminish the burden of societal stress.

See Also the Following Articles

Economic Factors and Stress; Social Status and Stress; Workplace Stress.

Further Reading

Gouldner, A. W. (1960). The norm of reciprocity. *American Sociological Review* **25**, 161–178.

Marmot, M., Siegrist, J. and Theorell, T. (2006). Health and the psychosocial environment at work. In: Marmot, M. & Wilkinson, R. G. (eds.) *Social determinants of health* (2nd edn., pp. 97–130). Oxford: Oxford University Press.

Siegrist, J. (1996). Adverse health effects of high effort – low reward conditions at work. *Journal of Occupational Health Psychology* **1**, 27–43.

Siegrist, J. (2005). Social reciprocity and health: new scientific evidence and policy implications. *Psychoneuroendocrinology* **30**, 1033–1038.

Siegrist, J., Starke, D., Chandola, T., et al. (2004). The measurement of effort-reward imbalance at work: European comparisons. *Social Science & Medicine* **58**, 1483–1499.

Tsutsumi, A. and Kawakami, N. (2004). A review of empirical studies on the model of effort – reward imbalance at work: reducing occupational stress by implementing a new theory. *Social Science & Medicine* **59**, 2335–2359.

Environmental Factors

W R Avison
University of Western Ontario, London, ON, Canada

This is a revised version of the article by W R Avison, Encyclopedia of Stress First Edition, volume 2, pp 53–59, © 2000, Elsevier Inc.

Glossary

Differential exposure hypothesis	The contention that specific statuses or roles are associated with greater or lesser levels of stressors that arise out of the conditions of life and which, in turn, affect levels of psychological distress.
Differential vulnerability hypothesis	Argument that elevated levels of distress among individuals in disadvantaged statuses reflect their greater responsiveness to stressors; that is, in two social groups exposed to the same levels of stressors, distress will be higher among those people in the disadvantaged statuses.
Environmental factors	Social or economic circumstances that affect exposure to stressors.
Social causation	A model that suggests that people in socially disadvantaged statuses will be exposed to more stressors that, in turn, result in more distress or disorder.
Social selection	A model that suggests that people with high levels of stress in their lives are more likely to experience mental health problems and consequently are more likely to occupy disadvantaged statuses.
Stress process paradigm	A model that describes how stressors manifest themselves in distress or disorder. It postulates the existence of three factors that either mediate or moderate the effects of stressors on distress or disorder: psychosocial resources, coping resources and strategies, and social supports. The model also specifies how environmental factors influence all other variables in the paradigm.

Historical Background

There is a vast body of research literature on the impact of social and economic factors on physical and mental health problems. In general, these studies have demonstrated that individuals' social locations in society, in terms of their social statuses and social roles, have important implications for both the kinds and levels of stressors to which they are exposed. Indeed, one of the most important contributions of the sociology of mental health has been to demonstrate conclusively that stressors are not experienced randomly by individuals but, rather, that there is a social distribution of stressors. This perspective has emerged out of a number of theoretical and empirical developments.

Much of the work on the social distribution of stressors has its intellectual origins in the work of Bruce and Barbara Dohrenwend in the 1970s. They observed that exposure to stressful life events was correlated positively with symptoms of mental illness. They argued that the higher rates of psychological impairment found among members of socially disadvantaged groups might be explained by their greater exposure to life events. The underlying assumption of this explanatory model was that social causation processes were operating: differences in social statuses and social roles produce variations in the experience of life events that result in different rates of mental health problems among these social groups.

For the next decade, social scientists exhaustively studied the relationships among environmental factors, stressful life events, and psychological distress and disorder. At least three major themes emerged from this work. First, a conceptual paradigm emerged for examining the interplay among environmental factors, stressors, mediators, and mental health outcomes. Second, it became clear that stressful life events constituted only one kind of stressor and that research needed to identify and study other types. Third, there was general agreement with the notion that the distribution of stressors is socially patterned.

The Stress Process

Several researchers working independently in the 1980s developed conceptual models that enable us to better understand how socially induced stressors manifest themselves in psychological distress, symptoms of psychiatric disorder, or in other dysfunctions or health problem. All of these models focus on the association between stressful life events and their distressful manifestations (psychological distress, psychiatric disorder, etc.). These models also postulate the existence of three important factors that either mediate or moderate the effects of stressors on distress or disorder. These include psychosocial resources, coping resources and strategies, and social supports. In recent years, this model has been elaborated by specifying the kinds of environmental factors – primarily social and economic variables associated with social statuses and roles – that influence all other variables in the paradigm. This paradigm has provided social scientists and epidemiologists with a conceptual framework for studying the effects of environmental factors on stressors as well as on all other components of the model.

The Stress Universe

Throughout the 1970s and early 1980s, most of the research on environmental sources of stressors focused on life-change events. The most widely used measures of life stress were events checklists that usually contained from 30 to 100 events that represented potential changes in people's lives. These included events such as the death of a loved one, marital separation or divorce, job loss, and geographical moves. Over time, however, two developments substantially altered the study of environmental stressors. First, it became clear to researchers who were studying the stress process that the association between eventful stressors and distress was modest at best. For many researchers, this suggested that stressors were not being measured comprehensively. Accordingly, they expanded life events inventories to include events that were not life changes, but which included other difficulties such as family conflicts, work conflicts, and financial difficulties. In part, the inclusion of these events reflected the realization among many researchers that stress often arises in the context of individuals' work and family roles. Second, investigations of intra-event variability in stressful life events revealed that life events inventories included ongoing or chronic stressors (such as family conflict, marital difficulties, and financial problems) as well as eventful stressors.

These considerations led researchers to develop more extensive strategies to measure a broader array of life stressors than had previously been the case. Perhaps the most comprehensive consideration of the many dimensions of life stress was presented by Wheaton. He distinguished among various concepts of stressors, including chronic stress, daily hassles, macro events, and traumatic events. In doing so, he presented a scheme for arraying these different stressors on a continuum ranging from sudden traumatic experiences and life change events at the discrete end to chronic stressors that are more continuous in nature. Wheaton demonstrated two important properties of these various dimensions of the stress universe: (1) they are relatively independent of one another and therefore are unlikely to be empirically confounded with one another and (2) they each have significant independent effects on various measures of physical and mental health outcomes. These findings suggest that any comprehensive attempt to estimate the impact of life stressors on health outcomes requires that we measure an array of stressors that includes both discrete life experiences and more chronic or ongoing stressors.

The Social Distribution of Stressors

Early research by Bruce and Barbara Dohrenwend and by George Brown and his colleagues on life events clearly established that socially induced stressors exerted important influences on various measures of mental health outcomes. What seemed particularly interesting was that the socially disadvantaged groups with the highest levels of distress and disorder also appeared to be exposed to the most stressful life events. This led to the hypothesis that social differences in distress and disorder might be accounted for by variations in either exposure or vulnerability to social stressors.

Subsequently, in a seminal article on the sociological study of stress, Pearlin argued for the need to systematically investigate the ways in which social structure affects individuals' exposure to stressors. Essentially, Pearlin asserted that the roles and statuses that people occupy in their everyday lives have important consequences for the kinds of stressors to which they are exposed and the frequency with which this occurs. In short, he argued that accounting for the impact of environmental factors is crucial for understanding the ways in which individuals experience social stressors.

This point has been made even more salient by Turner, Wheaton, and Lloyd in their paper on the epidemiology of social stress. Their findings from a large community study reveal that younger people are more exposed to a variety of stressors than are older respondents. They also find this pattern among women compared to men, unmarried people compared to married people, and individuals in lower socioeconomic status (SES) positions compared to those in higher SES positions. In their view, this clearly indicates that stressors are not experienced randomly in the population. Quite the contrary, they asserted that their results reveal that there is a social distribution of stressors that is characterized by greater exposure among members of disadvantaged social groups.

The Impact of Environmental Factors on Stressors

In thinking about the social distribution of stressors, social scientists have focused primarily on three major environmental determinants: social statuses, social roles, and the ambient environment. Most formulations of the stress process model take the view that individuals' locations in the structure of society place them at greater or lesser risk of encountering stressors. These locations are defined by the various statuses that individuals hold and by the various social roles they occupy. In addition, there are more ambient characteristics of the social environment that are not specific to statuses or roles but that may generate stressful experiences for individuals.

Social Statuses

In the literature, individuals' positions in the structure of society are often defined by six major status characteristics: age, gender, marital status, race/ethnicity, employment status, and SES. Each of these environmental factors is associated with differential exposure to stressful experiences.

Age There appears to be substantial agreement among researchers that exposure to stressful experiences declines with age. Whether the stressors in question are life events or chronic role strains, younger people report significantly more stress than do the elderly. Moreover, economic hardship tends to decline with age as does marital conflict in marriages that stay intact. Despite these findings, it is not yet clear whether the impact of age on exposure to stressors is a function of maturation processes, birth cohort or generational effects, or life-cycle processes.

Gender Studies of gender differences in exposure to stressors have generated inconsistent findings. Some research concludes that women experience more stressful life events than men, whereas other research finds no differences. Turner and Avison conducted one of the more comprehensive studies of gender exposure to various dimensions of stress. Women report more stressful life events than men, but they experience fewer lifetime traumatic events and less discrimination stress. Women and men do not differ in their exposure to chronic stressors. When these various dimensions of stress were considered cumulatively, they found that men experience greater exposure compared to women but that this difference is relatively small. Turner and Avison concluded that these small gender variations in exposure to stressors are unlikely to account for gender differences in psychological distress.

Although other researchers reported that women are more exposed than men to chronic strains due to financial hardship, workplace difficulties, and role overload associated with parenting and work, these differences are difficult to separate from the gendered roles that women and men play in the workplace and in the household division of labor. Indeed, one of the lessons of stress research in the sociology of mental health is that gender conditions the effects of a variety of roles and statuses on the exposure to stress.

Marital status One of the more robust findings in the study of social stress is the observation that married individuals experience considerably fewer stressors than either never married or formerly married individuals. This pattern can be observed for chronic strains as well as for stressful life events. Unlike age and gender, however, the causal direction of the relationship between marital status and stressful experience is open to competing interpretations. A social selection interpretation suggests that people with high levels of stress in their lives are less likely to marry or, if they do so, they are more likely to separate and divorce. A social causation interpretation suggests that people who have never married and those who have separated or divorced are more likely to experience an array of life events and chronic strains than are the married.

Some longitudinal research indicates that divorce leads to elevated levels of depression and that this change is accounted for by a decline in living standard, economic difficulties, and a reduction in social support. Even if the end of a marriage provides some escape from a stressful situation, divorce is accompanied by life stress that has depressive consequences. Other studies also report significant increases in psychological distress among the maritally disrupted over and above their predivorce levels, but find virtually no evidence that changes in financial stressors, changes in role demands, or changes in geographic location mediate the relationship between marital disruption and distress. These are reflective of longitudinal studies on marital disruption and remarriage insofar as they generate few consistent findings other than the observations that marital disruption is associated with elevated psychological distress and that remarriage results in only a partial reduction in this elevation.

Race and ethnicity Studies of racial and ethnic variations exposure to stressors are relatively recent in the literature. There is general agreement that experiences of discrimination constitute an important set of stressors for African Americans, Hispanic Americans, and American Indians. In addition, stressors arising out of the social disadvantages of these groups have also been observed. Among Asian Americans, the experience of discrimination and the stress of migration have been noted as important threats to their mental health.

Turner and Avison systematically examined differences between African Americans and Whites in the United States in exposure to stressors. Across five different dimensions (recent life events, chronic stressors, total lifetime major events, lifetime major discrimination, and daily discrimination), African Americans experience significantly more stress than do Whites. Indeed, the cumulative difference between African Americans and Whites in exposure to stress is more than 0.5 standard deviation.

It is interesting to note, however, that these elevated levels of stressors among racial and ethnic minority members do not necessarily translate into higher rates of distress or disorder for all groups. In their review of this issue, Williams and Harris-Reid concluded that African Americans have lower prevalence rates of psychiatric disorders than do Whites. The data are inconsistent when comparing Whites with Hispanic Americans or Asian Americans. What little data exist about the epidemiology of mental health among American Indians suggests that their rates of disorder, especially depression and alcohol abuse, are elevated.

It is difficult to interpret the meaning of these findings. Lower rates of disorder in the face of elevated levels of distress suggests that some racial and ethnic group may be less vulnerable than others to these stressors or that countervailing effects of psychosocial resources may reduce the impact of stressors on their mental health. Turner and Avison suggested that African Americans may exhibit a response tendency in which they underreport infrequent or mild experiences of distress, thus leading to an underestimation of their levels of distress. They demonstrate that once this tendency is taken into account, there is clear evidence that African Americans' elevated exposure to stress manifests itself in significantly higher distress.

Employment status Research leaves little doubt that the unemployed experience more negative mental health outcomes than do the employed. The evidence of this correlation is most clear for outcomes such as symptoms of depression and anxiety and measures of psychological distress. Longitudinal studies support the conclusion that job loss results in higher levels of mental health symptoms.

Studies of the factors that intervene between individuals' job losses and their health problems have identified at least two major sources of environmental stressors that mediate this relationship. Some researchers have shown that job loss and unemployment create financial strains that lead to mental health problems.

Others have examined the mediating role of marital and family conflict. These studies report that unemployment leads to increasing conflicts between the unemployed worker and other family members. Some researchers have suggested that the elevated levels of distress observed among women whose husbands are experiencing job-related stress may be consistent with the costs of caring hypothesis described earlier.

Socioeconomic status Although there is general agreement that SES and mental illness are inversely correlated and that exposure to stressors are a major determinant of mental health problems, there has been surprisingly little consensus among researchers about the SES–stress relationship. Whether SES is measured by some combination of education and income or by occupational prestige among those with jobs, contradictory results emerge. These inconsistent findings have led some researchers to argue that it is not stress exposure that produces higher rates of mental illness among individuals with lower SES. Rather, they suggest that the impact of stressors on mental illness is more substantial among low-SES than high-SES individuals. In other words, they argue that lower-class individuals are differentially vulnerable to stressors. It seems clear that this debate with respect to the influence of SES has not been resolved. Nevertheless, more recent studies suggest that when stressors are comprehensively measured, there is a significant social-class gradient in exposure to stress.

Some of the most compelling evidence of the effects of economic hardship on marital relationships has been presented in studies of families during the Great Depression of the 1930s. This work clearly indicates that economic difficulties increase marital tensions in most families and especially in those that were most vulnerable prior to the economic hardship. Similar findings have been reported in studies of families whose lives were affected by the farm crises of the 1980s.

Social Roles

A central focus of much research on the stress process has been on the ways in which the social roles that individuals occupy expose them to stressors. Pearlin described these role strains in rich detail. For Pearlin, several types of stress may arise from role occupancy: excessive demands of certain roles, inequities in rewards, the failure of reciprocity in roles, role conflict, role captivity, and role restructuring. These various types of stress are important sources of stress that may manifest themselves in symptoms of distress or disorder. These kinds of environmental stressors have been studied most intensively in investigations of family roles and work roles.

Family roles Recent research on the family and mental health has focused on family structure in terms of the intersection of marital status and parenthood. In this context, there has been intense interest in the impact of single parenthood on symptoms of distress. Results consistently show higher levels of distress among single mothers than among married mothers. These studies of single parenthood clearly reveal that family structure and the roles embedded in that structure are important determinants of women's mental health.

Research indicates that separation and divorce trigger chronic stressors such as income reduction and housing relocation. In addition, the divorced experienced more life events than the married, particularly negative events involving loss. When children are involved, there may be additional strains associated with separation or divorce. The custodial parent, usually the mother, assumes many household, financial, and emotional responsibilities previously shared by two parents.

The work role In addition to examining how differences in employment or work status influence exposure to stressors and subsequent mental health outcomes, social scientists have become aware of the importance of understanding how experiences in the work role are related to stress and health. Despite the observation that being employed generally has positive psychosocial consequences for individuals, not all employment circumstances are the same. Indeed, there are important variations in the stressors associated with any particular work situation. Work exposes individuals to various kinds of stressful experiences and provides different kinds of rewards for different people – financial rewards, self-esteem, a sense of control over one's life, and so on. It seems, then, that the net effect of paid employment for any individual will depend on the balance of these costs and benefits.

A number of recent contributions to the study of work and mental health have provided some useful models for this kind of research. In her comprehensive review of the literature on the interplay between work and family, Menaghan demonstrated clearly that work-related stressors are significantly associated with the mental health of family members. Other researchers have convincingly documented how role overload and the sense of personal power have important implications for the effects of women's employment on their mental health. Some investigations have shown how job characteristics such as full-time versus part-time work and substantive complexity have significant effects on mental health.

The intersection of work and family roles Research on work and family stress among women suggests a number of ways in which work and family roles interact in their effects on psychological distress and depression. These studies highlight the importance of considering both family stressors to which women are exposed and work-related stress.

Relatively few studies have examined how single parenthood and paid employment interact in their impact on mental health problems. The studies that have investigated this issue conclude that differences between single-parent families and two-parent families in role obligations and opportunities may have significant effects on the balance between work and family responsibilities. For married mothers, paid employment may be more easily integrated into daily family life. The presence of a spouse provides the opportunity to share some of the child-care responsibilities. Alternatively, dual-income families have more funds for outside child care or paid assistance in the home.

Employment for single-parent mothers may represent more of a pressing responsibility than an opportunity for achievement and development. Most single-parent families live in poverty or near poverty. In such circumstances, although paid employment may alleviate some of the most pressing financial strains, other strains persist. Moreover, when single mothers obtain employment, it is common for them to also bear the continued sole responsibility for the care and nurturance of their children. Such dual demands may generate a cost to employment – role overload.

Under these circumstances, it seems probable that fewer psychosocial rewards associated with employment (greater self-esteem, self-efficacy, or social support) will accrue to single mothers. This is all the more likely to be the case because single parents may be constrained to select jobs that are not their first choice but that, instead, are near their homes or have hours of work that fit with their children's schedules or with the availability of child care.

Ambient Strains

Not all stressors are associated with statuses and roles. Ambient strains that are not attributable to a specific role but, rather, are diffuse in nature and have a variety of sources. These include experiences such as living through an economic recession, living in unsafe housing, or living in a dangerous neighborhood. Some studies have demonstrated that ambient strains associated with the neighborhoods in which adolescents live magnify the impact of other stressors on their mental health. Other studies make the same point with respect to the ambient effect of economic environments.

Differential Exposure and Vulnerability to Environmental Stressors

An important issue has been to test the relative importance of differential exposure and differential vulnerability to stressors as explanations of the differences in psychological distress by social status or social role. The differential exposure hypothesis contends that specific statuses or roles are associated with greater or lesser levels of stressors that arise out of the conditions of life and which, in turn, affect levels of psychological distress. For example, applying this argument to marital status, the hypothesis is that the transition from marriage to separation or divorce brings with it significant increases in exposure to financial strains, role overload, and other types of stressors. This increase in the burden of stress experienced by the separated or divorced people translates into elevated levels of mental health problems. Conversely, individuals who remain married experience far fewer stressful circumstances and, accordingly, have lower levels of psychological distress.

The competing explanation, the differential vulnerability hypothesis, argues that elevated levels of distress among individuals in certain statuses reflect their greater responsiveness to stressors. Such increased responsiveness or vulnerability to stressors has been attributed to a number of different sources. These include dimensions of personal and social competence, such as self-efficacy, that contribute to individuals' greater or lesser resilience in the face of stress and access to coping resources that moderate stressful experiences. The most recent work on this debate has been conducted by Turner, Wheaton, and Lloyd. Their investigation of age, gender, marital status, and SES reveals little evidence that any of the differences associated with these social statuses in distress or disorder can be attributed to differential vulnerability. Instead, they found that observed variations in mental health outcomes are due largely to different levels of exposure to stressors. They and others argue that the use of a more comprehensive measure of stressors that includes live events and chronic strains is likely to better estimate actual exposure and to avoid the error of attributing unmeasured differential exposure to differential vulnerability.

See Also the Following Articles

Social Status and Stress; Workplace Stress; Work–Family Balance.

Further Reading

Aneshensel, C. S. and Phelan, J. C. (eds.) (1999). *Handbook of the sociology of mental health*. New York: Kluwer Academic/Plenum Publishers.

Brown, G. and Harris, T. (1989). *Life events and illness*. New York: Guilford Press.

Dohrenwend, B. S. and Dohrenwend, B. P. (eds.) (1974). *Stressful life events: Their nature and effects*. New York: John Wiley.

Menaghan, E. G. (1994). The daily grind: work stressors, family patterns, and intergenerational outcomes. In: Avison, W. R. & Gotlib, I. H. (eds.) *Stress and mental health: contemporary issues and prospects for the future*, pp. 115–147. New York: Plenum Press.

Mirowsky, J. and Ross, C. E. (2003). *Social causes of psychological distress*, 2nd ed. Hawthorne, NY: Aldine de Gruyter.

Pearlin, L. I. (1989). The sociological study of stress. *Journal of Health and Social Behavior* **30**, 241–256.

Pearlin, L. I., Lieberman, M. A., Menaghan, E. G. and Mullan, J. T. (1981). The stress process. *Journal of Health and Social Behavior* **22**, 337–356.

Turner, R. J. and Avison, W. R. (2003). Status variations in stress exposure: implications for the interpretation of research on race, socioeconomic status, and gender. *Journal of Health and Social Behavior* **44**, 488–505.

Turner, R. J., Wheaton, B. and Lloyd, D. A. (1995). The epidemiology of social stress. *American Sociological Review* **60**, 104–125.

Wheaton, B. (1994). Sampling the stress universe. In: Avison, W. R. & Gotlib, I. H. (eds.) *Stress and mental health: contemporary issues and prospects for the future*, pp. 77–114. New York: Plenum Press.

Williams, D. R. and Harris-Reid, M. (1999). Race and mental health: emerging patterns and promising approaches. In: Horwitz, A. V. & Scheid, T. L. (eds.) *A handbook for the study of mental health: social contexts, theories, and systems*, pp. 295–314. New York: Cambridge University Press.

Industrialized Societies

J Siegrist
University of Duesseldorf, Duesseldorf, Germany

This article is reproduced from Encyclopedia of Stress First Edition, volume 2, pp 565–569, © 2000, Elsevier Inc.

Glossary

Epidemiological transition — The changing pattern of most prevalent diseases from infectious to chronic degenerative diseases.

Formal rationality — The purposeful calculation of the most efficient means to achieve a goal where rational choices are made to maximize individual benefit.

Gender roles — The cluster of social expectations and norms guiding typically male vs. typically female behavior.

Health-related lifestyle — A collective pattern of health-promoting or health-damaging behavior based on routinized choices people make about food, exercise, hygiene, safety, relaxation, and so on. This pattern is structured by specific needs, social norms, and constraints.

Social disintegration — A weakening of social ties and an absence of cooperative exchange resulting in a lack of social rules and trust and, ultimately, in a breakdown of a social order.

Process of Industrialization and Epidemiological Transition

The industrial revolution started in Great Britain during the second half of the eighteenth century and has subsequently spread across a number of economically advanced countries. This revolution, together with the political revolution initiated in France, must be considered one of the most radical changes in human history. Within a very short time period, fundamental ways of living and working were transformed from a basically agricultural society to a society that is driven increasingly by technology and market economy. With the invention of engines and machines, productivity was increased in an unprecedented way. A large part of the workforce, employed formerly as peasants and craftsmen, moved to urban areas to engage in unskilled or semiskilled work. The rapid growth of cities and the formation of an industrial workforce contributed to two subsequent, most significant demographic trends: (1) a take-off period of population growth with declining infant mortality rates and (2) a decline in fertility with slow population growth in combination with increased life expectancy. At the same time, the social institutions of marriage and family underwent a marked transformation, and a new division of labor between the sexes started to develop.

After severe poverty and economic exploitation in the early stages of industrial capitalism, economic progress and the development of a welfare state were experienced by a growing proportion of industrial populations. This progress included the availability of healthier food, increased opportunities of energy consumption, better housing, transport, education, and general hygiene. In terms of population health, the process of industrialization was associated with a marked increase in life expectancy and a change in the pattern of prevailing diseases. Overall, 2 to 3 years are added to life expectancy at birth with each decade passing in advanced societies. This increase cannot be attributed to the fact that people, once becoming older, live substantially longer than in previous generations. Rather, increases in life expectancy were, and still are, mainly due to a reduction of death rates at earlier ages and, thus, to increased probabilities of survival. The most substantial decline has been in infant mortality, followed by reductions in childhood and midlife mortality. A dramatic reduction in mortality from infectious diseases played a major role in this process. The typical pattern of leading causes of disability and death in advanced societies is characterized by chronic conditions such as coronary heart disease, cancer, stroke, accidents, and metabolic and mental disorders. This change is referred to as the epidemiological transition.

While the development of modern medicine and related improvements of health care are a direct outflow of the broader processes of industrialization and modernization, it has been demonstrated that the impact of medicine on this major change in the pattern of morbidity and mortality has been limited. In fact, the bulk of the decline in mortality from infectious diseases came before medicine had developed effective forms of treatment and prevention. This means that public health measures and factors related to a general rise in living standards may have accounted for this change more significantly than medicine.

With this epidemiological transition from infectious to degenerative diseases, medicine and public health face new challenges. A substantial part of these challenges directly or indirectly concerns, the impact of stressful social environments on health. The following section discusses three different aspects of this impact in more detail.

Stressful Social Environments and Health

Stressful Experience and Health-Related Lifestyles

Many of the aforementioned degenerative diseases are considered diseases of affluence because they were prevalent to the extent that life became more comfortable. For instance, with technological advances and with the expansion of commercially available food and drugs, a number of behavioral health risks were programmed, e.g., access to a car reduced physical activity significantly, and, more importantly, it also increased the number of injuries and deaths from accidents. Frequent consumption of fat and meat, at first available to the wealthier groups, contributed to elevated blood lipids, overweight, and associated health risks. Spending money on drugs such as cigarettes or alcohol increased the risk of cancer and heart disease, among others. Consequently, during the first stage of the epidemiological transition, these behaviorally induced risks associated with a wealthier lifestyle were more prevalent among socially and economically privileged groups. At a later stage of the process of industrialization and modernization, however, this social pattern changed: diseases of affluence increasingly became the diseases of the poor. In contemporary societies, this is clearly the case in almost all northern, western, and central European countries, in the United States, and in Canada. The same pattern may be experienced in the near future in countries that are currently exposed to a process of rapid industrialization.

Hence, substantial social inequalities in health are observed, mainly due to higher rates of the former affluent diseases among lower socioeconomic groups.

To explain this shift in the social distribution of a broad range of degenerative diseases and their behavioral risk factors (e.g., smoking, alcohol consumption, overweight, hypertension, metabolic disorders, cardiovascular diseases, some manifestations of cancer, AIDS), the concept of health-related lifestyle needs to be described more precisely.

Health-related lifestyles are collective patterns of health-promoting or health-damaging behavior based on routinized choices people make about food, exercise, hygiene, safety, relaxation, and so on. In many cases, these choices form a coherent pattern that is structured by specific needs, attitudes, and social norms and by the constraints of a group's socioeconomic condition. Once established among a sociocultural group, such behavioral patterns may be transferred from one generation to the next through socialization processes or they may be adopted by model learning from peer groups during adolescence. Unfortunately, the latter is often the case with respect to health-damaging behaviors (smoking, alcohol and drug consumption, unsafe sex practices, etc.). As these behaviors are experienced as relief and reward in stressful psychosocial circumstances they may be reinforced easily and, thus, trigger careers of addiction later in life.

Alternatively, with higher levels of education and knowledge and with the availability of alternative means of coping with stressful psychosocial circumstances, health-damaging lifestyles may be abandoned more easily. This is most probably what happened to the wealthier populations in advanced societies in the recent past and what contributed, and still contributes, to the widening gap in life expectancy between socioeconomic groups.

To date, there are still powerful constraints toward maintaining health-damaging lifestyles among less privileged social groups. A major constraint concerns the exposure to adverse living and working environments. A large number of epidemiologic studies document associations between the amount of exposure to these unfavourable circumstances and the prevalence of unhealthy behavior. For instance, with respect to cigarette smoking, conditions such as heavy workload, shiftwork, social isolation at work, and job instability were identified. Moreover, people who suffer from unfavorable social comparison, e.g., regarding education, income, or general social standing, are at risk of exhibiting a health-damaging life-style. In all these cases, relief and reward experience in terms of some form of addictive behavior may be needed to mitigate a stressful experience.

Some of these processes operate in more subtle ways. It is well known that the processes of primary socialization vary considerably according to the parent's socioeconomic status. In particular, children born into families with a low educational level face more difficulties in deferring their gratifications and in pursuing long-lasting goals in future life. Their sense of self-efficacy and self-esteem is low, and they are more likely to experience their environment as uncontrollable and fateful. Thus, when facing frustrations, they may be less capable of coping in an active, effective way. Rather, they may seek relief in passive behavior, including drug consumption and related health risks.

This knowledge, derived from sociological and psychological research, has direct implications for health promotion activities and the design of preventive programs. It is evident that comprehensive approaches tackling structural and individual conditions are needed to change health lifestyles in a successful way.

Unfortunately, influential economic interests operate in almost all advanced societies to counteract these measures, most evidently the tobacco and alcohol industry. Advertising activities in mass medias and diffusion of new fashions through opinion leaders are effective means to maintain drug consumption. Efforts to equalize gender roles and to assimilate female attitudes and activities to behaviors that were typical attributes of the traditional male gender role resulted in an unprecedented increase in cigarette consumption among young women. Moreover, women in recent years, as compared to the 1950s, are more likely to work in occupations that were once almost exclusively male. As a consequence of these large-scale societal changes, some of the most advanced industrial societies, such as the United States, are moving toward greater equality in mortality between the sexes.

Impact of Social Disintegration on Health

Industrialized societies are characterized by a high level of mobility. A substantial part of this mobility is due to migration. Economic constraints and wars are the major causes of large migration waves that have shaped the life of many generations throughout the processes of industrialization and modernization. Social mobility is a second component of these secular trends. As mentioned briefly, the onset of early industrialization in Europe and the United States has been facilitated by a broader sociocultural development of modernization that promoted formal rationality and individualism as the dominant modes of thinking and behaving in western societies. Formal rationality is the purposeful calculation of the most efficient means to achieve a goal. Rational choices are made to maximize individual benefit. With the expansion of individual rights, duties, and life chances, traditional ways of maintaining group solidarity, social norms, and obligations lost their significance and attraction. Individual striving for an improved standard of living has become the dominant motivation overriding traditional social constraints. Thus, a large proportion of people was, and currently is, subject to intragenerational social upward (and downward) mobility in occupational life.

For a long time, social mobility and increased individualism were considered the ultimate benefits of modernization, as legitimized by substantial gains in the quality of life. However, more recently, awareness of the limits, risks, and possible health adverse effects of this development has been growing. One line of thinking along these lines concerns the negative effects on health produced by social disintegration.

Social disintegration is an often reported consequence of enhanced social mobility and related gain in individual freedom. It becomes manifest through a weakening of close social ties (e.g., among family members) and a decrease in reciprocal social exchange or solidarity. Under these conditions, the stability of social relationships is threatened, and commitments held among affiliates may lose their significance. Social disintegration is often associated with a state of social anomie, i.e., a lack of rules and orientations guiding interpersonal exchange. In a society characterized by anomie, individual behavior cannot be predicted by social norms any longer as these norms have lost their validity.

A growing number of investigations conducted by social epidemiologists and medical sociologists document adverse health effects among people who experience social disintegration. Lack of social cohesion or social support, shrinking social networks, and elevated proportions of societal members suffering from social isolation, social exclusion, or individual struggle are different facets of this general trend. For instance, in a cross-cultural perspective analyzing data from 84 different societies, one study concluded that with greater involvement in a money economy a systematic increase in mean blood pressure was evident, even after adjusting for important confounders such as salt consumption and body mass index. With greater involvement in modern money economy, individual competition and striving for benefit became dominant at the expense of cooperative social relationships. In a review of more recent investigations it was concluded that at least eight community-based prospective studies in industrialized societies reveal an association between social disintegration and mortality rates, usually death from all causes. In particular, mortality risks are elevated among people who lack social ties to others. Even at a more distant, macrosocial level, current evidence suggests that a decline in overall mortality, now familiar in most advanced societies, is prevented in an economy that is maximizing shareholder profit at the expense of investments into community life, culture, and social security.

Although the precise mechanisms that transform stressful experience resulting from social disintegration into increased susceptibility to fatal or nonfatal bodily disease are far from clear, impressive evidence is available from social experiments in mammals. It illustrates the critical role of rewarding and securing experiences that social exchange, affiliation, and affection play in regulating the body's basic physiological processes. It may well be that the cultural canon of modern industrialized societies heavily weighted toward formal rationality, control, and individual striving substantially diminishes the health gain associated with progress in human evolution. This latter conclusion is supported further by a third line of investigation focusing on the impact of modern working life on health.

Stress at Work and Health

The most profound change evoked by the process of industrialization concerns the nature of human work. For a large part of the workforce, work and home become two different places and two different types of social organization. In all economically advanced societies, work and occupation in adult life are accorded primacy for the following reasons. First, having a job is a principal prerequisite for continuous income and, thus, for independence from traditional support systems (family, community welfare, etc.). Increasingly, the level of income determines a wide range of life chances. Second, training for a job and achievement of occupational status are important goals of socialization. It is through education, job training, and status acquisition that personal growth and development are realized, that a core social identity outside the family is acquired, and that goal-directed activity in human life is shaped. At the same time, occupational settings produce the most pervasive continuous demands during one's lifetime, and exposure to harmful job conditions is an important determinant of disability and premature death in midlife.

The nature of work has changed dramatically over the past hundred years. Industrial mass production no longer dominates the labor market. This is due, in part, to technological progress, in part to a growing number of jobs available in the service sector, and, most importantly, in person-based service occupations and professions. In this latter case, unlike in the industrial sector, the potential of rationalization and related cut down in personnel is limited. However, even within industrial work, major changes have taken place. With less focus on physically strenuous work, with improved safety measures against chemical and physical hazards at work, and with more demands for psychomentally stressful jobs (e.g., information processing, controlling, coordinating activities, often performed under time pressure) new health risks emerged. Meanwhile, there has been a recognition that the importance of work for health goes beyond traditional occupational diseases as there is growing evidence of adverse health effects produced by psychomentally and socio-emotionally stressful jobs.

Before describing these health risks briefly, additional important changes in occupational life need to be mentioned. They are related to the structure of the labor market. There has been an increasing participation of women in the labor market, an increase in short term or part-time working and other forms of flexible job arrangements, and, most importantly, an increase in job instability and structural unemployment. This latter trend currently hits the economically most advanced societies as well as economies that lag behind. Overall, a substantial part of the economically active population is confined to insecure jobs, to premature retirement, or to job loss. Loss of job, as well as continued experience of job insecurity, was shown to be associated with an elevated risk of mortality in a number of prospective studies. In view of the rather high prevalence of these labor market conditions, the adverse effects on health produced by the economy are obvious.

Even within a continuously employed workforce, exposure to stressful psychosocial work environments carries the risk of ill health. Examples of this latter trend are shift work, irregular working hours and overwork, social isolation at work, conflicting demands, lack of control, and monotony. People working in jobs that are defined by a combination of at least some of these characteristics are at risk of developing chronic disease conditions such as hypertension, coronary heart disease, low back pain, or depression at least twice as often compared to people working in more favorable jobs. Additional evidence documents substantially elevated health risks among workers and employees who suffer from an imbalance between high efforts spent at work and low rewards received in terms of money, esteem, or promotion prospects. In many cases, such unfavorable job conditions are maintained, e.g., due to lack of alternatives in the labor market.

Concluding Remarks

In conclusion, despite substantial progress in life expectancy and the standard of living, the process of industrialization in technology, science, economy, and sociopolitical development has produced a substantial health burden that is attributable to an increasingly stressful social environment. Three aspects of this development were analyzed: (1) the impact of psychosocially adverse circumstances on health-damaging lifestyles; (2) health risks associated with social disintegration; and (3) afflictions of stressful working life and labor market conditions on well-being and health. It seems unlikely that these trends will be diminished in the near future as the process of economic and sociocultural globalization is progressing at a high pace. Moreover, pressures originating from population growth in rapidly developing parts of the world, new socioenvironmental risks, and man-made disasters may aggravate rather than moderate this burden. At the same time, with scientific progress in understanding the determinants and dynamics of stress-related health risks and with new worldwide public health efforts evolving, there is still hope that modernization and industrialization of human societies result in a sustainable humane and more healthy future.

See Also the Following Articles

Economic Factors and Stress; Indigenous Societies; Social Support; Workplace Stress.

Further Reading

Blaxter, M. (1990). *Health and lifestyles.* London: Routledge.

Cockerham, W. C. (1998). *Medical sociology* (7th edn.). Upper Saddle River, NJ: Prentice Hall.

Henry, J. P. (1997). *Cultural change and high blood pressure.* LIT Publishing, Germany: Münster.

Henry, J. P. and Stephens, P. M. (1977). *Stress, health, and the social environment.* Berlin: Springer.

Hobfoll, S. E. (1998). *Stress, culture, and community.* New York: Plenum.

Karasek, R. A. and Theorell, T. (1990). *Healthy work: stress, productivity, and the reconstruction of working life.* New York: Basic Books.

Marmot, M. G. and Wilkinson, R. (1999). *Social determinants of health.* Oxford: Oxford University Press.

Weber, M. (1958). *The protestant ethic and the spirit of capitalism.* New York: Scribner.

Community Studies

C J Holahan
University of Texas at Austin, Austin, TX, USA
R H Moos
Dept. of Veterans Affairs Health Care System and Stanford University Medical Center, Palo Alto, CA, USA
L M Groesz
University of Texas at Austin, Austin, TX, USA

This is a revised version of the article by C J Holahan, R H Moos, and J D Ragan, Encyclopedia of Stress First Edition, volume 1, pp 501–506, © 2000, Elsevier Inc.

Glossary

Chronic stressors Stressors that endure over time, such as ongoing problems in a marriage and long-term difficulties with a troublesome supervisor at work.

Coping strategies Cognitive and behavioral efforts to reduce or adapt to stressful conditions and associated emotional distress; most approaches distinguish between strategies oriented toward approaching and avoiding the problem.

Life change events Stressors that occur at a discrete point in time, such as the death of a family member or losing one's job.

Life crises and traumas Qualitatively more severe stressors, such as natural disasters or being the victim of a violent crime, such as rape.

Personal resources Relatively stable personality and cognitive characteristics that operate as stress moderators, such as dispositional optimism and self-efficacy.

Social resources Social factors that operate as stress moderators, such as emotional support and assistance from family members and friends.

Stress moderators Personal and social resources and coping strategies that function either as protective or vulnerability factors when stressors occur.

Stress resistance Individuals' adaptive capacity for resilience and constructive action in the face of challenge, emphasizing protective factors that can moderate the effects of stressors.

Conceptualizing Life Stressors

Community studies of life stressors investigate (1) life change events, (2) chronic stressors, and (3) major life crises and traumas (see **Table 1**). It should be noted that, although life change events and traumas have an acute onset, they often initiate chronic stressors, such as persistent economic and family problems. In fact, these enduring secondary stressors may account for many of the adverse effects of acute stressors.

Life Change Events

Initially, community studies of life stressors focused on acute life change events, which occur at a discrete point in time, such as the death of a close friend or losing one's job. Life change events generally are indexed by self-report questionnaires that may use objectively weighted life change units to reflect the relative level of adaptive demand associated with a particular life event. These weighted life change units are summed to reflect cumulative life change during a given period of time, typically the previous 12 months. Investigators also use in-depth interviews that, although time consuming, are able to assess the personal meaning of life changes. Although initial studies assumed that all life change, whether positive or negative, involved adaptive demands that were detrimental, later research revealed that the aderse health effects of life change are specific to negative life events. Later studies also showed that weighted life change units contributed little beyond an unweighted sum of events experienced in predicting illness. Based on these findings, most contemporary research on life change events uses the sum of negative events experienced during a given period of time.

Chronic Stressors

Early community studies of life stressors were limited by their narrow focus on acute stressors. Eventually, recognizing that many life stressors are ongoing, investigators began to examine chronic stressors, which endure over time, such as social role strains

Table 1 Major categories of life stressors with representative stressors[a]

Life change events	*Chronic stressors*	*Major crises and traumas*
Divorce	Family role strain	Victim of natural disaster
Death of a close friend	Work role strains	Life-threatening illness
Legal problem	Ongoing caregiving demands	Personal war exposure
Fired at work	Ongoing financial problems	Victim of violent crime

[a]Adapted from "Stress," Holahan, Ragan, & Moos, 2004, in Spielberger (Ed.), *Encyclopedia of Applied Psychology*, San Diego, CA: Academic Press. Copyright 2004 by Elsevier Science (USA).

and everyday hassles. Researchers studying social role strains often measure chronic family or work difficulties. Moreover, there has been a growing research interest in role strains associated with the interface between work and family life. Some stress studies have focused on additional burdens that often are associated with family life, such as caregiving for a chronically ill family member. For example, increasing interest is being devoted to caregivers of older family members suffering from Alzheimer's disease. Investigators have also studied minor life stressors that are experienced chronically, such as everyday hassles with troublesome neighbors or traffic problems. Increasingly, studies in this area also examine the health consequences of ongoing macrostressors, such as discrimination, national or regional economic recessions, and the ongoing threat of terrorism. As with acute stressors, the unweighted sum of these types of ongoing stressors provides an index of cumulative chronic stressors during a given period of time, typically the previous 12 months.

Major Life Crises and Traumas

In addition to indexes of cumulative stressors, community studies also focus on specific major life crises and traumas, which are qualitatively more severe than life events or role strains. For example, researchers have studied natural disasters, such as Hurricane Andrew in Florida; technological disasters, such as the Three Mile Island nuclear accident in Pennsylvania; and acts of terrorism, such as the destruction of the World Trade Center in New York. Current community studies also focus on how people cope with serious medical illnesses, such as heart disease, cancer, and diabetes. Interest in traumatic stressors is evidenced by a growing body of research on posttraumatic stress disorder (PTSD), a debilitating anxiety-based disorder caused by personal experience of a life-threatening stressor. Initially, PTSD research focused on stressors such as exposure to war as a civilian or soldier or being the victim of a violent crime such as rape. Over time, the definition of trauma has been broadened to encompass witnessing events that place others at risk of death or serious injury or witnessing individuals being badly injured or killed by such events.

Life Stressors and Adaptation

Initially community studies focused exclusively on the adverse health effects of life stressors. Eventually, however, the research focus broadened to encompass adaptive processes of stress resistance and stress-related growth.

Stressors and Illness

Findings with diverse community samples have shown that negative life change events are associated with psychological stress reactions that involve depression and anxiety. Interpersonal problems and losses are especially likely to be associated with depressive reactions and threatening events with anxiety. Even though chronic stressors may be less severe than acute life events, their effects may last longer and be more pervasive. Thus, chronic stressors generally are more strongly linked to psychological distress than are acute life change events. More severe trauma exposure produces a recognized pattern of PTSD symptoms, including psychologically reexperiencing the trauma through flashbacks and nightmares, emotional numbing, and heightened arousal.

Life stressors may elicit physiological stress reactions (e.g., circulatory, digestive, and musculoskeletal problems) that are mediated through the activation of the sympathetic nervous system. In addition, life stressors are associated with susceptibility to less serious infectious diseases (e.g., colds, influenza, and herpes) and possibly to the onset and exacerbation of autoimmune diseases (e.g., rheumatoid arthritis). Underlying these latter findings is an apparent correlation between life stressors and both cellular (e.g., reduced lymphocyte proliferation) and humoral (e.g., decreased antibody production) indices of immune suppression.

Stress Resistance

Despite the consistency of these stressor effects, they typically account for only a small portion of the variance in illness. Moreover, individuals showed highly variable reactions to stressors; many people remain healthy despite being exposed to stressful circumstances. These findings engendered a new approach to conceptualizing the stress and coping process, described as stress resistance. From an initial emphasis on people's deficits and vulnerabilities, contemporary community studies of life stressors have evolved to place increasing emphasis on protective factors that can counteract the potential adverse effects of life stressors.

A guiding assumption of stress resistance research is that personal and social resources and adaptive coping strategies can help individuals to manage stressful circumstances effectively and to remain healthy when stressors occur. Stress resistance research fundamentally changed the underlying assumptions that guided early investigators' conceptualization of the stress process. From initially placing an emphasis on people's deficits and vulnerabilities, stress research progressed to placing increasing emphasis on individuals' adaptive strengths and capacity for resilience and constructive action in the face of challenge.

Stress-Related Growth

Stress researchers have also come to recognize that life stressors can be constructive confrontations that challenge an individual and provide an opportunity for personal growth. Individuals may emerge from a stressful experience or life crisis with greater self-confidence, new coping skills, closer relationships with family and friends, and a richer appreciation of life. Stress-related growth can occur even when stressors involve profound adaptive demands, such as serious financial setbacks and the deaths of friends or family members. Of course, beneficial outcomes to life crises may emerge only after an initial stage of emotional distress and disorganization. Yet many people are able to grow stronger in the face of adversity.

Approximately half of women who experience a marital breakup show long-term improvements in psychological functioning. These women may become more assertive, develop more realistic views of themselves, and experience increased self-esteem with successful new careers. Similarly, survivors of serious illness often show more concern for and sense of community with others, a change in focus from the constant pressure of work to family relationships, and heightened awareness of religious and humanitarian values. Even in the context of stressors as profound as being a prisoner of war, a diagnosis of terminal illness, and the death of a close family member, some individuals are able to grow stronger, richer, and more caring.

Stress Moderators

Contemporary interest in adaptive outcomes in the stress process has encouraged efforts to identify factors that moderate the health effects of life stressors. Investigators have focused on the stress-moderating roles of personal and social resources, coping strategies, and personal agendas.

Personal and Social Resources

A variety of relatively stable personality characteristics operate as protective factors that can help individuals remain mentally and physically healthy when stressors occur. Personality characteristics that relate broadly to personal control, such as dispositional optimism and self-efficacy, are especially important. Individuals who are more optimistic about the eventual outcome of a stressful experience and those who are more confident in their ability to manage adaptive demands manage stressful episodes more successfully than individuals who lack these personal strengths. In contrast, negative personality characteristics, such as neuroticism and low self-esteem, can operate as vulnerability factors that increase health risk under high stressors.

Social resources also play a key role in protecting individuals from the potential adverse effects of life stressors. Social resources include guidance and assistance from one's family members, friends, and broader social network. Emotional support, such as the nurturance of a caring family member or attentive listening of a trusting confidant, is especially important as a protective factor during stressful times. Of course, social ties are complex and may entail criticism or competition as well as support. In fact, studies that consider both the positive and negative aspects of relationships show that negative aspects of relationships are at least as strongly related to poorer adjustment as positive aspects of relationships are related to better adjustment.

Box 1 The *Life Stressors and Social Resources Inventory* (LISRES) provides a comprehensive picture of the interrelated stressors and social resources in a person's life. The inventory includes nine indices of life stressors and seven indices of social resources. **Figure 1** shows an illustrative LISRES profile for a 66-year-old woman with rheumatoid arthritis (scores are standardized, with a mean of 50 and a standard deviation of 10). Although she reported well above-average physical health stressors, she had below-average stressors in six of the other seven domains. Moreover, she also had above-average social resources in her work setting and in her relationships with her spouse, extended family, and friends. At an 18-month follow-up, this favorable balance of moderate stressors and high resources enabled her to manage quite well; she reported high self-confidence and below-average depression.

Coping Strategies

A large number of community studies has examined the role of coping strategies in stress resistance. Coping encompasses cognitive and behavioral efforts to reduce or adapt to stressful conditions and associated emotional distress. Most conceptualizations distinguish between coping strategies that are oriented toward approaching and confronting the problem and strategies that are oriented toward reducing tension by avoiding dealing directly with the problem (see **Table 2**). People who rely more on approach coping strategies, such as problem solving and information seeking, tend to adapt better to life stressors.

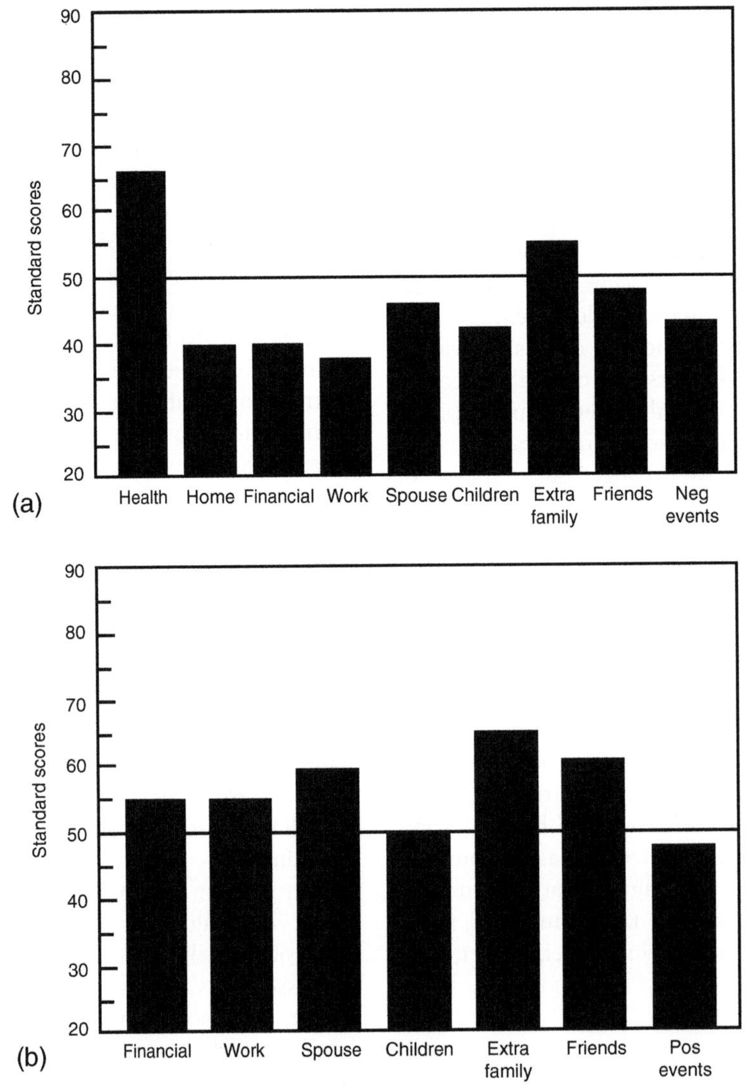

Figure 1 (a) Life stressors and (b) social resources profile for a 66-year-old woman with rheumatoid arthritis. Reproduced by special permission of the Publisher, Psychological Assessment Resources, Inc., 16204 N. Florida Avenue, Lutz, Florida 33549, from the LISRES-A by Rudolf H. Moos, Ph.D., Copyright 1994 by PAR, Inc. Further reproduction is prohibited without permission of PAR, Inc.

In contrast, avoidance coping strategies, such as denial and wishful thinking, generally are associated with more psychological distress.

Although we can draw overall conclusions about the relative efficacy of approach and avoidance coping strategies, such generalizations oversimplify the process of adaptation. Adaptation is best when coping efforts match situational demands. Individuals who are flexible in their choice of coping should show better adaptation than people who have a more restricted or rigid coping repertoire. Avoidance coping may be adaptive in the short term with time-limited stressors, such as pain, blood donation, and uncomfortable medical diagnostic procedures. However, avoidance generally is maladaptive as a long-term coping strategy. The manageability of a stressor also shapes coping effectiveness; approach coping processes are most effective in situations that are controllable.

Personal Agendas

An individual's personal agendas in the domain in which a stressor occurs shape the meaning and impact of the stressor. People function in multiple environments that often reflect different personal needs and commitments. Individuals appraise life stressors in the light of these personal agendas, and such appraisals can either enhance or reduce the stressfulness of a situation. For example, because chronic stressors provide a context within which new acute events are interpreted, they may alter the threshold at which events have negative impacts on health. Job loss during a period of bereavement may adversely affect health in part because it amplifies a more pervasive sense of personal loss.

Table 2 Four basic categories of coping strategies along with eight associated coping subtypes[a]

Basic coping categories	*Coping subtypes*
Cognitive approach	Logical analysis ("Did you think of different ways to deal with the problem?") Positive reappraisal ("Did you think about how you were much better off than other people with similar problems?")
Behavioral approach	Seeking guidance and support ("Did you talk with a friend about the problem?") Taking problem-solving action ("Did you make a plan of action and follow it?")
Cognitive avoidance	Cognitive avoidance ("Did you try to forget the whole thing?") Resigned acceptance ("Did you lose hope that things would ever be the same?")
Behavioral avoidance	Seeking alternative rewards ("Did you get involved in new activities?") Emotional discharge ("Did you yell or shout to let off steam?")

[a]Sample coping items are shown in parentheses. Adapted and reproduced by special permission of the Publisher, Psychological Assessment Resources, Inc., 16204 North Florida Avenue, Lutz, Florida 33549, from the Coping Responses Inventory by Rudolf Moos, Ph.D., Copyright 1993 by PAR, Inc. Further reproduction is prohibited without permission from PAR, Inc.

Similarly, when an event threatens or disrupts a domain in which a person has central commitments, that event is more likely to have an adverse outcome. For example, women who experience a new severe event in a life domain in which they have marked difficulties, or in a domain that matches an area of marked personal commitment, are more likely to develop depression than are women who experience a new severe event in some other domain. At the same time, strong commitments can sustain coping efforts in the face of profound obstacles, such as coping with bereavement or a life-threatening illness.

Integrative Models

Most recently, community studies have been examining integrative frameworks reflecting reciprocal links among stressors, resources, coping, and adaptation. Integrative models have addressed how maladaptive behavior generates life stressors, the role of stressors in eroding protective resources, and how protective factors operate together in a mutually supportive way.

Stress Generation

In a revision of traditional conceptualizations of the stress process, the stress generation model describes how depressed individuals, through their depression and related behaviors, generate life stressors, particularly interpersonal stressors. These stressors, in turn, are linked to increases in subsequent depressive symptoms. The stress generation model has been applied across diverse age groups to predict depressive outcomes in both clinical and nonclinical samples. An association between depression and subsequent stressors is evident for both acute events and chronic strains. In a similar way, avoidance coping is prospectively linked to both acute and chronic stressors, independent of depression. Cognitive avoidance may permit incipient stressors, such as financial problems, to worsen. Behavioral avoidance may actively promote new stressors, such as when emotional discharge aggravates strains in family relationships.

Resource Depletion

Another set of community studies has examined a support deterioration model that describes how life stressors can deplete psychosocial resources. Research on natural disasters, combat, and caregiving has shown that stressors can deplete both personal and social resources. Resource depletion may be tangible and intrinsically tied to a stressor; loss of income or loss of a loved one entail real reductions in resources. However, resource depletion also has a cognitive component; perceived support appears to be especially vulnerable to deterioration after crises. Support diminishes after the immediate crisis period even though crisis victims face enormous ongoing demands. Moreover, in community-level disasters, individuals who could potentially provide support are often crisis victims themselves. Resource loss may help to explain the association between life stressors and a decline in psychological functioning. For example, disaster-related stressors deplete perceived support; in turn, this loss in perceived support mediates the connection between initial stressors and later depression.

Coping Mediation

Resources models of coping examine how personal and social resources relate to better functioning under high stressors by fostering adaptive coping efforts. At one level, these models identify a key mechanism through which personal and social resources operate; at another level, they demonstrate that adaptive coping requires a strong underlying psychosocial foundation. Among community adults facing high stressors, adaptive personality characteristics and family support operate prospectively as coping resources; in turn, coping mediates between initial resources and later health status. Similarly, among women coping with breast cancer and students adjusting to law school, more adaptive coping efforts operate as a mediator through which optimism relates to better psychological adjustment. People with higher levels of self-efficacy, for instance, tend to approach challenging situations in an active and persistent style, whereas those with lower levels of self-efficacy are less active or tend to avoid such situations. Social resources can enhance coping efforts by bolstering feelings of self-confidence, as well as by providing informational guidance that aids in assessing threat and in planning coping strategies.

Acknowledgments

Preparation of this manuscript was supported in part by NIAAA grant AA12718 and by the Department of Veterans Affairs Health Services Research and Development Service. Opinions expressed herein are those of the authors and do not necessarily represent the views of the Department of Veterans Affairs.

Further Reading

Dohrenwend, B. P. (ed.) (1998). *Adversity, stress, and psychopathology.* New York: Oxford University Press.

Folkman, S. and Moskowitz, J. T. (2004). Coping: pitfalls and promise. *Annual Review of Psychology* **55**, 745–774.

Hammen, C. (1999). The emergence of an interpersonal approach to depression. In: Joiner, T. & Coyne, J. (eds.) *The interactional nature of depression: advances in interpersonal approaches*, pp. 21–35. Washington, DC: American Psychological Association.

Kaniasty, K. and Norris, F. H. (2001). Social support dynamics in adjustment to disasters. In: Sarason, B. R. & Duck, S. (eds.) *Personal relationships: implications for clinical and community psychology*, pp. 201–224. New York: John Wiley.

Kemeny, M. E. (2003). The psychobiology of stress. *Current Directions in Psychological Science* **12**, 124–129.

Kessler, R. C. (1997). The effects of stressful life events on depression. *Annual Review of Psychology* **48**, 191–214.

McNally, R. J. (2003). Progress and controversy in the study of posttraumatic stress disorder. *Annual Review of Psychology* **54**, 229–252.

Moos, R. H. and Moos, B. S. (1994). *The life stressors and social resources inventory.* Odessa, FL: Psychological Assessment Resources.

Moos, R. H. (2002). The mystery of human context and coping: an unraveling of cues. *American Journal of Community Psychology* **30**, 67–88.

Segerstrom, S. C. and Miller, G. E. (2004). Psychological stress and the human immune system: a meta-analytic study of 30 years of inquiry. *Psychological Bulletin* **130**, 601–630.

Snyder, C. R. (ed.) (1999). *Coping: the psychology of what works.* New York: Oxford University Press.

Taylor, R. D. and Wang, M. C. (eds.) (2000). *Resilience across contexts: family, work, culture, and community.* Mahwah, NJ: Lawrence Erlbaum.

Taylor, S. E., Repetti, R. L. and Seeman, T. (1997). Health psychology: what is an unhealthy environment and how does it get under the skin? *Annual Review of Psychology* **48**, 411–447.

Tedeschi, R. G., Park, C. L. and Calhoun, L. G. (eds.) (1998). *Posttraumatic growth: positive changes in the aftermath of crises.* Mahwah, NJ: Lawrence Erlbaum.

Yehuda, R. and McEwen, B. S. (2004). Protective and damaging effects of the biobehavioral stress response: cognitive, systemic and clinical aspects: ISPNE XXXIV meeting summary. *Psychoneuroendocrinology* **29**, 1212–1222.

Crime Victims

I Robbins
St. George's Hospital, London, UK

This article is reproduced from Encyclopedia of Stress First Edition, volume 1, pp 594–597, © 2000, Elsevier Inc.

Glossary

Acute stress disorder (ASD) — A disorder that may occur in the immediate aftermath of severe trauma. The diagnostic features include dissociation in the form of numbing, reduction in awareness, derealization, depersonalization, and dissociative amnesia. There is anxiety and increased arousal, which often accompanies reexperiencing of the trauma. As a consequence there is avoidance of reminders of the trauma and impairment in social or occupational functioning. The diagnosis of ASD requires three dissociative symptoms but only one symptom from the intrusion, avoidance, and arousal categories.

Posttraumatic stress disorder (PTSD) — Occurs following exposure to a traumatic event in which the person witnessed or was confronted with an event that involved actual or threatened death or serious injury to themselves or others and where their response involved intense fear, helplessness, or horror. It is characterized by persistent reexperiencing in the form of recurrent, intrusive thoughts or images and/or distressing dreams or flashbacks. There may be intense distress or arousal when confronted with reminders of the event. As a consequence there may be persistent avoidance of things associated with the trauma and numbing of general responsiveness. There may also be sleep disturbance, irritability or outbursts of anger, difficulty in concentration, hypervigilance, and exaggerated startle response. The symptoms result in significant impairment of social, occupational, or other important areas of functioning and need to last longer than 1 month for a diagnosis to be made.

Victimization

It is difficult to estimate the extent of criminal victimization in part because most victims of crime do not report the event to the police, resulting in an underrepresentation within the criminal statistics compiled from police data. Most crime differentially targets and damages victims who are poor, marginalized, and disempowered within society; individuals are usually targeted because of what they represent rather than because of who they are. Examples of this can include racially motivated attacks or sexual assaults. Within the United Kingdom the recent British Crime Survey of 1998 pointed to an 83% increase in crime since 1981, with the largest increase being in violent crime. Women are more likely to be at risk for sexual or domestic violence, whereas men are more likely to report physical violence from strangers.

Being the target of a crime may result in the individual feeling that he or she is a victim. Ochberg reported that victims feel diminished, pushed down, exploited, and invaded. There is a feeling of stigmatization and of being isolated by the experience, with a shattering of basic assumptions about the predictable orderly nature of the world where bad things are perceived as only happening to people who deserve it. Individuals lose their sense of autonomy, and their belief in being able to control their own lives is shattered, with a consequent increase in feelings of vulnerability. This is often associated with a belief that others do not understand unless they have experienced being a victim themselves. This feeling may be reinforced by the critical response they experience from friends or family when their recovery is not sufficiently rapid.

There may also be a considerable amount of self-blame, which may take one of two forms: behavioral or characterological. Behavioral self-blame is concerned with aspects of behavior that, if changed, could reduce the possibility of reoccurrence, whereas characterological self-blame implies that the victimization is attributable to the sort of person that the victim is. Clearly, behavioral self-blame, since it implies the possibility of increased control over events, is more healthy than characterological blame.

Psychological and Physical Health Consequences

Victims of violence may experience a sense of detachment or depersonalization at the time of the attack. While this may be a protective mechanism in the immediate aftermath of an attack, it may well hinder subsequent recovery, and recent evidence suggests that it may predict the subsequent development of posttraumatic stress disorder (PTSD). While dissociation is not a feature of PTSD, it is one of the major features of the diagnosis of acute stress disorder (ASD). Recent research has found that a diagnosis of ASD 1 month after experiencing a violent crime predicted the development of PTSD in 83% of cases at 6-month follow-up.

Many of the psychological consequences fit within the PTSD framework, with as many as 27% of all female crime victims meeting the criteria for diagnosis. Assaultive violence is more damaging than other types of crime, with higher rates of PTSD relating to increased perception of threat to life and extent of physical injury. In addition to PTSD, depression, anxiety, and substance abuse are common consequences of criminal victimization.

As well as the direct effects of the crime in terms of physical damage, victims are more likely to have poorer physical health and report increased drug and cigarette and alcohol consumption, health-care neglect, risky sexual behavior, and eating disorders.

Responses to Specific Crimes

Rape and Sexual Assault

Definitions as to what constitutes rape vary across countries. Within the United Kingdom the definition has recently been extended to include nonconsensual anal intercourse as well as vaginal intercourse. This change allows sexual attacks on men to be treated for the first time in law as rape, although it has to be acknowledged that the majority of victims of rape are women. Most sexual offences are unreported, and the rate of successful prosecution is low. Rape trauma syndrome was described by Burgess and Holstrom in 1974, but is now regarded as a variant of PTSD. Being the victim of a completed rape, being injured, and the extent of the perception of threat to life are predictive of increased rates of subsequent mental health problems in the longer term, as are prior victimization, previous psychological problems, and the lack of available social support. A third of women who report rape develop long-term psychological and social problems. A similar pattern was described in male victims of sexual assault by Mezey and King.

Stalking

Stalking has as yet been relatively poorly researched. Pathe and Mullen described severe social disruption and psychological distress with high levels of anxiety, persistent intrusive recollections and flashbacks, and suicidal thoughts. There are profound economic and social consequences of stalking, as victims often feel compelled to leave their employment or change their address. Over a third of victims in the Pathe and Mullen study met the criteria for PTSD.

Domestic Violence

Domestic violence, like sexual violence, is primarily but not exclusively directed against women. It is defined as an act carried out with intent to physically injure another person, usually an intimate partner. Recent surveys in the United Kingdom have suggested a lifetime prevalence of domestic violence of 1 in 4 women and an annual prevalence of 1 in 9 women. Battered woman syndrome, first described in the 1970s, contains within it many of the features of PTSD and describes the emotional, cognitive, and behavioral consequences. It is associated with apparent learned helplessness, whereby the victims of domestic violence appear to be unable to extricate themselves from abusive relationships. Rather than being helplessness, this unwillingness to leave an abusive partner may in fact be a rational appraisal of the danger involved in freeing themselves from an abusive partner. The degree of risk is seen in terms of the possibility that the domestic violence may end up causing severe physical injury and can progress to homicide. The consequences of domestic violence include depression, anxiety, suicidal behavior, substance abuse, and somatization. It is a frequent cause of divorce and homelessness and may be associated with child abuse.

Workplace Violence

Workplace assaults have increased in frequency and severity in recent years and are associated with increased job stress, reduced job satisfaction, and the likelihood of carrying weapons to work. Males are most likely to be involved in fatal workplace assaults, while women are more likely to be involved in nonfatal assaults. Health-care workers are particularly affected, with the rates for health- and social-care workers being 10 times those in non-health-care industries. Around a quarter of nurses and doctors report physical assaults in the course of their work.

Murder

Murder, unlike death by natural causes, disproportionately affects the young, leaving relatives, particularly parents, feeling as if their future has been taken from them. Relatives of murder victims often feel stigmatized and isolated, with a sense of shame and betrayal, which results in their being unable to communicate their distress or make emotional contact with others. The impact of traumatic bereavement may include physical symptoms, cognitive impairment, depression, and phobic avoidance as well as impaired work and social functioning. There is often a feeling of being let down by the criminal justice system, which compounds the sense of loss.

Robbery and Burglary

The effects of burglary may include PTSD but are generally less severe and long lasting. They may, however, include depression and anxiety and a sense of violation, which may be the most distressing and difficult aspect to resolve. Robbery, unlike burglary, involves direct contact with the perpetrator as well as a degree of threat to life and is therefore more likely to result in PTSD. Predictors of good recovery include a lower perception of threat to life, having had a preexisting view of the world as meaningful and orderly, and a rapid reduction of symptoms within the first month, whereas a depressive and avoidant coping style, fear of future violence, and increased somatic symptoms over time are associated with a poorer outcome.

Mass Shootings and Terrorist Crimes

While terrorist crimes are relatively infrequent, their social impact is much more widespread, inducing a climate of fear and uncertainty. For individuals caught up in terrorist attacks, the degree of threat to life and the extent of physical injury sustained during the attack are the best predictors of psychological problems, particularly PTSD, both in the immediate and the longer term. In the context of Northern Ireland a number of studies have found significant numbers of those with direct experience of terrorist incidents to be suffering from PTSD. This is in contrast to research on the impact of terrorist violence on the general population, which has been unable to detect a relationship between terrorist violence and resultant mental health problems in the population at large.

Studies that have looked at the impact of shootings tend by their very nature to be small scale but have found significant levels of distress and high rates of PTSD and other psychiatric disorders, with 33% or more being diagnosed as suffering from ASD in the immediate aftermath and this diagnosis being predictive of PTSD symptoms at follow-up several months later. Similarly, being held hostage has been related to high levels of subsequent distress both in victims and in their families. Victims of hostage taking may experience strong attachment and paradoxical gratitude toward the captors, with positive emotions including compassion and romantic love occurring. This may be expressed as profound gratitude for being allowed to live and has become referred to as Stockholm syndrome.

Support and Treatment Services

There are few culturally accepted rituals used to support victims of crime. This means that a major strategy in treatment and support services involves normalizing the process. In the first instance this may be best achieved by victim support schemes, which offer practical assistance such as accompanying people to court hearings, guiding them through the process of applying for compensation, and dealing with the complexities of the criminal justice system. They also offer emotional support and the opportunity to ventilate emotions following a crime. Referrals to schemes are often automatically made by the police but may also be made from mental health professionals or may be requested by victims themselves. Despite the high prevalence of PTSD in victims of crime who participate in the criminal justice system, there is still ample evidence that they do not have adequate access to mental health services. This occurs despite awareness that victims of serious crimes and the families of murder victims may develop psychiatric illnesses that require referral to mental health services for specialist treatment.

There has been an assumption that early intervention is more successful. There are few controlled studies of the impact of early intervention. Those that do exist seem to be evenly divided between three categories, i.e., bringing about improvement, having no impact, and resulting in deterioration, so as yet it is not possible to assume that early intervention is either effective or at least harmless. Research on victims of serious crimes such as rape suggests that in the immediate aftermath the majority of victims would meet the diagnostic criteria for PTSD but that by 4–5 months this decreases substantially to less than half. If recovery does not occur during this time then subsequent improvements may be slow, resulting in chronic problems. The fact that the majority of victims may recover spontaneously should not diminish the need for provision of adequate services for the significant minority who do not improve.

The effects of criminal victimization may be severe and incapacitating and may have long-term economic and social consequences. Victims of crime are rarely vocal on their own behalf, and as a consequence their needs may be unrecognized, both by the population at large and by health professionals in particular.

Further Reading

Brewin, C. J., Andrews, B., Rose, S. and Kirk, M. (1999). Acute stress disorder and posttraumatic stress disorder in victims of violent crime. *American Journal of Psychiatry* **156**, 360–366.

Burgess, A. W. and Holmstrom, L. L. (1974). Rape trauma syndrome. *American Journal of Psychiatry* **131**, 981–986.

Davis, R. C., Taylor, B. and Lurigio, A. J. (1996). Adjusting to criminal victimisation: the correlates of post crime distress. *Violence & Victims* **11**(1), 21–38.

Eisele, G. R., Watkins, J. P. and Mathews, K. O. (1998). Workplace violence at government sites. *American Journal of Industrial Medicine* **33**(5), 485–492.

Figley, C. R. (1985). *Trauma and its wake* (vol. 1). New York: Brunner Mazel.

Hilberman, E. (1976). *The rape victim.* New York: Basic Books.

Kilpatrick, D. G., Saunders, B. E., Amick-McMullan, A., Best, C. L., Veronen, L. J. and Resnick, H. (1989). Victim and crime factors associated with the development of crime-related post traumatic stress disorder. *Behavioral Therapy* **20**, 199–214.

Kilpatrick, D. G., Saunders, B. E., Veronen, L. J., Best, C. L. and Von, J. M. (1987). Criminal victimisation: lifetime prevalence, reporting to police and psychological impact. *Crime and Delinquency* **33**(4), 479–489.

Lees, S. (1996). *Carnal knowledge: rape on trial.* London: Hamish Hamilton.

Maguire, M. (1982). *Burglary in a dwelling.* London: Heinemann.

Mezey, G. C. and King, M. B. (1989). The effects of sexual assault on men: a survey of 22 victims. *Psychological Medicine* **19**, 205–209.

Mirlees-Black, C., Budd, T., Partridge, S. and Mayhew, P. (1998). *The 1998 British Crime Survey.* England and Wales: HMSO.

Ochberg, F. M. (1988). *Post traumatic therapy and victims of violence.* New York: Brunner Mazel.
Pathe, M. and Mullen, P. (1997). The impact of stalkers on their victims. *British Journal of Psychiatry* **170**, 12–17.
Resnick, H. S., Kilpatrick, D. G., Dansky, B. S., Saunders, B. E. and Best, C. L. (1993). Prevalence of civilian trauma and post traumatic stress in a representative national sample of women. *Journal of Consulting and Clinical Psychology* **61**(6), 984–991.
Van der Kolk, B. A., McFarlane, A. C. and Veisaeth, L. (eds.) (1996). *Traumatic stress: the effects of overwhelming experience of mind, body and society.* London: The Guildford Press.
Walker, L. E. (1979). *The battered woman.* New York: Harper and Row.

Crisis Intervention

D Hamaoka, D Benedek, T Grieger and R J Ursano
Uniformed Services University of the Health Sciences, Bethesda, MD, USA

Glossary

Crisis	The critical turning point of a situation or event; can be an individual crisis or a population-level/community crisis.
Psychological first aid	A group of evidence-informed interventions that can be helpful in the immediate aftermath of a crisis or traumatic event.
Resiliency	The dynamic process of healthy response and coping in the face of adversity.
Risk communication	Scientifically based method for communicating effectively under high-stress conditions.
Terrorism	Intentional acts of human malevolence with the primary goal of causing terror; implemented by those who wish to coerce societies by inducing fear, shock, horror, and revulsion, often with ideological, religious, and political agendas.

A crisis is defined as a critical turning point of a situation or event. Crises can occur at the individual or community levels and affect one person or an entire population. Typically crises arise for after severely stressful events. For example, stressful events include traumatic events (i.e., car accidents) affecting individuals and large-scale disasters (i.e., hurricane, earthquake, or terrorism) that have profound effects on communities and nations. Crises are of variable duration; they can be short-lived or persist for months and years. Over time, crises attenuate, resolve, or worsen, depending on the nature of the inciting event and its management. During severe crises, affected individuals often experience a period of stress, uncertainty, and anxiety and are concerned about their own safety or the safety of others. Each crisis often is followed by a series of crises (e.g., secondary crises such as loss of job, illness, or dislocation) that further stress the individual, group, and community.

Impact of Crises

Crises evoke a variety of reactions. Resilience and recovery are the rule, and most individuals do not develop chronic problems. For some, however, there are adverse psychological and behavioral responses. In crises precipitated by traumatic events such as disaster or terrorism, many people may experience sleeping difficulties; feel worried, sad, and anxious; increase alcohol and tobacco use; and change their regular behavior (e.g., alter their usual means of travel). Challenges to their faith and spiritual beliefs may also occur (**Figure 1**).

Many acute negative behavioral and emotional responses remit over time and do not require formal treatment. This tendency toward recovery is often credited to resiliency, a dynamic process of health recovery and coping in the face of adversity. Optimism, intelligence, humor, creativity, and active coping are related to resilience and positive outcomes after crises. Through active coping, individuals accept the impact of traumatic events and implement attainable, concrete measures to improve things.

Although many people experience distress after a crisis, some experience more persistent psychological sequelae, such as anxiety, insomnia, increased smoking, increased alcohol consumption, and bereavement.

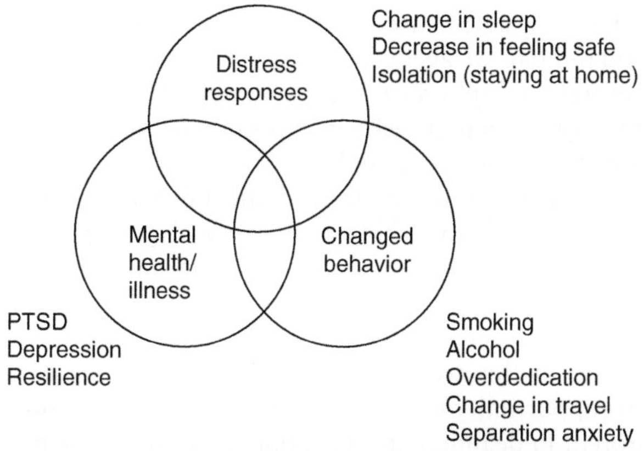

Figure 1 Psychological consequences of disasters, terrorism, and crises. PTSD, posttraumatic stress disorder. Adapted from Institute of Medicine (2003), *Preparing for the psychological consequences of terrorism: a public health strategy,* Washington, DC: National Academies Press.

This group may benefit from supportive psychological interventions, including psychological first aid and brief pharmacological interventions for sleep or anxiety. A still smaller group will develop psychiatric illness, including anxiety disorders (acute stress disorder, ASD; and posttraumatic stress disorder, PTSD), major depressive disorder, and substance use disorders. Such individuals require more formal (and perhaps more prolonged) interventions, including psychiatric treatment.

Individual responses to a crisis, which can include a traumatic event, a severe life stressor, or disaster, depend on a number of factors. Responses are influenced by proximity and involvement with the precipitating event. For a traumatic event, this means the severity of the trauma (e.g., degree of life threat). Responses are affected by psychological factors as well as interpersonal, family, and community stressors. In addition, research suggests social contexts, past experiences, future expectations, and genetic makeup interact with the characteristics of traumatic event to produce an individual's psychological response. Other identified risk factors that appear to increase the severity and/or duration of negative response include gender (e.g., women are more likely than men to develop acute PTSD), low level of social support, previous psychiatric illness, previous history of trauma, and ongoing negative life events after the trauma.

Groups and communities are also affected by crises, including the closing of a major community employer, the death of a beloved leader, and disasters. A community's response to a disaster often runs a predictable, but at times paradoxical, course. Communities temporarily coalesce immediately after a traumatic event. This is also known as the honeymoon period. During this time, individual heroics, a sense of working for a common cause, altruism, and "we will survive" attitude pervade the community. As time evolves, however, this optimism can change to disillusionment and often exposes the social fault lines of conflict, suspicion, and differential resources that are present along racial, ethnic, economic, and religious divides.

Community (as well as individual) responses to disasters are more pronounced when the trauma is intentional or the disaster humanmade. A relevant, modern-day example is terrorism. Here, acts of human malevolence are implemented with one primary goal – to cause terror. Terrorist acts are implemented by those who wish to coerce societies by inducing fear, shock, horror, and revulsion, often with ideological, religious, and political agendas. Although acts of terrorism may lead to death, injury, property damage, and the evacuation and displacement of communities, the main aim is to challenge a society's sense of well-being, cohesion, and security. The severity and length of the crisis may increase if chemical, biological, nuclear, radioactive, or high-yield explosives (CBNRE) agents are used because these agents are particularly effective in causing terror. The infectiousness of biological agents, the persistence of chemical weapons, and the delayed effects of radioactive agents, in particular, perpetuate fear and induce terror.

A variety of interventions are used to attenuate the course of and speed the recovery from a crisis. Although all such interventions have been developed to be helpful for those affected, it should be noted that some interventions are more helpful than others, and there are some interventions that may be harmful. The effectiveness of any crisis intervention depends on a number of factors, including timing and availability. Some interventions, for example, must take place immediately after the onset of a crisis (such as ensuring safety and basic needs). Others interventions take place weeks to months later, as the focus, concerns, and emphasis shift over the evolution of the crisis. Beyond life-saving actions, subsequent interventions can help mitigate the risk of or the degree of problems for those who survive. The principles of crisis intervention for large-scale disasters are discussed in the following sections.

Planning for Crisis

Large-scale community crises, such as a disaster, illustrate the range of principles important to crisis intervention. Although the term crisis intervention may seem to refer to actions taken only after disasters occur, steps that can be taken prior to the occurrence of such events should also be part of public health planning for crisis intervention. For example, an inventory of available resources (including personnel, material, and monetary) can be developed before a crisis. Important government and community leaders and spokespeople can be identified, at-risk populations accounted for (**Table 1**), and gaps in the current support and response systems can be examined. Educating leaders in the principles of risk communication may provide them with skills to assist in calming people, dispelling rumors, and maintaining the leaders' credibility after a disaster. Similarly, pre-event education of the populace about personal preparedness is also an important part of crisis intervention. Preparedness plans include forming a communication plan with loved ones, establishing and mapping out evacuation routes, having extra medical supplies, developing care plans for pets, and having extra necessities on hand in the event of an evacuation (e.g., at least a half tank of gas in the car at all times, extra batteries, plenty of bottled water, and nonperishable food items).

Interventions During and After the Crisis

In the immediate aftermath of a large-scale crisis such as a disaster, the most important interventions focus on medical emergencies and life-threatening emergencies. Although it is not known (and it is difficult to predict) how the public will react to a large-scale disaster such as the Madrid or London bombings or the anthrax attacks in the United States, previous responses to disasters have shown generally effective and collective action. Depending on the cause of the traumatic event, there may be a large number of people seeking medical care. These numbers will very likely increase and overwhelm medical capacity if CBRNE agents are involved. Biological, chemical, and radioactive agents (due to their invisible, odorless nature) tend to induce a great number of people who are not at actual risk of exposure to believe they might have been exposed.

Crisis intervention, from a mental health standpoint, includes working with medical personnel to perform initial triage. Those who are not reassured easily may benefit from a brief stay in an area that has been set aside, preferably close to the emergency room. In this way, acutely distressed patients have the opportunity to reconstitute while still being monitored. In dealing with this population, terms such as the worried well and psychological casualties should be avoided. These terms are pejorative and convey a message that it's all in their head. Recognizing that these individuals are experiencing distress and require caring responses can produce calm. The creation of a voluntary registry for individuals who are seen in the emergency room is not only a good public health intervention but can be therapeutic as well.

In addition to attending to the immediate medical needs, early crisis intervention addresses the basic needs of the survivors and includes safety from further harm as well as providing food, water, and shelter. As these needs are met, psychological first aid (PFA) can be employed. PFA is an evidenced-informed intervention that can be helpful in the immediate aftermath (hours to days) of an event (**Table 2**). The principles of PFA include establishing a sense of safety, facilitating social connectedness, fostering optimism, decreasing arousal, and restoring a sense of self-efficacy (e.g., the ability to take positive action). PFA can be thought of as flexible, supportive, and unlikely to cause harm; its main objectives are to limit distress, emphasize healthy behavior and activities, and minimize negative health behaviors. Although education and training in the PFA principles are required, the application of PFA can be accomplished by laypeople and does not require specific mental health expertise.

Table 1 Populations at risk for psychological problems after disaster

Previous exposure to trauma, particularly childhood
Direct exposure to the trauma/event (to include physically injured)
Those with premorbid psychiatric illness
Those experiencing acute losses
First responders (police, firefighters, emergency medical technicians)
Female gender
Those with minimal social support
Body handlers
Children
Elderly
Physically disabled
Those with negative life experiences after the trauma

Table 2 Principles of psychological first aid

Establish safety; identify safe areas and behaviors
Maximize individuals' ability to care for self and family and provide measures that allow individuals and families to be successful in their efforts
Teach calming skills and maintenance of natural body rhythms (e.g., nutrition, sleep, rest, exercise)
Maximize and facilitate connectedness to family and other social supports to the extent possible
Foster hope and optimism while not denying risk

Brief simple conversations and informal on-site talks with survivors and responders can be of great assistance. This early crisis intervention avoids mental health labeling, offers support, education, and problem-solving techniques. Later interventions include cognitive-behavioral therapy (CBT). CBT has demonstrated efficacy in the prevention of PTSD in those with acute stress disorder after trauma exposure. One well-publicized disaster intervention known as psychological debriefing has not been shown to prevent PTSD and may be harmful in certain settings. Supportive and educational groups should be conducted by experienced and well-trained personnel; should be accompanied by clear objectives, evaluation, and referral procedures; and should never be mandatory.

Crisis intervention also includes good risk communication, a scientifically based method for communicating effectively under high-stress conditions. The development of an effective risk communication strategy (as part of preevent intervention) is of vital importance in enabling leaders to inform and direct diverse populations. Individuals in the community look to their leaders for information, inspiration, a sense of control, optimism, and help during their period of grief. A major goal of the leaders should be to enlist the public as a partner. Information must be delivered frequently by credible and consistent sources. Messages should avoid speculation, never mix facts with reassurance, recommend specific steps people may take to protect themselves, and inform people when the next messages will be delivered. Good risk communication helps reduce negative psychological responses, encourage responsible safety behaviors, build trust, and minimize rumors and misinformation.

Critical Incident Needs Assessment Teams

Community crisis intervention that incorporates these principles in population health strategies must allocate and target resources at the individual, group, and community levels. Deploying critical incident needs assessment teams (CINATs) can be a helpful initial response to community disasters and crises. Such teams initiate planning, obtain on-site assessment, begin leadership consultation, and provide initial on-site guidance and support. CINATs thus are mental health-public health disaster response teams. CINATs are multidisciplinary and combine a public health approach and mental health knowledge to identify and respond to crisis. Teams initially quantify and identify needs in order to appropriately direct intervention and outreach resources.

CINATs recognize that interventions and responses are integrative, depend on a collaborative effort, and must use the community's inherent resiliency to help promote recovery. Teams can work effectively in responding to crises at workplaces (e.g., a shooting at a school or an airport after a crash). They target the individual and group levels that share a common task, mission, culture, structure, and/or physical proximity.

To be effective, CINATs require familiarity with the community or group they are deploying to assist. They may already be familiar with the given community or have received education and training about the community structure, culture, and leadership. These multidisciplinary groups include psychiatrists, psychologists, social workers, and mental health technicians. Additional individuals with particular areas of expertise, such as clergy and individuals responsible for security, communications, management, employee assistance, and human resources may be added.

In the aftermath of a community crisis, these pre-identified teams deploy to evaluate mental and behavioral health needs, identify high-risk groups, assist leadership function, and identify needed resources. CINATs avoid pathologizing appropriate responses to trauma and loss, and they identify those at greatest risk for subsequent problems. CINATs are a first population-level intervention. Subsequent care is arranged and distributed based on this epidemiological assessment. These teams also provide early support, education, PFA, and teaching about grief leadership (**Table 3**). CINATs may identify the need for additional supports including family support centers complete with legal assistance, casualty affairs assistance, Red Cross, and adult and child mental health counseling.

Table 3 Grief leadership actions after disasters[a]

Performs public announcements, appearances, and briefings
Presents calm demeanor
Organizes memorial services
Attends funerals, grieves
Endorses the various assistance programs
Attempts to describe loss in positive terms (acknowledging sacrifice and contributions)
Presents future goals and objectives

[a]Adapted from Wright K. M. and Bartone P. T. (1994), Community responses to disaster: the Gander plane crash. In: Ursano, R. J., McCaughey, & Fullerton C. S. (eds.) *Individual and community responses to trauma and disaster*, pp. 267–284, Cambridge, UK: Cambridge University Press.

Conclusion

Crises affect both individuals and communities. Disasters are a severe form of crisis. Interventions can foster resiliency and mitigate adverse responses and health risk behaviors for individual and community crises. Interventions include PFA for individuals, CINAT for community assessment and early intervention, and traditional health care for those more severely affected. With appropriate planning, proper implementation, considerate timing, and coordinated execution, an effective and efficient response can foster resiliency, limit impairment, and speed recovery.

Crisis intervention is not one size fits all approach and requires thoughtful consideration and planning. Crisis interventions must always be acceptable to the survivors and their culture. Even the most well-thought-out plans cannot account for every possibility. Leaders and helpers require flexibility in their approach and must meet disaster victims where they are – both literally and figuratively. Finally, those providing crisis intervention require support. They often do so with altruistic and noble intentions, and it is imperative that they take care of themselves as well as those they attempt to help.

Further Reading

Barbera, J., Macintyre, A., Gostin, L., et al. (2001). Large-scale quarantine following biological terrorism in the United States: scientific examination, logistic and legal limits, and possible consequences. *Journal of the American Medical Association* **286**(21), 2711–2717.

Benedek, D. M., Ursano, R. J., Fullerton, C. S., et al. (in press). Responding to workplace terrorism: applying military models of behavioral health and public health response. *Journal of Workplace Behavioral Health.*

Bisson, J. I., McFarlane, A. C. and Rose, A. (2000). Psychological debriefing. In: Foa, E. B., Keane, T. M. & Friedman, M. J. (eds.) *Effective treatments for PTSD: practice guidelines from the International Society of Traumatic Stress Studies*, pp. 317–319. New York: Guilford Press.

Bonanno, G. A. (2004). Loss, trauma, and human resilience: have we underestimated the human capacity to thrive after extremely aversive events? *American Psychologist* **59**(1), 20–28.

Bryant, R. A., Harvey, A. G., Dang, S. T., et al. (1998). Treatment of acute stress disorder: a comparison of cognitive-behavioral therapy and supportive counseling. *Journal of Consulting and Clinical Psychology* **66**(5), 862–866.

Department of Veterans Affairs and Department of Defense (2004). Medical response to weapons of mass destruction. Public Law 107–287, Section 3. Washington DC: Government Printing Office.

Galea, S., Ahern, J., Resnick, H., et al. (2002). Psychological sequelae of the September 11 terrorist attacks in New York City. *New England Journal of Medicine* **346**(13), 982–987.

Glass, T. A. and Schoch-Spana, M. (2002). Bioterrorism and the people: how to vaccinate a city against panic. *Clinical Infectious Diseases* **34**(2), 217–223.

Holloway, H. C., Norwood, A. E., Fullerton, et al. (1997). The threat of biological weapons: prophylaxis and mitigation of psychological and social consequences. *Journal of the American Medical Association* **278**(5), 425–427.

Institute of Medicine (2003). *Preparing for the psychological consequences of terrorism: a public health strategy.* Washington, DC: The National Academies Press.

North, C. S., Nixon, S. J., Shariat, S., et al. (1999). Psychiatric disorders among survivors of the Oklahoma City bombing. *Journal of the American Medical Association* **282**(8), 755–762.

Schlenger, W. E., Caddell, J. M., Ebert, L., et al. (2002). Psychological reactions to terrorist attacks: findings from the National Study of Americans' Reactions to September 11. *Journal of the American Medical Association* **288**(5), 581–588.

Tusaie, K. and Dyer, J. (2004). Resilience: a historical review of the construct. *Holistic Nursing Practice* **18**(1), 3–8, 9–10.

Wright, K. M. and Bartone, P. T. (1994). Community responses to disaster: the Gander plane crash. In: Ursano, R. J., McCaughey & Fullerton, C. S. (eds.) *Individual and community responses to trauma and disaster*, pp. 267–284. Cambridge, UK: Cambridge University Press.

Ursano, R. J., Kao, T. C. and Fullerton, C. S. (1992). Posttraumatic stress disorder and meaning: structuring human chaos. *Journal of Nervous and Mental Disease* **180**(12), 756–759.

Crowding Stress

L Kovács
Babes-Bolyai University, Clvj-Napoca, Romania
P Csermely
Semmelweis University, Budapest, Hungary

This is a revised version of the article by P Csermely, Encyclopedia of Stress First Edition, volume 1, pp 601–603, © 2000, Elsevier Inc.

Glossary

Amyloidosis — A severe pathological change of various organs and tissues during which aggregated amyloid fibers develop and induce the destruction of affected cells.

Channeling — Interaction of enzymes catalyzing consecutive enzyme reactions in which the product of the first reaction becomes the substrate of the second enzyme by a direct molecular transfer largely avoiding free diffusion.

Hypothalamic-pituitary-adrenocortical (HPA) axis — A major mechanism of the stress response, involving three major constituents: the corticotropin-releasing hormone (CRH), corticotropin (ACTH), and glucocorticoids.

Molecular crowding — A term to denote a dense population of molecules (usually macromolecules) where aggregation, diffusion, hydration, and other properties of the individual molecules are significantly altered.

Small and big phenotypes — Small and big phenotypes are well separated in most organisms. Smalls are optimized for low resources (crowded conditions), while bigs are optimized for high resources. These phenotypes are epigenetically inheritable, and their conversion often requires three generations.

Introduction

Studies on crowding stress consider an exceptionally high number of variables. Consequences of crowding stress may differ greatly, depending on whether population density is raised by an increased number of species living in the same area or by reducing their living space. If crowding is increased to such an extent that it leads to confinement, malnutrition, or an increased incidence of infections, other complications develop. Crowding stress may be acute (transient), i.e., the effects manifest after a few days, or chronic, i.e., changes occur after prolonged overcrowding lasting for weeks, months, or even years. Stress conditioning (or stress tolerance) can be observed in crowding stress: repeated stress exposure significantly diminishes the acute stress-induced effects occurring later. While mice or rats are the most commonly used species in crowding stress experiments, studies have been performed with almost all types of domesticated animals, various birds, fishes, and even humans. Though the conclusions of these studies can be directly compared only within the same species, some general trends can be observed. This article focuses on these general aspects of crowding stress.

Crowding Stress: Psychosocial Effects

Crowding as a chronic source of stress constitutes a major threat to psychological well-being. Crowding leads to anxiety and social instability. Dense populations are characterized by considerably increased aggressive behavior. Crowded monkeys (even well fed), including females and young, have brutal fights, wounding and killing each other. Crowding stress adversely affects gonadal functions, and if it occurs during pregnancy it may inhibit reproductive activity of even the second generation through masculinization of female pups. Chronic crowding leads to deficits in learning tasks and has been used in animal models to induce depression. In human populations, crowding stress evokes prominent psychosocial reactions: it is proposed to be an important factor in the development of increased urban insanity/schizophrenia. Moreover, substance abuse (alcohol, amphetamine, morphine, etc.) and addictive behavior are prompted by a stressful social environment, e.g., crowding stress.

Physiological Changes in Crowding Stress

Recently detailed studies were performed on the effect of crowding on birds. With increased brood size, nestlings of zebra finch *Taeniopygia guttata* grow less, and have decreased testosterone levels and a lower T cell response. These birds are significantly lighter and have shorter wing and tarsus length in adulthood. Females allocate less testosterone in the yolk of their eggs in crowded conditions. This hormone has a positive effect on the growth and muscular development of the embryos. Consequently, newborn birds already start with a growth deficit.

Crowding-related growth deficits can be observed and explained in a wider context. The average height of U.S. men becomes smaller by 1.75 inches (4.5 cm) as the population density increases from 55 persons per square mile to 60 000 persons per square mile. Obviously this change is affected by a large number of variables including the availability of health services, car use/abuse, pollution rates, and stress levels. However, small and big phenotypes seem to be well separated in several species including humans. Smalls are optimized for survival, while bigs were preferentially developed for proliferation. Smalls will develop and succeed under low resources (crowded conditions), while bigs prevail under ample resources (non-crowded conditions). Smalls and bigs properties are coded at the epigenetic level and are not readily interchangeable. As many as three generations may be needed for a phenotype switch from small to big or vice versa. A question for further exciting studies is how acute and prolonged crowding stress affect the switch between these phenotypes.

Crowding stress (especially if chronic) suppresses immune functions. Disturbed immune regulation leads to increased autoantibody levels and may be one of the factors behind the increased occurrence of childhood asthma. Various infections and increased susceptibility to poisoning are more likely to occur under crowded conditions. A widely established example indicates that household overcrowding is related to an increased prevalence of ulcer-inducing *Helicobacter pylori* infections. *H. pylori* infections and stress-induced gastric lesions significantly contribute to the development of ulcers and stomach cancer. Due to digestive problems and occasional appetite loss, chronic stress induces weight loss. In several organs, such as in kidneys and adrenals, chronic crowding stress induces intensive amyloidosis. Chronic overcrowding in many cases leads to hypertension in the resting state or to relative hypertension after exercise.

Possible Molecular Mechanisms of Crowding Stress

Crowding stress activates the hypothalamic-pituitary-adrenocortical axis (HPA axis) and enhances basal level or reactivity of plasma corticosterone secretion. This stress-related stimulation is triggered by the corticotropin-releasing hormone (CRH) system. HPA stimulation by other HPA-related biochemical factors, such as vasopressin, carbachol, and nicotine, is significantly diminished under crowded conditions. Moreover, crowding considerably impairs the HPA axis response to cholinergic and adrenergic stimulations. The mechanism of crowding-induced inhibition is best known in the case of nicotine: social stress affects signal transmission from membrane nicotinic receptors of different subtypes through ion channels into the cell. Crowding stress seems to induce an adaptive response to the non-CRH-induced HPA response to avoid the overstimulation of this important regulatory mechanism.

Repeated, short stresses induced by restraint or crowding attenuate the acute restraint stress-induced stimulatory action of the HPA axis. This indicates the occurrence of stress tolerance (stress conditioning) in the HPA axis response to acute stress. As a possible mechanism a short hypersecretion of corticosterone may induce a prolonged feedback inhibition of the HPA axis activity.

HPA stimulation is possibly the cause of decrease in appetite and consequent weight loss. HPA stimulation leads to compromised immune function and suppression of gonadal functions. The latter effect has an important role in regulation of population size, decreasing the chance of fertilization. Chronic HPA stimulation may lead to osteoporosis, chronic gastrointestinal pain, and retarded growth. Thus, prolonged activation of the HPA axis may explain many of the psychological effects of overcrowding, such as gastrointestinal problems, weight loss, sensitivity to infections, and decreased reproductive activity.

Additionally, crowding stress induces lipid peroxidation and impairs cellular signaling mechanisms, especially in elderly subjects. Impaired signaling may significantly contribute to immune suppression and decreased adaptive mechanisms.

Crowding of Flies and Worms

Signaling mechanisms can be studied more easily in simple organisms. Larval crowding in the fruit fly, *Drosophila melanogaster*, induces HSP (heat shock protein) expression and leads to increased adult longevity and adult thermal stress resistance. Flies that had been exposed to larval crowding exhibit greater starvation resistance and lipid content than populations that did not experience larval crowding. Crowding suffered in larval stage suspends the usual buffering of phenotypic variation: adults of crowded *D. melanogaster* larvae display an increased variability of thorax and wing length, as well as sternopleural and abdominal bristle number.

Food limitation and overcrowding also induce arrested development of the worm, *Caenorhabditis elegans*, leading to the formation of the so-called dauer larva. Daf-7, a homolog of the human transforming growth factor-β (TGF-β), prevents dauer larva commitment. Several other members of the dauer larva regulating Daf family are receptor serine-threonine kinases similar to the human TGF-β receptor. Mutations of another signaling pathway of *C. elegans* may quadruple the adult lifetime of the worm in addition to disturbing its dauer larva development. Thus, disturbances in signaling due to crowding stress may have profound consequences in the longevity of (simpler) organisms.

Cell Crowding

Experimenters often use cell cultures, where the cell density may be much smaller than under physiological conditions. During their proliferation, cells increase their density (in adherent cell lines the culture approaches confluency), and cell crowding may gradually develop. Cell crowding significantly alters the efficiency of autocrine and paracrine hormonal regulation and profoundly changes the influence of neighboring cells as well as the extracellular matrix on the individual cells. Cell crowding usually diminishes cell proliferation. However, tumor cells may escape from this control by expressing various molecules such as integrin $\alpha V\beta 6$ or lytic enzymes against components of the extracellular matrix. The extent of cell crowding should be always considered when interpreting the physiological relevance of experimental results with cell cultures.

Molecular Crowding

If the total volume of a macromolecular species occupies a significant fraction of the total volume of the solution, we refer to such a medium as crowded. Under experimental conditions molecular crowding is induced by polyethylene glycol or by dextrane. An intracellular environment, where the total amount of macromolecules usually occupies more than one-third of the total volume, is a typical example of molecular crowding.

Molecular crowding exerts profound quantitative effects on macromolecular interactions in living systems and induces an increased association of macromolecules. Crowding reduces diffusion rates. As a compensatory mechanism, it enhances channeling between enzymes catalyzing consecutive enzyme reactions as well as improves signaling efficiency in organized signaling cascades. By extending the range of intracellular conditions, where macromolecular interactions occur, crowding acts as a metabolic buffer.

Another potential outcome of molecular crowding is the effect on the properties of cellular water. The crowded environment in the cell results in a significant decrease of the proportion of cellular water being in contact with macromolecules such as proteins and DNA. Macromolecules begin to compete for water molecules, their hydration becomes compromised, and, consequently, osmotic stress occurs. The large amount of macromolecules and their immobilized hydrate shell constitute a large excluded volume. Thus, macromolecular crowding affects all those biochemical process in which a change of excluded volume occurs. Such a process is the collapse of newly synthesized polypeptide chain into compact functional proteins, the unfolding of proteins induced by stress, and the association of proteins into nonfunctional aggregates such as plaques in human amyloid diseases.

In conclusion, molecular crowding has a profound effect on the chemistry of life via its influence on association of macromolecules and on the cellular water properties.

Conclusions

Crowding may occur at various levels, from molecules through cells to organisms. Elements of crowded populations have an increased chance for extensive interactions, which increases community formation but may also lead to a high number of unspecific interactions, against which the elements have not previously developed an adaptive response. The unusual effects behave as perturbations of the elements and may lead to their destabilization – thus crowding stress occurs. Crowding stress profoundly affects the behavior of the element at all levels studied, be it a molecule, a cell, or a simple or higher organism up to humans. Crowding often leads to the reduction of the element number either by diminishing the birth of new elements or by destabilizing, segregating, and/or destroying previously existing elements. This article gave a number of examples of these changes.

Further Reading

Bar, J., Cohen-Noyman, E., Geiger, B. and Oren, M. (2004). Attenuation of the p53 response to DNA damage by high cell density. *Oncogene* **23**, 2128–2137.

Bateson, P., Barker, D., Clutton-Brock, T., et al. (2004). Developmental plasticity and human health. *Nature* **430**, 419–421.

Bugajski, J., Boricz, J., Gold, R. and Bugajski, A. J. (1995). Crowding stress impairs the pituitary-adrenocortical responsiveness to the vasopressin but not corticotropin-releasing hormone stimulation. *Brain Research* **618**, 223–228.

Csermely, P., Pénzes, I. and Tóth, S. (1995). Chronic overcrowding decreases cytoplasmic free calcium levels in the T lymphocytes of aged CBA/Ca mice. *Experientia* **51**, 976–979.

Ellis, R. J. (2001). Macromolecular crowding: obvious but underappreciated. *Trends in Biochemical Sciences* **26**, 597–604.

Galpin, O. P., Whitaker, C. J. and Dubiel, A. J. (1992). *Helicobacter pylori* infection and overcrowding in childhood. *Lancet* **339**, 619.

Gil, D., Heim, C., Bulmer, E., et al. (2004). Negative effects of early developmental stress on yolk testosterone levels in a passerine bird. *Journal of Experimental Biology* **207**, 2215–2220.

Goeckner, D. J., Greenough, W. T. and Mead, W. R. (1973). Deficits in learning tasks following chronic overcrowding in rats. *Journal of Personal and Social Psychology* **28**, 256–261.

Haller, J., Baranyi, J., Bakos, N. and Halász, J. (2004). Social instability in female rats: effects on anxiety and buspirone efficacy. *Psychopharmacology* **174**, 197–202.

Imasheva, A. G. and Bubliy, O. A. (2003). Quantitative variation of four morphological traits in *Drosophila melanogaster* under larval crowding. *Hereditas* **138**, 193–199.

Nagaraja, H. S. and Jeganathan, P. S. (2002). Voluntary alcohol drinking and caloric intake in rats exposed to crowding. *Indian Journal of Medical Research* **116**, 111–116.

Rohwer, J. M., Postma, P. W., Kholodenko, B. N. and Westerhoff, H. V. (1998). Implications of macromolecular crowding for signal transduction and metabolite channelling. *Proceedings of the National Academy of Sciences USA* **95**, 10547–10552.

Sørensen, J. G. and Loeschke, V. (2001). Larval crowding in *Drosophila melanogaster* induces Hsp70 expression, and leads to increased adult longevity and adult thermal stress resistance. *Journal of Insect Physiology* **47**, 1301–1307.

Xigeng, Z., Yonghui, L., Xiaojing, L., et al. (2004). Social crowding sensitizes high-responding rats to psychomotor-stimulant effects of morphine. *Pharmacology, Biochemistry, and Behavior* 79, 213–218.

Cultural Factors in Stress

J W Berry
Queen's University, Kingston, ONT, Canada
B Ataca
Bogazici University, Istanbul, Turkey

This is a revised version of the article by J W Berry and B Ataca, Encyclopedia of Stress First Edition, volume 1, pp 604–610, © 2000, Elsevier Inc.

Glossary

Acculturation — A process of cultural and psychological change that results from contact between two cultural groups.

Adaptation — A process of change that seeks to improve the fit between cultural groups and/or individuals and their habitat; it may result in outcomes that range from well-adapted to maladapted.

Culture — A shared way of life of a group of people, including their symbolic, social, and material products; cultures are transmitted to new members over generations.

Ecology — The study of relationships between human organisms and their physical habitats, including their biological, cultural, and psychological adaptations to these habitats.

Strategies — Various ways employed by cultures and individuals to adapt to their habitats, including adjustment, reaction, and withdrawal (e.g., coping strategies and acculturation strategies).

Stress — The cultural and psychological consequences that occur when changes exceed the capacity of groups and individuals to adapt.

Culture as Adaptation

Among the many approaches to understanding culture is the view that human groups develop a way of dealing with recurrent problems in their ecosystems; these solutions are widely shared among members of a society and transmitted to their offspring. That is, cultures are adaptive to context, and, to the extent that these adaptations are successful, their fit is enhanced and stress is reduced: "Culture is man's most important instrument of adaptation" (Cohen, 1968: 1). The empirical foundations for this conception of culture were laid by Forde and Kroeber, who demonstrated that in Africa and North America, culture areas generally mapped onto ecological areas; in both continents, broadly shared features of culture were associated with ecological features in a particular group's habitat. This conception of culture has permitted work in both anthropology and cross-cultural psychology to align with stress, coping, and adaptation frameworks that are widely used in psychology.

When ecological conditions are relatively stable and there is sufficient carrying capacity (i.e., support from the habitat), cultural adaptations are also stable. However, when there is ecosystem disturbance due to internal or external forces (such as natural disaster or invasion) or when there is a chronic shortfall in the ability of the habitat to sustain the cultural group, then new adaptations are required if the group is to survive. In these terms, ecosystem changes constitute stressors, attempts to find innovative ways to manage day-to-day existence constitute coping, and the solutions achieved (successful or not) constitute adaptation.

Concern with these two sources of influence (internal and external) has given rise to an ecocultural model that attempts to understand cultural and psychological phenomena as the result of adaptation to ecological factors and to those that arise from contact with other cultures (the process of acculturation). Both during the process and when there is limited adaptive success, two kinds of stress may result: cultural stress and acculturative stress.

For both kinds of stress, it is useful to consider some fundamental strategies of coping with these internal and external stressors. There are at least three ways to achieve adaptation: adjustment, reaction, and withdrawal. In the case of adjustment, behavioral changes are in a direction that reduces the conflict (that is, increases the congruence) between the environment and the behavior by changing the behavior to bring it into harmony with the environment. In general, this variety is the one most often intended by the term adaptation and may indeed be the most common form of adaptation. In the case of reaction, behavioral changes are in a direction that retaliates against the environment; these may lead to environmental changes that, in effect, increase the congruence between the two, but not by way of cultural or behavioral adjustment. In the case of withdrawal, behavior is in a direction that reduces the pressures from the environment; in a sense, it is a removal from the adaptive arena. These three varieties of adaptation are similar to the distinctions in the psychological literature made between moving with or toward, moving against, and moving away from a stimulus.

Cultural Stress

As noted previously, cultural stress occurs when extant or novel situations within the culture place demands on the group and its individual members that exceed their capacity to respond. Rather than maintaining or improving their fit, the responses of the group and individuals fail, and adaptation is unsuccessful. From the point of view of ecological anthropology, examples of successful adaptations are the most common; this is because those that are not successful fail to survive and are unavailable for contemporary observation. However, archaeology provides numerous examples of cultures that disappeared as a result of failure to adapt. Despite this imbalance in cases, there are examples of societies and individuals under cultural stress due to the extreme circumstances that they face at present. Two of these are the Ik of northern Uganda and the Mossi and Fulani of Burkina Faso.

The classic portrayal of the Ik was presented by Turnbull. This cultural group had lived for centuries as hunting and gathering nomads in a semidesert region at the intersection of Uganda, Sudan, and Kenya. Their main territory was a valley that had been taken over by the government to create a national park, from which they were excluded. With their old economic subsistence base taken away and agriculture impossible, they attempted to survive by raiding the cattle herds of neighboring groups. As the carrying capacity of their territory was reduced (exacerbated by failure of the rains), the social fabric of the Ik deteriorated. According to Turnbull, they "abandoned useless appendages . . . those basic qualities such as family, cooperative sociality, belief, love, hope and so forth, for the very good reason that in their context, these militated against survival" (1972: 289).

This portrait is one of extreme ecological change, one that was rather quickly followed by social, cultural, and psychological change, all of them maladaptive. In this extreme case, the stressors were so severe that the cultural resources were incapable of providing any coping strategies other than intense striving for individual survival. Severe hunger generated "loss of any community of interest, familial or economic, social or spiritual" (Turnbull, 1972: 157) and eventually resulted in a maladaptive "everyone for himself" strategy that in the end failed.

A second example of cultural stress, one that also resulted from ecological change, is that of two groups in the Sahel region of West Africa. Ongoing environmental degradation (deterioration of the soil, loss of nutrients, reduction in wildlife) has led to loss of food resources and income and constituted a major set of stressors in the lives of two societies in this region. The Fulani (pastoralists) and the Mossi (agriculturalists) had differentially adapted to this semi-arid ecosystem, one grazing their cattle over a large territory, the other enclosing small land areas for cultivation. In this study, coping with environmental change was directly assessed (by questionnaire), as was their locus of control and two psychological outcomes (feelings of marginality and of personal stress). With respect to coping, two factors emerged, the first representing a combination of problem solving and support seeking and the second mainly avoidance strategies; this split resembles the Lazarus and Folkman distinction between problem-focused and emotion-focused coping. For the locus of control measure, three factors were obtained: the first represented individual effort, the second nonpersonal control, and the third was uninterpretable. Both the marginality and stress scales produced single factors.

Structural analyses of the impact of ecological and cultural factors on the two psychological outcomes were carried out. The carrying capacity of the ecosystem was introduced as the latent variable, with four variables (environmental degradation, land use, cattle, and modernity) used as independent variables. The ecosystem provided a higher carrying capacity for the pastoralists than for the agriculturalists, and consequently the former were less marginalized and stressed. According to Van Haaften and Van de Vijver (1996: 426), "this finding is in agreement with the common observation that nomadic people (the pastoralists) are less susceptible to environmental stressors than are sedentary people (the agriculturalists). Unlike the latter, the former can move away from environmental stressors."

With these two examples, it is possible to identify links between ecological, cultural, and psychological changes in human populations. Evidence from these anthropological and psychological sources shows clearly that when cultural groups experience stressors, collective and individual coping sometimes leads to successful adaptation but sometimes does not, resulting in stress.

Acculturative Stress

When ecosystem and cultural changes are introduced from outside, the process of acculturation is initiated. In essence, acculturation refers to both the cultural and psychological changes that follow from contact between two or more cultural groups. At the cultural group level, these changes can occur in the physical, political, economic, or social domains (e.g., urbanization, loss of autonomy and livelihood, and the reorganization or even the destruction of social relationships). At the individual level, changes in the psychology of the individual take place.

It had been previously thought that acculturation inevitably brings social and psychological problems. However, such a negative and broad generalization no longer appears to be valid. Variability in psychological acculturation exists and is associated with three differing views about the degree of difficulty that is thought to exist during acculturation: behavioral shifts, acculturative stress, and psychopathology. The first is one in which changes in an individual's behavioral repertoire take place rather easily and are usually nonproblematic. This process encompasses three subprocesses: culture shedding, culture learning, and culture conflict. The first two involve the selective, accidental, or deliberate loss of behaviors and their replacement by behaviors that allow the individual a better fit with the larger society. Most often this process has been termed adjustment, since virtually all the adaptive changes take place in the acculturating individual, with few changes occurring among members of the larger society. These adjustments are typically made with minimal difficulty, in keeping with the appraisal of the acculturation experiences as nonproblematic. However, some degree of conflict may occur, in which incompatible behaviors create difficulties for the individual.

When greater levels of conflict are experienced, and the experiences are judged to be problematic but controllable and surmountable, then acculturative stress is the appropriate conceptualization. Drawing on the broader stress and adaptation paradigms, this approach advocates the study of the process of how individuals deal with acculturative problems on first encountering them, and over time. In this sense, acculturative stress is a stress reaction in response to life events that are rooted in intercultural contact. Within this orientation, depression (due to cultural loss) and anxiety (due to uncertainty about how to live) were the problems most frequently found in a series of studies in Canada. More recently, general and acculturation-related sources of immigrants' stress have been differentiated in the literature. It was found that acculturation-specific hassles, above and beyond general hassles, had a negative effect on psychological distress. In-group hassles of Vietnamese immigrant students, i.e., stressors that result from interactions with Vietnamese peers and family, and out-group hassles of Iranian immigrants, i.e., stressors that result from interactions or lack of interactions (perceived or real) with out-group members in Canada, were associated with depression.

When major difficulties are experienced, the psychopathology perspective is most appropriate. According to this perspective, changes in the cultural context exceed the individual's capacity to cope because of the magnitude, speed, or some other aspect of the change, leading to serious psychological disturbances such as clinical depression and incapacitating anxiety.

Long-term adaptation to acculturation is variable, ranging from a well to poorly-adapted situation in which individuals can manage their new lives very well to one in which they are unable to carry on in the new society. Short-term changes during acculturation are sometimes negative and often disruptive in character. For most acculturating individuals, however, after a period of time, some long-term positive adaptation to the new cultural context usually takes place.

Variations in adaptation result in part from the acculturation strategy adopted by individuals. These strategies derive from individuals orienting themselves to two fundamental issues faced during acculturation: (1) To what extent do individuals seek to maintain their heritage culture and identity? (2) To what extent do they seek to have contact with and participate in the larger society? These two issues can be responded to along two attitudinal dimensions, with generally positive or negative (yes or no) responses at opposite ends. Orientations to these issues intersect to define four acculturation strategies. From the point of view of nondominant groups, when individuals do not wish to maintain their cultural identity and seek daily interaction with other cultures, the assimilation strategy is defined. In contrast, when individuals place a value on holding on to their original culture and at the same time wish to avoid interaction with others, the separation alternative is defined. When there is an interest in maintaining one's original culture while in daily interactions with other groups, integration is the option; here, there is some degree of cultural integrity maintained while at the same time seeking, as a member of a cultural group, to participate as an integral part of the larger social network. Finally, when there is little possibility or interest in cultural maintenance (often for reasons of enforced cultural loss) and little interest in having relations with others (often for reasons of exclusion or discrimination), marginalization is defined. Acculturation strategies have been shown to have substantial relationships with positive adaptation: integration is usually the most successful, marginalization is the least, and assimilation and separation strategies are intermediate.

Adaptation is also multifaceted. It can be primarily internal or psychological (e.g., sense of well-being, self-esteem) or sociocultural, linking the individual to others in the new society (e.g., competence in the activities of daily intercultural living). Other forms of adaptation, including marital adaptation and economic adaptation, have also been proposed in the acculturation literature.

Each of these four domains of adaptation to acculturation may entail acculturative stress. In all four, the source of the stressors lies in the contact between groups and the resulting process of cultural change. It is important to note that acculturative stress is not a unique form of stress, but has unique antecedents (residing in the process of acculturation). Moreover, many of the outcomes are closely linked to the unique features of the acculturation process (such as experiencing cultural identity problems, acquiring culturally appropriate social skills, rearranging marital relations to take new cultural expectations into account, and experiencing difficulties due to employment discrimination in the new society). Thus, acculturative stress can be said to be a special kind of stress because of both its special set of stressors and its special set of outcomes. Following are examples of these four facets of acculturative stress.

The initial distinction between psychological and sociocultural adaptation was proposed and validated by Ward and colleagues. As noted earlier, psychological adaptation mostly involves one's psychological well-being and satisfaction in a new cultural context, whereas sociocultural adaptation refers to one's ability to acquire culturally appropriate knowledge and skills and to interact with the new culture and manage daily life. Conceptually, these two forms of adaptation reflect two distinct theoretical approaches to acculturation. Psychological adaptation is better interpreted in terms of a stress and coping model; sociocultural adaptation is better viewed from a social learning perspective. Stress and coping models are based on the notion that both positive and negative life changes are intrinsically stressful in that they require adaptive reactions. Acculturation has been viewed as entailing such stress-inducing life changes, which increase susceptibility to physical and mental illness. The second approach draws on a combination of social skills and culture learning models. Individuals experiencing culture change are socially unskilled in the new cultural setting. Social learning models emphasize the importance of the acquisition of social skills and knowledge appropriate to the new culture.

While conceptually distinct, psychological and sociocultural adaptation are empirically related to some extent (correlations between the two measures are in the 0.4 to 0.5 range). However, they are also empirically distinct in the sense that they usually have different experiential antecedents. Research has shown that psychological adaptation, defined in terms of well-being or mood states (e.g., depression, anxiety, stress), is predicted by personality, life changes, and social support variables. Locus of control, life changes, and personal relationship satisfaction accounted for a substantial portion of variance in psychological well-being in student and adult sojourners. In contrast, assessed in terms of social difficulty, sociocultural adaptation was predicted by variables that are related more strongly to cognitive factors and social skills acquisition, such as cultural knowledge, cultural distance, cultural identity, language ability, length of residence in the new culture, and amount of contact with hosts. Extending this framework to immigrant couples, Ataca and Berry also found that these two dimensions of adaptation were associated with different variables. Psychological adaptation of married

Turkish immigrant couples in Canada was associated with the personality variable of hardiness, social support, acculturation attitudes, and perceived discrimination, while sociocultural adaptation was mostly related to variables that are instrumental in acquiring social skills in the new culture, namely, English language proficiency and contact with Euro-Canadians.

Ataca and Berry also introduced the concept of marital adaptation, which relates to the accommodation of spouses in the process of acculturation when each is faced with the new culture and forms of behavior and different ways of acculturating. Their findings supported the distinctiveness of marital adaptation from psychological and sociocultural adaptation. Better marital adaptation was mostly associated with variables specific to marital life, namely, fewer marital stressors and greater marital support; yet, marital variables also displayed close relations with psychological adaptation. This is in line with the literature on the relationship between marital variables and psychological distress among immigrants. Marital stressors were found to have an impact on both the marital distress and the depressive and psychosomatic symptoms of Indo-Canadian women. Naidoo found that South Asian women in Canada who had supportive husbands were less stressed. While the marital life of Turkish immigrants was related to psychological well-being, it was unrelated to sociocultural adaptation. The social skill learning necessary to function in the new cultural context was neither impeded nor facilitated by the conjugal relationship.

A fourth aspect of adaptation, that of economic adaptation, refers to the process by which individuals cope with and reestablish sustainable work relationships in the new economic system (including problems of status loss, under- or unemployment, and status mobility). Immigrants typically suffer high rates of under or unemployment. Lack of knowledge of language, lack of training, and discrimination force many immigrants into low-skill jobs. Conversely, high levels of education, occupational skills, and professional training received in the home country are often not recognized by authorities in the new country, resulting in underemployment. Under- or unemployment, low incomes, and the concomitant loss in one's socioeconomic status constitute sources of stress and are related to psychological symptoms. Aycan and Berry found that a greater decline in present status in Canada compared to the departure status from Turkey was associated with high acculturative stress among Turkish immigrants. Those who experienced greater status loss were also less satisfied and less likely to describe themselves as accomplished in economic life. The longer the immigrants were unemployed, the more likely they suffered from acculturative stress, negative self-concept, alienation from the society, and adaptation difficulties.

Studying the adaptation of both professional and nonprofessional Turkish immigrants in Toronto, Ataca and Berry found that those of low socioeconomic status were more stressed yet more satisfied with their lives than those of high socioeconomic status. This finding again points to the consequence of status loss that professional immigrants experience. Immigrants of lower status make comparisons with what their economic condition used to be like and feel satisfied, while those of higher status make comparisons with their cohorts in Turkey and feel deprived. In this context, it was reported that low socioeconomic status and family income were also highly associated with high feelings of disturbance among South Asian women in Canada. Socioeconomic status is again an important predictor of stress in the studies with African American and Mexican American females and Korean American women.

Apart from personal factors, contextual factors are also important in the adaptation of immigrant and acculturating groups. Of utmost importance in the society of settlement are the attitudes of the dominant society. Perceptions and personal experiences of intolerance, hostility, and discrimination have been documented to serve as stressors and to have a negative impact on psychological adaptation.

In conclusion, stress does not take place in a vacuum: contextual factors, especially cultural ones that have been outlined here, clearly play a role. The importance of ecological and acculturative factors has been emphasized in order to provide a macro-level view of how stress and coping are shaped. Within these, micro-level experiences have been identified to illustrate the close links between culture and stress.

See Also the Following Articles

Cultural Transition; Economic Factors and Stress; Health and Socioeconomic Status; Indigenous Societies; Social Status and Stress.

Further Reading

Aldwin, C. M. (1994). *Stress, coping, and development.* New York: Guilford.

Ataca, B. and Berry (2002). Psychological, sociocultural, and marital adaptation of Turkish immigrants in Canada. *International Journal of Psychology* 37, 13–26.

Aycan, Z. and Berry, J. W. (1996). Impact of employment related experiences on immigrants' psychological well-being and adaptation to Canada. *Canadian Journal of Behavioural Science* 28, 240–251.

Berry, J. W. (1970). Marginality, stress and ethnic identification in an acculturated Aboriginal community. *Journal of Cross-Cultural Psychology* **1**, 239–252.
Berry, J. W. (1990). Psychology of acculturation. In: Berman, J. (ed.) *Cross-cultural perspectives,* (vol. 37), pp. 201–234. Lincoln, NE: University of Nebraska Press.
Berry, J. W. (1997). Immigration, acculturation, and adaptation. *Applied Psychology: An International Review* **46**, 5–68.
Berry, J. W. (2001). A psychology of immigration. *Journal of Social Issues* **57**, 615–631.
Berry, J. W. (2003). Conceptual approaches to acculturation. In: Chun, K., Balls-Organista, P. & Marin, G. (eds.) *Acculturation: advances in theory, measurement, and applied research*, pp. 17–37. Washington, D.C: American Psychological Association.
Berry, J. W. (2004). An ecocultural perspective on the development of competence. In: Sternberg, R. J. & Grigorenko, E. (eds.) *Culture and competence*, pp. 3–22. Washington, D.C: American Psychological Association.
Berry, J. W. (2005). Acculturative stress. In: Wong, P. & Wong, L. C. J. (eds.) *Handbook of multicultural perspectives on stress and coping*, pp. 283–294. New York: Springer.
Berry, J. W. and Kim, U. (1988). Acculturation and mental health. In: Dasen, P. R., Berry, J. W. & Sartorius, N. (eds.) *Health and cross cultural psychology: towards applications*, pp. 207–238. Newbury Park, CA: Sage.
Berry, J. W. and Sam, D. L. (2006). Cultural and ethnic factors in health. In: Ayers, S., et al. (eds.) *Cambridge handbook of psychology, health and medicine* (2nd edn.). Cambridge, UK: Cambridge University Press.
Berry, J. W., Kim, U., Minde, T. and Mok, D. (1987). Comparative studies of acculturative stress. *International Migration Review* **21**, 491–511.
Cohen, Y. (1968). Culture as adaptation. In: Cohen, Y. (ed.) *Man in adaptation*, pp. 40–60. Chicago, IL: Aldine.
Dion, K. L., Dion, K. K. and Pak, A. (1992). Personality-based hardiness as a buffer for discrimination-related stress in members of Toronto's Chinese community. *Canadian Journal of Behavioral Science* **24**, 517–536.
Dona, G. and Berry, J. W. (1994). Acculturation attitudes and acculturative stress of Central American refugees in Canada. *International Journal of Psychology* **29**, 57–70.
Dyal, J. A., Rybensky, L. and Somers, M. (1988). Marital and acculturative strain among Indo-Canadian and Euro-Canadian women. In: Berry, J. W. & Annis, R. C. (eds.) *Ethnic psychology: research and practice with immigrants, refugees, native peoples, ethnic groups, and sojourners*, pp. 80–95. Lisse, Netherlands: Swets and Zeitlinger.
Forde, D. (1934). *Habitat, economy and society.* London: Methuen.
Kroeber, A. (1939). *Cultural and natural areas of North America.* Berkeley, CA: University of California Press.
Lay, C. H. and Nguyen, T. (1998). The role of acculturation-related and acculturation non specific daily hassles: Vietnamese-Canadian students and psychological distress. *Canadian Journal of Behavioral Science* **30**, 172–181.
Lazarus, R. S. and Folkman, S. (1984). *Stress, appraisal and coping.* New York: Springer-Verlag.
Liebkind, K. (1996). Acculturation and stress: Vietnamese refugees in Finland. *Journal of Cross Cultural Psychology* **27**, 161–180.
Liebkind, K. and Jasinskaja-Lahti, I. (2000). The influence of experiences of discrimination on psychological stress: a comparison of seven immigrant groups. *Journal of Community and Applied Social Psychology* **10**, 1–16.
Naidoo, J. C. (1985). A cultural perspective on the adjustment of South Asian women in Canada. In: Lagunes, I. R. & Poortinga, Y. H. (eds.) *From a different perspective: studies of behavior across cultures*, pp. 76–92. Lisse, Netherlands: Swets and Zeitlinger.
Noh, S., Beiser, M., Kaspar, V., Hou, F. and Rummens, J. (1999). Perceived racial discrimination, depression and coping. *Journal of Health and Social Behavior* **40**, 193–207.
Safdar, A. F. and Lay, C. H. (2003). The relations of immigrant-specific and immigrant nonspecific daily hassles to distress controlling for psychological adjustment and cultural competence. *Journal of Applied Social Psychology* **33**, 299–320.
Sam, D. L. and Berry, J. W. (eds.) (2006). *Cambridge handbook of acculturation psychology.* Cambridge, UK: Cambridge University Press.
Turnbull, C. (1972). *The mountain people.* New York: Simon and Schuster.
Van Haaften, E. H. and Van de Vijver, F. J. R. (1996). Psychological consequences of environmental degradation. *Journal of Health Psychology* **1**, 411–429.
Ward, C. (1996). Acculturation. In: Landis, D. & Bhagat, R. (eds.) *Handbook of intercultural training* (2nd edn., pp. 124–147). Thousand Oaks, CA: Sage.
Ward, C. and Kennedy, A. (1993). Psychological and sociocultural adjustment during cross cultural transitions: A comparison of secondary school students overseas and at home. *International Journal of Psychology* **28**, 129–147.
Ward, C., Bochner, S. and Furnham, A. (2001). *The psychology of culture shock* (2nd edn.). East Sussek, UK: Routledge.

Cultural Transition

M S Kopp
Semmelweis University, Budapest, Hungary

This is a revised version of the article by M S Kopp, Encyclopedia of Stress First Edition, volume 1, pp 611–614, © 2000, Elsevier Inc.

Glossary

Chronic stress — According to the original concept of the general adaptation theory of Janos (Hans) Selye, the three phases of stress are alarm reaction, resistance phase, and, the physiologically most harmful phase, exhaustion, that is, chronic stress. Chronic stress theory incorporates the learned helplessness model, the psychosocial and psychiatric models of depression, the control theory of stress and health, and the concept of vital exhaustion.

Cognitive appraisal — The interpretation of an event or situation with respect to one's attitudes, values, and well-being.

Coping — Constantly changing cognitive and behavioral efforts to manage specific external and/or internal demands that are appraised as taxing or exceeding the resources of the person.

Depressive symptomatology — Symptoms of mood disturbances characterized by negative thoughts (for example, feelings of helplessness, inadequacy, loss of control, and low self-esteem), decreased motivation and interest in life, and such physical symptoms as sleep disturbances and fatigue. In civilized countries the prevalence of depressive symptomatology is around 20%.

Learned helplessness — A condition of loss of control created by being subjected to unavoidable trauma (such as shock and relative deprivation). Being unable to avoid or escape (flight or fight) an aversive situation produces a feeling of helplessness that generalizes to subsequent situations. Learned helplessness is the best animal model of human depressive symptomatology.

Social capital — Refers to features of social organization, such as trust, norms, and networks, that can improve the efficiency of society by facilitating coordinated actions. Indicators are levels of trust, perceived reciprocity, and density of membership in civic associations.

Social status — An individual's worth relative to other group members. This evaluation of worth must be at least tacitly understood and agreed upon by interacting individuals.

Sociocultural identification — Introjection of socially meaningful behavioral patterns (usually social roles), through significant persons, via nonverbal communication and contextual and situational cues, acquiring thereby also motivation to actualize the given behavior patterns in fantasy and in action. Learning by model, model following behavior, model learning, and imitation are behavioral descriptions of the same phenomenon. Identification is a psychoanalytic term, meaningful from a developmental and intrapsychic point of view.

Cultural Transition in the Central Eastern European (CEE) Countries as Field Experience

Cultural Transition and Health in CEE Countries

While in modern societies living conditions have improved in many respects, other aspects of life have been fundamentally damaged. Important factors of personality development, for instance, the mother–child relationship, social models of the extended family, and the order in which values are passed on, are being challenged. The accelerated pace of life and unpredictable environmental changes add to these factors. Therefore, it is understandable that in all developed countries the number of adults and children suffering from the symptoms of anxiety and depression has increased. Compared to other countries, more dramatic changes have been experienced in the suddenly changing CEE and Eastern European countries. For example, in Hungary the prevalence of severe depressive symptomatology increased from 2.9 to 7.1% between 1988 and 1995.

A unique field experience of cultural and socioeconomic transition has taken place in the CEE countries during the past several decades. Until the end of the 1970s, the mortality rates in the CEE countries, including Hungary, were better than those of Britain and Austria. Subsequently, whereas in Western Europe the life expectancy rose continuously, in the CEE countries, such as in Hungary, Poland, the Czech and Slovac Republics, and Romania, this tendency reversed. By 1990 the Hungarian mortality rate was the highest in Europe. This deterioration cannot be ascribed to deficiencies in health care, because during these years there was a significant decrease in infant mortality rate and improvements in other dimensions of health care. Until 1990 it was not due to a declining standard of living: between 1970 and 1988 the GDP rose by more than 200% in Hungary, and in 1988 the economic status of the lowest socioeconomic strata was even better than in 1970.

The changes in Hungary and other CEE countries since 1970 have been due to a gradually intensifying social and economic polarization. Whereas a large part of the population lived at nearly the same low level in 1970, by the end of the 1980s a large fraction of society had achieved a higher socioeconomic level, having obtained one or more cars, their own property, and substantially higher income. Gaps within society had consequently widened.

Multivariate analysis showed that it was not the relatively worse socioeconomic situation itself that resulted in the higher morbidity rates, but the subjective appraisal of the situation and the consequent chronic stress – not a difficult social situation itself, but the subjective experience of relative disadvantage was the most significant health risk factor. When, for example, an individual does not have a car and therefore feels disadvantaged and that he or she cannot properly provide for his or her family, this is the state of mind that intensifies deterioration of both mental and physical health.

Self-Destructive Cycles between Cultural and Socioeconomic Transition: Chronic Stress, Depressive Symptomatology, and Health

Returning to the original concept of the general adaptation theory of János Selye, the three phases of stress are alarm reaction, resistance phase, and, the physiologically most harmful phase, exhaustion, that is, chronic stress. Chronic stress theory could incorporate the learned helplessness model, the psychosocial and psychiatric models of depression, the control theory of stress and health, and the concept of vital exhaustion. Furthermore, such a unified stress model could best explain the morbidity and mortality crisis in the middle-aged male population in Central and Eastern Europe in the last decades. A self-destructive circle develops from the chronic stress of the enduring, relatively disadvantageous socioeconomic situation and depressive symptoms. This circle resulting in depressive symptoms plays a significant role in the increase of morbidity and mortality rates in the lower socioeconomic groups of the population. It is not the bad socioeconomic situation itself, but rather the subjective evaluation and cognitive appraisal of the relative disadvantage that seems to be the most significant risk factor of health deterioration, since at equal living standards, Hungarian and other health statistics were better than those of other European countries until the 1970s.

Amid rapid socioeconomic and cultural changes, those left behind can continually blame themselves or their environment, see their future as hopeless, and experience permanent loss of control and helplessness. Negative judgment of one's own situation and feelings of powerlessness and loss of control are the main background factors in the development of a chronic stress situation that might result in depressive symptomatology. This view of life at a time when society is rapidly polarizing, especially when the only goal of most of society is individual advancement, becomes very common.

Paralleling the increase in socioeconomic gaps within society there was an enormous decrease in perceived social support and social capital and increase in the sense of loss of control, not only in individuals, but in masses of people who felt rejected. The sudden transition of society continuously created situations in which the psychological and physiological balance could be maintained only with great difficulty; accordingly, there was a need for a change in attitudes and ways of coping. Only people with flexible coping resources adapted successfully.

Health Consequences of Chronic Stress and Depressive Symptomatology

There are many possible explanations for chronic stress and the consequent depressive symptomatology having an important role in higher morbidity and mortality rates during periods of cultural and socioeconomic transition.

The depressive condition affects perceived state of health and can lead to disability even without organic illness. Depression has a very close relationship with self-destructive behaviors, such as smoking and alcohol abuse, and suicidal behavior is especially common among depressive people. Those suffering from permanent mood disorder and depression are more vulnerable to various diseases and are less able to improve their social situation, so that they easily fall into a sustained vicious cycle. In recent decades, depression, vital exhaustion, and hopelessness have been identified as important independent risk factors for coronary disease. Learned helplessness or learned hopelessness, which can be regarded as the most appropriate model for depression, is associated with decreased immunological activity and affects tumor growth and vulnerability to various infections.

Mediating Role of Social Cohesion and Social Capital

In recent years, studies have suggested that cultural and social identity, sociocultural identification, social capital, and social cohesion are among the most important health protection factors in modern societies. Where they exist, wealthier people are prepared to make sacrifices for the community, and the disadvantaged do not feel that they have been completely left to themselves in a hostile world. Trust in each other, esteem for shared values, the acceptance and internalization of cultural and social identity result in a high level of social cohesion in the society, which is the foundation not only of health but also of economic wealth and prosperity.

Marmot, Kawachi, and Wilkinson, who drew attention to the fundamental risk of inequality within society, also considered the phenomena of social cohesion and social capital to be the most important factors behind differences between countries and regions. For a lower-level British civil servant, for example, it was not his or her relative poverty itself that was the cause of his or her bad health, because during German bombing the death rates of the London population greatly decreased despite difficult living circumstances. The weakening of social cohesion and social capital is a significant factor in the emergence of large social differences and the associated deterioration of health – not only in CEE countries, but also in the developed countries.

Changing Attitudes and Values and Cultural Transition

Psychological Definition of Freedom and Democracy

An important question is whether the crisis experienced in human communities nowadays is a necessary part of civilization. The latest results of behavioral science point out that, beyond the concomitant phenomenon of lifestyle, we can see the root cause of this crisis in the fact that in modern society new possibilities for arousing anxiety have taken place.

During previous centuries the basic optimization principles of life were survival, subsistence, and maintaining the family, which dominated people's behavior. As a result of technological development, focus on these principles are no longer fundamentally necessary in civilized countries. However, the previously fixed order and communal forms of passing on values have also ceased. A young person's self used to be formed on the basis of feedback from the family, the extended family, and contemporaries in the community of the village or small town in which he or she lived. Nowadays, this process takes places within a nuclear or broken family and through mass communication, which seemingly provides feelings of community, but in reality the person rarely receives the continuity of patterns and values with which they can identify themselves.

While there are undeniable benefits in the move away from more tight-knit, rule-bound traditional societies, under the conditions of continuous cultural and socioeconomic transition, the loss of balance in the human–environment system becomes more apparent. A solitary, anxious human being, deprived of relationships, values, goals, and self-esteem, can be used for the necessary functions of society and can be arbitrarily changed and manipulated. So we must recognize that technological developments have established the preliminary conditions for creating anxiety.

In order to maintain or increase their power, the person or group who possesses the most information can afford to either deprive others of information or give it as a reward, thereby creating anxiety in the environment. Arousing anxiety is not only a means, but also the essence of a dictatorship. The most effective tactic employed by a dictator is to create anxiety. A dictator wants to assure total decisional freedom for him- or herself. This is characteristic of all dependent relationships, in which the least dependent has the right to deprive the other person of information and thus keep the other in a situation over which he or she have no control. This not only occurs in totalitarian societies, but also can happen in families, schools, or jobs. Thus, we encounter the abuse of power and different ways of arousing anxiety every day, but we still do not give these situations enough attention, we do not recognize them in their embryonic forms, and we do not understand how this slow-action poison kills.

We can also arrive at the psychological definition of freedom and democracy through understanding the essence of anxiety. In a psychological sense, freedom means possessing the necessary, essential information needed to evaluate, solve, and control our situation, and being able to contribute actively to shaping our situation. Democracy means these rights – both the right and the responsibility of information and action.

Misuse of Anxiety in Cultural Transition

How does this apparently purely psychological and medical phenomenon, anxiety, become a basic concept that can shape society? We can ask whether anxiety has an adaptive function: is there any need for anxiety? Imagine a completely anxiety-free person: he or she does not recognize prospective danger and hence does not avoid dangerous situations and cannot be controlled by social sanctions. Some criminals and people with antisocial personality disorder belong to this type. In such cases, those in their environment suffer while they themselves follow their momentary drives.

Social co-existence requires a certain degree of anxiety. One learns as a child in which situations to expect punishment – a mother's frowning look or a bad mark in school. The avoidance of anxiety is a very important driving force from the first moments of life. If the rules of punishment are foreseeable and are commensurate with the mistakes made, then anxiety can have an adaptive function. But if the rules are opaque or do not exist, then the powerlessness and defenselessness can become a weapon in the hands of those who have power. If parents punish from a whim rather than for a reason, then the child will not understand and will not be able to understand when he is threatened by danger. If a teacher or university lecturer asks questions from material that the student could not learn, he or she hammers insufficiency and failure into the student. If leaders, managers, politicians, those who possess more information do not make the rules clear, then they assure their arbitrary authority by causing anxiety in deprived masses. The twentieth century has created the possibility of causing such total anxiety, spread by the mass communication media just as Hitler's or Stalin's radio speeches were transmitted by the loudspeakers of a whole empire.

It is obvious from the preceding that, since creating anxiety can involve issues of money, benefit, and power, there are enormous advantages in knowing how to deal with these powers effectively. Films, newspapers, magazines, and books infiltrate the community and human relationships and can belittle or deny values and mold people into a mass that can be led. This type of mass manipulation can occur even if the manipulator's aim differs from what actually takes place.

The ideology of the consumer society, to control human behavior through the liberation of instincts and search for pleasure, degrades human beings to the level of animals since an animal's decisions are influenced by its instincts to preserve its physiological balance. To achieve dominance by any means is a natural need in such a system.

On every level of society there is, day by day, a life-and-death struggle between two behaviors: either accepting and respecting other people, establishing agreement and a community of free people and bringing the value of democracy into being or arousing anxiety by withholding information from others. Not the slogans but the behavior classifies the participants.

The question is whether humans will be able to adapt themselves to the circumstances formed by history, or whether their lack of adaptive ability will lead the human race into extreme peril. This adaptation has to be realized on the level of both the individual and society.

See Also the Following Articles

Cultural Factors in Stress; Social Capital; Social Networks and Social Isolation; Social Status and Stress; Social Support.

Further Reading

Kawachi, I. and Berkman, L. F. (2000). Social cohesion, social capital, and health. In: Berkman, L. F. & Kawachi, I. (eds.) *Social epidemiology.* New York: Oxford University.

Kopp, M. S. and Réthelyi, J. (2004). Where psychology meets physiology: chronic stress and premature mortality-the Central-Eastern European health paradox. *Brain Research Bulletin* **62**, 351–367.

Marmot, M. (2004). *The status syndrome: how social standing affects our health and longevity.* New York: Times Books, Henry Holt and Company.

Skrabski, Á., Kopp, M. S. and Kawachi, I. (2004). Social capital and collective efficacy in Hungary: cross sectional associations with middle aged female and male mortality rates. *Journal of Epidemiology and Community Health* 58, 340–345.

Wilkinson, R. G. (1994). The epidemiological transition: from material scarcity to social disadvantage? *Daedalus* **123**(4), 61–77.

Economic Factors and Stress

R A Catalano
University of California, Berkeley, CA, USA

This is a revised version of the article by R A Catalano, Encyclopedia of Stress First Edition, volume 2, pp 9–14, © 2000, Elsevier Inc.

Glossary

Discount rate for pain A measurement of the difference between fear of pain experienced now and of that experienced in the future.

Expected value of pain The product of multiplying the likelihood of experiencing a painful event by the amount pain it would inflict.

Reservation wage The wage at which a worker with chronic illness will apply for disability benefits rather than compete for a job.

Social support Tangible and intangible help from family, friends, and social networks to cope with stressors.

Introduction: The Economy as a Population Stressor

We intuitively separate the stressors associated with physiological and behavioral disorders into several groups. These groups include undesirable as well as intuitively desirable job and financial events. As might be expected, the incidence of undesirable job and financial stressors increases during periods of economic contraction. The experience of undesirable job and financial events by a principal wage earner also increases the risk of disorder for his or her spouse and family. Undesirable job and financial experiences, moreover, increase the likelihood of subsequent stressful nonjob, nonfinancial experiences for the wage earner and his or her family. The contraction of a regional economy can, in other words, increase the experience of undesirable job and financial events that, in turn, increase the risk of experiencing yet other undesirable experiences not intuitively related to the economy. These undesirable events raise the risk of disorder not only for those who experience them, but also for spouses and other members of the family.

Researchers have focused on job loss more than any other economic stressor. While disagreement remains over the virulence of job loss as a pathogen, there is agreement that forced job loss increases the risk of depressed mood, alcohol abuse, and antisocial behavior. More controversy arises from claims of a connection with somatic illness, but job loss reportedly increases the risk of stress-related illnesses, including those associated with compromised endocrine and immune responses.

Persons exposed to undesirable job and financial events early in life may exhibit elevated risk of succumbing to future stressors, whether those are economic in nature or not. Research on those who experienced the Great Depression of the 1930s, for example, suggests that economic stressors can affect behavior well into the future.

Classic and recent theoretical literature concerned with the economy as a source of stressors posits that economies expanding more quickly than the rate to which a population has habituated should be pathogenic. This work argues that movements away from the expected value of macroeconomic performance, regardless of direction, should increase the incidence of stress-related illness. Individual-level research has not found desirable job and financial events to be as virulent or as contagious as undesirable events, but reports of ecological associations between rapid economic growth and the incidence of trauma and alcohol-related pathology appear in the literature. Fear of job loss, moreover, appears to reduce risk-taking behavior such as alcohol use and antisocial behavior. The pure income effects of changing economies could also affect the incidence of pathology in that more income makes risk taking more likely, while less income should suppress risk taking that requires outlay.

The known and suspected health effects of economic expansion raise an important issue for those who would estimate the health and behavioral cost of economic perturbations. Such estimates will be of the net effect of change and therefore require more empirical research than we now have into pathology induced by economic growth.

The Economy's Effect on Hazard Avoidance

The classic and contemporary stress literature connects environmental stressors to illness through the presumed effects of stressors on the endocrine and immune systems. Stressors, however, may affect health through other avenues, such as the effects of stressors on hazard avoidance.

We have a fixed capacity to assess, manage, or reduce hazards in our physical and social environments. We budget this capacity in that not all hazards receive equal attention. Candidates for less attention include hazards with the least potential for pain.

Potential for pain is the product of the expected value of pain and our discount rate. The expected value, in turn, is the product of the likelihood of succumbing to the hazard and the pain that doing so would inflict. The discount rate gauges the difference in fear of pain experienced now compared to that experienced in the future. We most likely neglect hazards that promise relatively little pain, have a low probability of occurring, and occur farthest in the future.

If a contracting economy confronts us with new and immediate hazards, those already low on our list for attention may fall off the list all together. Screening for the early signs of treatable disease or compliance with treatment regimens, for example, may decline among persons attending to hazards posed by lost income.

Attending to new hazards at the expense of old might not change the incidence of illness in a population if hazards came into and left our lives for reasons peculiar to each of us. Some of us would be experiencing new hazards while others were losing old ones, leaving the net effect in the population at or near zero. Incidence would, however, vary over time if the environments we share became more or less hazardous. We all share the constantly shifting economic environment.

The early detection of breast cancer provides an example of how the economic environment may affect the incidence of serious illness by causing shifts in attention across hazards. Ninety-three percent of women discovered with local breast cancer survive 5 or more years, but only 18% of those discovered with remote tumors do so. It appears that living in a contracting economy reduces the likelihood that women will discover tumors in the local stage. Women apparently seek less screening when coping with the sequelae of economic contraction. They do not, in other words, have sufficient capacity to attend to both the new hazards inflicted upon them by economic contraction and the old hazards farther down the list of priorities.

As noted earlier, changing economies have income effects such that expansion enables individuals to consume more while contraction tends to reduce consumption. Some individuals may use added income to pursue activities that expose them to more hazards than would otherwise be the case. Indeed, ecological associations between rapid economic growth and the incidence of trauma may reflect the risk taking enabled by economic expansion.

The Economy's Effect on Coping Assets

The stress literature posits, without great controversy, that coping assets mediate an individual's response to stressors. These assets can be genetic or acquired through interactions with the environment. The latter can be further separated into those that are unintentionally acquired (e.g., immunities induced by naturally occurring exposures to infectious pathogens) and those sought out (e.g., vaccines). Intentionally acquired coping assets include those purchased with money and those acquired through social arrangements analogous to mutual aid societies or insurance pools. While some have speculated regarding the effect of economic forces on unintentionally acquired, and even genetically endowed, coping assets, the empirical work focuses on those purchased with money or obtained through social arrangements.

Coping assets purchased with money include goods and services explicitly marketed as means to bolster one's capacity to deal with new or chronic stressors. These assets include professional medical care, leisure activities, organized exercise activity, and dietary supplements. Other goods and services can also help persons cope with stressors. Advertisers may not often cast nutritious food, decent housing, and entertainment, for example, as stress buffers, but much of the value of these products in the market may well arise from this function. The performance of the economy obviously affects our ability to acquire these resources because it affects how much money we have to spend. Money, in effect, is a generalized coping asset.

The performance of an economy also affects the availability of coping assets acquired outside the market. The literature pays much attention to social support and social capital as mediators of the stress response. These terms refer to all sorts of tangible and intangible resources obtained by stressed persons from their families, social networks, and public and private institutions.

The insurance pool metaphor conveys the effect of the economy on social support and capital. Social networks can be thought of as informal insurance pools to which participants not coping with stressors contribute surplus coping assets, and from which participants coping with stressors draw assets. As with all insurance pools, the arrangement works only if demands do not exceed the pooled resources. Participants in such pools often underestimate how many resources a pool needs because we intuitively make the actuarial assumption that the incidence of stressors remains relatively constant although those who suffer them may vary. If, however, an ambient shock stresses many persons in the pool, the demand for resources can be unexpectedly high and deplete the pool. A contracting economy acts as an ambient stressor that causes an unexpectedly large number of individuals and their families to suffer stressful losses and to resort to social networks for coping resources. Other members of the network who fear such a loss withdraw contributions to the pool, believing they themselves will need them. The incidence of stress-related illness therefore rises because social support cannot be gotten from an actuarially insufficient pool. Persons dealing with chronic stressors or stressful events unrelated to the economy also exhibit elevated incidence of illness because they cannot retrieve their usual support from a depleted pool. The effect of a contracting economy on the incidence of illness in populations embedded in contracting economies thereby grows beyond that expected from studies of individuals who, for example, are forced out of work.

Recent years have seen an increasing interest in the role of economic inequality on the coping process. Social reformers have traditionally drawn an analogy between income disparity and ambient pathogens such as air pollution. This disparity presumably emits a morally numbing pathogen that makes us not only less helpful to the needy, but also less willing to contribute to social support pools that include socioeconomic peers.

Contemporary reformers claim a causal chain in which widening income disparity erodes social cohesion. The loss of social cohesion makes it more difficult for everyone, not just the poor, to cope with biological and behavioral hazards. Failure to cope then manifests in illness and death itself.

The reformers' argument, although intended primarily to influence the policy debate over the distribution of wealth, has implications for the epidemiology of stress-related illness. If income disparity weakens social cohesion, it will likely reduce the effectiveness of social support networks. Less effective social support increases the likelihood that economic and other stressors will yield illness.

The Economy's Effect on Tolerance for Coping

The economy apparently affects the diagnosis of illness by affecting community tolerance for coping. Society applies the label illness to physical and behavioral characteristics that reduce a person's ability to perform day-to-day functions. The tolerance of a community for changes in performance, therefore, becomes an important determinant of whom it judges ill.

Sociologists and psychologists report that the economy affects tolerance for deviance from performance standards. Ecological psychologists have, for example, noted that understaffed organizations (i.e., those with a high ratio of roles, or functions, to participants) tolerate poor performance by members more than overstaffed organizations. Maintaining an understaffed organization supposedly requires members to be tolerant of the shortcomings, real or imagined, of the relatively few persons available to perform needed functions. Persons in understaffed organizations whose coping strategies include physiological and behavioral adaptations that could be labeled as illness (e.g., alcohol abuse) will go undiagnosed because the label may, by rule, disqualify them from positions for which less deviant candidates cannot be found.

Overstaffed organizations, on the other hand, can choose from among many candidates for positions and can set relatively high standards for acceptable functioning. Persons adapting to stressful events may not function as well as other candidates. This performance deficit makes them the least likely to find positions. Accepting the label ill gives them a socially acceptable explanation for their lack of a position.

Economists have developed the theory of reservation wage to describe the individual choice to seek work or income transfers. The theory implies a continuum of physical and behavioral fitness among those who compete for jobs. Society decides where on this continuum it will make income transfers. If too high on the continuum, otherwise productive workers will seek transfers rather than compete for work. If too low, persons with illness will be forced to compete for jobs and become even sicker.

Wherever on the continuum political institutions draw the income transfer line, workers near it have the option of competing for jobs or seeking benefits. Economists refer to the wage at which someone no longer competes and applies for income transfers as his or her reservation wage.

Sociologists have applied the staffing and reservation wage concepts to the community at large. A contracting economy implies relatively many overstaffed organizations, while an expanding economy implies the opposite. The fraction of the labor continuum that can exceed its reservation wage by holding a job goes up with understaffing and down with overstaffing. The number of persons seeking the label ill thereby changes with the ability of the economy to provide jobs with relatively high wages. The incidence of diagnosed illness moves inversely over time with the economy, not only because the labor market affects true incidence but also because it affects community tolerance for performance deficits.

Socioeconomic Status and Stress

The most frequently replicated findings in epidemiology include the inverse association between measures of socioeconomic status and health. Considerable controversy remains over the cause of this association. As might be expected, some argue that the relationship results from the fact that sick persons cannot compete well in the labor market with healthy persons. The argument that illness induces relative poverty justifies, in part, the extensive array of disability compensation programs in the industrial world. Ill persons unable to compete for jobs presumably need income transfers to avoid sinking into poverty.

The rival argument assumes that market economies create a distribution of income in which those with relatively little inherited wealth remain poor because gaining highly compensated skills and making investments requires wealth. Being relatively poor, moreover, means that a person can purchase relatively few of the goods and services that shelter us against stressors (e.g., decent housing in safe neighborhoods) or bolster our coping capacity (e.g., leisure, wholesome food). Being poor, therefore, increases the likelihood of becoming ill.

The relative contribution of each mechanism to the statistical association between socioeconomic status and health remains controversial. Researchers who study this issue also contribute to the economic stress literature because they document that persons most likely to avoid economic stressors also have coping assets and enjoy high community tolerance for their coping. We know from empirical study that persons with wealth suffer fewer stressful events during economic contraction than those in the middle and lower classes. It does not require empirical study to conclude that persons with more money can purchase more coping resources than can those with less money. It also appears that physical and behavioral deviance among the poor more likely leads to being labeled ill than similar deviance among the rich. Being relatively poor, therefore, makes a person particularly vulnerable to the stressors of economic contraction.

Policy Implications and Conclusions

Any discussion of economic stressors and their effects must at least allude to economic policy because such stressors result mostly from public and private decisions regulated by political institutions. Regulatory institutions intervene in these decisions only when costs appear to exceed benefits. While researchers may study the health effects of economic perturbations to satisfy their curiosity, they typically claim that the work has applied value in that it could help regulators better account the social costs of public and private decisions. The claim implies that public policy could, indeed, should reduce the frequency or virulence of economic stressors such as job loss.

Much controversy has arisen in Europe and North America over whether regulators have gone too far or not far enough in their attempts to reduce the stress of economic change. Policies now in place appear to assume that we previously went too far and discouraged private investment by depressing the return to capital. Defenders of the current policy acknowledge that increasing the return to private investment induces economic restructuring and its attendant pain in our personal and communal experience. They predict, however, that lowering the return to investors would drive capital to less regulated and less taxed economies. This would supposedly displace more labor in the developed world than restructuring, and inflict much unregulated stress and untreated illness in developing countries.

The assumptions underlying current policy remain controversial. The epidemiology of economic stress, therefore, will likely remain an important issue in public health as well as in the debate over economic policy.

In summary, the performance of an economy can affect the health of the population it supports. Economic contraction increases the number of persons coping with undesirable job and financial events. These events increase the risk of experiencing other stressors not intuitively connected to the economy. The adverse effects of these stressors spread to family and friends.

Rapid economic growth also induces adaptations that should, according to classic theory, increase the incidence of stress-related illness. Research on work-related trauma and alcohol consumption, for example, supports this connection.

A contracting economy affects our capacity to cope with stressors. Persons who lose income cannot purchase as many coping resources as they once did. This reduces their ability to deal not only with new economic stressors but also with chronic stressors previously buffered with purchased coping resources. The tangible and intangible coping resources gotten from social networks are also more difficult to obtain when the economy contracts. This is true because there are fewer surplus resources to contribute to the common pool at the same time that there are more demands upon it.

Economic stressors can also increase the incidence of illnesses not typically thought to be stress related, because coping with such stressors can leave us with fewer resources to avoid risk factors for, or detect early signs of, illnesses unrelated to stress. The economy can, moreover, affect the tolerance of society for persons coping with stressors. We know that overstaffed communities, as indicated by high unemployment rates, reduce competition for scarce jobs by increasing the diagnosis of disability.

Economic contraction inevitably increases the number of persons who are poor. Being poor is a risk factor for stressors of all sorts and, by definition, means that access to coping resources is relatively constrained.

See Also the Following Articles

Health and Socioeconomic Status; Industrialized Societies; Job Insecurity: The Health Effects of a Psychosocial Work Stressor; Social Status and Stress.

Further Reading

Brenner, M. (1973). *Mental illness and the economy.* Cambridge, MA: Harvard University Press.

Catalano, R. (1979). *Health, behavior and the community: an ecological perspective.* New York: Pergamon Press.

Catalano, R. (1991). The health effects of economic insecurity. *American Journal of Public Health* **81**, 1148–1152.

Catalano, R., Novaco, R. and McConnell, W. (1997). A model of the net effect of job loss on violence. *Journal of Personality and Social Psychology* **72**, 1440–1447.

Catalano, R., Satariano, W. and Ciemins, E. (2003). Unemployment and the detection of early stage breast tumors among African Americans and non-Hispanic whites. *Annals of Epidemiology* **13**, 8–16.

Catalano, R., Bruckner, T., Anderson, B. and Gould, J. (2005). Fetal death sex ratios: a test of the economic stress hypothesis. *International Journal of Epidemiology* **34**, 944–948.

Fryer, D. (1998). Special issue on mental health consequences of economic insecurity, relative poverty, and social exclusion: community psychological perspectives on recession. *Journal of Community and Applied Social Psychology* **8.**

Keiselbach, T. (1997). Special issue on job loss, unemployment, and social injustices. *Social Justice Research* **10.**

Neumayer, E. (2004). Recessions lower (some) mortality rates: evidence from Germany. *Social Science and Medicine* **58**(6), 1037–1047.

Ruhm, C. J. (2004). Healthy living in hard times. *Journal of Health Economics* **24**(2), 341–363.

Warr, P. (1987). *Work, unemployment, and mental health.* Fair Lawn, NY: Oxford University Press.

Wilkinson, R. (1996). *Unhealthy societies: the afflictions of inequality.* London: Routledge.

Education Levels and Stress

J Mirowsky and C E Ross
University of Texas at Austin, Austin, TX, USA

This is a revised version of the article by A V Ranchor and R Sanderman, Encyclopedia of Stress First Edition, volume 2, pp 15–18, © 2000, Elsevier Inc.

Glossary

Acute stressor — An undesirable and uncontrollable event or transition requiring personal adaptation.

Chronic stressor — A situation characterized by prolonged discrepancy between goals and means.

Human capital — Productive capacity developed, embodied, and stored in humans themselves.

Learned effectiveness — The ability to produce desired outcomes gained through study, practice, and experience.

Resource substitution — Using one thing in place of another, and finding ways to achieve ends with whatever materials, relationships, and circumstances present themselves.

Sense of control — A learned and generalized sense of directing one's own life, ranging by degrees from fatalism and a deep sense of helplessness to instrumentalism and a firm sense of mastery.

What Education Levels Indicate

Formal education serves three functions in modern societies: (1) developing abilities through progressive instruction and training, (2) grading individual levels of development and gating advancement, and (3) regulating access to occupations and jobs. Developed nations all measure attainment by years and degrees, in a manner increasingly comparable across nations. The years measure progressive levels, each attainable by most students within one school year of effort. The degrees certify the completion of specific multi-year programs. Education level refers both to years and degrees; it indicates the level of ability developed, the exposure to progression and selection, and the opportunities regulated as a consequence. Together these influence an individual's exposure and response to stressors throughout adulthood.

Lower Exposure to Stressful Situations

The abilities and opportunities provided by higher levels of education reduce exposure to stressful situations. Researchers generally categorize stressors as events (acute stressors) or conditions (chronic stressors.) Life-change events are transitions that require personal adaptation. They can be desirable (e.g., getting married) or undesirable (e.g., becoming widowed). They also can be controllable (e.g., quitting a job) or uncontrollable (e.g., getting fired). The more undesirable and uncontrollable the events, the more distress they produce. Higher levels of education shift the balance of events. Controllable and desirable ones become more likely; uncontrollable and undesirable ones become less likely. An event such as a job promotion produces some stress as the individual adapts to the new demands, but the positive implications moderate the stress and make it stimulating rather than disturbing. In addition, it marks a transition to new circumstances with a more favorable balance of events and greater social and economic resources. An event such as getting fired or laid off demands as much or more adaptation, but also has the demoralizing implications of inadequacy and impending hard times. In addition, it often marks a transition into prolonged unemployment, economic hardship, family strife, lower social standing, and diminished opportunity. Those situations are stressful, and they shift the likely balance of subsequent events unfavorably.

Higher levels of education help individuals avoid chronic stressors, characterized by a prolonged discrepancy between goals and means. Chronic stressors include prolonged unemployment; economic hardship and poverty; work that is repetitious, closely supervised, or boring; neighborhood disorder and decay; unsupportive or conflict-ridden relationships; parenting with no partner or an unhelpful one; solitary caring for an aging parent or other impaired dependent; and conflicting demands of work and family.

Chronic stressors are especially harmful to emotional and physical health. Their persistence erodes emotional, physical, and social resources and discourages corrective action. For example, when people are unemployed, they need or want paid work but are not able to find an acceptable position. Being unemployed for months can use up personal and household savings. The shortage of money can lead to economic hardship, which is not being able to buy things the household needs, such as food, clothes, transportation, medicine, and medical care, and not being able to pay the rent or other bills. Repeated failures to find a job become increasingly demoralizing and discouraging. Each failure makes people's emotional need for success greater while making success on the next try seem less likely. The need for comfort and relief can encourage people to overeat sugary and fatty foods, drink heavily, abuse drugs, engage in sexual indiscretions, or escape obsessively into television, movies, novels, games, and the like. Meanwhile, the economic shortfalls get larger with time.

Supportive relationships can ease the individuals' emotional and economic strains, but they do it by spreading the burden to others. The more intense and persistent the hardship, the greater the stain put on relationships. Tensions mount, expressed in irritation, blaming, anger, and strife that may include violence. The others become unsupportive and perhaps even hostile. Relationships break up.

The higher the level of education, the less likely individuals will get into situations of chronic stress, the better they cope if in them, and the quicker they get out of or correct the situation.

Better Response in Stressful Situations

Individuals with higher levels of education respond better in stressful situations. They solve problems better, control their neuroendocrine stress responses better, and use their mobilized energy more constructively. People with higher levels of education take a more pragmatic approach to problems, looking for solutions rather than just getting anxious, angry, or depressed. They also have greater cognitive flexibility, which is the ability to imagine and consider a variety of possible solutions or viewpoints. They are better at communicating and negotiating, have better sources of information, and have more skill at judging and applying information. These abilities make individuals more effective and also more self-assured, which reduces neuroendocrine reactivity.

Individuals with higher levels of education also make better use of the energy mobilized in the stress response. The mental and physical activity directed at problem solving helps use the energy constructively. In addition, adults with higher levels of education are more likely to have habits designed to channel the excess energy mobilized by stress constructively, such as jogging, bicycling, walking, gardening, weight lifting, swimming, playing active games such tennis, or taking fitness classes such as aerobics or yoga.

These better events, situations, and responses associated with higher levels of education result from its two primary consequences: socioeconomic status and learned effectiveness.

Higher Socioeconomic Status

Social scientists view education level as a major element of achieved social status, along with occupational status, management level, earnings, household income, and wealth. The level of education achieved acts as a structural element of a person's life, like a structural beam in a building. Many other aspects of life depend on a person's level of education and take shape with respect to it, including the other achieved statuses. In the advanced industrial nations, education level is increasingly important to status attainment (how high a person rises socially and economically) and status transmission (how many advantages in one generation are passed to the next). Higher status gives an individual more money, authority, influence, and freedom. It shifts life events toward more controllable and desirable ones, and it reduces the risk of a prolonged or severe discrepancy between goals and means.

The higher statuses achieved through education generally reduce stress. The chief exception is managerial responsibility. Management requires a responsibility to others for the performance of others; a manager is responsible to those above for the accomplishments of those below and is responsible to those below for the rewards and resources allocated by those above. But no one can completely control the behavior of others. This creates stress. Work organizations compensate for the stress of greater responsibility by reducing other strains on managers. Higher salaries reduce managers' household economic strains and allow the purchase of goods and services that relieve other demands on time and effort. More important, however, managers generally are given more freedom to decide what they do and how and when they do it, which reduces the stress associated with job demands. They also generally are given more resources and opportunities to do things they find challenging and interesting, which helps make job demands stimulating rather than distressing.

Learned Effectiveness and the Sense of Control

During the twentieth century, formal education came to be viewed as a system for developing human capital. Economists had long viewed capital as material wealth in the form of money or property that is or can be used to produce more material wealth. However, the growth of wealth in the United States and other nations exceeded what could be attributed solely to accumulating monetary and physical capital. Economists revived Adam Smith's concept of human capital as productive capacity developed, embodied, and stored in humans themselves. Levels of formal education are the most important measure of human capital, along with work experience. Formal education develops the skills and abilities of general productive value (such as reading ability or punctuality), as distinct from ones of value in a particular job (such as knowing which forms to fill out or how to operate a particular machine).

Education reduces stress partly by enhancing material productivity but mostly because it develops general problem-solving abilities. The learned effectiveness makes people better at avoiding or solving problems and more confident, reducing stress throughout life. Formal education teaches people to learn. It develops the skills and habits of communication: reading, writing, inquiring, discussing, looking things ups, and figuring things out. It develops analytic skills of broad use such as mathematics, logic, and, on a more basic level, observing, summarizing, synthesizing, interpreting, and experimenting. The more years of schooling, the greater the cognitive development, characterized by flexible, rational, complex strategies of thinking. Education teaches people to think logically and rationally, see many sides of an issue, analyze problems, and design strategies of personal action.

Education also develops broadly effective habits and attitudes such as dependability, good judgment, motivation, effort, trust, and confidence. It instills the habit of meeting problems with attention, thought, action, and persistence. In school, people encounter and solve problems that are progressively more difficult, complex, and subtle. This process develops persistence and self-assurance as well as skill.

When individuals control their own lives, this means they exercise authority and influence over it by directing and regulating it themselves. People vary in the control felt over their own lives. Some feel they can do just about anything they set their minds to. They see themselves as responsible for their own successes and failures and view misfortunes as the results of personal mistakes. Others feel that any good things that happen are mostly luck – fortunate outcomes they desire but do not design. They feel personal problems mostly result from bad breaks or the callous selfishness of others and feel little ability to regulate or avoid the bad things that happen. The sense of control varies by degree, ranging from fatalism and a deep sense of helplessness to instrumentalism and a firm sense of mastery.

The sense of personal control is a learned and generalized expectation. As such it acts as a cognitive-behavioral accumulator, integrating past experience and bringing it into the present. In many ways, a sense of control is to successful action as wealth is to profitable investment – an accumulated product returning subsequent advantage. Perceptions of control grow out of the interaction between intention and outcome. The occurrence of something desired, planned, or attempted reinforces a sense that individuals' choices and actions have consequences. This, in turn, encourages attention to setting goals, directing actions toward the goals, evaluating apparent consequences, and revising efforts.

The sense of control is more than seeing things occurring as individuals want. It is individuals seeing themselves as the authors and editors of the choices and actions that link their preference to occurrence. Within contexts that support its success, critical self-direction sharpens their ability and encourages effort. The resulting effectiveness and resilience strengthen the sense of control in a beneficial developmental spiral. The system of formal education serves as the chief social institution for developing this sense of control.

A number of social and behavioral sciences recognize the importance of a sense of personal control. The concept appears in a number of related forms with various names, including internal locus of control, mastery, instrumentalism, self-efficacy, and personal autonomy; at the other end of the continuum (lack of control), this is fatalism, perceived helplessness, and perceived powerlessness. A low or negative sense of control corresponds to learned helplessness, a behavioral state of suppressed attention and action that induces biological stress in mammals.

Life-Course Compounding

Many things in life produce effects that fade over time as individuals adjust to their circumstances, tastes and times change, enthusiasms wane, and new experiences intervene. Education's effects work the opposite way, growing with time. Education transforms people, putting individuals' lives on a different track. Because education develops resources that inhere in people, its consequences are present in all aspects of life throughout their entire lifetime. Education affects virtually all aspects of life, including habits, interpersonal relationships, family responsibilities, occupational exposures and opportunities, economic sufficiency and security, neighborhood qualities, autonomous and creative activities, and people's sense of controlling their own lives.

Education tends to speed or advance beneficial accumulations and to slow or delay detrimental ones. The consequences accumulate on many levels. They include job security, pay level, occupational status, and wealth on the socioeconomic level; habits such as exercise or smoking or relationships such as marriage on the behavioral level; body mass, atherosclerosis, or hippocampal mass on the anatomic level; aerobic capacity and blood pressure on the physiological level; and glucose tolerance or mitochondrial damage on the intracellular level. Undesirable accumulations typically can be reversed, even after a crisis, but generally only over a period of time as a result of concerted and multifaceted effort. Education helps individuals to avoid undesirable accumulations that need correction, to correct undesirable accumulations before they precipitate a crisis, and, failing that, to heed the implications of the crisis and take the difficult but necessary corrective action.

Many of education's consequences influence one another or regulate one another's effects. The feedback among accumulators amplifies the long-term effects of unchanging attributes such as sex, race, and year of birth and of persistent ones such as occupation and wealth. It also amplifies the effects of short-term random shocks to each accumulator.

Education makes individuals more adept at resource substitution (using one thing in place of another) and finding ways to achieve ends with whatever materials, relationships, and circumstances present themselves. Higher education makes individuals better at acquiring whatever they need and better at using whatever they find available. As a result, more education tends to increase an individual's store of the society's standard resources while improving the individual's ability to improvise resources. A greater capacity for resource substitution makes the absence of any one standard resource less harmful for the better educated. Conversely, less education leaves individuals less adept at acquiring and inventing resources, increasing the individuals' dependence on any standard resource they have.

Stressors often occur in cascading sequences. The relative lack of resources and resourcefulness among the poorly educated exacerbates the outcomes at each step. Ineffective individuals often move through a cascading sequence of corrosive situations made worse at each step by the predisposing traits and conditions that led to those situations. The capacity for resource substitution helps the better educated to avert problems or ameliorate outcomes at each step.

Signs of Lower Stress

A variety of observations indicate that people with higher levels of education generally have lower levels of stress. They encounter fewer undesirable events and situations, as summarized earlier. They also report fewer of the symptoms and health consequences of stress. They report fewer signs of autonomic arousal such as sweaty palms, queasy stomach, dry mouth, faintness, or short of breath and a racing heart when not exercising or working hard. They report fewer days of feeling worried, anxious, and tense. They also report less hostility and anger toward others. (However, when worried, anxious, or tense, they are more likely to report anger along with it.) The better educated have fewer symptoms of depression such as feeling sad, lonely, or worthless and being sleepless, listless, or unable to face the day. They have fewer stress-related health conditions such as high-blood pressure, poor blood sugar control, or frequent colds and influenzas; fewer of the stress-related diseases such as coronary artery disease or type 2 diabetes; and fewer of the stress-related medical crises such as heart attack or stroke.

The better educated have lower scores on biomarker indexes of allostatic load, which is the cumulative biological degradation from stress. There are two kinds of markers. One set measures blood, urine, or saliva levels of the hormones involved in the stress response, such as high overnight urinary excretion of cortisol, epinephrine, and norepinephrine and low serum dihydroepiandrosterone sulfate (DHEAS). The other set measures the cumulative effect of exposure to those hormones, such as high plasma levels of glycosylated hemoglobin (indicating chronic poor blood sugar control), high systolic and diastolic blood pressure, high serum levels of total and of high-density cholesterol, high waist-to-hip ratio (measuring central adiposity), low serum albumin and high fibrinogen and C-reactive protein (indicating chronic inflammation), and indicators of impaired organ function such as low creatinine clearance in the kidneys and low peak air flow in the lungs. Differences in allostatic load scores predict mortality risk in older Americans and statistically account for approximately one-third of the differences in mortality risk across degree levels of education.

See Also the Following Articles

Economic Factors and Stress; Health and Socioeconomic Status; Social Status and Stress; Social Support; Workplace Stress.

Further Reading

Kristenson, M., Eriksen, H. R., Sluiter, J. K., et al. (2004). Psychobiological mechanisms of socioeconomic differences in health. *Social Science and Medicine* **58**, 1511–1522.

Mirowsky, J. and Ross, C. E. (1998). Education, personal control, lifestyle and health: a human capital hypothesis. In: O'Rand, A. (ed.) *Special issue on education over the life course, Research on Aging*, 415–449.

Mirowsky, J. and Ross, C. E. (2003). *Education, social status and health.* Somerset, NJ: Aldine Transaction.

Mirowsky, J. and Ross, C. E. (2003). *Social causes of psychological distress* (2nd edn.). Somerset, NJ: Aldine Transaction.

Mirowsky, J. and Ross, C. E. (2005). Education, cumulative advantage and health. *Aging International* **30**, 27–62.

Ross, C. E. and Mirowsky, J. (1999). Refining the association between education and health: effects of quantity, credential, and selectivity. *Demography* **36**, 445–460.

Ross, C. E. and Mirowsky, J. (2001). Neighborhood disadvantage, disorder, and health. *Journal of Health and Social Behavior* **42**, 258–276.

Ross, C. E. and Van Willigen, M. (1997). Education and the subjective quality of life. *Journal of Health and Social Behavior* **38**, 275–297.

Ross, C. E. and Wu, C. (1995). The links between education and health. *American Sociological Review* **60**, 719–745.

Seeman, T. A., Crimmins, E., Huang, M.-H., et al. (2004). Cumulative biological risk and socio-economic differences in mortality: MacArthur Studies of Successful Aging. *Social Science & Medicine* **58**, 1985–1998.

Taylor, S. E. and Repetti, R. (1997). What is an unhealthy environment and how does it get under the skin? *Annual Review of Psychology* **48**, 411–447.

Turner, R. J. and Avison, W. R. (2003). Status variations in stress exposure: implications for the interpretation of research on race, socioeconomic status, and gender. *Journal of Health and Social Behavior* **44**, 488–505.

Turner, R. J., Wheaton, B. and Lloyd, D. A. (1995). The epidemiology of social stress. *American Sociological Review* **60**, 104–125.

Wheaton, B. (1985). Models for the stress-buffering functions of coping resources. *Journal of Health and Social Behavior* **24**, 208–229.

Employee Assistance and Counseling

M E Mor Barak
University of Southern California School of Social Work and Marshall School of Business, Los Angeles, CA, USA
D J Travis
University of Southern California School of Social Work, Los Angeles, CA, USA

Glossary

Counseling services The provision of professional advice and guidance utilizing psychological methods or various techniques of the personal interview to guide an employee in a constructive direction that will lead to the development and realization of the individual's potential.

Employee assistance program (EAP) Employer-sponsored counseling, educational, and mental health services that are available to all employees on a confidential and self- or supervisory referral basis.

In-house vs. external employee assistance program (EAP) Services provided by counselors who are employees of the company vs. those provided by an external firm.

Work–family conflict Incompatibility in some aspects of the simultaneous pressures from the work and family domains that makes it difficult to for employees to meet the demands of one or both domains.

Employee assistance and counseling are resources utilized by work organizations to manage employee stress and enhance workplace effectiveness through preventing, identifying, and resolving personal and work-related problems. Employee assistance programs (EAPs), specifically, are employer-sponsored counseling, educational, and mental health services that are available to all employees on a confidential and self- or supervisory referral basis. These programs can offer assessments, referrals, and clinical, preventive, and educational services to employees and their families to aid in managing work and life challenges.

History

EAPs grew out of the 1940s occupational alcoholism prevention programs (OAPs) that focused on alcohol abuse in the workplace. In the 1970s, the scope of services was broadened to include mental health and drug abuse problems (often referred to as broad brush services), hence the development of EAPs. During that time, employers began adopting measures to assess the costs at the individual and organizational level related to alcohol and drug abuse as well as occupational stress and individual and family problems.

In the late 1980s, work organizations also began to consider the overall mental, physical, and emotional well-being of their employees by incorporating preventive mechanisms into the structure of traditional EAPs as well as by developing employee enhancement programs (EEPs). Preventive models focused on stress management and other addictions such as overeating and smoking.

EAPs now tackle employees' work and life challenges and overall well-being involving workplace stress and conflict, relationships and family problems, financial and legal problems, childcare, eldercare, and career counseling. A recent estimate of EAP utilization indicates that more than 80 million individuals within the United States have access to an EAP, an approximate 250% increase from only a decade ago.

Rationale

Recent research reveals that workers' job performance and workplace productivity can be affected by work-related stress, family conflicts, and personal challenges. As an illustration, depression costs $44 billion annually in lost productivity, and substance abuse and mental illness cost $100 billion annually, or $3000 per employee. Hence, employee assistance and counseling provide supports to the employee and the employer, resulting in shared benefits including enhanced employee mental, emotional, and physical well-being, improved job performance, and improved organizational functioning (see **Figure 1**). Employees utilize EAPs and equivalent counseling programs as resources for managing work-related or family/personal stress. For the employer, EAPs help (1) contain health-care costs, (2) provide resources that supplement current organizational support services, (3) demonstrate care for their employees and enhance the work organization's image, (4) prevent or contain potential legal problems, and (5) address labor/organization relations.

EAPs and Stress

EAPs and Job Stress

Employee assistance and counseling services are available to aid in managing stress that is associated

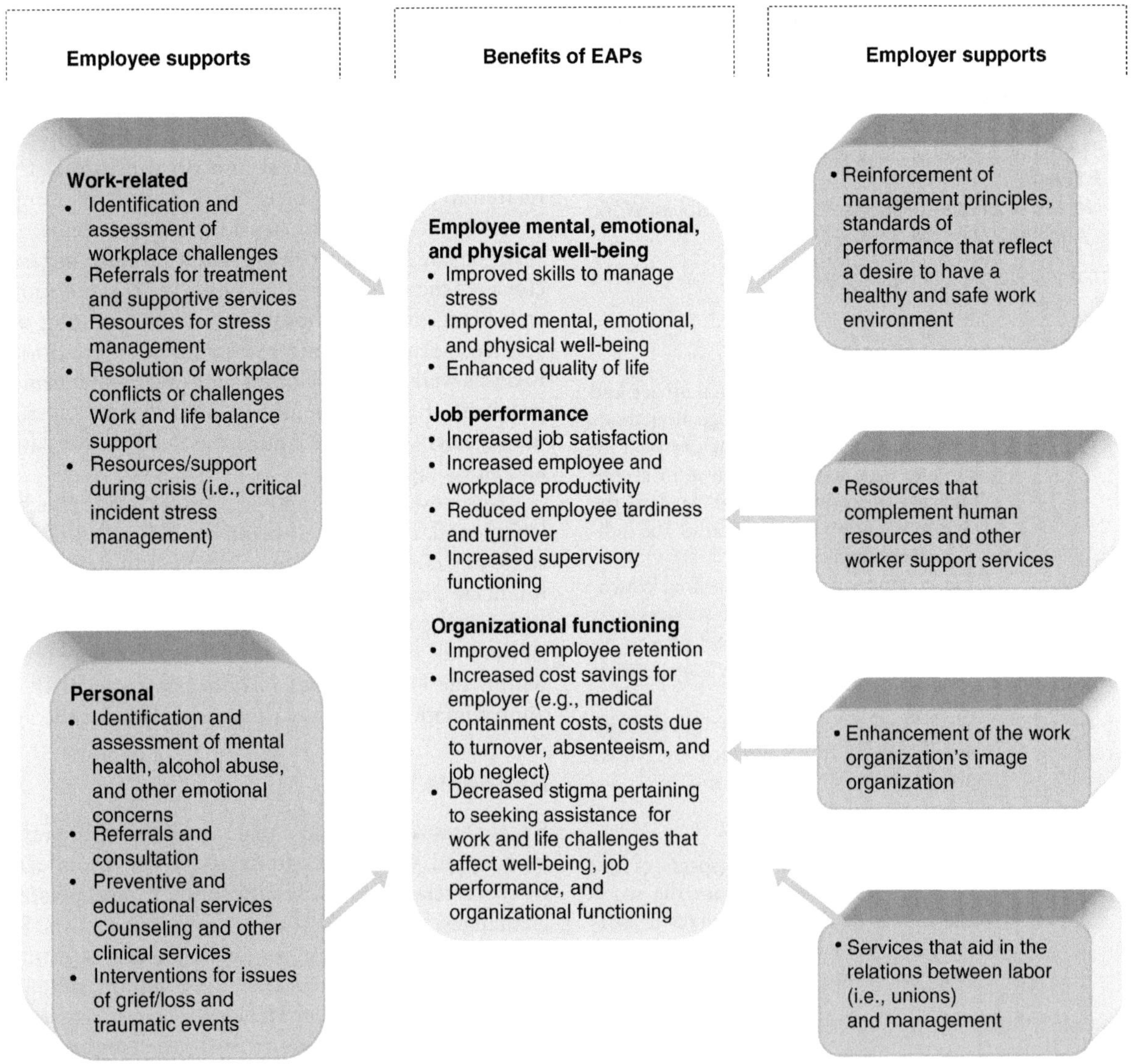

Employee supports
Benefits of EAPs
Employer supports
Work-related
• Identification and assessment of workplace challenges
• Referrals for treatment and supportive services
• Resources for stress management
• Resolution of workplace conflicts or challenges
Work and life balance support
• Resources/support during crisis (i.e., critical incident stress management)
Personal
• Identification and assessment of mental health, alcohol abuse, and other emotional concerns
• Referrals and consultation
• Preventive and educational services
Counseling and other clinical services
• Interventions for issues of grief/loss and traumatic events
Employee mental, emotional, and physical well-being
• Improved skills to manage stress
• Improved mental, emotional, and physical well-being
• Enhanced quality of life
Job performance
• Increased job satisfaction
• Increased employee and workplace productivity
• Reduced employee tardiness and turnover
• Increased supervisory functioning
Organizational functioning
• Improved employee retention
• Increased cost savings for employer (e.g., medical containment costs, costs due to turnover, absenteeism, and job neglect)
• Decreased stigma pertaining to seeking assistance for work and life challenges that affect well-being, job performance, and organizational functioning
• Reinforcement of management principles, standards of performance that reflect a desire to have a healthy and safe work environment
• Resources that complement human resources and other worker support services
• Enhancement of the work organization's image organization
• Services that aid in the relations between labor (i.e., unions) and management

Figure 1 Value of employee assistance and counseling.

with employees' work and life experiences. Counselors and therapists who provide those services (typically social workers, psychologists, and professional counselors) generally operate under the assumption that stress is not necessarily bad and that some stress is a normal part of work and life, but that excessive stress could be detrimental to both emotional and physical health. As such, employees can experience stress in the workplace in several areas, most notably in areas related to their job role and perception of social exclusion. These forms of work-related stress can adversely affect worker outcomes, such as lost job productivity, counterproductive work behaviors, and preventable turnover.

EAPs often address stress on the job by offering individual counseling, stress reduction seminars, or counseling management on how to restructure the work environment or work processes to reduce stress. The experience of job stress is the psychological state that represents an imbalance between peoples' perceptions of the demands placed on them and their ability to cope with those demands. Typically, employees experience too much work (role overload), a conflict between their expectations of their jobs and the actual reality of those jobs (role conflict), and lack of clarity regarding their supervisors' or management's expectations from them (role ambiguity). However, it is not only excessive demands that are the source of job stress but also understimulation, represented by work tasks that are boring, too simple, or not challenging.

Employee assistance services can also offer supportive resources to help employees negotiate perceived stress-related feelings of exclusion within the organization. The inclusion–exclusion continuum reflects the extent to which individuals feel part of important organizational processes that affect their jobs, have access to the organizational decision-making process, and have access to its information networks. Research over the past two decades indicates that exclusion from organizational information networks and from important decision-making processes is a significant problem facing today's diverse workforce. Perceptions of exclusion may play a critical role in explaining the connection between those employees who experience themselves as different from the corporate mainstream and their job stress, well-being, and other worker outcomes (e.g., job satisfaction, productivity, and turnover).

EAPs and Work–Family Life Stress

In the past two decades a new field of workplace service delivery, as well as a new field of scholarly inquiry, have emerged that focus on the stress associated with the need to balance work and family and, more generally, work and personal life. Many workers struggle to negotiate the demands of work with the expectations from their families and life outside of work, which include familial responsibilities such as child care and elder care, activities related to individuals' personal fulfillment, and activities related to community contributions and civic duty. Balancing or integrating the demands of work, family, and life can be associated with specific stress-related outcomes for workers, based on the presence and absence of conflict between their roles. The research on work–family and work–life balance has focused predominantly on the United States and Europe, but in recent years there has been more research on other countries and even some comparative studies that examine the similarity and differences in challenges faced by workers worldwide.

More and more work organizations are introducing work–family or work–life programs as part of, or in addition to, their EAP services. These services focus on the conflicts that employees experience in reconciling their work and family roles. They include individual and family counseling to help employees cope with the stresses associated with, for example, having to care for a sick parent or taking care of a new baby. In addition, work–family or work–life programs include new policies that allow employees to take periods of paid leave for family or personal reasons. More recently, workplace flexibility options have emerged as a way to address conflicts between work and life outside of work, including flexibility in scheduling full-time hours (e.g., compressed work weeks), flexibility in the number of hours worked (e.g., reduced work hours per week or working part of the year), career flexibility with multiple points of entry, exit, and re-entry into the workforce, and the ability to address unexpected and ongoing personal and family needs.

Program Characteristics

Service Delivery Models

There are several different EAP service delivery models, described in the following sections.

Alcohol and drug abuse prevention and treatment vs. broad brush Alcohol and drug abuse prevention programs focus on providing referrals and counseling for employees who are addressing substance abuse problems that can impact the workplace. Broad brush programs essentially focus on an expansive realm of services that aid employees in managing their marriage and family, emotional, financial, and legal problems.

In-house EAP vs. contracted EAP services Some companies choose to provide EAP services internally, by counselors who are themselves employees of the organization, while other companies choose to contract the services from external EAP providers. The latter are firms that provide the entire EAP staff. The advantages of the in-house service delivery model include the counselors having a greater familiarity with the organization's structure and the ability to provide organizational-level interventions when needed (e.g., when the cause of a problem is at the work unit or department level). The advantages of the external EAPs is that they provide a perceived (though not necessarily real) greater level of confidentiality, and sometimes they are less expensive than the in-house services.

Consortium and affiliate models When organizations lack the number of employees (typically fewer than 2000) to financially justify having their own EAP, a consortium model offers an alternative. An EAP consortium is a mutual agreement among organizations that collaborate to maximize resources as opposed to contracting individually. Affiliate models occur when a company has several offices and contracts services; the contractor may use affiliates and subcontractors. The affiliates, in this model, are those EAP providers based on a fee-for-service or case-by-case basis. The goal with the affiliate model is to ensure that all employees are covered as deemed necessary.

Types of Interventions

EAPs provide a range of services from traditional alcohol and drug abuse treatment to holistic interventions

Table 1 EAP interventions and services

Scope	*Examples of EAP interventions and services*
Assessment	Diagnosis of presented problems and treatment plan
Informational	Referrals to appropriate services outside of the EAP
	Consultation and suggestions of solutions
Therapeutic	Counseling
	Therapy (short-term or long-term and family, couple, or individual)
	Clinical services
Preventive	Stress management
	Health and fitness programs
Educational	Training
	Personal development
	Lunchtime seminars
	Newsletters, pamphlets, brochures
Crisis intervention	Critical incident stress debriefings
	Grief/loss/traumatic events
Organizational interventions	Trainings for work groups and leaders/supervisors
	Team building

geared toward stress management, other addictions (e. g.,. eating disorders, smoking cessation), work–life balance, and general well-being. These services can include assessment and referral models (one or two meetings), short-term intervention models (in which the number of meetings may be limited to 6–12 meetings per year), and long-term models (in which the number of meetings is not limited and depends on the needs of the client). Many of the services can be conducted in conjunction with other services to effectively address the employee's problems. **Table 1** provides examples of such interventions and services.

Challenges and Future Directions

The development, management, and delivery of employee assistance and counseling services continue to evolve and reflect the challenges of the contemporary workplace. Cultural and economic shifts, which influence the types and prevalence of employee problems, will affect the future configuration and operation of EAPs. Ultimately, these types of contemporary issues may affect worker productively and performance.

Employers are faced with new challenges related to the increased diversity in the workforce (e.g., gender, age, race, ethnicity, religion, sexual orientation, disability). This diverse workforce has the potential to be more creative and productive than a homogeneous one, but employers have to overcome potential problems related to distrust and miscommunication that are often associated with diversity. EAPs can help by offering organizational diversity assessment and training and team dispute resolution.

The exponential growth in global work arrangements such as international mergers, subsidiaries, call centers, and subcontracting in the past few decades has introduced yet another set of challenges: how do families and communities cope with these new stressful conditions? How do they adjust to the pressures presented by the 24/7 economy? How do individuals cope with the blurring boundaries between work and private time? EAPs will be challenged with expanding their services to adjust to the demands of rapidly changing family and work structures.

Finally, the future of EAPs will also be affected by two conflicting trends in health and mental health care. One trend is motivated by the urgent need to contain the ever-rising health-care costs through contracting out services and using managed care systems that work diligently to contain costs by limiting types of services and supervising the service provision process. The other trend advocates a holistic health-care approach that focuses on treating the whole person by attending to the individual's mental, emotional, and physical well-being. The latter may require more in-house services and, in the short term, may be more costly, though in the long term its preventive aspects may contribute to cost containment. The resolution of these two trends may affect the scope and methods of service delivery that EAPs will provide in the future.

See Also the Following Articles

Job Insecurity: The Health Effects of a Psychosocial Work Stressor; Work–Family Balance; Workplace Stress.

Further Reading

Akabas, S. H. and Kurzman, P. A. (2005). *Work and the workplace.* New York: Columbia Press.

Allen, T. D., Herst, D. E. L., Bruck, C. S. and Sutton, M. (2000). Consequences associated with work-to-family conflict: a review and agenda for future research. *Journal of Occupational Health Psychology* 5, 278–308.

Arthur, A. R. (2000). Employee assistance programmes: the emperor's new clothes of stress management? *British Journal of Guidance and Counseling* 28(4), 549–559.

Berridge, J., Cooper, C. I. and Highley-Marchington, C. (1997). *Employee assistance programmes and workplace counseling.* Chichester, UK: Wiley.

de Croon, E. M., Sluiter, J. K., Blonk, R. W., Broersen, J. P. and Frings-Dresen, M. H. (2004). Stressful work, psychological job strain, and turnover: a 2-year prospective cohort study of truck drivers. *Journal of Applied Psychology* 98(3), 442–454.

Emener, W. G., Hutchison, J. and Richards, M. A. (eds.) (2003). *Employee assistance programs: wellness enhancement programming* (3rd edn.) Springfield, IL: Charles C. Thomas Publisher, LTD.

Kossek, E. E. and Lambert, S. J. (eds.) (2005). *Work and life integration: organizational, cultural, and individual perspectives.* Mahwah, NJ: Lawrence Erlbaum Associates.

Mor Barak, M. E. (2005). *Managing diversity: toward a globally inclusive workplace.* Thousand Oaks, CA: Sage.

Mor Barak, M. E. and Bargal, D. (eds.) (2000). *Social services in the workplace.* New York: Haworth.

Mor Barak, M. E. and Cherin, D. A. (1998). A tool to expand organizational understanding of workforce diversity. *Administration in Social Work* 22(1), 47–65.

Mor Barak, M. E. and Levin, A. (2002). Outside of the corporate mainstream and excluded from the work community: a study of diversity, job satisfaction and well-being. *Community, Work & Family* 5(2), 133–157.

Mor Barak, M. E., Nissly, J. A. and Levin, A. (2001). Antecedents to retention and turnover among child welfare, social work, and other human service employees: what can we learn from past research? A review and meta-analysis. *Social Service Review* 625–661.

Spector, P. E., Cooper, C. L., Poelmans, S., Allen, T. D., O'Driscoll, M., Sanchez, J. I., et al. (2004). A cross-national comparative study of work-family stressors, working hours, and well-being: China and Latin America versus the Anglo world. *Personnel Psychology* 57, 119–142.

Stewart, W. F., Ricci, J. A., Chee, E., et al. (2003). Cost of lost productive work time among US workers with depression. *Journal of the American Medical Association* 289(23), 3135–3144.

Williams, E. S., Konrad, T. R., Scheckler, W. E., Pathman, D. R., et al. (2001). Understanding physicians' intentions to withdraw from practice: the role of job satisfaction, job stress, mental and physical health. *Health Care Management Review* 26(1), 7.

Environmental Stress, Effects on Human Performance

G R J Hockey
University of Sheffield, Sheffield, UK

This is a revised version of the article by G R J Hockey, Encyclopedia of Stress First Edition, volume 2, pp 60–65, © 2000, Elsevier Inc.

Glossary

Compensatory control — A general adaptive response to stress serving to protect high-priority goals from disruption.

Costs — Effort or other resources used to achieve task goals.

Environmental stressors — Identifiable external conditions that pose a threat to the performance of subjective state, such as noise, heat, and time pressure.

Human performance — The effectiveness of behavior in relation to specific task demands and goals, assumed to reflect the operation of underlying mental processes.

Latent degradation — The effects of performance impairment not necessarily manifested in disruption of primary task activities.

Short-term memory (STM) — General label used to describe memory for very recent events, referring to the storage of information over brief periods (typically 10–20 s).

Working memory (WM) — Cognitive system acting as a "mental workspace" for manipulating information necessary for carrying out current processing and problem solving tasks, comprising both storage and attention/control components.

Human performance refers to the effectiveness of task activity in relation to goals. This assumes a focus on the primary mental processes that underlie controlled human action, particularly in tasks requiring the use of memory, attention, decision making, and perceptual-motor skills. A concern with the effects of stress on human performance has a long history in psychology, driven by both practical and theoretical issues. It has been known since the 1970s that the nature of the task is a strong determinant of how performance will be affected; it has also recently become clear that there is a general problem that affects the performance of all tasks. The key to understanding this appears to be to consider the goals that underlie behavior. It is not surprising that goals change under extreme stress away from the current task and toward a concern with bodily states or emergency reactions. In more everyday contexts, this implies a need to examine the strategies used to manage goal-relevant information and the factors that determine changes in goals. This has not always been done in research in this area. In what follows, I discuss the theoretical background to research on stress and performance, review the evidence for different patterns of disruption across various task and performance criteria, and show how an adaptive regulatory perspective enhances our understanding of the nature of the problem.

Theories of Effects of Stressors on Performance

Stressors have traditionally been considered as having one of two kinds of effect on performance: distraction or arousal. Early research on the effects of what we now consider stressors (e.g., loud noises) assumed a broadly distraction kind of theory. In general, apart from transient effects, such experiments were spectacularly unsuccessful in demonstrating any effects on complex performance – including tests of intelligence, memory, and skill. Not until the mid-1950s, with the application of information processing concepts to psychology, did theory have much of a part to play in this kind of research. More recent treatments (triggered by the seminal work of Donald Broadbent and his colleagues) has recognized that the effects of stressors may be masked, or compensated for, by the built-in redundancy and strategy options available to the cognitive system. Broadbent argued that it should be possible to demonstrate the effects of stressors by designing tasks that effectively stretched this regulatory process, for example, by presenting information rapidly and without breaks or by making critical events rare and unpredictable in time and place (e.g., serial reaction and vigilance tasks).

In the distraction theory, environmental events were thought to compete for attention through either their strong stimulus qualities (noise or heat) or their impact on bodily states (causing anxiety and other emotional reactions). In its modern form, the distraction view was developed most fully in Broadbent's influential filter theory. For example, noise was thought to impair task-relevant operations by capturing selective attention. This involuntary attention to the noise source interrupted the effective intake of relevant task information and gave rise to processing errors. The distraction theory is best supported by studies of intermittent noise, which impairs performance in the few seconds following each burst. In general, however, the distraction view has been thought to offer a less convincing explanation of the effects of both continuous noise and of other stressors, such as sleep deprivation, not so readily identified with external events.

As an alternative to distraction theory, the arousal theory of stress and performance was developed in the 1960s following the generally accepted view of the day that arousal was a unitary, nonspecific brain process. The application of arousal theory to stress effects was based mainly on the systematic studies of combined effects of stressors carried out in Cambridge, UK. This made extensive use of the five-choice serial reaction task, in which subjects were required to respond to a continuous stream of lights coming on by tapping one of the five metal plates corresponding to the lights. This task showed impairment under noise and sleep deprivation and improvement when subjects were given incentives to do well. However, performance under noise improved somewhat when subjects were also sleep deprived, whereas incentives made their effects worse. These interactions between stressors were regarded as supporting the arousal theory of stressors because they appeared to show that impairment could be caused by both understimulation (sleep deprivation) and overstimulation (noise). However, the assumptions concerning the nature of arousal could not be convincingly demonstrated independently of the task itself. For example, there is no direct evidence that noise is arousing in a physiological sense, except in terms of the transient startle pattern at the onset. Increased arousal under noise is typically found only when people are carrying out cognitive tasks, and then only when they are concerned to prevent performance decrements occurring. In addition, it is clear from developments in physiological theory that arousal is more complex than previously assumed – more specific and linked to task processes. In sum, it has proved to be inadequate as a general theory of effects of stress.

Patterns of Stressor Impairment

The central approach to the understanding of stress effects presented in this article focuses on the problem of managing the general threat to task goals through adaptive changes in behavior. However, as I mentioned earlier, different stressors also appear to pose specific threats for tasks, depending on their information processing requirements. An analysis of stress effects on performance carried out in the 1980s found specific patterns of decrement across different indicators of performance and strategy. Some stressors were more likely to impairs performance on one kind of task and others on a different kind. For example, loud noise typically impairs performance on tasks that require accuracy, short-term memory (STM), or problem solving. Sleep deprivation causes impairment on tasks that require accuracy, speed, and a high level of selective attention, as well as having more general effects on memory. Both noise and sleep deprivation have effects that are more pronounced under fatigue conditions (when tasks involve long periods of work without breaks). Working in hot conditions has widespread effects on most aspects of performance, especially tasks involving more complex decision making. The effects are related to the exposure time and effective temperature, but, unlike noise, do not appear to increase with time at work.

The set of indicators used in this analysis included general alertness, selectivity of attention, speed versus accuracy, and STM. With changes in cognitive theory over the intervening period and the experience of the effects in real work tasks, some changes to this list are needed. General alertness no longer appears to have strong diagnostic value because it is likely to be involved in all active regulatory behavior. The mechanisms underlying STM have undergone considerable evolution with the development of working memory (WM) theory by Baddeley and colleagues. In addition, there is a need for a new analysis, which takes into account differential effects of regulatory activity. However, even with these caveats, changes in these performance indicators may be seen as a profile of the sorts of information-processing problems that different stress conditions may give rise to. The most general pattern of decrement is associated with environmental factors, such as noise, danger, or social evaluation, that give rise to subjective states of threat or anxiety. This may be regarded as the modal stress pattern involving a subjective state of high activation, high selectivity of attention, a preference for speed over accuracy, and reduced WM function. Decrements are more common on tasks of long duration, especially where the continued use of WM is central to maintaining the flow of the work. Selective attention is normally very effective, unless response is required to a number of different events or subtasks, in which case only the most important may be maintained. A familiar effect of such stressors is narrowed attention, in which the high-priority features of tasks are maintained and secondary aspects are neglected. Such an effect has been observed for a wide range of stress states, including noise, high workload, threat of shock, danger, and most forms of induced anxiety. Other stressors are associated with different kinds of changes. For example, WM appears relatively stable under hot working conditions or with extended work periods. In all cases, however, it has become clear that we cannot separate the underlying effects on cognitive processes from those relating to changes in performance goals or strategies. An increase in reliance on one kind of process may be the result of a strategic reduction in the use of another. Because of this, patterns of stressor effects cannot be discussed without reference to an understanding of what the performer is trying to do when carrying out a task and of what conflicts exist between different goals.

Compensatory Control under Stress

Modern treatments of psychological stress emphasize the cognitive transactions that mediate between stressful events and the adaptive response to them. This appraisal process evaluates the implications of the stressor for both current activities and personal well-being. In terms of performance tasks, this may mean focusing information processing resources more strongly on the task (performance protection) or withdrawing resources in order to combat the stressor itself. This latter reaction is likely to be more effective in reducing the effects on bodily or emotional states, but it inevitably leads to a loss of performance goals. Performance protection is the usual response in everyday situations in which the individual is highly skilled, the task sufficiently important, and the stressor familiar and manageable. Serious disruption is rare for high-priority activities and is usually associated with traumatic events. This is because a compensatory process operates to maintain the primary task goals under the increased threat of disruption, resulting in a reduced response to the control of the emotional state and other competing goals. The increased effort underlying compensatory control is considered to reflect the involvement of the central executive functions responsible for the maintenance of high-level cognitive behavior, as observed in problem solving, reasoning, and all goal maintenance activity. As such, it is a limited resource that inevitably attracts costs when it is overemployed.

On the other hand, we know that decrements are relatively common, especially in laboratory studies or where skill and motivation are low. Within this framework, the specific patterns of decrement outlined earlier may be considered a baseline or default pattern of decrement under different stressors – how performance might be expected to suffer in the absence of compensatory control activity. As an example, consider a pair of studies carried out in Stockholm in the 1980s. They showed that noise impaired performance on an arithmetic task on one occasion but not on another. How can this be understood? The answer is related to motivational factors such as compensatory effort. The investigators also measured the physiological and subjective costs associated with having to work on the task under noise. In the study in which performance was unimpaired, they observed a marked increase in adrenaline and ratings of subjective effort. However, in the case in which performance was disrupted by noise, no such changes were observed. The most satisfactory explanation of this (and other similar) findings is that noise imposes an additional load on our capacity to maintain adequate orientation toward the task. If we can make an additional effort under such circumstances, performance may be protected against disruption, although only at the cost of increased strain in other areas. Alternatively, we may be unwilling (or unable) to make such an effort, in which case we will experience less strain but inevitably suffer a decrement in task performance. Such trade-offs are the routine consequences of having to manage stress and other environmental demands while still carrying out our commitments to external task goals.

Latent Degradation under Stress

Although stress does not always result in any obvious reduction in performance, this should not be taken to mean that there is no threat to task goals. There is now considerable evidence of knock-on effects of performance protection to secondary aspects of behavior, related to both performance and costs; I have referred to these as latent degradation. By reducing the safe working margins of the adaptive control process, these may threaten the integrity of performance – for example, strategies that work only if there are no new problems to deal with. Four kinds of latent degradation may be identified: two performance indices (secondary task decrements and strategy changes) and two cost indices (psychophysiological activation and fatigue aftereffects).

Secondary Task Decrements

Decrements in the secondary aspects of performance are commonly observed in studies of the effects of high workload, providing an indirect measure of increasing load on primary tasks. Such effects have been studied less systematically in assessing threats from environmental stressors, although they are, in fact, also common. One of the best-documented forms of secondary task decrement under stress is the narrowing of attention found in spatially complex tasks. For example, although a central tracking task may be carried out effectively under noise, the detection of signals in the visual peripheral may be impaired. Similar attentional narrowing has been found under both laboratory and field conditions and for a wide range of environmental conditions (noise, heat, anxiety associated with deep sea diving, and threat of shock). This type of decrement may be related to strategy changes because they depend on a shift of priority between task elements.

Strategy Changes

Strategy changes are (usually adaptive) changes in the way that tasks are carried out under stress. One obvious way is to minimize the disruption to primary activities by reducing the time spent on secondary tasks. However, there may also be more subtle changes, involving a shift to less resource-intensive modes of task control, reducing dependency on effort-demanding processes such as WM, which is known to be impaired under stress conditions. Despite their obvious diagnostic value, such effects have not been well studied, partly because of the complex task environments necessary to analyze strategy changes. It has been known for some time that, under periods of difficulty or stress, industrial process operators may shift from an attention-demanding open-loop control (in which whole sequences of actions are guided mainly by the operator's internal mental model) to a simpler closed-loop strategy (in which actions are carried out one at a time, paying more attention to feedback). This may slow the process or fail to make optimal use of available options, but it minimizes the likelihood of serious errors.

A good example of this is a well-known study of French air-traffic controllers, carried out in the 1970s. The controllers adopted a simplified method of dealing with aircraft contacts when they exceeded a comfortable number, but under very high workload they switched from individual plane-by-plane routing instructions to a fixed procedure for all contacts. By minimizing the demands for planning and aircraft management, they reduced the need to involve the vulnerable WM system. The strategy change is adaptive in that secondary goals such as airport schedules and passenger comfort are compromised in the service of the primary goal of safety. A second example is the work of Schönpflug's group in Berlin, which used a simulated office environment to examine decision making in stock control. Under normal conditions, participants typically held background information (on prices, stock levels, etc.) in WM while making a sequence of decisions. However, under time pressure or loud noise, they tended to check lists containing such information before making each decision. Reducing the load on WM helped people to keep decision errors to a minimum, although at the expense of increased time costs. Again, the change is adaptive because accuracy matters more than speed in such work. However, in situations in which speed is also important, the hidden loss of efficiency represents a genuine stress-induced impairment.

Psychophysiological Activation

One of the most reliable costs of the use of increased effort to protect performance is the observation of increased levels of activation. This is particularly true of the physiological systems involved in emergency reactions (e.g., sympathetic and musculoskeletal responses, and responses of the neuroendocrine stress systems). These effects are typically accompanied by changes in subjective reports of emotional and mood states reflecting the affective response to emergency and sustained coping effort. These may be thought of as the unwanted side-effects of the compensatory behavior that helps to maintain primary performance under threat from environmental conditions.

The effect is illustrated in an early study of sleep deprivation, in which decrements in arithmetic computation following a night without sleep were smaller for participants found to have increased muscle tension (interpreted as evidence of greater effort to combat sleepiness and maintain orientation toward the task). This performance–cost trade-off is seen more clearly in several studies of noise effects using more meaningful psychophysiological measures. Noise has been shown to increase heart rate, blood pressure, adrenaline, and subjective effort in tasks in which performance decrement is forestalled. In the Swedish study referred to earlier, two different patterns of arithmetic performance and costs were observed in different experiments. In one, performance was impaired by noise, with no change in levels of adrenaline or effort. In the other, performance was maintained, but adrenaline and effort levels were both greater. Unfortunately, because of the difficulty of obtaining psychophysiological measures under such circumstances, there are few studies within real work contexts, although another Swedish study found that the absence of decrement in work output during an intense period of organizational change was, again, accompanied by a compensatory increase in adrenaline and cognitive effort.

Such effects illustrate the role of compensatory regulation in the protection of performance and may be seen as a trade-off between the protection of the primary performance goal and the level of mental effort that has to be invested in the task. They also indicate that the regulation of effort is at least partially under the control of the individual rather than being an automatic feature of task or environmental conditions.

Fatigue After Effects of Stress

A final form of latent degradation is one that appears only after set tasks have been completed, in terms of decrements on new (and less critical) tasks. Such aftereffects have also been studied very little, and then normally within a workload–fatigue paradigm. However, they are equally appropriate as a response to the sustained effort required to maintain effective levels of work under stressful environmental conditions.

Given its long-recognized importance, work fatigue has been studied extensively since the early days of psychology, although it has proved surprisingly difficult to demonstrate carry-over effects of this kind. Even intensive research programs carried out by the U.S. army failed to find any marked fatigue effects of periods of up to 60 h of continuous work. Holding and others have showed that there are methodological difficulties in the analysis of this apparently straightforward problem. As with the compensatory response to stressors, participants in such experiments appear able to work harder (make more effort) for brief periods to respond to the challenge of any new test, effectively compensating for any reduction in capacity. However, when tired people are provided with alternative ways of carrying out the postwork test they are more likely to choose one requiring low effort, even though it entails more risk of error. Similar results of high workload and stressful jobs have been found for driving examiners, bus drivers, and junior doctors. This approach to fatigue reveals it to be a state in which there is a shift toward preferring activities requiring less effort or use of WM. So far, there has been little direct research on this form of decrement with laboratory stressors, although similar effects have been found for noise and high workload.

The link between stress and fatigue is a very strong one. It is likely that actively managing stress in order to protect performance leads directly to fatigue, so that recovery is necessary before we can function even when the stressor is no longer present. Recent work carried out in the Netherlands suggests that fatigue impairs the effectiveness of the executive control system that maintains the activation of tasks in working memory, triggering both the withdrawal of effort and compensatory changes in information processing strategy. At present, we have no direct evidence of the brain processes involved in this stressor → control/effort → fatigue chain, but it is currently being addressed in a number of laboratories. Clearly, a better understanding of the physiological basis of the control of stress during task performance will help us manage work and other tasks more effectively, as well as informing our approach to the design and management of the working environment.

Further Reading

Frankenhaeuser, M. (1986). A psychobiological framework for research on human stress and coping. In: Appley, M. H. & Trumbell, R. (eds.) *Dynamics of stress: physiological, psychological and social perspectives*, pp. 101–116. New York: Plenum.

Hancock, P. A. and Desmond, P. A. (eds.) (2001). *Stress, workload, and fatigue*. Mahwah, NJ: Lawrence Erlbaum.

Hockey, G. R. J. (1986). Changes in operator efficiency as a function of environmental stress, fatigue and circadian rhythms. In: Boff, K., Kaufman, L. & Thomas, J. P. (eds.) *Handbook of perception and performance* (vol. 2), pp. 1–44. New York: John Wiley.

Hockey, G. R. J. (1997). Compensatory control in the regulation of human performance under stress and high workload: a cognitive energetical framework. *Biological Psychology* 45, 73–93.

Hockey, G. R. J., Gaillard, A. W. K. and Burov, O. (eds.) (2003). *Operator functional state: the assessment and prediction of human performance degradation in complex tasks*. Amsterdam: IOS Press.

Indigenous Societies

W W Dressler
University of Alabama, Tuscaloosa, AL, USA

This is a revised version of the article by W A Dessler, Encyclopedia of Stress First Edition, volume 2, pp 558–564, © 2000, Elsevier Inc.

Glossary

Acculturation — The process by which a society is culturally influenced by another society.

Culture-bound syndromes — Local idioms for the expression of distress, consisting of socially recognized illness categories that have no acknowledged counterpart in Western biomedicine.

Cultural consonance — The degree to which an individual approximates in his or her own behavior the prototypes for behavior encoded in shared cultural models.

Extended kin support systems — Systems in which help or assistance is most appropriately sought from individuals who are related by common ancestry or marriage.

Indigenous societies — Societies that are native to a particular locale, in which people speak a distinctive language and have a distinctive social heritage and which are often technologically less complex. Usually, the way of life of the people is on the periphery of the major world industrial societies. Indigenous societies can also be referred to as traditional societies.

Modernization — A special case of acculturation in which an indigenous society is undergoing economic change or development.

Status incongruence — A discrepancy between an individual's aspirations for social status or prestige and his or her resources for actually achieving those aspirations.

Introduction

An indigenous or traditional society is characterized as native to a specific region, with a distinctive language and way of life. Also, the way of life of the people is peripheral to global capitalist market systems. This does not mean that such a society is unaffected by global market systems; in fact, one major source of stress in indigenous societies is the impact of economic change emanating from those larger systems. Nor does this mean that an indigenous society cannot be embedded within a modern, industrial society (e.g., Native Americans). Rather, in an indigenous society, culture and related systems of social organization are structured more in terms of local context and local systems of meaning, and less in terms of the middle-class values of industrial society. Understanding stress and its effects in indigenous societies requires an examination of both social arrangements that generate stresses within the indigenous social structure and the way in which traditional culture and social structure interact with outside influences to generate stresses.

Stress in Unacculturated Indigenous Societies

Anthropologists conventionally describe the relative degree of external influence on a society or community along a continuum of acculturation. A society that is relatively unacculturated or traditional has been minimally influenced by processes of modernization. Usually this means that households tend to practice a mix of economic pursuits for subsistence (i.e., raising food directly for consumption within the household) and for exchange in local markets. With respect to material lifestyles, although there is some access to imported consumer goods, these often are primarily related to subsistence activities (e.g., agricultural implements, outboard motors). Most goods consumed by a household are produced locally. What wage labor exists is usually within the community, and there is little formal education. Social relationships tend to be dominated by kinship. Systems of kinship can range from large groups formed around descent from a common ancestor (or unilineal descent groups) to somewhat more loosely structured kindreds that are like large ego-centered social networks. Finally, belief systems reflect local meanings and understandings, even when there have been modernizing influences (e.g., missionaries).

Patterns of morbidity and mortality within traditional societies provide one clue to patterns of stress in those societies. Generally speaking, rates of high blood pressure, coronary artery disease, stroke, and cancer tend to be very low. In traditional societies, patterns of morbidity and mortality tend to be dominated by infectious and parasitic disease, especially in childhood, and by trauma in adulthood. Although any generalizations must be tempered by reference to local ecological conditions, in many traditional societies life expectancy beyond 5 years of age is comparable to life expectancy in industrial societies, and in the aged in these societies there is little evidence of the kind of pathologies (e.g., atherosclerosis) associated with aging in industrial societies.

What has been most illuminating in the study of stress in unacculturated societies is the study of culture-bound syndromes. Culture-bound syndromes are local idioms of distress. They can be thought of as culturally appropriate ways of experiencing and expressing distress arising from stressful social relationships. Some attempts have been made to equate the culture-bound syndromes with Western psychiatric diagnoses, but recent evidence indicates that there is not a direct correspondence between culture-bound syndromes and biomedical psychiatric diagnoses; it is probably more useful to think of culture-bound syndromes and Western psychiatric diagnoses as comorbid.

A classic example of a culture-bound syndrome is *susto* in Latino societies of Central and South America. The individual suffering from *susto* experiences a loss of energy, difficulty in maintaining customary activities, frequent spells of crying, and diffuse somatic symptoms such as loss of appetite and sleep disturbance. As the name in Spanish implies, *susto* is attributed to a sudden fright (e.g., seeing a snake), at which time the soul of the individual leaves the body and wanders freely.

Research has shown that the distribution of *susto* is socially patterned. The prevalence is higher in females, tends to increase with age, and tends to be higher in relatively poorer communities. Furthermore, the greatest risk of *susto* has been found among persons experiencing difficulty in enacting common social role expectations. This usually arises from a lack of specific kinds of social resources (e.g., not having a large kinship network) that can be called on in carrying out expected role obligations (such as contributions to community work groups). Similar findings have been obtained in research on other culture-bound syndromes such as *ataques de nervios* in Puerto Rico, *debilidad* in the Andean highlands, heart illness in Iran, and *nervos* in Brazil. Culture-bound syndromes occur when individuals are low in cultural consonance; that is, they are unable to approximate in their own behaviors the prototypes for behaviors that are encoded in widely shared cultural models.

The experience of a culture-bound syndrome is important in two respects. First, it makes meaningful and intelligible the experience of social stress both to the person suffering the stress and to his or her social network. Second, in many societies, there are cultural practices, including healing rituals and participation in religious organizations, that deal directly with the syndrome and the underlying difficulties in social relationships. The aim is to mend the tear in the fabric of social relationships and hence end the individual's suffering.

The existence of these beliefs and practices that are helpful in ameliorating cultural stresses may in part account for patterns of morbidity and mortality in indigenous societies. As noted previously, the diseases conventionally associated with stress in industrial societies are relatively less important in indigenous societies. Also, in most cases an increase of blood pressure with age is not observed in indigenous societies. Other patterns of disease distribution that are taken for granted in industrial societies are not observed in traditional societies. One of the more striking of these is the association of blood pressure with African descent ethnicity. While it is assumed that persons of African descent have higher blood pressures, in fact this is true primarily for those of African descent in the Western hemisphere, and more specifically in societies in which Africans had formerly been enslaved. So, for example, when communities of African descent are compared, communities in Africa have the lowest average blood pressures, communities in the West Indies have intermediate average blood pressures, and African American and African Brazilian communities have the highest average blood pressures. Recent findings show also that *quilombo* or refugee communities descended from escaped slaves in isolated areas of Brazil have low average blood pressures and exhibit little increase of blood pressure with age.

These patterns suggest two things. First, there may be a relatively higher level of social integration in indigenous societies, along with practices that help to moderate the impact of social stressors, that account for the lower prevalence of conditions and diseases associated with stress in industrial societies. Second, the process of social change leading to the modern industrial state may itself generate profound social stresses that contribute to the distinctive pattern of morbidity and mortality in those societies.

At the same time, it is important not to romanticize life in indigenous societies, in the sense of overemphasizing social integration and cohesion, because stresses will be generated within any system of social relationships. What is important to specify across different cultural contexts is the process by which social stresses are generated and the ability of indigenous support systems to deal with those stresses.

Promising results in this regard are emerging from research on hormones and neurotransmitters associated with the stress process. Newer techniques of data collection under difficult field conditions, along with techniques for the analysis of those data, are beginning to show how variation in social behavior within traditional societies is associated with inter- and intra-individual variation in stress hormones, which in turn is associated with acute illness. For example, research in a peasant village in the West Indies has shown that men who are perceived by their peers to emulate the ideals of manhood in this community have lower circulating levels of cortisol. Similarly, children growing up in families that are closer to the cultural ideal of the family have lower circulating cortisol levels and experience fewer acute illnesses. This research, coupled with research on local idioms of distress, suggests that stresses in unacculturated societies are deeply embedded in the system of social relationships that organizes everyday life.

Stress and Acculturation in Indigenous Societies

Societies that are undergoing acculturation are those that are being influenced by other social and cultural systems. In the study of stress and disease, the effect of modern industrial societies on local sociocultural systems has been of particular interest. There is considerable imbalance in this type of acculturation, because of the unequal power and influence that modern industrial states exert on traditional societies. The terms modernization and development have been used to describe this kind of influence.

Modernization in traditional societies was initiated by colonial expansion and has been particularly prominent since World War II and related processes of globalization. This influence has not been inadvertent. The aim has been to take advantage of both physical and social resources in developing societies.

These changes have had large effects on local social systems, including a transition from subsistence occupations to wage labor occupations, the replacement of indigenous languages by European languages, increased urbanization, increased emphasis on formal education, decreased emphasis on traditional social relationships, especially kinship, and substantial changes in indigenous belief systems. Everyday life can change at a rapid pace in modernizing contexts, the result being a stressful lack of consonance between traditional culture and the demands of modern life.

Specific and general aspects of this modernization process have been found to be associated with increasing rates of chronic diseases. Urbanization has been found to be associated with increasing rates of hypertension, independent of changes in diet and physical activity. Some investigators have used summary measures of acculturation both for individuals and for communities. When communities are ranked along a continuum of traditional, intermediate, and modern (depending on aggregate characteristics of the population by the variables noted previously), rates of hypertension, obesity, diabetes, and coronary artery disease consistently increase in communities with higher levels of acculturation or modernization. Also, daily circulating levels of hormones such as cortisol appear to increase in association with acculturative stress.

The results have been somewhat less consistent using measures of acculturation operationalized at the level of the individual. The pattern can still be observed in many studies, but the strength and the consistency of the associations are not as great. This has led some researchers to speculate that the linear model of stress and acculturation is not specified well enough to describe the process at the individual level.

Because the general model of stress and acculturation has not worked very well at the level of the individual, researchers have adapted the stress model, as it has been developed for European and American populations, and applied it to communities experiencing change and development. A major challenge in this research has been to identify factors that generalize across different cultural contexts and to distinguish those from factors that are culturally specific. There is emerging evidence to suggest that at least one set of social stressors generalizes across modernizing societies, primarily because these stressors are generated by the modernization process itself. In most societies undergoing modernization, there is an increased availability of Western consumer goods. Frequently the ownership of these goods becomes highly valued as symbols of status or prestige, often supplanting traditional indicators of higher status. This by itself contributes to the climate of change in a modernizing community. In addition, however, aspirations for the lifestyles of the Western middle class can quickly outstrip the ability of a developing economy to provide the kinds of jobs and salaries necessary to maintain such a lifestyle. Therefore, a kind of status incongruence can occur, in which the desire to attain and maintain a Western middle-class lifestyle exceeds an individual's economic resources for such a lifestyle. This kind of status incongruence has been found to be related to psychiatric symptoms, high blood pressure, elevated serum lipids, the risk of diabetes, and immunological status in developing societies in Latin America, the Caribbean, and Polynesia.

Resources for coping with stressors have been found to be more culturally variable. Social support systems are a good case in point. Social support can be defined as the emotional and practical assistance an individual believes is available to him or her during times of felt need; the social network in which this assistance is available is the social support system. In research in Europe and North America, generally speaking, emphasis has been placed on the nature of the assistance or social support transactions, rather than on who might provide that assistance. There is a growing body of cross-cultural research indicating that, in many societies, who provides the assistance is critical in determining the relationship between social support and health. This is probably a reflection of a continuing importance of kinship in defining who is and who is not an appropriate individual with whom to enter into a social relationship.

For example, in Latin American societies people have traditionally lived in large extended families organized around a father and his married sons (known as a patrilineal extended family). In addition to these extended family relationships, there is a social practice known as *compadrazgo*, through which individuals, especially men, establish formal, kinship-like relationships with unrelated persons (known as fictive kinship). The term *compadrazgo* literally means co-parenthood, and this carries the expectation of mutual support. These ties of fictive kinship are used to establish economically and politically important alliances. Research has shown that men who perceive greater amounts of support from both their extended and their fictive kin have lower blood pressures. Women are expected to restrict themselves to the household and domestic duties. Not surprisingly, with respect to health status, women benefit primarily from support available within the household. These studies show that the definition and effects of social supports are closely related to cultural and social structural factors and can only be understood within that context.

Other forms of stress resistance show similar differences cross-culturally, although the evidence is not quite as consistent as with social support. For example, in European and North American studies, a direct action coping style has been found to be helpful in moderating the effects of stressful events or circumstances. In this style of coping, attempting to directly confront and alter stressful circumstances contributes to better health status. In some research in traditional societies, this same relationship has been observed. In others, the opposite effect has been observed, i.e., a direct action coping style actually exacerbates distress and poor outcomes. In the specific case of this coping style, this probably has to do with the actual resources available to individuals and families in coping with stressors. When social and economic resources are meager at best, the belief that an individual can truly change the circumstances that are often thrust upon him- or herself may, in the long run, be deleterious.

A major source of stress in societies undergoing modernization is the increase in socioeconomic inequity that accompanies modernization. Generally speaking, the distribution of wealth becomes more unequal, resulting in marked social stratification, whereas previously such stratification was, if not absent, at least muted. Recent studies point to the effects of such stratification on cultural consonance as a potent source of stress. The capacity of an individual to achieve higher cultural consonance is severely compromised by lower socioeconomic status. Lower cultural consonance has been found to be associated with higher blood pressure and psychological distress and to mediate the effects of socioeconomic status in contexts of modernization. The inability to act on these widely shared cultural models is a potent source of stress in developing societies.

Stress and Migration

The other way in which social and cultural change can influence indigenous communities is through migration. This century has seen remarkable movements of people from traditional societies to North America and Western Europe, along with internal migration within developing societies that takes migrants into cosmopolitan urban centers in their own societies. Rarely can migration be considered an individual matter. Rather, it is much more common for entire communities of migrants to become established in their host country. This usually occurs because migration follows patterns established through social networks, especially kinship networks. Individuals and households take advantage of kin-based social support systems established in host countries in order to establish themselves there.

Research suggests that a similar pattern of stress and response develops in cases of migration like that observed in developing societies. That is, migrants come to the new setting with aspirations for a new life, aspirations that are reinforced in host countries through the depiction of middle-class lifestyles in advertising and other media forms. At the same time, migrants typically occupy the lowest levels of socioeconomic status in their host countries. Therefore, the ability of the migrant to amass the economic resources necessary to achieve a middle-class lifestyle is severely compromised. This status incongruence again has been found to be associated with chronic disease risk factors such as blood pressure and glucose levels.

Patterns of social support that can help an individual to cope with this kind of social stressor will often again be found in the kin support system. There are, however, several additional complications. First, kin support systems will often be fragmented. Only some people will migrate, not entire support systems. This can mean that some households and individuals are socially isolated, lacking even the most basic social supports. This can also mean that a large burden can be placed on a support system that is fragmented, and that the resulting demands for support are simply too much for the system to bear. Second, the migrant, especially to North America, is entering a highly competitive and individualistic society. The kinds of mutual rights and obligations entailed by kinship have ceased to be recognized as strongly, for example, in the United States as in traditional societies in Latin America or Southeast Asia. Therefore, in some specific situations, the kin support system can come to be a source of stress and tension, as opposed to a resource for resisting stress.

The complications entailed here are illustrated by migrants from Samoa to northern California. Traditionally organized into large extended kin groups represented by chiefs, Samoans have transplanted their social organization to some U.S. urban centers. Traditionally, the chief (or *matai*) controls economic decision making for the entire extended family. In the American urban setting, however, the economic demands of daily life for an individual household can conflict with the decisions made for the extended family, causing this traditional form of social organization to become a source of stress. At the same time, within the larger extended family, core systems of kin-based social support have emerged, especially involving networks of adult siblings. Individuals and households with a strong support system of this kind have better health status in spite of social stressors such as status incongruence. This specific case illustrates the importance of understanding the adaptation of migrants in a host society in relation to their traditional cultural context, as well as the demands of the new social setting.

Some research on migrants from the developing world has shown the long-term effects of major life events experienced by families in the society of origin. This has been observed in immigrants from Latin America and Southeast Asia who have been exposed to protracted civil war and related conflicts. For example, it was found that persons who had had relatives kidnapped or murdered by nonmilitary death squads in Guatemala had continuing high levels of anxiety and depression years after the event. Similarly, anxiety and depression levels in migrants from Southeast Asia to the United States were associated with time spent in refugee camps, independently from other stressors and demographic control variables. These major crises associated with large-scale political events and circumstances can have effects that continue well after the initial, acute stages.

Conclusion

The study of stress and indigenous societies has helped to illuminate various aspects of the stress process. Perhaps the most important has been the clear demonstration of the link between the stress process and the social and cultural context in which individuals and families live. When stressors and resistance resources are examined only within a single cultural context, it can appear as if individual differences in exposure to stressors or in access to resistance resources are the only key to understanding the process. What is lost is the recognition that what counts as a stressor or a resistance resource is itself a function of the cultural context and related social influences. Furthermore, the relationship between stressors, resources, and outcomes can also be modified by social and cultural context. Comparing the stress process in different cultural contexts has been integral to revealing this aspect of the process.

Future research must be explicitly comparative in scope in order to expand on findings produced thus far. For example, research in developing societies suggests that the most important stressors in those societies are actually a function of the development process itself, such as status incongruence. Put differently, this aspect of the stress process is comparable across different settings. On the other hand, the most important resources for resisting stress appear to be specific to the local setting, as in the way in which systems of social support are structured by the existing systems of social organization. Continuing to refine these studies, including better measurements of the physiological dimensions of stress, will increase our understanding of human adaptation.

See Also the Following Articles

Cultural Factors in Stress; Cultural Transition; Economic Factors and Stress; Health and Socioeconomic Status; Industrialized Societies; Minorities and Stress; Social Capital; Social Status and Stress; Social Support.

Further Reading

Decker, S., Flinn, M., England, B. G., et al. (2003). Cultural congruity and the cortisol stress response among Dominican men. In: Wilce, J. M., Jr. (ed.) *Social and cultural lives of immune systems*, pp. 147–169. London and New York: Routledge.

Dressler, W. W. (1994). Cross-cultural differences and social influences in social support and cardiovascular disease. In: Shumaker, S. A. & Czajkowski, S. M. (eds.) *Social support and cardiovascular disease*, pp. 167–192. New York: Plenum Publishing.

Dressler, W. W. (1999). Modernization, stress and blood pressure: new directions in research. *Human Biology* **71**, 583–605.

Dressler, W. W. (2004). Culture, stress and cardiovascular disease. In: Ember, C. R. & Ember, M. (eds.) *The encyclopedia of medical anthropology*, pp. 328–334. New York: Kluwer Academic/Plenum Publishers.

Dressler, W. W. and Bindon, J. R. (2000). The health consequences of cultural consonance. *American Anthropologist* **102**, 244–260.

Flinn, M. V. and England, B. G. (1997). Social economics of childhood glucocorticoid stress response and health. *American Journal of Physical Anthropology* **102**, 33–54.

Janes, C. R. (1990). *Migration, social change and health.* Stanford, CA: Stanford University Press.

McDade, T. W. (2001). Lifestyle incongruity, social integration, and immune function among Samoan adolescents. *Social Science and Medicine* **53**, 1351–1362.

Panter-Brick, C. and Worthman, C. W. (eds.) (1999). *Hormones, health, and behavior.* Cambridge: Cambridge University Press.

Rubel, A. J., O'Nell, C. W. and Ardon, R. C. (1984). *Susto: a folk illness.* Berkeley and Los Angeles, CA: University of California Press.

Minorities and Stress

I Mino
Harvard University, Cambridge, MA, USA
W E Profit
Los Angeles, CA, USA
C M Pierce
Harvard University, Cambridge, MA, USA

This is a revised version of the article by I Mino, W E Profit, and C M Pierce, Encyclopedia of Stress First Edition, volume 2, pp 771–776, © 2000, Elsevier Inc.

Glossary

Culture — Refers to the dominant set of symbolic codes (linguistic, moral, aesthetic) and material practices (dietary, behavioral) that characterize a group. Culture may refer to an entire society's codes and practices, as when reference is made to the American or Japanese culture.

Deculturated — When people lose their culture or cannot use it because of changed circumstances.

Discrimination — A negating selection and differential comparison not based on merit.

Ethnicity — Refers to the particular reference group for individuals with a shared heritage, e.g., Puerto Rican, American Jewish. Some reference groups may be voluntary, such as those based on religion. Others may be involuntarily ascribed to the persons, such as those based on race.

Minority — A part of a population, numerically less than 50%, differing from others in some characteristics and often subjected to different treatment.

Prejudice	An injurious and intolerant preconceived judgment.
Racism	Intentional or unintentional bias directed at individuals or groups based upon notions of the superiority or inferiority of skin color.
Stress	In minority communities, stress occurs when an individual or group's resources are overextended, even to the point of causing paralysis, apprehension, disintegration, and ineffectiveness from perceived and/or actual duress and assaults from the majority community.

Basic Issues

The basic issues in discussing minorities and stress include defining minority, differentiating the individual's stress from the stress of his or her minority group, and deciding which minority variables are best studied.

Who Is a Minority?

Everyone can claim multiple minority memberships. In fact, an individual may only or best be described in terms of such memberships. For instance, there are over 6000 languages in the world. Everyone's native language is a minority language. No one can claim majority status in terms of nationality, age, occupation, religion, avocation, or talent. Some minority memberships bring honor, others dishonor. Minority memberships may be forced or sought. They can be voluntary or involuntary. Many memberships are visible, often relating to appearance, including bodily features, uniforms, and insignia. Language usage can suggest a minority status. However, many minority memberships are invisible and can even be kept secret, such as migrant status, transnational allegiance, racial identity, and political and social affiliations.

Cultural and social forces determine the saliency of minority memberships. Humans create hierarchies, which in turn breed class distinctions, whereby minorities are made through a process of exclusion or inclusion. Rules of membership can be flexible or rigid, fluid or static. In a given community one might be in the most favored economic group but the least favored social group. Many minority memberships find favor or disfavor from legal regulations.

No matter which minority memberships one has, there are two conditions that must be negotiated for each minority membership. On the one hand, an accommodation for being acculturated and/or deculturated is made. On the other hand, some people or agency has to accept you as a member of the group. Such certification, written or unwritten, can be meticulous or arbitrary. The evaluation may not be accurate, complete, or satisfying to either the assessor or the assessed. Furthermore, certification of legitimacy may vary from the vantage point of various individuals, groups, and organizations.

Most individuals probably give little thought to most of their minority memberships. Therefore, they have not rank-ordered them. Yet, they are aware that the saliency and importance in their lives for any such membership is in a constant state of flux. The importance of a minority membership depends on the combination of specific, general, immediate, and far-flung circumstances at any moment and place.

These ever-shifting interpersonal interactions and intrapersonal considerations mean that in some sense an individual's minority status is situational. Furthermore, the situation depends both on what the individual perceives and on what other persons and groups perceive, even when there is agreement about exactly what minority membership is being scrutinized. Misperceptions between parties can range from being innocuous to being life-threatening. A common cause for misperceptions comes from different opinions about the speed, type, and quantity of acculturation. Also, views may differ significantly about how much a person or group is acculturated, should be acculturated, or can be acculturated.

Seldom is it possible to address these misperceptions among parties without the withering burden of stereotypical thinking by all participants. Thus, an obstacle in contemplating or negotiating a minority or majority issue is that all parties have confusion about what is unique to the individual versus what is a stereotype about a collective group.

The importance of and investment in any minority membership varies from person to person and even from time to time, whether or not one is a member of the in-group. Therefore, even with unequivocal certainty that one is a minority or one is dealing with a minority, the same stressors do not exert uniform force among the actors. Everyone attaches different valences to any minority status, even those that occupy his or her most intense concern. Furthermore, it is usually not possible to ascertain how much any participant identifies with, accepts, or knows about any minority membership that is under discussion.

Is Stress the Same for the Individual and the Group?

Stress results when resources are overextended and overwhelmed. There is the threat of dissolution with accompanying fears of abandonment and inability to escape. Stress is the reciprocal of support. Theoretically, perfect biological, sociological, and psychological support would equal no stress. Stress may be acute, chronic, or intermittent, with dimensions of intensity and duration.

Individuals in a group under stress will have varying perceptions and adjustments. These differences are mediated by both existing background factors and factors peculiar to the stress. For instance, age, state of health, prior relevant experience, and faith are examples of attributes that help govern response to stress.

The number and general condition of a group under stress, as well as the quality of its leadership and its ability to be cohesive and cooperative, are important determinants of the group's outcome. Resourcefulness and a fierce will to survive increase the odds for a favorable outcome. The ability to take decisive, independent action is important.

In groups under stress, behavior of individuals speaks to the important aspect of group morale. Among such behaviors are the willingness to share, carefulness never to endanger the group, and the ability to perform multiple tasks.

Some individuals in any group thrive better than others. This seems true even when all the participants have similar backgrounds and quality of health. These individuals, for whatever reasons, may have more tolerance for uncertainty and ambiguity. Likewise, they may be more able to consider the consequences of the uncontrollable, the unpredictable, and the unexpected, with a more sanguine philosophy. In a mundane extreme environment such as a racial group living under oppression, such individuals may be more accepting of high risk and low reward, as the price for their own and their group's survival. Such persons are the group's everyday heroes, who demonstrate the greatest hope in the group that relief and amelioration are in the future.

Stressful events, due to their limited duration and more discrete circumstances, may be easier to study than stressful backgrounds. Groups and individuals in a railroad crash may be more easily understood and supported than individuals undergoing daily stress. In stressful events the individuals are more conscious of and willing to work for the common survival of the group. This shared specific stressful event will become another minority membership for each participant.

However, individual minority background experiences are filled with so much randomness, variability, and strategy that they are not easily delineated for study. There is a wide range of responses by individual members exposed to the same general trauma. Proximate factors such as personal loss and pain, differences in exactly what was witnessed, and the quantity of available and accessible resources required are never identical. This alone determines a plethora of heterogeneous responses by minority individuals under stress.

Which Minority Variables Are Best Studied?

The great bulk of minority studies are performed on populations considered disadvantaged. They verify in detail that, in general, life is more terrible for these subjects. The data are abundant in this verification, whether addressing health disparities, inequalities in the law, unfair housing and employment, discrepancies in educational opportunity and achievement, harshness in the criminal justice system, insensitivity to the needs of children, etc. The studies focus on vulnerable populations and indicate negative patterns of service, response, and rates of problems. They document that under all manner of geographic, demographic, and political climates these minorities fare poorly.

There is an awareness of, but underpublished interest in, the strengths of individuals in these groups. The strengths the groups had to have in order to survive are less emphasized. Probably methodologies have not evolved that can capture the extensiveness of life events that permit and sustain the host of strengths that differentiate disadvantaged minority people.

A related issue is the huge thrust on aspects of resiliency in these populations, without much consideration of resistance. Studies of resilience imply posttraumatic phenomena. Resistance inquiries seek to understand the defenses against the offenses delivered to the disadvantaged populations, in which trauma continues to accumulate but is deflected, minimized, or diluted.

Disadvantaged Minorities

Social, cultural, economic, and political pressures determine what minority memberships are designated as disadvantaged. They may share features as the result of such designation, but each majority community would elect, in its own manner, which groups are targeted and what form of disenfranchisement and handicap is appropriate.

General Characteristics

A society may have written and unwritten rules that designate a group as disadvantaged. Such groups are disenfranchised in numerous ways. It is permitted and expected that the group will be abused and exploited. They occupy the margins of the society, often fractionated and segregated. The groups are likely to be the source of both amusement and wrath for the general population. While given substantially less in the community, it is demanded that they do more for less reward.

Petitions for succor by the disadvantaged prompt exasperation, perplexity, and astonishment. Social machinery is elaborated and sustained that is designed to control, dominate, and disrespect the unworthies. As such, the designated disenfranchised group struggles for its security, safety, and livelihood.

The disadvantaged are tyrannized and easily disregarded, discounted, and trivialized. Even so, they are feared as social or economic competitors. Regardless of their powerlessness, they are dismissed as unproductive noncontributors. They may be resented on grounds of their standards and values. They are given blame but little sympathy for an improper identity. Often they are accused of inviting their own catastrophe. In many cases, such as being female or having colored skin, there is no way the person can banish that identifier.

An individual member of a disadvantaged minority may live a lifetime with little or no direct, overt discrimination. Of course, many are victims of hatred, including physical assault, destruction of possessions, deliberate neglect, and even death.

More common are everyday minor, but cumulative, aggressions and insults. For instance, a White couple approaches a well-dressed Black male in a luxury hotel lobby and requests a taxi. They assume, incorrectly, that the man is an employee. The lifelong toll from these microaggressions, both physiologically and psychologically, remains unstudied.

An abundance of comparative data demonstrates the hardship and adversity suffered by disadvantaged minorities. For instance, between 1996 and 2002, the gap between American White and Black wealth grew from 10:1 to 14:1. In the United States, White family wealth now is 14 times the median net worth of Black families. Blacks make twice as many emergency room and outpatient visits as Whites. They make a third fewer visits to a doctor's office, however. In 2003, the percentage of Whites with advanced degrees was twice that of Blacks with advanced degrees. The same numbers hold in the comparison of White and Black college graduates.

There are clear burdens and risks imposed on groups designated as disadvantaged. In general, they are treated unfairly, and their efforts to improve their conditions generate a significant portion of the world's stress and violence.

The historical circumstances of each country determine which groups are disadvantaged and what efforts are made to promote intergroup peace and prosperity. In the United States, as elsewhere, there are numerous disadvantaged minorities. Due to demographic considerations, the most important issue for the United States in the twenty-first century may relate to disadvantaged minorities. It is expected that during this century Whites will become the minority population. The reduced proportion of Whites probably will be accompanied by significant alterations in the influence and hegemony of Whites. How Whites, especially White males, respond to this shift, may be the defining activity of the United States in this century.

Typological Classification

Any classification scheme is both arbitrary and limited. It follows that there can be no complete agreement, since every citizen can use his or her own system. Overall, in the United States, those generally considered by the general public to be disadvantaged minority groups meet a few broad criteria. First, there is evidence, usually with academic credibility, that the designated status does bring uncommon burdens to both the designated member and the general society. Second, the designated minority usually has a long and continuous history regarding getting legal relief from specified ills. Third, in the view of the public, sometimes including members of the minority itself, the designated group inspires fear, requires restraint, and often is deserving of mild to severe punitive actions.

There are those who are constitutionally handicapped. People are born into this category. These include women as well as selected racial/ethnic groups. The groups selected by the United States government include Blacks, Hispanics, Asians, and Native Americans.

The other large category, which most of the public considers disadvantaged, makes up a disparate miscellany. In this general group are migrants, the disabled, criminals, religious and cult community groups, especially those distant from core Christian organizations, and people with a variety of conditions in which there is some disagreement as to how much genetics is at fault. These conditions include obesity, homosexuality, alcohol and drug addiction, and sexual deviations.

All the groups in this classification scheme have been persecuted. For instance, Blacks were enslaved, Native Americans were objects for official genocide, and Hispanics lost large tracts of land to the United States. In general, in the United States, cross-racial interactions, particularly between White and colored races, has brought conflict and stress.

Special Obstacles

Designated minorities meet ongoing stress in an attempt to overcome obstacles in pursuing an occupation, finding adequate housing, and attracting political benefits. Always they remain sensitive as to whether they are welcome or merely tolerated. There is the ceaseless focus on how much, how fast, and in which ways the person and the group accommodate to or resist oppression.

All the separate disadvantaged minorities in the categorization have their own issues. For instance, in the racial/ethnic group there is enormous ambivalence about the cost of integration in such terms as increased intermarriage and loss of unity and leadership as segregated housing diminishes.

As another example, many migrants remain closely tied to their country of origin. The economy of entire countries would be seriously impaired without the input of dollars remitted by migrant workers in the United States. Some migrants in the United States exercise voting rights in other countries. Strong transnational loyalty has to be balanced against charges of diluted loyalty from host nationals.

In this age of wide and rapid communication, designated disenfranchised groups know, as studies show, that bad behavior by one of them has a disproportionate and negative impact on the memory and attitude of majority citizens. The problem of having little control over portrayal by the media becomes a vexing issue of some magnitude.

All the disadvantaged groups protest that the rules are constantly and covertly altered. The fundamental belief is that their space, time, energy, and mobility should be limited and serve majority purposes. This makes the quest for equality all the more elusive, since rules once learned and a system once understood become mystifying and obfuscating.

An advantaged population tends not to see any special, unmerited, or unjustified privilege in what it does. Similarly, it may not calculate any disadvantage from having privilege. Not counting the cost to themselves of disenfranchising whole groups brings serious consequences to the majority. However, if the police have permission to exercise tactics in the disadvantaged community that would not be allowed in the advantaged community, it means that the entire community has elements of a police state. Well over 25% of Americans are in a disadvantaged group. The United States operates under the stress of a huge disadvantage. Any body politic that functions at less than 100% potential is handicapped. The oppressing portion of a society has an obstacle to its own achievement when it does not count the cost of oppressive behavior in everything from total gross national product to intellectual, cultural, and technical achievement, as well as personal freedom.

Treatment Considerations

History teaches that minority groups do best when they themselves are unrelenting in seeking redress from wrongs inflicted upon them. The broad societal pressures are exerted on and felt by all members of a disadvantaged minority. Yet it is hard to imagine how any one-on-one process, even if achieved, could eliminate a minority group's stress. Accordingly, treatment possibilities must be conceived on a grand scale. Only a broad approach can be sketched.

In the foreseeable future, direct medical interventions seem less promising than possible sociological and psychological approaches. The aim in these approaches is to provide increased hope and increased esteem to both the whole disadvantaged group and its individual members. In order to accomplish this objective, the groups themselves must somehow articulate and agree upon who is in their group and what the group cherishes. It must decide what to preserve and what to relinquish in accomplishing intergroup amity. The tactics required to reach these goals involve decreasing stress and increasing adaptation. Political and social action is obligatory.

Decreasing Stress

The disadvantaged minorities and their allies will need to continue and enlarge concerted, dedicated, social, and political actions to decrease stress. Diverse, multiple means must be instituted to teach the group, especially its youngsters, to anticipate the future. To do this, the group will have to mobilize structures at home, in community organizations, at schools, and at churches. All media channels, especially the Internet, TV, and radio, must be enlisted to help. The substantive debate about the details of the subject matter needs participation by persons who will inform themselves, seek input from the community, and be mindful of the history of the group.

Stress research would predict that supplying ways to help oneself and securing more support would be curative. Among topics, for instance, for colored groups would be propaganda analysis to learn to modulate messages that promote defeatism, futility, and loss of self-respect; lifestyle education to indicate the available steps that need to be and can be taken to increase the quality and quantity of life; and cross-racial interactions to emphasize aspects of group dynamics that aid or hinder interpersonal relations.

Perhaps special focus for many groups needs to be on networking and applying demographic remedies. For instance, in the United States, the racially/ethnically disadvantaged compared to the general population tend to be younger, more segregated, and more urban. A firm command of information of this sort will allow framing the future in terms of possible strengths and weaknesses.

Increasing Adaptation

Hopelessness and helplessness are the chief enemies to those under stress. The overall need is to supply support. Corollary to this need is to maximize adaptation. That is, one must cope.

For members of disadvantaged groups and the group as a whole, adaptation, historically, has required education as the critical step toward opportunity. Acquisition of exploitable skills and unquestioned competency in these skills are more difficult to obtain by disadvantaged minorities. Therefore, much of their social action and networking has to be aimed at securing education.

Community members can facilitate adaptation for each other by countermeasures against noxious environmental stimuli: simple acts of encouragement, providing positive feedback, and giving credit for coping. Similarly, coping is facilitated by encouraging the members under stress, particularly youngsters, to explore options and to be cautious about foreclosing on any opportunity. Community members in a cohesive, cooperative community can augment coping by helping their community provide proper sites and environment for relaxation, another requirement for those in need of surcease. A community may underestimate its ability to contribute to coping. Yet by finding ways to make the community as stable as possible and by trying to reduce feelings of isolation the coping process is facilitated.

People cope better when they do not romanticize the past; when they have a present, clear, and certain mission; and when they appreciate the importance and urgency of that mission. Community members, by their positive attitudes and expectations, can contribute to the individual's enthusiasm for the direction of his or her future.

In coping, helplessness and hopelessness are to be avoided. Their presence may be manifested clinically, particularly by depression and anxiety. Furthermore, depression and anxiety may be comorbid with addiction, violence, obesity, diabetes, and cardiovascular disease. Medical surveillance to prevent illness and medical intervention to treat illness are important considerations in helping disadvantaged minorities to cope.

It is here that ongoing research holds promise to help disadvantaged populations. Advances in molecular biochemistry, endocrinology, genetics, and neurobiology can bring great relief to individuals and families of disadvantaged minorities. Being sure that medical care is accessible will depend somewhat on the political and social activities of the group itself.

See Also the Following Articles

Cultural Factors in Stress; Cultural Transition; Racial Harassment/Discrimination.

Further Reading

Bell, C. C. (2004). *The sanity of survival: reflections on community mental health and wellness.* Chicago, IL: Third World Press.

Cohen, S., Kessler, R. C. and Gordon, L. U. (eds.) (1995). *Measuring stress: a guide for health and social scientists.* New York: Oxford University Press.

Cornish, E. (2004). *Futuring: the exploration of the future.* Bethesda, MD: World Future Society.

Green, B. L., Lewis, R. K. and Bediako, S. M. (2005). Reducing and eliminating health disparities: a targeted approach. *Journal of the National Medical Association* 97, 25–30.

Gruenewald, T. L., Kemney, M. E., Aziz, H., et al. (2004). Acute threat to the social self: shame, social self-esteem and cortisol activity. *Psychosomatic Medicine* **66**, 915–924.

Hobfoll, S. E. (1998). *Stress, culture, and community: the psychology and philosophy of Stress.* New York: Plenum Press.

Jackson, J. S. and Volckens, J. (1998). Community stressors and racism: structural and individual perspectives on racial bias. In: Arriaga, X. B. & Oskamp, S. (eds.) *Addressing community problems: psychological research and interventions*, pp. 19–51. Thousand Oaks, CA: Sage Publications.

National Geographic Society. (2004). *Atlas of the world* (8th edn.). Washington, D.C: National Geographic Society Press.

Smedley, B. D., Stith, A. Y. and Nelson, A. R. (2003). *Unequal treatment: confronting racial and ethnic disparities in healthcare.* Washington, D.C.: National Academy Press.

Special Report. (2004). The state of African American health. *The Crisis* **111**, 17–35.

U.S. Census, Bureau. (2004). *Statistical abstract of the United States: 2004–2005* (124th edn.). Washington, D.C.: U.S. Government Printing Office.

Racial Harassment/Discrimination

D R Williams and S A Mohammed
University of Michigan Ann Arbor, MI, USA

Introduction: Discrimination Persists

Discrimination and Racial Harassment

Several lines of evidence converge to suggest that discrimination is an important feature of life in race-conscious societies in which race is an important determinant of access to a broad range of societal benefits and rewards. First, social psychological theory identifies discrimination as a key aspect of intergroup relationships that serve to reinforce the symbolic boundaries that separate one social group from another. Second, there is broad recognition that discrimination persists for socially disadvantaged populations. The American public acknowledges that a high level of discrimination and prejudice exists. National public opinion data reveal that most Americans concede that racial minorities suffer from a fairly high level of racial bias. Blacks are perceived as experiencing the most discrimination, followed by Hispanics and American Indians, and then Asians. They also perceive that some White ethnic/religious groups such as Jews, Italians, and Catholics experience more discrimination than Whites in general. In one national study, for example, two-thirds of the American population reported that blacks suffer a lot or a tremendous amount of discrimination.

Some of the best evidence of the persistence of discrimination comes from audit studies in which carefully matched Black and White applicants with identical qualifications apply for jobs or housing. Audit studies in employment, for example, find that discrimination favors the White over a Black applicant in one in five audits. Other audit studies suggest that discrimination persists for Blacks and other minorities in the purchase of a broad range of goods and services. For example, one carefully executed study found racial differences in the best price offered for the purchase of a new car. In this study, Black and White testers were sent to automobile dealerships to negotiate the price of a new car. Although all the testers were carefully trained to follow the same script, there were large racial and gender differences in the final price offered for the new car, with White males offered the lowest prices, followed by White females, African American males, and African American females. Similarly, a recent report from the Institute of Medicine documented systematic and pervasive discrimination in the quality and intensity of medical treatment received by Blacks and other minorities in the United States. Thus, there is abundant evidence that discrimination persists in contemporary society. However, not all experiences of discrimination are visible to their intended target. Frequently, victims of discrimination lack all of the details about an interpersonal transaction that they need to know in order to establish that discrimination has occurred. Although self-reports of bias understate the full extent of exposure to discrimination, they capture an important part of discriminatory experiences that are likely to be consequential for health.

Discrimination as a Stressor

This article focuses on aspects of discrimination that are perceived by individuals in society. Subjective experiences of discrimination or unfair treatment are viewed as an important type of stressful life experience that many traditional measures of stress fail to assess. Equity theory suggests that perceptions of unfair treatment can lead to negative emotional reactions and psychosomatic symptoms. Discrimination can also be stressful because it can reinforce negative social stigma and highlight low social regard. Qualitative descriptions of experiences of discrimination indicate that they can induce considerable levels of psychological distress. Laboratory studies have examined the experimental manipulation of unfair treatment and have found that it leads to elevated levels of psychological distress for a broad range of social groups. Other studies have directly measured physiological responses to racially stressful material in the laboratory setting. These studies have used mental imagery and videotaped vignettes of discriminatory behavior. Most, but not all, of these studies have found that exposure to discrimination leads to cardiovascular and psychological reactivity. An important methodological strength of laboratory studies is that they do not rely on respondents' self-reports of discrimination. However, observed effects in the laboratory are short term, making the extent to which acute physiological arousal under laboratory conditions generalizes to chronic elevation of stress processes and mechanisms in real life unclear. Some recent research documents that high reactivity to acute stressors in laboratory settings is predictive of elevated rates of hypertension several years later. Most of the early laboratory studies focused on Blacks. It is not clear from these studies, however, whether the physiological reactivity to racism-linked experiences is unique or enhanced in comparison to reactivity to other types of stressors.

Studies of Discrimination and Health

Mental health status is the most frequently used health measure in studies of discrimination. Multiple mental health indicators have been used. These include measures of well-being, self-esteem, perceptions of control, psychological distress, anger, and specific psychiatric disorders such as major depression, generalized anxiety, and substance use. These studies have found an inverse relationship between discrimination and mental health – higher levels of discrimination were associated with poorer mental health status. Most of the early research studies in this area were based in the United States and tended to focus on African Americans. Recent studies have documented similar patterns of associations for other minority groups in the United States. For example, studies of Mexican Americans, Chinese Americans, and American Indians have found that perceived discrimination is associated with higher levels of psychological distress. A growing number of international studies documented similar patterns. Studies of Asian immigrants in Canada; Iranians, Turks, and Moroccans in the Netherlands; immigrants in Finland; Blacks, Asians, and Arabs in Ireland; and multiple ethnic minority populations in the United Kingdom found that discrimination is positively associated with psychological distress. Ongoing research is also exploring these relationships in Australia, Brazil, New Zealand, and South Africa.

Measures of perceived discrimination have also been studied in relationship to multiple measures of physical health. Studies using a single-item global self-rated health measure and other self-ratings of health or checklists of chronic illnesses have also fairly consistently documented that discrimination is related to poorer health status. Two studies found that discrimination makes an incremental contribution above socioeconomic status (SES) in explaining Black-White differences in self-reported health status. Several studies have also examined the association between discrimination and blood pressure levels or hypertension. Some studies found a clear positive association between discrimination and elevated blood pressure, whereas others found that this effect varies with the coping style, sex, SES, or race. Still other studies found no association between discrimination and blood pressure.

Recent research has also paid attention to a broader range of health outcomes. Whereas perceptions of discrimination were unrelated to self-reported heart disease in some early studies, recent research documented a positive association between chronic discrimination and the onset of subclinical heart disease (intima media thickness and coronary calcification). Recent studies also found that maternal exposure to discrimination was associated with preterm deliver and low birth weight. Several studies have also examined the association between perceived racial bias and health behaviors. They have found a positive association between discrimination and cigarette use and alcohol consumption.

Understanding the Context of Discrimination and Responses to It

Some of the inconsistency in findings in studies of discrimination and health could be due to inadequate attention to characterizing the social and psychological context in which discrimination occurs as well as the specific characteristics of the discriminatory incident. First, personality characteristics could predict variations in the association between discrimination and health. Beliefs about the self, such as self-esteem, mastery, racial consciousness, and identity might affect an individual's appraisal and thus the potential threat of a discriminatory experience. Second, contextual variables such as social support could also enhance an individual's capacity to cope and respond to discriminatory experiences. At the present time, we do not have a clear understanding of the contextual factors that can foster either vulnerability or resilience to perceived bias.

Third, specific characteristics of the discriminatory experience and its particular context can be important determinants of its impact. Key aspects of discriminatory experiences include the type or domain in which it occurs, the magnitude of the incident, its temporal characteristics (acute versus chronic), and the nature of the relationship between this stressor and other race-related and non-race-related stressors. Inadequate attention has also been given to the extent to which the effects of discrimination may vary by the social characteristics of the perpetrator. For example, some limited evidence suggests that the negative health impact of perceived discrimination on African Americans is greater when the perpetrator is also African American than when the perpetrator is White.

Fourth, it is also likely that there are complex interactions between exposure to discrimination and particular coping strategies or styles. In addition to examining traditional problem-focused and emotion-focused measures of coping from the stress literature, research on discrimination needs to attend to discrimination-related measures. Heightened vigilance is one such measure. Because racism is often deeply embedded in the structure and culture of society, it can pose an ever-present threat for socially stigmatized groups. Some individuals respond to this by engaging in psychological and behavioral anticipatory coping strategies to mitigate the perceived dangers in the environment. This can lead to heightened physiological arousal that can adversely affect health. Using denial as a coping strategy is a theoretically important but difficult concept to measure. The literature suggests that, because experiences of discrimination can pose threats to the self, some individuals respond to its occurrence by minimizing or even denying its occurrence. There is also the suggestion in the literature that denying the occurrence of bias is damaging to health.

Measurement Issues

A prerequisite for understanding the association between discrimination and health is the development of valid and reliable measures that fully characterize exposure to discrimination. The literature identifies several issues that affect the appropriate assessment of discrimination.

Perceived Discrimination Is Subjective

An important issue in the assessment of discrimination is the challenge of obtaining valid and reliable indicators of subjective phenomena such as experiences of discrimination. It is possible that the salience of racial identity or perceived racism could lead some minority group members to perceive incidents as racist that may not be or, worse, could lead to the development of a mind-set in which they perceive experiences to be products of racism when in fact they were not. In fact, some limited evidence suggests that the use of discrimination terminology, in which race or gender is made salient in the assessment of discrimination, can induce respondent biases. This work emphasizes that questions with embedded terminology require both a description of an experience as well as an interpretation of that experience. Moreover, in the cooperative context of a research interview a respondent may make inferences about the questioner's intent and interests that could lead the respondent to try to provide information that is consistent with the questioner's perceived intent. All of this can lead to interpretive response bias that could produce higher estimates of discrimination, driven by the specific terminology used. Thus, questionnaires that ask repeated questions about "racial discrimination" or experiences "because of your race" could produce demand characteristics in which the respondent believes that it is desirable to the interviewer to report such experiences. This could lead to overreports of discrimination.

One promising approach in measuring discrimination seeks to reduce the salience of race by first asking respondents whether they have been treated "unfairly" in multiple domains of life. After respondents have endorsed an experience of unfair treatment, they are asked to attribute a reason. Potential reasons include race and ethnicity, but also allow for other factors such as gender, age, religion, weight, and sexual orientation. This approach enables respondents to report on all instances of unfair treatment, but allows the researcher to separate instances attributed to race from those linked to other reasons. Relatedly, this measurement approach allows for the evaluation of the extent that discrimination based on race is more deleterious to health than discrimination based on other social factors. Inadequate attention has been given to the relative impact of racial discrimination compared to other types of discrimination in the extant research to draw firm conclusions. However, some studies suggest that it is the generic perception of unfair treatment that is deleterious to health, irrespective of the specific attribution regarding the cause of the incident. Research is needed to identify the optimal approaches to the measurement of racial discrimination.

The available evidence suggests that concerns about the overreporting of discrimination may be overblown. First, making race salient in the assessment of discrimination can lead to underreporting of discrimination. Respondents vary in their thresholds of what constitutes discrimination and may fail to report as discriminatory incidents that were not perceived as very serious. Second, respondents appear to interpret the concept of discrimination as intended by researchers and self-reports of discrimination are consistent with objective experiences. Third, two studies have documented that baseline mental health status (psychological distress and major depression) is unrelated to subsequent reports of discrimination. Fourth, because reporting discrimination can negatively affect self-esteem and perceptions of control, at least some stigmatized group members are likely to minimize and deny experiences of discrimination. Thus, underreporting is as important a threat to the validity of self-reports of discrimination as overreporting. Nonetheless, it is important for researchers to adjust reports of discrimination for potentially confounding psychological characteristics such as social desirability, neuroticism, and other indicators of negative affect. Such adjustment strengthens the methodological rigor of a study and increases the likelihood that observed associations between perceived discrimination and health are not distorted by underlying psychological factors. Including such controls is especially important when the measure of health status is also based on self-report.

Several strategies that have been used to improve the accuracy of the reporting of stressors should also be applied to the study of discrimination. These include the use of cues to memory (such as visual representations and reminders of personally salient events), wording the questions in ways that clearly indicate the domain of the experience being captured, and using a life-events calendar to facilitate dating the onset and resolution of experiences of discrimination.

Perceived Discrimination Is Multidimensional

Capturing the exposure to discrimination in its full multidimensional complexity and assessing the cumulative burden of such exposure over the life course is also another major challenge. Some early studies of discrimination used single-item measures. Such assessment understates the actual level of discrimination. However, many current studies assess exposure to discrimination using retrospective recall to capture exposure within a 30-day, 1-year, 3-year or lifetime time frame.

Comprehensively capturing discrimination requires its assessment in multiple areas of social life. Like other stressors, discrimination is multidimensional and should be assessed in all relevant domains. The stress literature indicates that the most commonly measured types of stressors include life events, chronic stress, and daily hassles. Life events are major discrete stressors that are readily observable. Daily hassles are minor but often chronic irritations. Chronic stressors are ongoing problems that are typically role-related. There are analogues to all of these types of stressors in current measures of discrimination. Major acute experiences of racial bias are the most commonly assessed type of discriminatory experience. The literature on stress indicates that chronic stressors may be stronger predictors of the onset and course of illness than acute life events. Scales such as the Everyday Discrimination Scale attempt to capture persistent and recurring everyday chronic minor experiences. Future research needs to give more attention to capturing the frequency and duration of chronic discrimination in multiple social contexts, such as employment, educational, and public settings.

Other major types of stressors include traumas, nonevents, and macro-stressors. Developing analogs of these in the assessment of discrimination is a promising direction for future research. Traumas are acute stressors that are severe and overwhelming in impact, such as being kidnapped or raped. Macro-stressors are large-scale systems-related stressors such as economic recessions. Nonevents are desired and expected experiences that fail to occur. The stress literature indicates that the various types of stressors can have independent effects on health. Therefore, assessing all relevant types of stressors is a perquisite to an assessment of the full impact of stress on health.

A small but growing body of research on historical trauma and its intergenerational effects on the health of American Indians illustrates the benefit of expanding our definitions of race-related stressors. Historical trauma is viewed as a cumulative and collective psychological wounding over the life span and across generations as the result of the history of genocide and assimilation that American Indians experienced at the hands of Europeans. Studying historical trauma among American Indians is not unlike existing studies of other generational group traumas, such as studies of the effects of the Jewish Holocaust on the physical and mental health, as well as the social, economic, and political contexts, of descendants of Holocaust survivors. It has been argued that historical trauma contributes to a host of issues in the American Indian population, including unresolved grief, alcoholism, depression, anxiety, high rates of suicide, homicide, problematic gambling behaviors, domestic violence, child abuse, poverty, low education levels, and various physical diseases. The literature recognizes that although the concept of historical trauma is theoretically intuitive, there are challenges in distinguishing historical versus contemporary experiences, understanding how historical trauma is imparted across generations, and defining and measuring the levels of historical trauma. However, scales with good psychometric properties have been developed to assess historical trauma and find that as many as one-half of American Indians think regularly about these historical losses. Moreover, recent empirical studies have found support for an inverse association between historical trauma and health. Clinical interventions to address historical trauma have also been developed. A promising area of research would be to examine the generalizability of this pattern across health outcomes and American Indian cultures, as well as, seeing whether other highly visible traumatic historical events have similar effects for other groups.

Capturing Life Course Exposure

There are important measurement challenges in terms of identifying the appropriate questions that could capture the duration and frequency of discrimination over the life course. An isolated experience of discrimination, just like a random stressor, is unlikely to have long-term negative effects on health. The literature suggests that the key issue is being able to identify discriminatory experiences that are enduring and chronic. A life course perspective is critical in assessing the cumulative burden of discrimination over an individual's lifetime. Measures that do an excellent job of capturing exposure to all of the relevant types of discrimination do not currently exist. Overcoming the challenges linked to declines in the accuracy of recall with the passage of time will not be easy, but this is crucial to obtaining better measures of lifetime exposure to discrimination. Such data are necessary to begin to identify the lag times between exposure to discriminatory stressors and adverse changes in health. Life course assessment of discrimination must also be coupled with an equally comprehensive measurement of other types of stressors. The present-day literature does not provide a clear understanding of how experiences of discrimination relate to other stressors and combine, in additive and interactive ways, to affect specific health outcomes and trajectories of health status over time.

Attributional Ambiguity

Perceived discrimination is based on the perception of the individual. The subjective nature of discrimination and the ambiguity that occurs in much interpersonal interaction can lead to uncertainty regarding the attribution of specific incidents of bias or unfair treatment. It is possible that having to make sense of ambiguous social interactions can be physiologically stressful. The worry and rumination regarding the causes of experiences of discrimination may be an added burden that can be consequential for the health of nondominant group members. It is thus possible that the degree of ambiguity attending the perception of a discriminatory experience could negatively affect health. This issue deserves careful examination in future research.

Pathways from Discrimination to Health

Researchers have generally found a weaker association between discrimination and health for measures of physical health than for measures of mental health. Physical health outcomes typically assessed are chronic conditions involving complex etiological factors and varying patterns of development and progression over long periods of time. Greater attention needs to be given to the hypothesized pathways by which discrimination might affect health and to identifying the appropriate points along that pathway at which the individual is more vulnerable to exposure to discrimination and other stressors.

The stress literature reveals that one way that stressors can affect health is by giving rise to negative emotional states, such as anxiety and depression, which in turn can directly impact biological processes or patterns of behavior that affect disease risk. Accordingly, one of the pathways by which discrimination can affect physical health outcomes may be indirectly, through psychological distress. Thus, discrimination may lead to elevated psychological symptoms, which, in turn, may lead to chronic physiological arousal. In addition, the negative emotional states created by experiences of discrimination might lead to health behaviors that may ultimately affect disease risk, such as impaired sleep patterns, decreased physical activity, increased substance use, and consumption of more food than usual. It was noted earlier that prior research indicates that discrimination is positively associated with alcohol consumption and cigarette smoking. These and other health-related behaviors may be a pathway by which perceived bias has health consequences. The stress of discrimination and the negative emotional states created by it could also lead to lower levels of adherence to medical recommendations. This latter mechanism has not yet been explored in the literature. The potential effects of discrimination and other stressors on medical compliance emphasize the need to assess the contribution of discrimination not only to the onset of disease but also to its severity and course.

Our understanding is currently limited regarding how exposure to discrimination leads to changes in particular biological responses and health behaviors. Further research is needed to identify the physiological mediators of the effects of discrimination so that the specific biological pathways by which discrimination can adversely affect health may be studied. Such research should assess the conditions under which specific physiological systems, such as the cardiovascular, neuroendocrine, and immune systems, are affected by particular types of discrimination. We are presently unaware of the genetic and psychological factors that can lead some organ systems to be more vulnerable than others to the effects of discrimination on health.

Conclusion

Scientific research indicates that perceived discrimination is associated with poor health status, with the association being strongest for mental health. However, existing evidence does not clearly indicate the extent to which exposure to perceived discrimination leads to increased risk of disease, the conditions under which this is more or less likely to occur, or the underlying mechanisms and processes linking this stressor to health status. Advances have been made in the conceptualization and measurement of discrimination, but there is still more work to be done. The most urgent need is for the theoretical identification and the empirical verification of the plausible pathways by which experiences of bias can affect various health outcomes. At the same time, this field of research is clearly moving from infancy to childhood. The literature has now identified major gaps in this area, as well as promising conceptual, methodological, and analytic tools that are needed for the rigorous examination of the association between perceived discrimination and multiple indicators of health.

See Also the Following Articles

Cultural Factors in Stress.

Further Reading

Blank, R. M., Dabady, M. and Citro, C. F. (eds.) (2004). *Measuring racial discrimination: panel on methods for assessing discrimination.* National Research Council Committee on National Statistics, Division of Behavioral and Social Sciences and Education. Washington, DC: The National Academies Press.

Clark, R., Anderson, N. B., Clark, V. R., et al. (1999). Racism as a stressor for African Americans: a biopsychosocial model. *American Psychologist* **54**(10), 805–816.

Dion, K. J. (2001). The social psychology of perceived prejudice and discrimination. *Canadian Psychology* **43**(1), 1–10.

Fix, M. and Struyk, R. J. (1993). *Clear and convincing evidence: measurement of discrimination in America.* Washington, DC: Urban Institute Press.

Gomez, J. P. and Trierweiler, S. (2001). Does discrimination terminology create response bias in questionnaire studies of discrimination? *Personality and Social Psychology Bulletin* **27**(5), 630–638.

Harrell, J., Hall, S. and Taliaferro, J. (2003). Physiological responses to racism and discrimination: an assessment of the evidence. *American Journal of Public Health* **93**(2), 243–248.

Harrell, S. (2000). A multidimensional conceptualization of racism-related stress: implications for the well-being of people of color. *American Journal of Orthopsychiatry* **70**(1), 42–57.

Krieger, N. (1999). Embodying inequality: a review of concepts, measures, and methods for studying health consequences of discrimination. *International Journal of Health Services* **29**(2), 295–352.

Krieger, N., Smith, K., Naishadham, D., et al. (2005). Experiences of discrimination: validity and reliability of a self-report measure for population health research on racism and health. *Social Science and Medicine* **61**(7), 1576–1596.

Paradies, Y. (2006) A systematic review of empirical research on self-reported racism and health. *International Journal of Epidemiology* **35**, 888–901.

Whitbeck, L. B., Adams, G. W., Hoyt, D. R., et al. (2004). Conceptualizing and measuring historical trauma among American Indian people. *American Journal of Community Psychology* **33**(3–4), 119–130.

Williams, D. R. and Neighbors, H. W. (2002). Racism, discrimination, and hypertension: evidence and needed research. *Ethnicity and Disease* **11**, 800–816.

Williams, D. R., Neighbors, H. W. and Jackson, J. S. (2003). Racial/ethnic discrimination and health: findings from community studies. *American Journal of Public Health* **93**(2), 200–208.

School Stress and School Refusal Behavior

C A Kearney, L C Cook and G Chapman
University of Nevada, Las Vegas, NV, USA

This is a revised version of the article by C A Kearney and C Pursell, Encyclopedia of Stress First Edition, volume 3, pp 398–401, © 2000, Elsevier Inc.

Glossary

School refusal behavior — The substantial child-motivated refusal to attend school and/or difficulties remaining in classes for an entire day.

School stress — Unpleasant physical and cognitive symptoms in response to global and specific school-related stressors.

School Stress and Linkage to School Refusal Behavior

Children and adolescents become anxious about many things, but youths become particularly stressed by difficult family and school situations. School-related stressors may involve global and specific issues. Global school-related stressors include large class size, threats of victimization and violence, changes in academic and social status, excessive homework, and tedious curricula. Specific school-related stressors include teachers and other school officials, peer interactions, examinations, performances before others, social gatherings, and use of cafeterias and public restrooms.

School-related stressors are quite prevalent among youths, and many youths experience concomitant physiological and cognitive symptoms as a result. Common physiological symptoms include headaches, stomachaches, shortness of breath, trembling, dizziness, and heart palpitations. Common cognitive symptoms include catastrophic thoughts about losing control, going insane, suffering humiliation or harm, experiencing negative evaluation from others, appearing foolish, having few friends, having trouble concentrating, and lacking competence in various areas. If school-related stress becomes severe, then some youths may refuse to attend school to avoid these unpleasant symptoms.

Major Characteristics of School Refusal Behavior

School refusal behavior is the substantial child-motivated refusal to attend school and/or difficulties remaining in classes for an entire day. Specifically, the behavior involves youths ages 5–17 years who (1) are completely absent from school, (2) attend school but then leave school during the school day, (3) go to school following intense behavior problems such as tantrums in the morning, and/or (4) display unusual distress during the school day that leads to pleas for future nonattendance. School refusal behavior may also be defined by its timeline. For example, self-corrective school refusal behavior refers to absenteeism that remits spontaneously within 2 weeks. Acute school refusal behavior lasts from 2 weeks to 1 year, and chronic school refusal behavior lasts longer than 1 year. Greater chronicity is related to greater difficulty reintroducing a child to school.

Approximately 5–28% of school-age youths refuse school at some time in their lives. School refusal behavior is seen equally in boys and girls and among families of various income levels. The short-term consequences of school refusal behavior include declining academic status, social alienation, increased risk of legal trouble, family conflict, and severe disruption in a family's daily routine. The long-term consequences of school refusal behavior include school dropout and subsequent economic deprivation, occupational and marital problems, alcohol abuse and criminal behavior, and mental disorders.

School refusal behavior is marked by considerable symptom heterogeneity. Common internalizing problems include general and social anxiety/shyness, depression and social withdrawal, fear, fatigue, and somatic complaints such as stomachaches, headaches, nausea, and tremors. Common externalizing problems include tantrums, verbal and physical aggression, clinging, reassurance seeking, refusal to move, noncompliance, and running away from school or home.

School refusal behavior is also marked by many different diagnoses that could cause or be the result of problematic absenteeism. In this population, common comorbid diagnoses include separation anxiety disorder, generalized anxiety disorder, depression, and oppositional defiant disorder, among others. In addition, school refusal behavior has been linked to limited developmental disabilities such as learning disorders and pervasive developmental disabilities such as Asperger's disorder, autism, and mental retardation.

Etiology and Major Functions of School Refusal Behavior

The specific causes of school refusal behavior are often unclear for a particular case. However, common triggers include the onset of a new school year, entry into a new school building, school-related trauma, teacher or class changes, family illness or transition, parental psychopathology, and marital conflict or divorce. Child factors such as behavioral inhibition, excessive shyness, and association with deviant peers can also be influential. Unfortunately, identifying the etiology in this population is often a fruitless task. As such, clinicians may focus instead on the primary functions or reasons why youths refuse school:

1. To avoid school-related objects and situations that provoke a general sense of negative affectivity (dread, anxiety, depression, and physiological symptoms).
2. To escape aversive social and/or evaluative situations at school.
3. To receive attention from significant others outside of school.
4. To obtain tangible reinforcement outside of school.

The initial two functions refer to youths who refuse school for negative reinforcement, or to avoid something unpleasant at school. These functions are closely related to the concept of school stress. The latter two functions refer to youths who refuse school for positive reinforcement, or to pursue someone or something more alluring outside school. Some youths also refuse school for multiple reasons, and those who do often require complex and extended treatment.

Assessment of School Refusal Behavior

Assessing youths with school refusal behavior often involves defining a child's exact behavior problems, discovering primary and secondary functions for absenteeism, and identifying effective treatment. To do so, assessment methods may include interviews, child self-report and parent/teacher measures, direct observation, daily monitoring, and discussions with school officials. Interviews may be structured or unstructured in nature. A common structured interview for this population is the Anxiety Disorders Interview Schedule for Children, which has child and parent versions and helps clinicians identify various diagnoses. In addition, the interview contains a special section on school refusal behavior to help clinicians pinpoint the frequency and intensity of the behavior and related stress-based symptoms. Unstructured interviews may also be used to assess youths with school refusal behavior. Questions may relate to school-related stressors that affect a particular child, degree of avoidance, physiological and cognitive symptoms, attention-seeking, and pursuit of tangible reinforcers outside of school.

Several child self-report and parent and teacher measures also pertain to youths with school refusal behavior. The most common address negative affectivity, depression, general and social anxiety, somatic complaints, overactivity, aggression, noncompliance, demands for attention, social problems, fear, self-concept, family dynamics, and the function of school refusal behavior. Gathering information from multiple sources is recommended because school refusal behavior can include many subtle symptoms.

Direct observation of a child's and family's morning activities at home may also help define the primary symptoms and maintaining variables of school refusal behavior. Pertinent behaviors include:

1. Avoidance in the form of clinging, refusal to move, running away, and/or noncompliance to requests.
2. Physiological reactivity such as stomachaches, headaches, abdominal pain, tremors, and nausea/vomiting.
3. Cognitive distortions or verbalizations about discomfort related to school.
4. Sudden changes in behavior.
5. Pleas to stay home from school.
6. Increased family conflict, especially following a curtailment of the child's social activities.
7. Significant changes in parental behavior.
8. Teacher reports of differences in a child's behavior at school.

The daily assessment of a child's school refusal behaviors and attendance is also important. This helps gauge familial compliance to homework assignments, increase insight into a child's problem, and identify positive or negative changes in behavior across time. For example, family members may provide daily ratings with respect to a child's anxiety, depression, and overall distress (general feelings of dread or being upset). In addition, parents may rate a child's noncompliance (not listening to parent commands) and disruption to their daily routine. Parents can also list other child behavior problems and time missed from school.

Finally, school officials may be contacted for additional information, including course schedules, grades, written work, and required make-up work; goals and attitudes of school officials and peers regarding a child; procedures and timelines for reintegrating a child into school; potential obstacles to reintegrating a child into school; confirmation of past school refusal behavior; general social or other behaviors of a child in school; a map or outline of the school (e.g., lockers, cafeteria, library); feedback about treatment effectiveness; disciplinary procedures and procedures for contacting parents; and rules about absenteeism, conduct, or leaving school areas.

Treatment of School Refusal Behavior

Treatment for youths with school refusal behavior may be linked to the function of the behavior. For example, treatment for youths who refuse school to avoid stimuli provoking negative affectivity (i.e., school stress) often involves reducing unpleasant physiological symptoms and exposing a child to various school-related items and situations. Specifically, this involves psychoeducation about the nature and process of anxiety (i.e., linking feelings, thoughts and behaviors), developing an anxiety and avoidance hierarchy of situations and stimuli, teaching somatic management skills to decrease negative emotional arousal (i.e., relaxation training and breathing retraining), systematic imaginal and *in vivo* exposure to anxiety cues identified on a graded hierarchy (progressive reintroduction to the school setting), and having a child praise him- or herself for coping with transient negative emotions.

For youths who refuse school to escape aversive social and/or evaluative situations, treatment strategies involve building or refining social skills and reducing social anxiety in key interactive situations at school. Specifically, this involves psychoeducation about the nature and process of anxiety (i.e., linking feelings, thoughts, and behaviors), teaching a child to identify cognitive distortions (e.g., all-or-none thinking, catastrophization, and overgeneralization) and negative self-statements in anxiety-provoking situations, learning methods to change distorted thoughts to helpful coping thoughts, graduated exposure to anxiety-provoking social situations through in-session practice with a therapist (including modeling and role-play of different situations), and between-session practice of skills in real-life social situations.

For youths who refuse school for attention, treatment strategies involve parent-based techniques to shift parental attention away from school refusal behaviors and toward appropriate school attendance behaviors. Specifically, this involves restructuring parent commands, establishing fixed routines regarding a child throughout the day, implementing negative consequences for school refusal behaviors, implementing positive consequences for school attendance behaviors, and, in some cases, forced school attendance.

For youths who refuse school for tangible reinforcement outside school, treatment strategies involve improving a family's problem-solving abilities, reducing conflict, increasing rewards for school attendance, and decreasing rewards for school absenteeism. Specifically, this involves establishing times and places when family members can negotiate problem solutions, defining behavior problems specifically, designing written parent–child contracts to address problems, implementing contracts, training in communication skills, training in peer-refusal skills (i.e., helping a child refuse offers to miss school), and escorting a child to school or to each class. For all treatments, relapse-prevention training is also necessary.

Further Reading

Berg, I. and Nursten, J. (1996). *Unwillingly to school* (4th edn.). Washington, DC: American Psychiatric Press.

Kearney, C. A. (2001). *School refusal behavior in youth: a functional approach to assessment and treatment.* Washington, DC: American Psychological Association.

Kearney, C. A. and Albano, A. M. (2000). *When children refuse school: a cognitive-behavioral therapy approach/therapist's guide.* New York: Oxford.

Kearney, C. A. and Silverman, W. K. (1996). The evolution and reconciliation of taxonomic strategies for school refusal behavior. *Clinical Psychology: Science and Practice* 3, 339–354.

Kearney, C. A. and Silverman, W. K. (1999). Functionally-based prescriptive and nonprescriptive treatment for children and adolescents with school refusal behavior. *Behavior Therapy* 30, 673–695.

King, N. J., Ollendick, T. H. and Tonge, B. J. (1995). *School refusal: assessment and treatment.* Boston, MA: Allyn and Bacon.

Silverman, W. K. and Albano, A. M. (1996). *Anxiety disorders interview schedule for DSM-IV: child version.* New York: Oxford.

School Violence and Bullying

J Juvonen
University of California, Los Angeles,
Los Angeles, CA, USA

Bullying and school violence are significant sources of stress in American schools. In a recent national survey, children ages 8–15 rated bullying as one of the major concerns affecting their lives. Another survey indicated that almost two-thirds of public secondary school students thought that a shooting could take place in their school.

In contrast to violent behaviors that involve use of physical force, bullying entails the abuse of psychological strength, which can be achieved by various means. Bullies intimidate their victims by relying on name-calling, exclusion, threats, and/or spreading of rumors. Because the perpetrators of violent acts as well as bullying abuse their power, both forms of hostile behavior cause psychological distress in that the actual and potential victims of peer maltreatment or abuse experience anxiety. Repeated experiences of hostile behavior by schoolmates are, in turn, associated with increased feelings of depression and either withdrawn or aggressive behavior.

Hostile School Behavior: Prevalence and Concerns

According to the most recent national data, 14% of students ages 12–18 reported having been bullied in school during the previous 6 months. The estimates for bullying vary depending on how broadly the term is defined and the time frame provided. Using daily (as opposed to monthly or yearly) reports of bullying experiences, almost 50% of young teens reported at least one incident of bullying during a 2-week period in urban middle schools. Up to 70% of secondary students reported having experienced bullying at some point during their school careers. Although the experiences of bullying are fleeting for most students, an estimated 5–10% of students confront bullying on a weekly, if not daily, basis for 1 or more school years.

The prevalence estimates of bullying also vary by grade level and school type. Compared to other grade levels, middle school students reported the highest rates of bullying, and sixth-grade students were most fearful of their safety. Although girls reported being more concerned about their safety at school or on their way to and from school, boys reported more incidents of violence and bullying. Boys were also the perpetrators of the most violent incidents.

Approximately 70% of public schools reported one or more violent incidents during a school year. Although the most serious forms of violence are less common, one-fifth of public schools reported at least one incident involving aggravated assault, sexual assault, rape, or robbery per year. Violent incidents are most likely to take place during the high school years and in large urban schools.

Students in urban public schools are most likely to fear for their safety. Black and Latino students reported feeling more fearful of being attacked than did White students. Although some hostile incidents appeared to be racially motivated, this does not necessarily mean that students were worst off in ethnically mixed schools. Recent analyses of middle schools suggest that greater ethnic diversity (i.e., a larger number of ethnic groups and their relative balance) is associated with feelings of safety.

Connection between Bullying and Violent Offending

Children who bully in childhood are at risk of becoming violent offenders. Research conducted in Norway shows that boys identified as bullies in their teenage years were four times as likely to commit violent acts in their twenties than other boys. Long-term studies conducted in the United States reveal that when childhood bullying is associated with more serious subsequent fighting, the risk of committing assaults and rape significantly increases. Hence, at least the physical forms of bullying and violent offending among males reflect a spiral of increasingly serious hostile behaviors.

Both childhood bullying and school violence are predicted by personality dispositions (e.g., impulsivity), environmental factors beyond school (e.g., problematic relationships with parents), and school-related situations (e.g., perceptions of unfair treatment by teachers or peers). These risk factors often interact in that students with certain dispositions are more likely to encounter situations that prompt them to act aggressively. For example, impulsive students are likely to act in a way that increases their chances of someone's bumping into them in a hallway, and, after experiencing an unintended push, they are more likely to react with hostility. The hostile response is often promoted by a perception that the other person intended to cause harm.

Many aggressive students develop a generalized sense of mistrust. Hence, students commit hostile acts to protect themselves. For example, compared to nonbullied students, bullied students are more likely to carry a weapon to school. Fear for their safety is the most common reason provided by students who carry weapons to school.

Other students' hostile acts are motivated by a desire to maintain a sense of control and to show their power. These bullies or violent offenders enjoy at least temporary admiration among their peers because of their dominant status. Fellow students rarely challenge their mean and hurtful behaviors because they are fearful of the reactions of these dominant ringleaders. Passivity and acceptance of toughness, in turn, promote social norms that encourage and maintain bullying or even violent behavior. Thus, the school environment, including the reactions of fellow peers (victims or bystanders), plays a critical role in motivating hostile behavior in school.

Antecedents and Consequences of Hostile Experiences

Because of the low prevalence rates of serious violent incidents in school, little is known about the factors that increase the risk of being targeted. However, research on bullying shows that socially withdrawn and passive children are at risk of getting bullied. After repeated experiences of bullying, these submissive victims become even more withdrawn. These students most often suffer in silence, and teachers and parents are unaware of their plight or distress. Instructors may interpret the quiet signs of distress as a lack of interest in schoolwork. Indeed, teachers rate victims as being just as disengaged from schoolwork as bullies.

Students who respond to bullying with unregulated aggression (i.e., aggressive victims) are also at a high risk for continued peer maltreatment. In these cases, bullying experiences are related to extreme peer rejection and severe school difficulties. Aggressive victims are presumed to have underlying emotional difficulties, which are also used to help explain why their difficulties continue. Thus, in the cases of both submissive and aggressive victims, the causes and consequences of bullying form a vicious circle.

Although aggressive victims resemble violent offenders most closely, the victims of bullying are unlikely to resort to violence to get back at their tormentors. Nevertheless, the tragic school shooting incidents since the late 1990s highlight that chronic victims of bullying, like violent offenders, have trouble effectively dealing with social failures (e.g., public ridicule or rejection by a romantic partner). Some violence prevention and antibullying interventions are therefore specifically designed to help students better cope with bullying incidents.

The Effects of Witnessing Hostile Behaviors

The hostile behaviors of schoolmates affect not only those who are victimized but also those who witness peer abuse or maltreatment in school. For example, analyses of daily incidents of bullying in middle school show that social anxiety is increased when students see someone else being bullied. Students who witness violent incidents are likely to feel especially vulnerable and unsafe. Thus, although there may be relatively few hostile students in any one school, one or two can terrorize entire grade levels and a couple of violent events may cause widespread fear. In view of such exposure effects, the level of concern about bullying and violence in American schools is not unrealistically high.

Part of the distress caused by observed events is likely to be related to the school's response system (or lack thereof). Although the parents' concerns about the safety of their children at school may be alleviated by the presence of metal detectors and campus officers, students continue to worry about their safety because they know that someone can smuggle a weapon to campus or they are fearful of someone bullying them in sites lacking monitoring (e.g., restrooms and locker rooms). In addition to feeling vulnerable, an unsafe or noncaring school climate is likely to breed mistrust and alienation that, in turn, increase the risk of students carrying weapons and setting off a hostile response.

In summary, school violence and bullying cause, and are also partly caused by, feelings of vulnerability that reach beyond personal experiences of hostile acts. This can be depicted as a following process:

Perceived vulnerability of self → Hostile response to perceived threat → Unsafe school climate

To promote feelings of safety and trust, schools are relying more and more on prevention models that focus not only on at-risk youth but also on helping improve the school climate. A caring climate in schools, in which students feel they belong, are respected, and are listened to and in which teachers help mediate hostile incidents, can buffer the safety concerns and distress of the entire student body.

See Also the Following Articles

School Stress and School Refusal Behavior.

Further Reading

Jimerson, S. R. and Furlong, M. (eds.) (2006). *Handbook of school violence and school safety: from research to practice.* Mahwah, NJ: Lawrence Erlbaum.

Juvonen, J. and Graham, S. (eds.) (2001). *Peer harassment in school: the plight of the vulnerable and victimized.* New York: Guilford Press.

Juvonen, J., Nishina, A. and Graham, S. (2006). Ethnic diversity and perceptions of safety in urban middle schools. *Psychological Science* **17**, 393–400.

Leary, M. R., Kowalski, R. M., Smith, L., et al. (2003). Teasing, rejection, and violence: case studies of the school shootings. *Aggressive Behavior* **29**, 202–214.

Smith, P. K., Pepler, D. and Rigby, K. (eds.) (2004). *Bullying in schools: how successful can interventions be?* New York: Cambridge University Press.

Relevant Websites

U.S. Department of Education and U.S. Department of Justice. (2005). Indicators of school crime and safety: 2005. National Center of Education Statistics. http://nces.ed.gov.

Social Capital

I Kawachi
Harvard School of Public Health, Boston, MA, USA

This is a revised version of the article by I Kawachi, Encyclopedia of Stress First Edition, volume 3, pp 466–467, © 2000, Elsevier Inc.

Glossary

Bonding social capital — Social connections that exist within homogeneous groups, for example the strong ties that connect family members, close friends, or neighbors who are alike with respect to race/ethnicity, social class, and religion.

Bridging social capital — Social connections that cross race/ethnic, class, and other boundaries.

Social capital — The resources available to individuals and groups through their social connections and membership in community networks.

Forms and Functions of Social Capital

Social capital is the resources available to individuals through their social connections and membership in community networks. In contrast to financial capital, which resides in people's bank accounts, or human capital, which is embodied in individuals' investments in education and job training, social capital inheres in the structure and quality of social relationships between individuals.

The concept was originally developed in sociology and political science. According to James Coleman, social capital can take on several different forms, such as levels of trust within a social structure, norms and sanctions, information channels, and appropriable social organizations. An example of an appropriable social organization is the case of a residents' association in an urban housing project that formed initially for the purpose of pressuring builders to fix various problems (e.g., leaks and crumbling sidewalks). After the original problems were solved, the organization remained as available social capital within the community to improve the quality of life of residents in other ways.

In fields outside of health, social capital has been applied in a variety of settings ranging from the smooth and effective functioning of government institutions to the ability of communities to solve the problems of collective action, such as intervening to prevent the occurrence of juvenile delinquency. More recently, empirical studies have begun to link social capital to population health outcomes.

Measurement of Social Capital

Two approaches have been used to measure social capital: (1) surveys and (2) direct social observations. In the survey-based approach, researchers inquired about a range of attitudes (trust of others and expectations of reciprocity and mutual aid) as well as behaviors (e.g., membership in community organizations, levels of voluntarism, and intensity of informal social interactions with neighbors) that are thought to be indicative of social capital. By contrast, direct social observation may involve the use of experimental methods, such as the letter-drop experiment in which stamped addressed envelopes are deliberately dropped on street corners to determine the proportion of letters that are subsequently mailed to the addressee by strangers (an experimental indicator of reciprocity). More commonly, direct observational approaches emphasize the observable characteristics of communities that may serve as proxies for the extent of social capital, such as the density of voluntary associations within a given locality.

Given the well-established tradition in community psychology of studying the characteristics of cohesive communities, there is legitimate debate over the extent to which the concept of social capital represents old wine in new bottles. In community psychology, concepts such as the psychological sense of community, community competence, and neighboring all predate the current vogue for the term social capital. In addition, there is an extensive prior literature in health psychology and social epidemiology on the related constructs of social support and social integration. However, an important distinction between social support and social capital is that, whereas the former variable is measured at the individual level, the latter is most often conceptualized and measured at the community or area level. That is, social capital has most often been considered to be a property of the collective (neighborhoods, cities, or even regions).

If social capital is indeed a collective property, a critical question is whether aggregated responses to social surveys (e.g., in response to questions about trusting neighbors) genuinely represent a group characteristic or whether they are confounded by other characteristics of the individual respondents that correlate with perceptions of social capital. Some evidence suggests that aggregated survey responses actually capture genuine place-based differences. An analysis of the Community Survey of the Project on Human Development in Chicago Neighborhoods reported that even after controlling for the socio-demographic attributes of individual respondents (age, sex, race/ethnic status, income, and schooling), there were significant between-neighborhood variations in levels of social capital as measured by perceptions of trust.

Finally, research has increasingly pointed out the important distinction between bonding and bridging social capital. Bonding social capital refers to the social connections that exist within homogeneous groups, for example the strong ties that connect family members, close friends, or neighbors who are alike with respect to race/ethnicity, social class, and religion. By contrast, bridging social capital refers to social connections that cross race/ethnic, class, and other boundaries.

Social Capital and Population Health

Empirical studies have linked social capital to a growing number of population health outcomes, including mortality, mental health, health-related behaviors, self-rated health, and disability. In one of the first ecological analyses, indicators of social capital at the U.S. state level (levels of trust, perceptions of reciprocity, and density of civic associations) were strongly correlated with all-cause and cause-specific mortality rates. Subsequent investigations extended these findings down to the neighborhood level. In a study based in the 343 neighborhoods of Chicago, the levels of trust, reciprocity, and group membership were found to be significantly inversely correlated with mortality rates for residents, even after controlling for the degree of economic deprivation.

Increasingly, studies of social capital and health have used multilevel analysis, with interesting results. In one study of mental health among African American residents of a disadvantaged community in Alabama, higher bonding social capital was found to be associated with worse mental health outcomes, whereas bridging social capital was found to be associated with better mental health. In other words, within the context of a highly disadvantaged community, a greater level of social connection and involvement may be associated with worse health outcomes because of the strains associated with the obligation to help others in such settings. In another study analyzing self-rated health within the 2000 Social Capital Community Benchmark Survey (conducted in 40 U.S. communities), a complex interaction was found between community levels of social trust and individual levels of trust. Among individuals who expressed a high level of trust of others, there was a positive influence (on self-rated health) of living in communities with higher levels of trust. On the other hand, the opposite was found for individuals expressing mistrust of others in their community. For these individuals, the higher the community's level of trust, the worse they felt.

Mechanisms Linking Social Capital and Health

Several mechanisms have been hypothesized through which social capital can influence health. They include:

1. The ability of a community to undertake collective action (e.g., organizing to pass local ordnances that restrict smoking in public places or lobbying to fight the closure of local clinics).
2. The ability of a community to enforce healthy norms by exercising informal social control over deviant behaviors (e.g., underage drinking, smoking, and drug abuse).
3. The faster diffusion of innovation through information channels (e.g., new knowledge about a new cancer screening test).
4. The exchange of social support between members of the community (e.g., the provisions of emotional support and stress-buffering or the exchange of instrumental aid, such as cash loans, during emergencies).

It is important to emphasize, however, that not all kinds of social capital result in beneficial outcomes for health. Like any form of capital (e.g., financial capital), social capital can be used for pro-social as well as antisocial ends and can result in deleterious as well as beneficial health outcomes.

Negative Effects of Social Capital

Social capital is not a panacea for health promotion. Strong social ties within a group or a community (high bonding social capital) can imply a high level of social exchange, which in turn translates into role strain for certain members of the in-group (the support providers, who are often women). Strong bonding social capital can often coexist with conflict between the group and outside social groups low bridging social capital). In some instances, high social capital within a community has been channeled to exclude outsiders from entering the community – for example, by enforcing residential segregation. Strong levels of social cohesion can also imply restrictions on the freedom of individual expression as well as a downleveling of achievement norms. In addition, some forms of social capital, such as criminal gangs, may provide benefits to its members, but do very little to foster social cohesion with the rest of society. Finally, some have criticized the concept of social capital for encouraging the blaming of victims (or, in this case, the blaming of communities) for their problems. These criticisms emphasize the caution warranted in applying the concept of social capital in health promotion.

See Also the Following Articles

Community Studies; Social Support.

Further Reading

Coleman, J. S. (1990). *Foundations of social theory.* Cambridge, MA: Harvard University Press.

Kawachi, I., Kennedy, B. P., Lochner, K., et al. (1997). Social capital, income inequality, and mortality. *American Journal of Public Health* 87, 1491–1498.

Kawachi, I., Kim, D. J., Coutts, A., et al. (2004). Reconciling the three accounts of social capital. *International Journal of Epidemiology* 33(4), 682–690.

Lochner, K., Kawachi, I., Brennan, R. T., et al. (2003). Social capital and neighborhood mortality rates in Chicago. *Social Science & Medicine* 56(8), 1797–1805.

Lochner, K., Kawachi, I. and Kennedy, B. P. (1999). Social capital: a guide to its measurement. *Health and Place* 5, 259–270.

Mitchell, C. U. and LaGory, M. (2002). Social capital and mental distress in an impoverished community. *City & Community* 1(2), 195–215.

Szreter, S. and Woolcock, M. (2004). Health by association?: social capital, social theory, and the political economy of public health. *International Journal of Epidemiology* 33(4), 650–667.

Subramanian, S. V., Kim, D. J. and Kawachi, I. (2002). Social trust and self-rated health in US communities: a multilevel analysis. *Journal of Urban Health* 79(4, supplement 1), S21–S34.

Subramanian, S. V., Lochner, K. and Kawachi, I. (2003). Neighborhood differences in social capital in the US: compositional artifact or a contextual construct? *Health and Place* 9, 33–44.

Social Networks and Social Isolation

L F Berkman
Harvard School of Public Health, Boston, MA, USA

Glossary

Appraisal support	Help in decision making, giving appropriate feedback, or help deciding which course of action to take.
Emotional support	The amount of loving and caring, sympathy and understanding, and/or esteem and value available from others.
Instrumental support	Help, aid, or assistance with tangible needs such as getting groceries, getting to appointments, and cooking; aid in kind, money, or labor.
Social networks	The web of social relationships that surrounds an individual and the characteristics of those ties.
Social participation and engagement	The enactment or interaction of social ties in real-life activity. Meeting with friends and family, attending social or religious functions, and participating in occupational or social roles or in group recreation are examples.

Introduction

Over the last 25 years, there have been dozens of articles and books on issues related to social networks and social support. It is now widely recognized that social relationships and affiliation have powerful effects on physical and mental health for a number of reasons.

When investigators write about the impact of social relationships on health, many terms are used loosely and interchangeably, including social networks, social support, social ties and social integration. The aim of this article is to (1) discuss theoretical orientations from diverse disciplines that we believe are fundamental to advancing research in this area, (2) briefly review findings related to mortality and biological pathways leading to poor health, (3) provide a set of definitions of networks and aspects of networks and support, and (4) present an overarching model that integrates multilevel phenomena.

Theoretical Orientations

There are several sets of theories that form the bedrock for the empirical investigation of social relationships and their influence on health. The earliest theories came from sociologists such as Emile Durkheim, as well as from psychoanalysts such as John Bowlby, who first formulated attachment theory. A major wave of conceptual development also came from anthropologists, including Bott, Barnes, and Mitchell, and from quantitative sociologists, such as Fischer, Laumann, Wellman, and Marsden, who, along with others, developed social network analysis. This eclectic mix of theoretical approaches coupled with the contributions of epidemiolgists form the foundation of research on social ties and health.

Durkheim's contribution to the study of the relationship between society and health is immeasurable. Perhaps most important is his contribution to the understanding of how social integration and cohesion influence suicide. Durkheim's primary aim was to explain how individual pathology was a function of social dynamics. In light of recent attention to upstream determinants of health, Durkheim's work reemerges with great relevance today.

Social Network Theory: A New Way of Looking at Social Structure and Community

During the mid-1950s, a number of British anthropologists found it increasingly difficult to understand the behavior of either individuals or groups on the basis of traditional categories such as kin groups, tribes, or villages. Barnes and Bott developed the concept social networks to analyze ties that cut across traditional kinship, residential, and class groups and to explain behaviors they observed such as access to jobs, political activity, and marital roles. The development of social network models provided a way to view the structural properties of relationships among people.

Network analysis "focuses on the characteristic patterns of ties between actors in a social system rather than on characteristics of the individual actors themselves and use these descriptions to study how these social structures constrain network member's behavior" (Hall and Wellman, 1985: 26). Network analysis focuses on the structure and composition of the network and on the contents or specific resources that flow through those networks. The strength of social network theory rests on the testable assumption that the social structure of the network itself is largely responsible for determining individual behavior and attitudes by shaping the flow of resources that determine access to opportunities and constraints on behavior.

Health, Social Networks, and Social Integration

From the mid-1970s to the present, there have been a series of studies consistently showing that the lack of social ties or social networks predicts mortality from almost every cause of death. There are now a number of studies, relating outcomes to morbidity and biomarkers of stress or resilience to inflammation, metabolic and neuroendocrine functioning, and cardiovascular reactivity, that also support the hypothesis that social networks impact health and well-being directly through multiple pathophysiological mechanisms. Social networks and support may both directly affect health outcomes and buffer the effects of other stressful experiences.

Here, we briefly review the mortality studies. In the first of these studies from Alameda County, men and women who lacked ties to others (in this case, based on an index assessing contacts with friends and relatives, marital status, and church and group membership) were 1.9–3.1 times more likely to die in a 9-year follow-up period than those who had many more contacts. Another study, in Tecumseh, Michigan, showed a similar strength of positive association for men, but not for women, between social connectedness/social participation and mortality risk over a 10–12 year period; this study has the additional strength that it controlled for some biomedical predictors assessed from physical examination (e.g., cholesterol, blood pressure, and respiratory function).

Similar results have been reported from several studies in the United States and form three in Scandinavia. Investigators working on a study in Evans County, Georgia, found risks to be significant in older White men and women without social networks, even when biomedical and sociodemographic risk factors were controlled for, although some racial and gender differences were observed. Two studies in Sweden reported significantly increased risks among socially isolated adults, and a study of men and women in eastern Finland found that social connections were related to mortality risk for men, but not for women, independently of standard cardiovascular risk factors.

Studies of older men and women confirm the continued importance of these relationships into late life. Furthermore, two studies of large cohorts of men and women in a large health maintenance organization and 32,000 male health professionals suggested that social networks are, in general, more strongly related to mortality than to the incidence or onset of disease.

Two more recent studies in Danish men and in Japanese men and women further indicated that aspects of social isolation or social support are related to mortality. Virtually all these studies found that people who are socially isolated or disconnected from others are between two and five times more likely to die from all causes, compared to those who maintain strong ties to friends, family, and community.

Social networks and support have been found to predict a very broad array of other health outcomes from survival post-myocardial infarction to disease progression, functioning, and the onset and course of infectious diseases. Several studies suggested that social isolation is related to C-reactive protein (especially in men), measures of allostatic load, fibrinogen and cardiovascular reactivity, and neuroendocrine function. Although observational studies have been reasonably consistent in linking social isolation to outcome, psychosocial interventions have not been as successful at producing changes in social isolation or support that translate into better health outcomes.

A Conceptual Model Linking Social Networks to Health

Although the power of using measures of networks or social integration to predict health outcomes is indisputable, the interpretation of what the measures actually measure has been open to much debate. Hall and Wellman have appropriately commented that much of the work in social epidemiology has used the term social networks metaphorically because rarely have investigators conformed to more standard assessments used in network analysis. This criticism has been duly noted, and several calls have gone out to develop a second generation of network measures.

A second wave of research developed in reaction to this early work and as an outgrowth of work in health psychology, which has turned the orientation of the field in several ways. These social scientists focused on the qualitative aspects of social relations (i.e., their provision of social support or, conversely, the detrimental aspects of relationships) rather than on the elaboration of the structural aspects of social networks. Most of these investigators followed the assumption that what is most important about networks is the support functions they provide. Although social support is among the primary pathways by which social networks may influence physical and mental health status, it is not the only critical pathway. Moreover, the exclusive study of more proximal pathways detracts from the need to focus on the social context and structural underpinnings that may significantly influence the types and extent of social support provided.

In order to have a comprehensive framework in which to explain these phenomena, it is helpful to move upstream and return to a more Durkheimian orientation to network structure and social context. It is critical to maintain a view of social networks as lodged within those larger social and cultural contexts that shape the structure of networks.

Conceptually, social networks are embedded in a macro-social environment in which large-scale social forces may influence network structure, which in turn influences a cascading causal process beginning with the macro-social to psychobiological processes to impact health. In this framework, social networks are embedded in a larger social and cultural context in which upstream forces are seen to condition network structure.

Networks may operate at the behavioral level through at least five primary pathways: (1) provision of social support, (2) social influence, (3) social engagement and attachment, (4) person-to-person contact, and (5) access to resources and material goods. These psychosocial and behavioral processes may influence even more proximate pathways to health status, including direct physiological responses; psychological states, including self-esteem, self-efficacy, and depression; health-damaging behaviors such as tobacco consumption or high-risk sexual activity, health-promoting behavior such as appropriate health service use and exercise, and exposure to infectious disease agents such as human immunodeficiency virus (HIV), other sexually transmitted diseases (STDs), and tuberculosis.

The Assessment of Social Networks

Social networks might be defined as the web of social relationships that surround an individual and the characteristics of those ties. Network characteristics are:

- Range or size: the number of network members.
- Density: the extent to which the members are connected to each other.
- Boundedness: the degree to which they are defined on the basis of traditional structures such as kin, work, and neighborhood.
- Homogeneity: the extent to which individuals are similar to each other in a network.

Related to network structure, the characteristics of individual ties include:

- Frequency of contact.
- Multiplexity: the number of types of transactions or support flowing through ties.
- Duration: the length of time an individual knows another
- Reciprocity: the extent to which exchanges are reciprocal.

Downstream Social and Behavioral Pathways

We next briefly review the primary pathways by which networks may influence health.

Social support Moving downstream, we now consider the mediating pathways by which networks might influence health status. Most obviously, the structure of network ties influences health via the provision of many kinds of support. This framework immediately acknowledges that not all ties are supportive and that there is variation in the type, frequency, intensity, and extent of support provided. For example, some ties provide several types of support, whereas other ties are specialized and provide only one type. Social support is typically divided into emotional, instrumental, appraisal, and informational support.

Emotional support is related to the amount of "love and caring, sympathy and understanding and/or esteem or value available from others" (Thoits 1995: 64). Emotional support is most often provided by a confidant or intimate other, although less intimate ties can provide such support under circumscribed conditions. Instrumental support refers to help, aid, or assistance with tangible needs such as getting groceries, getting to appointments, phoning, cooking, cleaning, and paying bills. House identifies instrumental support as aid in kind, money, or labor. Appraisal support is help in decision making, help by giving appropriate feedback, or help in deciding which course of action to take. Informational support is the provision of advice or information in the service of particular needs. Emotional, appraisal, and informational support are often difficult to disaggregate and have various other definitions (e.g., self-esteem support).

Perhaps even deeper than support are the ways in which social relationships provide a basis for intimacy and attachment. Intimacy and attachment have meaning not only for relationships that we traditionally think of as intimate (e.g., between partners and between parents and children) but also for more extended ties. For instance, when relationships are solid at a community level, individuals feel strong bonds and attachment to places (e.g., neighborhood) and organizations (e.g., voluntary and religious).

Social influence Networks may influence health via several other pathways. One pathway increasingly recognized is social influence. Shared norms around health behaviors (e.g., alcohol and cigarette consumption, sexual practices, and health-care use) might be powerful sources of social influence with direct consequences for the behaviors of network members. For instance, the relationships of adolescent girls with both their male and female friends and with their parents are associated with pregnancy risk. The social influence that extends from the network's values and norms constitutes an important and underappreciated pathway through which networks impact health.

Social engagement and attachment A third and more difficult-to-define pathway by which networks may influence health status is by promoting social participation and social engagement. Participation and engagement result from the enactment of potential ties in real-life activity. Getting together with friends, attending social functions, participating in occupational or social roles, joining in group recreation, attending church are all instances of social engagement. Thus, through opportunities for engagement, social networks define and reinforce meaningful social roles, including parental, familial, occupational, and community roles, which in turn provide a sense of value, belonging, and attachment. Several recent studies suggest that social engagement is critical in maintaining cognitive ability and in reducing mortality.

In addition, network participation provides opportunities for companionship and sociability. Some have argued that these behaviors and attitudes are not the result of the provision of support *per se* but are the consequence of participation in a meaningful social context in and of itself. One reason measures of social integration or connectedness may be such powerful predictors of mortality over long periods of follow-up is that these ties give meaning to individuals' lives by virtue of enabling them to participate fully, to be obligated (in fact, often to be the providers of support), and to feel attached to their community.

Person-to-person contact Another behavioral pathway by which networks influence disease is by restricting or promoting exposure to infectious disease agents. In this regard, the methodological links between epidemiology and networks are striking. What is perhaps most remarkable is that the same network characteristics that can be health-promoting can at the same time be health-damaging if they serve as vectors for the spread of infectious disease. Efforts to link mathematical models applying network approaches to epidemiology are in their infancy and have started to appear over the last 10 years.

The contribution of social network analysis to model of disease transmission is the understanding that in many, if not most cases, disease transmission is not spread randomly throughout a population. Social network analysis is well suited to the development of models in which exposure between individuals is not random but rather is based on geographic location, sociodemographic characteristics (e.g., age, race, and gender), or other important characteristics of the individual such as socioeconomic position, occupation, and sexual orientation. Furthermore, because social network analysis focuses on characteristics of the network rather than on characteristics of the individual, it is ideally suited to the study of the diffusion of transmissible diseases through populations via bridging ties between networks or to uncovering the characteristics of ego-centered networks that promote the spread of disease.

Access to resources and material goods Surprisingly little research has sought to examine differential access to material goods, resources, and services as a mechanism through which social networks might operate. This, in our view, is unfortunate given the work of sociologists showing that social networks operate by regulating an individual's access to life opportunities by virtue of the extent to which networks overlap with other networks. In this way, networks operate to provide access or to restrict opportunities in much the same way as the social status does. Perhaps the most important among studies exploring this tie is Granovetter's classic study of the power of weak ties that, on the one hand, lack intimacy but, on the other hand, facilitate the diffusion of influence and information and provide opportunities for mobility.

Conclusion

This article has reviewed the ways in which social isolation, lack of support, and disengagement may be chronically stressful social experiences and are linked to poor health outcomes. With the development of multilevel framework, we are struck by two issues of profound importance. The first is the upstream question of identifying the conditions that influence the development and structure of social networks. Such questions have been the substantive focus of much of social network research, especially in relationship to urbanization, social stratification, and culture change. Yet little of this work has been integrated with health issues in a way that might guide us in the development of policies or interventions to improve public health. Recent work relating social cohesion to economic inequality has begun to help us decipher the complex interrelationships between these social experiences. Of particular interest are the ways in which social policies may impact the form and function of social networks. For instance, work/family policies and housing policies may impact network and supportive relationships in important ways, ultimately having a health impact.

The second major issue relates to the downstream question. Many investigators have assumed that networks influence health via social support functions. Our framework makes clear that this is but one pathway linking networks to health outcomes. Furthermore, the work on conflict and stress points out not only that are not all relationships positive in valence but that some of the most powerful impacts on health that social relationships may have are through acts of abuse, violence, and trauma. Fully elucidating these downstream experiences and how they are linked to health and via which biological mechanisms remains a major challenge in the field.

Acknowledgments

This paper is adapted from Berkman, L. F. and Glass, T. (2000), Social integration, social networks, social support and health, In Berkman, L. F. & Kawachi, I. (eds) *Social epidemiology.* New York: Oxford University Press; and Berkman, L. F. (2001), Social integration, social networks, and health. In Smelser, N. J. & Baltes, P. B. (eds), *International encyclopedia of the social and behavioral sciences.* New York: Elsevier.

See Also the Following Article

Social Support.

Further Reading

Bassuk, S., Glass, T. and Berkman, L. F. (1999). Social disengagement and incident cognitive decline in community-dwelling elderly persons. *Annals of Internal Medicine* **131**, 165–173.

Berkman, L. (2001). Social integration, social networks and health. In: Smelser, N. J. & Baltes, P. B. (eds.) *International encyclopedia of the social and behavioral sciences* (vol. 21), pp. 14327–14332. New York: Elsevier.

Berkman, L. F. and Glass, T. (2000). Social integration, social networks, social support and health. In: Berkman, L. F. & Kawachi, I. (eds.) *Social epidemiology*, pp. 137–173. New York: Oxford University Press.

Berkman, L. F. and Syme, S. (1979). Social networks, host resistance, and mortality: a nine-year follow-up of Alameda County residents. *American Journal of Epidemiology* **109**, 186–204.

Bearman, P. and Bruckner, H. (1999). Peer effects on adolescent sexual debut and pregnancy: an analysis of a national survey of adolescent girls. The National Campaign for the Prevention of Teen Pregnancy.

Cohen, S., Underwood, S. and Gottlieb, B. (2000). *Social support measures and intervention.* New York: Oxford University Press.

Durkheim, E. (1897). *Suicide.* New York: Free Press.

Fischer, C. S., Jackson, R. M., Steuve, C. A., et al. (1977). *Networks and places.* New York: Free Press.

Glass, T., Mendes de Leon, C., Marottoli, R., et al. (1999). Population based study of social and productive activities

as predictors of survival among elderly Americans. *British Medical Journal* **319**, 478–483.
Granovetter, M. (1973). The strength of weak ties. *American Journal of Sociology* **78**, 1360–1380.
Hall, A. and Wellman, B. (1985). Social networks and social support. In: Cohen, S. & Syme, S. L. (eds.) *Social support and health*, pp. 23–41. Orlando, FL: Academic Press.
Kawachi, I., Colditz, G. A., Ascherio, A., et al. (1996). A prospective study of social networks in relation to total mortality and cardiovascular disease in men in the U.S.A. *Journal of Epidemiology Community Health* **50**, 245–251.
Pennix, B. W., van Tilburg, T., Kriegsman, D. M., et al. (1997). Effects of social support and personal coping resources on mortality in older age: the Longitudinal Aging Study, Amsterdam. *American Journal of Epidemiology* **146**, 510–519.
Seeman, T. (1996). Social ties and health: the benefits of social integration. *Annals of Epidemiology* **6**, 442–451.
Sugisawa, H., Liang, J. and Liu, X. (1994). Social networks, social support and mortality among older peoplein Japan. *Journal of Gerontology* **49**, S3–S13.
Thoits, P. (1995). Stress, coping, and social support processes: where are we? What next? *Journal of Health and Social Behavior* (extra issue), 53–79.

Social Status and Stress

D de Ridder
Utrecht University, Utrecht, The Netherlands

This is a revised version of the article by D de Ridder, Encyclopedia of Stress First Edition, volume 3, pp 468–473, © 2000, Elsevier Inc.

Glossary

Coping resources — The personal (e.g., self-esteem and sense of control) and social (most notably, social support) resources an individual has at his or her disposal to counter the adverse effects of the experience of distress.

Coping strategies — The cognitive and behavioral attempts an individual may employ when faced with the experience of distress.

Exposure — The actual confrontation with stressful situations (events) of chronic stressful conditions.

Social status — Any attribute indicating the social position of an individual in a group or in the society. The most important attribute is socioeconomic status, comprising income, education, and occupation.

Vulnerability — The lack of personal and social coping resources, which increases the risk of a greater adverse impact of stressful conditions.

Social Status, Health, and Stress

The relationship between social status and health is intriguing because it challenges existing models of how a distal variable such as social status might affect health. Research in the past decades focused on explaining the association between low social status, especially low socioeconomic status (SES), and poor health, assuming that the greater distress of living in deprived social and material conditions is an important factor in the strong and consistent association between health and social status. The extensive literature on SES and health provides some indications why the theoretical framework of stress should be considered an interesting candidate in furthering our understanding of the association between SES and health. First, the linearity of the relationship between SES and health implies better health outcomes as individuals ascend the SES continuum, so that even relatively affluent groups exhibit worse health than their higher SES counterparts. This suggests that factors other than the obvious role of inadequate financial resources or poor living conditions are involved and that SES might also affect psychosocial factors. Identifying these factors may be considered a search for more health-proximal processes so as to bridge the gap between indicators of social status and the associated health outcomes. Second, the analysis of potential measurement artifacts shows that the association between social status and health is robust and is little affected by social selection factors, which would be the case if those who are in poor health were at a higher risk of getting a lower social status. Social selection effects are rare, however, and limited to young children who are unable to attend school as a result of a serious and disabling disease. The absence of social selection effects suggests that the strong association between social status and health is explained by social causation mechanisms – social status affects health instead of the other way around. Particular elements of the stress-coping paradigm offer a framework to study the causal chain between social status at one end of the continuum and health at the other one, particularly those elements that deal with conceptualizing environmental risk for health (exposure to stressors) and individual responses to explain the impact of these stressors (vulnerability to stress).

Indicators of Social Status

Traditionally, most social-epidemiological research has employed the criteria of income, occupation, and education for assessing social status. Less frequently, indicators of material wealth such as car ownership, house ownership, the number of computers in the house, or the number of annual holidays have been used. Interestingly, the sociocultural component of SES expressed in educational attainment appears to have a stronger impact than the more socioeconomic elements of income and occupational status. Recent research indicates that the relationship between income and health varies substantially by level of education. Education improves health, and its effects are larger at low levels of income; education also reduces the strength of the income–health relationship. The linear gradient relationship between income and health is thus more characteristic of groups with higher levels of education, suggesting that education might improve skills needed to cope effectively with stress. This is shown, for example, in the finding that the mother's educational status is a better predictor of family stress than both family income or the occupational status of the father.

Recently, it has been argued that it is not the absolute level of SES that is important for understanding its association with health and distress but rather inequality from relative standing. There is suggestive evidence that subjective social status (assessed by a ladder with 10 rungs representing where people stand in society in terms of who are the best off, have the most money, have most education, and have the best jobs) is more strongly linked to health in terms of self-rated health, heart rate, and cortisol habituation to repeated stress than the traditional objective measures of SES (education, income, and occupation). The so-called hierarchy stress perspective argues that the gradient-like association between SES and health reflects social ordering rather than material deprivation *per se*. According to this perspective, higher income leads to less stress, less status anxiety, and more perceived control. These underlying mechanisms are psychological and related to relative rather than absolute material deprivation. Social ordering has effects that are no less substantial than absolute deprivation because relative deprivation leads to worse health both directly through physiological pathways (e.g., cortisol levels) and indirectly through maladaptive coping behaviors (e.g., smoking or alcohol consumption). It is noteworthy that in countries with a high degree of income inequality (e.g., the United States) the SES–health gradient is steeper than in economically more egalitarian European countries. Thus, although SES is a reliable and robust indicator of health, SES as such provides few cues for understanding its relationship with stress. In the words of the social epidemiologists Brown and Harris (1978; p. 10), "It is not that the 'demographic type' measures are of no use, it is that they are not enough. What is required is their combination with concepts and measures dealing directly and in detail with the immediate . . . experience of the individual."

Such an approach is found in social role research, advancing the hypothesis that the lower social status of, for example, the nonemployed affects their sense of meaning and purpose in life and has much less to do with the direct material consequences of their income and employment status. Striking findings in this area have been reported 30 years ago on the disadvantaged social role of nonemployed married women, who generally reported poorer health than both employed married women and men – although it is not clear to what extent social changes since the 1970s concerning the role of women make those observations still valid. These studies revealed that women who confront the double role of parent and employee reported lower levels of psychological distress than women who are devoted to the role of homemaker. These findings suggest that regardless the actual level of stressful experiences due to overload, the social status of worker is somehow beneficial for the employed women's health. It should be noted, however, that, although working women may be more protected from distress than nonemployed women, they are still confronted with more distress than employed men.

The results from social role studies are corroborated by findings on particular social groups in our Western community who cannot claim high social status regardless of their income, education, or employment status. Research on the elderly, the unmarried, and nonwhites puts results from social role studies in a somewhat different perspective, suggesting that it is not only the meaning associated with particular roles that accounts for the greater distress of those low in social status but also their ranking order in the social group. Individuals from disadvantaged social groups have been reported to be in poorer health and facing more distress, which may be accounted for by their lower social ranking, although direct tests of this assumption in humans are not available. Animal studies have shown that subordination tends to be associated with a chronically overactive stress response (e.g., higher blood pressure). This pattern is believed to reflect the classic picture of dominance hierarchies as linear pecking orders in which resources are unevenly distributed, inequalities are maintained through aggression and intimidation, and subordinates are subject to the most severe resource limitations, the fewest opportunities for coping, and the greatest physical and social stressors. However, recent studies suggest that the relationship between social rank and patterns of the stress response may be more diverse than has been assumed hitherto. More specifically, it appears that the negative effects of low ranking on stress responses may be attenuated by complex affiliative relationships that may help low-status stressed individuals to cope. It is unknown, however, to what extent these studies on social ranking in animals are directly relevant for humans because humans often belong to multiple hierarchies and tend to value most the one in which they rank highest.

Social Status and Exposure to Stressful Conditions

The common approach to social status and psychological distress suggests that those who are in a disadvantaged social position are confronted with more stressors than their more privileged counterparts, either as a result of exposure to more frequent or more intense negative life events or of living in chronic stressful conditions associated with continuous exposure to daily hassles. Thus, this approach reflects the notion that poorer health associated with lower social status results from social causation, emphasizing the role of structural and material conditions in causing distress. The life event approach to stress dictates that major life events (e.g., divorce or being fired) impose a breach in behavioral routines, cause distress, and therefore require adaptive efforts, eventually exhausting the system. The chronic stress approach takes a somewhat different perspective and states that is the repeated exposure to minor events or daily hassles (e.g., refused services or poor transportation facilities) that ultimately causes wear and tear on the individual.

Life Events

The assumption that people with low social status report more life events than those with higher status is corroborated only weakly by empirical research. Insofar as individuals of lower SES have reported higher numbers or life events, most of these events are directly related to financial problems. There is also a higher report of uncontrollable life events, reflecting to some extent the conditions of poverty and deprivation (e.g., discharge due to becoming obsolete) in individuals with lower social status. Still, even when a higher frequency of life events is reported, this generally fails to account for the higher levels of self-reported distress; no more than 10% of the variance in distress is explained by exposure to life events. Adopting an approach that allows for a contextual evaluation of events shows slightly different results, demonstrating that it is not so much the number of events or even their quality (e.g., uncontrollability) that counts but their potential influence on a number of crucial life areas. Research by social epidemiologists Brown and Harris describing the onset of depression in working-class women clearly demonstrated that these women were confronted with life events that had the potential of generating a chain of other stressful events. The most typical event these women reported involved a teenage pregnancy, which caused these young women to drop out of school and engage in an untimely and unwanted marriage, eventually leaving them divorced, socially isolated, financially deprived, and without a significant chance of entering the labor market or controlling their future in another way – leaving them in a state of hopelessness that is characteristic of depression. Other studies of lower-class women have demonstrated that the lives of these women are fraught with a large number of network events, meaning that they consider the life events experienced by significant others in their social network as if they concerned them directly, which may further explain the higher levels of distress reported by these women. Nevertheless, it is clear that, although the number of major life events appears to be somewhat higher in those occupying low social status, the higher levels of exposure to major life events are not a sufficient explanation to account for the higher levels of distress.

Daily Hassles and Chronic Stressful Conditions

It appears that it is not so much the incidence of particular major life events that is causing high levels of distress in low-social-status individuals but the continuous confrontation with a large number of repetitive small events that mark living in deprived circumstances. The lower an individual is on the SES continuum, the greater the amount of hassles and the greater the time needed to address the basic tasks of living, including shopping in poorly provided facilities, lack of good transportation, poor access to social and health-care facilities, and refused services. Of course, such difficulties in accomplishing daily routines have their echo in social relations. It is not surprising, therefore, that minor conflicts in relationships in work, marriage, and parenting appear to be more common in low-SES individuals. Still, it is hard to imagine that the experience of minor stress is a simple question of individual exposure. Improving the understanding of how chronic stress affects individuals of lower SES may not so much lie in the study of individual experience of these minor stressors but in identifying the environmental features of low-SES neighborhoods themselves, implying that low SES may have an impact on a community level too. Interestingly, research shows that neighborhood-level indicators predict distress above the effects of individual-level indicators. This suggests that the more proximal environment in which people live may provide important information for identifying the environmental features that cause distress. Those in the lower ends of the social-class distribution disproportionally live in deprived neighborhoods, occupy jobs characterized by high demands and low control, and live in social environments in which they are exposed to violence, conflict, abuse, crowding, and noise. All these environmental features may be considered to increase the experience of distress, although it remains to be answered how these unhealthy environments get under an individual's skin (Taylor & Repetti, 1997). Adopting a perspective that conceptualizes social status as a proxy to understanding the stressful features of particular environments raises the issue of how situational demands should be distinguished from subjective appraisals of these objective demands. This issue constitutes a classic problem in the cognitive approach to stress formulated by Richard Lazarus and deals with the important question of how demands in the environment are appraised and handled by the individual.

Social Status and Vulnerability to Stressful Conditions

No matter how unhealthy and environment is, not all individuals sharing the same environment are affected by that environment in a similar way, suggesting that factors concerning individual susceptibility to these environmental threats are at work. The approach highlighting a differential vulnerability to stressful conditions may improve our understanding of why individuals of lower social status experience more distress. Vulnerability is reflected in the availability of resources that may be helpful in countering the adverse effects of exposure to stress, including the repertoire of coping strategies, social support, and beliefs about control and competence. Because exposure to environmental threats fails to offer a sufficient explanation for the experience of greater distress in low-SES individuals, it has been hypothesized that the availability of coping resources varies with social status. The question is whether and why lower SES is associated with lower availability of these and other coping resources.

Coping

The employment of adequate cognitive and behavioral coping efforts constitutes one of the most important resources for buffering the adverse effects of psychological distress. Individuals who find constructive ways of coping with stress, such as taking direct action or finding meaning in their experience, are better able to withstand the negative effects of stressful circumstances than individuals who believe their coping resources to be minimal or who believe that the situation is beyond their control and rely on avoidance coping strategies, which in the long run often turn out to compromise their health. Generally, people of low social status are more inclined to adopt avoiding and emotion-focused strategies when they are confronted with stress than are their more advantaged peers. Education level and family income directly relate to the frequency of problem-focused coping for dealing with financial strain and other hassles, with those of low social status reporting less problem-focused coping. Why low SES promotes generally ineffective coping strategies is unknown, although it has been suggested that the acquisition of coping strategies may to some extent be shaped by the continuous confrontation with few possibilities to control their environment. Although research that directly links social status and coping is rare, it has been shown that individuals of low social status are more sensitive to stress and think of it as unpleasant, disruptive and beyond their control. In contrast, individuals with higher social status appear to be less bothered by distressing events and more often regard it as a challenge to do something about it. It thus seems that the appraisal of potentially upsetting situations as uncontrollable and overwhelming may activate dysfunctional coping patterns. More generally, it seems that low-SES environments reduce individuals' reserve capacity to manage stress, thereby increasing negative emotions and cognitions with subsequent effects for dealing with these stressful conditions themselves.

Social Support

The adverse effect of chronic exposure to stressful environments may be partially offset if an individual has at least one supportive person in his or her neighborhood. Living in low-SES communities may compromise the effective use of social contacts, however. Although the social network of low-SES individuals generally is not smaller than the network of those with better education and higher incomes, the networks of low-SES individuals tend to be more homogeneous, with a large proportion of kin, which may affect the type of support provided and its perceived helpfulness. If an individual is not willing to share particular problems with family members, the possibilities for social support decrease dramatically. The larger proportion of kin in the social networks of low-social-status individuals also has consequences for mutual dependency. Asking for help on one occasion implies some kind of obligation to provide support when a family member asks for it on another occasion. The larger proportion of family in the network also bears costs because it may promote the experience of stress when a family member experiences distress. In addition, the rare prospective research in this area demonstrates that the experience of distress may affect the availability of social support. Studies of economic stressors such as financial hardship or unemployment confirm a pattern in which economic stressors lead to increased marital stress and decreased social support.

Social Distribution of Coping Resources

It is not clear why low-SES individuals are at a disadvantage with regard to the availability of coping resources. Vulnerability is thought to be partly genetically determined and partly acquired during childhood and adolescence by accumulating negative experiences, which may be difficult to compensate for. Lack of financial resources and poor material conditions are, of course, more common in low-SES individuals, but these factors do not appear to be the most important determinants of vulnerability. No evidence is available that limited access to coping resources is a direct result of deficient life conditions. Low self-esteem and low personal control are acquired during repetitive and accumulating negative events causing a negative spiral in which an individual learns to be helpless and hopeless. Low chances of employment or low educational attainment do not by themselves cause vulnerability to distress, but this does not mean that vulnerability does not operate at a social level. Particular resources and coping strategies may be distributed differently among the social classes and also particular beliefs about stress and health may be socially shaped and transmitted. The employment of ineffective coping strategies seems to depend on strong beliefs about what constitutes stress and what can be done about it. Beliefs reflect, at least in part, socially shared assumptions about stress, coping, and health and may be considered cultural models of the individual and his or her social group. A significant example concerns cigarette smoking as a way of coping. Although smoking is widely recognized as a health-threatening habit in both low-SES and high-SES individuals, in low-social-status individuals smoking has often turned into one of their few available coping options and creates a feeling of rest and control when faced with distress. Further research on the social distribution of coping resources is certainly required.

See Also the Following Articles

Cultural Factors in Stress; Economic Factors and Stress; Education Levels and Stress; Minorities and Stress; Social Capital.

Further Reading

Abbott, D. H., Keverne, E. B., Bercovich, G. B., et al. (2003). Are subordinates always stressed?: a comparative analysis of rank differences in cortisol levels among primates. *Hormones and Behavior* **43**, 67–82.

Adler, N. E., Boyce, T., Chesney, M. A., et al. (1994). Socioeconomic status and health: the challenge of the gradient. *American Psychologist* **49**, 15–25.

Adler, N. E., Epel, E. S., Castellazzo, G., et al. (2000). Relationship of subjective and objective social status with psychological and physiological functioning: preliminary data in healthy white women. *Health Psychology* **19**, 586–592.

Antonovsky, A. (1967). Social class, life expectancy and overall mortality. *Millbank Quarterly* **45**, 31–73.

Brown, G. W. and Harris, T. (1978). *Social origins of depression: a study of psychiatric disorder in women.* London: Tavistock.

Chen, E., Matthews, K. A. and Boyce, W. T. (2002). Socioeconomic differences in children's health: how and why do these relationships change with age? *Psychological Bulletin* **128**, 295–329.

Cohen, S., Kaplan, G. A. and Salonen, J. T. (1999). The role of psychological characteristics in the relation between socioeconomic status and perceived health. *Journal of Applied Social Psychology* **29**, 445–468.

Feldman, P. J. and Steptoe, A. (2004). How neighborhoods and physical functioning are related: the roles of neighborhood socioeconomic status, perceived neighborhood strain, and individual health risk factors. *Annals of Behavioral Medicine* **27**, 91–99.

Gallo, L. C. and Matthews, K. A. (2003). Understanding the association between socioeconomic status and health: do negative emotions play a role? *Psychological Bulletin* **129**, 10–51.

Sapolsky, R. M. (2004). Social status and health in humans and other animals. *Annual Review of Anthropology* **33**, 393–418.

Taylor, S. E. and Repetti, R. L. (1997). Health psychology: what is an unhealthy environment and how does it get under the skin? *Annual Review of Psychology* **48**, 411–447.

Wilkinson, R. G. (1999). Health, hierarchy, and social anxiety. In: Adler, N. E., Marmot, M., McEwen, B. & Stewart, J. (eds.) *Special issue on socioeconomic status and health in industrial nations: social, psychological, and biological pathways, Annals of the New York Academy of Sciences*, 48–63.

Social Support

T C Antonucci
University of Michigan, Ann Arbor, MI, USA
J E Lansford
Duke University, Durham, NC, USA
K J Ajrouch
Eastern Michigan University, Ypsilanti, MI, USA

This is a revised version of the article by T C Antonucci, J E Lansford and K J Ajrouch, Encyclopedia of Stress First Edition, volume 3, pp 479–482, © 2000, Elsevier Inc.

Glossary

Anticipated support	Support perceived to be available if the need for it arises in the future.
Appraisal support	Feedback relevant to self-evaluation.
Emotional support	The provision of empathy, reassurance, liking, and respect.
Informational support	Help with problem solving and advice.
Instrumental support	Aid with services and the tasks of daily living.
Social network	The group of individuals with whom an individual may exchange support.

This article examines the concept of social support and its relationship to stress. A brief review of several illustrative theoretical perspectives of social support is presented first. Next, an outline and overview of the research focusing on social support as a coping mechanism is provided, followed by a discussion of social support as a source of stress and a brief summary and conclusion.

Theoretical Perspectives

Social support has received a great deal of attention in the last several decades. There are some points that are now relatively well accepted: social support tends to be cumulative over the life course; it is often multigenerational; it is best when an individual both provides and receives support, although not necessarily in the context of the same relationship; and it can include exchanges between family and friends and between formal and informal providers.

Research thus far has offered interesting and sometimes quite useful evidence for how social relations affect the individual's socialization, development, coping, and general well-being. The concept of social support has been attractive to researchers in a wide variety of disciplines, including epidemiology, sociology, psychology, social work, and health care. The related theoretical perspectives or frameworks offered by each of these disciplines are too numerous to mention here; instead, illustrative examples are provided.

Epidemiologists offered some of the earliest theorizing about the role of social support and health. Researchers in this field suggested that social relations help protect the individual from disease. This perspective was initially considered quite revolutionary because these researchers claimed that physical as well as mental health could be influenced by social relations. More recently, other researchers have found empirical support for this perspective.

Kahn and Antonucci extended this notion by suggesting that individuals are surrounded by convoys of family and friends. The resulting interaction and socialization processes teach them the roles and responsibilities of childhood, adulthood, and old age. This convoy of relations is assumed to have a positive effect, helping the individual successfully meet the challenges of life. However, it is recognized that convoys may not always be positive and sometimes can expose individuals to stress rather than serve as protection. This theoretical framework suggests that social support is best understood within a life course perspective and that social interactions are cumulative and developmental.

These theoretical frameworks were general and broad; other theories have taken a more practical approach to understanding social support. Cantor's hierarchical theory of social support suggests that a natural hierarchy of people exists from whom an individual prefers to receive support. People prefer to receive support from a spouse and children first and then turn to friends and neighbors if the former are unavailable. Only if all of these informal sources of support are unavailable are people likely to seek support from a formal provider (e.g., government and community institutions). A somewhat complementary theory was offered by Litwak, who suggested that people turn to those who are most able to provide the specific goods or services they need rather than to those to whom they feel closest. Both of these theoretical perspectives have a practical task-oriented focus.

Some theories have been more psychologically focused. For example, Pearlin argued that others step in when needed and help the individual achieve his or her goal. This provides the individual with a feeling of ability or personal achievement, which not only aids in coping with a specific event but also provides the individual with a more generalizeable sense of mastery. This theoretical perspective is similar to that offered by Antonucci and Jackson, who suggested that there is a life-span developmental benefit to the constant repetition of supportive interactions. Receiving support over time leads to viewing oneself as worthy, cared for, and loved. Under optimal conditions, this exchange provides the individual with a sense of personal efficacy that is critical as the individual faces the challenges or crises of life.

The types of theoretical perspectives that have guided research in this area can be summarized as follows: (1) general broad-based theories suggesting that social relations affect an individual's ability to resist stress and disease; (2) more practical, task- or person-specific theoretical frameworks that provide guidelines for determining who is the logical choice for helping a person cope with a specific problem, task, or crisis; and finally (3) more global, developmental perspectives that are designed to explain how an individual develops the ability to cope with stress over time. We turn now to a consideration of the evidence that examines how social support influences the individual's experience of stress.

Social Support as a Mechanism for Coping with Stress

It is well established that social relationships influence individuals' psychological well-being by providing love, intimacy, reassurance of worth, tangible assistance, and guidance. Across the life span, the lack of high-quality relationships is associated with negative physical and psychological consequences such as anxiety, depression, loneliness, and poor health. Studies of social support and well-being generally reflect two lines of research. First, support is thought to have direct effects on health maintenance and recovery, enhancing well-being regardless of the level of stress experienced. Second, support has been conceptualized as having indirect effects on well-being by acting as a buffer against stress. According to this second approach, during stressful events social support mediates the association between stress and adjustment so individuals who have high-quality support are not as negatively affected by stress as those who have less adequate support. Research provides evidence for both models. In this section, however, we focus on conceptualizing support as a buffer against stress.

Empirical studies provide evidence that social support can reduce the negative impact of stress associated with physical illness, unwanted or unexpected life events, and developmental transitions. For example, supportive relationships with family members and friends can help children cope with stress associated with school transitions, young adults adjust to the birth of a child, or older adults negotiate retirement. In particular, having a confidant appears to be an especially helpful resource in coping with stress. Recent evidence highlights race, ethnicity, and culture as important factors in links between stress and social support. For example, studies suggest that social support can buffer ethnic minorities from the stress associated with discrimination.

Social support is most effective as a buffer against stress when the support matches the needs elicited by the stressor. Researchers discuss four main types of support: emotional, appraisal, informational, and instrumental. Different types of support are more appropriate as buffers against some stressful experiences than others. For example, bereavement may call for emotional support, and illness may call for instrumental support.

Researchers also distinguish between the perceived availability of support and the actual receipt of support. Available or anticipated support is the belief that social network members are willing to provide support if the need for it arises in the future. Anticipated support and received support have different effects on psychological well-being. It appears that the perception that support is available if needed has direct positive effects on well-being but that actually receiving support is not always beneficial. In particular, received support may not act as a buffer against stress because receiving support may be a signal that an individuals' own coping resources have been inadequate in resolving the stressful situation. Individuals are likely to try to deal with stress on their own before turning to others for help. Thus, receiving support may indicate that their own efforts have failed and in some sense counteract the beneficial effects of the support. In addition, receiving support may place burdens on the support network and lead to conflicts among members. Anticipated support, on the other hand, promotes individuals' own coping efforts, helps individuals maintain hope that others are available if needed, and reflects a sense of caring and commitment from the social network.

It is important to recognize that the presence of a social relationship does not necessarily indicate that the relationship is supportive. The overall quality of the relationship is more important than its mere existence. For example, Major and colleagues found that supportive relationships could help women cope with the stressful experience of having an abortion. If these supportive relationships were also perceived as being high in conflict, however, the women showed more distress than if the relationships were low in conflict. Among women who did not perceive their relationships as supportive, there was no association between conflict in these relationships and distress. Thus, in considering whether relationships can act as buffers against stress, it is important to consider their negative as well as supportive characteristics.

To summarize, a great deal of evidence suggests that social support can help individuals cope with stress. To be most beneficial, this support should match the needs elicited by the stressor and be provided or expected in the context of a high quality relationship.

Social Support as a Source of Stress

The fact that social support can have negative consequences for the individual has only recently been addressed, and researchers are now openly calling for more attention to this issue. Social networks can become a source of conflict, stress, and sometimes health-damaging effects. One important dimension to this approach is the finding that larger social networks do not guarantee happiness, nor do they necessarily create a buffer from stress. For example, larger social networks are associated with greater stress among women, especially due to role strain. A case in point is role overload, a situation in which demands are placed on an individual that exceed his or her capacities to cope with them. For example, the responsibilities of informal caregivers to seriously impaired relatives may compete with other demands of a social network, resulting in a significant amount of stress for the individual. Having more social contacts "not only provides more potential resources but also may create additional demands on time and increase the probability of interpersonal conflicts" (Cohen and Syme, 1985: 12). Nevertheless, role theorists, such as Coontz, have noted that multiple roles are also associated with multiples sources of satisfactions, reward and accomplishments, thus suggesting the picture is not a simple one.

The most recent findings about social relations as a source of stress provide some insight into biopsychosocial links. When social relations are negative in nature, physiological reactivity becomes heightened. For instance, hostile spousal interactions increase heart rate, blood pressure, and neuroendocrine reactivity, as well as compromising immune functions. Moreover, negative social relations earlier in the life course directly affect physiological reactions later in life, contributing to allostatic load, which in turn may accelerate disease and poor mental health. This new body of research suggests that social relations influence physiological stress indicators and that, furthermore, the effects may be lifelong and cumulative.

Assistance from family is often thought to be the most reliable and consistent source of social support, yet family members who provide social support during times of crisis are themselves the sources of stress at other times. Moreover, negative interactions are more likely to involve kin than nonkin. Family also tends to make up the majority of individuals' social networks as they age. Thus, the source of stress is often found through the relationships that unfold within the confines of family support situations. For example, divorced women with social networks dominated by family may be more criticized for their failed marriage and thus experience significantly more, rather than less, stress.

Morgan conducted focus group discussions with recently widowed women and men to explore whether social networks actually ease adjustment to widowhood. The discussions revealed that a significant portion of negative outcomes derived from relationships with family members. Morgan stated that his findings may generate useful hypotheses about the role of family and friends as sources of support by suggesting that a distinction be made between positive and negative aspects of relationships. Support from family often produces stress when discrepancies exist between expectations and actual performance.

High levels of social support have also been found to cause stress. For example, research with the elderly demonstrates that such high levels of support from caregivers may cause stress and thus be harmful to the elder's well-being. Similarly, research has shown that family assistance to adolescent mothers helps them cope with many stressful aspects of their experience, but this support often is accompanied by conflict, frustration, disappointment, and stress. Too much support may foster dependency, causing the receiver to lose autonomy and hence develop low self-esteem. Another example is chronic financial strain. Stack found that survival in a poverty-ridden community depended on financial support from social network members. Support of this type, although generally positive, could under certain conditions be problematic. Having others expect support can also limit the success of the support provider. The network members they turn to for support in the face of chronic financial stress are likely to be facing financial difficulties of their own. The issue is complex. Social support can help minorities cope with the harmful mental and physical health consequences of racial discrimination. Jackson, Williams, and Torres hypothesize that, although negative health outcomes are associated with the stress of discrimination and the related experience of social inequality and racism, these effects can be successfully buffered by social support. At the same time, it has been noted that having a strong group identity may elevate individuals' perceptions of discrimination and in some ways make them more vulnerable to its effects.

Summary and Conclusion

Many theorists from several different disciplines have developed frameworks regarding the association between social support and stress. Empirical investigations of these theories have revealed that social support can help individuals cope with stress but that social support also can be a source of stress. These theories and research suggest that social support can be a complicated matter with both positive and negative implications for individuals and their ability to cope with the stress and challenges of everyday life.

See Also the Following Articles

Health and Socioeconomic Status; Social Capital.

Further Reading

Antonucci, T. C. and Jackson, J. S. (1987). Social support, interpersonal efficacy, and health: a life course perspective. In: Carstensen, L. L. & Edelstein, B. A. (eds.) *Handbook of clinical gerontology*, pp. 291–311 New York: Pergamon.

Cantor, M. H. (1979). Neighbors and friends: an overlooked resource in the informal support system. *Research on Aging* **1**, 434–463.

Cohen, S. and Syme, S. L. (1985). Issues in the study and application of social support. In: Cohen, S. & Syme, S. L. (eds.) *Social support and health*, pp. 3–22 New York: Academic Press.

Coontz, S. (1992). *The way we never were: American families and the nostalgia trap*. New York: BasicBooks.

Jackson, J. S., Williams, D. R. and Torres, M. (2003). Discrimination, health and mental health: the social stress process. In: Maney, A. (ed.) *Socioeconomic conditions, stress and mental disorders: toward a new synthesis of research and public policy*, pp. 86–146. Bethesda, MD: NIH Office of Behavioral and Social Research.

Kahn, R. L. and Antonucci, T. C. (1980). Convoys over the life course: attachment, roles and social support. In: Baltes, P. B. & Brim, O. (eds.) *Life-span development and behavior* (vol. 3), pp. 254–283. Boston: Lexington.

Kiecolt-Glaser, J. K. and Newton, T. L. (2001). Marriage and health: his and hers. *Psychological Bulletin* **127**, 472–503.

Litwak, E. (1985). *Helping the elderly: the complementary roles of informal networks and formal systems.* New York: Guilford.

Major, B., Zubek, J. M., Cooper, M. L., et al. (1997). Mixed messages: implications of social conflict and social support within close relationships for adjustment to a stressful life event. *Journal of Personality and Social Psychology* **72**, 1349–1363.

McEwen, B. S. (2000). Allostasis and allostatic load: implications for neuropsychopharmacology. *Neuropsychopharmacology* **22**, 108–124.

Morgan, D. L. (1989). Adjusting to widowhood: do social networks really make it easier? *The Gerontologist* **29**, 101–107.

Pearlin, L. I. (1985). Social structure and processes of social support. In: Cohen, S. & Syme, S. L. (eds.) *Social support and health*, pp. 43–60 New York: Academic Press.

Seeman, T. E. and Crimmins, E. (2001). Social and environmental effects on health and aging: integrating epidemiologic and demographic perspectives. In: Seeman, T. E. (ed.) *Special issue on population heath and aging: strengthening the dialogue between epidemiology and demography. Annals of the New York Academy of Sciences,* 954), pp. 88–117. 88–117.

Sellers, R. M. and Shelton, J. N. (2003). The role of racial identity in perceived racial discrimination. *Journal of Personality and Social Psychology* **84**, 1079–1092.

Stack, C. B. (1974). *All our kin*. New York: Harper and Row.

Transport-Related Stress

R G Smart
Centre for Addiction and Mental Health,
Toronto, Canada

Glossary

Acute stress disorder	Severe stress resulting from a dangerous situation and lasting up to 4 weeks.
Driver stress	Stress that is not trait stress but relates specifically to the problems and challenge of driving.
Posttraumatic stress	Severe stress resulting from a dangerous situation, marked by anxiety, threat, fear, and helplessness; role impairment; and a preoccupation with the situation. This stress lasts more than 4 weeks.
Road rage	Situations in which drivers or passengers attempt to kill, injure, or intimidate another driver, another passenger, or a pedestrian.
Trait stress	Stress that is not situational but is related to ongoing personality and lifestyle factors and is an enduring feature of a person's life.

The Natural Stress of Driving

Advertisements for new cars often show drivers racing along an open road, luxuriating in the comfort and phenomenal speed of the car. There are no other cars about, no backseat drivers, and no children crying, "Are we there yet?" The reality of driving can be very different. Driving is often done in small cars with restricted space and difficult passengers. The environment is frequently noisy because of horns honking and the din of traffic. Attentional overload because of the complexity of modern cars may also create stress. There are often time restrictions: getting to work on time, picking up children, or making it to appointments. Many roads are congested, under repair, or closed altogether. There are strict performance demands – we must pay attention, avoid accidents, and cope with some other drivers' wrath. Driving in heavy rain and in the winter in northern countries creates more stress.

Drivers are usually immobile and cannot get out, especially on freeways. Driving can also be dangerous because traffic lights change quickly and other drivers tailgate, cut in and out, or express their anger in other ways.

Many roads in or around cities are congested, and the levels of congestion are increasing in most North American cities. Highway building has not kept pace with car ownership. In North America, there are, on average, two vehicles per family, whereas there was only one vehicle per family for the previous generation. People are spending longer times in their cars and making longer commutes to work or school. Hence, they expose themselves to greater stress on the road.

Driving is often seen as stressful and difficult. In a recent Canadian study, 55% of drivers said that some of their driving was stressful and 15.7% said that half or more was stressful. Approximately 75% said that half or more of their driving was on busy roads and approximately 50% said that most or all of it was on busy roads. Considerable research shows that most drivers find driving on congested roads to be more stressful.

Some drivers have physical limitations that make driving more stressful for them. These include people with arthritis, with neurological or serious psychological problems, and who are elderly or disabled. Cars are not well designed to suit the needs of such people, and driving demands are difficult for them to fulfill. Elderly people often stop driving for physical or psychological reasons. However, the loss of driving capabilities often causes more stress and can lead to depression and social isolation for the elderly.

Driver Stress and Driver Behavior

Particular driving events cause stress among drivers, but many drivers have high levels of stress before they get in the car. Trait stress, or ongoing nonsituational stress, has been much studied and several scales have been developed to measure it. Driver stress is greater in situations in which there is a lot of congestion and in which there is time urgency. Daily hassles contribute to driver stress. Drivers who recently had an illness, personal conflict, or bereavement are more likely to be in serious accidents.

Total driver stress varies because of the driving situation, personal disposition or trait stress levels, and nondriving events such as daily hassles. High levels of stress in drivers cause attention lapses, errors, and traffic violations. In several studies, driver stress has also been related to aggression and to involvement in accidents. However, most driver stress dissipates quickly once the driver gets out of the car.

Several methods of reducing driver stress have been investigated. Commuters who worked at a job with flextime had less driver stress than those who always traveled during rush hours. Drivers on flextime also felt less time urgency. Experimental studies have shown that drivers who viewed computerized highway drives that had more vegetation than human-made structures had less stress. Also, listening to music may reduce driver stress.

Stress after Motor Vehicle Accidents

Many drivers experience long-term stress after an injury in a motor vehicle accident (MVA). This stress can last many months or even years. The proportion of MVA victims having serious postaccident stress varies from study to study. Accident-induced stress is often assessed using the criteria from the *Diagnostic and Statistical Manual of Mental Disorders*. Acute stress disorder (ASD) is diagnosed within 1 month of the accident, and posttraumatic stress disorder (PTSD) is not diagnosed until after stress has lasted more than 1 month. Both involve subjective feelings of anxiety, fear, and helplessness; role impairment; and a preoccupation with the accident and its consequences.

Most studies of ASD and PTSD involve victims who were injured in accidents and assessed in emergency wards. In such samples, the rate of ASD varies from 10 to 40% and the rate of PTSD from 10 to more than 70%. The highest rates have typically been found in children injured in traffic accidents and people involved in litigation after an accident. Usually, victims with ASD are far more likely than others to develop the long-term stress syndromes seen in PTSD. However, some victims do not develop PTSD after having ASD. Most, but not all, studies found little correlation between PTSD and the severity of the injury.

In children, the likelihood of PTSD often relates to the seriousness that they attribute to the accident. Children after accidents are often afflicted with anger, alienation, thought suppression, and intensive memories of the accident. Most studies show that PTSD is much more common among female than male victims. PTSD may be also more common among those with lower socioeconomic status.

Postaccident stress is not found only among the victims of accidents. Parents also experience considerable stress if their children have PTSD. Also, PTSD, guilt and shame have been found among drivers who caused deaths in motor vehicle accidents. In that group PTSD and guilt were associated with the degree of responsibility the driver assumes for the accident and the severity of their punishment.

Post accident stress can last a long time and can also be related to other negative life events. Among PTSD victims, events such as loss of job or income, broken relationships, and serious illnesses were more common than among accident victims without PTSD. Because of legal liability and compensation issues, some postaccident stress may be faked or exaggerated. Some studies have shown that actors can fool evaluators of stress, especially if little corroborative evidence is available.

Aggressive Driving and Stress

Aggressive driving often causes stress for other drivers as well as for the aggressive driver. Aggressive driving typically involves tailgating; cutting in and out of traffic; preventing other drivers from passing; not moving forward on green lights; and shouting, gesticulating, or criticizing other drivers. If there is an attempt to threaten or intimidate other drivers or to damage their vehicle, this is referred to as road rage, but the two terms often overlap.

Angry or aggressive drivers are more likely to be male and young. Scales for measuring trait driver anger have been devised. Drivers who score high on these scales have more anger and anxiety and show less control over their aggression; they have more minor accidents and close calls but probably not more major accidents.

Driver anger is common and probably comes from feelings of stress during driving. Approximately one in four college student drivers reported being angry with another driver once or more per day. They rated stress from other drivers as equal to the stress of college examinations; traffic congestion, road construction, and finding a parking place were seen as less stressful.

Driving Stress and Road Rage

Road rage may appear to be a new cause of stress for drivers. However, it has been around for a long time. Sophocles in his play *Oedipus the King,* written in about 420 BCE, made road rage the reason that Oedipus kills his father. Also, the poet Byron was engaged in several incidents of road rage in the early 1700s. There are other historical cases as well. It is clear that mass media reports of road rage have recently increased in several countries, although one survey shows that incidents of road rage have been decreasing recently.

Road rage has no accepted definition; it has been defined as a situation in which a driver or passenger attempts to kill, injure, or intimidate another driver, another passenger or a pedestrian in a driving incident. Cases have been described in many countries in North America and Europe, and many have led to death or serious injury. A national study in the United States found that 30% of respondents had complained about other drivers; 17% had yelled at other drivers; 3% had chased other drivers; and 1–2% had gotten out of their cars to hurt other drivers, deliberately hit other drivers, or had carried a weapon. A study in Arizona found that 28% of respondents had aggressively blocked other drivers or followed them to retaliate. Approximately 11% always (4%) or sometimes (7%) carried a gun in their car, and hostile driving behavior was much more common for those with guns.

A Canadian study found that almost half of drivers each year were cursed at or had gestures made to them. Approximately 7.2% were threatened with personal injury or damage to their cars. This study and several others found that perpetrators of road rage are more likely to be younger and male. The victims and perpetrators of road rage are often the same people. However, there is a group of frequent perpetrators of road rage that accounts for almost all of the serious cases involving injury.

Road rage can be a very stressful event for its victims, especially if there is an injury. These victims may remember the event for long periods, modifying their driving behaviors to avoid later incidents. Victims of road rage often feel trapped and unable to get to safety. The immediate effects of road rage are fear, anxiety, anger, and annoyance. Victims report being shaken by it and sometimes being confused. Some victims have lingering thoughts and negative emotions after road rage, but most of this disappears in a few weeks unless there is a serious injury. Being the victim of road rage does make some drivers more cautious about driving.

Road rage is often associated with psychiatric morbidity and distress. In several studies, frequent perpetrators of road rage were found to have high rates of psychiatric distress and, more significant, stressful life events. It may be that frequent perpetrators of road rage bring their stress into the driving situation and, because of their high trait stress, are easily upset in traffic, lashing out at other drivers frequently.

Some studies have also shown that victims of road rage have high levels of psychiatric distress (i.e., anxiety, depression, and stress). Being a victim in a serious incident of road rage is likely to be traumatic for many drivers. The direct casual relationship between serious, injurious incidents of road rage and stress levels has not been examined, but such a relationship is highly plausible given what we know about stress after traffic accidents.

Road rage has been found to be more common among drivers who have more stressful driving experiences. Studies in Canada found that road rage was more frequent for drivers who often drove in congested driving conditions, whose driving was mostly done on busy roads, and who drove longer distances. Road rage was also more common for truck drivers; they drive in stressful situations with tight time schedules, and they are often tired.

Bus drivers have been found in several studies to be both the victims and perpetrators of road rage. They are often victimized by angry passengers, and such conflicts often lead to burnout and the desire to leave the job.

What Can Be Done to Reduce Stress in Driving?

Some of the stress drivers experience is trait stress that they had when they entered the car, and some comes from the experiences they have when driving. Reducing trait stress may require drivers to change relationships, work, and life styles and get better control over their lives. Reviewing these changes is beyond our scope here and we address only the stress that is directly related to driving.

Much stress in driving relates to traffic congestion, and most large cities are experiencing greater congestion. Fully automated transportation systems may eventually divert traffic from congested areas. A few cities are attempting to reduce congestion by increasing public transit, limiting rush-hour traffic, charging motorists for using certain roadways, and the like. Whether and how these measures reduce stress to reasonable levels is unclear at this time. More could be done to allow flextime and reduce rush-hour travel. Roads could be built to be less complex for drivers, perhaps through traffic calming or other engineering changes.

Much of the serious stress from driving derives from involvement in accidents, especially those with injuries. In North America, the rates of fatal and injury-causing accidents have been declining for many years. The reasons for these declines are the greater use of seat belts and air bags, reduction in alcohol-related accidents because of strict enforcement, better licensing programs for young drivers, and engineering changes to make car crashes more survivable. The extension of these policy changes to other geographic areas could further reduce serious accident levels; so could more technical developments in cars and highways to make them safer.

Some driving stress comes from road rage and aggressive driving. Methods for reducing road rage include better education programs and anger management for convicted drivers as well as changes to vehicles. Some vehicle manufacturers such as Jaguar and Mercedes make cars that have radar systems to prevent tailgating, a common cause of road rage. These systems could be made more available. Cars could be redesigned to have voice-activated warnings when drivers raise their voices. Also cars could have lights that signal when drivers are becoming victims of road rage. Further modifications could also be made to track the perpetrators of road rage with global positioning systems (GPSs) and provide warnings to them. Much driver aggression relates to traffic congestion, and anything that reduces it will lower road rage, aggressive driving, and stress levels for drivers.

Acknowledgment

This research was supported by a grant from Auto21, one of the Networks of Centres of Excellence.

Further Reading

Blanchard, E. B. and Hickling, E. J. (2004). *After the crash: psychological assessment and treatment of survivors of motor vehicle accidents.* Washington, DC: American Psychological Association.

Hancock, P. A. and Desmond, P. A. (2001). *Stress, workload and fatigue: human factors in transportation.* Mahwah, NJ: Lawrence Erlbaum.

Hennessy, D. A. and Wiesenthal, D. L. (2001). Gender, driver aggression and other driver violence: an applied evaluation. *Sex Roles* **44**(11–12), 661–676.

Hennessy, D. A., Wiesenthal, D. L. and Kohn, P. M. (2000). The influence of traffic congestion, daily hassles and trait stress susceptibility on state driver stress: an interactive perspective. *Journal of Applied Biobehavioural Research* 5(2), 162–179.

Lowinger, T. and Salomon, Z. (2004). PTSD, guilt and shame among reckless drivers. *Journal of Loss and Trauma* 9(4), 327–344.

Mather, F. J., Tate, R. L. and Hannon, T. J. (2003). Post-traumatic stress disorder in children following road traffic accidents: a comparison of those with and without mild traumatic brain injury. *Brain Injury* **17**(12), 1077–1087.

Mizell, L. (1997). *Aggressive driving.* Washington, DC: Automobile Association for Traffic Safety.

Smart, R. G., Asbridge, M., Mann, R. E., et al. (2003). Psychiatric distress among road rage victims and perpetrators. *Canadian Journal of Psychiatry* **48**(10), 681–688.

Smart, R. G. and Mann, R. E. (2002). Is road rage a serious traffic problem? *Traffic Injury Research* 3(3), 183–189.

Smart, R. G., Mann, R. E., Zhao, J., et al. (2005). Is road rage increasing: results of a repeated survey. *Journal of Safety Research* 36(1), 195–201.

Unemployment, Stress, and Health

M Bartley
University College London Medical School, London, UK

Glossary

Cohort study A cohort study is one in which a group of individuals is followed over time. A birth cohort consists of a group whose members were all born at around the same time and are therefore the same age. The advantage of this for research on unemployment and health is that it allows us to see whether those who become unemployed differ in any health-relevant manner from those who do not, even before they experience unemployment.

Economically active The employed and self-employed plus all those looking actively for paid employment.

Economically inactive Persons who neither have a job nor are currently actively seeking one.

Employment Work that either is paid by an employer or yields income from self-employment or a small business.

Latent consequences of employment The idea that employment has benefits other than providing a wage, such as the opportunity to use skills, social integration, and self-esteem.

Life course perspective A relatively new approach to understanding health differences between people in different social groups that takes account of experiences over time. For example, the approach looks at whether people who experience more unemployment tend to have had different experiences in childhood than those who have experienced little or no unemployment.

Mac-job — Employment that requires little education or training, is very low paid, and is accompanied by no career prospects, low autonomy, and low job security.

Parasuicide — This term does not mean attempted suicide that did not succeed, but refers to serious self-harm that is, however, not thought to be intended to result in death.

Reservation wage — The rate of pay at which an unemployed person will consider taking on a new job.

Selection — The possibility that pre-existing health may have resulted in unemployment.

Unemployment — Defined by the International Labour Organisation as "neither employed nor self employed and actively seeking employment." Practices in different nations vary as to the period of time during which an individual must have looked for a job in order to be regarded as unemployed; a common usage is within the last 2 weeks.

Unemployment rate — Calculated as the number of those seeking employment divided by the economically active population. Those not seeking paid work are not included in the denominator.

Work — Not synonymous with employment. It has been calculated that at least half of the work that is done in a society is unpaid. Most unpaid work is carried out by women.

Introduction

From levels in 1977 of around 4.5% in the UK and 6.5% in the US for men over the age of 16 in the mid-1970s, the unemployment rates of these nations rose sharply to around 11–12% in the early 1980s. In the UK, unemployment rose again to another peak, over 12% in men, in the early 1990s, while in the United States it fell more steadily. **Figures 1** and **2** show both similarities and differences in the trends in these two nations. Although unemployment is now far lower than its highest level, conditions are very different from those of the 1970s, which preceded the 1980s recession and restructuring of labor markets. The labor market has to some extent polarized. On the one hand, there are more jobs that require high levels of education and skill in new high-technology industries and, even more, in services such as banking, law, and health care. On the other hand, the jobs available to those without further post-school education and training have increasingly become what are known as Mac-jobs (after the McDonalds catering empire). The paradigmatic Mac-job is in the fast food industry and consists of relatively unskilled forms of preparing and serving of meals. Another job typical of the new labor market is the call center. Working in a call center does not require specific qualifications or skills, but is only possible for those capable of clear, grammatical speech, without a heavy regional dialect, and who have sufficient social skills to deal with many different (often dissatisfied) customers in a series of intensive remote encounters.

In many mainland European nations, however, large-scale replacement of unemployment by low-paid work has not yet taken place. Unemployment rates in Germany and France, for example, are still very high, at 10–11%. To some extent it could be said that mainland Europe and Scandinavia lag behind the United States and UK, in that the economic crisis of the 1980s in the latter nations occurred in mainland Europe and Scandinavia about 10 years later. It is, therefore, still relevant to consider whether there may be effects of unemployment on health.

Health Effects of Unemployment

Research has repeatedly shown a higher prevalence of ill health and excess mortality in men and women who are unemployed. Men who are unemployed, and women who are either unemployed or keeping house full time, are more likely than those with paid employment to describe their health as generally fair or poor. Damage to psychological health is also found by the vast majority of studies, an effect that appears to be independent of pre-existing health and to be reversed on re-employment in many cases.

However, it is not a simple step from this observation to a causal relationship between unemployment and health. In aggregate level studies, increases in unemployment in nations or areas are not consistently found to be related to increases in mortality or morbidity. The increase of unemployment in industrialized nations took place during a period when life expectancy was rising steadily. This is not too great a mystery, as even what would be regarded as a very high unemployment rate would be no more than 10–15% of the economically active population of a nation. A typical rate of economic activity in an industrial nation would be 65–75% of those regarded as of working age, which is usually between around 18 and 65 years old (the rest of the population comprising children, the retired, and those looking after home and family). It is also typical of observed patterns of unemployment that the risk of job loss is not randomly spread throughout the population. In general, there will be a group characterized by having worked in a declining industry, having few skills relevant to other industries, and living in an economically

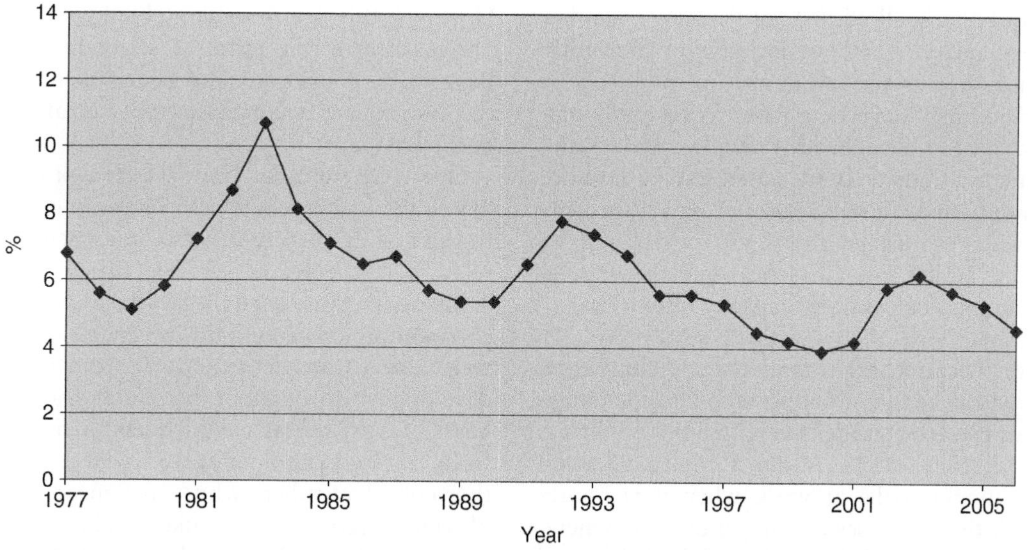

Figure 1 Trends in unemployment of working-age men (16 years and over), United States, 1977–2006 (January). From http://data.bls.gov.

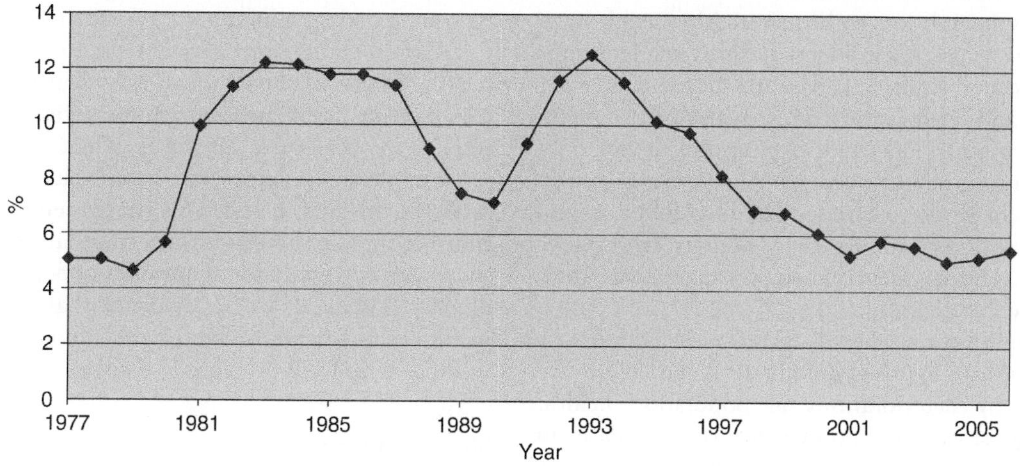

Figure 2 Trends in unemployment of working-age men (16 years and over), UK, 1977–2006 (January). From http://www.statistics.com.

declining region, who experience long-term and/or multiple spells of unemployment. This group will carry most of the total burden of unemployment for the society as a whole. This needs to be remembered when we examine the evidence on the health effects of unemployment. It is more or less impossible to find a group of workers who become and remain unemployed for any appreciable period of time who do not also suffer from one or more other burdens of socioeconomic disadvantage.

The reason we need to be cautious about studies showing that people who report that they are unemployed also report worse mental or physical health is that those who are ill may be more likely to lose their jobs and find it harder to regain employment Or there may be indirect effects whereby men and women with other characteristics such as lower levels of education, which are known to be related to health risks, are also less likely to be employed. This type of relationship, in which certain people are more at risk of both unemployment and ill health is known as selection.

Selection

There are very few studies that have examined relationships of unemployment to health over a long time period. Convincing evidence of a causal effect would be present if long-term studies showed that healthy people who became unemployed subsequently experienced a deterioration in their health. Early studies of unemployed people in the 1970s and 1980s indicated that their physical health did not necessarily decline during a spell of unemployment; a number of studies failed to find an increase in morbidity among those who were continuously unemployed for up to 18 months. However, a more recent study of a representative sample of healthy people over a period of 10 years did observe an increased risk of developing a limiting illness in the year after having become unemployed. Another careful study carried out by occupational health specialists measured a clear deterioration in physical working capacity after a year of unemployment.

However, because of the scarcity of good long-term evidence on the health of people who become unemployed, we need to consider the possibility of what is called a selection effect. A direct health selection effect is thought to be at work when it is poorer health itself that increases the risk of unemployment. Ill health may be a risk for both initial job loss and subsequent chances of re-employment. However, studies in which an entire workplace closes down and all workers are dismissed so that there is no possibility for job loss to be affected by health have also shown increases in illness in those made redundant. Research using linked census-based data from England and Wales and from the Nordic countries has shown that higher risk of mortality is not only present among unemployed people who were already ill. A recent study in Sweden has also found excess risk of mortality among twin siblings who experienced unemployment when compared to their siblings who did not.

Although most studies of increases in national or regional unemployment do not find that these are followed by deteriorations in population health, there is most certainly no evidence that increases in unemployment happen because people's health gets worse. The large increases in unemployment during the 1980s in the Anglo-Saxon nations and during the 1990s in many European nations were not due to worsening health of workers in these countries (indeed, this will seem rather an absurd statement to make). In fact, unemployment rates increased dramatically in different nations during the 1980s and 1990s, at the same time that levels of health in the population actually improved. So there is no possibility that an increase in unemployment overall can be blamed on some kind of general deterioration in the health of the working-age population.

There may still be some tendency for those who remain unemployed for longer periods to be different from those who do not, even if this difference does not take the form of a life-threatening disease. Perhaps people at high risk of unemployment may also have certain personality characteristics, for example, an external locus of control or a weak coping ability. However, this is a more complex hypothesis, and is not necessarily the same as selection. These ideas have to be considered alongside other evidence on the life course accumulation of social and health disadvantage.

One study that has been able to ask the question "How far is the poor health of the unemployed due to their health before they became unemployed?" in relation to mental health is a British birth cohort study of everyone born in the second week of March 1958 and followed until the present time. Researchers were able to use data on health and psychological development throughout the school years and young adult life, as well as complete employment histories from leaving school to age 33. These data showed that cohort members who experienced more unemployment were also more likely to have grown up in economically disadvantaged and overcrowded households. The study also addressed the possibility that the high level of psychological morbidity found in unemployed men and women might have been due to a pre-existing vulnerability to poor mental health. Even after taking into account pre-existing mental health, recent unemployment was clearly related to the onset of psychiatric symptoms severe enough to require medical care. However, when those with a prior tendency to depression were excluded from the analysis, this had the effect of strengthening the relationship between longer term accumulation of unemployment and the onset of episodes of depression and anxiety. This adds to the evidence that longer term unemployment causes deterioration in mental health in those who were previously healthy.

Mechanisms

What might be the reasons for the relationship between unemployment and health? Several have been put forward, and the following sections consider three of these: poverty, the fact that unemployment is a stressful life event, and changes in health-related behaviors at the time of unemployment.

Poverty

Low living standards are not an inevitable consequence of unemployment; this is a result of the levels at which benefits are set, which results from political decisions. During the 1980s and 1990s, levels of income replacement for the unemployed were lowered in many nations. It was argued that under conditions of increasing automation of unskilled and semi-skilled work, levels of benefits available to the unemployed exceeded the market worth of their labor, that is, the wage rate that employers were willing to pay. If the level of pay at which an unemployed person will accept new employment – the reservation wage – is too high, employers will not take them on. If benefit levels are too high, the state is raising the reservation wage and therefore may be contributing to the problem of high unemployment.

On becoming unemployed, most people will experience a decrease in income. The extent of this decrease varies between nations, from around 20% in some Nordic countries to approximately 60–70% or more in the UK and United States. Many studies link the health effects of unemployment directly to financial problems. In modern welfare states, state benefits available to those unable to undertake paid employment are thought to avoid starvation and severe physical privation. However, recent research on the financial cost of what medical evidence has shown to be a healthy lifestyle, which includes a diet adequate in essential nutrients, warm housing, and a level of social participation consistent with mental health, costs approximately double the level of social security benefit in the UK. It is therefore inevitable that once savings are exhausted, unemployed people will be forced to borrow money in order to sustain health. Debt, in its turn, has been shown to increase the risk to mental health and the risk of stress-related deterioration in physical health. In several studies, long-term unemployed people who had gone into debt or had to borrow money in the past year had a risk of depression that was more than double that of those who did not have to borrow money. These studies also found that those obliged to borrow were also more likely to report deterioration in physical health. Others have documented the ways in which increasing financial pressures, as savings are used up and worn-out items need to be replaced, are responsible for the growing inactivity and social isolation of many unemployed people.

These British findings are echoed in other countries, such as the United States and the Netherlands, where financial problems were shown to be the main reason why unemployed people's mental and physical health were worse than that of the employed. However, it seems that eventually many of the unemployed adapt to straitened financial and social circumstances. Several studies agree that there appears to be no further deterioration in psychological well-being after a period of between 1 year and 18 months (but no improvement, either, so that unemployed people remain two to three times more likely than the employed to be in poor mental health). This adds weight to the argument for providing early assistance to those who become unemployed. Other evidence suggests that adaptation to unemployment is accompanied by lowered expectations of oneself, and perhaps by a degree of alienation and cynicism. This process has been compared to the adaptive process found in institutionalized inmates of prisons or psychiatric hospitals.

Unemployment as a Stressful Life Event

Research on the ways in which people react to job loss shows it to be a highly stressful life event, which has been characterized as a form of bereavement. International studies provide consistent evidence of the importance of stress. Many researchers have suggested that employment has a number of nonfinancial benefits to the individual, the so-called latent consequences, and it is the loss of these that results in the threatening character of unemployment. These latent consequences of employment include giving a time structure to the day, self-esteem, and the respect of others; physical and mental activity; use of skills; and interpersonal contact. It may be that the loss of these psychosocial benefits of employment is at least as important as loss of income to the health of unemployed people.

Evidence of the importance of stress for the relationship between unemployment and health comes from studies in Scandinavian nations. In these nations, cash benefits to the unemployed are relatively generous, and therefore the financial effects might not be expected to be as great as in the United States or the UK; however, similar relationships between unemployment and a range of health indicators are seen. A study in Stockholm of men with irregular work histories and a variety of problems that required frequent social service assistance found that those who were employed, even in low-paid casual jobs, were all more active and integrated (and psychologically healthier) than the unemployed. Among unemployed industrial workers in Finland, those who regained paid work experienced a considerable improvement in psychological health regardless of their financial circumstances either before or after re-employment. Italian workers laid off from their jobs experienced raised amounts of both psychological and physical illness despite receiving the whole of their normal wage. These studies provide evidence of the nonfinancial benefits of employment for psychological health. Stress may affect physical health as well as psychological health as a result perhaps of chronically increased levels of anxiety and the relationship this may have to the functioning of the endocrine system.

Health-Related Behavior

There is evidence that unemployment is associated with some forms of health-damaging behavior, although previous research has yielded inconsistent findings on the relationship. Associations between unemployment and health behaviors need to be seen in the context of the longer term development of these behaviors. The little research that exists on this topic seems to indicate not so much that people who become unemployed take up new, health-damaging activities such as smoking and drinking, not least because the costs of these pursuits could be ill-afforded. Rather, it seems that the experience of unemployment makes it harder for individuals to carry through their intentions to improve their health behaviors. For example, in one study, after taking account of adolescent health risk behaviors, even well-educated and intelligent young men who experienced 12 months of more without a job between the ages of 23 and 33 were less likely than their peers with no unemployment experience to have a healthy lifestyle in their mid-30s.

Self-destructive behavior among unemployed men has been widely investigated. In the UK and in Scandinavian nations, suicide has been found to be more likely in unemployed people. Parasuicide (attempted suicide) has also been found to be higher in unemployed men. Unemployment seems to increase the likelihood of other adverse life events and to reduce the psychological and social resources needed to cope with these. There is, for example, a higher risk of partnership and marriage breakdown among unemployed men. Many of the unemployed also lose contact with their social networks due to the stigma of their situation.

Unemployment and Health in the Life Course

Perhaps the best way to approach the study of the relationship between health and labor market status is from the perspective that unemployment and work insecurity are part of a process through which health disadvantage is accumulated over the life course. Research taking this perspective turns away from any simple opposition between selection and causation and shows that unemployment occurs as part of a much longer term sequence of events in the life of the individual. It is now becoming possible to look at these processes using cohort studies that follow individuals from childhood to middle age. We can see, for example, that those most likely to experience unemployment may also be more vulnerable to excess mortality and morbidity because of earlier experiences of other kinds of hardship and disadvantage. Their experience of unemployment itself therefore contributes to a process of accumulation of health risks. There is little research conducted along these lines. One such analysis showed that while those with disadvantaged childhoods had the highest risk of later unemployment during the recession of the 1980s, young men who had experienced over 12 months of unemployment seemed to be on a less healthy track in terms of both social and behavioral risk, even if they were from more advantaged social origins. It seems as though unemployment also tends to wipe out some of the health advantages built up over the period from childhood to young adulthood in those who had come from socially advantaged homes and done relatively well in education.

Recent longitudinal research has made it possible to understand the relationship between unemployment and health in a more dynamic way. Biological endowment and material and emotional experiences during childhood confer varying amounts of health resources or health potential to the young person. In the real world, people from less secure and advantaged backgrounds are more likely to enter occupations with more adverse working conditions and lower rates of pay. It is of no surprise, therefore, that the aging process itself is known to take place at differential rates according to the employment history of the individual, with more arduous work being associated with faster aging. The physical resources the individual brings to the labor market when he or she must look for a new job will in many cases have already been damaged by these experiences at work, even before any spell of unemployment he or she may suffer. Many of the most hazardous (and least well paid) occupations also tend to be less secure, which means that there will be some degree of coincidence between poor health and the risk of job loss, not just because of the individual's own characteristics but also because of social structure. In contrast to physical resources, psychological and social resources are more likely to be enhanced by the experiences of activity, companionship, and cooperation involved in (even hazardous) employment. Deterioration in psychological health during unemployment is therefore more immediate and visible than deteriorations in physical health, and improvement on re-employment happens quickly.

For young people, employment forms part of the process of establishing an independent identity, so that stable employment may in fact be even more important for younger than for middle-aged or older people. For many, entry into stable employment is now preceded by long periods of job insecurity. The process of identity formation is therefore far more at risk, with accompanying rises in rates of relationship breakdown, poor mental health, addiction, and accidental and self-inflicted harm. Employment is known to aid the development of secure identity and self-esteem and to facilitate the formation of stable relationships. Accordingly, as the British economy shifted from one in which there were larger numbers of stable jobs to one in which employment conditions were more insecure, British birth cohort studies showed that levels of mental health problems in those of young working age increased sharply. Although rates of major diseases of middle age have continued to decline during the period of labor market change, rates of suicide in young men have continued to rise.

Policy Implications

A growing body of international comparative research suggests that societies with higher levels of unemployment and job insecurity may actually produce different sorts of life histories in individual members than those that provide larger numbers of secure jobs. It has been all too easy to take for granted some of the effects of quasi-full employment on the wider society. When jobs were plentiful, in order to recruit and retain workers most large firms undertook extensive training, recruiting school leavers at an early age into apprenticeships. Schools therefore had far fewer restless and unmotivated youth to deal with than would otherwise have been the case, benefiting all children in the school. Internal labor markets (the availability of promotion within a firm based on experience rather than on qualifications) offered people the chance to advance in their jobs even in the absence of school qualifications, from a later starting point. Increasing numbers of firms offered occupational pensions, thus raising the living standards of the retired population at little cost to the state. As part of the McDonaldization of the labor market, the costs of training and of supporting those who are no longer able to work for payment are now increasingly being borne by the individual (the disappearance of apprenticeships and the appearance of student loans, critical illness policies, and private pensions are examples). There has also been an increase in the numbers of persons who become economically inactive, which in many countries far exceeds the increase in the numbers of those officially unemployed and seeking employment.

Increasing the number of low-paid, low-skilled Mac-jobs is often advocated as a solution to the problem of unemployment. However, the evidence on the success of such a policy is mixed, and the impact on population health has not as yet been fully investigated.

During the 1990s, new data from birth cohort studies (studies of large numbers of people all born in the same year) added a considerable amount to our understanding of why unemployment is associated with poor health. We began to see that unemployment takes place as part of a process of accumulation of disadvantage that may begin in childhood, and that a spell of unemployment often occurs as part of a more general pattern of hazardous and insecure work. The old assumptions behind the notion of a social insurance or welfare state safety net are seen to be too simple. The people most likely to fall into the net bear a heavier weight of disadvantage than those who are less likely to need its support. The idea that benefit levels for the unemployed should be set no higher than mere subsistence, in order not to encourage voluntary unemployment, is therefore becoming discredited. On the contrary, both the taxpayer and the unemployed person (who is of course a past and potential taxpayer him- or herself) benefits more from a generous provision of both material and psychosocial support for those who find themselves without employment.

See Also the Following Articles

Job Insecurity: The Health Effects of a Psychosocial Work Stressor.

Further Reading

Allmendinger, J. and Hinz, T. (1998). Occupational careers under different welfare regimes: West Germany, Britain and Sweden. In: Leisering, L. & Walker, R. (eds.) *The dynamics of modern society*, pp. 64–84. Bristol, UK: Policy Press.

Bethune, A. (1996). Economic activity and mortality of the 1981 Census cohort in the OPCS Longitudinal Study. *Population Trends* **83**, 37–42.

Burchell, B. (1996). Who is affected by unemployment? In: Gallie, D., Marsh, C. & Vogler, C. (eds.) *Unemployment & social change*, pp. 45–58. Oxford, UK: Oxford University Press.

Catalano, R., Dooley, D., Wilson, G. and Hough, R. (1993). Job loss and alcohol abuse: a test using data from the Epidemiologic Catchment Area project. *Journal of Health Society and Behavior* **34**, 215–225.

Catalano, R., Dooley, D., Novaco, R. W., Wilson, G. and Hough, R. (1993). Using ECA survey data to examine the effect of job layoffs on violent behavior. *Hospital and Community Psychiatry* **44**, 874–879.

Dooley, D. and Catalano, R. (1991). Unemployment as a stressor: findings and implications of a recent study. *WHO Regional Publications European Series* **37**, 313–339.

Dooley, D., Fielding, J. and Levi, L. (1996). Health and unemployment. *Annual Reviews of Public Health* **17**, 449–465.

Kessler, R. C., Turner, J. B. and House, J. S. (1987). Intervening processes in the relationship between unemployment and health. *Psychological Medicine* **17**, 949–961.

Levenstein, S., Smith, M. W. and Kaplan, G. A. (2001). Psychosocial predictors of hypertension in men and women. *Archives of Internal Medicine* **161**, 1341–1346.

Montgomery, S. M., Bartley, M. J., Cook, D. G. and Wadsworth, M. E. (1996). Health and social precursors of unemployment in young men in Great Britain. *Journal of Epidemiology and Community Health* **50**, 415–422.

Montgomery, S. M., Cook, D. G., Bartley, M. J. and Wadsworth, M. E. J. (1998). Unemployment, cigarette smoking, alcohol consumption and body weight in young British men. *European Journal of Public Health* **8**, 21–27.

Montgomery, S. M., Cook, D. G., Bartley, M. J. and Wadsworth, M. E. (1999). Unemployment pre-dates symptoms of depression and anxiety resulting in medical consultation in young men. *International Journal of Epidemiology* **28**, 95–100.

Morris, J. N., Donkin, A. J. M., Wonderling, D., Wilkinson, P. and Dowler, E. A. (2000). A minimum income for healthy living. *Journal of Epidemiology and Community Health* **54**, 885–889.

Moser, K., Goldblatt, P. O., Fox, A. J. and Jones, D. R. (1987). Unemployment and mortality. *British Medical Journal* **294**, 509–512.

Moser, K., Goldblatt, P., Fox, J. and Jones, D. (1990). Unemployment and mortality. In: Goldblatt, P. O. (ed.) *Longitudinal study: mortality and social organisation*, pp. 77–102. London: HMSO.

Ostry, A. S. (2001). Effects of de-industrialization on unemployment, re-employment, and work conditions in a manufacturing workforce. *BMC Public Health* **1**, 15.

Ritzer, G. (1993). *The McDonaldization of society.* Oakland, CA: Pine Forge Press.

Wadsworth, M. E., Montgomery, S. M. and Bartley, M. J. (1999). The persisting effect of unemployment on health and social well-being in men early in working life. *Social Science and Medicine* **48**, 1491–1499.

Warr, P. (1987). *Work, unemployment and mental health.* London: Oxford University Press.

Work–Family Balance

J G Grzywacz
Wake Forest University School of Medicine, Winston-Salem, NC, USA
A B Butler
University of Northern Iowa, Cedar Falls, IA, USA

Glossary

Family Responsibilities and activities that arise from shared goals, values, and long-term commitments among two or more people who are related by common ancestry, adoption, marriage, and other legal or socially recognized unions.

Work Responsibilities and activities inherent in an individual's trade, profession, vocation, or other means of livelihood.

Work–family conflict The extent to which an individual's work interferes with his or her family or an individual's family interferes with his or her work.

Work–family facilitation The extent to which an individual's work benefits his or her family or an individual's family benefits his or her work.

Work–family interface Areas of physical, psychological, social, or temporal overlap in which an individual's work and family affect each other.

Defining Work–Family Balance

Work–family balance remains largely undefined despite its frequent use in both the popular and scholarly vernacular. One influential definition characterizes work–family balance in terms of equal engagement in both work and family responsibilities. This definition of work–family balance is influential because it is clearly grounded in theory and is consistent with the balance metaphor. Despite these strengths, however, the definition overlooks several important complexities such as the multiple forms or ways in which individuals can engage in their work and family lives, and whether or not different forms of engagement are functionally equivalent. Recognizing these complexities, more recent definitions of work–family balance continue to highlight notions of equality, but they also emphasize comparable levels of satisfaction within each domain and the relative absence of conflict between the domains. Work–family balance, therefore, generally refers to a work and family life that is well integrated and a situation in which the individual is actively engaged in both domains.

Prevalence and Emergence of Interest in Work–Family Balance

Difficulty maintaining work–family balance is reported by the majority of working adults. Estimates from the U.S. General Social Survey suggest that fewer than 40% of adults believe that they are successfully balancing their work and family lives. The widespread difficulty in achieving work–family balance, and subsequent scholarly and popular interest, results from significant socioeconomic shifts in the constitution of the labor force as well as in the nature of work itself. In the final quarter of the twentieth century, women's labor force participation increased dramatically, particularly among women with children. The proportion of children being raised in a single-parent household increased, as did the rate of employment among single parents. Concomitantly, substantial job growth in the service-producing sector coupled with increased global competition created new demands on the labor force, such as increased use of contingent labor and other flexible staffing models, as well as greater need for work that occurs outside the bounds of traditional business hours.

The shifts in work and family in the later portion of the twentieth century made navigating daily work and family life more complex for many adults. Growth in women's labor force participation challenged the gender-based division of labor and brought basic issues related to household management and childcare to the forefront. Securing high-quality and affordable childcare is an ongoing challenge, as is care for sick children and elder care. The transition to a service-based economy was accompanied by a fall in real wages, particularly among lower and working-class families. Globalization and the increased reliance on contract and contingent employment arrangements elevated concerns over job insecurity and raised new questions about the nature of the employer–employee relationship. Technology and the 24/7 economy has redefined when, where, and how work is performed for a substantially larger portion of workers. The increased complexity of daily work and family life for many adults has fueled widespread interest in the causes and consequences of work–family balance.

Work–Family Balance and the Stress Process

Work–family balance has been applied and studied at two major points in the stress process. Work–family balance or, more typically, imbalance, is frequently conceptualized as a primary stressor. The basic theoretical rationale for viewing imbalance between work and family as a primary stressor is that the social roles of employee/worker, spouse, and parent have substantial social and cultural value and, therefore, play a central role in adults' identity and sense of self. Indeed, some researchers suggest that successful integration of work and family life is a central task of adult development. If work and family are out of balance, there is substantial social and personal pressure placed on individuals to better manage their responsibilities.

Multiple lines of research support the view of work–family imbalance as a primary stressor. Adults seek to maintain work–family balance through a variety of strategies such as changing jobs, reducing hours, renegotiating household responsibilities, cutting back on personal leisure pursuits, and modifying standards or expectations for their work and family life. Individuals who do not have a well-balanced work and family life – typically operationalized in terms of high levels of work–family conflict – have less life satisfaction as well as elevated levels of depression and somatic complaints, conditions frequently implicated in the stress response. Corroborating this research is more recent evidence linking indicators of work–family balance to common physiological stress responses such as elevated blood pressure, heart rate, and cortisol. Social support from co-workers, supervisors, or family members has been found to buffer the effects of poor work–family balance on stress-related outcomes such as levels of distress and domains of life satisfaction. In summary, there is a wide evidence base suggesting that work–family balance behaves like a primary stressor.

Other research situates work–family imbalance as a secondary stressor, or a downstream consequence of other circumstances or events. This research exists in two largely separate streams of inquiry. In the first stream, work–family balance is studied as a consequence resulting from the relative availability of work- and family-related resources to meet the demands of work and family life. This research focuses on work-related demands such as the time and timing of when work is performed, features of the work such as the amount of authority and variety workers are given, the availability of family-friendly policies such as flexible work schedules or on-site childcare centers, and the supportiveness of co-workers and supervisors. On the family side, research tends to focus on the number and ages of children, the employment status of adults in the family (e.g., dual-earner versus single-earner), qualities of intrafamily relations such as levels of conflict among partners, and the division of household labor. In the second stream of research, work–family balance is seen as a mechanism through which broader social forces exert influence on individual outcomes. For example, some investigators argue that observed health disparities, particularly in child health and development, result (at least in part) from the social allocation of demands and resources necessary for successfully balancing work and family. Racial and ethnic minorities as well as individuals with a low education, for example, are overrepresented in jobs requiring nonstandard schedules that provide few (if any) formal programs that assist workers in balancing their work and family responsibilities. Despite these arguments and the fact that the current focus on work–family balance is a consequence of profound sociostructural changes in work and family, the literature is dominated by views of balance as a personal challenge confronted by individuals.

Promoting Work–Family Balance

Given the stress-related consequences of work–family imbalance, both individuals and organizations may be motivated to take action to restore or maintain balance. Individuals who set goals and employ adaptive strategies to reach those goals are less likely to experience conflict between work and family. An active coping style and social support are also associated with greater work–family balance. Organizational interventions to improve balance typically focus on offering family-friendly benefits designed to facilitate management of conflicting role demands. Such benefits are broad and varied, including flexible scheduling, on-site daycare, and eldercare assistance. These benefits tend to be underutilized by workers, and evidence regarding their efficacy for improving balance is equivocal. Family-supportive organizational cultures, of which family-friendly benefits are but one feature, are also widely believed to be essential to promoting work–family balance.

Gaps and Needed Research

Understanding of work–family balance is undermined by several conceptual and methodological gaps in the literature. Conceptually, although most researchers agree that work–family balance represents some vague notion of equality and harmony in an individual's work and family life, it is not clear what work–family balance is or whether the balance metaphor is appropriate. Moreover, there is very little theoretical work underlying work–family balance research. Methodologically, measurement of work–family balance remains encumbered. Most studies rely on single-item measures (e.g., How successful do you feel at balancing your paid work and your family life?). There is currently a division in the literature regarding how to measure work–family balance: some scholars advocate the use of individuals' overall appraisals of balance, whereas others suggest that work–family balance is a latent construct best measured indirectly using indicators of work–family conflict and work–family facilitation. Future research needs to systematically evaluate the strengths and weaknesses of each approach and develop recommendations. Although there are notable exceptions, work–family balance research is also overly reliant on cross-sectional cohort designs, convenience samples, and self-report measures. Research is needed that clarifies the conceptual meaning of work–family balance, develops valid and innovative measures of work–family balance, and studies the phenomenon using multiple methods.

See Also the Following Articles

Burnout; Environmental Stress, Effects on Human Performance; Social Status and Stress; Social Support; Workplace Stress.

Further Reading

Clark, S. C. (2000). Work/family border theory: a new theory of work/family balance. *Human Relations* 53, 747–770.

Eckenrode, J. and Gore, S. (eds.) (1990). *Stress between work and family.* New York: Plenum.

Frone, M. R. (2003). Work-family balance. In: Quick, J. C. & Tetrick, L. E. (eds.) *Handbook of occupational health psychology*, pp. 143–162. Washington, D.C.: American Psychological Association.

Greenhaus, J. H., Collins, K. M. and Shaw, J. D. (2003). The relation between work-family balance and quality of life. *Journal of Vocational Behavior* 63, 510–531.

Heymann, J. (2000). *The widening gap: why America's working families are in jeopardy, and what can be done about it.* New York: Basic Books.

Marks, S. R. and MacDermid, S. M. (1996). Multiple roles and the self: a theory of role balance. *Journal of Marriage and the Family* 58, 417–432.

Voydanoff, P. (2005). Toward a conceptualization of perceived work-family fit and balance: a demands and resources approach. *Journal of Marriage and Family* 67, 822–836.

Workplace Stress

U Lundberg
Stockholm University, Stockholm, Sweden

This is a revised version of the article by U Lundberg, Encyclopedia of Stress First Edition, volume 3, pp 684–692, © 2000, Elsevier Inc.

Glossary

Allostatic load — The cost of adaptation (allostasis), reflecting wear and tear on the body systems and processes that increases the risk for disease.

Cardiovascular illness — Circulatory disturbances such as hypertension, myocardial infarction, and stroke.

Demand–control model — Defines work strain as a combination of high workload and low control. The dimension of social support has been added to this model.

Effort–reward imbalance model — Stress and health risks are created by an imbalance between high effort and lack of adequate rewards (money, status, support).

Musculoskeletal disorders — Degenerative processes, damage, inflammation, and pain in muscles and joints in the body (neck, shoulder, arms, lower back, etc.).

Sympathetic-adrenal-medullary system and the hypothalamic-pituitary-adrenocortical axis — These form the two major neuroendocrine stress systems in the body.

Introduction

Work has a very central role in most people's lives. In industrialized countries, there have been quite dramatic changes in the conditions at work during the past decades, caused by economic, social, and technical development. Today, as a consequence, people at work are exposed to high quantitative as well as high qualitative demands and to hard competition, caused by a global economy, multinational companies, lean production, downsizing, and increased demands for efficiency. Fewer employed people are expected to produce more, and experiences of stress due to overstimulation have become a serious problem. At the same time, a considerable part of the population is unemployed or only temporarily employed, because no jobs are available or because they have an inadequate or insufficient education. These people experience stress mainly due to lack of economic resources and understimulation. This polarization of the labor market is likely to have contributed to the social gradient in health and well-being, which has increased in recent years. This article summarizes present knowledge regarding how the modern work environment may contribute to stress and negative health outcomes.

The Role of Work

Most adults spend a large part of their daily life at work. As a consequence, conditions at the workplace are likely to be of considerable importance for people's mental as well as physical well-being. Work has a central role in people's lives, and a stimulating job may contribute to a more meaningful life, a higher sense of self-esteem, social ties, and economic independence – conditions that characterize positive human health. Work also creates a time structure in daily life and is a major determinant of the individual's socioeconomic status. Negative psychosocial conditions at work, such as a low job satisfaction and lack of influence and control, are known to be associated with various health risks.

Changing Work Conditions

During the past century, the work situation in industrialized countries has undergone profound changes. For women in particular, these changes have been quite dramatic. At the beginning of the twentieth century, women were often involved in heavy physical work (e.g., working in the fields as a farmer's wife). As urbanization increased in the middle of this century, a married woman was generally expected to assume the role of homemaker, with the primary duty of taking care of her children, husband, and home or household. In the last part of this century, an increasing number of women entered the labor market, and in the Scandinavian countries (as well as in many big cities all over the world) the labor force today comprises practically the same number of women as men. However, despite women's greater involvement in paid work and their importance for the family economy, their responsibility for unpaid work at home does not seem to have been reduced accordingly. In keeping with this, employed women often report stress from work overload and role conflicts.

In the modern work environment, physical hazards and demands have been reduced, whereas psychosocial stress, caused by a very high work pace, competition and efficiency, and successive readjustment to organizational changes, has increased. This can be seen as part of a general and accelerating trend in modern society toward a more rapid pace of life, more frequent introduction of new technology, and continuous demands for coping with new conditions. Major improvements in physical conditions at work during the past decades have thus contributed to a switch in health focus, specifically to the role of psychosocial factors such as stress.

Developments in communication technology (faxes, e-mail, Internet, mobile phones, etc.) have enabled greater flexibility and mobility (e.g., teleworking) and have removed traditional boundaries between different roles in life (work, family, leisure). In addition, temporary employment and work on short-term projects have become more common. These new trends are likely to involve the potential for beneficial effects in terms of greater variation and flexibility, but also an increased risk of stress due to work overload, role conflicts, and lack of time for rest and recovery. The individual, rather than the company, has to set the boundaries between work and his or her other roles in life.

Impact of the Work Environment

Conditions at the workplace may influence the individual in different ways. Physical conditions, such as noise, light, cold, heat, and so on are sensorily mediated by the individual and directly perceived as, for example, harmful or pleasant. In contrast, the individual cannot directly perceive exposure to many other physical conditions, such as radiation, certain chemicals and heavy metals, air and water pollution, and radioactive fallout, as harmful. The health risks associated with such work conditions are mainly based on information obtained from education, mass media, personal communication, or earlier experiences. In such cases, it is not often clear to what extent the stress and health problems associated with these occupational hazards are caused by the actual exposure or by the individual's own fear and anxiety from having been exposed.

Health problems can be caused by the effects of stress on various bodily systems, functions, and organs, such as blood pressure, secretion of stress hormones, immune functions, metabolism, the heart, the brain, and the gastrointestinal system. Health risks can also be caused by the effects of stress on various health-related behaviors, such as cigarette smoking, alcohol and drug abuse, poor eating habits, and lack of physical activity. Additional health risks at work are associated with violence or accidents caused by the greater risk of making mistakes under stress, or being reluctant (or neglecting) to use protective means (e.g., seat belts, helmets, hearing protection) when under time pressure.

Associations between work stress and cardiovascular illness (e.g., hypertension, myocardial infarction) have been reported repeatedly for a long time. However, there is also increasing evidence for strong associations between psychosocial work conditions and a great number of other health problems. A major work-related health problem today is that of musculoskeletal disorders. Neck, shoulder, and lower back pain are the most common reasons for absenteeism from work and for early retirement in Europe and North America, and also affect younger workers. In addition to the pain and suffering caused by these disorders, the economic costs are enormous.

Epidemiological studies have demonstrated dramatic and very consistent relationships between socioeconomic status and health. Social status is usually defined by type of occupation and educational level, and higher status is consistently linked to better health. The social gradient in health can only partly be explained by differential exposure to physical hazards at work, poor material conditions (food, housing), genetic factors, or health-related behaviors. Other factors must also be involved, and there is strong evidence that psychosocial factors at work and income inequality are important for the social differences in health.

Models of Work Stress

Several models have been proposed to explain the causes of work-related stress. Frankenhaeuser and colleagues and other investigators have described a model in which stress is defined in terms of the imbalance between the perceived demands from the environment and the individual's perceived resources to meet those demands. This imbalance can be caused by quantitative overload (a very high pace of work, too much work to do, etc.) or qualitative overload (too much responsibility, problems too complex to solve, conflicts, etc.). However, an interesting feature of this model is that it also proposes that stress may be due to an imbalance caused by understimulation, for example, by work tasks that are too simple, that do not allow individuals to use their education, skills, and experiences, and that do not allow them to learn new skills and develop their abilities. This situation can be found in monotonous and repetitive work, such as traditional assembly line work and in data entry work at video display units, and among people who are unemployed. It is also common among highly educated immigrants, who often have to accept very simple jobs due to insufficient knowledge of the new language or discrimination, which means that their training and experience cannot be used.

Another well-known model describing work stress or strain is the demand–control model, proposed by Karasek and Theorell and developed and expanded by others. According to this model, the combination of high demands and lack of control and influence (low job discretion) over the work situation causes high work strain. High demands combined with a high degree of control, which characterizes many high-status jobs, are described as an active work situation and are not associated with enhanced health risks.

The demand–control model has been tested in numerous studies that, in general, show that occupations characterized by high job strain, for instance, a waiter or an assembly worker, are associated with elevated health risks compared with low-strain jobs, such as being a forester or a scientist. Although most studies are cross-sectional, thus excluding the possibility of making causal inferences, the few prospective studies that have been performed report similar findings. In the late 1980s, a third dimension – social support – was added to the demand–control model. High job strain combined with low social support at work contributes to even more elevated health risks.

The control dimension describes a wide range of factors typical of a positive and healthy work situation. It involves the individual's possibilities for developing and using his or her skills, knowledge, education, and experience to be able to work out new methods and ways of doing the job, learning new skills, taking responsibility, being independent, and experiencing variation at work. Low scores on this dimension have consistently been linked to various negative health outcomes, whereas the results regarding the dimension demands are less conclusive. A possible explanation for the inconsistent findings regarding high demands could be that this dimension does not distinguish between physical and mental demands or between quantitative (e.g., high work pace) and qualitative demands (e.g., too much responsibility). For example, individuals in high-ranking positions often report both high demands and good health.

Social support is generally considered to protect against stress at work or to serve as a buffer against health risks under stressful conditions. It is defined by factors such as having close social ties and someone to share emotional experiences with, good collaboration with colleagues and superiors, the possibility of getting help when needed, and adequate feedback about one's effort and performance. The number of social contacts is less important than the quality of these relationships. In a literature review, low social support was consistently found to be associated with higher morbidity and mortality.

Siegrist proposed a new model for stress at work called the effort–reward imbalance model. According to this model, lack of adequate reward in response to the individual's achievement efforts is considered to contribute to high stress levels and elevated health risks. Reward could be obtained in terms of economic benefits such as a higher income, but also in terms of appreciation and adequate support from colleagues and superiors, or by obtaining better career chances and a higher social rank at the job. A personality characteristic, overachievement, is also an important part of this model; individuals high in overachievement are at particular risk for health problems. In a recent prospective study, this model was found to significantly predict elevated risk of myocardial infarction.

Type A Behavior

A stress- and work-related behavior pattern termed type A behavior has attracted a considerable amount of attention over the past decades. This attention was based, to a large extent, on findings from the prospective Western Collaborative Group Study, in which about 3000 middle-aged employed men were classified either as type A individuals or as their more relaxed type B counterparts on the basis of a standardized interview technique (the structured interview). At the 8.5-year follow-up, it was found that the prevalence of myocardial infarction was about twice as high among type A as among type B individuals, after controlling for traditional risk factors (blood pressure, blood lipids, cigarette smoking, etc.). This study initiated a great number of investigations and experiments aimed at revealing factors that contribute to the development of this behavior pattern and the psychophysiological mechanisms that could create a link to myocardial infarction. Work-related stress was found to play an important role in this context.

Type A behavior is defined in terms of an extreme sense of time urgency, impatience, competitiveness, and aggression/hostility. Work conditions in industrialized countries, emphasizing the importance of efficiency, productivity, a high work pace, and competitiveness, are considered to contribute to the development of this behavior pattern. In addition, individuals classified as type A have been found to be particularly responsive to challenges at work (obstacles to keeping up the pace of work, lack of control, competition, harassment, etc.) in terms of blood pressure, heart rate, blood lipids, and catecholamine output. Intensive, frequent, and/or sustained activation ofthese physiological stress responses contributes to the atherosclerotic process and to blood clotting and are, thus, likely to form a pathway between type A behavior and the elevated risk of myocardial infarction. Results for women are in general less consistent than they are for men, which could be explained by the fact that the structured interview was developed using male subjects.

The high work pace and competitiveness associated with the type A behavior pattern are usually reinforced at work by giving the individual a higher income, appreciation, and a successful occupational career (higher rank). Consequently, efforts to modify this behavior pattern in healthy individuals have not been particularly successful. However, after a myocardial infarction individuals tend to be more motivated to change their lifestyle, and, indeed, a prospective intervention study has shown a reduced risk of reinfarction among individuals who were able to modify their type A behavior.

Interest in the global type A behavior has diminished in favor of one specific component of this behavior pattern – the aggression-hostility component, which seems to be the most toxic factor in terms of myocardial risk. The important role played by hostility in cardiovascular disease was first demonstrated in a longitudinal study by Barefoot and colleagues, which found that medical students with high scores on the Cook-Medley hostility scale of the Minnesota Multiphasic Personality Inventory (MMPI) had a sixfold increase in mortality when followed up 25 years later, mainly due to coronary heart disease (CHD). Subsequent studies have consistently supported this finding by showing that individuals who are high in hostility have a significantly increased risk of myocardial infarction. As medication to prevent and treat cardiovascular disease has improved considerably during the past decades and the incidence rate of myocardial infarction has declined steadily since 1980, interest in performing large prospective studies on type A behavior and CHD has diminished accordingly.

Gender Differences in Response to Work Stress

As the number of women in the labor force approaches that of men but the traditional female responsibility for home and family mainly remains the same, stress from work overload and role conflicts has become an increasing problem for many women. Although women generally live longer than men, women tend to report more health problems than men. Women's longevity is associated with behavioral factors (e.g., men use more drugs and alcohol, men commit suicide more often, men expose themselves to greater risks at work and in traffic), environmental factors (men perform more dangerous jobs, are more violent, and engage in criminal behavior more often) and biological factors (women contract fatal cardiovascular disorders such as myocardial infarction and stroke about 10 years later in life than men, mainly due to the protective effects of female sex hormones before menopause). However, musculoskeletal and gastrointestinal disorders, headache, chronic fatigue, and psychiatric disorders are reported more frequently by women than by men.

Women's employment, even in low-status jobs, seems to be associated with better health compared to the role of a homemaker. To some extent this could be explained by the fact that it is easier for women in good health to get and keep a job, compared with women with poorer health. However, a paid job is also likely to contribute to better health and well-being by increasing the possibilities for social relations, higher self-esteem, and economic independence. Provided that men and women are matched for education and occupational level, physiological stress responses at work seem to be quite similar. However, consistent gender differences have been found off the job. Frankenhaeuser and colleagues compared stress responses during and after work in male and female white collar workers, matched for age and occupational level, and found that men's physiological arousal rapidly returned to baseline after work, whereas women's stress levels remained high several hours after work. These findings have been replicated in recent studies of men and women in high-ranking positions. A likely explanation for these gender differences is that women were unable to unwind and relax due to their greater responsibility for unpaid work at home (e.g., household chores, child care).

Several studies show that women's work stress is reflected not only at work but also in terms of their physiological arousal in non-work conditions. Men seem to respond more specifically to the acute stress exposure at work, and their work stress does not seem to spill over into non-work conditions.

In a prospective study of approximately 600 000 men and 400 000 women in Sweden, Alfredsson and colleagues found that overtime at work (10 h or more per week) was associated with a significantly elevated risk of myocardial infarction during a 1-year follow-up in women but not in men. Men's overtime was even associated with a significantly reduced risk of infarction.

One possible explanation for this gender difference, which is supported by psychophysiological data in other studies, is that women's CHD risk is related to elevated and sustained physiological stress levels caused by work overload and their more pronounced role conflicts, when they are trying to combine overtime at work with responsibility for various unpaid duties at home. Another possible explanation is that women, more often than men, are employed in low-status jobs, in which high demands are combined with little influence over the work situation, including overtime. Such high-strain jobs, according to the demand–control model, are known to increase the risk of CHD in both men and women.

A paid job as well as the unpaid work of household chores and child care is likely to contribute to the greater total workload of full-time employed women, compared with men. This could be relevant for women's greater health problems, but it also reduces their chances of having a professional career on the same terms as men. A study of about 1000 male and 1000 female full-time employed white collar workers, matched for age and type of occupation, confirmed that a greater proportion of women compared to men reported having the main responsibility for most unpaid duties at home. In terms of number of working hours in paid and unpaid productive activity, the total workload of men and women seems to be about the same in families having no children at home, whereas the workload increases more rapidly for women than for men depending on the number of children at home.

Psychobiological Mechanisms Linking Work Stress to Health Problems

Allostatic Load

A new stress model, the allostatic load model, refers to the ability to achieve stability through change. A normal and economic response to stress means activation of physiological systems in order to cope with the stressor, followed by a shut-off of the allostatic response as soon as the stress is terminated, whereas over- or underactivity of the allostatic systems may add to the wear and tear of the organism. Examples are frequent and intensive activation of physiological systems (cardiovascular, hormonal, metabolic, immune function) without enough time for rest and recovery or an inability to shut off the stress response after the stress exposure, which may cause overactivity and exhaustion of the systems. Overexposure to stress hormones increases the risk of cardiovascular illness and immune deficiency, as well as cognitive impairment. Lack of adequate response in one system, due to exhaustion, may cause compensatory overactivation of other systems.

The allostatic load associated with blue collar jobs is usually higher than that associated with white collar jobs. Manual jobs involve mental as well as physical stress and are associated with more pronounced physiological responses. In addition, repetitive work associated with many blue collar jobs seems to contribute to sustained levels of stress after work, which further adds to the allostatic load. In women, the unpaid work responsibilities of household chores and child care may further contribute to a lack of opportunity for unwinding and to sustained stress levels in non-work situations.

Health problems are consistently more common among blue collar workers with low education, responsibility for monotonous and repetitive tasks, and low income than among white collar workers with more stimulation and variation at work.

Work Stress and Activity of the Hypothalamic-Pituitary-Adrenocortical Axis

Negative psychosocial and socioeconomic factors are associated not only with increased morbidity and mortality but also with elevated activity of the hypothalamic-pituitary-adrenocortical (HPA) system and increased cortisol secretion. Additionally, a very high workload, such as regularly working more than 10 h of overtime per week, has been associated with markedly elevated cortisol levels, at least in women. Sustained activity of the HPA system is related to a series of endocrine and metabolic effects, causing, among other things, increased storage of fat in the abdominal region. The amount of central fat accumulation indicates long-term overactivity of the HPA system and can be measured as the relationship between the waist and the hip circumference, the waist–hip ratio (WHR). An association has been demonstrated between high WHR and a series of negative socioeconomic factors, such as low education and income, poor housing and/or living alone, psychiatric problems and use of antidepressive drugs, and high absenteeism from work. The relationship between low socioeconomic status and high WHR is enhanced by the fact that health-related behaviors, such as cigarette smoking, alcohol and drug abuse, and lack of exercise, also contribute to increasing the activity of the HPA system. High WHR has been shown to increase the risk of diabetes and cardiovascular disease, and, through its anti-inflammatory effects, cortisol also has an important role in the functioning of the immune system. It has been concluded that chronic or long-term stress is associated with compromised immune functions and, thus, increased risk for infections and slower healing of wounds. Elevated cortisol levels have recently also been related to cognitive functions, such as explicit memory deficiency and low hippocampal volume.

Thus, in summary, the pattern of results suggests that individuals exposed to negative psychosocial work conditions (low income, low education, risk of unemployment, etc.) are more likely to have elevated cortisol secretion, more central fat accumulation, and greater health risks.

Work Stress and Musculoskeletal Disorders

Musculoskeletal disorders increased dramatically during the 1980s and have become one of the most important work-related health problems in Europe and North America today. Research indicates that psychosocial work stress is an important factor contributing to this development.

The association between such factors as bad ergonomic conditions at work, heavy lifting, and physically monotonous or repetitive work and an increase in shoulder, neck, and lower back pain problems has been well documented. However, considerable ergonomic improvements of the work environment have not resulted in a lower incidence of musculoskeletal disorders, and musculoskeletal disorders are frequent not only in physically demanding jobs but also in light physical work. An increasing number of studies report an association between psychosocial factors at the workplace and neck, shoulder, and lower back pain problems. Conditions typical of many low-status jobs, such as low work satisfaction, time pressure, lack of influence over one's work, and constant involvement in repetitive tasks of short duration, often characterize jobs associated with a high risk for muscular problems.

Musculoskeletal disorders differ from many other major health problems, such as cardiovascular disease and cancer, in that symptoms often appear very early in life and after a relatively short exposure to adverse environmental conditions. In repetitive work, pain syndromes are often reported after only 6–12 months on the job, and it has been documented that even very low levels of muscle activation (less than 1% of maximal voluntary contraction) may contribute to the development of chronic pain syndromes.

So far it has been difficult to explain the high incidence of musculoskeletal disorders in light physical work. However, it has been suggested that sustained low-level muscle activity, induced by physical and/or psychological demands, may initiate a pathogenetic mechanism resulting in muscle pain and thus form a link to musculoskeletal disorders. In a recent experimental study, it was demonstrated that the smallest functional units of the muscle, the motor units, can be activated by physical as well as mental stress. Psychological and psychosocial factors on and off the job, muscle pain, and illness behavior may also form a vicious circle with increasing sensitization and pain symptoms. Eventually, the individual will become chronically ill.

An important feature of psychological stress, which could be relevant to its role in the etiology of muscle pain, is that it is more lasting or chronic than physical demands at work. Stressful conditions such as low job satisfaction, low income, low status, an irritating boss, and fear of losing one's job influence the individual more or less continuously, whereas physical demands terminate at the end of the workday and during breaks at work.

Support for the assumption that work stress contributes to muscle tension and pain has been obtained inseveral studies. For example, in an interesting prospective study of female packing workers, it was found that women who contracted clinically diagnosed trapezius myalgia within the first year of employment had significantly higher muscle activity during breaks at work but not during actual work and, in addition, had fewer periods of very low muscular electrical activity (electromyographic [EMG] gaps). These findings indicate that, in the modern work environment, lack of relaxation during breaks at work and after work may be an even more important health problem than the actual level of stress or the intensity of muscle activation during work.

The prevalence of musculoskeletal disorders is markedly higher among women than among men. One would generally expect that this gender difference could be explained by women's lower physical capacity compared with men. However, because several studies show that the physical characteristics of the individual do not seem to predict future musculoskeletal disorders and that the physical load in white collar jobs, where the gender difference is most pronounced, is usually quite low, a more likely explanation is that women are often employed in stressful, emotionally demanding, monotonous, and repetitive jobs, where the risk of developing neck and shoulder disorders is high. Additional explanations could be that the physical work environment is better suited for men than for women, so that chairs and desks are too high for shorter women and tools are too big and heavy for women's smaller hands. Also the work organization is usually designed by men and may be less adequate for women. Lack of unwinding after work may further contribute to the higher health risks for women.

Concluding Remarks

Numerous studies suggest an important role not only for physical but also for psychosocial stress at work in major health problems, and several plausible psychobiological mechanisms have been proposed. Two important neuroendocrine stress systems – the sympathetic adrenal medullary and the HPA systems – seem to play an important role for these relationships.

Information on psychobiological pathways between psychosocial stress at work and symptoms and illness is of great importance for the possibility of preventing and treating work-related ill health. Such knowledge could also help individual workers to better understand their own health problems and find ways of breaking vicious circles that form between work stress, behavior, and symptoms. It may also help to create a more understanding attitude in general toward people who, under stressful work conditions, have developed somatic symptoms. However, most important is that knowledge about these mechanisms is a strong incentive for implementing structural and organizational changes at work in order to protect people from mental and physical disorders. The psychobiological parameters may be used as warning signals but may also offer new possibilities for evaluating improvement of work conditions before they are reflected in somatic illness patterns, which usually (but not always) take a long time to develop. With regard to the enormous costs and suffering associated with musculoskeletal disorders, actions leading even to a moderate or small reduction of these problems would be extremely cost efficient.

The new forms of work that have become possible through the development of communication technology and that allow maximal flexibility and mobility have the potential for beneficial as well as harmful stress effects. The balance between negative and positive consequences of this type of boundaryless work is likely to be determined by factors such as the organization of work, the creation of new boundaries between different roles, and individual factors. An adequate balance between activation (energy mobilization) and rest and recovery (e.g., recreation, healing, growth) is necessary for long-term health.

Acknowledgment

Financial support has been obtained from the Swedish Council for Work Life Research, the Swedish Research Council, and the Bank of Sweden Tercentenary Foundation.

See Also the Following Articles

Economic Factors and Stress; Education Levels and Stress; Industrialized Societies; Work–Family Balance.

Further Reading

Bongers, P. M., de Winter, C. R., Kompier, M. A. J. and Hildebrandt, V. H. (1993). Psychosocial factors at work and musculoskeletal disease. *Scandinavian Journal of Work Environment and Health* **19**, 297–312.

Bosma, H., Peter, R., Siegrist, J. and Marmot, M. (1998). Alternative job stress models and risk of coronary heart disease. The effort-reward imbalance model and the job strain model. *American Journal of Public Health* **88**, 68–74.

Frankenhaeuser, M., Lundberg, U. and Chesney, M. (eds.) (1991). *Women, work and stress* New York: Plenum.

House, J. S., Landis, K. R. and Umberson, D. (1988). Social relationships and health. *Science* **241**, 540–545.

Karasek, R. A. and Theorell, T. (1990). *Healthy work. Stress, productivity, and the reconstruction of working life.* New York: Basic Books.

Lundberg, U. (1996). The influence of paid and unpaid work on psychophysiological stress responses of men and women. *Journal of Occupational Health and Psychology* **1**, 117–130.

Lundberg, U. and Hellström, B. (2002). Workload and morning salivary cortisol in women. *Work and Stress* **16**, 356–363.

Lundberg, U. and Johansson, G. (2000). Stress and health risks in repetitive work and supervisory monitoring work. In: Backs, R. & Boucsein, W. (eds.) *Engineering psychophysiology: issues and applications*, pp. 339–359, Hillsdale, NJ: Lawrence Erlbaum Associates.

Lundberg, U., Mårdberg, B. and Frankenhaeuser, M. (1994). The total workload of male and female white collar workers as related to occupational level, number of and age. *Scandinavian Journal of Psychology* **35**, 315–327.

Marmot, M. G., Davey Smith, G., Stansfeld, S., Patel, C., North, F., Head, J., et al. (1991). Health inequalities among British civil servants: the Whitehall II study. *Lancet* **337**, 1387–1393.

McEwen, B. S. and Lasley, E. N. (2002). *The end of stress as we know it.* Washington DC: Joseph Henry Press.

Ryff, C. D. and Singer, B. (1998). The contours of positive human health. *Psychological Inquiry* **9**, 1–28.

Sapolsky, R. M. (1998). *Why zebras don't get ulcers. An update guide to stress, stress-related diseases, and coping.* New York: W.H. Freeman and Co.

Siegrist, J. (1996). Adverse health effects of high-effort/low-reward conditions. *Journal of Occupational Health and Psychology* **1**, 27–41.

Williams, R. B., Barefoot, J. C. and Shekelle, R. B. (1985). The health consequences of hostility. In: Chesney, M. A. & Rosenman, R. H. (eds.) *Anger and hostility in cardiovascular and behavioral disorders*, pp 173–185. New York: McGraw-Hill.

Burnout

C Maslach
University of California, Berkeley, CA, USA
M P Leiter
Acadia University, Wolfville, Nova Scotia, Canada

This is a revised version of the article by C Maslach and M P Leiter, Encyclopedia of Stress First Edition, volume 1, pp 358–362, © 2000, Elsevier Inc.

Glossary

Burnout	A psychological syndrome of exhaustion, cynicism, and inefficacy, which is experienced in response to chronic job stressors.
Cynicism	A negative, callous, or excessively detached response to various aspects of the job.
Engagement with work	The positive antithesis of burnout, which is characterized by energy, involvement, and efficacy.
Exhaustion	Feelings of being overextended and depleted of one's emotional and physical resources.
Inefficacy	Feelings of incompetence and lack of achievement in work.

Definition and Assessment

Burnout is a psychological syndrome of exhaustion, cynicism, and inefficacy in the workplace. It is considered to be an individual stress experience embedded in a context of complex social relationships, and it involves the person's conception of both self and others on the job. Unlike unidimensional models of stress, this multidimensional model conceptualizes burnout in terms of its three core components.

Burnout Components

Exhaustion refers to feelings of being overextended and depleted of one's emotional and physical resources. Workers feel drained and used up, without any source of replenishment. They lack enough energy to face another day or another person in need. The exhaustion component represents the basic individual stress dimension of burnout.

Cynicism refers to a negative, hostile, or excessively detached response to the job, which often includes a loss of idealism. It usually develops in response to the overload of emotional exhaustion and is self-protective at first – an emotional buffer of detached concern. But the risk is that the detachment can turn into dehumanization. The cynicism component represents the interpersonal dimension of burnout.

Inefficacy refers to a decline in feelings of competence and productivity at work. People experience a growing sense of inadequacy about their ability to do the job well, and this may result in a self-imposed verdict of failure. The inefficacy component represents the self-evaluation dimension of burnout.

What has been distinctive about burnout is the interpersonal framework of the phenomenon. The centrality of relationships at work – whether it be relationships with clients, colleagues, or supervisors – has always been at the heart of descriptions of burnout. These relationships are the source of both emotional strains and rewards, they can be a resource for coping with job stress, and they often bear the brunt of the negative effects of burnout. Thus, if one were to look at burnout out of context and simply focus on the individual exhaustion component, one would lose sight of the phenomenon entirely.

The principal measure of burnout is the Maslach Burnout Inventory (MBI), which provides distinct assessments of each of the three burnout components. Different forms of the MBI have been developed for different types of occupations: the human services survey (MBI-HSS), the educators survey (MBI-ES), and the general survey (MBI-GS). As a result of international interest in burnout research, the MBI has been translated into many languages.

Burnout Correlates

Unlike acute stress reactions, which develop in response to specific critical incidents, burnout is a cumulative stress reaction to ongoing occupational stressors. With burnout, the emphasis has been more on the process of psychological erosion and the psychological and social outcomes of this chronic exposure, rather than just the physical ones. Because burnout is a prolonged response to chronic interpersonal stressors on the job, it tends to be fairly stable over time.

Health Symptoms Of the three burnout components, exhaustion is the closest to an orthodox stress variable, and therefore is more predictive of stress-related health outcomes than the other two components. Exhaustion is typically correlated with such stress symptoms as headaches, chronic fatigue, gastrointestinal disorders, muscle tension, hypertension, cold/flu episodes, and sleep disturbances. These physiological correlates mirror those found with other indices of prolonged stress. Similarly parallel findings have been found for the link between burnout and various forms of substance abuse.

In terms of mental, as opposed to physical, health, the link with burnout is more complex. It has been assumed that burnout may result in subsequent mental disabilities, and there is some evidence to link burnout with greater anxiety, irritability, and depression. However, an alternative argument is that burnout is itself a form of mental illness, rather than a cause of it. Much of this discussion has focused on depression, and whether or not burnout is a different phenomenon. Research has demonstrated that the two constructs are indeed distinct: burnout is job-related and situation-specific, as opposed to depression, which is general and context-free.

Job Behaviors Burnout has been associated with various forms of job withdrawal – absenteeism, intention to leave the job, and actual turnover. However, for people who stay on the job, burnout leads to lower productivity and effectiveness at work. To the extent that burnout diminishes opportunities for satisfying experiences at work, it is associated with decreased job satisfaction and a reduced commitment to the job or the organization.

People who are experiencing burnout can have a negative impact on their colleagues, both by causing greater personal conflict and by disrupting job tasks. Thus, burnout can be contagious and perpetuate itself through informal interactions on the job. There is also some evidence that burnout has a negative spillover effect on people's home life.

Engagement: The Opposite of Burnout

The opposite of burnout is not a neutral state, but a definite state of mental health within the occupational domain. Engagement with work is a productive and fulfilling state, and is defined in terms of the same three dimensions as burnout, but the positive end of those dimensions rather than the negative. Thus, engagement consists of a state of high energy (rather than exhaustion), strong involvement (rather than cynicism), and a sense of efficacy (rather than inefficacy).

One important implication of the burnout–engagement continuum is that strategies to promote engagement may be just as important for burnout prevention as strategies to reduce the risk of burnout. A workplace that is designed to support the positive development of the three core qualities of energy, involvement, and effectiveness should be successful in promoting the well-being and productivity of its employees, and thus the health of the entire organization. From this perspective, health is not limited to the physical or emotional well-being of individuals but is evident in enduring patterns of social interactions among people.

A Mediation Model of Burnout and Engagement

Inherent to the fundamental concept of stress is the problematic relationship between the individual and the situation. Thus, prior research has tried to identify both the key personal and job characteristics that put individuals at risk for burnout. In general, far more evidence has been found for the impact of job variables than for personal ones. These job factors fall into six key domains within the workplace: workload, control, reward, community, fairness, and values.

However, more recent theorizing has argued that personal and job characteristics need to be considered jointly within the context of the organizational environment. The degree of fit, or match, between the person and the job within the six areas of work life, will determine the extent to which the person experiences engagement or burnout, which in turn will determine various outcomes, such as personal health, work behaviors, and organizational measures. In other words, the burnout–engagement continuum (with its three dimensions) mediates the impact of the six areas of work life on important personal and organizational outcomes (see **Figure 1**).

Job Characteristics: Six Areas of Work Life

An analysis of the research literature on organizational risk factors for burnout has led to the identification of six major domains. Both workload and control are reflected in the demand–control model of job stress, and reward refers to the power of reinforcements to shape behavior. Community captures all of the work on social support and interpersonal conflict, while fairness emerges from the literature on equity and social justice. Finally, the area of values picks up the cognitive-emotional power of job goals and expectations.

Workload Both qualitative and quantitative work overload contribute to burnout by depleting the capacity of people to meet the demands of the job. When this kind of overload is a chronic job condition, there is little opportunity to rest, recover, and restore balance. A sustainable workload, in contrast, provides opportunities to use and refine existing skills as well as to become effective in new areas of activity.

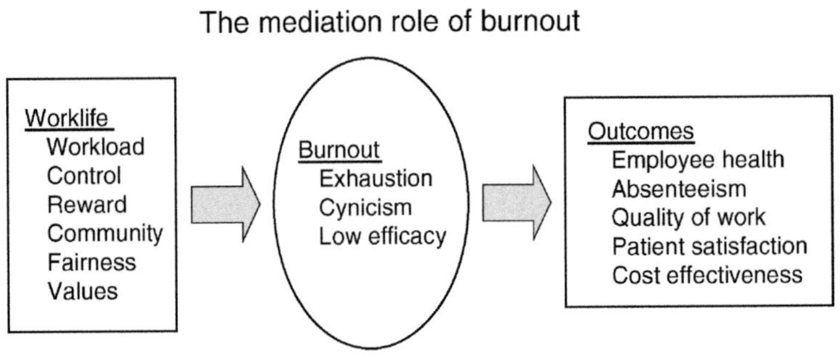

Figure 1 The role of burnout in mediating the impact of work life on personal and organizational outcomes.

Control Research has identified a clear link between a lack of control and high levels of stress and burnout. However, when employees have the perceived capacity to influence decisions that affect their work, to exercise professional autonomy, and to gain access to the resources necessary to do an effective job, they are more likely to experience job engagement.

Reward Insufficient recognition and reward (whether financial, institutional, or social) increases people's vulnerability to burnout, because it devalues both the work and the workers, and is closely associated with feelings of inefficacy. In contrast, consistency in the reward dimension between the person and the job means that there are both material rewards and opportunities for intrinsic satisfaction.

Community Community has to do with the ongoing relationships that employees have with other people on the job. When these relationships are characterized by a lack of support and trust and by unresolved conflict, then there is a greater risk of burnout. However, when these job-related relationships are working well, there is a great deal of social support, employees have effective means of working out disagreements, and they are more likely to experience job engagement.

Fairness Fairness is the extent to which decisions at work are perceived as being fair and equitable. People use the quality of the procedures and their own treatment during the decision-making process as an index of their place in the community. Cynicism, anger, and hostility are likely to arise when people feel they are not being treated with the respect that comes from being treated fairly.

Values Values are the ideals and motivations that originally attracted people to their job, and thus they are the motivating connection between the worker and the workplace, which goes beyond the utilitarian exchange of time for money or advancement. When there is a values conflict on the job and thus a gap between individual and organizational values, employees will find themselves making a trade-off between work they want to do and work they have to do, and this can lead to greater burnout.

Personal Characteristics

Although job variables and the organizational context are the prime predictors of burnout and engagement, a few personality variables have shown some consistent correlational patterns. In general, burnout scores are higher for people who have a less hardy personality, who have a more external locus of control, and who score as neurotic on the Five-Factor Model of personality. There is also some evidence that people who exhibit type A behavior (which tends to predict coronary heart disease) are more prone to the exhaustion dimension of burnout.

There are few consistent relationships of burnout with demographic characteristics. Although higher age seems to be associated with lower burnout, it is confounded with both years of experience and with survival bias (i.e., those who survive early job stressors and do not quit). Thus, it is difficult to derive a clear explanation for this age pattern. The only consistent gender difference is a tendency for men to score slightly higher on cynicism. These weak demographic relationships are congruent with the view that the work environment is of greater significance than personal characteristics in the development of burnout.

Implications for Interventions

The personal and organizational costs of burnout have led to the development of various intervention strategies. Some try to treat burnout after it has occurred, while others focus on how to prevent burnout by promoting engagement. Intervention may occur on the level of the individual, workgroup, or entire organization. At each level, the number of people affected by an intervention and the potential for enduring change increase.

The primary emphasis has been on individual strategies to prevent burnout, rather than social or organizational ones. This is particularly paradoxical given that research has found that situational and organizational factors play a bigger role in burnout than individual ones. Also, individual strategies are relatively ineffective in the workplace, where the person has much less control of stressors than in other domains of his or her life. There are both philosophical and pragmatic reasons underlying the predominant focus on the individual, including notions of individual causality and responsibility and the assumption that it is easier and cheaper to change people instead of organizations.

Recently, the range of options for intervention has expanded, given the recognition of (1) aiming for the positive goal of promoting engagement and (2) using the six areas of work life to better identify the critical intervention targets. These options have now been incorporated into both individual and organizational strategies, all of which focus on the job context and its impact on the people who work within it.

See Also the Following Articles

Workplace Stress.

Further Reading

Bakker, A. B., Schaufeli, W. B., Sixma, H. J., Bosveld, W. and Van Dierendonck, D. (2000). Patient demands, lack of reciprocity, and burnout: a five-year longitudinal study among general practitioners. *Journal of Organizational Behavior* **21**, 425–441.

Burke, R. J. and Greenglass, E. (2000). A longitudinal study of teacher burnout and perceived self-efficacy in classroom management. *Teaching and Teacher Education* **16**, 239–253.

Cherniss, C. (1995). *Beyond burnout.* New York: Routledge.

Cordes, C. L. and Dougherty, T. W. (1993). A review and integration of research on job burnout. *Academy of Management Review* **18**, 621–656.

Leiter, M. P. and Maslach, C. (2000). *Preventing burnout and building engagement: a complete program for organizational renewal.* San Francisco, CA: Jossey Bass.

Leiter, M. P. and Maslach, C. (2005). *Banishing burnout: six strategies for improving your relationship with work.* San Francisco, CA: Jossey Bass.

Maslach, C. and Leiter, M. P. (1997). *The truth about burnout.* San Francisco, CA: Jossey-Bass.

Maslach, C., Jackson, S. E. and Leiter, M. P. (1996). *Maslach burnout inventory manual* (3rd ed.). Palo Alto, CA: Consulting Psychologists Press.

Maslach, C., Schaufeli, W. B. and Leiter, M. P. (2001). Job burnout. *Annual Review of Psychology* **52**, 397–422.

Schaufeli, W. and Enzmann, D. (1998). *The burnout companion for research and practice.* Washington, D.C.: Taylor & Francis.

Schaufeli, W., Maslach, C. and Marek, T. (eds.) (1993). *Professional burnout: recent developments in theory and research.* Washington, D.C.: Taylor & Francis.

Shirom, A. (2003). Job-related burnout: a review. In: Quick, J. C. & Tetrick, L. E. (eds.) *Handbook of occupational health psychology*, pp. 245–265. Washington, D.C.: APA.

Toppinen-Tanner, S., Kalimo, R. and Mutanen, P. (2002). The process of burnout in white-collar and blue-collar jobs: eight-year prospective study of exhaustion. *Journal of Organizational Behavior* **23**, 555–570.

van Dierendonck, D., Schaufeli, W. B. and Buunk, B. P. (1998). The evaluation of an individual burnout intervention program: the role of inequity and social support. *Journal of Applied Psychology* **83**, 392–407.

SUBJECT INDEX

NOTES

Cross-reference terms in italics are general cross-references, or refer to subentry terms within the main entry (the main entry is not repeated to save space). Readers are also advised to refer to the end of each article for additional cross-references – not all of these cross-references have been included in the index cross-references.

The index is arranged in set-out style with a maximum of three levels of heading. Major discussion of a subject is indicated by bold page numbers. Page numbers suffixed by *t* and *f* refer to Tables and Figures respectively; *vs.* indicates a comparison.

Nomenclature used within the index reflects that used in the text

This index is in letter-by-letter order, whereby hyphens and spaces within index headings are ignored in the alphabetization. Prefixes and terms in parentheses are excluded from the initial alphabetization.

Common abbreviations used in subentries:

ACTH – adrenocorticotropic hormone

ADHD – attention deficit hyperactivity disorder

CRF – corticotropin-releasing factor

CRH – corticotropin-releasing hormone

HPA axis – hypothalamic–pituitary–adrenal axis

HPG axis – hypothalamic–pituitary–gonadal axis

HPT axis – hypothalamic–pituitary–thyroid axis

PTSD – posttraumatic stress disorder

SNP – single nucleotide polymorphism

A

B

C

D

E

F

G

H

I

N

O

P

Q

R

S

Printed and bound by CPI Group (UK) Ltd, Croydon, CR0 4YY
08/05/2025
01865033-0001